2nd Edition

HARRISON'S™

PULMONARY AND CRITICAL CARE MEDICINE

Derived from Harrison's Principles of Internal Medicine, 18th Edition

Editors

DAN L. LONGO, MD

Professor of Medicine, Harvard Medical School; Senior Physician, Brigham and Women's Hospital; Deputy Editor, New England Journal of Medicine, Boston, Massachusetts

DENNIS L. KASPER, MD

William Ellery Channing Professor of Medicine, Professor of Microbiology and Molecular Genetics, Harvard Medical School; Director, Channing Laboratory, Department of Medicine, Brigham and Women's Hospital, Boston, Massachusetts

J. LARRY JAMESON, MD, PhD

Robert G. Dunlop Professor of Medicine; Dean, University of Pennsylvania School of Medicine; Executive Vice-President of the University of Pennsylvania for the Health System, Philadelphia, Pennsylvania

ANTHONY S. FAUCI, MD

Chief, Laboratory of Immunoregulation; Director, National Institute of Allergy and Infectious Diseases, National Institutes of Health, Bethesda, Maryland

STEPHEN L. HAUSER, MD

Robert A. Fishman Distinguished Professor and Chairman, Department of Neurology, University of California, San Francisco, San Francisco, California

JOSEPH LOSCALZO, MD, PhD

Hersey Professor of the Theory and Practice of Medicine, Harvard Medical School; Chairman, Department of Medicine; Physician-in-Chief, Brigham and Women's Hospital, Boston, Massachusetts

2nd Edition

HARRISON'S™

PULMONARY AND CRITICAL CARE MEDICINE

EDITOR

Joseph Loscalzo, MD, PhD
Hersey Professor of the Theory and Practice of Medicine,
Harvard Medical School; Chairman, Department of Medicine;
Physician-in-Chief, Brigham and Women's Hospital, Boston, Massachusetts

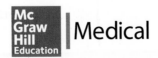

New York   Chicago   San Francisco   Lisbon   London   Madrid   Mexico City
Milan   New Delhi   San Juan   Seoul   Singapore   Sydney   Toronto

Harrison's Pulmonary and Critical Care Medicine, Second Edition

3 4 5 6 7 8 9 0   CTP/CTP   18 17 16 15

ISBN 978-0-07-181494-2
MHID 0-07-181494-9

This book was set in Bembo by Cenveo® Publisher Services. The editors were James F. Shanahan and Kim J. Davis. The production supervisor was Catherine H. Saggese. Project management was provided by Tania Andrabi, Cenveo Publisher Services. The cover design was by Thomas DePierro. Cover illustration, x-ray of the lungs, from BSIP/Science Source.

China Translation & Printing Services, Ltd. was the printer and binder.

Library of Congress Cataloging-in-Publication Data

Harrison's pulmonary and critical care medicine/editor,
Joseph Loscalzo. -- 2nd ed.
    p. ; cm.
    Pulmonary and critical care medicine
    Comprises the key pulmonary and critical care medicine chapters in Harrison's principles of internal medicine, 18th ed.
    Includes bibliographical references and index.
    ISBN 978-0-07-181494-2 (pbk. : alk. paper) −   ISBN 0-07-181494-9 (pbk. : alk. paper)
    I. Loscalzo, Joseph.   II. Harrison, Tinsley Randolph, 1900-1978.   III. Harrison's principles of internal medicine.   IV. Title: Pulmonary and critical care medicine.
    [DNLM: 1. Respiratory Tract Diseases. 2. Critical Care. 3. Critical Illness. WF 140]
616—dc23

                                                                                2012041262

McGraw-Hill Education books are available at special quantity discounts to use as premiums and sales promotions, or for use in corporate training programs. To contact a representative please e-mail us at bulksales@mcgraw-hill.com.

CONTENTS

SECTION IV
COMMON CRITICAL ILLNESSES AND SYNDROMES

SECTION V
DISORDERS COMPLICATING CRITICAL ILLNESSES AND THEIR MANAGEMENT

Appendix

Numbers in brackets refer to the chapter(s) written or co-written by the contributor.

Elliott M. Antman, MD
Professor of Medicine, Harvard Medical School; Brigham and Women's Hospital; Boston, Massachusetts [33]

Gordon L. Archer, MD
Professor of Medicine and Microbiology/Immunology; Senior Associate Dean for Research and Research Training, Virginia Commonwealth University School of Medicine, Richmond, Virginia [40]

Valder R. Arruda, MD, PhD
Associate Professor of Pediatrics, University of Pennsylvania School of Medicine; Division of Hematology, The Children's Hospital of Philadelphia, Philadelphia, Pennsylvania [39]

Lindsey R. Baden, MD
Associate Professor of Medicine, Harvard Medical School; Dana-Farber Cancer Institute, Brigham and Women's Hospital, Boston, Massachusetts [41]

John R. Balmes, MD
Professor of Medicine, San Francisco General Hospital, San Francisco, California [10]

Peter J. Barnes, DM, DSc, FMedSci, FRS
Head of Respiratory Medicine, Imperial College, London, United Kingdom [8]

Rebecca M. Baron, MD
Assistant Professor, Harvard Medical School; Associate Physician, Department of Pulmonary and Critical Care Medicine, Brigham and Women's Hospital, Boston, Massachusetts [16]

John G. Bartlett, MD
Professor of Medicine and Chief, Division of Infectious Diseases, Department of Medicine, Johns Hopkins School of Medicine, Baltimore, Maryland [16]

Robert C. Basner, MD
Professor of Clinical Medicine, Division of Pulmonary, Allergy, and Critical Care Medicine, Columbia University College of Physicians and Surgeons, New York, New York [Appendix]

Richard C. Boucher, MD
Kenan Professor of Medicine, Pulmonary and Critical Care Medicine; Director, Cystic Fibrosis/Pulmonary Research and Treatment Center, University of North Carolina at Chapel Hill, Chapel Hill, North Carolina [17]

Eugene Braunwald, MD, MA (Hon), ScD (Hon) FRCP
Distinguished Hersey Professor of Medicine, Harvard Medical School; Founding Chairman, TIMI Study Group, Brigham and Women's Hospital, Boston, Massachusetts [32]

Cynthia D. Brown
Assistant Professor of Medicine, Division of Pulmonary and Critical Care Medicine, University of Virginia, Charlottesville, Virginia [Review and Self-Assessment]

Christopher P. Cannon, MD
Associate Professor of Medicine, Harvard Medical School; Senior Investigator, TIMI Study Group, Brigham and Women's Hospital, Boston, Massachusetts [32]

Agustin Castellanos, MD
Professor of Medicine, and Director, Clinical Electrophysiology, Division of Cardiology, University of Miami Miller School of Medicine, Miami, Florida [31]

Bartolome R. Celli, MD
Lecturer on Medicine, Harvard Medical School; Staff Physician, Division of Pulmonary and Critical Care Medicine, Brigham and Women's Hospital, Boston, Massachusetts [26]

Glenn M. Chertow, MD, MPH
Norman S. Coplon/Satellite Healthcare Professor of Medicine; Chief, Division of Nephrology, Stanford University School of Medicine, Palo Alto, California [36]

Augustine M. K. Choi, MD
Parker B. Francis Professor of Medicine, Harvard Medical School; Chief, Division of Pulmonary and Critical Care Medicine, Brigham and Women's Hospital, Boston, Massachusetts [1, 6, 29]

Raphael Dolin, MD
Maxwell Finland Professor of Medicine (Microbiology and Molecular Genetics), Harvard Medical School; Beth Israel Deaconess Medical Center; Brigham and Women's Hospital, Boston, Massachusetts [13, 14, 41]

Neil J. Douglas, MD, MB ChB, DSc, Hon MD, FRCPE
Professor of Respiratory and Sleep Medicine, University of Edinburgh, Edinburgh, Scotland, United Kingdom [23]

Thomas D. DuBose, Jr., MD, MACP
Tinsley R. Harrison Professor and Chair, Internal Medicine; Professor of Physiology and Pharmacology, Department of Internal Medicine, Wake Forest University School of Medicine, Winston-Salem, North Carolina [38]

Janice Dutcher, MD
Department of Oncology, New York Medical College, Montefiore, Bronx, New York [43]

John E. Edwards, Jr,. MD
Chief, Division of Infectious Diseases, Harbor/University of California, Los Angeles (UCLA) Medical Center, Torrance, California; Professor of Medicine, David Geffen School of Medicine at UCLA, Los Angeles, California [42]

Andrew J. Einstein, MD, PhD
Assistant Professor of Clinical Medicine, Columbia University College of Physicians and Surgeons; Department of Medicine, Division of Cardiology, Department of Radiology, Columbia University Medical Center and New York-Presbyterian Hospital, New York, New York [Appendix]

Christopher Fanta, MD
Associate Professor of Medicine, Harvard Medical School; Member, Pulmonary and Critical Care Division, Brigham and Women's Hospital, Boston, Massachusetts [3]

Anne L. Fuhlbrigge, MD, MS
Assistant Professor, Harvard Medical School; Pulmonary and Critical Care Division, Brigham and Women's Hospital, Boston, Massachusetts [6]

Alicia K. Gerke, MD
Associate, Division of Pulmonary and Critical Care Medicine,
University of Iowa, Iowa City, Iowa [9]

Samuel Z. Goldhaber, MD
Professor of Medicine, Harvard Medical School; Director, Venous
Thromboembolism Research Group, Cardiovascular Division,
Brigham and Women's Hospital, Boston, Massachusetts [20]

Daryl R. Gress, MD, FAAN, FCCM
Professor of Neurocritical Care and Stroke; Professor of Neurology,
University of California, San Francisco, San Francisco, California [35]

Rasim Gucalp, MD
Professor of Clinical Medicine, Albert Einstein College of Medicine;
Associate Chairman for Educational Programs, Department of
Oncology; Director, Hematology/Oncology Fellowship, Monte-
fiore Medical Center, Bronx, New York [43]

Jesse B. Hall, MD, FCCP
Professor of Medicine, Anesthesia and Critical Care; Chief, Section
of Pulmonary and Critical Care Medicine, University of Chicago,
Chicago, Illinois [25]

Anna R. Hemnes
Assistant Professor, Division of Allergy, Pulmonary, and Critical
Care Medicine, Vanderbilt University Medical Center, Nashville,
Tennessee [Review and Self-Assessment]

J. Claude Hemphill, III, MD, MAS
Professor of Clinical Neurology and Neurological Surgery,
Department of Neurology, University of California, San Francisco;
Director of Neurocritical Care, San Francisco General Hospital,
San Francisco, California [35]

Katherine A. High, MD
Investigator, Howard Hughes Medical Institute; William H. Bennett
Professor of Pediatrics, University of Pennsylvania School of Medi-
cine; Director, Center for Cellular and Molecular Therapeutics,
Children's Hospital of Philadelphia, Philadelphia, Pennsylvania [39]

Judith S. Hochman, MD
Harold Snyder Family Professor of Cardiology; Clinical Chief, Leon
Charney Division of Cardiology; Co-Director, NYU-HHC Clinical
and Translational Science Institute; Director, Cardiovascular Clinical
Research Center, New York University School of Medicine,
New York, New York [30]

Gary W. Hunninghake, MD
Professor, Division of Pulmonary and Critical Care Medicine, University of Iowa, Iowa City, Iowa [9]

David H. Ingbar, MD
Professor of Medicine, Pediatrics, and Physiology; Director, Pulmonary Allergy, Critical Care and Sleep Division, University of Minnesota School of Medicine, Minneapolis, Minnesota [30]

Talmadge E. King, Jr., MD
Julius R. Krevans Distinguished Professor in Internal Medicine;
Chair, Department of Medicine, University of California, San
Francisco, San Francisco, California [19]

Alexander Kratz, MD, PhD, MPH
Associate Professor of Pathology and Cell Biology, Columbia University
College of Physicians and Surgeons; Director, Core Laboratory, Columbia
University Medical Center, New York, New York [Appendix]

John P. Kress, MD
Associate Professor of Medicine, Section of Pulmonary and Critical
Care, University of Chicago, Chicago, Illinois [25]

Patricia Kritek, MD, EdM
Associate Professor, Division of Pulmonary and Critical Care Medicine, University of Washington, Seattle, Washington [1, 3, 7]

Bruce D. Levy, MD
Associate Professor of Medicine, Harvard Medical School; Pulmo-
nary and Critical Care Medicine, Brigham and Women's Hospital,
Boston, Massachusetts [29]

Richard W. Light, MD
Professor of Medicine, Division of Allergy, Pulmonary, and Critical
Care Medicine, Vanderbilt University, Nashville, Tennessee [21]

Kathleen D. Liu, MD, PhD, MAS
Assistant Professor, Divisions of Nephrology and Critical Care
Medicine, Departments of Medicine and Anesthesia, University of
California, San Francisco, San Francisco, California [36]

Joseph Loscalzo, MD, PhD
Hersey Professor of the Theory and Practice of Medicine,
Harvard Medical School; Chairman, Department of Medicine;
Physician-in-Chief, Brigham and Women's Hospital, Boston,
Massachusetts [4, 33]

Ronald V. Maier, MD
Jane and Donald D. Trunkey Professor and Vice-Chair, Surgery,
University of Washington; Surgeon-in-Chief, Harborview Medical
Center, Seattle, Washington [27]

Lionel A. Mandell, MD, FRCP(C), FRCP(LOND)
Professor of Medicine, McMaster University, Hamilton, Ontario,
Canada [11]

John F. McConville, MD
Assistant Professor of Medicine, University of Chicago, Chicago,
Illinois [22]

David B. Mount, MD, FRCPC
Assistant Professor of Medicine, Harvard Medical School, Renal
Division, VA Boston Healthcare System; Brigham and Women's
Hospital, Boston, Massachusetts [37]

Robert S. Munford, MD
Bethesda, Maryland [28]

Robert J. Myerburg, MD
Professor, Departments of Medicine and Physiology, Division of
Cardiology; AHA Chair in Cardiovascular Research, University of
Miami Miller School of Medicine, Miami, Florida [312]

Edward T. Naureckas, MD
Associate Professor of Medicine, Section of Pulmonary and Critical
Care Medicine, University of Chicago, Chicago, Illinois [5]

Richard J. O'Brien, MD
Head, Product Evaluation and Demonstration, Foundation for Inno-
vative and New Diagnostics (FIND), Geneva, Switzerland [12]

Michael A. Pesce, PhD
Professor Emeritus of Pathology and Cell Biology, Columbia
University College of Physicians and Surgeons; Columbia
University Medical Center, New York, New York [Appendix]

Ronald E. Polk, PharmD
Professor of Pharmacy and Medicine; Chairman, Department of
Pharmacy, School of Pharmacy, Virginia Commonwealth University/
Medical College of Virginia Campus, Richmond, Virginia [40]

Mario C. Raviglione, MD
Director, Stop TB Department, World Health Organization,
Geneva, Switzerland [12]

John J. Reilly, Jr., MD
Executive Vice Chairman; Department of Medicine; Professor of Medicine, University of Pittsburgh, Pittsburgh, Pennsylvania [7, 18]

Allan H. Ropper, MD
Professor of Neurology, Harvard Medical School; Executive Vice Chair of Neurology, Raymond D. Adams Distinguished Clinician, Brigham and Women's Hospital, Boston, Massachusetts [34]

Richard M. Schwartzstein, MD
Ellen and Melvin Gordon Professor of Medicine and Medical Education; Associate Chief, Division of Pulmonary, Critical Care, and Sleep Medicine, Beth Israel Deaconess Medical Center, Harvard Medical School, Boston, Massachusetts [1]

Steven D. Shapiro, MD
Jack D. Myers Professor and Chair, Department of Medicine, University of Pittsburgh, Pittsburgh, Pennsylvania [18]

Edwin K. Silverman, MD, PhD
Associate Professor of Medicine, Harvard Medical School; Channing Laboratory, Pulmonary and Critical Care Division, Department of Medicine, Brigham and Women's Hospital, Boston, Massachusetts [18]

Wade S. Smith, MD, PhD
Professor of Neurology, Daryl R. Gress Endowed Chair of Neurocritical Care and Stroke; Director, University of California, San Francisco Neurovascular Service, San Francisco, San Francisco, California [35]

A. George Smulian, MBBCh
Associate Professor of Medicine, University of Cincinnati College of Medicine; Chief, Infectious Disease Section, Cincinnati VA Medical Center, Cincinnati, Ohio [15]

Julian Solway, MD
Walter L. Palmer Distinguished Service Professor of Medicine and Pediatrics; Associate Dean for Translational Medicine, Biological Sciences Division; Vice Chair for Research, Department of Medicine; Chair, Committee on Molecular Medicine, University of Chicago, Chicago, Illinois [5, 22]

Frank E. Speizer, MD
E. H. Kass Distinguished Professor of Medicine, Channing Laboratory, Harvard Medical School; Professor of Environmental Science, Harvard School of Public Health, Boston, Massachusetts [10]

Elbert P. Trulock, MD
Rosemary and I. Jerome Flance Professor in Pulmonary Medicine, Washington University School of Medicine, St. Louis, Missouri [24]

Peter D. Walzer, MD, MSc
Professor of Medicine, University of Cincinnati College of Medicine; Associate Chief of Staff for Research, Cincinnati VA Medical Center, Cincinnati, Ohio [15]

Charles M. Wiener, MD
Dean/CEO Perdana University Graduate School of Medicine, Selangor, Malaysia; Professor of Medicine and Physiology, Johns Hopkins University School of Medicine, Baltimore, Maryland [Review and Self-Assessment]

Richard Wunderink, MD
Professor of Medicine, Division of Pulmonary and Critical Care, Northwestern University Feinberg School of Medicine, Chicago, Illinois [11]

PREFACE

Harrison's Principles of Internal Medicine has been a respected information source for more than 60 years. Over time, the traditional textbook has evolved to meet the needs of internists, family physicians, nurses, and other health care providers. The growing list of *Harrison's* products now includes *Harrison's* for the iPad, *Harrison's Manual of Medicine*, and *Harrison's Online*. This book, *Harrison's Pulmonary and Critical Care Medicine*, now in its second edition, is a compilation of chapters related to respiratory disorders, respiratory diseases, general approach to the critically ill patient, common critical illnesses and syndromes, and disorders complicating critical illnesses and their management.

Our readers consistently note the sophistication of the material in the specialty sections of *Harrison's*. Our goal was to bring this information to our audience in a more compact and usable form. Because the topic is more focused, it is possible to enhance the presentation of the material by enlarging the text and the tables. We have also included a Review and Self-Assessment section that includes questions and answers to provoke reflection and to provide additional teaching points.

Pulmonary diseases are major contributors to morbidity and mortality in the general population. Although advances in the diagnosis and treatment of many common pulmonary disorders have improved the lives of patients, these complex illnesses continue to affect a large segment of the global population. The impact of cigarette smoking cannot be underestimated in this regard, especially given the growing prevalence of tobacco use in the developing world. Pulmonary medicine is, therefore, of critical global importance to the field of internal medicine.

Pulmonary medicine is a growing subspecialty and includes a number of areas of disease focus, including reactive airways diseases, chronic obstructive lung disease, environmental lung diseases, and interstitial lung diseases. Furthermore, pulmonary medicine is linked to the field of critical care medicine, both cognitively and as a standard arm of the pulmonary fellowship training programs at most institutions. The breadth of knowledge in critical care medicine extends well beyond the respiratory system, of course, and includes selected areas of cardiology, infectious diseases, nephrology, and hematology. Given the complexity of these disciplines and the crucial role of the internist in guiding the management of patients with chronic lung diseases and in helping to guide the management of patients in the intensive care setting, knowledge of the discipline is essential for competency in the field of internal medicine.

The scientific basis of many pulmonary disorders and intensive care medicine is rapidly expanding. Novel diagnostic and therapeutic approaches, as well as prognostic assessment strategies, populate the published literature with great frequency. Maintaining updated knowledge of these evolving areas is, therefore, essential for the optimal care of patients with lung diseases and critical illness.

In view of the importance of pulmonary and critical care medicine to the field of internal medicine and the speed with which the scientific basis of the discipline is evolving, this sectional was developed. The purpose of this book is to provide the readers with an overview of the field of pulmonary and critical care medicine. To achieve this end, this sectional comprises the key pulmonary and critical care medicine chapters in *Harrison's Principles of Internal Medicine*, 18th edition, contributed by leading experts in the fields. This sectional is designed not only for physicians-in-training, but also for medical students, practicing clinicians, and other health care professionals who seek to maintain adequately updated knowledge of this rapidly advancing field. The editors believe that this book will improve the reader's knowledge of the discipline, as well as highlight its importance to the field of internal medicine.

The first section of the book, "Diagnosis of Respiratory Disorders," provides a systems overview, beginning with approach to the patient with disease of the respiratory system. The integration of pathophysiology with clinical management is a hallmark of *Harrison's*, and can be found throughout each of the subsequent disease-oriented chapters. The book is divided into five main sections that reflect the scope of pulmonary and critical care medicine: (I) Diagnosis of Respiratory Disorders; (II) Diseases of the Respiratory System; (III) General Approach to the Critically Ill Patient; (IV) Common Critical Illnesses and Syndromes; and (V) Disorders Complicating Critical Illnesses and Their Management.

Our access to information through web-based journals and databases is remarkably efficient. Although these sources of information are invaluable, the daunting body of data creates an even greater need for synthesis by experts in the field. Thus, the preparation of these chapters is a special craft that requires the ability to distill core information from the ever-expanding knowledge base. The editors are, therefore, indebted to our authors, a group of internationally recognized authorities who are masters at providing a comprehensive overview while being able to distill a topic into a concise and interesting chapter. We are indebted to our colleagues at McGraw-Hill. Jim Shanahan is a champion for *Harrison's* and these books were impeccably produced by Kim Davis. We hope you will find this book useful in your effort to achieve continuous learning on behalf of your patients

Joseph Loscalzo, MD, PhD

Review and self-assessment questions and answers were taken from Wiener CM, Brown CD, Hemnes AR (eds). *Harrison's Self-Assessment and Board Review*, 18th ed. New York, McGraw-Hill, 2012, ISBN 978-0-07-177195-5.

 The global icons call greater attention to key epidemiologic and clinical differences in the practice of medicine throughout the world.

 The genetic icons identify a clinical issue with an explicit genetic relationship.

SECTION I

DIAGNOSIS OF RESPIRATORY DISORDERS

CHAPTER 1

APPROACH TO THE PATIENT WITH DISEASE OF THE RESPIRATORY SYSTEM

Patricia Kritek ■ Augustine Choi

The majority of diseases of the respiratory system fall into one of three major categories: (1) obstructive lung diseases; (2) restrictive disorders; and (3) abnormalities of the vasculature. Obstructive lung diseases are most common and primarily include disorders of the airways such as asthma, chronic obstructive pulmonary disease (COPD), bronchiectasis, and bronchiolitis. Diseases resulting in restrictive pathophysiology include parenchymal lung diseases, abnormalities of the chest wall and pleura, as well as neuromuscular disease. Disorders of the pulmonary vasculature are not always recognized and include pulmonary embolism, pulmonary hypertension, and pulmonary venoocclusive disease. Although many specific diseases fall into these major categories, both infective and neoplastic processes can affect the respiratory system and may result in myriad pathologic findings, including obstruction, restriction, and pulmonary vascular disease (see Table 1-1).

The majority of respiratory diseases present with abnormal gas exchange. Disorders can also be grouped into the categories of gas exchange abnormalities, including hypoxemic, hypercarbic, or combined impairment. Importantly, many diseases of the lung do not manifest gas exchange abnormalities.

As with the evaluation of most patients, the approach to a patient with disease of the respiratory system begins with a thorough history. A focused physical examination is helpful in further categorizing the specific pathophysiology. Many patients will subsequently undergo pulmonary function testing, chest imaging, blood and sputum analysis, a variety of serologic or microbiologic studies, and diagnostic procedures, such as bronchoscopy. This step-wise approach is discussed in detail later.

HISTORY

DYSPNEA AND COUGH

The cardinal symptoms of respiratory disease are dyspnea and cough (Chaps. 2 and 3). Dyspnea can result from many causes, some of which are not predominantly caused by lung pathology. The words a patient uses to describe breathlessness or shortness of breath can suggest certain etiologies of the dyspnea. Patients with obstructive lung disease often complain of "chest tightness" or "inability to get a deep breath," whereas patients with congestive heart failure more commonly report "air hunger" or a sense of suffocation.

The tempo of onset and duration of a patient's dyspnea are helpful in determining the etiology. Acute shortness of breath is usually associated with sudden physiological changes, such as laryngeal edema, bronchospasm, myocardial infarction, pulmonary embolism, or pneumothorax. Patients with underlying lung disease commonly have progressive shortness of breath or episodic dyspnea. Patients with COPD and idiopathic pulmonary fibrosis (IPF) have a gradual progression of dyspnea on exertion, punctuated by acute exacerbations of shortness of breath. In contrast, most asthmatics have normal breathing the majority of the time and have recurrent episodes of dyspnea usually associated with specific triggers, such as an upper respiratory tract infection or exposure to allergens.

Specific questioning should focus on factors that incite the dyspnea, as well as any intervention that helps resolve the patient's shortness of breath. Of the obstructive lung diseases, asthma is most likely to have specific triggers related to sudden onset of dyspnea, although this can also be true of COPD. Many patients with

2

TABLE 1-1

CATEGORIES OF RESPIRATORY DISEASE

CATEGORY	EXAMPLES
Obstructive lung disease	Asthma
	COPD
	Bronchiectasis
	Bronchiolitis
Restrictive pathophysiology—parenchymal disease	Idiopathic pulmonary fibrosis (IPF)
	Asbestosis
	Desquamative interstitial pneumonitis (DIP)
	Sarcoidosis
Restrictive pathophysiology—neuromuscular weakness	Amyotrophic lateral sclerosis (ALS)
	Guillain-Barré syndrome
Restrictive pathophysiology—chest wall/pleural disease	Kyphoscoliosis
	Ankylosing spondylitis
	Chronic pleural effusions
Pulmonary vascular disease	Pulmonary embolism
	Pulmonary arterial hypertension (PAH)
Malignancy	Bronchogenic carcinoma (non-small-cell and small cell)
	Metastatic disease
Infectious diseases	Pneumonia
	Bronchitis
	Tracheitis

Abbreviation: COPD, chronic obstructive pulmonary disease.

lung disease report dyspnea on exertion. It is useful to determine the degree of activity that results in shortness of breath as it gives the clinician a gauge of the patient's degree of disability. Many patients adapt their level of activity to accommodate progressive limitation. For this reason it is important, particularly in older patients, to delineate the activities in which they engage and how they have changed over time. Dyspnea on exertion is often an early symptom of underlying lung or heart disease and warrants a thorough evaluation.

Cough is the other common presenting symptom that generally indicates disease of the respiratory system. The clinician should inquire about the duration of the cough, whether or not it associated with sputum production, and any specific triggers that induce it. Acute cough productive of phlegm is often a symptom of infection of the respiratory system, including processes affecting the upper airway (e.g., sinusitis, tracheitis) as well as the lower airways (e.g., bronchitis, bronchiectasis) and lung parenchyma (e.g., pneumonia). Both the quantity and quality of the sputum, including whether it is blood-streaked or frankly bloody, should be determined. Hemoptysis warrants an evaluation as delineated in Chap. 3.

Chronic cough (defined as persisting for more than 8 weeks) is commonly associated with obstructive lung diseases, particularly asthma and chronic bronchitis, as well as "nonrespiratory" diseases, such as gastroesophageal reflux (GERD) and postnasal drip. Diffuse parenchymal lung diseases, including idiopathic pulmonary fibrosis, frequently present with a persistent, nonproductive cough. As with dyspnea, all causes of cough are not respiratory in origin, and assessment should consider a broad differential, including cardiac and gastrointestinal diseases as well as psychogenic causes.

ADDITIONAL SYMPTOMS

Patients with respiratory disease may complain of wheezing, which is suggestive of airways disease, particularly asthma. Hemoptysis, which must be distinguished from epistaxis or hematemesis, can be a symptom of a variety of lung diseases, including infections of the respiratory tract, bronchogenic carcinoma, and pulmonary embolism. Chest pain or discomfort is also often thought to be respiratory in origin. As the lung parenchyma is not innervated with pain fibers, pain in the chest from respiratory disorders usually results from either diseases of the parietal pleura (e.g., pneumothorax) or pulmonary vascular diseases (e.g., pulmonary hypertension). As many diseases of the lung can result in strain on the right side of the heart, patients may also present with symptoms of cor pulmonale, including abdominal bloating or distention, and pedal edema.

ADDITIONAL HISTORY

A thorough social history is an essential component of the evaluation of patients with respiratory disease. All patients should be asked about current or previous cigarette smoking as this exposure is associated with many diseases of the respiratory system, most notably COPD and bronchogenic lung cancer but also a variety of diffuse parenchymal lung diseases (e.g., desquamative interstitial pneumonitis [DIP] and pulmonary Langerhans cell histiocytosis). For most disorders, the duration and intensity of exposure to cigarette smoke increases the risk of disease. There is growing evidence that "second-hand smoke" is also a risk factor for respiratory tract pathology; for this reason, patients should be asked about parents, spouses, or housemates who smoke. It is becoming less common for patients to be exposed to cigarette smoke on the job, but for older patients, an occupational history should include the potential for heavy cigarette smoke exposure (e.g., flight attendants working prior to prohibition of smoking on airplanes).

Possible inhalational exposures should be explored, including those at the work place (e.g., asbestos, wood smoke) and those associated with leisure (e.g., pigeon excrement from pet birds, paint fumes) (Chap. 10). Travel predisposes to certain infections of the respiratory tract, most notably the risk of tuberculosis. Potential exposure to fungi found in specific geographic regions or climates (e.g., *Histoplasma capsulatum*) should be explored.

Associated symptoms of fever and chills should raise the suspicion of infective etiologies, both pulmonary and systemic. Some systemic diseases, commonly rheumatologic or autoimmune, present with respiratory tract manifestations. Review of systems should include evaluation for symptoms that suggest undiagnosed rheumatologic disease. These may include joint pain or swelling, rashes, dry eyes, dry mouth, or constitutional symptoms. Additionally, carcinomas from a variety of primary sources commonly metastasize to the lung and cause respiratory symptoms. Finally, therapy for other conditions, including both radiation and medications, can result in diseases of the chest.

PHYSICAL EXAMINATION

The clinician's suspicion for respiratory disease often begins with a patient's vital signs. The respiratory rate is often informative, whether elevated (tachypnea) or depressed (hypopnea). In addition, pulse oximetry should be measured as many patients with respiratory disease will have hypoxemia, either at rest or with exertion.

Simple observation of the patient is informative. Patients with respiratory disease may be in distress, often using accessory muscles of respiration to breathe. Severe kyphoscoliosis can result in restrictive pathophysiology. Inability to complete a sentence in conversation is generally a sign of severe impairment and should result in an expedited evaluation of the patient.

AUSCULTATION

The majority of the manifestations of respiratory disease present with abnormalities of the chest examination. Wheezes suggest airway obstruction and are most commonly a manifestation of asthma. Peribronchial edema in the setting of congestive heart failure, often referred to as "cardiac asthma," can also result in diffuse wheezes as can any other process that causes narrowing of small airways. For this reason, clinicians must take care not to attribute all wheezing to asthma.

Rhonchi are a manifestation of obstruction of medium-sized airways, most often with secretions. In the acute setting, this may be a sign of viral or bacterial bronchitis. Chronic rhonchi suggest bronchiectasis or COPD. Bronchiectasis, or permanent dilation and irregularity of the bronchi, often causes what is referred to as a "musical chest" with a combination of rhonchi, pops, and squeaks. Stridor or a low-pitched, focal inspiratory wheeze usually heard over the neck, is a manifestation of upper airway obstruction and should result in an expedited evaluation of the patient as it can precede complete upper airway obstruction and respiratory failure.

Crackles, or rales, are commonly a sign of alveolar disease. A variety of processes that fill the alveoli with fluid result in crackles. Pneumonia, or infection of the lower respiratory tract and air spaces, may cause crackles. Pulmonary edema, of cardiogenic or noncardiogenic cause, is associated with crackles, generally more prominent at the bases. Interestingly, diseases that result in fibrosis of the interstitium (e.g., IPF) also result in crackles often sounding like Velcro being ripped apart. Although some clinicians make a distinction between "wet" and "dry" crackles, this has not been shown to be a reliable way to differentiate among etiologies of respiratory disease.

One way to help distinguish between crackles associated with alveolar fluid and those associated with interstitial fibrosis is to assess for egophony. Egophony is the auscultation of the sound "AH" instead of "EEE" when a patient phonates "EEE." This change in note is due to abnormal sound transmission through consolidated lung and will be present in pneumonia but not in IPF. Similarly, areas of alveolar filling have increased whispered pectoriloquy as well as transmission of larger airway sounds (i.e., bronchial breath sounds in a lung zone where vesicular breath sounds are expected).

The lack of breath sounds or diminished breath sounds can also help determine the etiology of respiratory disease. Patients with emphysema often have a quiet chest with diffusely decreased breath sounds. A pneumothorax or pleural effusion may present with an area of absent breath sounds, although this is not always the case.

REMAINDER OF CHEST EXAMINATION

In addition to auscultation, percussion of the chest helps distinguish among pathologic processes of the respiratory system. Diseases of the pleural space are often suggested by differences in percussion note. An area of dullness may suggest a pleural effusion, whereas hyperresonance, particularly at the apex, can indicate air in the pleural space (i.e., pneumothorax).

Tactile fremitus will be increased in areas of lung consolidation, such as pneumonia, and decreased with pleural effusion. Decreased diaphragmatic excursion can suggest neuromuscular weakness manifesting as respiratory disease or hyperinflation associated with COPD.

Careful attention should also be paid to the cardiac examination with particular emphasis on signs of right heart failure as it is associated with chronic hypoxemic lung disease and pulmonary vascular disease. The clinician should feel for a right ventricular heave and listen for a prominent P2 component of the second heart sound, as well as a right-sided S4.

OTHER SYSTEMS

Pedal edema, if symmetric, may suggest cor pulmonale, and if asymmetric may be due to deep venous thrombosis and associated pulmonary embolism. Jugular venous distention may also be a sign of volume overload associated with right heart failure. Pulsus paradoxus is an ominous sign in a patient with obstructive lung disease as it is associated with significant negative intrathoracic (pleural) pressures required for ventilation, and impending respiratory failure.

As stated earlier, rheumatologic disease may manifest primarily as lung disease. Owing to this association, particular attention should be paid to joint and skin examination. Clubbing can be found in many lung diseases, including cystic fibrosis, IPF, and lung cancer, although it can also be associated with inflammatory bowel disease or as a congenital finding of no clinical importance. Patients with COPD do not usually have clubbing; thus, this sign should warrant an investigation for second process, most commonly an unrecognized bronchogenic carcinoma, in these patients. Cyanosis is seen in hypoxemic respiratory disorders that result in more than 5 g/dL deoxygenated hemoglobin.

DIAGNOSTIC EVALUATION

The sequence of studies is dictated by the clinician's differential diagnosis determined by the history and physical examination. Acute respiratory symptoms are often evaluated with multiple tests obtained at the same time in order to diagnose any life threatening diseases rapidly (e.g., pulmonary embolism or multilobar pneumonia). In contrast, chronic dyspnea and cough can be evaluated in a more protracted, step-wise fashion.

PULMONARY FUNCTION TESTING

(See also Chap. 6) The initial pulmonary function test obtained is spirometry. This study is used to assess for obstructive pathophysiology as seen in asthma, COPD, and bronchiectasis. A diminished forced expiratory volume in 1 second (FEV_1)/forced vital capacity (FVC) (often defined as less than 70% of predicted value) is diagnostic of obstruction. History as well as further testing can help distinguish among different obstructive diseases. COPD is almost exclusively seen in cigarette smokers. Asthmatics often show an acute response to inhaled bronchodilators (e.g., albuterol). In addition to the measurements of FEV_1 and FVC, the clinician should examine the flow-volume loop. A plateau of the inspiratory or expiratory curves suggests large airway obstruction in extrathoracic and intrathoracic locations, respectively.

Normal spirometry or spirometry with symmetric decreases in FEV_1 and FVC warrants further testing, including lung volume measurement and the diffusion capacity of the lung for carbon monoxide (D_LCO). A total lung capacity (TLC) less than 80% of the predicted value for a patient's age, race, gender, and height defines restrictive pathophysiology. Restriction can result from parenchymal disease, neuromuscular weakness, or chest wall or pleural diseases. Restriction with impaired gas exchange, as indicated by a decreased D_LCO, suggests parenchymal lung disease. Additional testing, such as maximal expiratory pressure (MEP) and maximal inspiratory pressure (MIP), can help diagnose neuromuscular weakness. Normal spirometry, normal lung volumes, and a low D_LCO should prompt further evaluation for pulmonary vascular disease.

Arterial blood gas testing is often also helpful in assessing respiratory disease. Hypoxemia, while usually apparent with pulse oximetry, can be further evaluated with the measurement of arterial PO_2 and the calculation of an alveolar gas and arterial blood oxygen tension difference $[(A-a)DO_2]$. It should also be noted that at times, most often due to abnormal hemoglobins or non-oxygen hemoglobin-ligand complexes, pulse oximetry can be misleading (such as observed with carboxyhemoglobin). Diseases that cause ventilation-perfusion mismatch or shunt physiology will have an increased (A-a) DO_2 at rest. Arterial blood gas testing also allows for the measurement of arterial PCO_2. Most commonly, acute or chronic obstructive lung disease presents with hypercarbia; however, many diseases of the respiratory system can cause hypercarbia if the resulting increase in work of breathing is greater than that which allows a patient to sustain an adequate minute ventilation.

CHEST IMAGING

(See Chap. 7) Most patients with disease of the respiratory system will undergo imaging of the chest as part of initial evaluation. Clinicians should generally begin with a plain chest radiograph, preferably posterior-anterior (PA) and lateral films. Several findings, including opacities of the parenchyma, blunting of the costophrenic angles, mass lesions, and volume loss, can be very helpful in determining an etiology. It should be noted that many diseases of the respiratory system, particularly those of the airways and pulmonary vasculature, are associated with a normal chest radiograph.

Subsequent computed tomography of the chest (CT scan) is often obtained. The CT scan allows better delineation of parenchymal processes, pleural disease, masses or nodules, and large airways. If administered with contrast, the pulmonary vasculature can be assessed with particular utility for determination of pulmonary emboli. Intravenous contrast also allows lymph nodes to be delineated in greater detail.

FURTHER STUDIES

Depending on the clinician's suspicion, a variety of other studies may be obtained. Concern for large airway lesions may warrant bronchoscopy. This procedure may also be used to sample the alveolar space with bronchoalveolar lavage (BAL) or to obtain nonsurgical lung biopsies. Blood testing may include assessment for hypercoagulable states in the setting of pulmonary vascular disease, serologic testing for infectious or rheumatologic disease, or assessment of inflammatory markers or leukocyte counts (e.g., eosinophils). Sputum evaluation for malignant cells or microorganisms may be appropriate. An echocardiogram to assess right- and left-sided heart function is often obtained. Finally, at times, a surgical lung biopsy is needed to diagnose certain diseases of the respiratory system. All of these studies will be guided by the preceding history, physical examination, pulmonary function testing, and chest imaging.

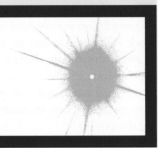

CHAPTER 2

DYSPNEA

Richard M. Schwartzstein

DYSPNEA

The American Thoracic Society defines *dyspnea* as a "subjective experience of breathing discomfort that consists of qualitatively distinct sensations that vary in intensity. The experience derives from interactions among multiple physiological, psychological, social, and environmental factors and may induce secondary physiological and behavioral responses." Dyspnea, a symptom, must be distinguished from the signs of increased work of breathing.

MECHANISMS OF DYSPNEA

Respiratory sensations are the consequence of interactions between the *efferent*, or outgoing, motor output from the brain to the ventilatory muscles (feed-forward) and the *afferent*, or incoming, sensory input from receptors throughout the body (feedback), as well as the integrative processing of this information that we infer must be occurring in the brain **(Fig. 2-1)**. In contrast to painful sensations, which can often be attributed to the stimulation of a single nerve ending, dyspnea sensations are more commonly viewed as holistic, more akin to hunger or thirst. A given disease state may lead to dyspnea by one or more mechanisms, some of which may be operative under some circumstances, e.g., exercise, but not others, e.g., a change in position.

Motor efferents

Disorders of the ventilatory pump, most commonly increase airway resistance or stiffness (decreased compliance) of the respiratory system, are associated with increased work of breathing or a sense of an increased effort to breathe. When the muscles are weak or fatigued, greater effort is required, even though the mechanics of the system are normal. The increased neural output from the motor cortex is sensed via a corollary discharge, a neural

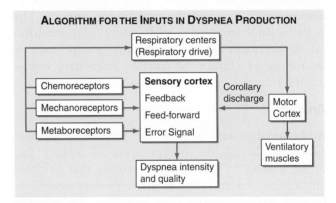

FIGURE 2-1

Hypothetical model for integration of sensory inputs in the production of dyspnea. Afferent information from the receptors throughout the respiratory system projects directly to the sensory cortex to contribute to primary qualitative sensory experiences and provide feedback on the action of the ventilatory pump. Afferents also project to the areas of the brain responsible for control of ventilation. The motor cortex, responding to input from the control centers, sends neural messages to the ventilatory muscles and a corollary discharge to the sensory cortex (feed-forward with respect to the instructions sent to the muscles). If the feed-forward and feedback messages do not match, an error signal is generated and the intensity of dyspnea increases. (*Adapted from MA Gillette, RM Schwartzstein: Mechanisms of Dyspnea, in Supportive Care in Respiratory Disease, SH Ahmedzai and MF Muer [eds]. Oxford, U.K., Oxford University Press, 2005.*)

signal that is sent to the sensory cortex at the same time that motor output is directed to the ventilatory muscles.

Sensory afferents

Chemoreceptors in the carotid bodies and medulla are activated by hypoxemia, acute hypercapnia, and acidemia. Stimulation of these receptors, as well as others that lead to an increase in ventilation, produce a sensation of air hunger. Mechanoreceptors in the lungs, when stimulated by bronchospasm, lead to a sensation of chest tightness. J-receptors, sensitive to interstitial edema, and pulmonary vascular receptors, activated by acute changes in pulmonary artery pressure, appear to contribute to air hunger. Hyperinflation is associated with the sensation of increased work of breathing and an inability to get a deep breath or of an unsatisfying breath. Metaboreceptors, located in skeletal muscle, are believed to be activated by changes in the local biochemical milieu of the tissue active during exercise and, when stimulated, contribute to the breathing discomfort.

Integration: Efferent-reafferent mismatch

A discrepancy or mismatch between the feed-forward message to the ventilatory muscles and the feedback from receptors that monitor the response of the ventilatory pump increases the intensity of dyspnea. This is particularly important when there is a mechanical derangement of the ventilatory pump, such as in asthma or chronic obstructive pulmonary disease (COPD).

Anxiety

Acute anxiety may increase the severity of dyspnea either by altering the interpretation of sensory data or by leading to patterns of breathing that heighten physiologic abnormalities in the respiratory system. In patients with expiratory flow limitation, for example, the increased respiratory rate that accompanies acute anxiety leads to hyperinflation, increased work and effort of breathing, and a sense of an unsatisfying breath.

ASSESSING DYSPNEA

Quality of sensation

As with pain, dyspnea assessment begins with a determination of the quality of the discomfort (Table 2-1). Dyspnea questionnaires, or lists of phrases commonly used by patients, assist those who have difficulty describing their breathing sensations.

Sensory intensity

A modified Borg scale or visual analogue scale can be utilized to measure dyspnea at rest, immediately following exercise, or on recall of a reproducible physical task, e.g., climbing the stairs at home. An alternative approach is to inquire about the activities a patient can do, i.e., to gain a sense of the patient's disability. The Baseline Dyspnea Index and the Chronic Respiratory Disease Questionnaire are commonly used tools for this purpose.

Affective dimension

For a sensation to be reported as a symptom, it must be perceived as unpleasant and interpreted as abnormal.

TABLE 2-1

ASSOCIATION OF QUALITATIVE DESCRIPTORS AND PATHOPHYSIOLOGIC MECHANISMS OF SHORTNESS OF BREATH

DESCRIPTOR	PATHOPHYSIOLOGY
Chest tightness or constriction	Bronchoconstriction, interstitial edema (asthma, myocardial ischemia)
Increased work or effort of breathing	Airway obstruction, neuromuscular disease (COPD, moderate to severe asthma, myopathy, kyphoscoliosis)
Air hunger, need to breathe, urge to breathe	Increased drive to breathe (CHF, pulmonary embolism, moderate to severe airflow obstruction)
Cannot get a deep breath, unsatisfying breath	Hyperinflation (asthma, COPD) and restricted tidal volume (pulmonary fibrosis, chest wall restriction)
Heavy breathing, rapid breathing, breathing more	Deconditioning

Abbreviations: CHF, congestive heart failure; COPD, chronic obstructive pulmonary disease.
Source: From RM Schwartzstein, D Feller-Kopman: Shortness of breath, in *Primary Cardiology*, 2nd ed, E Braunwald and L Goldman (eds). Philadelphia, WB Saunders, 2003.

Laboratory studies have demonstrated that air hunger evokes a stronger affective response than does increased effort or work of breathing. Some therapies for dyspnea, such as pulmonary rehabilitation, may reduce breathing discomfort, in part, by altering this dimension.

DIFFERENTIAL DIAGNOSIS

Dyspnea is the consequence of deviations from normal function in the cardiopulmonary systems. These deviations produce breathlessness as a consequence of increased drive to breathe; increased effort or work of breathing; and/or stimulation of receptors in the heart, lungs, or vascular system. Most diseases of the respiratory system are associated with alterations in the mechanical properties of the lungs and/or chest wall, frequently as a consequence of disease of the airways or lung parenchyma. In contrast, disorders of the cardiovascular system more commonly lead to dyspnea by causing gas exchange abnormalities or stimulating pulmonary and/or vascular receptors (Table 2-2).

Respiratory system dyspnea

▬▬ Diseases of the airways

Asthma and COPD, the most common obstructive lung diseases, are characterized by expiratory airflow obstruction, which typically leads to dynamic hyperinflation of the lungs and chest wall. Patients with moderate to severe disease have increased resistive and elastic loads

TABLE 2-2

MECHANISMS OF DYSPNEA IN COMMON DISEASES

DISEASE	↑ WORK OF BREATHING	↑ DRIVE TO BREATHE	HYPOXEMIA[a]	ACUTE HYPERCAPNIA[a]	STIMULATION OF PULMONARY RECEPTORS	STIMULATION OF VASCULAR RECEPTORS	METABORECEPTORS
COPD	•		•	•			
Asthma	•	•	•	•	•		
ILD	•	•	•	•	•		
PVD		•	•			•	
CPE	•	•	•		•	•	•
NCPE	•	•	•		•		
Anemia							•
Decond							•

[a]Hypoxemia and hypercapnia are not always present in these conditions. When hypoxemia is present, dyspnea usually persists, albeit at a reduced intensity, with correction of hypoxemia by the administration of supplemental oxygen.

Abbreviations: COPD, chronic obstructive pulmonary disease; CPE, cardiogenic pulmonary edema; Decond, deconditioning; ILD, interstitial lung disease; NCPE, noncardiogenic pulmonary edema; PVD, pulmonary vascular disease.

(a term that relates to the stiffness of the system) on the ventilatory muscles and increased work of breathing. Patients with acute bronchoconstriction also complain of a sense of tightness, which can exist even when lung function is still within the normal range. These patients commonly hyperventilate. Both the chest tightness and hyperventilation are probably due to stimulation of pulmonary receptors. Both asthma and COPD may lead to hypoxemia and hypercapnia from ventilation-perfusion ($\dot{V}/\dot{Q}$) mismatch (and diffusion limitation during exercise with emphysema); hypoxemia is much more common than hypercapnia as a consequence of the different ways in which oxygen and carbon dioxide bind to hemoglobin.

Diseases of the chest wall

Conditions that stiffen the chest wall, such as kyphoscoliosis, or that weaken ventilatory muscles, such as myasthenia gravis or the Guillain-Barré syndrome, are also associated with an increased effort to breathe. Large pleural effusions may contribute to dyspnea, both by increasing the work of breathing and by stimulating pulmonary receptors if there is associated atelectasis.

Diseases of the lung parenchyma

Interstitial lung diseases, which may arise from infections, occupational exposures, or autoimmune disorders, are associated with increased stiffness (decreased compliance) of the lungs and increased work of breathing. In addition, $\dot{V}/Q$ mismatch, and destruction and/or thickening of the alveolar-capillary interface may lead to hypoxemia and an increased drive to breathe. Stimulation of pulmonary receptors may further enhance the hyperventilation characteristic of mild to moderate interstitial disease.

Cardiovascular system dyspnea

Diseases of the left heart

Diseases of the myocardium resulting from coronary artery disease and nonischemic cardiomyopathies result in a greater left-ventricular end-diastolic volume and an elevation of the left-ventricular end-diastolic, as well as pulmonary capillary pressures. These elevated pressures lead to interstitial edema and stimulation of pulmonary receptors, thereby causing dyspnea; hypoxemia due to $\dot{V}/Q$ mismatch may also contribute to breathlessness. Diastolic dysfunction, characterized by a very stiff left ventricle, may lead to severe dyspnea with relatively mild degrees of physical activity, particularly if it is associated with mitral regurgitation.

Diseases of the pulmonary vasculature

Pulmonary thromboemoblic disease and primary diseases of the pulmonary circulation (primary pulmonary hypertension, pulmonary vasculitis) cause dyspnea via increased pulmonary-artery pressure and stimulation of pulmonary receptors. Hyperventilation is common, and hypoxemia may be present. However, in most cases, use of supplemental oxygen has minimal effect on the severity of dyspnea and hyperventilation.

Diseases of the pericardium

Constrictive pericarditis and cardiac tamponade are both associated with increased intracardiac and pulmonary vascular pressures, which are the likely cause of dyspnea in these conditions. To the extent that cardiac output is limited, at rest or with exercise, stimulation of metaboreceptors and chemoreceptors (if lactic acidosis develops) contribute as well.

Dyspnea with normal respiratory and cardiovascular systems

Mild to moderate anemia is associated with breathing discomfort during exercise. This is thought to be related to stimulation of metaboreceptors; oxygen saturation is normal in patients with anemia. The breathlessness associated with obesity is probably due to multiple mechanisms, including high cardiac output and impaired ventilatory pump function (decreased compliance of the chest wall). Cardiovascular deconditioning (poor fitness) is characterized by the early development of anaerobic metabolism and the stimulation of chemoreceptors and metaboreceptors.

APPROACH TO THE PATIENT: Dyspnea

(Fig. 2-2) In obtaining a *history*, the patient should be asked to describe in his/her own words what the discomfort feels like, as well as the effect of position, infections, and environmental stimuli on the dyspnea. Orthopnea is a common indicator of congestive heart failure (CHF), mechanical impairment of the diaphragm associated with obesity, or asthma triggered by esophageal reflux. Nocturnal dyspnea suggests CHF or asthma. Acute, intermittent episodes of dyspnea are more likely to reflect episodes of myocardial ischemia, bronchospasm, or pulmonary embolism, while chronic persistent dyspnea is typical of COPD, interstitial lung disease, and chronic thromboembolic disease. Risk factors for occupational lung disease and for coronary artery disease should be elicited. Left atrial myxoma or hepatopulmonary syndrome should be considered when the patient complains of *platypnea*, defined as dyspnea in the upright position with relief in the supine position.

The *physical examination* should begin during the interview of the patient. Inability of the patient to speak in full sentences before stopping to get a deep breath suggests a condition that leads to stimulation of the controller or an impairment of the ventilatory pump with reduced vital capacity. Evidence for increased work of breathing (supraclavicular retractions, use of accessory muscles of ventilation, and the tripod position, characterized by sitting with one's hands braced on the knees) is indicative of increased airway resistance or stiff lungs and chest wall. When measuring the vital signs, one should accurately assess the respiratory rate and measure the pulsus paradoxus; if it is >10 mmHg, consider the presence of COPD or acute asthma. During the general examination, signs of anemia (pale conjunctivae), cyanosis, and cirrhosis (spider angiomata, gynecomastia) should be sought. Examination of the chest should focus on symmetry of movement; percussion (dullness indicative of pleural effusion, hyperresonance a sign of emphysema); and auscultation (wheezes, rales, rhonchi, prolonged expiratory phase, diminished breath sounds, which are clues to disorders of the airways, and interstitial edema or fibrosis). The cardiac examination should focus on signs of elevated right heart pressures (jugular venous distention, edema, accentuated pulmonic component to the second heart sound); left ventricular dysfunction (S3 and S4 gallops); and valvular disease (murmurs). When examining the abdomen with the patient in the supine position, it should be noted whether there is paradoxical movement of the abdomen (inward motion during inspiration), a sign of diaphragmatic weakness; rounding of the abdomen during exhalation is suggestive of pulmonary edema. Clubbing of the digits may be an indication of interstitial pulmonary fibrosis, and the presence of joint swelling or deformation as well as changes consistent with Raynaud's disease may be indicative of a collagen-vascular process that can be associated with pulmonary disease.

Patients with exertional dyspnea should be asked to walk under observation in order to reproduce the symptoms. The patient should be examined for new findings that were not present at rest and for oxygen saturation.

Following the history and physical examination, a *chest radiograph* should be obtained. The lung volumes should be assessed (hyperinflation indicates obstructive lung disease; low lung volumes suggest interstitial edema or fibrosis, diaphragmatic dysfunction, or impaired chest wall motion). The pulmonary parenchyma should be examined for evidence of interstitial disease and emphysema. Prominent pulmonary vasculature in the upper zones indicates pulmonary venous hypertension, while enlarged central pulmonary arteries suggest pulmonary artery hypertension. An enlarged cardiac silhouette suggests a dilated cardiomyopathy or valvular disease. Bilateral pleural effusions are typical of CHF and some forms of collagen vascular disease. Unilateral effusions raise the specter of carcinoma and pulmonary embolism but may also occur in heart failure. *Computed tomography* (CT) *of the chest* is generally reserved for further evaluation of the lung parenchyma (interstitial lung disease) and possible pulmonary embolism.

Laboratory studies should include an electrocardiogram to look for evidence of ventricular hypertrophy and prior myocardial infarction. Echocardiography is indicated in patients in whom systolic dysfunction, pulmonary hypertension, or valvular heart disease is suspected. Bronchoprovocation testing is useful in patients with intermittent symptoms suggestive of asthma but normal physical examination and lung function; up to one-third of patients with the clinical diagnosis of asthma do not have reactive airways disease when formally tested.

Distinguishing Cardiovascular From Respiratory System Dyspnea If a patient has evidence of both pulmonary and cardiac disease, a cardiopulmonary exercise test should be carried out to determine

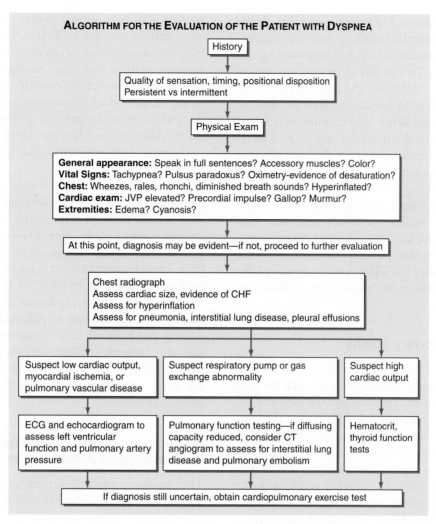

ALGORITHM FOR THE EVALUATION OF THE PATIENT WITH DYSPNEA

History

Quality of sensation, timing, positional disposition
Persistent vs intermittent

Physical Exam

General appearance: Speak in full sentences? Accessory muscles? Color?
Vital Signs: Tachypnea? Pulsus paradoxus? Oximetry-evidence of desaturation?
Chest: Wheezes, rales, rhonchi, diminished breath sounds? Hyperinflated?
Cardiac exam: JVP elevated? Precordial impulse? Gallop? Murmur?
Extremities: Edema? Cyanosis?

At this point, diagnosis may be evident—if not, proceed to further evaluation

Chest radiograph
Assess cardiac size, evidence of CHF
Assess for hyperinflation
Assess for pneumonia, interstitial lung disease, pleural effusions

Suspect low cardiac output, myocardial ischemia, or pulmonary vascular disease

Suspect respiratory pump or gas exchange abnormality

Suspect high cardiac output

ECG and echocardiogram to assess left ventricular function and pulmonary artery pressure

Pulmonary function testing—if diffusing capacity reduced, consider CT angiogram to assess for interstitial lung disease and pulmonary embolism

Hematocrit, thyroid function tests

If diagnosis still uncertain, obtain cardiopulmonary exercise test

FIGURE 2-2

An algorithm for the evaluation of the patient with dyspnea.
JVP, jugular venous pulse; CHF, congestive heart failure; ECG, electrocardiogram; CT, computed tomography. (*Adapted from* *RM Schwartzstein, D Feller-Kopman: Shortness of breath, in Primary Cardiology, 2nd ed, E Braunwald and L Goldman [eds]. Philadelphia, WB Saunders, 2003.*)

which system is responsible for the exercise limitation. If, at peak exercise, the patient achieves predicted maximal ventilation, demonstrates an increase in dead space or hypoxemia, or develops bronchospasm, the respiratory system is probably the cause of the problem. Alternatively, if the heart rate is >85% of the predicted maximum, if anaerobic threshold occurs early, if the blood pressure becomes excessively high or decreases during exercise, if the O_2 pulse (O_2 consumption/heart rate, an indicator of stroke volume) falls, or if there are ischemic changes on the electrocardiogram, an abnormality of the cardiovascular system is likely the explanation for the breathing discomfort.

the patient's quality of life. Supplemental O_2 should be administered if the resting O_2 saturation is ≤89% or if the patient's saturation drops to these levels with activity. For patients with COPD, pulmonary rehabilitation programs have demonstrated positive effects on dyspnea, exercise capacity, and rates of hospitalization. Studies of anxiolytics and antidepressants have not demonstrated consistent benefit. Experimental interventions—e.g., cold air on the face, chest-wall vibration, and inhaled furosemide—to modulate the afferent information from receptors throughout the respiratory system are being studied.

TREATMENT Dyspnea

The first goal is to correct the underlying problem responsible for the symptom. If this is not possible, one attempts to lessen the intensity of the symptom and its effect on

PULMONARY EDEMA

MECHANISMS OF FLUID ACCUMULATION

The extent to which fluid accumulates in the interstitium of the lung depends on the balance of hydrostatic and oncotic forces within the pulmonary capillaries and in the surrounding tissue. Hydrostatic pressure favors movement of fluid from the capillary into the interstitium. The oncotic pressure, which is determined by the protein concentration in the blood, favors movement of fluid into the vessel. Albumin, the primary protein in the plasma, may be low in conditions such as cirrhosis and nephrotic syndrome. While hypoalbuminemia favors movement of fluid into the tissue for any given hydrostatic pressure in the capillary, it is usually not sufficient by itself to cause interstitial edema. In a healthy individual, the tight junctions of the capillary endothelium are impermeable to proteins, and the lymphatics in the tissue carry away the small amounts of protein that may leak out; together, these factors result in an oncotic force that maintains fluid in the capillary. Disruption of the endothelial barrier, however, allows protein to escape the capillary bed and enhances the movement of fluid into the tissue of the lung.

Cardiogenic pulmonary edema

(See also Chap. 30) Cardiac abnormalities that lead to an increase in pulmonary venous pressure shift the balance of forces between the capillary and the interstitium. Hydrostatic pressure is increased and fluid exits the capillary at an increased rate, resulting in interstitial and, in more severe cases, alveolar edema. The development of pleural effusions may further compromise respiratory system function and contribute to breathing discomfort.

Early signs of pulmonary edema include exertional dyspnea and orthopnea. Chest radiographs show peribronchial thickening, prominent vascular markings in the upper lung zones, and Kerley B lines. As the pulmonary edema worsens, alveoli fill with fluid; the chest radiograph shows patchy alveolar filling, typically in a perihilar distribution, which then progresses to diffuse alveolar infiltrates. Increasing airway edema is associated with rhonchi and wheezes.

Noncardiogenic pulmonary edema

In noncardiogenic pulmonary edema, lung water increases due to damage of the pulmonary capillary lining with leakage of proteins and other macromolecules into the tissue; fluid follows the protein as oncotic forces are shifted from the vessel to the surrounding lung tissue. This process is associated with dysfunction of the surfactant lining the alveoli, increased surface forces, and a propensity for the alveoli to collapse at low lung volumes. Physiologically, noncardiogenic pulmonary edema is characterized by intrapulmonary shunt with hypoxemia and decreased pulmonary compliance. Pathologically, hyaline membranes are evident in the alveoli, and inflammation leading to pulmonary fibrosis may be seen. Clinically, the picture ranges from mild dyspnea to respiratory failure. Auscultation of the lungs

may be relatively normal despite chest radiographs that show diffuse alveolar infiltrates. CT scans demonstrate that the distribution of alveolar edema is more heterogeneous than was once thought. Although normal intracardiac pressures are considered by many to be part of the definition of noncardiogenic pulmonary edema, the pathology of the process, as described earlier, is distinctly different, and one can observe a combination of cardiogenic and noncardiogenic pulmonary edema in some patients.

It is useful to categorize the causes of noncardiogenic pulmonary edema in terms of whether the injury to the lung is likely to result from direct, indirect, or pulmonary vascular causes (Table 2-3). Direct injuries are mediated via the airways (e.g., aspiration) or as the consequence of blunt chest trauma. Indirect injury is the consequence of mediators that reach the lung via the blood stream. The third category includes conditions that may be the consequence of acute changes in pulmonary vascular pressures, possibly the result of sudden autonomic discharge in the case of neurogenic and high-altitude pulmonary edema, or sudden swings of pleural pressure, as well as transient damage to the pulmonary capillaries in the case of reexpansion pulmonary edema.

Distinguishing cardiogenic from noncardiogenic pulmonary edema

The *history* is essential for assessing the likelihood of underlying cardiac disease as well as for identification of

TABLE 2-3

COMMON CAUSES OF NONCARDIOGENIC PULMONARY EDEMA

Direct Injury to Lung

Chest trauma, pulmonary contusion
Aspiration
Smoke inhalation
Pneumonia
Oxygen toxicity
Pulmonary embolism, reperfusion

Hematogenous Injury to Lung

Sepsis
Pancreatitis
Nonthoracic trauma
Leukoagglutination reactions
Multiple transfusions
Intravenous drug use, e.g., heroin
Cardiopulmonary bypass

Possible Lung Injury Plus Elevated Hydrostatic Pressures

High-altitude pulmonary edema
Neurogenic pulmonary edema
Reexpansion pulmonary edema

one of the conditions associated with noncardiogenic pulmonary edema. The *physical examination* in cardiogenic pulmonary edema is notable for evidence of increased intracardiac pressures (S3 gallop, elevated jugular venous pulse, peripheral edema), and rales and/or wheezes on auscultation of the chest. In contrast, the physical examination in noncardiogenic pulmonary edema is dominated by the findings of the precipitating condition; pulmonary findings may be relatively normal in the early stages. The *chest radiograph* in cardiogenic pulmonary edema typically shows an enlarged cardiac silhouette, vascular redistribution, interstitial thickening, and perihilar alveolar infiltrates; pleural effusions are common. In noncardiogenic pulmonary edema, heart size is normal, alveolar infiltrates are distributed more uniformly throughout the lungs, and pleural effusions are uncommon. Finally, the *hypoxemia* of cardiogenic pulmonary edema is due largely to $\dot{V}/Q$ mismatch and responds to the administration of supplemental oxygen. In contrast, hypoxemia in noncardiogenic pulmonary edema is due primarily to intrapulmonary shunting and typically persists despite high concentrations of inhaled O_2.

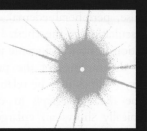

CHAPTER 3

COUGH AND HEMOPTYSIS

Patricia Kritek ■ Christopher Fanta

COUGH

Cough provides an essential protective function for human airways and lungs. Without an effective cough reflex, we are at risk for retained airway secretions and aspirated material, predisposing to infection, atelectasis, and respiratory compromise. At the other extreme, excessive coughing can be exhausting; can be complicated by emesis, syncope, muscular pain, or rib fractures; and can aggravate abdominal or inguinal hernias and urinary incontinence. Cough is often a clue to the presence of respiratory disease. In many instances, cough is an expected and accepted manifestation of disease, such as during an acute respiratory tract infection. However, persistent cough in the absence of other respiratory symptoms commonly causes patients to seek medical attention, accounting for as many as 10–30% of referrals to pulmonary specialists.

COUGH MECHANISM

Spontaneous cough is triggered by stimulation of sensory nerve endings that are thought to be primarily rapidly adapting receptors and C-fibers. Both chemical (e.g., capsaicin) and mechanical (e.g., particulates in air pollution) stimuli may initiate the cough reflex. A cationic ion channel, called the type-1 vanilloid receptor, is found on rapidly adapting receptors and C-fibers; it is the receptor for capsaicin, and its expression is increased in patients with chronic cough. Afferent nerve endings richly innervate the pharynx, larynx, and airways to the level of terminal bronchioles and into the lung parenchyma. They may also be found in the external auditory meatus (the auricular branch of the vagus nerve, called the Arnold nerve) and in the esophagus. Sensory signals travel via the vagus and superior laryngeal nerves to a region of the brainstem in the nucleus tractus solitarius, vaguely identified as the "cough center." Mechanical

stimulation of bronchial mucosa in a transplanted lung (in which the vagus nerve has been severed) does not produce cough.

The cough reflex involves a highly orchestrated series of involuntary muscular actions, with the potential for input from cortical pathways as well. The vocal cords adduct, leading to transient upper-airway occlusion. Expiratory muscles contract, generating positive intrathoracic pressures as high as 300 mmHg. With sudden release of the laryngeal contraction, rapid expiratory flows are generated, exceeding the normal "envelope" of maximal expiratory flow seen on the flow-volume curve **(Fig. 3-1)**. Bronchial smooth muscle contraction together with dynamic compression of airways narrows airway lumens and maximizes the velocity of exhalation (as fast as 50 miles per hour). The kinetic energy available to dislodge mucus from the inside of airway walls is directly proportional to the square of the velocity

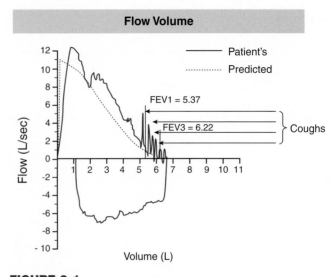

FIGURE 3-1

Flow-Volume Loop. Flow-volume curve with spikes of high expiratory flow achieved with cough.

14

of expiratory airflow. A deep breath preceding a cough optimizes the function of the expiratory muscles; a series of repetitive coughs at successively lower lung volumes sweeps the point of maximal expiratory velocity progressively further into the lung periphery.

IMPAIRED COUGH

Weak or ineffective cough compromises the ability to clear lower respiratory tract infections, predisposing to more serious infections and their sequelae. Weakness, paralysis, or pain of the expiratory (abdominal and intercostal) muscles is foremost on the list of causes of impaired cough (Table 3-1). Cough strength is generally assessed qualitatively; peak expiratory flow or maximal expiratory pressure at the mouth can be used as a surrogate marker for cough strength. A variety of assistive devices and techniques have been developed to improve cough strength, spanning the gamut from simple (splinting the abdominal muscles with a tightly-held pillow to reduce post-operative pain while coughing) to complex (a mechanical cough-assist device applied via face mask or tracheal tube that applies a cycle of positive pressure followed rapidly by negative pressure). Cough may fail to clear secretions despite a preserved ability to generate normal expiratory velocities, either due to abnormal airway secretions (e.g., bronchiectasis due to cystic fibrosis) or structural abnormalities of the airways (e.g., tracheomalacia with expiratory collapse during cough).

SYMPTOMATIC COUGH

The cough of chronic bronchitis in long-term cigarette smokers rarely leads the patient to seek medical advice. It lasts only seconds to a few minutes, is productive of benign-appearing mucoid sputum, and is not discomforting. Similarly, cough may occur in the context of other respiratory symptoms that, together, point to a diagnosis, such as when cough is accompanied by wheezing, shortness of breath, and chest tightness after exposure to a cat or other sources of allergens. At times, however, cough is the dominant or sole symptom of disease, and it may be of

TABLE 3-1

CAUSES OF IMPAIRED COUGH
Decreased expiratory-muscle strength
Decreased inspiratory-muscle strength
Chest-wall deformity
Impaired glottic closure or tracheostomy
Tracheomalacia
Abnormal airway secretions
Central respiratory depression (e.g., anesthesia, sedation, or coma)

sufficient duration and severity that relief is sought. The duration of cough is a clue to its etiology. Acute cough (<3 weeks) is most commonly due to a respiratory tract infection, aspiration event, or inhalation of noxious chemicals or smoke. Subacute cough (3–8 weeks duration) is frequently the residuum from a tracheobronchitis, such as in pertussis or "post-viral tussive syndrome." Chronic cough (>8 weeks) may be caused by a wide variety of cardiopulmonary diseases, including those of inflammatory, infectious, neoplastic, and cardiovascular etiologies. When initial assessment with chest examination and radiograph is normal, cough-variant asthma, gastroesophageal reflux, nasopharyngeal drainage, and medications (angiotensin converting enzyme [ACE] inhibitors) are the most common causes of chronic cough. Cough of less than 8 weeks' duration may be the early manifestation of a disease causing chronic cough.

ASSESSMENT OF CHRONIC COUGH

Details as to the sound, time of occurrence during the day, and pattern of coughing infrequently provide useful etiology clues. Regardless of cause, cough often worsens when one first lies down at night or with talking or in association with the hyperpnea of exercise; it frequently improves with sleep. Exceptions might include the characteristic inspiratory whoop after a paroxysm of coughing that suggests pertussis or the cough that occurs only with certain allergic exposures or exercise in cold air, as in asthma. Useful historical questions include the circumstances surrounding the onset of cough, what makes the cough better or worse, and whether or not the cough produces sputum.

The physical examination seeks clues to the presence of cardiopulmonary disease, including findings such as wheezing or crackles on chest examination. Examination of the auditory canals and tympanic membranes (for irritation of the tympanic membrane resulting in stimulation of Arnold's nerve), the nasal passageways (for rhinitis), and nails (for clubbing) may also provide etiologic clues. Because cough can be a manifestation of a systemic disease, such as sarcoidosis or vasculitis, a thorough general examination is equally important.

In virtually all instances, evaluation of chronic cough merits a chest radiograph. The list of diseases that can cause persistent coughing without other symptoms and without detectable abnormality on physical examination is long. It includes serious illnesses such as Hodgkin's disease in young adults and lung cancer in an older population. An abnormal chest film leads to evaluation of the radiographic abnormality to explain the symptom of cough. A normal chest image provides valuable reassurance to the patient and the patient's family, who may have imagined the direst explanation for the cough.

In a patient with chronic productive cough, examination of expectorated sputum is warranted. Purulent-appearing sputum should be sent for routine bacterial culture and, in certain circumstances, mycobacterial culture as well. Cytologic examination of mucoid sputum may be useful to assess for malignancy and to distinguish neutrophilic from eosinophilic bronchitis. Expectoration of blood—whether streaks of blood, blood mixed with airway secretions, or pure blood—deserves a special approach to assessment and management, as discussed later.

CHRONIC COUGH WITH A NORMAL CHEST RADIOGRAPH

It is commonly held that use of an angiotensin-converting enzyme inhibitor; post-nasal drainage; gastroesophageal reflux; and asthma, alone or in combination, account for more than 90% of patients who have chronic cough and a normal or noncontributory chest radiograph. However, clinical experience does not support this contention, and strict adherence to this concept discourages the search for alternative explanations by both clinicians and researchers. On the one hand, chronic idiopathic cough is common and its management deserves study and discussion. On the other hand, serious pulmonary diseases, including inflammatory lung diseases, chronic infections, and neoplasms, may remain occult on plain chest imaging and require additional testing for detection.

ACE inhibitor-induced cough occurs in 5–30% of patients taking ACE inhibitors and is not dose-dependent. Any patient with chronic unexplained cough who is taking an ACE inhibitor should be given a trial period off the medication, regardless of the timing of the onset of cough relative to the initiation of ACE inhibitor therapy. In most instances, a safe alternative is available; angiotensin-receptor blockers do not cause cough. Failure to observe a decrease in cough after one month off medication argues strongly against this diagnosis. ACE metabolizes bradykinin and other tachykinins, such as substance P. The mechanism of ACE inhibitor cough may involve sensitization of sensory nerve endings due to accumulation of bradykinin. In support of this hypothesis, polymorphisms in the neurokinin-2 receptor gene are associated with ACE inhibitor–induced cough.

Post-nasal drainage of any etiology can cause cough as a response to stimulation of sensory receptors of the cough-reflex pathway in the hypopharynx or aspiration of draining secretions into the trachea. Clues to this etiology include symptoms of post-nasal drip, frequent throat clearing, and sneezing and rhinorrhea. On speculum examination of the nose, one may see excess mucoid or purulent secretions, inflamed and edematous nasal mucosa, and/or nasal polyps; in addition, one might visualize secretions or a cobblestoned appearance of the mucosa along the posterior pharyngeal wall. Unfortunately, there is no means by which to quantitate post-nasal drainage. In many instances, one is left to rely on a qualitative judgment based on subjective information provided by the patient. This assessment must also be counterbalanced by the fact that many people who have chronic post-nasal drainage do not experience cough.

Linking gastroesophageal reflux to chronic cough poses similar challenges. It is thought that reflux of gastric contents into the lower esophagus may trigger cough via reflex pathways initiated in the esophageal mucosa. Reflux to the level of the pharynx with consequent aspiration of gastric contents causes a chemical bronchitis and possible pneumonitis that can elicit cough for days after the aspiration event. Retrosternal burning after meals or on recumbency, frequent eructation, hoarseness, and throat pain are potential clues to gastroesophageal reflux. Reflux may also elicit no or minimal symptoms. Glottic inflammation may be a clue to recurrent reflux to the level of the throat, but it is a nonspecific finding and requires direct or indirect laryngoscopy for detection. Quantification of the frequency and level of reflux requires a somewhat invasive procedure to measure esophageal pH directly (a catheter with pH probe placed nasopharyngeally in the esophagus for 24 h, or pH monitoring using a radiotransmitter capsule placed endoscopically into the esophagus). Precise interpretation of test results enabling one to link reflux and cough in a causative way remains debated. Again, assigning the cause of cough to gastroesophageal reflux must be weighed against the observation that many people with chronic reflux (such as frequently occurs during pregnancy) do not experience chronic cough.

Cough alone as a manifestation of asthma is common in children, but not in adults. Cough due to asthma in the absence of wheezing, shortness of breath, and chest tightness is referred to as "cough-variant asthma." A history suggestive of cough-variant asthma ties the onset of cough to typical triggers for asthma and resolution of cough upon withdrawal from exposure to them. Objective testing can establish the diagnosis of asthma (airflow obstruction on spirometry that varies over time or reverses in response to bronchodilator) or exclude it with certainty (negative response to bronchoprovocation challenge, such as with methacholine). In a patient capable of making reliable measurements, home expiratory peak flow monitoring can be used as a cost-effective method to support or discount a diagnosis of asthma.

Chronic eosinophilic bronchitis causes chronic cough with a normal chest radiograph. This condition is characterized by sputum eosinophilia in excess of 3% without airflow obstruction or bronchial hyperresponsiveness and is successfully treated with inhaled glucocorticoids.

Treatment of chronic cough in a patient with a normal chest radiograph is often empiric and is targeted at the most likely cause or causes of cough as determined by history, physical examination, and possibly pulmonary-function testing. Therapy for post-nasal drainage depends on the presumed etiology (infection, allergy, or vasomotor rhinitis) and may include systemic antihistamines; antibiotics; nasal saline irrigation; and nasal pump sprays with corticosteroids, antihistamines, or anticholinergics. Antacids, histamine type-2 (H2) receptor antagonists, and proton-pump inhibitors are used to neutralize or decrease production of gastric acid in gastroesophageal reflux disease; dietary changes, elevation of the head and torso during sleep, and medications to improve gastric emptying are additional therapies. Cough-variant asthma typically responds well to inhaled glucocorticoids and intermittent use of inhaled beta-agonist bronchodilators.

Patients who fail to respond to treatment of the common causes of cough or who have had these causes excluded by appropriate diagnostic testing should undergo chest CT. Examples of diseases causing cough that may be missed on chest x-ray include carcinoid tumor, early interstitial lung disease, bronchiectasis, and atypical mycobacterial pulmonary infection. On the other hand, patients with chronic cough who have normal chest examination, lung function, oxygenation, and chest CT imaging can be reassured as to the absence of serious pulmonary pathology.

SYMPTOMATIC TREATMENT OF COUGH

Chronic idiopathic cough is distressingly common. It is often experienced as a tickle or sensitivity in the throat area, occurs more often in women, and is typically "dry" or at most productive of scant amounts of mucoid sputum. It can be exhausting, interfere with work, and cause social embarrassment. Once serious underlying cardiopulmonary pathology has been excluded, an attempt at cough suppression is appropriate. Most effective are narcotic cough suppressants, such as codeine or hydrocodone, which are thought to act in the "cough center" in the brainstem. The tendency of narcotic cough suppressants to cause drowsiness and constipation and their potential for addictive dependence limit their appeal for long-term use. Dextromethorphan is an over-the-counter, centrally acting cough suppressant with fewer side effects and less efficacy compared to the narcotic cough suppressants. It is thought to have a different site of action than narcotic cough suppressants and can be used in combination with them if necessary. Benzonatate is thought to inhibit neural activity of sensory nerves in the cough-reflex pathway. It is generally free of side effects; however, its effectiveness in suppressing cough is variable and unpredictable. Novel

cough suppressants without the limitations of currently available therapies are greatly needed. Approaches that are being explored include development of neurokinin receptor antagonists, type-1 vanilloid receptor antagonists, and novel opioid and opioidlike receptor agonists.

HEMOPTYSIS

Hemoptysis is the expectoration of blood from the respiratory tract. It can arise from any part of the respiratory tract, from the alveoli to the glottis. It is important, however, to distinguish hemoptysis from epistaxis (i.e., bleeding from the nasopharynx) and hematemesis (i.e., bleeding from the upper gastrointestinal tract). Hemoptysis can range from blood-tinged sputum to life-threatening large volumes of bright red blood. For most patients, any degree of hemoptysis can be anxiety-producing and often prompts medical evaluation.

While precise epidemiologic data are lacking, the most common etiology of hemoptysis is infection of the medium-sized airways. In the United States, this is usually due to a viral or bacterial bronchitis. Hemoptysis can arise in the setting of either acute bronchitis or during an exacerbation of chronic bronchitis. Worldwide, the most common cause of hemoptysis is tuberculous infection presumably owing to the high prevalence of the disease and its predilection for cavity formation. While these are the most common causes, there is an extensive differential diagnosis for hemoptysis, and a step-wise approach to the evaluation of this symptom is appropriate.

ETIOLOGY

One way to approach the source of hemoptysis is systematically to assess for potential sites of bleeding from the alveolus to the mouth. Diffuse bleeding in the alveolar space, often referred to as diffuse alveolar hemorrhage (DAH), may present with hemoptysis, although this is not always the case. Causes of DAH can be divided into inflammatory and noninflammatory types. Inflammatory DAH is due to small vessel vasculitis/capillaritis from a variety of diseases, including granulomatosis with polyangiitis (Wegener's) and microscopic polyangiitis. Similarly, systemic autoimmune disease, such as systemic lupus erythematosus (SLE), can manifest as pulmonary capillaritis and result in DAH. Antibodies to the alveolar basement membrane, as are seen in Goodpasture's disease, can also result in alveolar hemorrhage. In the early time period after a bone marrow transplant (BMT), patients can also develop a form of inflammatory DAH, which can be catastrophic and life-threatening. The exact pathophysiology of this process is not well understood, but DAH should be suspected in patients with sudden-onset dyspnea and hypoxemia in the first 100 days after a BMT.

Alveoli can also bleed due to noninflammatory causes, most commonly due to direct inhalational injury. This category includes thermal injury from fires, inhalation of illicit substances (e.g., cocaine), and inhalation of toxic chemicals. If alveoli are irritated from any process, patients with thrombocytopenia, coagulopathy, or anti-platelet or anticoagulant use will have an increased risk of developing hemoptysis.

As already noted, the most common site of hemoptysis is bleeding from the small- to medium-sized airways. Irritation and injury of the bronchial mucosal can lead to small-volume bleeding. More significant hemoptysis can also occur because of the proximity of the bronchial artery and vein to the airway, running together in what is often referred to as the "bronchovascular bundle." In the smaller airways, these blood vessels are close to the airspace and, therefore, lesser degrees of inflammation or injury can result in rupture of these vessels into the airways. Of note, while alveolar hemorrhage arises from capillaries that are part of the low-pressure pulmonary circulation, bronchial bleeding is generally from bronchial arteries, which are under systemic pressure and, therefore, predisposed to larger-volume bleeding.

Any infection of the airways can result in hemoptysis, although, most commonly, acute bronchitis is caused by viral infection. In patients with a history of chronic bronchitis, bacterial super infection with organisms such as *Streptococcus pneumoniae*, *Hemophilus influenzae*, or *Moraxella catarrhalis* can also result in hemoptysis. Patients with bronchiectasis, a permanent dilation and irregularity of the airways, are particularly prone to hemoptysis due to anatomic abnormalities that bring the bronchial arteries closer to the mucosal surface and the associated chronic inflammatory state. One common presentation of patients with advanced cystic fibrosis, the prototypical bronchiectatic lung disease, is hemoptysis, which, at times, can be life-threatening.

Pneumonias of any sort can cause hemoptysis. Tuberculous infection, which can lead to bronchiectasis or cavitary pneumonia, is a very common cause of hemoptysis worldwide. Community-acquired pneumonia and lung abscess can also result in bleeding. Once again, if the infection results in cavitation, there is a greater likelihood of bleeding due to erosion into blood vessels. Infections with *Staphylococcus aureus* and gram-negative rods (e.g., *Klebsiella pneumoniae*) are more likely to cause necrotizing lung infections and, thus, are more often associated with hemoptysis. Previous severe pneumonias can cause scarring and abnormal lung architecture, which may predispose a patient to hemoptysis with subsequent infections.

While it is not commonly seen in North America, pulmonary paragonimiasis (i.e., infection with the lung fluke *Paragonimus westermani*) often presents with fever, cough, and hemoptysis. This infection is a public health issue in Southeast Asia and China and is commonly confused with active tuberculosis, because the clinical pictures can be similar. Paragonimiasis should be considered in recent immigrants from endemic areas with new or recurrent hemoptysis. In addition, there are reports of pulmonary paragonimiasis in the United States secondary to ingestion of crayfish or small crabs.

Other causes of irritation of the airways resulting in hemoptysis include inhalation of toxic chemicals, thermal injury, direct trauma from suctioning of the airways (particularly in intubated patients), and irritation from inhalation of foreign bodies. All of these etiologies should be suggested by the individual patient's history and exposures.

Perhaps the most feared cause of hemoptysis is bronchogenic lung cancer, although hemoptysis is not a particularly common presenting symptom of this disease with only approximately 10% of patients having frank hemoptysis on initial assessment. Cancers arising in the proximal airways are much more likely to cause hemoptysis, although any malignancy in the chest can do so. Because both squamous cell carcinoma and small cell carcinoma are more commonly central and large at presentation, they are more often a cause of hemoptysis. These cancers can present with large-volume and life-threatening hemoptysis because of erosion into the hilar vessels. Carcinoid tumors, which are almost exclusively found as endobronchial lesions with friable mucosa, can also present with hemoptysis.

In addition to cancers arising in the lung, metastatic disease in the pulmonary parenchyma can also bleed. Malignancies that commonly metastasize to the lungs include renal cell, breast, colon, testicular, and thyroid cancers as well as melanoma. While they are not a common way for metastatic disease to present, multiple pulmonary nodules and hemoptysis should raise the suspicion for this etiology.

Finally, disease of the pulmonary vasculature can cause hemoptysis. Perhaps most commonly, congestive heart failure with transmission of elevated left atrial pressures, if severe enough, can lead to rupture of small alveolar capillaries. These patients rarely present with bright red blood but more commonly have pink, frothy sputum or blood-tinged secretions. Patients with a focal jet of mitral regurgitation can present with an upper-lobe infiltrate on chest radiograph together with hemoptysis. This is thought to be due to focal increases in pulmonary capillary pressure due to the regurgitant jet. Pulmonary arterio-venous malformations are prone to bleeding. Pulmonary embolism can also lead to the development of hemoptysis, which is generally associated with pulmonary infarction. Pulmonary arterial hypertension from other causes rarely results in hemoptysis.

EVALUATION

As with most symptoms, the initial step in the evaluation of hemoptysis is a thorough history and physical examination **(Fig. 3-2)**. As already mentioned, questioning should begin with determining if the bleeding is truly from the respiratory tract and not the nasopharynx or gastrointestinal tract, because these sources of bleeding require different evaluation and treatment approaches.

HISTORY AND PHYSICAL EXAM

The nature of the hemoptysis, whether they are blood-tinged, purulent secretions; pink, frothy sputum; or frank blood, may be helpful in determining an etiology. Specific triggers of the bleeding, such as recent inhalation exposures as well as any previous episodes of hemoptysis, should be elicited during history-taking. Monthly hemoptysis in a woman suggests catamenial hemoptysis from pulmonary endometriosis. The volume of the hemoptysis is also important not only in determining the cause, but in gauging the urgency for further diagnostic and therapeutic maneuvers. Patients rarely exsanguinate from hemoptysis but can effectively "drown" in aspirated blood. Large-volume hemoptysis, referred to as *massive hemoptysis*, is variably defined as

hemoptysis of greater than 200–600 cc in 24 h. Massive hemoptysis should be considered a medical emergency. The medical urgency related to hemoptysis depends on both the amount of bleeding and the severity of underlying pulmonary disease.

All patients should be asked about current or former cigarette smoking; this behavior predisposes to both chronic bronchitis and increases the likelihood of bronchogenic cancer. Symptoms suggestive of respiratory tract infection— including fever, chills, and dyspnea— should be elicited. The practitioner should inquire about recent inhalation exposures or use of illicit substances as well as risk factors for venous thromboembolism.

Past medical history of malignancy or treatment thereof, rheumatologic disease, vascular disease, or underlying lung disease such as bronchiectasis may be relevant to the cause of hemoptysis. Because many of the causes of DAH can be part of a pulmonary-renal syndrome, specific inquiry into a history of renal insufficiency also is important.

The physical examination begins with an assessment of vital signs and oxygen saturation to gauge whether there is evidence of life-threatening bleeding. Tachycardia, hypotension, and decreased oxygen saturation should dictate a more expedited evaluation of hemoptysis. Specific focus on respiratory and cardiac

Cough and Hemoptysis

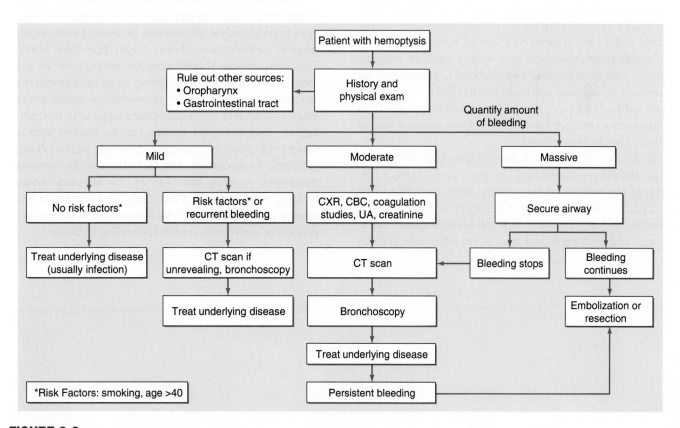

FIGURE 3-2

Flowchart—evaluation of hemoptysis. Decision tree for evaluation of hemoptysis. CBC, complete blood count; CT, computed tomography; CXR, chest x-ray; UA, urinalysis.

examinations are important and should include inspection of the nares, auscultation of the lungs and heart, assessment of the lower extremities for symmetric or asymmetric edema, and evaluation for jugular venous distention. Clubbing of the digits may suggest underlying lung diseases such as bronchogenic carcinoma or bronchiectasis, which predispose to hemoptysis. Similarly, mucocutaneous telangiectasias should raise the specter of pulmonary arterial-venous malformations.

DIAGNOSTIC EVALUATION

For most patients, the next step in evaluation of hemoptysis should be a standard chest radiograph. If a source of bleeding is not identified on plain film, a CT of the chest should be obtained. CT allows better delineation of bronchiectasis, alveolar filling, cavitary infiltrates, and masses than does chest x-ray; it also gives further information on mediastinal lymphadenopathy, which may support a diagnosis of thoracic malignancy. The practitioner should consider a CT protocol to assess for pulmonary embolism if the history or examination suggests venous thromboembolism as a cause of the bleeding.

Laboratory studies should include a complete blood count to assess both the hematocrit as well as platelet count and coagulation studies. Renal function and urinalysis should be assessed because of the possibility of pulmonary-renal syndromes presenting with hemoptysis. Acute renal insufficiency, or red blood cells or red blood cell casts on urinalysis should increase suspicion for small-vessel vasculitis, and studies such as antineutrophil cytoplasmic antibody (ANCA), antiglomerular basement membrane antibody (anti-GBM), and antinuclear antibody (ANA), should be considered. If a patient is producing sputum, Gram and acid-fast stains as well as culture should be obtained.

If all of these studies are unrevealing, bronchoscopy should be considered. In any patient with a history of cigarette smoking, airway inspection should be part of the evaluation of new hemoptysis. Because these patients are at increased risk of bronchogenic carcinoma, and endobronchial lesions are often not reliably visualized on computed tomogram, bronchoscopy should be seriously considered to add to the completeness of the evaluation.

TREATMENT	Hemoptysis

For the most part, the treatment of hemoptysis will vary based on its etiology. However, large-volume, life-threatening hemoptysis generally requires immediate intervention regardless of the cause. The first step is to establish a patent airway usually by endotracheal intubation and subsequent mechanical ventilation. As most large-volume hemoptysis arises from an airway lesion, it is ideal if the site of the bleeding can be identified either by chest imaging or bronchoscopy (more commonly rigid than flexible). The goal is then to isolate the bleeding to one lung and not allow the preserved airspaces in the other lung to be filled with blood, further impairing gas exchange. Patients should be placed with the bleeding lung in a dependent position (i.e., bleeding-side down) and, if possible, dual lumen endotracheal tubes or an airway blocker should be placed in the proximal airway of the bleeding lung. These interventions generally require the assistance of anesthesiologists, interventional pulmonologists, or thoracic surgeons.

If the bleeding does not stop with therapies of the underlying cause and passage of time, severe hemoptysis from bronchial arteries can be treated with angiographic embolization of the culprit bronchial artery. This intervention should only be entertained in the most severe and life-threatening cases of hemoptysis because there is a risk of unintentional spinal-artery embolization and consequent paraplegia with this procedure. Endobronchial lesions can be treated with a variety of bronchoscopically directed interventions, including cauterization and laser therapy. In extreme conditions, surgical resection of the affected region of lung is considered. Most cases of hemoptysis will resolve with treatment of the infection or inflammatory process or with removal of the offending stimulus.

CHAPTER 4

HYPOXIA AND CYANOSIS

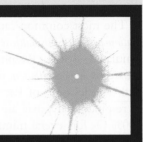

Joseph Loscalzo

HYPOXIA

The fundamental purpose of the cardiorespiratory system is to deliver O_2 and nutrients to cells and to remove CO_2 and other metabolic products from them. Proper maintenance of this function depends not only on intact cardiovascular and respiratory systems but also on an adequate number of red blood cells and hemoglobin and a supply of inspired gas containing adequate O_2.

RESPONSES TO HYPOXIA

Decreased O_2 availability to cells results in an inhibition of oxidative phosphorylation and increased anaerobic glycolysis. This switch from aerobic to anaerobic metabolism, the Pasteur effect, maintains some, albeit reduced, adenosine 5'-triphosphate (ATP) production. In severe hypoxia, when ATP production is inadequate to meet the energy requirements of ionic and osmotic equilibrium, cell membrane depolarization leads to uncontrolled Ca^{2+} influx and activation of Ca^{2+}-dependent phospholipases and proteases. These events, in turn, cause cell swelling and, ultimately, cell death.

The adaptations to hypoxia are mediated, in part, by the upregulation of genes encoding a variety of proteins, including glycolytic enzymes such as phosphoglycerate kinase and phosphofructokinase, as well as the glucose transporters Glut-1 and Glut-2; and by growth factors, such as vascular endothelial growth factor (VEGF) and erythropoietin, which enhance erythrocyte production. The hypoxia-induced increase in expression of these key proteins is governed by the hypoxia-sensitive transcription factor, hypoxia-inducible factor-1 (HIF-1).

During hypoxia, systemic arterioles dilate, at least in part, by opening of K_{ATP} channels in vascular smooth-muscle cells due to the hypoxia-induced reduction in ATP concentration. By contrast, in pulmonary vascular smooth-muscle cells, inhibition of K^+ channels causes depolarization which, in turn, activates voltage-gated Ca^{2+} channels raising the cytosolic $[Ca^{2+}]$ and causing smooth-muscle cell contraction. Hypoxia-induced pulmonary arterial constriction shunts blood away from poorly ventilated portions toward better ventilated portions of the lung; however, it also increases pulmonary vascular resistance and right ventricular afterload.

Effects on the central nervous system

Changes in the central nervous system (CNS), particularly the higher centers, are especially important consequences of hypoxia. Acute hypoxia causes impaired judgment, motor incoordination, and a clinical picture resembling acute alcohol intoxication. High-altitude illness is characterized by headache secondary to cerebral vasodilation, gastrointestinal symptoms, dizziness, insomnia, fatigue, or somnolence. Pulmonary arterial and sometimes venous constriction cause capillary leakage and high-altitude pulmonary edema (HAPE) (Chap. 2), which intensifies hypoxia, further promoting vasoconstriction. Rarely, high-altitude cerebral edema (HACE) develops, which is manifest by severe headache and papilledema and can cause coma. As hypoxia becomes more severe, the regulatory centers of the brainstem are affected, and death usually results from respiratory failure.

CAUSES OF HYPOXIA

Respiratory Hypoxia

When hypoxia occurs from respiratory failure, PaO_2 declines, and when respiratory failure is persistent, the hemoglobin-oxygen (Hb-O_2) dissociation curve is displaced to the right, with greater quantities of O_2 released at any level of tissue PO_2. Arterial hypoxemia, i.e., a reduction of O_2 saturation of arterial blood (SaO_2), and consequent cyanosis are likely to be more marked when such depression of PaO_2 results from pulmonary disease than when the depression occurs as the result of a decline in the fraction of oxygen in inspired air (FiO_2). In this latter situation, $PaCO_2$ falls secondary to anoxia-induced hyperventilation and the Hb-O_2 dissociation curve is displaced to the left, limiting the decline in SaO_2 at any level of PaO_2.

The most common cause of respiratory hypoxia is *ventilation-perfusion mismatch* resulting from perfusion of poorly ventilated alveoli. Respiratory hypoxemia may also be caused by *hypoventilation*, in which case it is then associated with an elevation of $PaCO_2$ (Chap. 5). These two forms of respiratory hypoxia are usually correctable by inspiring 100% O_2 for several minutes. A third cause of respiratory hypoxia is shunting of blood across the lung from the pulmonary arterial to the venous bed (*intrapulmonary right-to-left shunting*) by perfusion of nonventilated portions of the lung, as in pulmonary atelectasis or through pulmonary arteriovenous connections. The low PaO_2 in this situation is only partially corrected by an FiO_2 of 100%.

Hypoxia secondary to high altitude

As one ascends rapidly to 3000 m (~10,000 ft), the reduction of the O_2 content of inspired air (FiO_2) leads to a decrease in alveolar PO_2 to approximately 60 mmHg, and a condition termed *high-altitude illness* develops (see earlier). At higher altitudes, arterial saturation declines rapidly and symptoms become more serious; and at 5000 m, unacclimated individuals usually cease to be able to function normally owing to the changes in CNS function described earlier.

Hypoxia secondary to right-to-left extrapulmonary shunting

From a physiologic viewpoint, this cause of hypoxia resembles intrapulmonary right-to-left shunting but is caused by congenital cardiac malformations, such as tetralogy of Fallot, transposition of the great arteries, and Eisenmenger's syndrome. As in pulmonary right-to-left shunting, the PaO_2 cannot be restored to normal with inspiration of 100% O_2.

Anemic hypoxia

A reduction in hemoglobin concentration of the blood is accompanied by a corresponding decline in the O_2-carrying capacity of the blood. Although the PaO_2 is normal in anemic hypoxia, the absolute quantity of O_2 transported per unit volume of blood is diminished. As the anemic blood passes through the capillaries and the usual quantity of O_2 is removed from it, the PO_2 and saturation in the venous blood decline to a greater extent than normal.

Carbon monoxide (CO) intoxication

Hemoglobin that binds with CO (carboxyhemoglobin, COHb) is unavailable for O_2 transport. In addition, the presence of COHb shifts the Hb-O_2 dissociation curve to the left so that O_2 is unloaded only at lower tensions, contributing further to tissue hypoxia.

Circulatory hypoxia

As in anemic hypoxia, the PaO_2 is usually normal, but venous and tissue PO_2 values are reduced as a consequence of reduced tissue perfusion and greater tissue O_2 extraction. This pathophysiology leads to an increased arterial-mixed venous O_2 difference (a-v-O_2 difference), or gradient. Generalized circulatory hypoxia occurs in heart failure and in most forms of shock (Chap. 27).

Specific organ hypoxia

Localized circulatory hypoxia may occur as a result of decreased perfusion secondary to arterial obstruction, as in localized atherosclerosis in any vascular bed, or as a consequence of vasoconstriction, as observed in Raynaud's phenomenon. Localized hypoxia may also result from venous obstruction and the resultant expansion of interstitial fluid causing arteriolar compression and, thereby, reduction of arterial inflow. Edema, which increases the distance through which O_2 must diffuse before it reaches cells, can also cause localized hypoxia. In an attempt to maintain adequate perfusion to more vital organs in patients with reduced cardiac output secondary to heart failure or hypovolemic shock, vasoconstriction may reduce perfusion in the limbs and skin, causing hypoxia of these regions.

Increased O_2 requirements

If the O_2 consumption of tissues is elevated without a corresponding increase in perfusion, tissue hypoxia ensues and the PO_2 in venous blood declines. Ordinarily, the clinical picture of patients with hypoxia due to an elevated metabolic rate, as in fever or thyrotoxicosis, is quite different from that in other types of hypoxia: the skin is warm and flushed owing to increased cutaneous blood flow that dissipates the excessive heat produced, and cyanosis is usually absent.

Exercise is a classic example of increased tissue O_2 requirements. These increased demands are normally met by several mechanisms operating simultaneously: (1) increase in the cardiac output and ventilation and, thus, O_2 delivery to the tissues; (2) a preferential shift in blood flow to the exercising muscles by changing vascular resistances in the circulatory beds of exercising tissues, directly and/or reflexly; (3) an increase in O_2 extraction from the delivered blood and a widening of the arteriovenous O_2 difference; and (4) a reduction in the pH of the tissues and capillary blood, shifting the Hb-O_2 curve to the right, and unloading more O_2 from hemoglobin. If the capacity of these mechanisms is exceeded, then hypoxia, especially of the exercising muscles, will result.

Improper oxygen utilization

Cyanide and several other similarly acting poisons cause cellular hypoxia. The tissues are unable to utilize O_2, and, as a consequence, the venous blood tends to have a high O_2 tension. This condition has been termed *histotoxic hypoxia*.

ADAPTATION TO HYPOXIA

An important component of the respiratory response to hypoxia originates in special chemosensitive cells in the carotid and aortic bodies and in the respiratory center in the brainstem. The stimulation of these cells by hypoxia increases ventilation, with a loss of CO_2, and can lead to respiratory alkalosis. When combined with the metabolic acidosis resulting from the production of lactic acid, the serum bicarbonate level declines (Chap. 38).

With the reduction of PaO_2, cerebrovascular resistance decreases and cerebral blood flow increases in an attempt to maintain O_2 delivery to the brain. However, when the reduction of PaO_2 is accompanied by hyperventilation and a reduction of $PaCO_2$, cerebrovascular resistance rises, cerebral blood flow falls, and tissue hypoxia intensifies.

The diffuse, systemic vasodilation that occurs in generalized hypoxia increases the cardiac output. In patients with underlying heart disease, the requirements of peripheral tissues for an increase of cardiac output with hypoxia may precipitate congestive heart failure. In patients with ischemic heart disease, a reduced PaO_2 may intensify myocardial ischemia and further impair left ventricular function.

One of the important compensatory mechanisms for chronic hypoxia is an increase in the hemoglobin concentration and in the number of red blood cells in the circulating blood, i.e., the development of polycythemia secondary to erythropoietin production. In persons with chronic hypoxemia secondary to prolonged residence at a high altitude (>13,000 ft, 4200 m), a condition termed *chronic mountain sickness* develops. This disorder is characterized by a blunted respiratory drive, reduced ventilation, erythrocytosis, cyanosis, weakness, right ventricular enlargement secondary to pulmonary hypertension, and even stupor.

CYANOSIS

Cyanosis refers to a bluish color of the skin and mucous membranes resulting from an increased quantity of reduced hemoglobin (i.e., deoxygenated hemoglobin) or of hemoglobin derivatives (e.g., methemoglobin or sulfhemoglobin) in the small blood vessels of those tissues. It is usually most marked in the lips, nail beds, ears, and malar eminences. Cyanosis, especially if developed recently, is more commonly detected by a family member than the patient. The florid skin characteristic of polycythemia vera must be distinguished from the true cyanosis discussed here. A cherry-colored flush, rather than cyanosis, is caused by COHb.

The degree of cyanosis is modified by the color of the cutaneous pigment and the thickness of the skin, as well as by the state of the cutaneous capillaries. The accurate clinical detection of the presence and degree of cyanosis is difficult, as proved by oximetric studies. In some instances, central cyanosis can be detected reliably when the SaO_2 has fallen to 85%; in others, particularly in dark-skinned persons, it may not be detected until it has declined to 75%. In the latter case, examination of the mucous membranes in the oral cavity and the conjunctivae rather than examination of the skin is more helpful in the detection of cyanosis.

The increase in the quantity of reduced hemoglobin in the mucocutaneous vessels that produces cyanosis may be brought about either by an increase in the quantity of venous blood as a result of dilation of the venules and venous ends of the capillaries or by a reduction in the SaO_2 in the capillary blood. In general, cyanosis becomes apparent when the concentration of reduced hemoglobin in capillary blood exceeds 40 g/L (4 g/dL).

It is the *absolute*, rather than the *relative*, quantity of reduced hemoglobin that is important in producing cyanosis. Thus, in a patient with severe anemia, the *relative* quantity of reduced hemoglobin in the venous blood may be very large when considered in relation to the total quantity of hemoglobin in the blood. However, since the concentration of the latter is markedly reduced, the *absolute* quantity of reduced hemoglobin may still be small, and, therefore, patients with severe anemia and even *marked* arterial desaturation may not display cyanosis. Conversely, the higher the total hemoglobin content, the greater the tendency toward cyanosis; thus, patients with marked polycythemia tend to be cyanotic at higher levels of SaO_2 than patients with normal hematocrit values. Likewise, local passive congestion, which causes an increase in the total quantity of reduced hemoglobin in the vessels in a given area, may cause cyanosis. Cyanosis is also observed when nonfunctional hemoglobin, such as methemoglobin or sulfhemoglobin, is present in blood.

Cyanosis may be subdivided into central and peripheral types. In *central* cyanosis, the SaO_2 is reduced or an abnormal hemoglobin derivative is present, and the mucous membranes and skin are both affected. *Peripheral* cyanosis is due to a slowing of blood flow and abnormally great extraction of O_2 from normally saturated arterial blood; it results from vasoconstriction and diminished peripheral blood flow, such as occurs in cold exposure, shock, congestive failure, and peripheral vascular disease. Often in these conditions, the mucous membranes of the oral cavity or those beneath the tongue may be spared. Clinical differentiation between central and peripheral cyanosis may not always be simple, and in conditions such as cardiogenic shock with pulmonary edema there may be a mixture of both types.

DIFFERENTIAL DIAGNOSIS

Central cyanosis

(Table 4-1) Decreased SaO_2 results from a marked reduction in the PaO_2. This reduction may be brought about by a decline in the FiO_2 without sufficient compensatory alveolar hyperventilation to maintain alveolar PO_2. Cyanosis usually becomes manifest in an ascent to an altitude of 4000 m (13,000 ft).

Seriously *impaired pulmonary function*, through perfusion of unventilated or poorly ventilated areas of the lung or alveolar hypoventilation, is a common cause of central cyanosis (Chap. 5). This condition may occur acutely, as in extensive pneumonia or pulmonary edema, or chronically, with chronic pulmonary

TABLE 4-1

CAUSES OF CYANOSIS
Central Cyanosis
Decreased arterial oxygen saturation
Decreased atmospheric pressure—high altitude
Impaired pulmonary function
Alveolar hypoventilation
Uneven relationships between pulmonary ventilation and perfusion (perfusion of hypoventilated alveoli)
Impaired oxygen diffusion
Anatomic shunts
Certain types of congenital heart disease
Pulmonary arteriovenous fistulas
Multiple small intrapulmonary shunts
Hemoglobin with low affinity for oxygen
Hemoglobin abnormalities
Methemoglobinemia—hereditary, acquired
Sulfhemoglobinema—acquired
Carboxyhemoglobinemia (not true cyanosis)
Peripheral Cyanosis
Reduced cardiac output
Cold exposure
Redistribution of blood flow from extremities
Arterial obstruction
Venous obstruction

diseases (e.g., emphysema). In the latter situation, secondary polycythemia is generally present and clubbing of the fingers (see later) may occur. Another cause of reduced SaO_2 is *shunting of systemic venous blood into the arterial circuit*. Certain forms of congenital heart disease are associated with cyanosis on this basis (see earlier).

Pulmonary arteriovenous fistulae may be congenital or acquired, solitary or multiple, microscopic or massive. The severity of cyanosis produced by these fistulae depends on their size and number. They occur with some frequency in hereditary hemorrhagic telangiectasia. SaO_2 reduction and cyanosis may also occur in some patients with cirrhosis, presumably as a consequence of pulmonary arteriovenous fistulae or portal vein–pulmonary vein anastomoses.

In patients with cardiac or pulmonary right-to-left shunts, the presence and severity of cyanosis depend on the size of the shunt relative to the systemic flow as well as on the Hb-O_2 saturation of the venous blood. With increased extraction of O_2 from the blood by the exercising muscles, the venous blood returning to the right side of the heart is more unsaturated than at rest, and shunting of this blood intensifies the cyanosis. Secondary polycythemia occurs frequently in patients in this setting and contributes to the cyanosis.

Cyanosis can be caused by small quantities of circulating methemoglobin (Hb Fe^{3+}) and by even smaller quantities of sulfhemoglobin; both of these hemoglobin derivatives are unable to bind oxygen. Although they are uncommon causes of cyanosis, these abnormal hemoglobin species should be sought by spectroscopy when cyanosis is not readily explained by malfunction of the circulatory or respiratory systems. Generally, digital clubbing does not occur with them.

Peripheral cyanosis

Probably the most common cause of peripheral cyanosis is the normal vasoconstriction resulting from exposure to cold air or water. When cardiac output is reduced, cutaneous vasoconstriction occurs as a compensatory mechanism so that blood is diverted from the skin to more vital areas such as the CNS and heart, and cyanosis of the extremities may result even though the arterial blood is normally saturated.

Arterial obstruction to an extremity, as with an embolus, or arteriolar constriction, as in cold-induced vasospasm (Raynaud's phenomenon), generally results in pallor and coldness, and there may be associated cyanosis. Venous obstruction, as in thrombophlebitis or deep venous thrombosis, dilates the subpapillary venous plexuses and thereby intensifies cyanosis.

APPROACH TO THE PATIENT	Cyanosis

Certain features are important in arriving at the cause of cyanosis:

1. It is important to ascertain the time of onset of cyanosis. Cyanosis present since birth or infancy is usually due to congenital heart disease.
2. Central and peripheral cyanosis must be differentiated. Evidence of disorders of the respiratory or cardiovascular systems are helpful. Massage or gentle warming of a cyanotic extremity will increase peripheral blood flow and abolish peripheral, but not central, cyanosis.
3. The presence or absence of clubbing of the digits (see later) should be ascertained. The combination of cyanosis and clubbing is frequent in patients with congenital heart disease and right-to-left shunting and is seen occasionally in patients with pulmonary disease, such as lung abscess or pulmonary arteriovenous fistulae. In contrast, peripheral cyanosis or acutely developing central cyanosis is *not* associated with clubbed digits.
4. Pao_2 and Sao_2 should be determined, and, in patients with cyanosis in whom the mechanism is obscure, spectroscopic examination of the blood performed to look for abnormal types of hemoglobin (critical in the differential diagnosis of cyanosis).

CLUBBING

The selective bulbous enlargement of the distal segments of the fingers and toes due to proliferation of connective tissue, particularly on the dorsal surface, is termed *clubbing*; there is also increased sponginess of the soft tissue at the base of the clubbed nail. Clubbing may be hereditary, idiopathic, or acquired and associated with a variety of disorders, including cyanotic congenital heart disease (see earlier), infective endocarditis, and a variety of pulmonary conditions (among them primary and metastatic lung cancer, bronchiectasis, asbestosis, sarcoidosis, lung abscess, cystic fibrosis, tuberculosis, and mesothelioma), as well as with some gastrointestinal diseases (including inflammatory bowel disease and hepatic cirrhosis). In some instances, it is occupational, e.g., in jackhammer operators.

Clubbing in patients with primary and metastatic lung cancer, mesothelioma, bronchiectasis, or hepatic cirrhosis may be associated with *hypertrophic osteoarthropathy*. In this condition, the subperiosteal formation of new bone in the distal diaphyses of the long bones of the extremities causes pain and symmetric arthritis-like changes in the shoulders, knees, ankles, wrists, and elbows. The diagnosis of hypertrophic osteoarthropathy may be confirmed by bone radiograph or MRI. Although the mechanism of clubbing is unclear, it appears to be secondary to humoral substances that cause dilation of the vessels of the distal digits as well as growth factors released from unfragmented platelet precursors in the digital circulation.

ACKNOWLEDGMENT

Dr. Eugene Braunwald authored this chapter in the previous edition. Some of the material from the 17th edition of Harrison's Principles of Internal Medicine has been carried forward.

CHAPTER 5

DISTURBANCES OF RESPIRATORY FUNCTION

Edward T. Naureckas ■ Julian Solway

INTRODUCTION

The primary function of the respiratory system is to oxygenate blood and eliminate carbon dioxide, which requires that blood come into virtual contact with fresh air to facilitate diffusion of respiratory gases between blood and gas. This process occurs in the lung alveoli, where blood flowing through alveolar wall capillaries is separated from alveolar gas by an extremely thin membrane of flattened endothelial and epithelial cells, across which respiratory gases diffuse and equilibrate. Blood flow through the lung is unidirectional via a continuous vascular path, along which venous blood absorbs oxygen from and loses CO_2 to inspired gas. The path for airflow, in contrast, reaches a dead end at the alveolar walls; as such, the alveolar space must be ventilated tidally, with inflow of fresh gas and outflow of alveolar gas alternating periodically at the respiratory rate (RR). To achieve an enormous alveolar surface area (typically 70 m^2) for blood-gas diffusion within the modest volume of a thoracic cavity (typically 7 L), nature has distributed both blood flow and ventilation among millions of tiny alveoli through multigenerational branching of both pulmonary arteries and bronchial airways. As a consequence of variations in tube lengths and calibers along these pathways, and of the effects of gravity, tidal pressure fluctuations, and anatomic constraints from the chest wall, there is variation among alveoli in their relative ventilations and perfusions. Not surprisingly, for the lung to be most efficient in exchanging gas, the fresh gas ventilation of a given alveolus must be matched to its perfusion.

For the respiratory system to succeed in oxygenating blood and eliminating carbon dioxide, it must be able to ventilate the lung tidally to freshen alveolar gas; it must provide for perfusion of the individual alveolus in a manner proportional to its ventilation; and it must allow for adequate diffusion of respiratory gases between alveolar gas and capillary blood. Furthermore, it must be able to accommodate severalfold increases in the demand for oxygen uptake or CO_2 elimination imposed by metabolic

needs or acid-base derangement. Given these multiple requirements for normal operation, it is not surprising that many diseases disturb respiratory function. Here, we consider in greater detail the physiologic determinants of lung ventilation and perfusion, and how their matching distributions and rapid gas diffusion allow for normal gas exchange. We also discuss how common diseases derange these normal functions, and thereby impair gas exchange—or at least raise the work of the respiratory muscles or heart to maintain adequate respiratory function.

VENTILATION

It is useful to think about the respiratory system as having three independently functioning components—the lung including its airways, the neuromuscular system, and the chest wall; the latter includes everything that is not lung or active neuromuscular system. As such, the mass of the respiratory muscles is part of the chest wall, while the force they generate is part of the neuromuscular system; the abdomen (especially an obese abdomen) and the heart (especially an enlarged heart) are, for these purposes, part of the chest wall. Each of these three components has mechanical properties that relate to its enclosed volume, or in the case of the neuromuscular system, the respiratory system volume at which it is operating, and to the rate of change of its volume (i.e., flow).

VOLUME-RELATED MECHANICAL PROPERTIES—STATICS

Figure 5-1 shows the volume-related properties of each component of the respiratory system. Due both to surface tension at the air-liquid interface between alveolar wall lining fluid and alveolar gas and to elastic recoil of the lung tissue itself, the lung requires a positive transmural pressure difference between alveolar gas and its

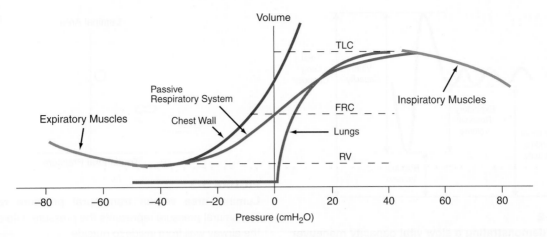

FIGURE 5-1

Pressure-volume curves of the isolated lung, isolated chest wall, combined respiratory system, inspiratory **muscles, and expiratory muscles.** FRC, functional residual capacity; RV, residual volume; TLC, total lung capacity.

pleural surface to stay inflated; this difference is called the elastic recoil pressure of the lung, and it increases with lung volume. Importantly, the lung becomes rather stiff at high lung volumes, so that relatively small volume changes are accompanied by large changes in transpulmonary pressure; in contrast, the lung is compliant at lower lung volumes, including those at which tidal breathing normally occurs. Note that at zero inflation pressure, even normal lungs retain some air in the alveoli. This occurs because the small peripheral airways of the lung are tethered open by radially outward pull from inflated lung parenchyma attached to adventitia; as the lung deflates during exhalation, those small airways are pulled open progressively less, and eventually they close, trapping some gas in the alveoli. This effect can be exaggerated with age and especially with obstructive airways diseases, resulting in gas trapping at quite large lung volumes.

The elastic behavior of the passive chest wall (i.e., in the absence of neuromuscular activation) differs markedly from that of the lung. Whereas the lung tends toward full deflation with no distending (transmural) pressure, the chest wall encloses a large volume when pleural pressure equals body surface (atmospheric) pressure. Furthermore, the chest wall is compliant at high enclosed volumes, readily expanding even further in response to increases in transmural pressure. The chest wall also remains compliant at small negative transmural pressures (i.e., when pleural pressure falls slightly below atmospheric pressure), but as the volume enclosed by the chest wall becomes quite small in response to large negative transmural pressures, the passive chest wall becomes stiff due to squeezing together of ribs and intercostal muscles, diaphragm stretch, displacement of abdominal contents, and straining of ligaments and bony articulations. Under normal circumstances, the lung and the passive chest wall enclose essentially the same volume, the only difference between these being

the volumes of the pleural fluid and of the lung parenchyma (both quite small). As such, and because the lung and chest wall function in mechanical series, the pressure required to displace the passive respiratory system (lungs + chest wall) at any volume is simply the sum of the elastic recoil pressure of the lungs and the transmural pressure across the chest wall. When plotted against respiratory system volume, this relationship assumes a sigmoid shape, exhibiting stiffness at high lung volumes (imparted by the lung), stiffness at low lung volumes (imparted by the chest wall, or sometimes by airway closure), and compliance in the middle range of lung volumes. There is also a passive resting point of the respiratory system, attained when alveolar gas pressure equals body surface pressure (i.e., the transrespiratory system pressure is zero). At this volume (called *functional residual capacity* [FRC]), the outward recoil of the chest wall is balanced exactly by the inward recoil of the lung. As these recoils are transmitted through the pleural fluid, the latter is pulled both outward and inward simultaneously at FRC, and, thus, its pressure falls below atmospheric pressure (typically, −5 cmH$_2$O).

The normal passive respiratory system would equilibrate at FRC and remain there were it not for the actions of respiratory muscles. The inspiratory muscles act on the chest wall to generate the equivalent of positive pressure across the lungs and passive chest wall, while the expiratory muscles generate the equivalent of negative transrespiratory pressure. The maximal pressures these sets of muscles can generate varies with the lung volume at which they operate, due to length-tension relationships in striated muscle sarcomeres and to changes in mechanical advantage as the angles of insertion change with lung volume (Fig. 5-1). Nonetheless, under normal conditions the respiratory muscles are substantially "overpowered" for their roles, and generate more than adequate force to drive the respiratory system to its stiffness extremes, as determined

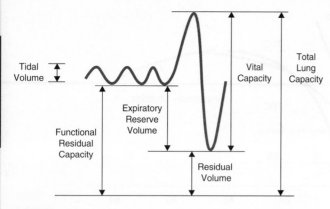

FIGURE 5-2

Spirogram demonstrating a slow vital capacity maneuver and various lung volumes.

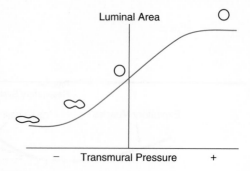

FIGURE 5-3

Luminal area versus transmural pressure relationship. Transmural pressure represents the pressure difference across the airway wall from inside to outside.

by the lung (total lung capacity [TLC]) or chest wall or airway closure (residual volume [RV]) importantly, the latter always prevents the adult lung from emptying completely under normal circumstances. The excursion between full and minimal lung inflation is called vital capacity (VC; **Fig. 5-2**), and is readily seen to be the difference between volumes at two unrelated stiffness extremes—one determined by the lung (TLC) and the other determined by the chest wall or airways (RV). Thus, although VC is easy to measure (see below), it tells one little about the intrinsic properties of the respiratory system. It is much more useful, as we shall see, for the clinician to know TLC and RV individually.

FLOW-RELATED MECHANICAL PROPERTIES—DYNAMICS

The passive chest wall and active neuromuscular system do exhibit mechanical behaviors related to the rate of change of volume, but these become quantitatively important only at markedly supraphysiologic breathing frequencies (e.g., during high-frequency mechanical ventilation), and, thus, we shall not address these here. In contrast, the dynamic airflow properties of the lung substantially determine the ability to ventilate and contribute importantly to the work of breathing, and are often deranged by disease. Understanding these properties is, therefore, well worthwhile.

As with flow of any fluid (gas or liquid) in any tube, maintenance of airflow within the pulmonary airways requires a pressure gradient that falls along the direction of flow, the magnitude of which is determined by the flow rate and the frictional resistance to flow. During quiet tidal breathing, the pressure gradients driving inspiratory or expiratory flow are small owing to the very low frictional resistance of normal pulmonary airways (normally <2 cmH_2O/L per second). However, during rapid exhalation another phenomenon reduces flow below that which would have been

expected were frictional resistance the only impediment to flow. This phenomenon is called dynamic airflow limitation, and it occurs because the bronchial airways through which air is exhaled are collapsible rather than rigid (**Fig. 5-3**). An important anatomic feature of the pulmonary airways is its treelike branching structure. While the individual airways in each successive generation, from most proximal (trachea) to most distal (respiratory bronchioles), are smaller than those of the parent generation, their number increases exponentially such that the summed cross-sectional area of the airways becomes very large toward the lung periphery. Because flow (volume/time) is constant along the airway tree, the velocity of airflow (flow/summed cross-sectional area) is much greater in the central airways than in the peripheral airways. During exhalation, gas leaving the alveoli must therefore gain velocity as it proceeds toward the mouth. The energy required for this "convective" acceleration is drawn from the component of gas energy manifested as its local pressure, thereby reducing intraluminal gas pressure (the Bernoulli effect), reducing airway transmural pressure, reducing airway size (Fig. 5-3), and reducing flow. If one tries to exhale more forcefully, the local velocity increases further and reduces airway size further, resulting in no net increase in flow. Under these circumstances, flow has reached its maximum possible value, or its flow limit. Lungs normally exhibit such dynamic airflow limitation. The maximum value of flow is related to the gas density, airway cross-section and distensibility, the elastic recoil pressure of the lung, and the frictional pressure loss to the flow-limiting airway site. Under normal conditions, maximal expiratory flow falls with lung volume (**Fig. 5-4**), due primarily to the dependence of lung recoil pressure on lung volume (Fig. 5-1). In pulmonary fibrosis, lung recoil pressure is increased at any lung volume, and, thus, the maximum expiratory flow is relatively elevated when considered in relation to lung volume. Conversely, in emphysema, lung recoil pressure is reduced, which is a principal mechanism by which maximal expiratory flows fall. Diseases that narrow the airway lumen

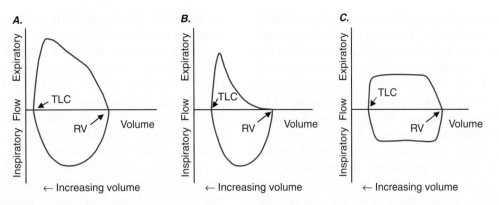

FIGURE 5-4
Flow-volume loops. *A.* Normal. ***B.*** Airflow obstruction. ***C.*** Fixed central airway obstruction. RV, residual volume; TLC, total lung capacity.

at any transmural pressure, such as asthma or chronic bronchitis, or which cause excessive airway collapsibility, like tracheomalacia, also reduce maximal expiratory flow.

The Bernoulli effect also acts during inspiration, but the more negative pleural pressures during inspiration lower the pressure outside of airways, thereby increasing transmural pressure and promoting airway expansion. Thus, inspiratory airflow limitation seldom occurs due to diffuse pulmonary airway disease. Conversely, extra-thoracic airway narrowing (as due to a tracheal adenoma or post-tracheostomy stricture) can lead to inspiratory airflow limitation (Fig. 5-4).

The phenomenon of flow limitation and the importance of airway size and distensibility and of upstream pressure (lung elastic recoil pressure for forced exhalation) can easily be appreciated by sniffing through one's nose with low, medium, or substantial effort. If one keeps the nostrils relaxed, increasing from low to medium inspiratory effort raises inspiratory flow through the nose somewhat, but inhaling even harder will likely not increase inspiratory nasal airflow more but, rather, will just collapse the nares, a manifestation of dynamic airflow limitation. One can increase inspiratory nasal airflow, however, by flaring one's nostrils using the alae nasi muscles. This increases nostril area (reducing velocity for a given flow through the nares) and stiffens the nostril walls (reducing their narrowing in response to negative transmural pressure). Spring-like nasal strips sometimes used by football players have the same effect. In patients with obstructive sleep apnea (OSA), a narrowed and excessively compliant pharyngeal airway also collapses in response to negative transmural pressure generated by the Bernoulli effect and by inspiratory frictional pressure loss in the nose (which is why an upper respiratory infection often worsens OSA). Increasing the upstream driving pressure from which these phenomena lower intrapharyngeal gas pressure with positive nasal airway pressure keeps pharyngeal transmural pressure positive, preventing inspiratory airflow limitation. Inspiratory airflow limitation in the

nose or in the pharynx of patients with OSA closely parallels expiratory flow limitation in the lung.

WORK OF BREATHING

In health, the elastic (volume change–related) and dynamic (flow-related) loads that must be overcome to ventilate the lungs at rest are small, and the work required of the respiratory muscles is minimal. However, the work of breathing can increase considerably, due either to requirement for substantially increased ventilation, an abnormally increased mechanical load, or both. As discussed below, the rate of ventilation is primarily set by the need to eliminate carbon dioxide, and, thus, ventilation increases during exercise (sometimes more than 20-fold) and during metabolic acidosis as a compensatory response. Naturally, the work rate required to overcome the elasticity of the respiratory system increases with both the depth and frequency of tidal breaths, while the work required to overcome the dynamic load increases with total ventilation. A modest increase of ventilation is most efficiently achieved by increasing tidal volume but not respiratory rate, which is the normal ventilatory response to lower level exercise. At high levels of exercise, deep breathing persists, but respiratory rate also increases. The pattern chosen by the respiratory controller minimizes the work of breathing.

Work of breathing also increases when disease reduces the compliance of the respiratory system or increases the resistance to airflow. The former occurs commonly in diseases of the lung parenchyma (interstitial processes or fibrosis, alveolar filling diseases such as pulmonary edema or pneumonia, or substantial lung resection), and the latter occurs in obstructive airways diseases such as asthma, chronic bronchitis, emphysema, and cystic fibrosis. Furthermore, severe airflow obstruction can functionally reduce the compliance of the respiratory system by leading to dynamic hyperinflation. In this scenario, expiratory flows slowed by the obstructive airways disease may be insufficient to allow for complete exhalation during the expiratory phase of tidal breathing; as a result, the "functional residual capacity" from which the next breath is inhaled is greater than the static FRC. With repetition of incomplete exhalations of each tidal breath, the operating FRC becomes dynamically elevated, sometimes to a level that approaches TLC. At these high lung volumes, the respiratory system is much less compliant than at normal breathing volumes, and, thus, the elastic work of each tidal breath is also increased. The dynamic pulmonary hyperinflation that accompanies severe airflow obstruction causes patients to sense difficulty in breathing in—even though the pathophysiologic abnormality at root cause is expiratory airflow obstruction.

ADEQUACY OF VENTILATION

As noted earlier, the respiratory control system that sets the rate of ventilation responds to chemical signals, including arterial carbon dioxide and oxygen tensions and blood pH, and to volitional needs, such as the need to inhale deeply before playing a long phrase on the trumpet. Disturbances in ventilation are discussed in Chap. 22. Here, we focus on the relationship between ventilation of the lung and carbon dioxide elimination.

At the end of each tidal exhalation, the conducting airways are filled with alveolar gas that had not reached the mouth when expiratory flow stopped. During the ensuing inhalation, fresh gas immediately enters the airway tree at the mouth, but the gas first entering the alveoli at the start of inhalation is that same alveolar gas in the conducting airways that had just left the alveoli. As such, fresh gas does not enter the alveoli until the volume of the conducting airways has been inspired. This volume is called the anatomic dead space. Quiet breathing with tidal volumes smaller than the anatomic dead space introduces no fresh gas into the alveoli at all; only that part of the inspired tidal volume (V_T) that is greater than the dead space (V_D) introduces fresh gas into the alveoli. Importantly, the dead space can be further increased functionally if some of the inspired tidal volume is delivered to a part of the lung that receives no pulmonary blood flow, and, thus, cannot contribute to gas exchange, as can occur in the portion of the lung distal to a large pulmonary embolus. As such, exhaled minute ventilation ($\dot{V}_E = V_T \times RR$) includes a component of dead space ventilation ($\dot{V}_D = V_D \times RR$) and a component of fresh gas alveolar ventilation ($\dot{V}_A = [V_T - V_D] \times RR$). Carbon dioxide elimination from the alveoli is equal to $\dot{V}_A$ times the difference in CO_2 fraction between inspired air (essentially zero) and alveolar gas (typically ~5.6%, after correcting for humidification of inspired air, corresponding to 40 mmHg). In the steady state, the alveolar fraction of CO_2 is equal to the metabolic CO_2 production divided by the alveolar ventilation. Because,

as discussed below, alveolar and arterial CO_2 tensions are equal, and because the respiratory controller normally strives to maintain arterial P_{CO_2} (Pa_{CO_2}) at ~40 mmHg, the adequacy of alveolar ventilation is reflected in Pa_{CO_2}. If Pa_{CO_2} falls much below 40 mmHg, alveolar hyperventilation is present, and if Pa_{CO_2} exceeds 40 mmHg, then alveolar hypoventilation is present. Ventilatory failure is characterized by extreme alveolar hypoventilation.

As a consequence of oxygen uptake of alveolar gas into capillary blood, alveolar oxygen tension falls below that of inspired gas. The rate of oxygen uptake (determined by the body's metabolic oxygen consumption) is related to the average rate of metabolic carbon dioxide production and their ratio, called the "respiratory quotient" ($R = \dot{V}_{CO_2}/\dot{V}_{O_2}$), depends largely on the fuel being metabolized. For a typical American diet, R is usually around 0.85, and more oxygen is absorbed than CO_2 is excreted. Together, these phenomena allow the estimation of alveolar oxygen tension, according to the following relationship, known as the alveolar gas equation:

$$Pa_{O_2} = Fi_{O_2} \times (P_{bar} - P_{H_2O}) - Pa_{CO_2}/R$$

The alveolar gas equation also highlights the influences of inspired oxygen fraction (Fi_{O_2}), barometric pressure (P_{bar}), and vapor pressure of water ($P_{H_2O} = 47$ mmHg at 37°C) in addition to alveolar ventilation (which sets Pa_{CO_2}) in determining Pa_{O_2}. An implication of the alveolar gas equation is that severe arterial hypoxemia rarely occurs as a pure consequence of alveolar hypoventilation at sea level while breathing air. The potential for alveolar hypoventilation to induce severe hypoxemia with otherwise normal lungs increases as P_{bar} falls with increasing altitude.

GAS EXCHANGE

DIFFUSION

For oxygen to be delivered to the peripheral tissues, it must pass from alveolar gas into alveolar capillary blood by diffusing through alveolar membrane. The aggregate alveolar membrane is highly optimized for this process, with a very large surface area and minimal thickness. Diffusion through the alveolar membrane is so efficient in the human lung that in most circumstances its hemoglobin becomes fully oxygen saturated by the time a red blood cell has traveled just one-third the length of the alveolar capillary. As such, uptake of alveolar oxygen is ordinarily limited by the amount of blood transiting the alveolar capillaries rather than how rapidly oxygen can diffuse across the membrane; thus, oxygen uptake from the lung is said to be "perfusion limited."

Carbon dioxide also equilibrates rapidly across the alveolar membrane. Thus, the oxygen and CO_2 tensions in capillary blood leaving a normal alveolus are essentially equal to those in alveolar gas. In only rare circumstances is oxygen uptake from normal lungs diffusion-limited, which can occur at high altitude and/or by high-performance athletes exerting maximum effort. Diffusion limitation can also occur in interstitial lung disease if substantially thickened alveolar walls remain perfused.

VENTILATION-PERFUSION HETEROGENEITY

As noted earlier, for gas exchange to be most efficient, the ventilation to each individual alveolus should be matched to the perfusion to its accompanying capillaries for each of millions of alveoli. Due to the differential effects of gravity on lung mechanics and blood flow throughout the lung, and due to differences of airway and vascular architecture among various respiratory paths, there is minor ventilation/perfusion heterogeneity even in the normal lung; however, $\dot{V}/\dot{Q}$ heterogeneity can be particularly marked in disease. Two extreme examples are (1) ventilation of unperfused lung distal to a pulmonary embolus, in which ventilation of the physiologic dead space is "wasted" in the sense that it does not contribute to gas exchange; and (2) perfusion of nonventilated lung, a condition known as a "shunt." The latter allows venous blood to pass through the lung unaltered; when mixed with fully oxygenated blood leaving other well-ventilated lung units, shunted venous blood disproportionately lowers the mixed arterial Pa_{O_2}, due to the nonlinear oxygen content versus the P_{O_2} relationship of hemoglobin **(Fig. 5-5)**. Furthermore, the resulting arterial hypoxemia is refractory to supplemental inspired oxygen. This is because raising inspired Fi_{O_2} has no effect on alveolar gas tensions in nonventilated alveoli, and while raising inspired Fi_{O_2} does increase Pa_{O_2} in ventilated alveoli, the oxygen content of blood exiting ventilated units increases only slightly as hemoglobin will already have been nearly fully saturated and the solubility of oxygen in plasma is quite small.

More commonly occurring than the two extreme examples given earlier is a widening of the distribution of ventilation/perfusion ratios; such $\dot{V}/\dot{Q}$ heterogeneity is a common consequence of lung disease. In this circumstance, perfusion of relatively underventilated alveoli results in the incomplete oxygenation of exiting blood. When mixed with well-oxygenated blood leaving higher $\dot{V}/\dot{Q}$ regions, this partially preoxygenated blood disproportionately lowers arterial Pa_{O_2}, although to a lower extent than does a similar perfusion fraction of blood leaving regions of pure shunt. In addition, in contrast to shunt regions, inhalation of supplemental oxygen does raise the Pa_{O_2} even in relatively underventilated

low $\dot{V}/\dot{Q}$ regions, and so the arterial hypoxemia induced by $\dot{V}/\dot{Q}$ heterogeneity is typically responsive to oxygen therapy (Fig. 5-5).

In sum, arterial hypoxemia can be caused by substantial reduction of inspired oxygen tension, by severe alveolar hypoventilation, or by perfusion of relatively underventilated (low $\dot{V}/\dot{Q}$) or completely unventilated (shunt) lung regions, and, in unusual circumstances, by limitation of gas diffusion.

APPROACH TO THE PATIENT | **Disturbances of Respiratory Function**

There are many diseases that injure the respiratory system, but there are relatively few ways in which it responds to that injury. For this reason, the pattern of physiologic abnormalities may or may not provide sufficient information to discriminate among conditions. The following studies are commonly used to characterize a patient's respiratory function and often lead to a better understanding of the underlying disorder.

MEASUREMENT OF VENTILATORY FUNCTION

Lung Volumes Figure 5-2 demonstrates a spirometry tracing in which the volume of air entering or exiting the lung is plotted over time. In a slow vital capacity maneuver, the subject inhales from FRC, fully inflating the lungs to TLC, and then the patient exhales slowly to RV; VC is the difference between TLC and RV, and represents the maximum excursion of the respiratory system. Spirometry discloses relative volume changes during these maneuvers, but cannot reveal the absolute volumes at which they occur. To determine absolute lung volumes, two approaches are commonly used—inert gas dilution and body plethysmography. In the former, a known amount of a nonabsorbable inert gas (usually helium or neon) is inhaled in a single large breath or is rebreathed from a closed circuit; the inert gas is diluted by the gas resident in the lung at the time of inhalation, and its final concentration reveals the volume of resident gas contributing to the dilution. A drawback of this method is that regions of the lung that ventilate poorly (e.g., due to airflow obstruction) may not receive much inspired inert gas and so do not contribute to its dilution. As such, inert gas dilution often underestimates true lung volumes.

In the second approach, FRC is determined by measuring the compressibility of gas within the chest, which is proportional to the volume of gas being compressed. The patient sits in a body plethysmograph, a chamber usually made of transparent plastic to minimize claustrophobia, and at the end of a normal tidal breath (i.e., when lung volume is FRC) is instructed to pant against a closed shutter, thus, periodically compressing air within the lung slightly. Pressure fluctuations at the mouth

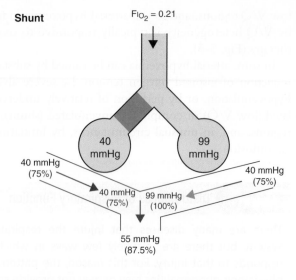

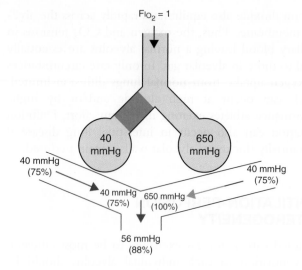

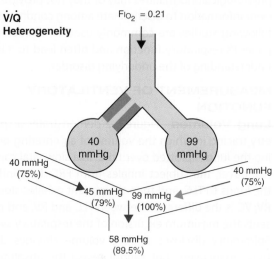

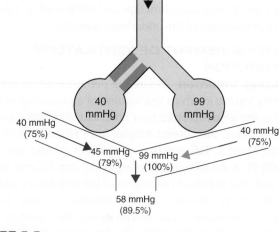

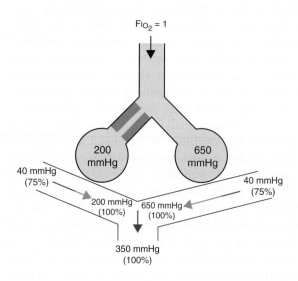

FIGURE 5-5

Influence of air vs oxygen breathing on mixed arterial oxygenation in shunt and ventilation/perfusion heterogeneity. Partial pressure of oxygen (mmHg) and oxygen saturations are shown for mixed venous blood, end capillary blood for normal versus affected alveoli, and for mixed arterial blood.

and volume fluctuations within the body box (equal but opposite to those of the chest) are measured, and from these the thoracic gas volume is calculated using Boyle's law. Once FRC is obtained, TLC and RV are calculated by adding the inspiratory capacity or subtracting expiratory reserve volume, respectively, values determined during spirometry (Fig. 5-2). The most important determinants of healthy individuals' lung volumes are height, age, and gender, but there is considerable additional normal variation beyond that accounted for by these parameters. In addition, race influences lung volumes; on average TLC values are about 12% smaller in African Americans and 6% smaller in Asian Americans when compared with those of white Americans. In practice, a mean "normal" value is predicted by multivariate regression equations using height, age, and gender, and the patient's value is divided by the predicted value

(often with "race correction" applied) to determine "percent predicted." For most measures of lung function, 85–115% of the predicted value can be normal, but in health the various lung volumes tend to scale together. For example, if one is "normal big" with TLC 110% of the predicted value, then all other lung volumes and spirometry values will also approximate 110% of their respective predicted values. This pattern is particularly helpful in evaluating airflow, as discussed below.

Air Flow As noted earlier, spirometry plays a key role in lung volume determination. But even more often, spirometry is used to measure air flow, which reflects the dynamic properties of the lung. During a forced vital capacity maneuver, the patient inhales to TLC and then exhales rapidly and forcefully to RV; this ensures that flow limitation has been achieved, so that the precise effort made has little influence on actual flow. The total amount of air exhaled is the forced vital capacity (FVC) and the amount of air exhaled in the first second is the forced expiratory volume in one second (FEV_1); note that FEV_1 is a flow rate, as it reveals volume change per time. As with lung volumes, an individual's maximal expiratory flows should be compared to predicted values based on height, age, and gender. While the FEV_1/FVC ratio is typically reduced in airflow obstruction, airflow obstruction can also reduce FVC by raising RV. If this occurs, the FEV_1/FVC ratio may be "artifactually normal," erroneously suggesting that airflow obstruction is absent. To circumvent this problem, it is useful to compare FEV_1 as a fraction of its predicted value with TLC as a fraction of its predicted value. In health, these are usually similar. In contrast, even an FEV_1 value that is 95% of its predicted value may actually be relatively low if TLC is 110% of its respective prediction. In this case, airflow obstruction might be present, despite the "normal" value for FEV_1.

The relationships among volume, flow, and time during spirometry are best displayed in two plots—the spirogram (volume vs. time) and the flow-volume loop (flow vs. volume) (Fig. 5-4). In conditions that cause airflow obstruction, the site of obstruction can sometimes be correlated with the shape of the flow-volume loop. In diseases that cause lower airway obstruction such as asthma or emphysema, flows decrease more rapidly with declining lung volumes leading to a characteristic scooping of the flow-volume loop. In contrast, fixed upper airway obstruction typically leads to inspiratory and/or expiratory flow plateaus (Fig. 5-4).

Airways Resistance The total resistance of the pulmonary and upper airways is measured in the same body plethysmography used to measure FRC. The patient is asked once again to pant, but this time against a closed and then opened shutter. Panting against the closed shutter reveals the thoracic gas volume as above. When the shutter is opened, flow is now directed to and from the body box, so that volume fluctuations in the box reveal the extent of thoracic gas compression, which in turn reveals the pressure fluctuations driving flow. Flow is measured simultaneously, allowing the calculation of lung resistance (as flow divided by pressure). In health, airways resistance is very small, <2 cmH$_2$O/L per second, and half of this resides within the upper airway. Of the lung's contribution, most of the resistance originates in the central airways. For this reason, airways resistance measurement tends to be insensitive to peripheral airflow obstruction.

Respiratory Muscle Strength To measure respiratory muscle strength, the patient is instructed to exhale or inhale with maximum effort against a closed shutter while pressure is monitored at the mouth. Pressures greater than ±60 cmH$_2$O at FRC are considered adequate,

making unlikely the possibility that respiratory muscle weakness accounts for any other ventilatory dysfunction that might be identified.

MEASUREMENT OF GAS EXCHANGE

Diffusing Capacity This test uses a small (and safe) amount of carbon monoxide to measure gas exchange across the alveolar membrane during a 10-second breath hold. Carbon monoxide in exhaled breath is analyzed to determine the quantity of CO absorbed by crossing the alveolar membrane and combining with hemoglobin in red blood cells. This "single-breath diffusing capacity" (diffusion capacity of the lung for carbon monoxide [$D_{L_{CO}}$]) value increases with the surface area available for diffusion and the amount of hemoglobin within the capillaries, and varies inversely with alveolar membrane thickness. Thus, $D_{L_{CO}}$ decreases in diseases that thicken or destroy alveolar membranes (e.g., pulmonary fibrosis, emphysema), curtail the pulmonary vasculature (e.g., pulmonary hypertension), or reduce alveolar capillary hemoglobin (e.g., anemia). Single-breath diffusing capacity may be elevated in acute congestive heart failure, asthma, polycythemia, and pulmonary hemorrhage.

Arterial Blood Gases The effectiveness of gas exchange can be assessed by measuring the partial pressures of oxygen and carbon dioxide in a sample of blood obtained by arterial puncture. The oxygen content of blood (Ca_{O_2}) depends upon arterial saturation ($\%O_2$Sat), which is set by Pa_{O_2}, pH, and Pa_{CO_2} according to the oxyhemoglobin dissociation curve; Ca_{O_2} can also be measured by oximetry (see below):

$$Ca_{O_2}\ (mL/dL) = 1.34(mL/dL/g) \times [hemoglobin]\,(g)$$
$$\times\ \%O_2 Sat + 0.003(mL/dL/mmHg) \times Pa_{O_2}\ (mmHg)$$

Pulse Oximetry Continuous monitoring of arterial blood gases requires either repeated arterial punctures or an indwelling arterial catheter, and so may be difficult in many circumstances. Instead, the oxygen saturation fraction of hemoglobin can be measured continuously using pulse oximetry, a tool that measures the absorbance by hemoglobin of several wavelengths of light transmitted across a finger, toe, or ear by a noninvasive probe. However, since oxygen content varies relatively little with Pa_{O_2} at saturations above 90%, it is difficult to know the precise Pa_{O_2} using this device. In addition, as noted earlier, Pa_{CO_2} is needed to fully assess the mechanism of hypoxemia, a value that is not revealed by pulse oximetry.

CLINICAL CORRELATIONS: TYPICAL EXAMPLES

This chapter has highlighted the physiologic processes underlying respiratory system function and the techniques used by clinicians to assess them. **Figure 5-6** lists

	Restriction due to increased lung elastic recoil (pulmonary fibrosis)	Restriction due to chest wall abnormality (moderate obesity)	Restriction due to respiratory muscle weakness (myasthenia gravis)	Obstruction due to airway narrowing (acute asthma)	Obstruction due to decreased elastic recoil (severe emphysema)
TLC	60%	95%	75%	100%	130%
FRC	60%	65%	100%	104%	220%
RV	60%	100%	120%	120%	310%
FVC	60%	92%	60%	90%	60%
FEV$_1$	75%	92%	60%	35% pre-b.d. 75% post-b.d.	35% pre-b.d. 38% post-b.d.
R$_{aw}$	1.0	1.0	1.0	2.5	1.5
DL$_{CO}$	60%	95%	80%	120%	40%

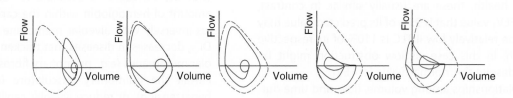

FIGURE 5-6

Commonly seen abnormalities of pulmonary function (see text). Pulmonary function values are expressed as percent of normal predicted values, except for R$_{aw}$, which is expressed as cmH$_2$O/L/s (normal <2 cmH$_2$O/L/s). The figures at the bottom of each column show typical configuration of flow-volume loops in each condition, including the flow-volume relationship during tidal breathing. b.d., bronchodilator; DL$_{CO}$, diffusion capacity of lung for carbon monoxide; FEV$_1$, forced expiratory volume in one second; FRC, functional residual capacity; FVC, forced vital capacity; R$_{aw}$, airways resistance; RV, residual volume; TLC, total lung capacity.

abnormalities in pulmonary function testing typically found in a number of common respiratory disorders and highlights the simultaneous occurrence of multiple physiologic abnormalities. Importantly, some of these respiratory disorders can coexist, which results in more complex superposition of these abnormalities.

VENTILATORY RESTRICTION DUE TO INCREASED ELASTIC RECOIL—EXAMPLE: IDIOPATHIC PULMONARY FIBROSIS

Idiopathic pulmonary fibrosis raises lung recoil at all lung volumes, thereby lowering TLC, FRC, and RV, as well as FVC. Maximal expiratory flows are also reduced compared with normal values, but are relatively elevated when considered in relation to lung volumes. The latter occurs both because the increased lung recoil drives greater maximal flow at any lung volume and because airway diameters are relatively increased due to greater radially outward traction exerted on bronchi by the stiff lung parenchyma. Airway resistance is also normal, for the same reason. Pulmonary capillaries are destroyed by the fibrotic process resulting in marked reduction in diffusing capacity. Oxygenation is often severely reduced due to persistent perfusion of alveolar units that are relatively underventilated due to fibrosis of nearby (and mechanically linked) lung. The flow-volume loop looks like a miniature version of a normal loop but is shifted toward lower absolute lung volumes and displays maximum expiratory flows that are increased for any given volume when compared to the normal tracing.

VENTILATORY RESTRICTION DUE TO CHEST WALL ABNORMALITY—EXAMPLE: MODERATE OBESITY

As the size of the average American continues to increase, this pattern may become the most commonly seen of pulmonary function abnormalities. In moderate obesity, the outward recoil of the chest wall is blunted due to the weight of chest wall fat and to the space occupied by intraabdominal fat. As such, preserved inward recoil of the lung now overbalances the reduced outward recoil of the chest wall, and FRC falls. Because respiratory muscle strength and lung recoil remain normal, TLC is typically unchanged (although TLC may fall in massive obesity) and RV is normal (but may be reduced in massive obesity). Mild hypoxemia may be present, due to perfusion of alveolar units that are poorly ventilated because of airway closure that occurs in dependent portions of the lung while breathing near the reduced FRC. Flows remain normal, as does DL$_{CO}$, unless obstructive sleep apnea (which often accompanies obesity) and associated chronic intermittent hypoxemia have induced pulmonary arterial hypertension, in which case $D_{L_{CO}}$ may be low.

VENTILATORY RESTRICTION DUE TO REDUCED MUSCLE STRENGTH—EXAMPLE: MYASTHENIA GRAVIS

FRC remains normal, as both lung recoil and passive chest wall recoil are normal. However, TLC is low and RV is elevated, as respiratory muscle strength is insufficient to push the passive respiratory system fully toward either volume extreme. Caught between the low TLC and the elevated RV, FVC and FEV_1 are reduced as "innocent bystanders." As airway size and the lung vasculature are unaffected, both airways resistance (R_{aw}) and $D_{L_{CO}}$ are normal. Oxygenation is normal unless weakness becomes so severe that the patient has insufficient strength to reopen collapsed alveoli during sighs, with resulting atelectasis.

AIRFLOW OBSTRUCTION DUE TO DECREASED AIRWAY DIAMETER—EXAMPLE: ACUTE ASTHMA

During an episode of acute asthma, luminal narrowing due to smooth muscle constriction and inflammation and thickening within the small- and medium-sized bronchi raise frictional resistance and reduce airflow. Scooping of the flow-volume loop is caused by reduction of airflow, especially at lower lung volumes. Often, airflow obstruction can be reversed by inhalation of β_2-adrenergic agonists acutely or by treatment with inhaled steroids chronically. Total lung capacity (TLC) usually remains normal (although elevated TLC is sometimes seen in long-standing asthma), but FRC may be dynamically elevated. RV is often increased due to exaggerated airway closure at low lung volumes, and this elevation of RV reduces FVC. Because central airways are narrowed, airways resistance is usually elevated. Mild arterial hypoxemia is often present due to perfusion of relatively underventilated alveoli distal to obstructed airways (and is responsive to oxygen supplementation), but $D_{L_{CO}}$ is normal or mildly elevated.

AIRFLOW OBSTRUCTION DUE TO DECREASED ELASTIC RECOIL—EXAMPLE: SEVERE EMPHYSEMA

Loss of lung elastic recoil in severe emphysema results in pulmonary hyperinflation, of which elevated TLC is the hallmark. FRC is more severely elevated due both to loss of lung elastic recoil and to dynamic hyperinflation (the same phenomenon as autoPEEP, which is the unintended positive end-expiratory pressure). Residual volume is very severely elevated due to airway closure and because exhalation toward RV may take so long that RV cannot be reached before the patient must inhale again. Both FVC and FEV_1 are markedly decreased, the former due to the severe elevation of RV, and the latter because loss of lung elastic recoil reduces the pressure driving maximal expiratory flow and also reduces tethering open of small intrapulmonary airways. The flow-volume loop demonstrates marked scooping of the flow-volume loop, with an initial transient spike of flow attributable largely to expulsion of air from collapsing central airways at the onset of forced exhalation. Otherwise, the central airways remain relatively unaffected, so R_{aw} is normal in "pure" emphysema. Loss of alveolar surface and capillaries in the alveolar walls reduces $D_{L_{CO}}$, but because poorly ventilated emphysematous acini are also poorly perfused (due to loss of their capillaries), arterial hypoxemia is usually not seen at rest until emphysema becomes very severe. However, during exercise, Pa_{O_2} may fall precipitously if extensive destruction of the pulmonary vasculature prevents a sufficient increase in cardiac output and mixed venous oxygen content falls substantially. Under these circumstances, any venous admixture through low $\dot{V}/\dot{Q}$ units has a particularly marked effect in lowering mixed arterial oxygen tension.

ACKNOWLEDGMENT

The authors wish to acknowledge the contribution of Dr. Steven E. Weinberger and Irene M. Rosen to this chapter in previous edits and the helpful contributions of Drs. Mary Strek and Jeff Jacobson.

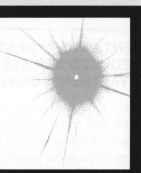

CHAPTER 6

DIAGNOSTIC PROCEDURES IN RESPIRATORY DISEASE

Anne L. Fuhlbrigge ■ Augustine M. K. Choi

The diagnostic modalities available for assessing the patient with suspected or known respiratory system disease include imaging studies and techniques for acquiring biologic specimens, some of which involve direct visualization of part of the respiratory system. Methods to characterize the functional changes developing as a result of disease, including pulmonary function tests and measurements of gas exchange, are discussed in Chap. 5.

IMAGING STUDIES

ROUTINE RADIOGRAPHY

Routine chest radiography, generally including both posteroanterior (PA) and lateral views, is an integral part of the diagnostic evaluation of diseases involving the pulmonary parenchyma, the pleura, and, to a lesser extent, the airways and the mediastinum (see Chaps. 1 and 7). Lateral decubitus views are often useful for determining whether pleural abnormalities represent freely flowing fluid, whereas apical lordotic views can often visualize disease at the lung apices better than the standard PA view. Portable equipment is often used for acutely ill patients who either cannot be transported to a radiology suite or cannot stand for PA and lateral views. Portable films are more difficult to interpret owing to several limitations: (1) the single antero posterior (AP) projection obtained; (2) variability in over- and under-exposure of film; (3) a shorter focal spot-film distance leading to lack of edge sharpness, and loss of fine detail; and (4) magnification of the cardiac silhouette and other anterior structures by the AP projection. Common radiographic patterns and their clinical correlates are reviewed in Chap. 7.

Advances in computer technology and the availability of reusable radiation detectors have allowed the development of digital or computed radiography. The images obtained in this format can be subjected to significant postprocessing analysis to improve diagnostic information. In addition, the benefit of immediate availability of the images, the ability to store images electronically, and the facility of transfer within or between health care systems have led many hospital systems to convert to digital systems.

COMPUTED TOMOGRAPHY

Computed tomography (CT) offers several advantages over routine chest radiography (**Figs. 6-1A, B** and **6-2A, B**; see also Figs. 19-3, 19-4, and 29-4). First, the use of cross-sectional images allows distinction between densities that would be superimposed on plain radiographs. Second, CT is far better than routine radiographic studies at characterizing tissue density, distinguishing subtle density differences between adjacent structures, and providing accurate size assessment of lesions.

CT is particularly valuable in assessing hilar and mediastinal disease (which is often poorly characterized by plain radiography), in identifying and characterizing disease adjacent to the chest wall or spine (including pleural disease), and in identifying areas of fat density or calcification in pulmonary nodules (Fig. 6-2). Its utility in the assessment of mediastinal disease has made CT an important tool in the staging of lung cancer, as an assessment of tumor involvement of mediastinal lymph nodes is critical to proper staging. With the additional use of contrast material, CT also makes it possible to distinguish vascular from nonvascular structures, which is particularly important in distinguishing lymph nodes and masses from vascular structures primarily in the mediastinum, and vascular disorders such as pulmonary embolism.

In high-resolution CT (HRCT), the thickness of individual cross-sectional images is ~1–2 mm, rather than the

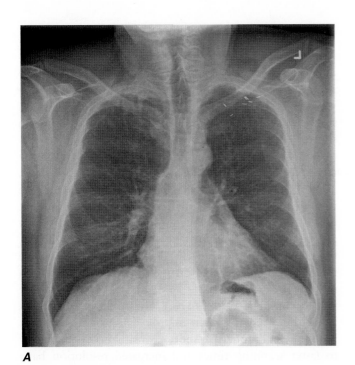

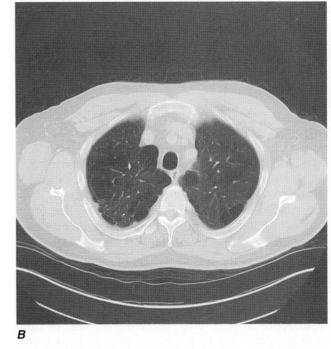

A *B*

FIGURE 6-1
Chest x-ray (*A*) and CT scan (*B*) from a patient with emphysema. The extent and distribution of emphysema are

not well appreciated on plain film but clearly evident on CT scan obtained.

usual 7–10 mm in conventional CT. The visible detail on HRCT scans allows better recognition of subtle parenchymal and airway disease, thickened interlobular septa,

ground-glass opacification, small nodules, and the abnormally thickened or dilated airways seen in bronchiectasis. Using HRCT, characteristic patterns are recognized for

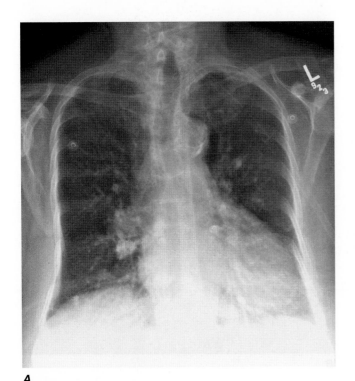

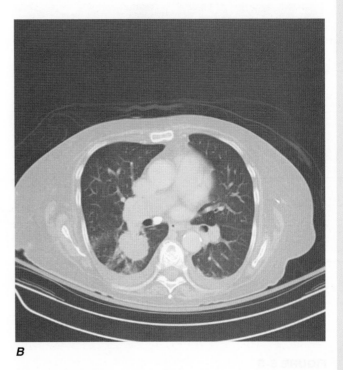

A *B*

FIGURE 6-2
Chest x-ray (*A*) and CT scan (*B*) demonstrating a right lower-lobe mass. The mass is not well appreciated on the plain film because of the hilar structures and known calcified

adenopathy. CT is superior to plain radiography for the detection of abnormal mediastinal densities and the distinction of masses from adjacent vascular structures.

many interstitial lung diseases such as lymphangitic carcinoma, idiopathic pulmonary fibrosis, sarcoidosis, and eosinophilic granuloma. However, there is debate about, the settings in which the presence of a characteristic pattern on HRCT eliminates the need for obtaining lung tissue to make a diagnosis.

HELICAL CT SCANNING

Recent advances in computer processing have allowed the development of helical CT scanning. Helical CT technology results in faster scans with improved contrast enhancement and thinner collimation. The image is obtained during a single breath-holding maneuver that allows less motion artifact. In addition, helical CT scanning allows the collection of continuous data over a larger volume of lung than is possible with conventional CT. Data from the imaging procedure can be reconstructed as images in planes other than the traditional cross-sectional (axial) view, including coronal, or sagittal planes (**Fig. 6-3A**). Finally, sophisticated volumetric "3D" representations of structures can be produced (**Fig. 6-3B**) including the ability to perform a *virtual bronchoscopy,* mimicking direct visualization through a bronchoscope (**Fig. 6-4**).

MULTIDETECTOR CT (MDCT)

Refinements in detector technology have allowed production of scanners with additional detectors along the scanning axis (z-axis). These scanners, called *multidetector CT* (MDCT) scanners, can obtain multiple slices in a single rotation that are thinner and can be acquired in a shorter period of time. This results in enhanced resolution and increased image reconstruction ability. As the technology has progressed, higher numbers (2, 4, 6, 8, 10, 16, 32, 40 and currently up to 64) of detectors are used to produce clearer final images. The development of MDCT allows for even shorter breath holds, which are beneficial for all patients but especially children, the elderly, and the critically ill. However, it should be noted that despite the advantages of MDCT, there is an increase in radiation dose compared to single-detector CT to consider. With MDCT, the additional detectors along the z-axis result in improved use of the contrast bolus. In addition, the shorter breath holds secondary to faster scanning times and increased resolution have all led to improved imaging of the pulmonary vasculature and the ability to detect segmental and subsegmental emboli. In contrast to pulmonary angiography, CT pulmonary angiography (CTPA) also allows simultaneous detection of parenchymal abnormalities that may be contributing to a patient's clinical presentation. Secondary to these advantages and increasing availability,

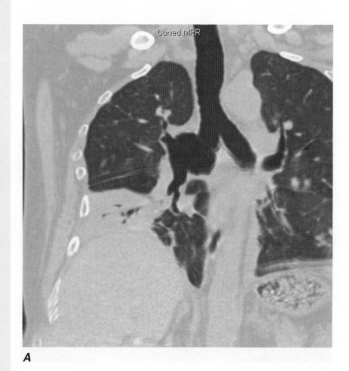

A

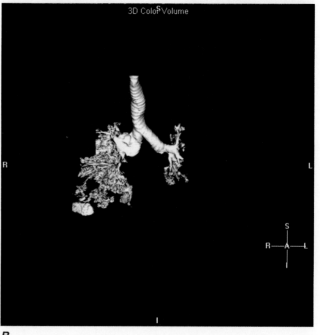

B

FIGURE 6-3

Spiral CT with reconstruction of images in planes other than axial view. Spiral CT in a lung transplant patient with a dehiscence and subsequent aneurysm of the anastomosis. CT images were reconstructed in the sagittal view (**A**) and using digital subtraction to view images of the airways only (**B**), which demonstrate the exact location and extent of the abnormality.

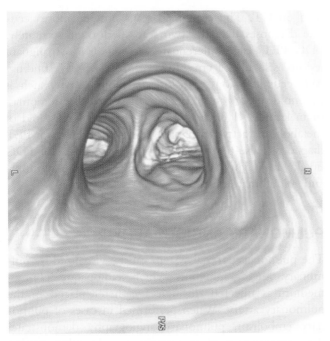

FIGURE 6-4
Virtual bronchoscopic image of the trachea. The view projected is one that would be obtained from the trachea looking down to the carina. The left and right main stem airways are seen bifurcating from the carina.

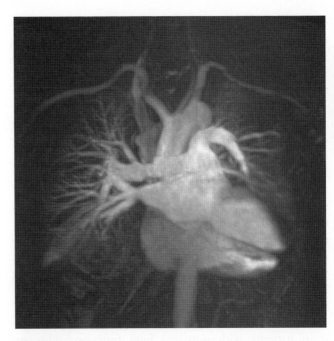

FIGURE 6-5
MRA image of the vasculature of a patient after lung transplant. The image demonstrates the detailed view of the vasculature that can be obtained using digital subtraction techniques. Images from a patient after lung transplant show the venous and arterial anastomosis on the right; a slight narrowing is seen at the site of the anastomosis, which is considered within normal limits and not suggestive of obstruction.

CTPA has rapidly become the test of choice for many clinicians in the evaluation of pulmonary embolism; it is considered equal to pulmonary angiography in terms of accuracy, and with less associated risks.

MAGNETIC RESONANCE IMAGING

The role of magnetic resonance (MR) imaging in the evaluation of respiratory system disease is less well-defined than that of CT. Magnetic resonance provides poorer spatial resolution and less detail of the pulmonary parenchyma, and for these reasons is currently not considered a substitute for CT in imaging the thorax. However, the use of hyperpolarized gas in conjunction with MR has led to the investigational use of MR for imaging the lungs, particularly in obstructive lung disease. Of note, MR examinations are difficult to obtain among several subgroups of patients. Patients who cannot lie still or who cannot lie on their backs may have MR images that are of poor quality; some tests require patients to hold their breaths for 15 to 25 s at a time in order to get good MR images. MR is generally avoided in unstable and/or ventilated patients and those with severe trauma because of the hazards of the MR environment and the difficulties in monitoring patients within the MR room. The presence of metallic foreign bodies, pacemakers, and intracranial aneurysm clips also preclude use of MR.

An advantage of MR is the use of nonionizing electromagnetic radiation. Additionally, MR is well suited to distinguish vascular from nonvascular structures without the need for contrast. Blood vessels appear as hollow tubular structures because flowing blood does not produce a signal on MR imaging. Therefore, MR can be useful in demonstrating pulmonary emboli, defining aortic lesions such as aneurysms or dissection, or other vascular abnormalities (Fig. 6-5) if radiation and IV contrast medium cannot be used. Gadolinium can be used as an intravascular contrast agent for MR angiography (MRA); however, synchronization of data acquisition with the peak arterial bolus is one of the major challenges of MRA; the flow of contrast medium from the peripheral injection site to the vessel of interest is affected by a number of factors including heart rate, stroke volume, and the presence of proximal stenotic lesions.

NUCLEAR MEDICINE TECHNIQUES

Nuclear imaging depends on the selective uptake of various compounds by organs of the body. In thoracic imaging, these compounds are concentrated by one of three mechanisms: blood pool or compartmentalization (e.g., within the heart), physiologic incorporation (e.g., bone or thyroid) and capillary blockage (e.g., lung scan). Radioactive isotopes can be administered by either the IV or inhaled routes or both. When injected intravenously, albumin macroaggregates labeled with [^{99m}Tc] become lodged in pulmonary capillaries; the distribution of the trapped radioisotope follows the distribution of blood flow. When inhaled, radiolabeled xenon gas can be used to demonstrate the distribution of ventilation. Using these techniques, ventilation-perfusion lung scanning was a commonly used technique for the evaluation of pulmonary embolism. Pulmonary thromboembolism produces one or more regions of ventilation-perfusion mismatch (i.e., regions in which there is a defect in perfusion that follows the distribution of a vessel and that is not accompanied by a corresponding defect in ventilation [Chap. 20]). However, with advances in CT scanning, scintigraphic imaging has been largely replaced by CT angiography in patients with suspected pulmonary embolism.

Another common use of ventilation-perfusion scans is in patients with impaired lung function, who are being considered for lung resection. Because many patients with bronchogenic carcinoma have coexisting chronic obstructive pulmonary disease (COPD), the question arises as to whether or not a patient can tolerate lung resection. The distribution of the isotope(s) can be used to assess the regional distribution of blood flow and ventilation, allowing the physician to estimate the level of postoperative lung function.

POSITRON EMISSION TOMOGRAPHIC SCANNING

Positron emission tomographic (PET) scanning is commonly used to identify malignant lesions in the lung, based on their increased uptake and metabolism of glucose. The technique involves injection of a radiolabeled glucose analogue, [^{18}F]-fluoro-2-deoxyglucose (FDG), which is taken up by metabolically active malignant cells. However, FDG is trapped within the cell following phosphorylation, and the unstable [^{18}F] decays by emission of positrons, which can be detected by a specialized PET camera or by a gamma camera that has been adapted for imaging of positron-emitting nuclides. This technique has been used in the evaluation of solitary pulmonary nodules and in staging lung cancer through the detection or exclusion of mediastinal lymph node involvement and identification of extrathoracic disease. The limited anatomical definition of radionuclide imaging has been improved by the development of hybrid imaging that allows the superimposition of nuclear medicine and CT images, a technique known as functional–anatomical mapping. Today, most PET scans are performed using instruments with combined PET and CT scanners. The hybrid PET/CT scans provide images that help pinpoint the abnormal metabolic activity to anatomical structures

seen on CT. The combined scans provide more accurate diagnoses than the two scans performed separately. FDG–PET can differentiate benign from malignant lesions as small as 1 cm. However, false-negative findings can occur in lesions with low metabolic activity such as carcinoid tumors and bronchioloalveolar cell carcinomas, or in lesions <1 cm in which the required threshold of metabolically active malignant cells is not present for PET diagnosis. False-positive results can be seen due to FDG uptake in inflammatory conditions such as pneumonia and granulomatous diseases.

PULMONARY ANGIOGRAPHY

The pulmonary arterial system can be visualized by pulmonary angiography, in which radiopaque contrast medium is injected through a catheter placed in the pulmonary artery. When performed in cases of pulmonary embolism, pulmonary angiography demonstrates the consequences of an intravascular thrombus—either a defect in the lumen of a vessel (a filling defect) or an abrupt termination (cutoff) of the vessel. Other, less common indications for pulmonary angiography include visualization of a suspected pulmonary arteriovenous malformation and assessment of pulmonary arterial invasion by a neoplasm. The risks associated with modern arteriography are extremely small, generally of greatest concern in patients with severe pulmonary hypertension. With advances in CT scanning, MDCT angiography (MDCTA) is replacing conventional angiography for the diagnosis of pulmonary embolism.

ULTRASOUND

Diagnostic ultrasound (US) produces images using echoes or reflection of the ultrasound beam from interfaces between tissues with differing acoustic properties. US is nonionizing and safe to perform on pregnant patients and children. It is helpful in the detection and localization of pleural abnormalities, and a quick and effective way of guiding percutaneous needle biopsy of peripheral lung, pleural, or chest wall lesions. US is also helpful in identifying septations within loculated collections and can facilitate placement of a needle for sampling of pleural liquid (i.e., for thoracentesis), improving the yield and safety of the procedure. Bedside availability makes it valuable in the intensive care setting. Real-time imaging can be used to assess the movement of the diaphragm. Using the Doppler mode, patterns of blood flow in both large and small vessels can be visualized. Because US energy is rapidly dissipated in air, it is not useful for evaluation of the pulmonary parenchyma and cannot be used if there is any aerated lung between the US probe and the abnormality of interest.

Endobronchial US, in which the US probe is passed through a bronchoscope, is emerging as a valuable adjunct to bronchoscopy, allowing identification and localization of pathology adjacent to airway walls or within the mediastinum, discussed further later.

VIRTUAL BRONCHOSCOPY

The three-dimensional (3D) image of the thorax obtained by MDCT can be digitally stored, reanalyzed, and displayed as 3D reconstructions of the airways down to the sixth- to seventh-generation. Using these computed generated reconstructions, a "virtual" bronchoscopy can be performed (Fig. 6-5). Virtual bronchoscopy has been proposed as an adjunct to conventional bronchoscopy in several clinical situations: It can allow accurate assessment of the extent and length of an airway stenosis, including the airway distal to the narrowing; it can provide useful information about the relationship of the airway abnormality to adjacent mediastinal structures; and it allows preprocedure planning for therapeutic bronchoscopy to help ensure the appropriate equipment is available for the procedure. Virtual bronchoscopy can also be used to perform noninvasive follow-up of patients with treated airway lesions. Navigational systems using virtual bronchoscopy have been developed to allow pathfinding to guide the bronchoscopist to a peripheral region within the lung, allowing peripheral lung lesions to be sampled more efficiently. Finally, with the advent of endobronchial lung volume reduction surgery in the management of pulmonary emphysema, virtual bronchoscopy may be able to help target the area of peripheral lung for endobronchial valve procedures. The extent of emphysema in each segmental region together with other anatomic details may help in choosing the most appropriate subsegments. However, software packages for the generation of virtual bronchoscopic images are relatively early in development and their utilization and potential impact on patient care are still unknown. In addition to allowing virtual bronchoscopy, advances in computing capabilities and digital imaging allow the bronchoscopic images obtained through a real bronchoscopic examination to be stored as digital images and reviewed after completion of the procedure.

MEDICAL TECHNIQUES FOR OBTAINING BIOLOGIC SPECIMENS

COLLECTION OF SPUTUM

Sputum can be collected either by spontaneous expectoration or after inhalation of an irritating aerosol such as hypertonic saline. The latter method, called *sputum induction,* is commonly used to obtain sputum for diagnostic studies, either because sputum is not spontaneously being produced or because of an expected higher yield of certain types of findings. Knowledge of the appearance and quality of the sputum specimen obtained is especially important when one is interested in Gram's method and culture. Because sputum consists mainly of secretions from the tracheobronchial tree rather than the upper airway, the finding of alveolar macrophages and other inflammatory cells is consistent with a lower respiratory tract origin of the sample, whereas the presence of squamous epithelial cells in a "sputum" sample indicates contamination by secretions from the upper airways.

In addition to processing for routine bacterial pathogens by Gram's method and culture, sputum can be processed for a variety of other pathogens, including staining and culture for mycobacteria or fungi, culture for viruses, and staining for *Pneumocystis jiroveci.* In the specific case of sputum obtained for evaluation of *P. jiroveci* pneumonia in a patient infected with HIV, for example, sputum should be collected by induction rather than spontaneous expectoration, and an immunofluorescent stain should be used to detect the organisms. Cytologic staining of sputum for malignant cells, using the traditional Papanicolaou method, allows noninvasive evaluation for suspected lung cancer. Traditional stains and cultures are now also being supplemented in some cases by immunologic techniques and by molecular biologic methods, including the use of polymerase chain reaction amplification and DNA probes.

PERCUTANEOUS NEEDLE ASPIRATION (TRANSTHORACIC)

A needle can be inserted through the chest wall into a pulmonary lesion to aspirate material for analysis by cytologic or microbiologic techniques. Aspiration can be performed to obtain a diagnosis or to decompress and/or drain a fluid collection. The procedure is usually carried out under CT or ultrasound guidance to assist positioning of the needle and assure localization in the lesion. The low potential risk of this procedure (intrapulmonary bleeding or creation of a pneumothorax with collapse of the underlying lung) in experienced hands is usually acceptable owing to the information obtained. However, a limitation of the technique is sampling error due to the small size of the tissue sample. Thus, findings other than a specific cytologic or microbiologic diagnosis are of limited clinical value.

THORACENTESIS

Sampling of pleural liquid by thoracentesis is commonly performed for diagnostic purposes or, in the case of a large effusion, for palliation of dyspnea. Diagnostic sampling, either by blind needle aspiration or after localization by US, allows the collection of liquid for microbiologic and cytologic studies. Analysis of the fluid obtained for its cellular composition and chemical constituents, including glucose, protein, and lactate dehydrogenase, allows the effusion to be classified as either exudative or transudative (Chap. 21).

BRONCHOSCOPY

Bronchoscopy is the process of direct visualization of the tracheobronchial tree. Although bronchoscopy is now performed almost exclusively with flexible fiberoptic instruments, rigid bronchoscopy, generally performed in an operating room on a patient under general anesthesia, still has a role in selected circumstances, primarily because of a larger suction channel and the fact that the patient can be ventilated through the bronchoscope channel. These situations include the retrieval of a foreign body and the suctioning of a massive hemorrhage, for which the small suction channel of the bronchoscope may be insufficient.

FLEXIBLE FIBEROPTIC BRONCHOSCOPY

This outpatient procedure is usually performed in an awake but sedated patient (conscious sedation). The bronchoscope is passed through either the mouth or the nose, between the vocal cords, and into the trachea. The ability to flex the scope makes it possible to visualize virtually all airways to the level of subsegmental bronchi. The bronchoscopist is able to identify endobronchial pathology, including tumors, granulomas, bronchitis, foreign bodies, and sites of bleeding. Samples from airway lesions can be taken by several methods, including washing, brushing, and biopsy. Washing involves instillation of sterile saline through a channel of the bronchoscope and onto the surface of a lesion. A portion of the liquid is collected by suctioning through the bronchoscope, and the recovered material can be analyzed for cells (cytology) or organisms (by standard stains and cultures). Brushing or biopsy of the surface of the lesion, using a small brush or biopsy forceps at the end of a long cable inserted through a channel of the bronchoscope, allows recovery of cellular material or tissue for analysis by standard cytologic and histopathologic methods.

The bronchoscope can be used to sample material not only from the regions that can be directly visualized (i.e., the airways) but also from the more distal pulmonary parenchyma. With the bronchoscope wedged into a subsegmental airway, aliquots of sterile saline can be instilled through the scope, allowing sampling of cells and organisms even from alveolar spaces. This procedure, called *bronchoalveolar lavage,* has been particularly useful for the recovery of organisms such as *P. jiroveci* in patients with HIV infection.

Brushing and biopsy of the distal lung parenchyma can also be performed with the same instruments that are used for endobronchial sampling. These instruments can be passed through the scope into small airways, where they penetrate the airway wall, allowing biopsy of peribronchial alveolar tissue. This procedure, called *transbronchial biopsy,* is used when there is either relatively diffuse disease or a localized lesion of adequate size. With the aid of fluoroscopic imaging, the bronchoscopist is able to determine not only whether and when the instrument is in the area of abnormality, but also the proximity of the instrument to the pleural surface. If the forceps are too close to the pleural surface, there is a risk of violating the visceral pleura and creating a pneumothorax; the other potential complication of transbronchial biopsy is pulmonary hemorrhage. The incidence of these complications is less than several percent.

TRANSBRONCHIAL NEEDLE ASPIRATION (TBNA)

Another procedure involves use of a hollow-bore needle passed through the bronchoscope for sampling of tissue adjacent to the trachea or a large bronchus. The needle is passed through the airway wall (transbronchial), and cellular material can be aspirated from mass lesions or enlarged lymph nodes, generally in a search for malignant cells. Other promising new techniques that are not yet widely available include fluorescence bronchoscopy (to detect early endobronchial malignancy) and endobronchial ultrasound (to better identify and localize peribronchial and mediastinal pathology). Mediastinoscopy has been considered the gold standard for mediastinal staging; however, TBNA allows sampling from the lungs and surrounding lymph nodes without the need for surgery or general anesthesia.

ENDOBRONCHIAL ULTRASOUND (EBUS)– TRANSBRONCHIAL NEEDLE ASPIRATION (TBNA)

Further advances in needle aspiration techniques have been accomplished with the development of endobronchial ultrasound (EBUS). The technology uses an ultrasonic bronchoscope fitted with a probe that allows for needle aspiration of mediastinal and hilar lymph nodes guided by real-time US images. This procedure offers access to more difficult-to-reach areas and smaller lymph nodes in the staging of malignancies. EBUS–TBNA has the potential to access the same paratracheal and subcarinal lymph node stations as mediastinoscopy, but also extends out to the hilar lymph nodes (levels 10 and 11). The usefulness of EBUS for clinical indications other than lung cancer is unclear, although studies on sarcoidosis point to the effectiveness of endobronchial ultrasonography in diagnosing this disease.

INTERVENTIONAL PULMONOLOGY (IP)

Interventional pulmonology was initially developed to focus on procedures to help palliate patients with advanced thoracic malignancies. However, the availability of advanced bronchoscopic and pleuroscopic techniques is enabling interventional pulmonologists to provide alternatives to surgery for patients with a wide variety of thoracic disorders and problems. IP can be defined as "the art and science of medicine as related to the performance of diagnostic and invasive therapeutic procedures that which require additional training and expertise beyond that which required in a standard pulmonary medicine training program."

A central role for an IP physician is the acquisition of tissue for diagnosing mass lesions within the thorax. Several techniques already discussed are part of the day-to-day procedural armamentarium used by an IP physician. TBNA to obtain cytologic, histologic, or microbiologic sampling of lesions within the airway wall, the lung parenchyma, and mediastinum. TBNA is frequently performed in combination with EBUS to improve diagnostic yield. Transthoracic needle aspiration and biopsy (TTNA/B) refers to the percutaneous sampling of lesions involving the chest wall, lung parenchyma, and mediastinum for cytologic, histopathologic, or microbiologic examinations.

AUTOFLUORESCENCE BRONCHOSCOPY

Autofluorescence bronchoscopy (AFB) uses bronchoscopes with an additional light source that allows an experienced operator (interventional pulmonologist or surgeon) to distinguish between normal and abnormal tissue. This technique can be used as a screening tool in high-risk individuals to inspect the tracheobronchial tree in order to identify premalignant lesions (airway dysplasia) and carcinoma in situ.

MEDICAL THORACOSCOPY

Medical thoracoscopy (or pleuroscopy) focuses on the diagnosis of pleural-based problems. The procedure is performed with a conventional rigid or a semirigid pleuroscope (similar in design to a bronchoscope and enabling the operator to inspect the pleural surface, sample and/or drain pleural fluid, or perform targeted biopsies of the parietal pleura). Medical thoracoscopy

can be performed in the endoscopy suite or operating room with the patient under conscious sedation and local anesthesia. In contrast, video-assisted thoracoscopic surgery (VATS) requires general anesthesia and is only performed in the OR. A common diagnostic indication for medical thoracoscopy is the evaluation of a pleural effusion or biopsy of presumed parietal pleural carcinomatosis. It can also be used to place a chest tube under visual guidance, or perform chemical or talc pleurodesis, a therapeutic intervention to prevent a recurrent pleural effusion (usually malignant) or recurrent pneumothorax.

THERAPEUTIC BRONCHOSCOPY

The bronchoscope may provide the opportunity for treatment as well as diagnosis. A central role of the IP physican is the performance of therapeutic bronchoscopy. For example, an aspirated foreign body may be retrieved with an instrument passed through the bronchoscope (either flexible or rigid), and bleeding may be controlled with a balloon catheter similarly introduced. Newer interventional techniques performed through a bronchoscope include methods for achieving and maintaining patency of airways that are partially or completely occluded, especially by tumors. These techniques include laser therapy, cryotherapy, argon plasma coagulation, electrocautery, balloon bronchoplasty and dilation, and stent placement. Many IP physicians are also trained in performing percutaneous tracheotomy.

SURGICAL TECHNIQUES FOR OBTAINING BIOLOGIC SPECIMENS

Evaluation and diagnosis of disorders of the chest commonly involve collaboration between pulmonologists and thoracic surgeons. While procedures such as mediastinoscopy, VATS, and thoracotomy are performed by thoracic surgeons, there is overlap in many minimally invasive techniques that can be performed by a pulmonologist or a thoracic surgeon.

MEDIASTINOSCOPY AND MEDIASTINOTOMY

Proper staging of lung cancer is of paramount concern when determining a treatment regimen. Although CT and PET scanning are useful for determining the size and nature of mediastinal lymph nodes as part of the staging of lung cancer, tissue biopsy and histopathologic examination are often critical for the diagnosis of mediastinal masses or enlarged mediastinal lymph nodes. The two major surgical procedures used to obtain specimens from masses or nodes in the mediastinum are mediastinoscopy (via a suprasternal approach) and mediastinotomy (via a parasternal approach). Both procedures are performed under general anesthesia by a qualified surgeon. In the case of suprasternal mediastinoscopy, a rigid mediastinoscope is inserted at the suprasternal notch and passed into the mediastinum along a pathway just anterior to the trachea. Tissue can be obtained with biopsy forceps passed through the scope, sampling masses or nodes that are in a paratracheal or pretracheal position (levels 2R, 2L, 3, 4R, 4L). Aortopulmonary lymph nodes (levels 5, 6) are not accessible by this route and thus are commonly sampled by parasternal mediastinotomy (the Chamberlain procedure). This approach involves a parasternal incision and dissection directly down to a mass or node that requires biopsy.

As an alternative to surgery, a bronchoscope can be used to perform TBNA (discussed earlier) to obtain tissue from the mediastinum, and, when combined with EBUS, can allow access to the same lymph node stations associated with mediastinoscopy, but also extend access out to the hilar lymph nodes (levels 10, 11). Finally, endoscopic ultrasound (EUS)–fine-needle aspiration (FNA) is a second procedure that complements EBUS–FNA in the staging of lung cancer. EUS–FNA is performed via the esophagus and is ideally suited for sampling lymph nodes in the posterior mediastinum (levels 7, 8, 9). Because US imaging cannot penetrate air filled spaces, the area directly anterior to the trachea cannot accurately be assessed and is a "blind spot" for EUS–FNA. However, EBUS–FNA can visualize the anterior lymph nodes and can complement EUS–FNA. The combination of EUS–FNA and EBUS–FNA is a technique that is becoming an alternative to surgery for staging the mediastinum in thoracic malignancies.

VIDEO-ASSISTED THORACIC SURGERY

Advances in video technology have allowed the development of thoracoscopy, or VATS, for the diagnosis and management of pleural as well as parenchymal lung disease. This procedure is performed in the operating room using single-lung ventilation with double-lumen endotracheal intubation and involves the passage of a rigid scope with a distal lens through a trocar inserted into the pleura. A high-quality image is shown on a monitor screen, allowing the operator to manipulate instruments passed into the pleural space through separate small intercostal incisions. With these instruments the operator can biopsy lesions of the pleura under direct visualization. In addition, this procedure is now used commonly to biopsy peripheral lung tissue or to remove peripheral nodules for both diagnostic and therapeutic purposes. This much less invasive procedure has largely supplanted the traditional "open lung biopsy" performed via thoracotomy. The decision to use a VATS technique versus performing an open thoracotomy is made by the thoracic surgeon and is based on whether a patient can tolerate the single-lung ventilation that is required to allow adequate visualization of the lung. With further advances in instrumentation and experience, VATS can be used to perform procedures previously requiring thoracotomy, including stapled lung biopsy, resection of pulmonary nodules, lobectomy, pneumonectomy, pericardial window, or other standard thoracic surgical procedures; but allows them to be performed in a minimally invasive manner.

THORACOTOMY

Although frequently replaced by VATS, thoracotomy remains an option for the diagnostic sampling of lung tissue. It provides the largest amount of material, and it can be used to biopsy and/or excise lesions that are too deep or too close to vital structures for removal by VATS. The choice between VATS and thoracotomy needs to be made on a case-by-case basis.

ACKNOWLEDGMENT

We wish to acknowledge Dr. Scott Manaker and Dr. Steven Weinberger for their contributions to prior versions of this chapter.

CHAPTER 7

ATLAS OF CHEST IMAGING

Patricia Kritek ■ John J. Reilly, Jr.

This atlas of chest imaging is a collection of interesting chest radiographs and computed tomograms of the chest. The readings of the films are meant to be illustrative of specific, major findings. The associated text is not intended as a comprehensive assessment of the images.

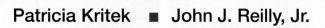

EXAMPLES OF NORMAL IMAGING

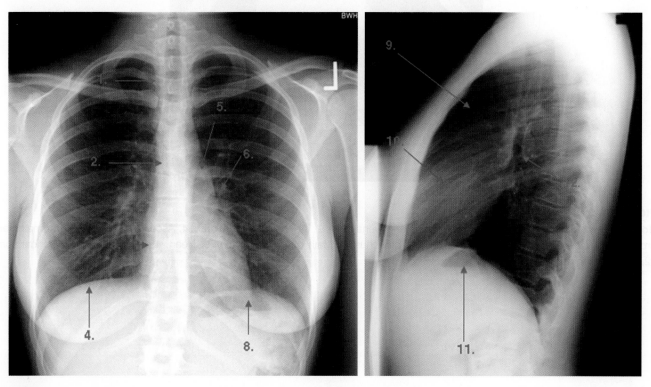

FIGURE 7-1
Normal chest radiograph—review of anatomy. 1. Trachea. 2. Carina. 3. Right atrium. 4. Right hemidiaphragm. 5. Aortic knob. 6. Left hilum. 7. Left ventricle. 8. Left hemidiaphragm (with stomach bubble). 9. Retrosternal clear space. 10. Right ventricle. 11. Left hemidiaphragm (with stomach bubble). 12. Left upper lobe bronchus.

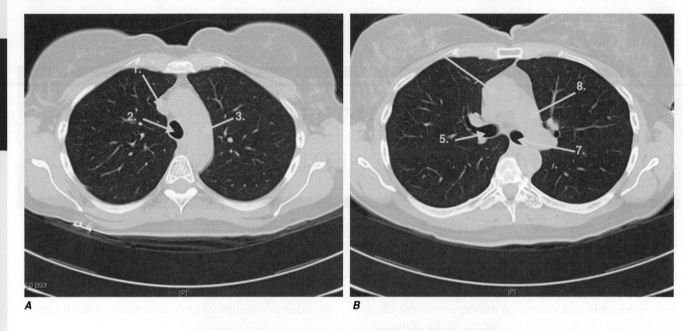

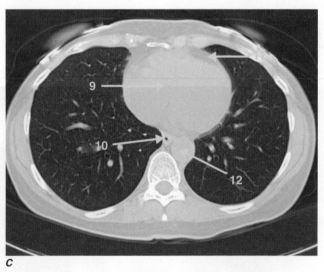

FIGURE 7-2

Normal chest tomogram—note anatomy. 1. Superior vena cava. 2. Trachea. 3. Aortic arch. 4. Ascending aorta. 5. Right mainstem bronchus. 6. Descending aorta. 7. Left mainstem bronchus. 8. Main pulmonary artery. 9. Heart. 10. Esophagus. 11. Pericardium. 12. Descending aorta.

VOLUME LOSS

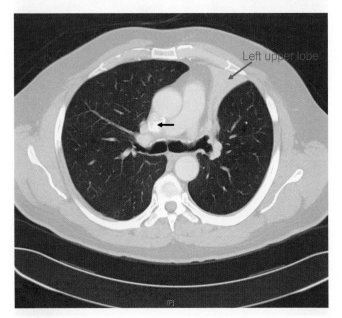

FIGURE 7-3

CT scan demonstrating left upper lobe collapse. The patient was found to have an endobronchial lesion (not visible on the CT scan) resulting in this finding. The superior vena cava (*black arrow*) is partially opacified by intravenous contrast.

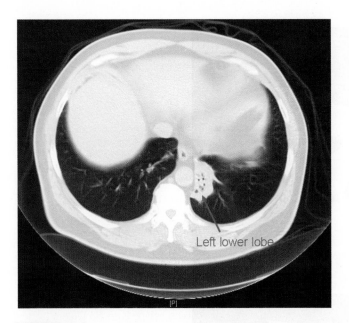

FIGURE 7-4

CT scan revealing chronic left lower lobe collapse. Note dramatic volume loss with minimal aeration. There is subtle mediastinal shift to the left.

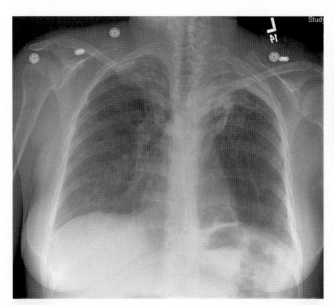

FIGURE 7-5

Left upper lobe scarring with hilar retraction with less prominent scarring in right upper lobe as well. Findings consistent with previous tuberculosis infection in an immigrant from Ecuador.

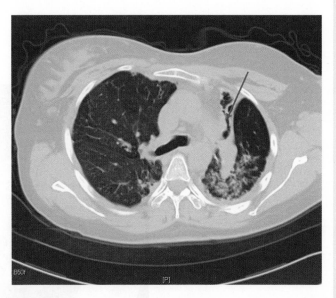

FIGURE 7-6

Apical scarring, traction bronchiectasis (*red arrow*), and decreased lung volume consistent with previous tuberculosis infection. Findings most significant in left lung.

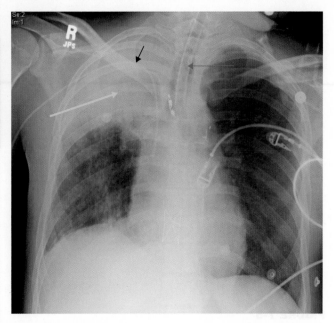

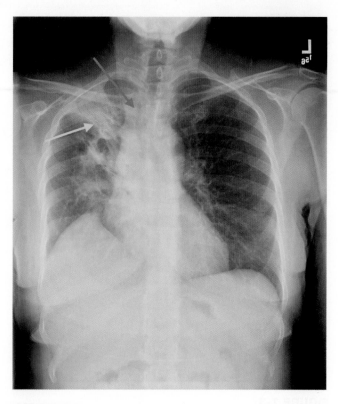

FIGURE 7-7

Chest x-ray (CXR) demonstrating right upper lobe collapse (*yellow arrow*). Note the volume loss as demonstrated by the elevated right hemidiaphragm as well as mediastinal shift to the right. Also apparent on the film are an endotracheal tube (*red arrow*) and a central venous catheter (*black arrow*).

FIGURE 7-8

Opacity in the right upper lobe. Note the volume loss as indicated by the elevation of the right hemidiaphragm, elevation of minor fissure (*yellow arrow*) and deviation of the trachea to the right (*blue arrow*).

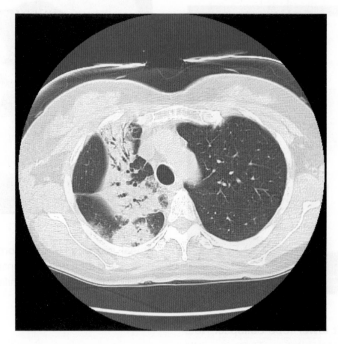

FIGURE 7-9

CT scan of the same right upper lobe opacity. Note the air bronchograms and areas of consolidation.

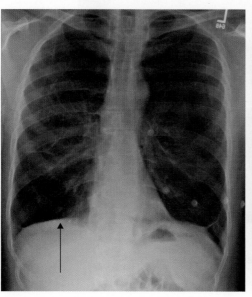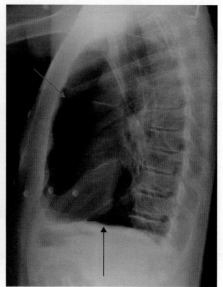

FIGURE 7-10

Emphysema with increased lucency, flattened diaphragms (*black arrows*), increased AP diameter, and increased retrosternal clear space (*red arrow*).

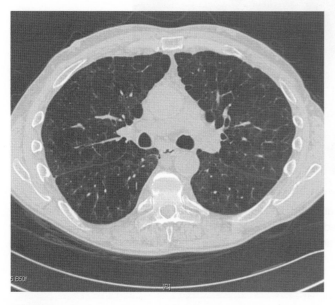

FIGURE 7-11
CT scan of diffuse, bilateral emphysema.

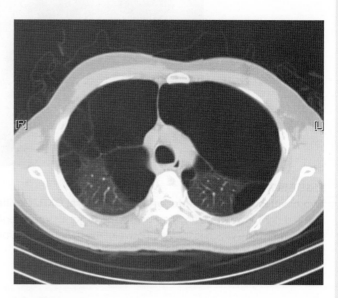

FIGURE 7-12
CT scan of bullous emphysema.

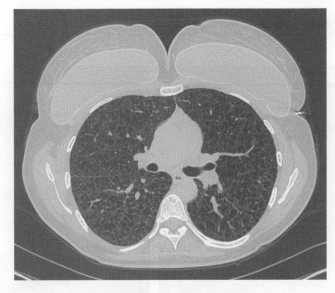

FIGURE 7-13

Lymphangioleiomyomatosis—note multiple thin-walled parenchymal cysts.

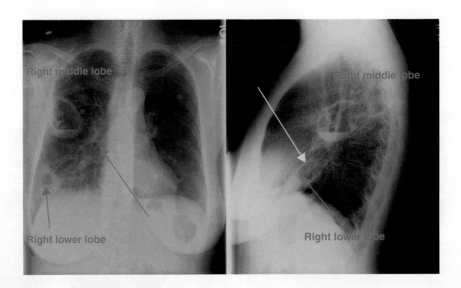

FIGURE 7-14

Two cavities on posteroanterior (PA) and lateral CXR. Cavities and air-fluid levels identified by *blue arrows*. The smaller cavity is in the right lower lobe (located below the major fissure, identified with the *yellow arrow*) and the larger cavity is located in the right middle lobe which is located between the minor (*blue arrow*) and major fissures. There is an associated opacity surrounding the cavity in the right lower lobe.

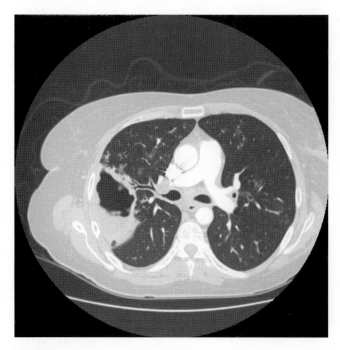

FIGURE 7-15
CT scan of parenchymal cavity.

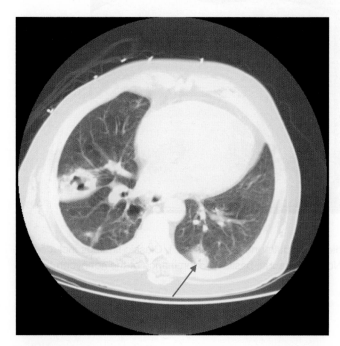

FIGURE 7-16
Thick-walled cavitary lung lesions. The mass in the right lung has thick walls and advanced cavitation, while the smaller nodule on the left has early cavitary changes (*arrow*). This patient was diagnosed with Nocardia infection.

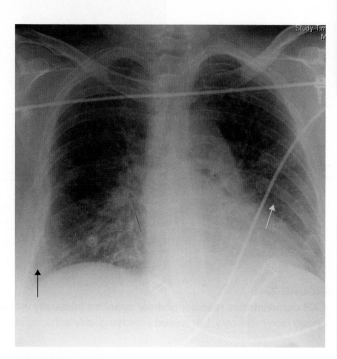

FIGURE 7-17
Mild congestive heart failure. Note the Kerley B lines (*black arrow*) and perivascular cuffing (*yellow arrow*) as well as the pulmonary vascular congestion (*red arrow*).

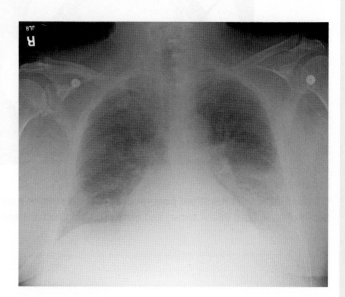

FIGURE 7-18
Pulmonary edema. Note indistinct vasculature, perihilar opacities, and peripheral interstitial reticular opacities. While this is an anteroposterior film making cardiac size more difficult to assess, the cardiac silhouette still appears enlarged.

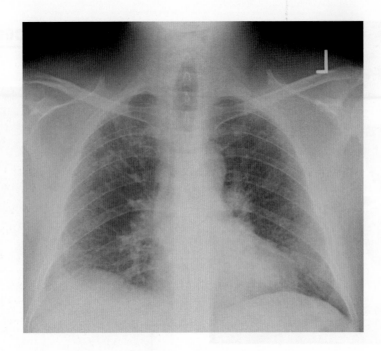

FIGURE 7-19

CXR demonstrates reticular nodular opacities bilaterally with small lung volumes consistent with usual interstitial pneumonitis (UIP) on pathology. Clinically, UIP is used interchangeably with idiopathic pulmonary fibrosis (IPF).

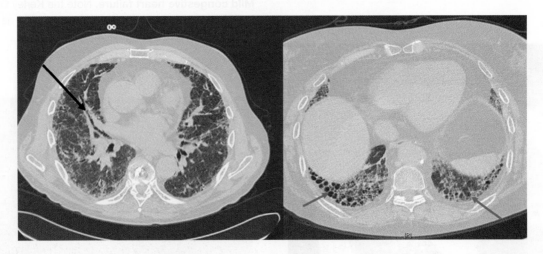

FIGURE 7-20

CT scan of usual interstitial pneumonitis (UIP), also known as idiopathic pulmonary fibrosis (IPF). Classic findings include traction bronchiectasis (*black arrow*) and honeycombing (*red arrows*). Note subpleural, basilar predominance of the honeycombing.

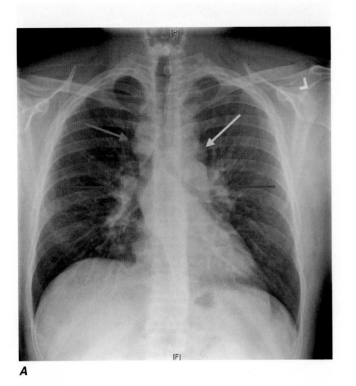

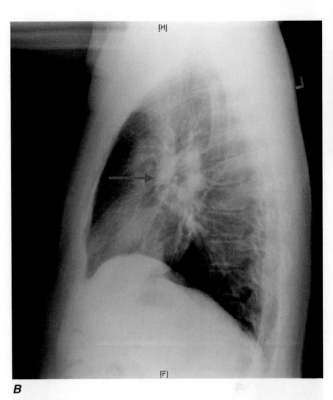

A

B

FIGURE 7-21

(**A**) PA chest film—note presence of paratracheal (*blue arrow*), aortopulmonary window (*yellow arrow*) and hilar (*purple arrows*) lymphadenopathy. (**B**) Lateral film—note hilar lymphadenopathy (*purple arrow*).

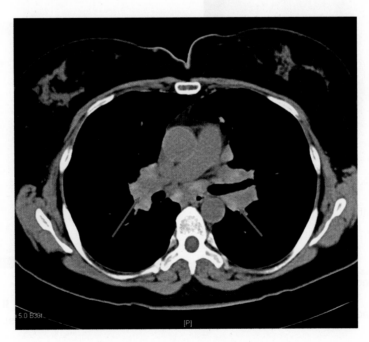

FIGURE 7-22

Sarcoid—CT scan of stage I demonstrating bulky hilar and mediastinal lymphadenopathy (*red arrows*).

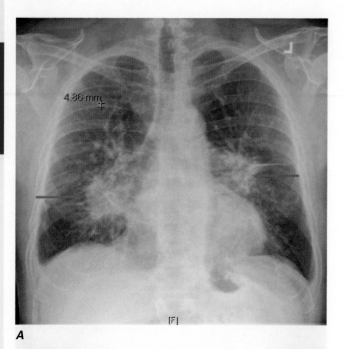

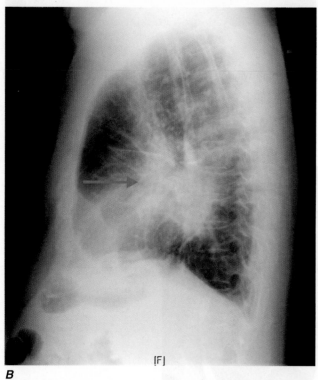

FIGURE 7-23
Sarcoid—CXR of stage II.
(*A*) PA film with hilar lymphadenopathy (*green arrows*) and parenchymal changes.
(*B*) Lateral film with hilar adenopathy (*green arrow*) and parenchymal changes.

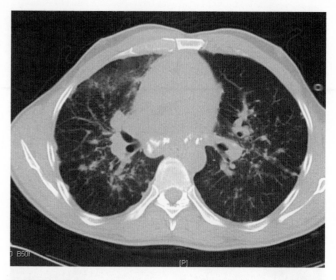

FIGURE 7-24
Sarcoid—CT scan of stage II (calcified lymphadenopathy, parenchymal infiltrates).

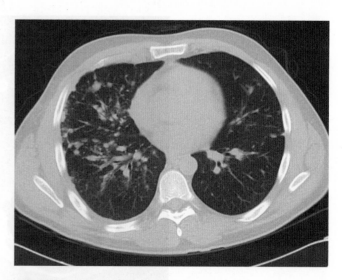

FIGURE 7-25
Sarcoid—CT scan of stage II (nodular opacities tracking along bronchovascular bundles).

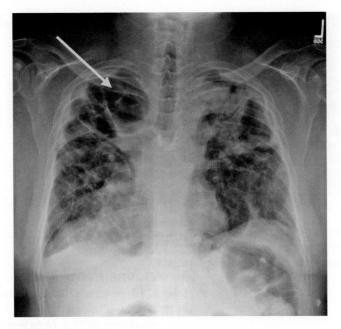

FIGURE 7-26
Sarcoid—stage IV with fibrotic lung disease and cavitary areas (*yellow arrow*).

ALVEOLAR PROCESSES

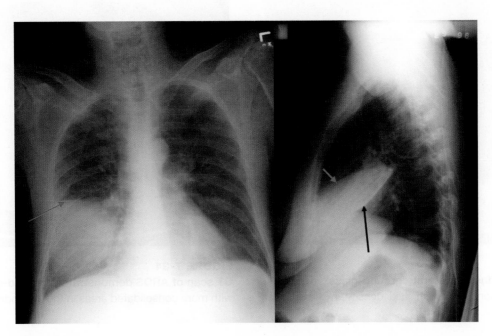

FIGURE 7-27
Right middle lobe opacity illustrates major (*black arrow*) and minor fissures (*red arrows*) as well as the "silhouette sign" on the right heart border.

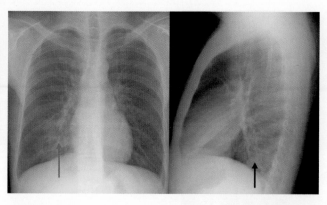

FIGURE 7-28
Right lower lobe pneumonia—subtle opacity on PA film (*red arrow*), while the lateral film illustrates the "spine sign" (*black arrow*) where the lower spine does not become more lucent.

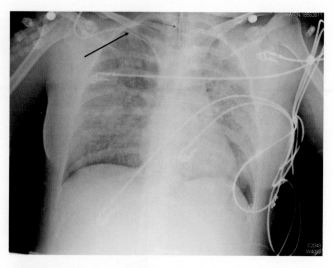

FIGURE 7-30
CXR reveals diffuse, bilateral alveolar opacities without pleural effusions, consistent with acute respiratory distress syndrome (ARDS). Note that the patient has an endotracheal tube (*red arrow*) and a central venous catheter (*black arrow*).

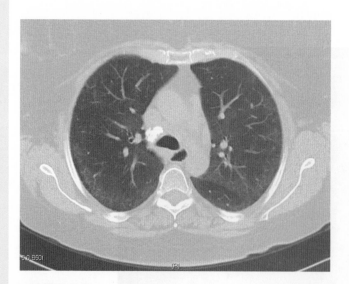

FIGURE 7-29
CT scan of diffuse, bilateral "ground-glass" opacities. This finding is consistent with fluid density in the alveolar space.

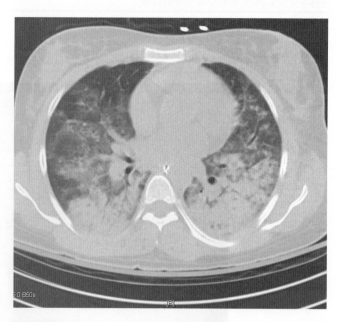

FIGURE 7-31
CT scan of ARDS demonstrates "ground-glass" opacities with more consolidated areas in the dependent lung zones.

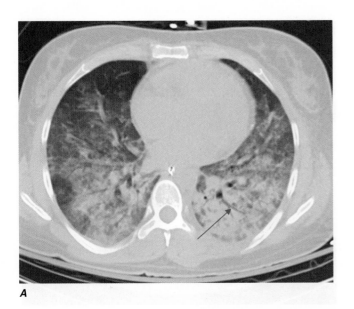

A

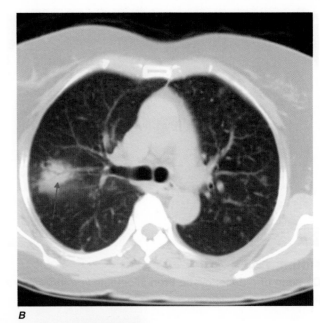

B

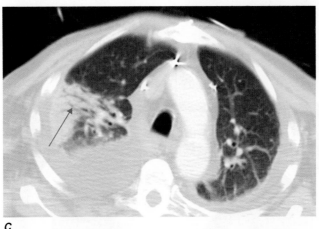

C

FIGURE 7-32
Three examples of air bronchograms (*red arrows*) on chest CT.

BRONCHIECTASIS

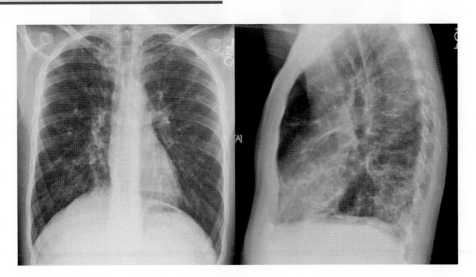

FIGURE 7-33
Cystic fibrosis with bronchiectasis, apical disease.

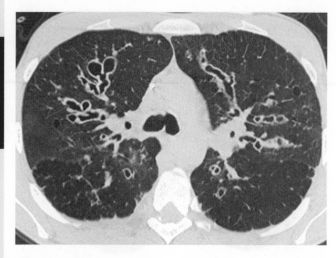

FIGURE 7-34
CT scan of diffuse, cystic bronchiectasis (*red arrows*) in a patient with cystic fibrosis.

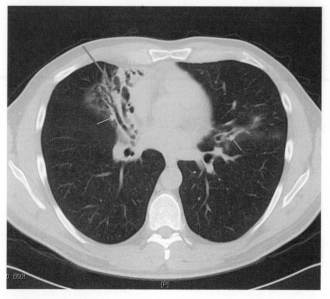

FIGURE 7-35
CT scan of focal right middle lobe and lingular bronchiectasis (*yellow arrows*). Note that there is near total collapse of the right middle lobe (*red arrow*).

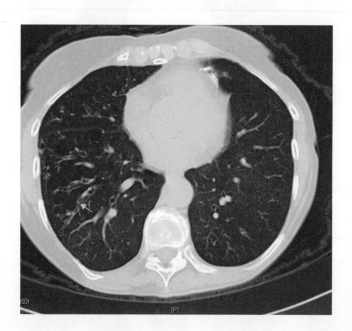

FIGURE 7-36
"Tree in bud" opacities (*red arrows*) and bronchiectasis (*yellow arrow*) consistent with atypical mycobacterial infection. "Tree in bud" refers to small nodules clustered around the centrilobular arteries as well as increased prominence of the centrilobular branching. These findings are consistent with bronchiolitis.

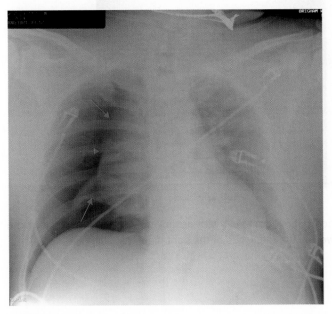

FIGURE 7-37
Large right pneumothorax with near complete collapse of right lung. Pleural reflection highlighted with *red arrows*.

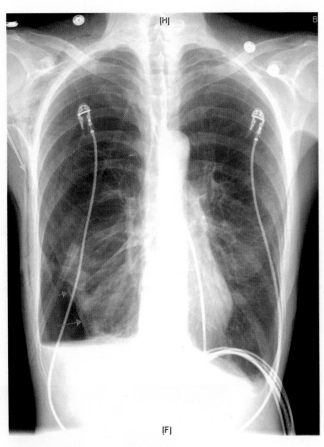

FIGURE 7-38
Basilar pneumothorax with visible pleural reflection (*red arrows*). Also note, patient has subcutaneous emphysema (*yellow arrow*).

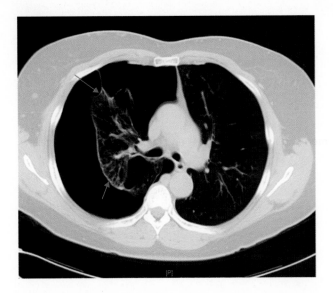

FIGURE 7-39
CT scan of large right-sided pneumothorax. Note significant collapse of right lung with adhesion to anterior chest wall. Pleural reflection highlighted with *red arrows*. The patient has severe underlying emphysema.

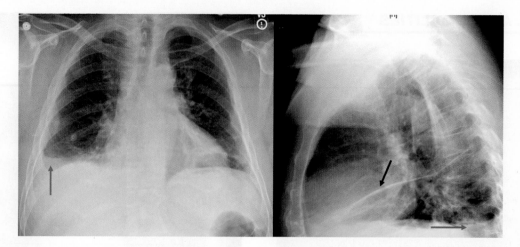

FIGURE 7-40
Small right pleural effusion (*red arrows* highlight blunted right costophrenic angles) with associated pleural thickening. Note fluid in the major fissure (*black arrow*) visible on the lateral film as well as the meniscus of the right pleural effusion.

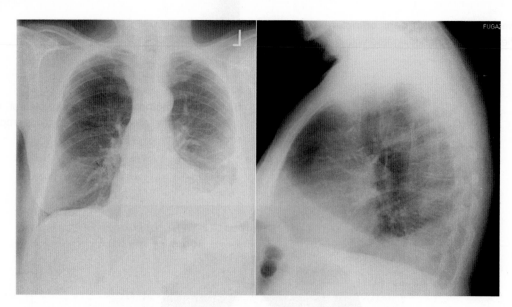

FIGURE 7-41
Left pleural effusion with clear meniscus seen on both PA and lateral chest radiographs.

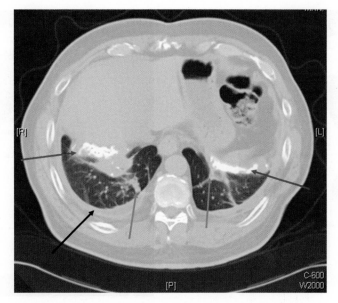

FIGURE 7-42
Asbestosis. Note calcified pleural plaques (*red arrows*), pleural thickening (*black arrow*), and subpleural atelectasis (*green arrows*).

NODULES AND MASSES

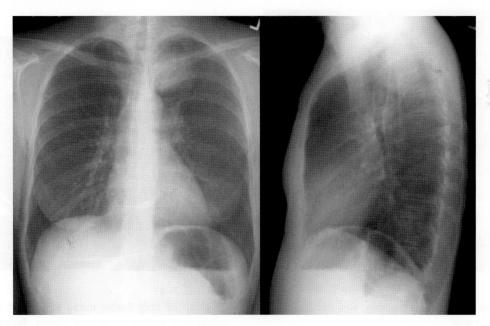

FIGURE 7-43
Left upper lobe mass, which biopsy revealed to be squamous cell carcinoma.

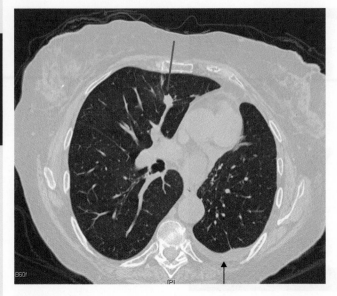

FIGURE 7-44
Solitary pulmonary nodule on the right (*red arrow*) with a spiculated pattern concerning for lung cancer. Note also that the patient is status-post left upper lobectomy with resultant volume loss and associated effusion (*black arrow*).

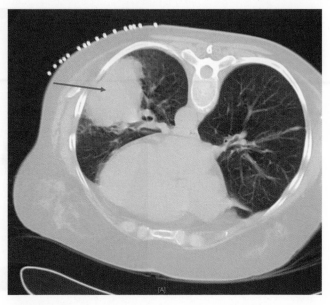

FIGURE 7-46
Left lower lobe lung mass (*red arrow*) abutting pleura. Biopsy demonstrated small cell lung cancer.

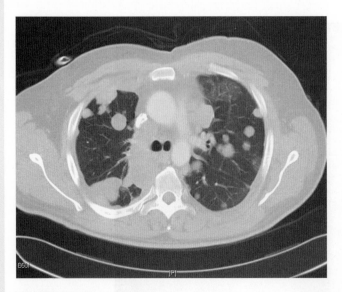

FIGURE 7-45
Metastatic sarcoma. Note the multiple, well-circumscribed nodules of different size.

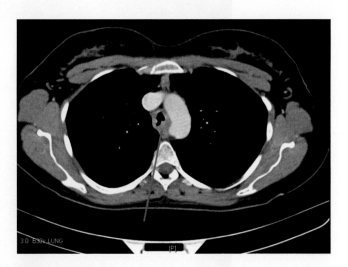

FIGURE 7-47
CT scan of soft tissue mass encircling the trachea (*red arrow*) and invading tracheal lumen. Biopsy demonstrated adenoid cystic carcinoma (cylindroma).

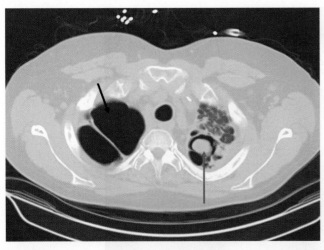

FIGURE 7-48
Mycetoma. Fungal ball (*red arrow*) growing in preexisting cavity on the left. Right upper lobe has a large bulla (*black arrow*).

PULMONARY VASCULAR ABNORMALITIES

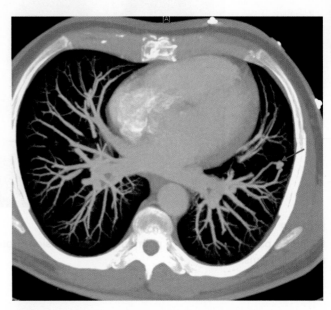

FIGURE 7-49
Pulmonary arteriovenous malformation (AVM) demonstrated on reformatted CT angiogram (*red arrow*).

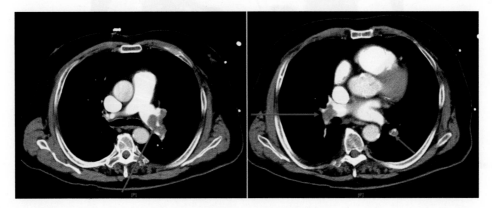

FIGURE 7-50
Large bilateral pulmonary emboli (intravascular filling defects in contrast scan identified by *red arrows*).

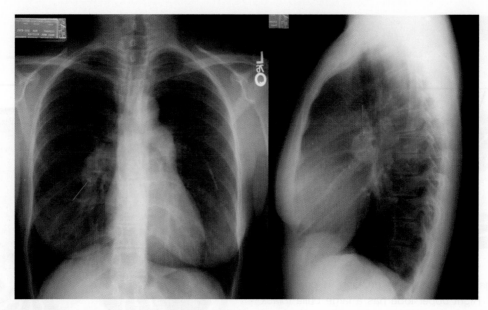

FIGURE 7-51
CXR of a patient with severe pulmonary hypertension. Note the enlarged pulmonary arteries (*red arrows*) visible on both PA and lateral films.

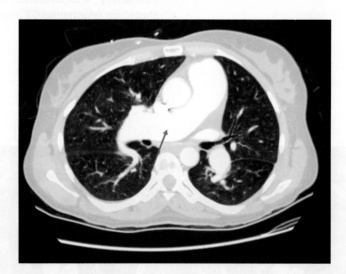

FIGURE 7-52
CT scan of the same patient as in Fig. 7-51. Note the markedly enlarged pulmonary arteries (*red arrow*).

SECTION II

DISEASES OF THE RESPIRATORY SYSTEM

CHAPTER 8

ASTHMA

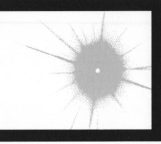

Peter J. Barnes

Asthma is a syndrome characterized by airflow obstruction that varies markedly, both spontaneously and with treatment. Asthmatics harbor a special type of inflammation in the airways that makes them more responsive than nonasthmatics to a wide range of triggers, leading to excessive narrowing with consequent reduced airflow and symptomatic wheezing and dyspnea. Narrowing of the airways is usually reversible, but in some patients with chronic asthma there may be an element of irreversible airflow obstruction. The increasing global prevalence of asthma, the large burden it now imposes on patients, and the high health care costs have led to extensive research into its mechanisms and treatment.

PREVALENCE

Asthma is one of the most common chronic diseases globally and currently affects approximately 300 million people worldwide. The prevalence of asthma has risen in affluent countries over the last 30 years but now appears to have stabilized, with approximately 10–12% of adults and 15% of children affected by the disease. In developing countries where the prevalence of asthma had been much lower, there is a rising prevalence, which is associated with increased urbanization. The prevalence of atopy and other allergic diseases has also increased over the same time, suggesting that the reasons for the increase are likely to be systemic rather than confined to the lungs. This epidemiologic observation suggests that there is a maximum number of individuals in the community, who are likely to be affected by asthma, most likely by genetic predisposition. Most patients with asthma in affluent countries are atopic, with allergic sensitization to the house dust mite *Dermatophagoides pteronyssinus* and other environmental allergens.

Because asthma is both common and frequently complicated by the effects of smoking on the lungs, it is difficult to be certain about the natural history of the disease in adults. Asthma can present at any age, with a peak age of 3 years. In childhood, twice as many males as females are asthmatic, but by adulthood the sex ratio has equalized. The commonly held belief that children "grow out of their asthma" is justified to some extent. Long-term studies that have followed children until they reach the age of 40 years suggest that many with asthma become asymptomatic during adolescence, but that asthma returns in some during adult life, particularly in those with persistent symptoms and severe asthma. Adults with asthma, including those with onset during adulthood, rarely become permanently asymptomatic. The severity of asthma does not vary significantly within a given patient; those with mild asthma rarely progress to more severe disease, whereas those with severe asthma usually have severe disease at the onset.

Deaths from asthma are uncommon, and in many affluent countries have been steadily declining over the last decade. A rise in asthma mortality seen in several countries during the 1960s was associated with increased use of short-acting β_2-adrenergic agonists (as rescue therapy), but there is now compelling evidence that the more widespread use of inhaled corticosteroids (ICS) in patients with persistent asthma is responsible for the decrease in mortality in recent years. Major risk factors for asthma deaths are poorly controlled disease with frequent use of bronchodilator inhalers, lack of corticosteroid therapy, and previous admissions to hospital with near-fatal asthma.

It has proved difficult to agree on a definition of asthma, but there is good agreement on the description of the clinical syndrome and disease pathology. Until the etiologic mechanisms of the disease are better understood, it will be difficult to provide an accurate definition.

ETIOLOGY

Asthma is a heterogeneous disease with interplay between genetic and environmental factors. Several risk factors have been implicated (Table 8-1).

ATOPY

Atopy is the major risk factor for asthma, and nonatopic individuals have a very low risk of developing asthma. Patients with asthma commonly suffer from other atopic diseases, particularly allergic rhinitis, which may be found in over 80% of asthmatic patients, and atopic dermatitis (eczema). Atopy may be found in 40–50% of the population in affluent countries, with only a proportion of atopic individuals becoming asthmatic. This observation suggests that some other environmental or genetic factor(s) predispose to the development of asthma in atopic individuals. The allergens that lead to sensitization are usually proteins that have protease activity, and the most common allergens are derived from house dust mites, cat and dog fur, cockroaches (in inner cities), grass and tree pollens, and rodents (in laboratory workers). Atopy is due to the genetically determined production of specific IgE antibody, with many patients showing a family history of allergic diseases.

TABLE 8-1

RISK FACTORS AND TRIGGERS INVOLVED IN ASTHMA	
ENDOGENOUS FACTORS	**ENVIRONMENTAL FACTORS**
Genetic predisposition	Indoor allergens
Atopy	Outdoor allergens
Airway hyperresponsiveness	Occupational sensitizers
Gender	Passive smoking
Ethnicity?	Respiratory infections
Obesity?	
Early viral infections?	
Triggers	
Allergens	
Upper respiratory tract viral infections	
Exercise and hyperventilation	
Cold air	
Sulfur dioxide and irritant gases	
Drugs (β-blockers, aspirin)	
Stress	
Irritants (household sprays, paint fumes)	

INTRINSIC ASTHMA

A minority of asthmatic patients (approximately 10%) have negative skin tests to common inhalant allergens and normal serum concentrations of IgE. These patients, with nonatopic or intrinsic asthma, usually show later onset of disease (adult-onset asthma), commonly have concomitant nasal polyps, and may be aspirin-sensitive. They usually have more severe, persistent asthma. Little is understood about mechanism, but the immunopathology in bronchial biopsies and sputum appears to be identical to that found in atopic asthma. There is recent evidence for increased local production of IgE in the airways, suggesting that there may be common IgE-mediated mechanisms; staphylococcal enterotoxins, which serve as "superantigens," have been implicated.

INFECTIONS

Although viral infections are common as triggers of asthma exacerbations, it is uncertain whether they play a role in etiology. There is some association between respiratory syncytial virus infection in infancy and the development of asthma, but the specific pathogenesis is difficult to elucidate, as this infection is very common in children. More recently, atypical bacteria such as *Mycoplasma* and *Chlamydophila,* have been implicated in the mechanism of severe asthma, but thus far, the evidence is not very convincing of a true association.

GENETIC CONSIDERATIONS

The familial association of asthma and a high degree of concordance for asthma in identical twins indicate a genetic predisposition to the disease; however, whether or not the genes predisposing to asthma are similar or in addition to those predisposing to atopy is not yet clear. It now seems likely that different genes may also contribute to asthma specifically, and there is increasing evidence that the severity of asthma is also genetically determined. Genetic screens with classical linkage analysis and single-nucleotide polymorphisms of various candidate genes indicate that asthma is polygenic, with each gene identified having a small effect that is often not replicated in different populations. This observation suggests that the interaction of many genes is important, and these may differ in different populations. The most consistent findings have been associations with polymorphisms of genes on chromosome 5q, including the T helper 2 (T_h2) cells interleukin (IL)-4, IL-5, IL-9, and IL-13, which are associated with atopy. There is increasing evidence for a complex interaction between genetic polymorphisms and environmental factors that will require very large population studies to unravel. Novel genes that have been associated with asthma, including

ADAM-33, DPP-10, and *GPRA,* have also been identified by positional cloning, but their function in disease pathogenesis is not yet clear. Recent genome-wide association studies have identified further novel genes, although, again, their functional role is not yet clear. Genetic polymorphisms may also be important in determining the response to asthma therapy. For example, the Arg-Gly-16 variant in the β_2-receptor has been associated with reduced response to β_2-agonists, and repeats of an Sp1 recognition sequence in the promoter region of 5-lipoxygenase may affect the response to antileukotrienes. However, these effects are small and inconsistent and do not yet have any implications for asthma therapy.

ENVIRONMENTAL FACTORS

It is likely that environmental factors in early life determine which atopic individuals become asthmatic. The increasing prevalence of asthma, particularly in developing countries, over the last few decades also indicates the importance of environmental mechanisms interacting with a genetic predisposition.

Hygiene hypothesis

The observation that allergic sensitization and asthma were less common in children with older siblings first suggested that lower levels of infection may be a factor in affluent societies that increase the risks of asthma. This "hygiene hypothesis" proposes that lack of infections in early childhood preserves the T_H2 cell bias at birth, whereas exposure to infections and endotoxin results in a shift toward a predominant protective T_H1 immune response. Children brought up on farms who are exposed to a high level of endotoxin are less likely to develop allergic sensitization than children raised on dairy farms. Intestinal parasite infection may also be associated with a reduced risk of asthma. While there is considerable epidemiologic support for the hygiene hypothesis, it cannot account for the parallel increase in T_H1-driven diseases such as diabetes mellitus over the same period.

Diet

The role of dietary factors is controversial. Observational studies have shown that diets low in antioxidants such as vitamin C and vitamin A, magnesium, selenium, and omega-3 polyunsaturated fats (fish oil) or high in sodium and omega-6 polyunsaturates are associated with an increased risk of asthma. Vitamin D deficiency may also predispose to the development of asthma. However, interventional studies with supplementary diets have not supported an important role for these dietary factors. Obesity is also an independent risk factor for asthma, particularly in women, but the mechanisms are thus far unknown.

Air pollution

Air pollutants such as sulfur dioxide, ozone, and diesel particulates, may trigger asthma symptoms, but the role of different air pollutants in the etiology of the disease is much less certain. Most evidence argues against an important role for air pollution as asthma is no more prevalent in cities with a high ambient level of traffic pollution than in rural areas with low levels of pollution. Asthma had a much lower prevalence in East Germany compared to West Germany despite a much higher level of air pollution, but since reunification these differences have decreased as eastern Germany has become more affluent. Indoor air pollution may be more important with exposure to nitrogen oxides from cooking stoves and exposure to passive cigarette smoke. There is some evidence that maternal smoking is a risk factor for asthma, but it is difficult to dissociate this association from an increased risk of respiratory infections.

Allergens

Inhaled allergens are common triggers of asthma symptoms and have also been implicated in allergic sensitization. Exposure to house dust mites in early childhood is a risk factor for allergic sensitization and asthma, but rigorous allergen avoidance has not shown any evidence for a reduced risk of developing asthma. The increase in house dust mites in centrally heated poorly ventilated homes with fitted carpets has been implicated in the increasing prevalence of asthma in affluent countries. Domestic pets, particularly cats, have also been associated with allergic sensitization, but early exposure to cats in the home may be protective through the induction of tolerance.

Occupational exposure

Occupational asthma is relatively common and may affect up to 10% of young adults. Over 200 sensitizing agents have been identified. Chemicals such as toluene diisocyanate and trimellitic anhydride, may lead to sensitization independent of atopy. Individuals may also be exposed to allergens in the workplace such as small animal allergens in laboratory workers and fungal amylase in wheat flour in bakers. Occupational asthma may be suspected when symptoms improve during weekends and holidays.

OTHER FACTORS

Several other factors have been implicated in the etiology of asthma, including lower maternal age, duration of breast-feeding, prematurity and low birthweight, and inactivity, but are unlikely to contribute to the recent global increase in asthma prevalence. There is also an association with acetaminophen (paracetamol) consumption in childhood, which remains unexplained.

PATHOGENESIS

Asthma is associated with a specific chronic inflammation of the mucosa of the lower airways. One of the main aims of treatment is to reduce this inflammation.

PATHOLOGY

The pathology of asthma has been revealed through examining the lungs at autopsy of patients who have died of asthma and from bronchial biopsies in patients with usually mild asthma. The airway mucosa is infiltrated with activated eosinophils and T lymphocytes, and there is activation of mucosal mast cells. The degree of inflammation is poorly related to disease severity and may be found in atopic patients without asthma symptoms. The inflammation is reduced by treatment with ICS. A characteristic finding is thickening of the basement membrane due to subepithelial collagen deposition. This feature is also found in patients with eosinophilic bronchitis presenting as cough who do not have asthma and is, therefore, likely to be a marker of eosinophilic inflammation in the airway as eosinophils release fibrogenic factors. The epithelium is often shed or friable, with reduced attachments to the airway wall and increased numbers of epithelial cells in the lumen. The airway wall itself may be thickened and edematous, particularly in fatal asthma. Another common finding in fatal asthma is occlusion of the airway lumen by a mucous plug, which is comprised of mucous glycoproteins secreted from goblet cells and plasma proteins from leaky bronchial vessels (Fig. 8-1). There is also vasodilation and increased numbers of blood vessels (angiogenesis). Direct observation by bronchoscopy indicates that the airways may be narrowed, erythematous, and edematous. The pathology of asthma is remarkably uniform in different types of asthma, including atopic, nonatopic, occupational, aspirin-sensitive, and pediatric asthma. These pathologic changes are found in all airways, but do not extend to the lung parenchyma; peripheral airway inflammation is found particularly in patients with severe asthma. The involvement of airways may be patchy and this is consistent with bronchographic findings of uneven narrowing of the airways.

INFLAMMATION

There is inflammation in the respiratory mucosa from the trachea to terminal bronchioles, but with a predominance in the bronchi (cartilaginous airways). Considerable research has identified the major cellular components of inflammation, but it is still uncertain how inflammatory cells interact and how inflammation translates into the symptoms of asthma (Fig. 8-2). There is good evidence that the specific pattern of airway inflammation in asthma is associated with airway hyperresponsiveness (AHR), the physiologic abnormality of asthma, which is correlated with variable airflow obstruction. The pattern of inflammation in asthma is characteristic of allergic diseases, with similar inflammatory cells seen in the nasal mucosa in rhinitis. However, an indistinguishable pattern of inflammation is found in intrinsic asthma, and this may reflect local rather than systemic IgE production. Although most attention

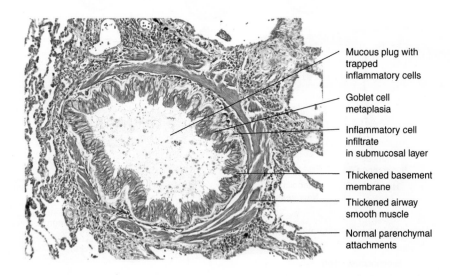

Mucous plug with trapped inflammatory cells

Goblet cell metaplasia

Inflammatory cell infiltrate in submucosal layer

Thickened basement membrane

Thickened airway smooth muscle

Normal parenchymal attachments

FIGURE 8-1

Histopathology of a small airway in fatal asthma. The lumen is occluded with a mucous plug, there is goblet cell metaplasia, and the airway wall is thickened, with an increase in basement membrane thickness and airway smooth muscle. (*Courtesy of Dr. J. Hogg, University of British Colombia.*)

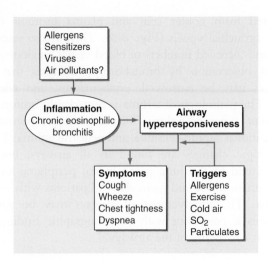

FIGURE 8-2

Inflammation in the airways of asthmatic patients leads to airway hyperresponsiveness and symptoms. SO_2, sulfur dioxide.

has focused on the acute inflammatory changes seen in asthma, this is a chronic condition, with inflammation persisting over many years in most patients. The

mechanisms involved in persistence of inflammation in asthma are still poorly understood. Superimposed on this chronic inflammatory state are acute inflammatory episodes, which correspond to exacerbations of asthma. Many inflammatory cells are known to be involved in asthma with no key cell that is predominant **(Fig. 8-3)**.

Mast cells

Mast cells are important in initiating the acute bronchoconstrictor responses to allergens and several other indirectly acting stimuli such as exercise and hyperventilation (via osmolality or thermal changes), as well as fog. Activated mast cells are found at the airway surface in asthma patients and also in the airway smooth-muscle layer, whereas this is not seen in normal subjects or patients with eosinophilic bronchitis. Mast cells are activated by allergens through an IgE-dependent mechanism, and binding of specific IgE to mast cells renders them more sensitive to activation. The importance of IgE in the pathophysiology of asthma has been highlighted by clinical studies with humanized anti-IgE antibodies, which inhibit IgE-mediated effects, reduce asthma symptoms,

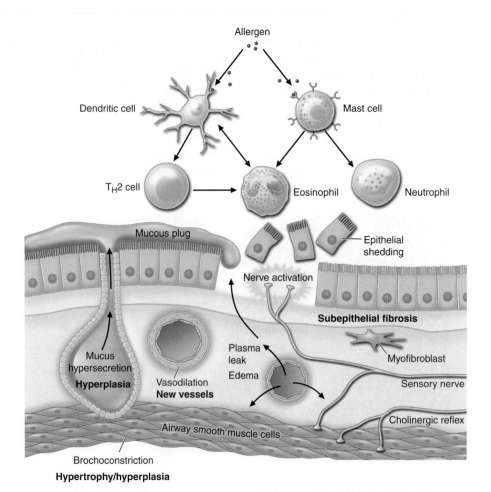

FIGURE 8-3

The pathophysiology of asthma is complex with participation of several interacting inflammatory cells, which result in acute and chronic inflammatory effects on the airway.

and reduce exacerbations. There are, however, uncertainties about the role of mast cells in more chronic allergic inflammatory events. Mast cells release several bronchoconstrictor mediators, including histamine, prostaglandin D_2, and cysteinyl-leukotrienes, but also several cytokines, chemokines, growth factors, and neurotrophins.

Macrophages and dendritic cells

Macrophages, which are derived from blood monocytes, may traffic into the airways in asthma and may be activated by allergens via low affinity IgE receptors ($Fc_\varepsilon RII$). Macrophages have the capacity to initiate a type of inflammatory response via the release of a certain pattern of cytokines, but these cells also release anti-inflammatory mediators (e.g., IL-10) and, thus, their roles in asthma are uncertain. Dendritic cells are specialized macrophage-like cells in the airway epithelium, which are the major antigen-presenting cells. Dendritic cells take up allergens, process them to peptides, and migrate to local lymph nodes where they present the allergenic peptides to uncommitted T-lymphocytes to program the production of allergen-specific T cells. Immature dendritic cells in the respiratory tract promote T_H2 cell differentiation and require cytokines such as IL-12 and tumor necrosis factor α (TNF-α), to promote the normally preponderant T_H1 response. The cytokine thymic stromal lymphopoietin (TSLP) released from epithelial cells in asthmatic patients instructs dendritic cells to release chemokines that attract T_H2 cells into the airways.

Eosinophils

Eosinophil infiltration is a characteristic feature of asthmatic airways. Allergen inhalation results in a marked increase in activated eosinophils in the airways at the time of the late reaction. Eosinophils are linked to the development of AHR through the release of basic proteins and oxygen-derived free radicals. Eosinophil recruitment involves adhesion of eosinophils to vascular endothelial cells in the airway circulation due to interaction between adhesion molecules, migration into the submucosa under the direction of chemokines, and their subsequent activation and prolonged survival. Blocking antibodies to IL-5 causes a profound and prolonged reduction in circulating and sputum eosinophils, but is not associated with reduced AHR or asthma symptoms, although in selected patients with steroid-resistant airway eosinophils, there is a reduction in exacerbations. Eosinophilic inflammation is also found in patients with chronic cough (eosinophilic bronchitis) who do not have AHR or clinical features of asthma. Increasing evidence suggests that eosinophils may be important in release of growth factors involved in airway remodeling, in exacerbations but not in AHR.

Neutrophils

Increased numbers of activated neutrophils are found in sputum and airways of some patients with severe asthma and during exacerbations, although there is a proportion of patients even with mild or moderate asthma who have a predominance of neutrophils. The roles of neutrophils in asthma that are resistant to the anti-inflammatory effects of corticosteroids are currently unknown.

T lymphocytes

T lymphocytes play a very important role in coordinating the inflammatory response in asthma through the release of specific patterns of cytokines, resulting in the recruitment and survival of eosinophils and in the maintenance of a mast cell population in the airways. The naïve immune system and the immune system of asthmatics are skewed to express the T_H2 phenotype, whereas in normal airways T_H1 cells predominate. T_H2 cells, through the release of IL-5, are associated with eosinophilic inflammation and, through the release of IL-4 and IL-13, are associated with increased IgE formation. Recently, bronchial biopsies have demonstrated a preponderance of natural killer CD4$^+$ T lymphocytes that express high levels of IL-4. Regulatory T cells play an important role in determining the expression of other T cells, and there is evidence for a reduction in a certain subset of regulatory T cells (CD4+CD25+) in asthma that is associated with increased T_H2 cells.

Structural cells

Structural cells of the airways, including epithelial cells, fibroblasts, and airway smooth-muscle cells, are also important sources of inflammatory mediators such as cytokines and lipid mediators, in asthma. Indeed, because structural cells far outnumber inflammatory cells, they may become the major sources of mediators driving chronic inflammation in asthmatic airways. In addition, epithelial cells may have key roles in translating inhaled environmental signals into an airway inflammatory response, and are probably major target cells for ICS.

INFLAMMATORY MEDIATORS

Many different mediators have been implicated in asthma, and they may have a variety of effects on the airways that could account for the pathologic features of asthma (Fig. 8-4). Mediators such as histamine, prostaglandin D_2, and cysteinyl-leukotrienes contract airway smooth muscle, increase microvascular leakage, increase airway mucus secretion, and attract other inflammatory cells. Because each mediator has many effects, the role of individual mediators in the pathophysiology of asthma is not yet clear. Although the multiplicity of

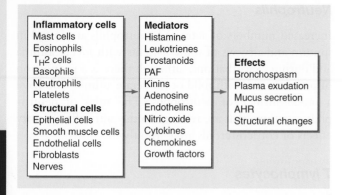

FIGURE 8-4

Many cells and mediators are involved in asthma and lead to several effects on the airways.

mediators makes it unlikely that preventing the synthesis or action of a single mediator will have a major impact in clinical asthma, recent clinical studies with antileukotrienes suggest that cysteinyl-leukotrienes have clinically important effects.

Cytokines

Multiple cytokines regulate the chronic inflammation of asthma. The TH2 cytokines IL-4, IL-5, and IL-13 mediate allergic inflammation, whereas proinflammatory cytokines such as TNF-α and IL-1β, amplify the inflammatory response and play a role in more severe disease. Thymic stromal lymphopoietin is an upstream cytokine released from epithelial cells of asthmatics that orchestrates the release of chemokines that selectively attract T_H2 cells. Some cytokines such as IL-10 and IL-12 are anti-inflammatory and may be deficient in asthma.

Chemokines

Chemokines are involved in attracting inflammatory cells from the bronchial circulation into the airways. Eotaxin (CCL11) is selectively attractant to eosinophils via CCR3 and is expressed by epithelial cells of asthmatics, whereas CCL17 (TARC) and CCL22 (MDC) from epithelial cells attract T_H2 cells via CCR4 **(Fig. 8-5)**.

Oxidative stress

There is increased oxidative stress in asthma as activated inflammatory cells such as macrophages and eosinophils that produce reactive oxygen species. Evidence for increased oxidative stress in asthma is provided by the increased concentrations of 8-isoprostane (a product of oxidized arachidonic acid) in exhaled breath condensates and increased ethane (a product of lipid peroxidation) in the expired air of asthmatic patients. Increased oxidative stress is related to disease severity, may amplify the inflammatory response, and may reduce responsiveness to corticosteroids.

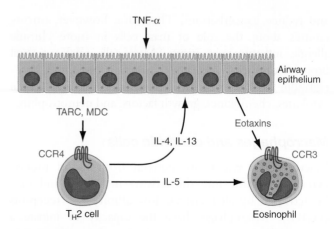

FIGURE 8-5

Chemokines in asthma. Tumor necrosis factor α (TNF-α) and other triggers of airway epithelial cells release thymus and activationregulated chemokine (TARC, CCL17) and macrophage-derived chemokine (MDC, CCL22) from epithelial cells that attract T_H2 cells via activation of their CCR4 receptors. These promote eosinophilic inflammation directly through the release of interleukin (IL)-5 and indirectly via the release of IL-4 and IL-13, which induce eotaxin (CCL11) formation in airway epithelial cells.

Nitric oxide

Nitric oxide (NO) is produced by several cells in the airway by NO synthases, particularly airway epithelial cells and macrophages. The level of NO in the expired air of patients with asthma is higher than normal and is related to the eosinophilic inflammation. Increased NO may contribute to the bronchial vasodilation observed in asthma. Exhaled NO is increasingly used in the diagnosis and monitoring of asthmatic inflammation, although it is not yet used routinely in clinical practice.

Transcription factors

Proinflammatory transcription factors such as nuclear factor-κB (NF-κB) and activator protein-1, are activated in asthmatic airways and orchestrate the expression of multiple inflammatory genes. More specific transcription factors that are involved include nuclear factor of activated T cells and GATA-3, which regulate the expression of T_H2 cytokines in T cells.

EFFECTS OF INFLAMMATION

The chronic inflammatory response has several effects on the target cells of the airways, resulting in the characteristic pathophysiologic changes associated with asthma. Asthma may be regarded as a disease with continuous inflammation and repair proceeding simultaneously. Important advances continue to be made in our understanding of these changes, but, despite these new insights, the relationship between chronic inflammatory processes and asthma symptoms is often not clear.

Airway epithelium

Airway epithelial shedding may be important in contributing to AHR and may explain how several mechanisms, such as ozone exposure, virus infections, chemical sensitizers, and allergen exposure, can lead to its development, as all of these stimuli may lead to epithelial disruption. Epithelial damage may contribute to AHR in a number of ways, including loss of its barrier function to allow penetration of allergens; loss of enzymes (such as neutral endopeptidase) that degrade certain peptide inflammatory mediators; loss of a relaxant factor (so called epithelial-derived relaxant factor); and exposure of sensory nerves, which may lead to reflex neural effects on the airway.

Fibrosis

In all asthmatic patients, the basement membrane is apparently thickened due to subepithelial fibrosis with deposition of types III and V collagen below the true basement membrane and is associated with eosinophil infiltration, presumably through the release of profibrotic mediators such as transforming growth factor-β. Mechanical manipulations can alter the phenotype of airway epithelial cells in a profibrotic fashion. In more severe patients, there is also fibrosis within the airway wall, which may contribute to irreversible narrowing of the airways.

Airway smooth muscle

There is still debate about the role of abnormalities in airway smooth muscle in asthmatic airways. In vitro airway smooth muscle from asthmatic patients usually shows no increased responsiveness to constrictors. Reduced responsiveness to β-agonists has also been reported in postmortem or surgically removed bronchi from asthmatics, although the number of β-receptors is not reduced, suggesting that β-receptors have been uncoupled. These abnormalities of airway smooth-muscle may be secondary to the chronic inflammatory process. Inflammatory mediators may modulate the ion channels that serve to regulate the resting membrane potential of airway smooth-muscle cells, thus altering the level of excitability of these cells. In asthmatic airways there is also a characteristic hypertrophy and hyperplasia of airway smooth muscle, which is presumably the result of stimulation of airway smooth-muscle cells by various growth factors such as platelet-derived growth factor (PDGF) or endothelin-1 released from inflammatory or epithelial cells.

Vascular responses

There is increased airway mucosal blood flow in asthma. The bronchial circulation may play an important role in regulating airway caliber, since an increase in the vascular volume may contribute to airway narrowing. Increased airway blood flow may be important in removing inflammatory mediators from the airway, and may play a role in the development of exercise-induced asthma. There is an increase in the number of blood vessels in asthmatic airways as a result of angiogenesis in response to growth factors, particularly vascular-endothelial growth factor. Microvascular leakage from postcapillary venules in response to inflammatory mediators is observed in asthma, resulting in airway edema and plasma exudation into the airway lumen.

Mucus hypersecretion

Increased mucus secretion contributes to the viscid mucous plugs that occlude asthmatic airways, particularly in fatal asthma. There is evidence for hyperplasia of submucosal glands that are confined to large airways and of increased numbers of epithelial goblet cells. IL-4 and IL-13 induce mucus hypersecretion in experimental models of asthma.

Neural effects

Various defects in autonomic neural control may contribute to AHR in asthma, but these are likely to be secondary to the disease, rather than primary defects. Cholinergic pathways, through the release of acetylcholine acting on muscarinic receptors, cause bronchoconstriction and may be activated reflexly in asthma. Inflammatory mediators may activate sensory nerves, resulting in reflex cholinergic bronchoconstriction or release of inflammatory neuropeptides. Inflammatory products may also sensitize sensory nerve endings in the airway epithelium such that the nerves become hyperalgesic. Neurotrophins, which may be released from various cell types in airways, including epithelial cells and mast cells, may cause proliferation and sensitization of airway sensory nerves. Airway nerves may also release neurotransmitters, such as substance P, which have inflammatory effects.

AIRWAY REMODELING

Several changes in the structure of the airway are characteristically found in asthma, and these may lead to irreversible narrowing of the airways. Population studies have shown a greater decline in lung function over time than in normal subjects; however, most patients with asthma preserve normal or near-normal lung function throughout life if appropriately treated. This observation suggests that the accelerated decline in lung function occurs in a smaller proportion of asthmatics, and these are usually patients with more severe disease. There is some evidence that the early use of ICS may reduce the decline in lung function. The characteristic structural changes are increased airway smooth muscle, fibrosis, angiogenesis, and mucus hyperplasia.

ASTHMA TRIGGERS

Several stimuli trigger airway narrowing, wheezing, and dyspnea in asthmatic patients. While the previous view held that these should be avoided, it is now seen as evidence for poor control and an indicator of the need to increase controller (preventive) therapy.

ALLERGENS

Inhaled allergens activate mast cells with bound IgE directly leading to the immediate release of bronchoconstrictor mediators, resulting in the early response that is reversed by bronchodilators. Often, experimental allergen challenge is followed by a late response when there is airway edema and an acute inflammatory response with increased eosinophils and neutrophils that are not very reversible with bronchodilators. The most common allergens to trigger asthma are *Dermatophagoides* species, and environmental exposure leads to low-grade chronic symptoms that are perennial. Other perennial allergens are derived from cats and other domestic pets, as well as cockroaches. Other allergens, including grass pollen, ragweed, tree pollen, and fungal spores, are seasonal. Pollens usually cause allergic rhinitis rather than asthma, but in thunderstorms the pollen grains are disrupted and the particles that may be released can trigger severe asthma exacerbations (thunderstorm asthma).

VIRUS INFECTIONS

Upper respiratory tract virus infections such as rhinovirus, respiratory syncytial virus, and coronavirus are the most common triggers of acute severe exacerbations and may invade epithelial cells of the lower as well as the upper airways. The mechanism whereby these viruses cause exacerbations is poorly understood, but there is an increase in airway inflammation with increased numbers of eosinophils and neutrophils. There is evidence for reduced production of type I interferons by epithelial cells from asthmatic patients, resulting in increased susceptibility to these viral infections and a greater inflammatory response.

PHARMACOLOGIC AGENTS

Several drugs may trigger asthma. Beta-adrenergic blockers commonly acutely worsen asthma, and their use may be fatal. The mechanisms are not clear but are likely mediated through increased cholinergic bronchoconstriction. All beta blockers need to be avoided and even selective β_2 blocker or topical application (e.g., timolol eye drops) may be dangerous. Angiotensin-converting enzyme inhibitors are theoretically detrimental as they inhibit breakdown of kinins, which are bronchoconstrictors; however, they rarely worsen asthma, and the characteristic cough is no more frequent in asthmatics than in nonasthmatics. Aspirin may worsen asthma in some patients (aspirin-sensitive asthma is discussed later under "Special Considerations").

EXERCISE

Exercise is a common trigger of asthma, particularly in children. The mechanism is linked to hyperventilation, which results in increased osmolality in airway lining fluid and triggers mast cell mediator release, resulting in bronchoconstriction. Exercise-induced asthma (EIA) typically begins after exercise has ended, and recovers spontaneously within about 30 min. EIA is worse in cold, dry climates than in hot, humid conditions. It is, therefore, more common in sports such as cross-country running in cold weather, overland skiing, and ice hockey than in swimming. It may be prevented by prior administration of β_2-agonists and antileukotrienes, but is best prevented by regular treatment with ICS, which reduce the population of surface mast cells required for this response.

PHYSICAL FACTORS

Cold air and hyperventilation may trigger asthma through the same mechanisms as exercise. Laughter may also be a trigger. Many patients report worsening of asthma in hot weather and when the weather changes. Some asthmatics become worse when exposed to strong smells or perfumes, but the mechanism of this response is uncertain.

FOOD

There is little evidence that allergic reactions to food lead to increased asthma symptoms, despite the belief of many patients that their symptoms are triggered by particular food constituents. Exclusion diets are usually unsuccessful at reducing the frequency of episodes. Some foods such as shellfish and nuts may induce anaphylactic reactions that may include wheezing. Patients with aspirin-induced asthma may benefit from a salicylate-free diet, but these are difficult to maintain. Certain food additives may trigger asthma. Metabisulfite, which is used as a food preservative, may trigger asthma through the release of sulfur dioxide gas in the stomach. Tartrazine, a yellow food-coloring agent, was believed to be a trigger for asthma, but there is little convincing evidence for this.

AIR POLLUTION

Increased ambient levels of sulfur dioxide, ozone, and nitrogen oxides are associated with increased asthma symptoms.

OCCUPATIONAL FACTORS

Several substances found in the workplace may act as sensitizing agents, as discussed earlier, but may also act as triggers of asthma symptoms. Occupational asthma is characteristically associated with symptoms at work with relief on weekends and holidays. If removed from exposure within the first 6 months of symptoms, there is usually complete recovery. More persistent symptoms lead to irreversible airway changes, and, thus, early detection and avoidance are important.

HORMONAL FACTORS

Some women show premenstrual worsening of asthma, which can occasionally be very severe. The mechanisms are not completely understood, but are related to a fall in progesterone and in severe cases may be improved by treatment with high doses of progesterone or gonadotropin-releasing factors. Thyrotoxicosis and hypothyroidism can both worsen asthma, although the mechanisms are uncertain.

GASTROESOPHAGEAL REFLUX

Gastroesophageal reflux is common in asthmatic patients as it is increased by bronchodilators. Although acid reflux might trigger reflex bronchoconstriction, it rarely causes asthma symptoms, and antireflux therapy fails to reduce asthma symptoms in most patients.

STRESS

Many asthmatics report worsening of symptoms with stress. There is no doubt that psychological factors can induce bronchoconstriction through cholinergic reflex pathways. Paradoxically, very severe stress such as bereavement usually does not worsen, and may even improve, asthma symptoms.

PATHOPHYSIOLOGY

Limitation of airflow is due mainly to bronchoconstriction, but airway edema, vascular congestion, and luminal occlusion with exudate may also contribute. This results in a reduction in forced expiratory volume in 1 second (FEV_1), FEV_1/forced vital capacity (FVC) ratio, and peak expiratory flow (PEF), as well as an increase in airway resistance. Early closure of peripheral airway results in lung hyperinflation, (air trapping) and increased residual volume, particularly during acute exacerbations and in severe persistent asthma. In more severe asthma, reduced ventilation and increased pulmonary blood flow result in mismatching of ventilation and perfusion and in bronchial hyperemia. Ventilatory failure is very uncommon, even in patients with severe asthma, and arterial P_{CO_2} tends to be low due to increased ventilation.

AIRWAY HYPERRESPONSIVENESS

AHR is the characteristic physiologic abnormality of asthma and describes the excessive bronchoconstrictor response to multiple inhaled triggers that would have no effect on normal airways. The increase in AHR is linked to the frequency of asthma symptoms, and, thus, an important aim of therapy is to reduce AHR. Increased bronchoconstrictor responsiveness is seen with *direct* broncho constrictors such as histamine and methacholine, which contract airway smooth muscle, but is characteristically also seen with many *indirect* stimuli, which release bronchoconstrictors from mast cells or activate sensory nerves. Most of the triggers for asthma symptoms appear to act indirectly, including allergens, exercise, hyperventilation, fog (via mast cell activation), irritant dusts, and sulfur dioxide (via a cholinergic reflex).

CLINICAL FEATURES AND DIAGNOSIS

The characteristic symptoms of asthma are wheezing, dyspnea, and coughing, which are variable, both spontaneously and with therapy. Symptoms may be worse at night and patients typically awake in the early morning hours. Patients may report difficulty in filling their lungs with air. There is increased mucus production in some patients, with typically tenacious mucus that is difficult to expectorate. There may be increased ventilation and use of accessory muscles of ventilation. Prodromal symptoms may precede an attack, with itching under the chin, discomfort between the scapulae, or inexplicable fear (impending doom).

Typical physical signs are inspiratory, and to a greater extent expiratory, rhonchi throughout the chest, and there may be hyperinflation. Some patients, particularly children, may present with a predominant nonproductive cough (cough-variant asthma). There may be no abnormal physical findings when asthma is under control.

DIAGNOSIS

The diagnosis of asthma is usually apparent from the symptoms of variable and intermittent airways obstruction, but is usually confirmed by objective measurements of lung function.

Lung function tests

Simple spirometry confirms airflow limitation with a reduced FEV_1, FEV_1/FVC ratio, and PEF. Reversibility is demonstrated by a >12% and 200-mL increase in FEV_1 15 min after an inhaled short-acting β_2-agonist or in some patients by a 2 to 4 week trial of oral corticosteroids (OCS) (prednisone or prednisolone 30–40 mg daily). Measurements of PEF twice daily may confirm the diurnal variations in airflow obstruction. Flow-volume loops show reduced peak flow and reduced maximum expiratory flow. Further lung function tests are rarely necessary, but whole body plethysmography shows increased airway resistance and may show increased total lung capacity and residual volume. Gas diffusion is usually normal, but there may be a small increase in gas transfer in some patients.

Airway responsiveness

The increased AHR is normally measured by methacholine or histamine challenge with calculation of the provocative concentration that reduces FEV_1 by 20% (PC_{20}). This is rarely useful in clinical practice, but can be used in the differential diagnosis of chronic cough and when the diagnosis is in doubt in the setting of normal pulmonary function tests. Occasionally exercise testing is done to demonstrate the postexercise bronchoconstriction if there is a predominant history of EIA. Allergen challenge is rarely necessary and should only be undertaken by a specialist if specific occupational agents are to be identified.

Hematologic tests

Blood tests are not usually helpful. Total serum IgE and specific IgE to inhaled allergens (radioallergosorbent test [RAST]) may be measured in some patients.

Imaging

Chest roentgenography is usually normal but in more severe patients may show hyperinflated lungs. In exacerbations, there may be evidence of a pneumothorax. Lung shadowing usually indicates pneumonia or eosinophilic infiltrates in patients with bronchopulmonary aspergillosis. High-resolution CT may show areas of bronchiectasis in patients with severe asthma, and there may be thickening of the bronchial walls, but these changes are not diagnostic of asthma.

Skin tests

Skin prick tests to common inhalant allergens are positive in allergic asthma and negative in intrinsic asthma, but are not helpful in diagnosis. Positive skin responses may be useful in persuading patients to undertake allergen avoidance measures.

Exhaled nitric oxide

Exhaled NO is now being used as a noninvasive test to measure eosinophilic airway inflammation. The typically elevated levels in asthma are reduced by ICS, so this may be a test of compliance with therapy. It may also be useful in demonstrating insufficient anti-inflammatory therapy.

DIFFERENTIAL DIAGNOSIS

It is usually not difficult to differentiate asthma from other conditions that cause wheezing and dyspnea. Upper airway obstruction by a tumor or laryngeal edema can mimic severe asthma, but patients typically present with stridor localized to large airways. The diagnosis is confirmed by a flow-volume loop that shows a reduction in inspiratory as well as expiratory flow, and bronchoscopy to demonstrate the site of upper airway narrowing. Persistent wheezing in a specific area of the chest may indicate endobronchial obstruction with a foreign body. Left ventricular failure may mimic the wheezing of asthma but basilar crackles are present in contrast to asthma.

Eosinophilic pneumonias and systemic vasculitis, including Churg-Strauss syndrome and polyarteritis nodosa, may be associated with wheezing. Chronic obstructive pulmonary disease (COPD) is usually easy to differentiate from asthma as symptoms show less variability, never completely remit, and show much less (or no) reversibility to bronchodilators. Approximately 10% of COPD patients have features of asthma, with increased sputum eosinophils and a response to oral corticosteroids; these patients probably have both diseases concomitantly.

TREATMENT   Asthma

The treatment of asthma is straightforward and the majority of patients are now managed by internists and family doctors with effective and safe therapies. There are several aims of therapy (Table 8-2). Most emphasis has been placed on drug therapy, but several nonpharmacologic approaches have also been used. The main drugs for asthma can be divided into bronchodilators, which give rapid relief of symptoms mainly through relaxation of airway smooth muscle,

TABLE 8-2

AIMS OF ASTHMA THERAPY

- Minimal (ideally no) chronic symptoms, including nocturnal
- Minimal (infrequent) exacerbations
- No emergency visits
- Minimal (ideally no) use of a required β_2-agonist
- No limitations on activities, including exercise
- Peak expiratory flow circadian variation <20%
- (Near) normal PEF
- Minimal (or no) adverse effects from medicine

Abbreviation: PEF, peak expiratory flow.

TABLE 8-3

EFFECTS OF β-ADRENERGIC AGONISTS ON AIRWAYS

- Relaxation of airway smooth muscle (proximal and distal airways)
- Inhibition of mast cell mediator release
- Inhibition of plasma exudation and airway edema
- Increased mucociliary clearance
- Increased mucus secretion
- Decreased cough
- No effect on chronic inflammation

and controllers, which inhibit the underlying inflammatory process.

BRONCHODILATOR THERAPIES Bronchodilators act primarily on airway smooth muscle to reverse the bronchoconstriction of asthma. This gives rapid relief of symptoms but has little or no effect on the underlying inflammatory process. Thus, bronchodilators are not sufficient to control asthma in patients with persistent symptoms. There are three classes of bronchodilators in current use: β_2-adrenergic agonists, anticholinergics, and theophylline; of these, β_2-agonists are by far the most effective.

β_2-Agonists β_2-Agonists activate β_2-adrenergic receptors, which are widely expressed in the airways. β_2-Receptors are coupled through a stimulatory G protein to adenylyl cyclase, resulting in increased intracellular cyclic adenosine monophosphate (AMP), which relaxes smooth muscle cells and inhibits certain inflammatory cells, particularly mast cells.

Mode of Action The primary action of β_2-agonists is to relax airway smooth-muscle cells of all airways, where they act as functional antagonists, reversing and preventing contraction of airway smooth-muscle cells by all known bronchoconstrictors. This generalized action is likely to account for their great efficacy as bronchodilators in asthma. There are also additional nonbronchodilator effects that may be clinically useful, including inhibition of mast cell mediator release, reduction in plasma exudation, and inhibition of sensory nerve activation (Table 8-3). Inflammatory cells express small numbers of β_2-receptors, but these are rapidly downregulated with β_2-agonist activation so that, in contrast to corticosteroids, there are no effects on inflammatory cells in the airways and there is no reduction in AHR.

Clinical Use β_2-Agonists are usually given by inhalation to reduce side effects. Short-acting β_2-agonists (SABAs) such as albuterol and terbutaline have a duration of action of 3–6 h. They have a rapid onset of bronchodilation and are, therefore, used as needed for

symptom relief. Increased use of SABAs indicates that asthma is not controlled. They are also useful in preventing EIA if taken prior to exercise. SABAs are used in high doses by nebulizer or via a metered-dose inhaler with a spacer. Long-acting β_2-agonists (LABAs) include salmeterol and formoterol, both of which have a duration of action over 12 h and are given twice daily by inhalation. LABAs have replaced the regular use of SABAs, but LABAs should not be given in the absence of ICS therapy as they do not control the underlying inflammation. They do, however, improve asthma control and reduce exacerbations when added to ICS, which allows asthma to be controlled at lower doses of corticosteroids. This observation has led to the widespread use of fixed combination inhalers that contain a corticosteroid and a LABA, which have proved to be highly effective in the control of asthma.

Side Effects Adverse effects are not usually a problem with β_2-agonists when given by inhalation. The most common side effects are muscle tremor and palpitations, which are seen more commonly in elderly patients. There is a small fall in plasma potassium due to increased uptake by skeletal muscle cells, but this effect does not usually cause any clinical problem.

Tolerance Tolerance is a potential problem with any agonist given chronically, but while there is down-regulation of β_2-receptors, this does not reduce the bronchodilator response as there is a large receptor reserve in airway smooth-muscle cells. By contrast, mast cells become rapidly tolerant, but their tolerance may be prevented by concomitant administration of ICS.

Safety The safety of β_2-agonists has been an important issue. There is an association between asthma mortality and the amount of SABA used, but careful analysis demonstrates that the increased use of rescue SABAs reflects poor asthma control, which is a risk factor for asthma death. The slight excess in mortality that has been associated with the use of LABAs is related to the lack of use of concomitant ICS, as the LABA therapy fails to suppress the underlying inflammation. This highlights the importance of always using an ICS when LABAs are given, which is most conveniently achieved by using a combination inhaler.

Anticholinergics Muscarinic receptor antagonists such as ipratropium bromide, prevent cholinergic nerve-induced bronchoconstriction and mucus secretion. They are much less effective than β_2-agonists in asthma therapy as they inhibit only the cholinergic reflex component of bronchoconstriction, whereas β_2-agonists prevent all bronchoconstrictor mechanisms. Anticholinergics are, therefore, only used as an additional bronchodilator in patients with asthma that is not controlled by other inhaled medications. High doses may be given by nebulizer in treating acute severe asthma but should only be given following β_2-agonists, as they have a slower onset of bronchodilation.

Side effects are not usually a problem as there is little or no systemic absorption. The most common side effect is dry mouth; in elderly patients, urinary retention and glaucoma may also be observed.

Theophylline Theophylline was widely prescribed as an oral bronchodilator several years ago, especially as it was inexpensive. It has now fallen out of favor as side effects are common and inhaled β_2-agonists are much more effective as bronchodilators. The bronchodilator effect is due to inhibition of phosphodiesterases in airway smooth-muscle cells, which increases cyclic AMP, but doses required for bronchodilation commonly cause side effects that are mediated mainly by phosphodiesterase inhibition. There is increasing evidence that theophylline at lower doses has anti-inflammatory effects, and these are likely to be mediated through different molecular mechanisms. There is evidence that theophylline activates the key nuclear enzyme histone deacetylase-2, which is a critical mechanism for switching off activated inflammatory genes.

Clinical Use Oral theophylline is usually given as a slow-release preparation once or twice daily as this gives more stable plasma concentrations than normal theophylline tablets. It may be used as an additional bronchodilator in patients with severe asthma when plasma concentrations of 10–20 mg/L are required, although these concentrations are often associated with side effects. Low doses of theophylline, giving plasma concentrations of 5–10 mg/L, have additive effects to ICS and are particularly useful in patients with severe asthma. Indeed, withdrawal of theophylline from these patients may result in marked deterioration in asthma control. At low doses, the drug is well tolerated. IV aminophylline (a soluble salt of theophylline) was used for the treatment of severe asthma but has now been largely replaced by high doses of inhaled SABAs, which are more effective and have fewer side effects. Aminophylline is occasionally used (via slow IV infusion) in patients with severe exacerbations that are refractory to SABAs.

Side Effects Oral theophylline is well absorbed and is largely inactivated in the liver. Side effects are related to plasma concentrations; measurement of plasma theophylline may be useful in determining the correct dose. The most common side effects are nausea, vomiting, and headaches and are due to phosphodiesterase inhibition. Diuresis and palpitations may also occur, and at high concentrations cardiac arrhythmias, epileptic seizures, and death may occur due to adenosine A_1-receptor antagonism. Theophylline side effects are related to plasma concentration and are rarely observed at plasma concentrations below 10 mg/L. Theophylline is metabolized by CYP450 in the liver, and, thus, plasma concentrations may be elevated by drugs that block CYP450 such as erythromycin and allopurinol. Other drugs may also reduce clearance by other mechanisms leading to increased plasma concentrations (Table 8-4).

CONTROLLER THERAPIES

Inhaled Corticosteroids ICS are by far the most effective controllers for asthma, and their early use has revolutionized asthma therapy.

Mode of Action ICS are the most effective anti-inflammatory agents used in asthma therapy, reducing inflammatory cell numbers and their activation in the airways. ICS reduce eosinophils in the airways and sputum,

TABLE 8-4

FACTORS AFFECTING CLEARANCE OF THEOPHYLLINE
Increased Clearance
• Enzyme induction (rifampicin, phenobarbitone, ethanol)   • Smoking (tobacco, marijuana)   • High-protein, low-carbohydrate diet   • Barbecued meat   • Childhood
Decreased Clearance
• Enzyme inhibition (cimetidine, erythromycin, ciprofloxacin, allopurinol, zileuton, zafirlukast)   • Congestive heart failure   • Liver disease   • Pneumonia   • Viral infection and vaccination   • High carbohydrate diet   • Old age

and numbers of activated T lymphocytes and surface mast cells in the airway mucosa. These effects may account for the reduction in AHR that is seen with chronic ICS therapy.

The molecular mechanism of action of corticosteroids involves several effects on the inflammatory process. The major effect of corticosteroids is to switch off the transcription of multiple activated genes that encode inflammatory proteins such as cytokines, chemokines, adhesion molecules, and inflammatory enzymes. This effect involves several mechanisms, including inhibition of the transcription factors NF-κB and activator protein (AP)-1, but an important mechanism is recruitment of histone deacetylase-2 to the inflammatory gene complex, which reverses the histone acetylation associated with increased gene transcription. Corticosteroids also activate anti-inflammatory genes such as mitogen-activated protein (MAP) kinase phosphatase-1, and increase the expression of β_2-receptors. Most of the metabolic and endocrine side effects of corticosteroids are also mediated through transcriptional activation.

Clinical Use ICS are by far the most effective controllers in the management of asthma and are beneficial in treating asthma of any severity and age. ICS are usually given twice daily, but some may be effective once daily in mildly symptomatic patients. ICS rapidly improve the symptoms of asthma, and lung function improves over several days. They are effective in preventing asthma symptoms, such as EIA and nocturnal exacerbations, but also prevent severe exacerbations. ICS reduce AHR, but maximal improvement may take several months of therapy. Early treatment with ICS appears to prevent irreversible changes in airway function that occur with chronic asthma. Withdrawal of ICS results in slow deterioration of asthma control, indicating that they suppress inflammation and symptoms, but do not cure the underlying condition. ICS are now given as first-line therapy for patients with persistent asthma, but if they do not control symptoms at low doses, it is usual to add a LABA as the next step.

Side Effects Local side effects include hoarseness (dysphonia) and oral candidiasis, which may be reduced with the use of a large-volume spacer device. There has been concern about systemic side effects from lung absorption, but many studies have demonstrated that ICS have minimal systemic effects (Fig. 8-6). At the highest recommended doses, there may be some suppression of plasma and urinary cortisol concentrations, but there is no convincing evidence that long-term treatment leads to impaired growth in children or to osteoporosis in adults. Indeed effective control of asthma with ICS reduces the number of courses of OCS that are needed and, thus, reduces systemic exposure to ICS.

Systemic Corticosteroids Corticosteroids are used intravenously (hydrocortisone or methylprednisolone) for the treatment of acute severe asthma, although several studies now show that OCS are as effective and easier to administer. A course of OCS (usually prednisone or prednisolone 30–45 mg once daily for 5–10 days) is used to treat acute exacerbations of asthma; no tapering of the dose is needed. Approximately 1% of asthma patients may require maintenance treatment with OCS; the lowest dose necessary to maintain control needs to be determined. Systemic side effects, including truncal obesity, bruising, osteoporosis, diabetes, hypertension, gastric ulceration, proximal myopathy, depression, and cataracts, may be a major problem, and steroid–sparing therapies may be considered if side effects are a significant problem. If patients require maintenance treatment with OCS, it is important to monitor bone density so that preventive treatment with bisphosphonates or estrogen in postmenopausal women may be initiated if bone density is low. Intramuscular triamcinolone acetonide is a depot preparation that is occasionally used in noncompliant patients, but proximal myopathy is a major problem with this therapy.

Antileukotrienes Cysteinyl-leukotrienes are potent bronchoconstrictors, cause microvascular leakage, and increase eosinophilic inflammation through the activation of cys-LT$_1$-receptors. These inflammatory mediators are produced predominantly by mast cells and, to a lesser extent, eosinophils in asthma. Antileukotrienes such as montelukast and zafirlukast, block cys-LT$_1$-receptors and provide modest clinical benefit in asthma. They are less effective than ICS in controlling asthma and have less effect on airway inflammation, but are useful as an add-on therapy in some patients not controlled with low doses of ICS, although they are less effective than LABAs. They are given orally once or twice daily and are well tolerated. Some patients show a better response than others to antileukotrienes, but this has not been convincingly linked to any genomic differences in the leukotriene pathway.

Cromones Cromolyn sodium and nedocromil sodium are asthma controller drugs that appear to inhibit mast cell and sensory nerve activation and are, therefore, effective in blocking trigger-induced asthma such as EIA and allergen- and sulfur dioxide–induced symptoms. Cromones have relatively little benefit in the long-term control of asthma due to their short duration of action (at least four times daily by inhalation). They are very safe and were popular in the treatment of childhood asthma, although now low doses of ICS are preferred as they are more effective and have a proven safety profile.

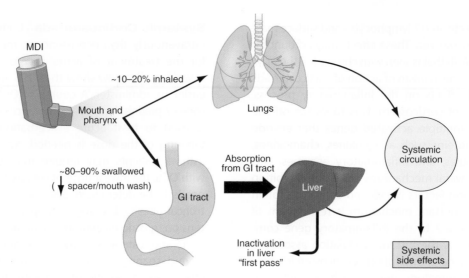

FIGURE 8-6
Pharmacokinetics of inhaled corticosteroids.

Steroid-Sparing Therapies Various immuno-modulatory treatments have been used to reduce the requirement for OCS in patients with severe asthma, who have serious side effects with this therapy. Methotrexate, cyclosporin A, azathioprine, gold, and IV gamma globulin have all been used as steroid-sparing therapies, but none of these treatments has any long-term benefit and each is associated with a relatively high risk of side effects.

Anti-IgE Omalizumab is a blocking antibody that neutralizes circulating IgE without binding to cell-bound IgE and, thus, inhibits IgE-mediated reactions. This treatment has been shown to reduce the number of exacerbations in patients with severe asthma and may improve asthma control. However, the treatment is very expensive and is only suitable for highly selected patients who are not controlled on maximal doses of inhaler therapy and have a circulating IgE within a specified range. Patients should be given a 3 to 4-month trial of therapy to show objective benefit. Omalizumab is usually given as a subcutaneous injection every 2–4 weeks and appears not to have significant side effects, although anaphylaxis is very occasionally seen.

Immunotherapy Specific immunotherapy using injected extracts of pollens or house dust mites has not been very effective in controlling asthma and may cause anaphylaxis. Side effects may be reduced by sublingual dosing. It is not recommended in most asthma treatment guidelines because of lack of evidence of clinical efficacy.

Alternative Therapies Nonpharmacologic treatments, including hypnosis, acupuncture, chiropraxis, breathing control, yoga, and speleotherapy, may be popular with some patients. However, placebo-controlled studies have shown that each of these treatments lacks efficacy and cannot be recommended. However, they are not detrimental and may be used as long as conventional pharmacologic therapy is continued.

Future Therapies It has proved very difficult to discover novel pharmaceutical therapies, particularly as current therapy with corticosteroids and β_2-agonists is so effective in the majority of patients. There is, however, a need for the development of new therapies for patients with refractory asthma who have side effects with systemic corticosteroids. Antagonists of specific mediators have little or no benefit in asthma, apart from antileukotrienes, which have rather weak effects, presumably reflecting the fact that multiple mediators are involved. Blocking antibodies against IL-5 may reduce exacerbations in highly selected patients who have sputum eosinophils despite high doses of corticosteroids, whereas anti-TNF-α antibodies are not effective in severe asthma. Novel anti-inflammatory treatments that are in clinical development include inhibitors of phosphodiesterase-4, NF-κB and p38 MAP kinase. However, these drugs, which act on signal transduction pathways common to many cells, are likely to have troublesome side effects, necessitating their delivery by inhalation. Safer and more effective immunotherapy using T-cell peptide fragments of allergens or DNA vaccination are also being investigated. Bacterial products, such as CpG oligonucleotides that stimulate T_h1 immunity or regulatory T cells, are also currently under evaluation.

MANAGEMENT OF CHRONIC ASTHMA There are several aims of chronic therapy in asthma (Table 8-2). It is important to establish the diagnosis objectively using spirometry or PEF measurements at home. Triggers that worsen asthma control, such as allergens or occupational

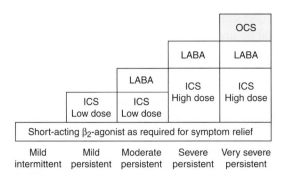

				OCS
			LABA	LABA
		LABA	ICS High dose	ICS High dose
ICS Low dose	ICS Low dose	ICS High dose		

Short-acting β₂-agonist as required for symptom relief

Mild intermittent	Mild persistent	Moderate persistent	Severe persistent	Very severe persistent

FIGURE 8-7

Stepwise approach to asthma therapy according to the severity of asthma and ability to control symptoms. ICS, inhaled corticosteroids; LABA, long-acting β₂-agonist; OCS, oral corticosteroid.

agents, should be avoided, whereas triggers, such as exercise and fog, which result in transient symptoms, provide an indication that more controller therapy is needed.

Stepwise Therapy For patients with mild, intermittent asthma, a short-acting β₂-agonist is all that is required (Fig. 8-7). However, use of a reliever medication more than three times a week indicates the need for regular controller therapy. The treatment of choice for all patients is an ICS given twice daily. It is usual to start with an intermediate dose (e.g., 200 [μg] bid of [beclomethasone dipropionate] BDP) or equivalent and to decrease the dose if symptoms are controlled after three months. If symptoms are not controlled, a LABA should be added, which is most conveniently given by switching to a combination inhaler. The dose of controller should be adjusted accordingly, as judged by the need for a rescue inhaler. Low doses of theophylline or an antileukotriene may also be considered as an add-on therapy, but these are less effective than LABAs. In patients with severe asthma, low-dose oral theophylline is also helpful, and when there is irreversible airway narrowing, the long-acting anticholinergic tiotropium bromide may be tried. If asthma is not controlled despite the maximal recommended dose of inhaled therapy, it is important to check compliance and inhaler technique. In these patients, maintenance treatment with an OCS may be needed and the lowest dose that maintains control should be used. Occasionally omalizumab may be tried in steroid-dependent asthmatics who are not well controlled. Once asthma is controlled, it is important to slowly decrease therapy in order to find the optimal dose to control symptoms.

Education Patients with asthma need to understand how to use their medications and the difference between reliever and controller therapies. Education may improve compliance, particularly with ICS. All patients should be taught how to use their inhalers correctly. In particular, they need to understand how to recognize worsening

of asthma and how to step up therapy. Written action plans have been shown to reduce hospital admissions and morbidity rates in adults and children, and are recommended particularly in patients with unstable disease who have frequent exacerbations.

ACUTE SEVERE ASTHMA

Exacerbations of asthma are feared by patients and may be life threatening. One of the main aims of controller therapy is to prevent exacerbations; in this respect, ICS and combination inhalers are very effective.

CLINICAL FEATURES

Patients are aware of increasing chest tightness, wheezing, and dyspnea that are often not or poorly relieved by their usual reliever inhaler. In severe exacerbations patients may be so breathless that they are unable to complete sentences and may become cyanotic. Examination usually shows increased ventilation, hyperinflation, and tachycardia. Pulsus paradoxus may be present, but this is rarely a useful clinical sign. There is a marked fall in spirometric values and PEF. Arterial blood gases on air show hypoxemia and P_{co_2} is usually low due to hyperventilation. A normal or rising P_{co_2} is an indication of impending respiratory failure and requires immediate monitoring and therapy. A chest roentgenogram is not usually informative, but may show pneumonia or pneumothorax.

TREATMENT Acute Severe Asthma

A high concentration of oxygen should be given by face mask to achieve oxygen saturation of >90%. The mainstay of treatment are high doses of SABAs given either by nebulizer or via a metered-dose inhaler with a spacer. In severely ill patients with impending respiratory failure, IV β₂-agonists may be given. An inhaled anticholinergic may be added if there is not a satisfactory response to β₂-agonists alone, as there are additive effects. In patients who are refractory to inhaled therapies, a slow infusion of aminophylline may be effective, but it is important to monitor blood levels, especially if patients have already been treated with oral theophylline. Magnesium sulfate given intravenously or by nebulizer has also been shown to be effective when added to inhaled β₂-agonists, and is relatively well tolerated but is not routinely recommended. Prophylactic intubation may be indicated for impending respiratory failure, when the p_{co_2} is normal or rises. For patients with respiratory failure, it is necessary to intubate and institute ventilation. These patients may benefit from an anesthetic such as halothane if they have not responded to conventional bronchodilators. Sedatives should never be given as they may depress ventilation. Antibiotics should not be used routinely unless there are signs of pneumonia.

REFRACTORY ASTHMA

Although most patients with asthma are easily controlled with appropriate medication, a small proportion of patients (approximately 5% of asthmatics) are difficult to control despite maximal inhaled therapy. Some of these patients will require maintenance treatment with OCS. In managing these patients, it is important to investigate and correct any mechanisms that may be aggravating asthma. There are two major patterns of difficult asthma: some patients have persistent symptoms and poor lung function, despite appropriate therapy, whereas others may have normal or near normal lung function but intermittent, severe (sometimes life-threatening) exacerbations.

MECHANISMS

The most common reason for poor control of asthma is noncompliance with medication, particularly ICS. Compliance with ICS may be low because patients do not feel any immediate clinical benefit or may be concerned about side effects. Compliance with ICS is difficult to monitor as there are no useful plasma measurements that can be made. Compliance may be improved by giving the ICS as a combination with a LABA that gives symptom relief. Compliance with OCS may be measured by suppression of plasma cortisol and the expected concentration of prednisone/prednisolone in the plasma. There are several factors that may make asthma more difficult to control, including exposure to high, ambient levels of allergens or unidentified occupational agents. Severe rhinosinusitis may make asthma more difficult to control; upper airway disease should be vigorously treated. Gastroesophageal reflux is common among asthmatics due to bronchodilator therapy, but there is little evidence that it is a significant factor in worsening asthma, and treatment of the reflux is not usually effective at improving asthma symptoms. Some patients may have chronic infection with *Mycoplasma pneumoniae* or *Chlamydophila pneumoniae* and benefit from treatment with a macrolide antibiotic. Drugs such as beta-adrenergic blockers, aspirin, and other cyclooxygenase (cox) inhibitors may worsen asthma. Some women develop severe premenstrual worsening of asthma, which is unresponsive to corticosteroids and requires treatment with progesterone or gonadotropin-releasing factors. Few systemic diseases make asthma more difficult to control, but hyper- and hypothyroidism may increase asthma symptoms and should be investigated if suspected.

Relatively little is known about the pathology of refractory asthma, as biopsy studies are more difficult in these patients. Some patients show the typical eosinophilic pattern of inflammation, whereas others have a predominantly neutrophilic pattern. There may be an increase in T_H1 cells and CD8 lymphocytes compared to mild asthma and increased expression of TNF-α. Structural changes in the airway, including fibrosis, angiogenesis, and airway smoothmuscle thickening, are more commonly seen in these patients.

DIFFERENTIAL DIAGNOSIS

Some patients who apparently have difficult-to-control asthma have vocal cord dysfunction, resulting in wheezing or stridor. This symptom is thought to be an attention-seeking hysterical conversion syndrome and may lead to escalating doses of asthma therapy with some patients taking high doses of oral corticosteroids. It may be recognized by the characteristic discrepancy between tests of forced expiration, such as FEV_1 and PEF, and relatively normal airway resistance. Direct inspection by laryngoscopy may confirm adduction of the vocal cords at the time of symptoms. This condition is usually difficult to manage, but it is important that patients be weaned off OCS and ICS. Speech therapy is sometimes beneficial. Some patients with COPD may be diagnosed as asthmatic and may show the characteristic poor response to corticosteroids and bronchodilators, but this situation is complicated by the fact that some patients with COPD also have concomitant asthma.

CORTICOSTEROID-RESISTANT ASTHMA

A few patients with asthma show a poor response to corticosteroid therapy and may have various molecular abnormalities that impair the anti-inflammatory action of corticosteroids. Complete resistance to corticosteroids is extremely uncommon and affects less than 1 in 1000 patients. It is defined by a failure to respond to a high dose of oral prednisone/prednisolone (40 mg once daily over 2 weeks), ideally with a 2-week run-in with matched placebo. More common is reduced responsiveness to corticosteroids where control of asthma requires OCS (corticosteroid-dependent asthma). In all patients with poor responsiveness to corticosteroids, there is a reduction in the response of circulating monocytes and lymphocytes to the anti-inflammatory effects of corticosteroids in vitro and reduced skin blanching in response to topical corticosteroids. There are several mechanisms that have been described, including an excess of the transcription factor AP-1, an increase in the alternatively spliced form of the glucocorticoid receptor (GR)-β, an abnormal pattern of histone acetylation in response to corticosteroids, a defect in IL-10 production, and a reduction in histone deacetylase activity (as in COPD). These observations suggest that there are likely to be heterogeneous mechanisms for corticosteroid resistance; whether these mechanisms are genetically determined has yet to be decided.

BRITTLE ASTHMA

Some patients show chaotic variations in lung function despite taking appropriate therapy. Some show a persistent pattern of variability and may require oral corticosteroids or, at times, continuous infusion of β₂-agonists (type I brittle asthma), whereas others have generally normal or near-normal lung function but precipitous, unpredictable falls in lung function that may result in death (type 2 brittle asthma). These latter patients are difficult to manage as they do not respond well to corticosteroids, and the worsening of asthma does not reverse well with inhaled bronchodilators. The most effective therapy is subcutaneous epinephrine, which suggests that the worsening is likely to be a localized airway anaphylactic reaction with edema. In some of these patients, there may be allergy to specific foods. These patients should be taught to self-administer epinephrine and should carry a medical warning accordingly.

TREATMENT   Refractory Asthma

Refractory asthma is difficult to control, by definition. It is important to check compliance and the correct use of inhalers and to identify and eliminate any underlying triggers. Low doses of theophylline may be helpful in some patients, and theophylline withdrawal has been found to worsen in many patients. Most of these patients will require maintenance treatment with oral corticosteroids, and the minimal dose that achieves satisfactory control should be determined by careful dose titration. Steroid-sparing therapies are rarely effective. In some patients with allergic asthma, omalizumab is effective, particularly when there are frequent exacerbations. Anti-TNF therapy is not effective in severe asthma and should not be used. A few patients may benefit from infusions of β₂-agonists. New therapies are needed for these patients, who currently consume a disproportionate amount of health care spending.

SPECIAL CONSIDERATIONS

Although asthma is usually straightforward to manage, there are some situations that may require additional investigation and different therapy.

ASPIRIN-SENSITIVE ASTHMA

A small proportion (1–5%) of asthmatics become worse with aspirin and other COX inhibitors, although this is much more commonly seen in severe cases and in those patients with frequent hospital admission. Aspirin-sensitive asthma is a well defined subtype of asthma that is usually preceded by perennial rhinitis and nasal polyps in nonatopic patients with a late onset of the disease. Aspirin, even in small doses, characteristically provokes rhinorrhea, conjunctival irritation, facial flushing, and wheezing. There is a genetic predisposition to increased production of cysteinyl-leukotrienes with functional polymorphism of cys-leukotriene C synthase. Asthma is triggered by COX inhibitors, but is persistent even in their absence. All nonselective COX inhibitors should be avoided, but selective COX2 inhibitors are safe to use when an anti-inflammatory analgesic is needed. Aspirin-sensitive asthma responds to usual therapy with ICS. Although antileukotrienes should be effective in these patients, they are no more effective than in allergic asthma. Occasionally, aspirin desensitization is necessary, but this should only be undertaken in specialized centers.

ASTHMA IN THE ELDERLY

Asthma may start at any age, including in elderly patients. The principles of management are the same as in other asthmatics, but side effects of therapy may be a problem, including muscle tremor with β₂-agonists and more systemic side effects with ICS. Comorbidities are more frequent in this age group, and interactions with drugs such as β₂-blockers, COX inhibitors, and agents that may affect theophylline metabolism need to be considered. COPD is more likely in elderly patients and may coexist with asthma. A trial of OCS may be very useful in documenting the steroid responsiveness of asthma.

PREGNANCY

Approximately one-third of asthmatic patients who are pregnant improve during the course of a pregnancy, one-third deteriorate, and one-third are unchanged. It is important to maintain good control of asthma as poor control may have adverse effects on fetal development. Compliance may be a problem as there is often concern about the effects of antiasthma medications on fetal development. The drugs that have been used for many years in asthma therapy have now been shown to be safe and without teratogenic potential. These drugs include short-acting β₂-agonists, ICS, and theophylline; there is less safety information about newer classes of drugs such as LABAs, antileukotrienes, and anti-IgE. If an OCS is needed, it is better to use prednisone rather than prednisolone as it cannot be converted to the active prednisolone by the fetal liver, thus protecting the fetus from systemic effects of the corticosteroid. There is no contraindication to breast-feeding when patients are using these drugs.

CIGARETTE SMOKING

Approximately 20% of asthmatics smoke, which may adversely affect asthma in several ways. Smoking asthmatics have more severe disease, more frequent hospital admissions, a faster decline in lung function, and a higher risk of death from asthma than nonsmoking asthmatics. There is evidence that smoking interferes with the anti-inflammatory actions of corticosteroids, necessitating higher doses for asthma control. Smoking cessation improves lung function and reduces the steroid resistance, and, thus, vigorous smoking cessation strategies should be used. Some patients report a temporary worsening of asthma when they first stop smoking, which could be due to the loss of the bronchodilating effect of no in cigarette smoke.

SURGERY

If asthma is well controlled, there is no contraindication to general anesthesia and intubation. Patients who are treated with OCS will have adrenal suppression and should be treated with an increased dose of OCS immediately prior to surgery. Patients with FEV_1 <80% of their normal levels should also be given a boost of OCS prior to surgery. High-maintenance doses of corticosteroids may be a contraindication to surgery because of increased risks of infection and delayed wound healing.

BRONCHOPULMONARY ASPERGILLOSIS

Bronchopulmonary aspergillosis (BPA) is uncommon and results from an allergic pulmonary reaction to inhaled spores of *Aspergillus fumigatus* and, occasionally, other *Aspergillus* species. A skin prick test to *A. fumigatus* is always positive, whereas serum *Aspergillus* precipitins are low or undetectable. Characteristically, there are fleeting eosinophilic infiltrates in the lungs, particularly in the upper lobes. Airways become blocked with mucoid plugs rich in eosinophils, and patients may cough up brown plugs and have hemoptysis. BPA may result in bronchiectasis, particularly affecting central airways, if not suppressed by corticosteroids. Asthma is controlled in the usual way by ICS, but it is necessary to give a course of OCS if any sign of worsening or pulmonary shadowing is found. Treatment with the oral antifungal itraconazole is beneficial in preventing exacerbations.

CHAPTER 9

HYPERSENSITIVITY PNEUMONITIS AND PULMONARY INFILTRATES WITH EOSINOPHILIA

Alicia K. Gerke ■ Gary W. Hunninghake

HYPERSENSITIVITY PNEUMONITIS

First described in 1874, hypersensitivity pneumonitis (HP), or extrinsic allergic alveolitis, is an inflammatory disorder of the lung involving alveolar walls and terminal airways that is induced by repeated inhalation of a variety of organic agents in a susceptible host. The expression of HP depends on factors related to the host susceptibility and the inciting agent. The frequency of HP varies with the environmental exposure and the specific antigen involved, which often depends on season, geographic location, or presence of certain industries.

ETIOLOGY

Agents implicated as causes of HP are diverse and include those listed in Table 9-1. The common name of each disease often reflects the occupational or avocational risk associated with that disease. In the United States, the most common types of HP are farmer's lung, bird fancier's lung, and chemical worker's lung. In *farmer's lung*, inhalation of proteins, such as thermophilic bacteria and fungal spores that are present in moldy bedding and feed, are most commonly responsible for the development of HP. These antigens are probably also responsible for the etiology of *mushroom worker's disease* (moldy composted growth medium), bagassosis (moldy sugar cane), and water-related exposure (molds in air conditioners or humidifiers). *Hot tub lung* refers to a hypersensitivity reaction to *Mycobacterium avium complex*, which is present in hot tubs or whirlpools and is differentiated from actual infection. *Bird fancier's lung* (and the related disorders of duck fever, turkey handler's lung, and dove pillow's lung) is a response to inhalation of proteins from feathers and droppings. *Chemical worker's lung* is an example of how simple chemicals, such as isocyanates, may also cause immune-mediated diseases. Interestingly,

cigarette smoking has been associated with decreased incidence of HP; however, smoking may lead to a more progressive or severe course of HP once the disease is present.

PATHOGENESIS

The finding that precipitating antibodies against extracts of moldy hay were demonstrable in most patients with farmer's lung led to the early conclusion that HP was an immune complex–mediated reaction. Subsequent investigations of HP in human beings and animal models provided evidence for the importance of cell-mediated hypersensitivity. The very early (acute) reaction is characterized by an increase in polymorphonuclear leukocytes in the alveoli and small airways. This early lesion is followed by an influx of mononuclear cells into the lung and the formation of granulomas that appear to be the result of a classic delayed (T cell–mediated) hypersensitivity reaction to repeated inhalation of antigen and adjuvant-active materials. Studies in animal models suggest that the disease is a T_H1-mediated immune response to antigen, with interferon γ, interleukin (IL)-12, and possibly IL-18 contributing to disease expression. Most likely, multiple cytokines (including also IL-1β, transforming growth factor β [TGF-β], tumor necrosis factor α [TNF-α] and others) interact to promote HP; their source includes both alveolar macrophages and T lymphocytes in the lung. Data support a genetic predisposition to the development of HP; certain polymorphisms of the TNF-α promoter region and major histocompatibility complex reportedly confer an enhanced susceptibility to pigeon breeder's disease.

After inhalation of an antigenic particle, the attraction and accumulation of inflammatory cells in the lung may be due to one or more of the following mechanisms: induction of the adhesion molecules L-selectin and

85

TABLE 9-1

SELECTED EXAMPLES OF HYPERSENSITIVITY PNEUMONITIS (HP)

DISEASE	ANTIGEN	SOURCE OF ANTIGEN
Bagassosis	Thermophilic actinomycetes[a]	"Moldy" bagasse (sugar cane)
Bird fancier's, breeder's, or handler's lung[b]	Parakeet, pigeon, chicken, turkey proteins	Avian droppings or feathers
Cephalosporium HP	Contaminated basement (sewage)	*Cephalosporium*
Cheese washer's lung	*Penicillium casei*	Moldy cheese
Chemical worker's lung[b]	Isocyanates	Polyurethane foam, varnishes, lacquer
Coffee worker's lung	Coffee bean dust	Coffee beans
Compost lung	*Aspergillus*	Compost
Detergent worker's disease	*Bacillus subtilis enzymes* (subtilisins)	Detergent
Familial HP	*Bacillus subtilis*	Contaminated wood dust in walls
Farmer's lung[b]	Thermophilic actinomycetes[a]	"Moldy" hay, grain, silage
Fish food lung	Unknown	Fish food
Fish meal worker's lung	Fish meal dust	Fish meal
Furrier's lung	Animal fur dust	Animal pelts
Hot tub lung	*Cladosporium* spp., *Mycobacterium avium* complex	Mold on ceiling; contaminated water
Humidifier or air conditioner lung (ventilation pneumonitis)	*Aureobasidium pullulans, Candida albicans,* Thermophilic actinomycetes,[a] *Mycobacterium* spp., other microorganisms	Contaminated water in humidification or forced-air air conditioning systems
Japanese summer-type HP	*Trichosporon cutaneum, T. asahii,* and *T. mucoides*	House dust, bird droppings
Laboratory worker's HP	Male rat urine	Laboratory rat
Lycoperdonosis	*Lycoperdon* puffballs	Puffball spores
Malt worker's lung	*Aspergillus fumigatus* or *A. clavatus*	Moldy barley
Maple bark disease	*Cryptostroma corticale*	Maple bark
Metalworking fluid lung	*Mycobacterium* spp., *Pseudomonas* spp.	Contaminated metalworking fluid
Miller's lung	*Sitophilus granarius* (wheat weevil)	Infested wheat flour
Miscellaneous medication	Amiodarone, bleomycin, efavirenz, gemcitabine, hydralazine, hydroxyurea, isoniazid, methotrexate, paclitaxel, penicillin, procarbazine, propranolol, riluzole, sirolimus, sulfasalazine	Medication
Mushroom worker's lung	Thermophilic actinomycetes,[a] *Hypsizygus marmoreus, Bunashimeji,* and other exotic mushrooms	Mushroom compost; mushrooms
Pituitary snuff taker's lung	Animal proteins	Heterologous pituitary snuff
Potato riddler's lung	Thermophilic actinomycetes,[a] *Aspergillus*	"Moldy" hay around potatoes
Sauna taker's lung	*Aureobasidium* spp., other	Contaminated sauna water
Sausage worker's lung	*Penicillium nalgiovense*	Dry sausage mold
Sequoiosis	*Aureobasidium, Graphium* spp.	Redwood sawdust
Streptomyces albus HP	*Streptomyces albus*	Contaminated fertilizer
Suberosis	*Penicillium glabrum* and *Chrysonilia sitophila*	Cork dust

(continued)

TABLE 9-1

DISEASE	ANTIGEN	SOURCE OF ANTIGEN
Tap water lung	*Mycobacteria* spp.	Contaminated tap water
Thatched roof disease	*Saccharomonospora viridis*	Dried grasses and leaves
Tobacco worker's disease	*Aspergillus* spp.	Mold on tobacco
Winegrower's lung	*Botrytis cinerea*	Mold on grapes
Wood trimmer's disease	*Rhizopus* spp., *Mucor* spp.	Contaminated wood trimmings
Woodman's disease	*Penicillium* spp.	Oak and maple trees
Woodworker's lung	Wood dust, *Alternaria*	Oak, cedar, pine, and mahogany dusts

SELECTED EXAMPLES OF HYPERSENSITIVITY PNEUMONITIS (HP) (*CONTINUED*)

[a]Thermophilic actinomycetes species include *Micropolyspora faeni, Thermoactinomyces vulgaris, T. saccharri, T. viridis,* and *T. candidus.*
[b]Most common causes of hypersensitivity pneumonitis in the United States.

E-selectin, elaboration by dendritic cells of CC chemokine 1 (DC-CK-1/CCL18), or increased expression of CXCR3/CXCL10 by $CD4^+$ and $CD8^+$ lymphocytes. Increased levels of Fas protein and FasL in the lung (which would be expected to suppress inflammation by induction of T cell apoptosis) is counterbalanced by increased expression of the inducible antiapoptotic gene *Bcl-xL*, resulting in a lower overall level of pulmonary lymphocyte apoptosis in HP patients.

Bronchoalveolar lavage (BAL) in patients with HP consistently demonstrates an increase in T lymphocytes in lavage fluid (a finding that is also observed in patients with other granulomatous lung disorders). Patients with recent or continual exposure to antigen may have an increase in polymorphonuclear leukocytes in lavage fluid, which has been associated with lung fibrosis. A role for oxidant injury has been proposed in HP. Several markers of oxidative stress are reported to be increased during exacerbation of HP and are reduced by treatment with glucocorticoids.

CLINICAL PRESENTATION

The clinical picture is that of an interstitial pneumonitis, which varies from patient to patient and seems related to the frequency and intensity of exposure to the causative antigen and, perhaps, other host factors. The presentation can be acute, subacute, or chronic. In the *acute* form, symptoms such as cough, fever, chills, malaise, and dyspnea may occur 6 to 8 h after exposure to the antigen and usually clear within a few days if there is no further exposure to antigen; it often closely resembles an influenza-like illness. The *subacute* form often appears insidiously over a period of weeks marked by cough and dyspnea and may progress to cyanosis and severe dyspnea, requiring hospitalization. In some patients, a subacute form of the disease may persist after an acute presentation of the disorder, especially if there is continued exposure to antigen. In most patients with the acute or subacute form of HP, the symptoms, signs, and other manifestations of HP disappear within days, weeks, or months if the causative agent is no longer inhaled. Transformation to a chronic form of the disease may occur, but the frequency of such progression is uncertain.

Continuous low-level antigen exposure or repeated episodes can also lead to chronic disease with more subtle symptoms, accounting for delayed or uncertain diagnosis over a long period of time. This may occur without a prior history of acute or subacute manifestations. The *chronic* form of HP may be clinically indistinguishable from pulmonary fibrosis in its later stages. Symptoms include cough, weight loss, malaise, and gradual increase in dyspnea. Physical examination may reveal inspiratory crackles and digital clubbing. Imaging shows interstitial fibrosis or emphysema. Progressive worsening may result in dependence on supplemental oxygen, pulmonary hypertension, or respiratory failure. Pulmonary fibrosis is the clinical manifestation of HP with the greatest predictive value for mortality. Fibrosis appears most prominent in hypersensitivity pneumonitis associated with birds, while emphysema is often more common in farmer's lung.

DIAGNOSIS

All forms of the disease may be associated with elevations in erythrocyte sedimentation rate, C-reactive protein, rheumatoid factor, lactate dehydrogenase, or serum immunoglobulins. Following acute exposure to an antigen, neutrophilia and lymphopenia are frequently present. Eosinophilia is not a feature. Examination for *serum precipitins* against suspected antigens, such as those listed in Table 9-1, is an important part of the diagnostic workup and should be performed on any patient with interstitial lung disease, especially if a suggestive exposure history is elicited. The occurrence of precipitins indicates sufficient exposure to the causative agent for generation of an immunologic response and is one of the major diagnostic criteria; however, the diagnosis of HP is not established solely by the presence of precipitins, as they are found in sera of many individuals exposed to appropriate antigens who demonstrate no other evidence of HP. False-negative results may occur because of unreliable testing techniques or an inappropriate choice of antigens. Extraction of antigens from the suspected source may at times be helpful.

Chest x-ray shows no specific or distinctive changes in HP. It can be normal even in symptomatic patients. The acute or subacute phases may be associated with poorly defined, patchy, or diffuse infiltrates; with discrete, nodular infiltrates; or with air-space consolidation. In the chronic phase, the chest x-ray usually shows a diffuse reticulonodular infiltrate. Honeycombing may eventually develop as the condition progresses. Apical sparing is common, suggesting that disease severity correlates with inhaled antigen load, but no particular distribution or pattern is classic for HP. Abnormalities rarely seen in HP include pleural effusion or thickening and significant hilar adenopathy.

High-resolution chest CT has become the procedure of choice for imaging of HP. Although pathognomonic features have not been identified, acute HP may appear with diffuse "ground-glass" infiltrates, a reticulonodular pattern, or confluent alveolar opacification. In subacute disease, centrilobular nodules and "ground-glass" changes predominate, and expiratory views may demonstrate air trapping or mosaic perfusion **(Fig. 9–1)**. This pattern is more common in individuals whose exposure to antigen

continues rather than in those in whom removal from antigen exposure has occurred. In chronic HP, diffuse changes include patchy emphysema and interstitial fibrosis; subpleural linear opacities and honeycombing are also common. The findings are often similar (but not identical) to idiopathic pulmonary fibrosis.

Pulmonary function studies in all forms of HP may show a restrictive or an obstructive pattern with loss of lung volumes, impaired diffusing capacity, and decreased compliance. Resting or exercise-induced hypoxemia may be seen. Bronchospasm and bronchial hyperreactivity are sometimes found in acute HP. With antigen avoidance, the pulmonary function abnormalities are usually reversible in acute and subacute disease.

BAL is used in some centers to aid in diagnostic evaluation. A marked lymphocytic alveolitis on BAL is almost universal, although not pathognomonic. Lymphocytes are typically activated and show a decreased helper/suppressor ratio, although this ratio can be variable depending on dose and duration of exposure. Alveolar neutrophilia is also prominent acutely, but tends to fade in the absence of recurrent exposure. Bronchoalveolar mastocytosis may correlate with disease activity.

Lung biopsy, obtained through flexible bronchoscopy, open-lung procedures, or thoracoscopy, may be diagnostic. Although the histopathology is distinctive, it may not be pathognomonic of HP **(Fig. 9–2)**. When the biopsy is taken during the active phase of disease, typical findings include an interstitial alveolar infiltrate consisting of plasma cells, lymphocytes, and occasional eosinophils and neutrophils, usually accompanied by

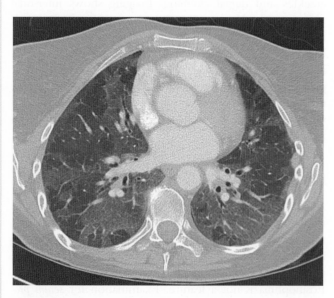

FIGURE 9-1
Chest CT scan of a patient with subacute hypersensitivity pneumonitis in which scattered regions of ground-glass infiltrates in a mosaic pattern consistent with air trapping are seen bilaterally. This patient had *bird fancier's lung. (Courtesy of TJ Gross; with permission.)*

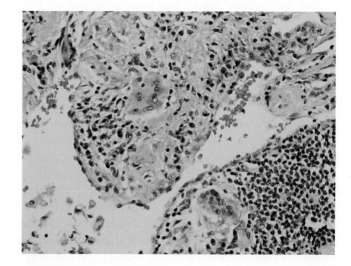

FIGURE 9-2
Open-lung biopsy from a patient with subacute hypersensitivity pneumonitis demonstrating a loose, nonnecrotizing granuloma made up of histiocytes and multinucleated giant cells. Peribronchial inflammatory infiltrate made up of lymphocytes and plasma cells is also seen. *(Courtesy of TJ Gross; with permission.)*

loose, noncaseating peribronchial granulomas. Some degree of bronchiolitis is found in about one-half the cases. Rarely, bronchiolitis obliterans with organizing pneumonia (BOOP) (Chap. 19) may be present. In subacute disease, the triad of mononuclear bronchiolitis; interstitial infiltrates of lymphocytes and plasma cells; and single, nonnecrotizing, randomly scattered parenchymal granulomas without mural vascular involvement is consistent with HP. Interstitial fibrosis may be present, but most often is mild in earlier stages of the disease. Chronic HP has variable pathology and may resemble nonspecific interstitial pneumonia, organizing pneumonia, or usual interstitial pneumonia; granulomas may or may not be present. Centrilobular fibrosis, peribronchial inflammation with fibrosis, bridging fibrosis, and emphysema are common.

A *prediction rule* for the clinical diagnosis of HP has been developed by the International HP Study Group. Six significant predictors of HP (exposure to a known antigen, positive predictive antibodies to the antigen, recurrent episodes of symptoms, inspiratory crackles, symptoms developing 4–8 h after exposure, and weight loss) were retrospectively developed then validated in a separate cohort. This diagnostic paradigm has a high predictive value in the diagnosis of HP, without the need for invasive testing. In cases where only a subset of the criteria is fulfilled, the diagnosis is less certain. It is clear, however, that the diagnosis of HP is established by (1) consistent symptoms, physical findings, pulmonary function tests, and radiographic tests; (2) a history of exposure to a recognized antigen; and (3) ideally, identification of an antibody to that antigen. Symptoms upon re-exposure to the suspected antigen also support the diagnosis. In some circumstances, BAL and/or lung biopsy may be needed. The most important tool in diagnosing HP continues to be a high index of suspicion.

DIFFERENTIAL DIAGNOSIS

Chronic HP may often be difficult to distinguish from a number of other interstitial lung disorders (Chap. 19). A negative history for use of relevant drugs and no evidence of a systemic disorder usually exclude the presence of drug-induced lung disease or a collagen vascular disorder. BAL often shows predominance of neutrophils in idiopathic pulmonary fibrosis and a predominance of CD4+ lymphocytes in sarcoidosis. Hilar/paratracheal lymphadenopathy or evidence of multisystem involvement also favors the diagnosis of sarcoidosis. In some patients, a lung biopsy may be required to differentiate chronic HP from other interstitial diseases. The lung disease associated with acute or subacute HP may clinically resemble other disorders that present with systemic symptoms and recurrent pulmonary infiltrates, including the allergic bronchopulmonary mycoses and other eosinophilic pneumonias.

Eosinophilic pneumonia is often associated with asthma and is typified by peripheral eosinophilia; neither of these is a feature of HP. Allergic bronchopulmonary aspergillosis (ABPA) is the most common example of the allergic bronchopulmonary mycoses and is sometimes confused with HP because of the presence of precipitating antibodies to *Aspergillus fumigatus*. ABPA is associated with allergic (atopic) asthma. Acute HP may be confused with *organic dust toxic syndrome* (ODTS), a condition that is more common than HP. ODTS follows heavy exposure to organic dusts and is characterized by transient fever and muscle aches, with or without dyspnea and cough. Serum precipitins are absent, and the chest x-ray is usually normal. This distinction is important, as ODTS is a self-limited disorder without significant long-term sequelae, whereas continued antigen exposure in HP can result in permanent disability. Massive exposure to moldy silage may result in a syndrome termed *pulmonary mycotoxicosis*, with fever, chills, and cough and the presence of pulmonary infiltrates within a few hours of exposure. No previous sensitization is required, and precipitins are absent to *Aspergillus*, the suspected causative agent.

TREATMENT Hypersensitivity Pneumonitis

Because effective treatment depends largely on avoiding the antigen, identification of the causative agent and its source is essential. This is usually possible if the physician takes a detailed environmental and occupational history or, if necessary, visits the patient's environment. The simplest way to avoid the incriminated agent is to remove the patient from the environment or remove the source of the agent from the patient's environment. This recommendation cannot be taken lightly when it completely changes the lifestyle or livelihood of the patient. In many cases, the source of exposure (birds, humidifiers, molds, etc.) can be removed. Pollen masks, personal dust respirators, airstream helmets, and ventilated helmets with a supply of fresh air are increasingly efficient means of purifying inhaled air. If symptoms recur or physiologic abnormalities progress in spite of these measures, more effective measures to avoid antigen exposure must be pursued. The chronic form of HP typically results from low-grade or recurrent exposure over many months to years, and the lung disease may already be partially or completely irreversible. These patients are usually advised to avoid all possible contact with the offending agent.

Patients with the *acute*, recurrent form of HP usually recover without need for glucocorticoids. *Subacute* HP may be associated with severe symptoms and marked physiologic impairment and may continue to progress for several days despite hospitalization. Urgent establishment of the diagnosis and prompt institution of glucocorticoid treatment are indicated in such patients. Prednisone at a dosage of 1 mg/kg per d or its equivalent is continued for 7 to 14 days and then tapered over the ensuing 2 to 6 weeks at a rate that depends on the patient's clinical status. Patients with *chronic* HP may gradually recover without therapy following environmental control. In many patients, however, a trial of prednisone may be useful to obtain maximal reversibility of the lung disease. Following initial prednisone therapy (1 mg/kg per d for 2 to 4 weeks), the drug is tapered to the lowest dosage that will maintain the functional status of the patient. Many patients will not require or benefit from long-term therapy if there is no further exposure to antigen. Although a short course of corticosteroids has been shown to accelerate recovery from the acute stage, glucocorticoid therapy does not appear to have an effect on long-term prognosis of farmer's lung. Improvement of lung function may continue over a few months to years.

PULMONARY INFILTRATES WITH EOSINOPHILIA

Pulmonary infiltrates with eosinophilia (PIE, eosinophilic pneumonias) include distinct individual syndromes characterized by eosinophilic pulmonary infiltrates and, commonly, peripheral blood eosinophilia. Since Loeffler's initial description of a transient, benign syndrome of migratory pulmonary infiltrates and peripheral blood eosinophilia of unknown cause, this group of disorders has been enlarged to include several diseases of both known and unknown etiology (Table 9–2). These diseases may be considered as immunologically mediated lung diseases, but are not to be confused with HP, in which eosinophilia is *not* a feature. In differentiating the

etiologies of this heterogeneous group of lung disorders, an extensive history and full examination of all organ systems are essential.

When an eosinophilic pneumonia is associated with bronchial asthma, it is important to determine if the patient has atopic asthma and has wheal–and–flare skin reactivity to *Aspergillus* or other relevant fungal antigens. If so, other criteria should be sought for the diagnosis of ABPA (Table 9–3) or other, rarer examples of allergic bronchopulmonary mycosis such as those caused by *Penicillium, Candida, Curvularia,* or *Helminthosporium* spp. *A. fumigatus* is the most common cause of ABPA. The chest roentgenogram in ABPA may show transient, recurrent infiltrates or may suggest the presence of proximal bronchiectasis. High-resolution chest CT is a sensitive, noninvasive technique for the recognition of proximal bronchiectasis. The bronchial asthma of ABPA likely involves an IgE-mediated hypersensitivity, whereas the bronchiectasis associated with this disorder is thought to result from a deposition of immune complexes in proximal airways. Adequate treatment usually requires the long-term use of systemic glucocorticoids. Another eosinophilic process associated with asthma is Churg-Strauss syndrome, or allergic angiitis granulomatosis, which presents with necrotizing eosinophilic vasculitis and eosinophilic infiltration of multiple organs, including the lung.

A travel history or evidence of recent immigration should prompt the consideration of parasite-associated disorders. *Tropical eosinophilia* is usually caused by filarial infection; however, eosinophilic pneumonias also occur with other parasites such as *Ascaris* spp., *Ancyclostoma* spp., *Toxocara* spp., and *Strongyloides stercoralis*. Tropical eosinophilia due to *Wuchereria bancrofti* or *W. malayi* occurs most commonly in southern Asia, Africa, and South

TABLE 9-2

PULMONARY INFILTRATES WITH EOSINOPHILIA
Etiology Known
Allergic bronchopulmonary mycoses
Parasitic infestations
Drug reactions
Eosinophilia-myalgia syndrome
Idiopathic
Loeffler's syndrome
Acute eosinophilic pneumonia
Chronic eosinophilic pneumonia
Allergic granulomatosis of Churg and Strauss
Hypereosinophilic syndrome

TABLE 9-3

DIAGNOSTIC FEATURES OF ALLERGIC BRONCHOPULMONARY ASPERGILLOSIS (ABPA)
Main Diagnostic Criteria
Bronchial asthma
Pulmonary infiltrates
Peripheral eosinophilia (>1000/μL)
Immediate wheal-and-flare response to *Aspergillus fumigatus*
Serum precipitins to *A. fumigatus*
Elevated serum IgE
Central bronchiectasis
Other Diagnostic Features
History of brownish plugs in sputum
Culture of *A. fumigatus* from sputum
Elevated IgE (and IgG) class antibodies specific for *A. fumigatus*

America and is treated successfully with diethylcarbamazine. In the United States, *Strongyloides* is endemic to the Southeastern and Appalachian regions. Even in cases of known foreign travel, identification of the causative agent is not always possible, as exemplified by 18 cases (2 fatal) of acute eosinophilic pneumonia reported amongst U.S. military personnel deployed in Iraq.

In the United States, *drug-induced eosinophilic pneumonias* are the most common cause of eosinophilic pulmonary infiltrates. These are exemplified by acute reactions to nitrofurantoin, which may begin 2 h to 10 days after nitrofurantoin is started, with symptoms of dry cough, fever, chills, and dyspnea; an eosinophilic pleural effusion accompanying patchy or diffuse pulmonary infiltrates may also occur. Other drugs associated with eosinophilic pneumonias include sulfonamides, penicillin, chlorpropamide, thiazides, tricyclic antidepressants, hydralazine, gold salts, isoniazid, indomethacin, and others. One report has identified anti-TNF-α monoclonal antibody therapy as a cause of eosinophilic pneumonitis. Treatment consists of withdrawal of the incriminated drugs or toxins and the use of glucocorticoids, if necessary.

The group of primary (idiopathic) eosinophilic pneumonias consists of diseases of varying severity. *Loeffler's syndrome* was originally reported as a benign, acute eosinophilic pneumonia of unknown cause characterized by migrating pulmonary infiltrates and minimal clinical manifestations. In some patients, these clinical characteristics prove to be secondary to parasites or drugs. *Acute eosinophilic pneumonia* is an idiopathic acute febrile illness of <7 days' duration with severe hypoxemia, pulmonary infiltrates, pleural effusions, and no history of asthma. BAL fluid reveals greater than 25% eosinophils (normally less than 2% in nonsmokers); however, the peripheral eosinophilia tends to develop later in the course and may not be apparent on initial presentation. *Chronic eosinophilic pneumonia* presents with significant systemic symptoms including fever, chills, night sweats, cough, anorexia, and weight loss of several weeks' to months' duration. The chest x-ray classically shows peripheral infiltrates, and pulmonary function testing reveals obstruction. Peripheral blood and BAL eosinophilia is more pronounced than in the acute form. Some patients also have bronchial asthma of the intrinsic or nonallergic type. For both acute and chronic disease, dramatic clearing of symptoms and chest x-ray is often noted after initiation of glucocorticoid therapy In contrast to acute eosinophilic pneumonia, chronic eosinophilic pneumonia tends to recur and may require repeated treatment.

The *hypereosinophilic syndrome* is characterized by presence of >1500 eosinophils per microliter of peripheral blood for 6 months or longer; lack of evidence for parasitic, allergic, or other known causes of eosinophilia;

and signs or symptoms of multisystem organ dysfunction. Consistent features are blood and bone marrow eosinophilia with tissue infiltration by relatively mature eosinophils. The heart may be involved with tricuspid valve abnormalities or endomyocardial fibrosis and a restrictive, biventricular cardiomyopathy. Other organs affected typically include the lungs, liver, spleen, skin, and nervous system. Therapy of the disorder consists of glucocorticoids and/or hydroxyurea, plus therapy as needed for cardiac dysfunction, which is frequently responsible for much of the morbidity and mortality in this syndrome. Pulmonary eosinophilia has also been associated with T cell lymphoma and has been reported following *lung* and *bone marrow transplantation*.

GLOBAL PICTURE OF HYPERSENSITIVITY PNEUMONITIS AND PULMONARY INFILTRATES WITH EOSINOPHILIA

 HP is more prevalent outside of the United States than within, and the range of antigen responses is somewhat different. Internationally, bird breeder's lung is the most common form of HP. Rather than being associated with avocational exposures, bird-raising practices, highlighted by the emerging threat of avian influenza, lead to substantial exposure to workers involved in poultry husbandry and processing. This increases antigen exposure enormously, in comparison to U.S. workers, and enhances the risk of HP. Importantly, it is the most common cause of pediatric HP and has been reported in individuals as young as 4 years, presenting as a chronic cough.

Farmer's lung, one of the earliest reported causes of HP, appears to be waning worldwide. This is likely in response to changing agricultural practices; increased use of masks and impermeable barriers in hay storage has reduced the exposure and proliferation of thermophilic bacteria, and thus HP.

The international manifestations of HP resemble those of the U.S. disease. Many industrialized nations have increasingly reported HP due to mycobacteria and pseudomonads in contaminated metalworking fluids. The prevalence of these environmental contaminants greatly depends on workplace hygiene practices. Some forms of HP are almost exclusively geographically limited, such as summer-type hypersensitivity pneumonitis in Japan from exposure to *Trichosporon cutaneum* associated with birds. Likewise, cork worker's pneumonitis (suberosis), caused by exposure to contaminated corks, is almost exclusively seen in Spain and southern Europe because of the regional cork industry. However, one of the causative antigens (*Chrysonilia sitophila*) is also reported to be an antigen in lung diseases associated with logging in Canada. In Spain, esparto, a member of the grass family, is used as a fiber for the weaving of mats, baskets, and ropes; it is also incorporated into traditional plaster construction. In both of its uses, it has been associated with HP (most likely due to contamination with *A. fumigatus*), again geographically limited because of the utility of the product, though not of the underlying fungal antigen. Exposure to exotic mushrooms is greater in Asia than in the United States, and this has recently been linked to cases of HP.

Pulmonary infiltrates with eosinophilia are also a greater international than U.S. health burden. In this case, parasitic infestation is far more common than drug-induced lung disease, but the manifestations are similar.

ACKNOWLEDGMENT

We acknowledge the contribution of Dr. Joel N. Kline to this chapter in the 17th edition of Harrison's Principles of Internal Medicine.

CHAPTER 10

OCCUPATIONAL AND ENVIRONMENTAL LUNG DISEASE

John R. Balmes   ■   Frank E. Speizer

Occupational and environmental lung diseases are difficult to distinguish from those of nonenvironmental origin. Virtually all major categories of pulmonary disease can be caused by environmental agents, and environmentally related disease usually presents clinically in a manner indistinguishable from that of disease not caused by such agents. In addition, the etiology of many diseases may be multifactorial; occupational and environmental factors may interact with other factors (such as smoking and genetic risk). It is often only after a careful exposure history is taken that the underlying workplace or general environmental exposure is uncovered.

Why is knowledge of occupational or environmental etiology so important? Patient management and prognosis are affected significantly by such knowledge. For example, patients with occupational asthma or hypersensitivity pneumonitis often cannot be managed adequately without cessation of exposure to the offending agent. Establishment of cause may have significant legal and financial implications for a patient who no longer can work in his or her usual job. Other exposed people may be identified as having the disease or prevented from getting it. In addition, new associations between exposure and disease may be identified (e.g., nylon flock worker's lung disease and diacetyl-induced bronchiolitis obliterans).

Although the exact proportion of lung disease due to occupational and environmental factors is unknown, a large number of individuals are at risk. For example, 15–20% of the burden of adult asthma and chronic obstructive pulmonary disease (COPD) has been estimated to be due to occupational factors.

HISTORY AND PHYSICAL EXAMINATION

The patient's history is of paramount importance in assessing any potential occupational or environmental exposure. Inquiry into specific work practices should include questions about the specific contaminants involved, the presence of visible dusts, chemical odors, the size and ventilation of workspaces, the use of respiratory protective equipment, and whether co-workers have similar complaints. The temporal association of exposure at work and symptoms may provide clues to occupation-related disease. In addition, the patient must be questioned about alternative sources of exposure to potentially toxic agents, including hobbies, home characteristics, exposure to secondhand smoke, and proximity to traffic or industrial facilities. Short-term and long-term exposures to potential toxic agents in the distant past also must be considered.

Workers in the United States have the right to know about potential hazards in their workplaces under federal Occupational Safety and Health Administration (OSHA) regulations. Employers must provide specific information about potential hazardous agents in products being used through Material Safety Data Sheets as well as training in personal protective equipment and environmental control procedures. Reminders posted in the workplace may warn workers about hazardous substances. However, the introduction of new processes and/or new chemical compounds may change exposure significantly, and often only the employee on the production line is aware of the change. For the physician caring for a patient with a suspected work-related illness, a visit to the work site can be very instructive. Alternatively, an affected worker can request an inspection by OSHA.

The physical examination of patients with environmentally related lung diseases may help determine the nature and severity of the pulmonary condition but usually does not contribute information that points to a specific etiology.

PULMONARY FUNCTION TESTS AND CHEST IMAGING

Exposures to inorganic and organic dusts can cause interstitial lung disease that presents with a restrictive pattern and a decreased diffusing capacity (Chap. 5). Similarly, exposures to a number of organic dusts or chemical agents may result in occupational asthma or COPD that is characterized by airway obstruction. Measurement of change in forced expiratory volume (FEV_1) before and after a working shift can be used to detect an acute bronchoconstrictive response. For example, an acute decrement of FEV_1 over the first work shift of the week is a characteristic feature of cotton textile workers with byssinosis (an obstructive airway disorder with features of both asthma and chronic bronchitis).

The chest radiograph is useful in detecting and monitoring the pulmonary response to mineral dusts, certain metals, and organic dusts capable of inducing hypersensitivity pneumonitis. The International Labour Organisation (ILO) International Classification of Radiographs of Pneumoconioses classifies chest radiographs by the nature and size of opacities seen and the extent of involvement of the parenchyma. In general, small rounded opacities are seen in silicosis or coal worker's pneumoconiosis and small linear opacities are seen in asbestosis. The profusion of such opacities is rated by using a 12-point scheme. Although useful for epidemiologic studies and screening large numbers of workers, the ILO system can be problematic when applied to an individual worker's chest radiograph. With dusts causing rounded opacities, the degree of involvement on the chest radiograph may be extensive, whereas pulmonary function may be only minimally impaired. In contrast, in pneumoconiosis causing linear, irregular opacities like those seen in asbestosis, the radiograph may lead to underestimation of the severity of the impairment until relatively late in the disease. For patients with a history of asbestos exposure, conventional computed tomography (CT) is more sensitive for the detection of pleural thickening and high-resolution CT (HRCT) improves the detection of asbestosis.

Other procedures that may be of use in identifying the role of environmental exposures in causing lung disease include evaluation of heavy metal concentrations in urine (cadmium in battery plant workers), skin prick testing or specific IgE antibody titers for evidence of immediate hypersensitivity to agents capable of inducing occupational asthma (flour antigens in bakers), specific IgG precipitating antibody titers for agents capable of causing hypersensitivity pneumonitis (pigeon antigen in bird handlers), and assays for specific cell-mediated immune responses (beryllium lymphocyte proliferation testing in nuclear workers or tuberculin skin testing in health care workers). Sometimes a bronchoscopy to obtain transbronchial biopsies of lung tissue may be required for histologic diagnosis (chronic beryllium disease). Rarely, video-assisted thoracoscopic surgery to obtain a larger sample of lung tissue may be required to determine the specific diagnosis of environmentally induced lung disease (hypersensitivity pneumonitis or giant cell interstitial pneumonitis due to cobalt exposure).

EXPOSURE ASSESSMENT

If reliable environmental sampling data are available, that information should be used in assessing a patient's exposure. Since many of the chronic diseases result from exposure over many years, current environmental measurements should be combined with work histories to arrive at estimates of past exposure.

In situations in which individual exposure to specific agents—either in a work setting or via ambient air pollutants—has been determined, the chemical and physical characteristics of those agents affect both the inhaled dose and the site of deposition in the respiratory tract. Water-soluble gases such as ammonia and sulfur dioxide are absorbed in the lining fluid of the upper and proximal airways and thus tend to produce irritative and bronchoconstrictive responses. In contrast, nitrogen dioxide and phosgene, which are less soluble, may penetrate to the bronchioles and alveoli in sufficient quantities to produce acute chemical pneumonitis that can be life-threatening.

Particle size of air contaminants must also be considered. Because of their settling velocities in air, particles >10–15 μm in diameter do not penetrate beyond the nose and throat. Particles <10 μm in size are deposited below the larynx. These particles are divided into three size fractions on the basis of their size characteristics and sources. Particles ~2.5–10 μm (coarse-mode fraction) contain crustal elements such as silica, aluminum, and iron. These particles mostly deposit relatively high in the tracheobronchial tree. Although the total mass of an ambient sample is dominated by these larger respirable particles, the number of particles, and therefore the surface area on which potential toxic agents can deposit and be carried to the lower airways, is dominated by particles <2.5 μm (fine-mode fraction). These fine particles are created primarily by the burning of fossil fuels or high-temperature industrial processes resulting in condensation products from gases, fumes, or vapors. The smallest particles, those <0.1 μm in size, represent the ultrafine fraction and make up the largest number of particles; they tend to remain in the airstream and deposit in the lung only on a random basis as they come into contact with the alveolar walls. If they do deposit, however, particles of this size range may penetrate into the circulation and be carried to extrapulmonary sites. New technologies create particles of this size ("nanoparticles") for use in many commercial applications. Besides the size characteristics of particles and the solubility of gases, the actual chemical composition, mechanical properties, and immunogenicity or infectivity of inhaled material determine in large part the nature of the diseases found among exposed persons.

OCCUPATIONAL EXPOSURES AND PULMONARY DISEASE

Table 10-1 provides broad categories of exposure in the workplace and diseases associated with chronic exposure in those industries.

ASBESTOS-RELATED DISEASES

Asbestos is a generic term for several different mineral silicates, including chrysolite, amosite, anthophyllite, and crocidolite. In addition to workers involved in the production of asbestos products (mining, milling, and manufacturing), many workers in the shipbuilding and construction trades, including pipe fitters and boiler-makers, were occupationally exposed because asbestos was widely used during the twentieth century for its thermal and electrical insulation properties. Asbestos also was used in the manufacture of fire-resistant textiles, in cement and floor tiles, and in friction materials such as brake and clutch linings.

TABLE 10-1

CATEGORIES OF OCCUPATIONAL EXPOSURE AND ASSOCIATED RESPIRATORY CONDITIONS		
OCCUPATIONAL EXPOSURES	**NATURE OF RESPIRATORY RESPONSES**	**COMMENT**
Inorganic Dusts		
Asbestos: mining, processing, construction, ship repair	Fibrosis (asbestosis), pleural disease, cancer, mesothelioma	Virtually all new mining and construction with asbestos done in developing countries
Silica: mining, stone cutting, sandblasting, quarrying	Fibrosis (silicosis), progressive massive fibrosis (PMF), cancer, tuberculosis, chronic obstructive pulmonary disease (COPD)	Improved protection in United States, persistent risk in developing countries
Coal dust: mining	Fibrosis (coal worker's pneumoconiosis), PMF, COPD	Risk persists in certain areas of United States, increasing in countries where new mines open
Beryllium: processing alloys for high-tech industries	Acute pneumonitis (rare), chronic granulomatous disease, lung cancer (highly suspect)	Risk in high-tech industries persists
Other metals: aluminum, chromium, cobalt, nickel, titanium, tungsten carbide, or "hard metal" (contains cobalt)	Wide variety of conditions from acute pneumonitis to lung cancer and asthma	New diseases appear with new process development
Organic Dusts		
Cotton dust: milling, processing	Byssinosis (an asthma-like syndrome), chronic bronchitis, COPD	Increasing risk in developing countries with drop in United States as jobs shift overseas
Grain dust: elevator agents, dock workers, milling, bakers	Asthma, chronic bronchitis, COPD	Risk shifting more to migrant labor pool
Other agricultural dusts: fungal spores, vegetable products, insect fragments, animal dander, bird and rodent feces, endotoxins, microorganisms, pollens	Hypersensitivity pneumonitis (farmer's lung), asthma, chronic bronchitis	Important in migrant labor pool but also resulting from in-home exposures
Toxic chemicals: wide variety of industries, see Table 10-2	Asthma, chronic bronchitis, COPD, hypersensitivity pneumonitis, pneumoconiosis, and cancer	Reduced risk with recognized hazards; increasing risk for developing countries where controlled labor practices are less stringent
Other respiratory environmental agents: uranium and radon daughters, secondhand tobacco smoke, polycyclic hydrocarbons, biomass smoke, diesel exhaust, welding fumes, wood finishing	Occupational exposures estimated to contribute to up to 10% of all lung cancers; chronic bronchitis, COPD, and fibrosis	In-home exposures important; in developing countries biomass smoke is a major risk factor for COPD among women

Exposure to asbestos is not limited to persons who directly handle the material. Cases of asbestos-related diseases have been encountered in individuals with only bystander exposure, such as painters and electricians who worked alongside insulation workers in a shipyard. Community exposure resulted from the use of asbestos-containing mine and mill tailings as landfill, road surface, and playground material (e.g., Libby, MT, the site of a vermiculite mine in which the ore was contaminated with asbestos). Finally, exposure can occur from the disturbance of naturally occurring asbestos (e.g., from increasing residential development in the foothills of the Sierra Mountains in California).

Asbestos has largely been replaced in the developed world with synthetic mineral fibers such as fiberglass and refractory ceramic fibers, but it continues to be used increasingly in the developing world. Despite current OSHA regulations mandating adequate training for any worker potentially exposed to asbestos, exposure continues among inadequately trained and protected demolition workers. The major health effects from exposure to asbestos are pleural and pulmonary fibrosis, cancers of the respiratory tract, and pleural and peritoneal mesothelioma.

Asbestosis is a diffuse interstitial fibrosing disease of the lung that is directly related to the intensity and duration of exposure. The disease resembles other forms of diffuse interstitial fibrosis (Chap. 19). Usually, moderate to severe exposure has taken place for at least 10 years before the disease becomes manifest, and it may occur after exposure to any of the asbestiform fiber types. The mechanisms by which asbestos fibers induce lung fibrosis are not completely understood but are known to involve oxidative injury due to the generation of reactive oxygen species by the transition metals on the surface of the fibers as well as from cells engaged in phagocytosis.

The chest radiograph can be used to detect the pulmonary manifestations of asbestos exposure. Past exposure is specifically indicated by pleural plaques, which are characterized by either thickening or calcification along the parietal pleura, particularly along the lower lung fields, the diaphragm, and the cardiac border. Without additional manifestations, pleural plaques imply only exposure, not pulmonary impairment. Benign pleural effusions also may occur. The fluid is typically a serous or bloody exudate. The effusion may be slowly progressive or may resolve spontaneously. Irregular or linear opacities, evidence of asbestosis that usually are first noted in the lower lung fields and spreading into the middle and upper lung fields, occur as the disease progresses. An indistinct heart border or a "ground-glass" appearance in the lung fields is seen in some cases. In cases in which the x-ray changes are less obvious, HRCT may show distinct changes of subpleural curvilinear lines 5–10 mm in length that appear to be parallel to the pleural surface **(Fig. 10-1)**.

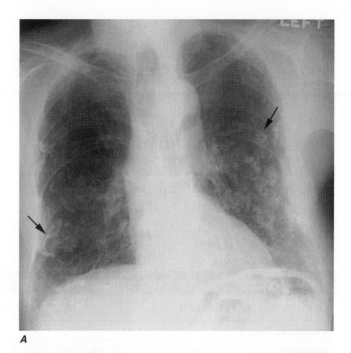

A

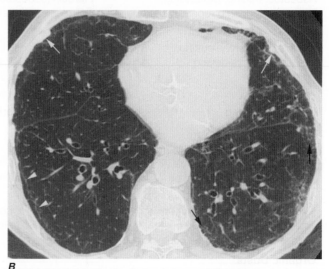

B

FIGURE 10-1
Asbestosis: A. Frontal chest radiograph shows bilateral calcified pleural plaques consistent with asbestos-related pleural disease. Poorly defined linear and reticular abnormalities are seen in the lower lobes bilaterally. **B.** Axial high-resolution computed tomography of the thorax obtained through the lung bases shows bilateral, subpleural reticulation (*black arrows*), representing fibrotic lung disease due to asbestosis. Subpleural lines are also present (*arrowheads*), characteristic of, though not specific for, asbestosis. Calcified pleural plaques representing asbestos-related pleural disease (*white arrows*) are also evident.

Pulmonary function testing in asbestosis reveals a restrictive pattern with a decrease in both lung volumes and diffusing capacity. There may also be evidence of mild airflow obstruction (due to peribronchiolar fibrosis).

No specific therapy is available for the management of patients with asbestosis. The supportive care is the same as that given to any patient with diffuse interstitial fibrosis of any cause. In general, newly diagnosed cases will have resulted from exposures that occurred many years before.

Lung cancer is the most common cancer associated with asbestos exposure. The excess frequency of lung cancer (all histologic types) in asbestos workers is associated with a minimum latency of 15–19 years between first exposure and development of the disease. Persons with more exposure are at greater risk of disease. In addition, there is a significant interactive effect of smoking and asbestos exposure that results in greater risk than what would be expected from the additive effect of each factor.

Mesotheliomas (Chap. 21), both pleural and peritoneal, are also associated with asbestos exposure. In contrast to lung cancers, these tumors do not appear to be associated with smoking. Relatively short-term asbestos exposures of ≤1–2 years or less, occurring up to 40 years in the past, have been associated with the development of mesotheliomas (an observation that emphasizes the importance of obtaining a complete environmental exposure history). Although the risk of mesothelioma is much less than that of lung cancer among asbestos-exposed workers, over 2000 cases were reported in the United States per year at the start of the twenty-first century.

Although ~50% of mesotheliomas metastasize, the tumor generally is locally invasive, and death usually results from local extension. Most patients present with effusions that may obscure the underlying pleural tumor. In contrast to the findings in effusion due to other causes, because of the restriction placed on the chest wall, no shift of mediastinal structures toward the opposite side of the chest will be seen. The major diagnostic problem is differentiation from peripherally spreading pulmonary adenocarcinoma or adenocarcinoma that has metastasized to pleura from an extrathoracic primary site. Although cytologic examination of pleural fluid may suggest the diagnosis, biopsy of pleural tissue, generally with video-assisted thoracic surgery, and special immunohistochemical staining usually are required. There is no effective therapy.

Since epidemiologic studies have shown that >80% of mesotheliomas may be associated with asbestos exposure, documented mesothelioma in a patient with occupational or environmental exposure to asbestos may be compensable.

SILICOSIS

In spite of being one of the oldest known occupational pulmonary hazards, *free silica* (SiO$_2$), or crystalline quartz, is still a major cause of disease. The major occupational exposures include mining; stonecutting; employment in abrasive industries such as stone, clay, glass, and cement manufacturing; foundry work; packing of silica flour; and quarrying, particularly of granite. Most often, pulmonary fibrosis due to silica exposure (silicosis) occurs in a dose-response fashion after many years of exposure.

Workers heavily exposed through sandblasting in confined spaces, tunneling through rock with a high quartz content (15–25%), or the manufacture of abrasive soaps may develop acute silicosis with as little as 10 months of exposure. The clinical and pathologic features of acute silicosis are similar to those of pulmonary alveolar proteinosis (Chap. 19). The chest radiograph may show profuse miliary infiltration or consolidation, and there is a characteristic HRCT pattern known as "crazy paving" **(Fig. 10-2)**. The disease may be quite severe and progressive despite the discontinuation of exposure. Whole-lung lavage may provide symptomatic relief and slow the progression.

With long-term, less intense exposure, small rounded opacities in the upper lobes may appear on the chest radiograph after 15–20 years of exposure (*simple silicosis*). Calcification of hilar nodes may occur in as many as 20% of cases and produces a characteristic "eggshell" pattern. Silicotic nodules may be identified more readily

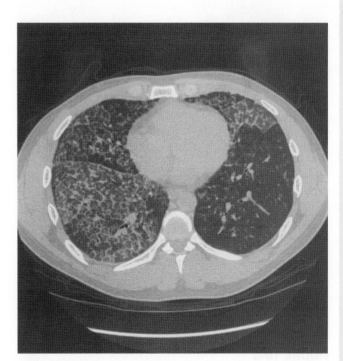

FIGURE 10-2

Acute silicosis. This high-resolution computed tomography scan shows multiple small nodules consistent with silicosis but also diffuse ground-glass densities with thickened intralobular and interlobular septa producing polygonal shapes. This has been referred to as "crazy paving."

by HRCT (**Fig. 10-3**). The nodular fibrosis may be progressive in the absence of further exposure, with coalescence and formation of nonsegmental conglomerates of irregular masses >1 cm in diameter (*complicated silicosis*). These masses can become quite large, and when this occurs, the term *progressive massive fibrosis* (PMF) is applied. Significant functional impairment with both restrictive and obstructive components may be associated with this form of silicosis.

Because silica is cytotoxic to alveolar macrophages, patients with silicosis are at greater risk of acquiring lung infections that involve these cells as a primary defense (*Mycobacterium tuberculosis*, atypical mycobacteria and fungi). Because of the increased risk of active tuberculosis, the recommended treatment of latent tuberculosis in these patients is longer. Another potential clinical complication of silicosis is autoimmune connective tissue disorders such as rheumatoid arthritis and scleroderma. In addition, there are sufficient epidemiologic data that

the International Agency for Research on Cancer lists silica as a probable lung carcinogen.

Other, less hazardous silicates include fuller's earth, kaolin, mica, diatomaceous earths, silica gel, soapstone, carbonate dusts, and cement dusts. The production of fibrosis in workers exposed to these agents is believed to be related either to the free silica content of these dusts or, for substances that contain no free silica, to the potentially large dust loads to which these workers may be exposed.

Other silicates, including *talc dusts*, may be contaminated with asbestos and/or free silica. Fibrosis and/or pleural or lung cancer have been associated with chronic exposure to commercial talc.

COAL WORKER'S PNEUMOCONIOSIS (CWP)

Occupational exposure to *coal dust* can lead to CWP, which has enormous social, economic, and medical significance in every nation in which coal mining is an important industry. Simple radiographically identified CWP is seen in ~10% of all coal miners and in as many as 50% of anthracite miners with more than 20 years' work on the coal face. The prevalence of disease is lower in workers in bituminous coal mines.

With prolonged exposure to coal dust (i.e., 15–20 years), small, rounded opacities similar to those of silicosis may develop. As in silicosis, the presence of these nodules (*simple CWP*) usually is not associated with pulmonary impairment. Much of the symptomatology associated with simple CWP appears to be due to the effects of coal dust on the development of chronic bronchitis and COPD (Chap. 18). The effects of coal dust are additive to those of cigarette smoking.

Complicated CWP is manifested by the appearance on the chest radiograph of nodules ranging from 1 cm in diameter to the size of an entire lobe, generally confined to the upper half of the lungs. As in silicosis, this condition can progress to PMF that is accompanied by severe lung function deficits and associated with premature mortality. Despite improvements in technology to protect coal miners, cases of PMF still occur in the United States at a disturbing rate.

Caplan's syndrome, first described in coal miners but subsequently found in patients with silicosis, includes seropositive rheumatoid arthritis with characteristic pneumoconiotic nodules. Silica has immunoadjuvant properties and is often present in anthracitic coal dust.

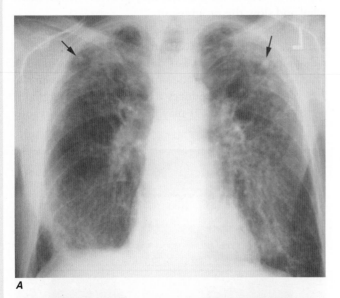

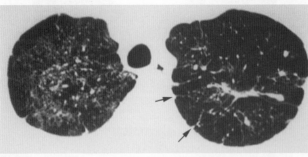

FIGURE 10-3
Chronic silicosis. *A.* Frontal chest radiograph in a patient with silicosis shows variably sized, poorly defined nodules (*arrows*) predominating in the upper lobes, ***B.*** Axial thoracic computed tomography image through the lung apices shows numerous small nodules, more pronounced in the right upper lobe. A number of the nodules are subpleural in location (*arrows*).

CHRONIC BERYLLIUM DISEASE

Beryllium is a lightweight metal with tensile strength that has good electrical conductivity and is valuable in the control of nuclear reactions through its ability to quench neutrons. Although beryllium may produce an acute pneumonitis, it is far more commonly associated with a chronic granulomatous inflammatory disease that is similar to sarcoidosis. Unless one inquires specifically about occupational exposures to beryllium in the manufacture of alloys, ceramics, or high-technology electronics in a patient with sarcoidosis, one may miss entirely the etiologic relationship to the occupational exposure. What distinguishes chronic beryllium disease (CBD) from sarcoidosis is evidence of a specific cell-mediated immune response (i.e., delayed hypersensitivity) to beryllium.

The test that usually provides this evidence is the beryllium lymphocyte proliferation test (BeLPT). The BeLPT compares the in vitro proliferation of lymphocytes from blood or bronchoalveolar lavage in the presence of beryllium salts with that of unstimulated cells. Proliferation is usually measured by lymphocyte uptake of radiolabeled thymidine.

Chest imaging findings are similar to those of sarcoidosis (nodules along septal lines) except that hilar adenopathy is somewhat less common. As with sarcoidosis, pulmonary function test results may show restrictive and/or obstructive ventilatory deficits and decreased diffusing capacity. With early disease, both chest imaging studies and pulmonary function tests may be normal. Fiberoptic bronchoscopy with transbronchial lung biopsy usually is required to make the diagnosis of CBD. In a beryllium-sensitized individual, the presence of noncaseating granulomas or monocytic infiltration in lung tissue establishes the diagnosis. Accumulation of beryllium-specific CD4+ T cells occurs in the granulomatous inflammation seen on lung biopsy. CBD is one of the best studied examples of gene-environment interaction. Susceptibility to CBD is highly associated with human leukocyte antigen DP (HLA-DP) alleles that have a glutamic acid in position 69 of the β chain.

Other metals, including aluminum and titanium dioxide, have been rarely associated with a sarcoid-like reaction in lung tissue. Exposure to dust containing tungsten carbide, also known as "hard metal," may produce giant cell interstitial pneumonitis. Cobalt is a constituent of tungsten carbide and is the likely etiologic agent of both the interstitial pneumonitis and the occupational asthma that may occur. The most common exposures to tungsten carbide occur in tool and dye, saw blade, and drill bit manufacture. Diamond polishing may also involve exposure to cobalt dust. The same Glu69 polymorphism of the HLA-DP β chain that confers increased risk of CBD also appears to increase the risk of cobalt-induced giant cell interstitial pneumonitis.

In patients with interstitial lung disease, one should always inquire about exposure to metal fumes and/or dusts. Especially when sarcoidosis appears to be the diagnosis, one should always consider possible CBD.

OTHER INORGANIC DUSTS

Most of the inorganic dusts discussed thus far are associated with the production of either dust macules or interstitial fibrotic changes in the lung. Other inorganic and organic dusts (see categories in Table 10-1), along with some of the dusts previously discussed, are associated with chronic mucus hypersecretion (chronic bronchitis), with or without reduction of expiratory flow rates. Cigarette smoking is the major cause of these conditions, and any effort to attribute some component of the disease to occupational and environmental exposures must take cigarette smoking into account. Most studies suggest an additive effect of dust exposure and smoking. The pattern of the irritant dust effect is similar to that of cigarette smoking, suggesting that small airway inflammation may be the initial site of pathologic response in those cases and continued exposure may lead to chronic bronchitis and COPD.

ORGANIC DUSTS

Some of the specific diseases associated with organic dusts are discussed in detail in the chapters on asthma (Chap. 8) and hypersensitivity pneumonitis (Chap. 9). Many of these diseases are named for the specific setting in which they are found, e.g., farmer's lung, malt worker's disease, and mushroom worker's disease. Often the temporal relation of symptoms to exposure furnishes the best evidence for the diagnosis. Three occupational exposures are singled out for discussion here because they affect the largest proportions of workers.

Cotton dust (byssinosis)

Workers occupationally exposed to cotton dust (but also to flax, hemp, or jute dust) in the production of yarns for textiles and rope making are at risk for an asthma-like syndrome known as byssinosis. Exposure occurs throughout the manufacturing process but is most pronounced in the portions of the factory involved with the treatment of the cotton before spinning, i.e., blowing, mixing, and carding (straightening of fibers). The risk of byssinosis is associated with both cotton dust and endotoxin levels in the workplace environment.

Byssinosis is characterized clinically as occasional (early-stage) and then regular (late-stage) chest tightness toward the end of the first day of the workweek ("Monday chest tightness"). In epidemiologic studies, depending on the level of exposure via the carding room air, up to 80% of employees may show a significant drop in FEV_1 over the course of a Monday shift.

Initially the symptoms do not recur on subsequent days of the week. However, in 10–25% of workers, the disease may be progressive, with chest tightness recurring or persisting throughout the workweek. After >10 years of exposure, workers with recurrent symptoms are more likely to have an obstructive pattern on pulmonary function testing. The highest grades of impairment generally are seen in smokers.

Reduction of dust exposure is of primary importance to the management of byssinosis. Dust levels can be controlled by the use of exhaust hoods, general increases in ventilation, and wetting procedures, but respiratory protective equipment appears to be required during certain operations to prevent workers from being exposed to levels of cotton dust that exceed the current OSHA-permissible exposure level. Regular surveillance of pulmonary function in cotton dust–exposed workers using spirometry before and after the workshift is required by OSHA. All workers with persistent symptoms or significantly reduced levels of pulmonary function should be moved to areas of lower risk of exposure.

Grain dust

Worldwide, many farmers and workers in grain storage facilities are exposed to grain dust. The presentation of obstructive airway disease in grain dust–exposed workers is virtually identical to the characteristic findings in cigarette smokers, i.e., persistent cough, mucus hypersecretion, wheeze and dyspnea on exertion, and reduced FEV_1 and FEV_1/FVC (forced vital capacity) ratio (Chap. 5).

Dust concentrations in grain elevators vary greatly but can be >10,000 $\mu g/m^3$; approximately one-third of the particles, by weight, are in the respirable range. The effect of grain dust exposure is additive to that of cigarette smoking, with ~50% of workers who smoke having symptoms. Among nonsmoking grain elevator operators, approximately one-quarter have mucus hypersecretion, about five times the number that would be expected in unexposed nonsmokers. Smoking grain dust–exposed workers are more likely to have obstructive ventilatory deficits on pulmonary function testing. As in byssinosis, endotoxin may play a role in grain dust–induced chronic bronchitis and COPD.

Farmer's lung

This condition results from exposure to moldy hay containing spores of thermophilic actinomycetes that produce a hypersensitivity pneumonitis (Chap. 9). A patient with acute farmer's lung presents 4–8 h after exposure with fever, chills, malaise, cough, and dyspnea without wheezing. The history of exposure is obviously essential to distinguish this disease from influenza or pneumonia with similar symptoms. In the chronic form of the disease, the history of repeated attacks after similar exposure is important in differentiating this

syndrome from other causes of patchy fibrosis (e.g., sarcoidosis).

A wide variety of other organic dusts are associated with the occurrence of hypersensitivity pneumonitis (Chap. 9). For patients who present with hypersensitivity pneumonitis, specific and careful inquiry about occupations, hobbies, and other home environmental exposures is necessary to uncover the source of the etiologic agent.

TOXIC CHEMICALS

Exposure to toxic chemicals affecting the lung generally involves gases and vapors. A common accident is one in which the victim is trapped in a confined space where the chemicals have accumulated to toxic levels. In addition to the specific toxic effects of the chemical, the victim often sustains considerable anoxia, which can play a dominant role in determining whether the individual survives.

Table 10-2 lists a variety of toxic agents that can produce acute and sometimes life-threatening reactions in the lung. All these agents in sufficient concentrations have been demonstrated, at least in animal studies, to affect the lower airways and disrupt alveolar architecture, either acutely or as a result of chronic exposure. Some of these agents may be generated acutely in the environment (see later).

Firefighters and fire victims are at risk of *smoke inhalation*, an important cause of acute cardiorespiratory failure. Smoke inhalation kills more fire victims than does thermal injury. Carbon monoxide poisoning with resulting significant hypoxemia can be life-threatening. Synthetic materials (plastic, polyurethanes), when burned, may release a variety of other toxic agents (such as cyanide and hydrochloric acid), and this must be considered in evaluating smoke inhalation victims. Exposed victims may have some degree of lower respiratory tract inflammation and/or pulmonary edema.

Exposure to certain highly reactive, low-molecular-weight agents used in the manufacture of synthetic polymers, paints, and coatings (*diisocyanates* in polyurethanes, *aromatic amines* and *acid anhydrides* in epoxies) are associated with a high risk of occupational asthma. Although this occupational asthma manifests clinically as if sensitization has occurred, an IgE antibody–mediated mechanism is not necessarily involved. Hypersensitivity pneumonitis–like reactions also have been described in diisocyanate and acid anhydride–exposed workers.

Fluoropolymers such as Teflon, which at normal temperatures produce no reaction, become volatilized upon heating. The inhaled agents cause a characteristic syndrome of fever, chills, malaise, and occasionally mild wheezing, leading to the diagnosis of *polymer fume fever*. A similar self-limited, influenza-like syndrome—*metal*

TABLE 10-2   101

SELECTED COMMON TOXIC CHEMICAL AGENTS THAT AFFECT THE LUNG

AGENT(S)	SELECTED EXPOSURES	ACUTE EFFECTS FROM HIGH OR ACCIDENTAL EXPOSURE	CHRONIC EFFECTS FROM RELATIVELY LOW EXPOSURE
Acid anhydrides	Manufacture of resin esters, polyester resins, thermoactivated adhesives	Nasal irritation, cough	Asthma, chronic bronchitis, hypersensitivity pneumonitis
Acid fumes: H_2SO_4, HNO_3	Manufacture of fertilizers, chlorinated organic compounds, dyes, explosives, rubber products, metal etching, plastics	Mucous membrane irritation, followed by chemical pneumonitis 2–3 days later	Bronchitis and suggestion of mildly reduced pulmonary function in children with lifelong residential exposure to high levels
Acrolein and other aldehydes	By-product of burning plastics, woods, tobacco smoke	Mucous membrane irritant, decrease in lung function	Upper respiratory tract irritation
Ammonia	Refrigeration; petroleum refining; manufacture of fertilizers, explosives, plastics, and other chemicals	Same as for acid fumes, but bronchiectasis also has been reported	Upper respiratory tract irritation, chronic bronchitis
Cadmium fumes	Smelting, soldering, battery production	Mucous membrane irritant, acute respiratory distress syndrome (ARDS)	Chronic obstructive pulmonary disease (COPD)
Formaldehyde	Manufacture of resins, leathers, rubber, metals, and woods; laboratory workers, embalmers; emission from urethane foam insulation	Same as for acid fumes	Nasopharyngeal cancer
Halides and acid salts (Cl, Br, F)	Bleaching in pulp, paper, textile industry; manufacture of chemical compounds; synthetic rubber, plastics, disinfectant, rocket fuel, gasoline	Mucous membrane irritation, pulmonary edema; possible reduced FVC 1–2 yrs after exposure	Upper respiratory tract irritation, epistaxis, tracheobronchitis
Hydrogen sulfide	By-product of many industrial processes, oil, other petroleum processes and storage	Increase in respiratory rate followed by respiratory arrest, lactic acidosis, pulmonary edema, death	Conjunctival irritation, chronic bronchitis, recurrent pneumonitis
Isocyanates (TDI, HDI, MDI)	Production of polyurethane foams, plastics, adhesives, surface coatings	Mucous membrane irritation, dyspnea, cough, wheeze, pulmonary edema	Upper respiratory tract irritation, cough, asthma, hypersensitivity pneumonitis, reduced lung function
Nitrogen dioxide	Silage, metal etching, explosives, rocket fuels, welding, by-product of burning fossil fuels	Cough, dyspnea, pulmonary edema may be delayed 4–12 h; possible result from acute exposure: bronchiolitis obliterans in 2–6 wks	Emphysema in animals, ?chronic bronchitis, associated with reduced lung function in children with lifelong residential exposure
Ozone	Arc welding, flour bleaching, deodorizing, emissions from copying equipment, photochemical air pollutant	Mucous membrane irritant, pulmonary hemorrhage and edema, reduced pulmonary function transiently in children and adults, and increased hospitalization with exposure to summer haze	Excess cardiopulmonary mortality rates
Phosgene	Organic compound, metallurgy, volatilization of chlorine-containing compounds	Delayed onset of bronchiolitis and pulmonary edema	Chronic bronchitis
Sulfur dioxide	Manufacture of sulfuric acid, bleaches, coating of nonferrous metals, food processing, refrigerant, burning of fossil fuels, wood pulp industry	Mucous membrane irritant, epistaxis, bronchospasm (especially in people with asthma)	Chronic bronchitis

fume fever—results from acute exposure to fumes or smoke containing zinc oxide. The syndrome may begin several hours after work and resolves within 24 h, only to return on repeated exposure. Welding of galvanized steel is the most common exposure leading to metal fume fever.

Two other agents have been recently associated with potentially severe interstitial lung disease. Occupational exposure to nylon flock has been shown to induce a lymphocytic bronchiolitis, and workers exposed to diacetyl used to provide "butter" flavor in the manufacture of microwave popcorn and other foods have developed bronchiolitis obliterans (Chap. 19).

World Trade Center disaster

A consequence of the attack on the World Trade Center (WTC) on September 11, 2001, was relatively heavy exposure of a large number of firefighters and other rescue workers to the dust generated by the collapse of the buildings. Environmental monitoring and chemical characterization of WTC dust has revealed a wide variety of potentially toxic constituents, although much of the dust was pulverized cement. Possibly because of the high alkalinity of WTC dust, significant cough, wheeze, and phlegm production occurred among firefighters and cleanup crews. New cough and wheeze syndromes also occurred among local residents. Initial longitudinal follow-up of New York firefighters suggests that heavier exposure to WTC dust is associated with accelerated decline of lung function. Ongoing follow-up will provide data on whether massive exposure to this irritant dust has led to the development of chronic respiratory disease.

OCCUPATIONAL RESPIRATORY CARCINOGENS

Exposures at work have been estimated to contribute to 10% of all lung cancer cases. In addition to asbestos, other agents either proven or suspected to be respiratory carcinogens include acrylonitrile, arsenic compounds, beryllium, bis (chloromethyl) ether, chromium (hexavalent), formaldehyde (nasal), isopropanol (nasal sinuses), mustard gas, nickel carbonyl (nickel smelting), polyaromatic hydrocarbons (coke oven emissions and diesel exhaust), secondhand tobacco smoke, silica (both mining and processing), talc (possible asbestos contamination in both mining and milling), vinyl chloride (sarcomas), wood (nasal cancer only), and uranium. Workers at risk of radiation-related lung cancer include not only those involved in mining or processing uranium but also those exposed in underground mining operations of other ores where radon daughters may be emitted from rock formations.

ASSESSMENT OF DISABILITY

Patients who have lung disease may not be able to continue to work in their usual jobs because of respiratory symptoms. *Disability* is the term used to describe the decreased ability to work due to the effects of a medical condition. Physicians are generally able to assess physiologic dysfunction, or *impairment*, but the rating of disability for compensation of loss of income also involves nonmedical factors such as the education and employability of the individual. The disability rating scheme differs with the compensation-granting agency. For example, the U.S. Social Security Administration requires that an individual be unable to do any work (i.e., *total* disability) before he or she will receive income replacement payments. Many state workers' compensation systems allow for payments for *partial* disability. In the Social Security scheme no determination of cause is done, whereas work-relatedness must be established in workers' compensation systems.

For respiratory impairment rating, resting pulmonary function tests (spirometry and diffusing capacity) are used as the initial assessment tool, with cardiopulmonary exercise testing (to assess maximal oxygen consumption) used if the results of the resting tests do not correlate with the patient's symptoms. Methacholine challenge (to assess airway reactivity) can also be useful in patients with asthma who have normal spirometry when evaluated. Some compensation agencies (e.g., Social Security) have proscribed disability classification schemes based on pulmonary function test results. When no specific scheme is proscribed, the *Guidelines of the American Medical Association* should be used.

Evaluating relation to work exposure requires a detailed work history, as previously discussed in this chapter. Occasionally, as with some cases of suspected occupational asthma, challenge to the putative agent in the work environment with repeated pulmonary function measures may be required.

GENERAL ENVIRONMENTAL EXPOSURES

OUTDOOR AIR POLLUTION

In 1971, the U.S. government established national air quality standards for several pollutants believed to be responsible for excess cardiorespiratory diseases. Primary standards regulated by the U.S. Environmental Protection Agency (EPA) designed to protect the public health with an adequate margin of safety exist for sulfur dioxide, particulates matter, nitrogen dioxide, ozone, lead, and carbon monoxide. Standards for each of these pollutants are updated regularly through an extensive review process conducted by the EPA. (For details on current standards, go to *http://www.epa.gov/air/criteria.html.*)

Pollutants are generated from both stationary sources (power plants and industrial complexes) and mobile sources (automobiles), and none of the regulated pollutants occurs in isolation. Furthermore, pollutants may be changed by chemical reactions after being emitted. For example, sulfur dioxide and particulate matter emissions from a coal-fired power plant may react in air to produce acid sulfates and aerosols, which can be transported long distances in the atmosphere. Oxidizing substances such as oxides of nitrogen and volatile organic compounds from automobile exhaust may react with sunlight to produce ozone. Although originally thought to be confined to Los Angeles, photochemically derived pollution ("smog") is now known to be a problem throughout the United States and in many other countries. Both acute and chronic effects of these exposures have been documented in large population studies.

The symptoms and diseases associated with air pollution are the same as conditions commonly associated with cigarette smoking. In addition, decreased growth of lung function and asthma have been associated with chronic exposure to only modestly elevated levels of traffic-related gases and respirable particles. Multiple population-based time-series studies within cities have demonstrated excess health care utilization for asthma and other cardiopulmonary conditions and mortality rates. Cohort studies comparing cities that have relatively high levels of particulate exposures with less polluted communities suggest excess morbidity and mortality rates from cardiopulmonary conditions in long-term residents of the former. The strong epidemiologic evidence that fine particulate matter is a risk factor for cardiovascular morbidity and mortality has prompted toxicologic investigations into the underlying mechanisms. The inhalation of fine particles from combustion sources probably generates oxidative stress followed by local injury and inflammation in the lungs that in turn lead to autonomic and systemic inflammatory responses that can induce endothelial dysfunction and/or injury. Recent research findings on the health effects of air pollutants have led to stricter U.S. ambient air quality standards for ozone, oxides of nitrogen, and particulate matter as well as greater emphasis on publicizing pollution alerts to encourage individuals with significant cardiopulmonary impairment to stay indoors during high-pollution episodes.

INDOOR EXPOSURES

Secondhand tobacco smoke, radon gas, wood smoke, and other biologic agents generated indoors must be considered. Several studies have shown that the respirable particulate load in any household is directly proportional to the number of cigarette smokers living in that home. Increases in prevalence of respiratory illnesses, especially asthma, and reduced levels of pulmonary function measured with simple spirometry have been found in the children of smoking parents in a number of studies. Recent meta-analyses for lung cancer and cardiopulmonary diseases, combining data from multiple secondhand tobacco smoke epidemiologic studies, suggest an ~25% increase in relative risk for each condition, even after adjustment for major potential confounders.

Exposure to *radon gas* in homes is a risk factor for lung cancer. The main radon product (radon 222) is a gas that results from the decay series of uranium 238, with the immediate precursor being radium 226. The amount of radium in earth materials determines how much radon gas will be emitted. Outdoors, the concentrations are trivial. Indoors, levels are dependent on the sources, the ventilation rate of the space, and the size of the space into which the gas is emitted. Levels associated with excess lung cancer risk may be present in as many as 10% of the houses in the United States. When smokers reside in the home, the problem is potentially greater, since the molecular size of radon particles allows them to attach readily to smoke particles that are inhaled. Fortunately, technology is available for assessing and reducing the level of exposure.

Other indoor exposures of concern are bioaerosols that contain antigenic material (fungi, cockroaches, dust mites, and pet danders) associated with an increased risk of atopy and asthma. Indoor chemical agents include strong cleaning agents (bleach, ammonia), formaldehyde, perfumes, pesticides, and oxides of nitrogen from gas appliances. Nonspecific responses associated with "tight-building syndrome," perhaps better termed "building-associated illness," in which no particular agent has been implicated, have included a wide variety of complaints, among them respiratory symptoms that are relieved only by avoiding exposure in the building in question. The degree to which "smells" and other sensory stimuli are involved in the triggering of potentially incapacitating psychological or physical responses has yet to be determined, and the long-term consequences of such environmental exposures are unknown.

PORTAL OF ENTRY

The lung is a primary point of entry into the body for a number of toxic agents that affect other organ systems. For example, the lung is a route of entry for benzene (bone marrow), carbon disulfide (cardiovascular and nervous systems), cadmium (kidney), and metallic mercury (kidney, central nervous system). Thus, in any disease state of obscure origin, it is important to consider the possibility of inhaled environmental agents. Such consideration can sometimes furnish the clue needed to identify a specific external cause for a disorder that might otherwise be labeled "idiopathic."

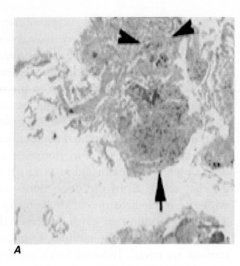

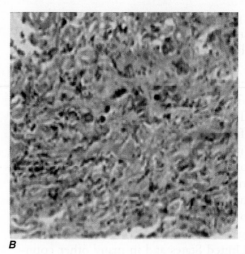

FIGURE 10-4

Histopathologic features of biomass smoke–induced interstitial lung disease. **A.** Anthracitic pigment is seen accumulating along alveolar septae (*arrowheads*) and within a pigmented dust macule (*single arrow*). **B.** A high-power photomicrograph contains a mixture of fibroblasts and carbon-laden macrophages.

Global considerations

Indoor exposure to *biomass smoke* (wood, dung, crop residues, charcoal) is estimated to be responsible for ~3% of worldwide disability-adjusted life-years (DALYs) lost, due to acute lower respiratory infections in children and COPD and lung cancer in women. This burden of disease places indoor exposure to biomass smoke as the second leading environmental hazard for poor health, just behind unsafe water, sanitation, and hygiene, and is 3.5 times larger than the burden attributed to outdoor air pollution.

More than one-half of the world's population uses biomass fuel for cooking, heating, or baking. This occurs predominantly in the rural areas of developing countries. Because many families burn biomass fuels in open stoves, which are highly inefficient, and inside homes with poor ventilation, women and young children are exposed on a daily basis to high levels of smoke. In these homes, 24-h mean levels of fine particulate matter, a component of biomass smoke, have been reported to be 2–30 times higher than the National Ambient Air Quality Standards set by the U.S. EPA.

Epidemiologic studies have consistently shown associations between exposure to biomass smoke and both chronic bronchitis and COPD, with odds ratios ranging between 3 and 10 and increasing with longer exposures. In addition to the common occupational exposure to biomass smoke of women in developing countries, men from such countries may be occupationally exposed. Because of increased migration to the United States from developing countries, clinicians need to be aware of the chronic respiratory effects of exposure to biomass smoke, which can include interstitial lung disease (Fig. 10-4). Evidence is beginning to emerge that improved stoves with chimneys can reduce biomass smoke–induced respiratory illness in both children and women.

CHAPTER 11

PNEUMONIA

Lionel A. Mandell ■ Richard Wunderink

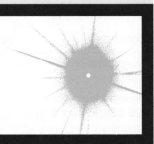

DEFINITION

Pneumonia is an infection of the pulmonary parenchyma. Despite being the cause of significant morbidity and mortality, pneumonia is often misdiagnosed, mistreated, and underestimated. In the past, pneumonia was typically classified as community-acquired (CAP), hospital-acquired (HAP), or ventilator-associated (VAP). Over the past two decades, however, some persons presenting as outpatients with onset of pneumonia have been found to be infected with the multidrug-resistant (MDR) pathogens previously associated with HAP. Factors responsible for this phenomenon include the development and widespread use of potent oral antibiotics, earlier transfer of patients out of acute-care hospitals to their homes or various lower-acuity facilities, increased use of outpatient IV antibiotic therapy, general aging of the population, and more extensive immunomodulatory therapies. The potential involvement of these MDR pathogens has led to a new category of pneumonia—termed *health care–associated pneumonia* (HCAP)—distinct from CAP. Conditions associated with HCAP and the likely pathogens are listed in **Table 11-1**.

Although the new classification system has been helpful in designing empirical antibiotic strategies, it is not without disadvantages. Not all MDR pathogens are associated with all risk factors (Table 11-1). Moreover, HCAP is a distillation of multiple risk factors, and each patient must be considered individually. For example, the risk of infection with MDR pathogens for a nursing home resident who has dementia but can independently dress, ambulate, and eat is quite different from the risk for a patient who is in a chronic vegetative state with a tracheostomy and a percutaneous feeding tube in place. In addition, risk factors for MDR infection do not preclude the development of pneumonia caused by the usual CAP pathogens.

This chapter deals with pneumonia in patients who are not considered to be immunocompromised.

PATHOPHYSIOLOGY

Pneumonia results from the proliferation of microbial pathogens at the alveolar level and the host's response to those pathogens. Microorganisms gain access to the lower respiratory tract in several ways. The most common is by aspiration from the oropharynx. Small-volume aspiration occurs frequently during sleep (especially in the elderly) and in patients with decreased levels of consciousness. Many pathogens are inhaled as contaminated droplets. Rarely, pneumonia occurs via hematogenous spread (e.g., from tricuspid endocarditis) or by contiguous extension from an infected pleural or mediastinal space.

Mechanical factors are critically important in host defense. The hairs and turbinates of the nares capture larger inhaled particles before they reach the lower respiratory tract. The branching architecture of the tracheobronchial tree traps particles on the airway lining, where mucociliary clearance and local antibacterial factors either clear or kill the potential pathogen. The gag reflex and the cough mechanism offer critical protection from aspiration. In addition, the normal flora adhering to mucosal cells of the oropharynx, whose components are remarkably constant, prevents pathogenic bacteria from binding and thereby decreases the risk of pneumonia caused by these more virulent bacteria.

When these barriers are overcome or when the microorganisms are small enough to be inhaled to the alveolar level, resident alveolar macrophages are extremely efficient at clearing and killing pathogens. Macrophages are assisted by local proteins (e.g., surfactant proteins A and D) that have intrinsic opsonizing

TABLE 11-1

CLINICAL CONDITIONS ASSOCIATED WITH AND LIKELY PATHOGENS IN HEALTH CARE–ASSOCIATED PNEUMONIA

		PATHOGEN		
CONDITION	MRSA	*PSEUDOMONAS AERUGINOSA*	*ACINETOBACTER* SPP.	MDR ENTEROBACTERIACEAE
Hospitalization for ≥48 h	X	X	X	X
Hospitalization for ≥2 days in prior 3 months	X	X	X	X
Nursing home or extended-care-facility residence	X	X	X	X
Antibiotic therapy in preceding 3 months		X		X
Chronic dialysis	X			
Home infusion therapy	X			
Home wound care	X			
Family member with MDR infection	X			X

Abbreviations: MDR, multidrug-resistant; MRSA, methicillin-resistant *Staphylococcus aureus*.

properties or antibacterial or antiviral activity. Once engulfed by the macrophage, the pathogens—even if they are not killed—are eliminated via either the mucociliary elevator or the lymphatics and no longer represent an infectious challenge. Only when the capacity of the alveolar macrophages to ingest or kill the microorganisms is exceeded does clinical pneumonia become manifest. In that situation, the alveolar macrophages initiate the inflammatory response to bolster lower respiratory tract defenses. The host inflammatory response, rather than the proliferation of microorganisms, triggers the clinical syndrome of pneumonia. The release of inflammatory mediators, such as interleukin (IL)-1 and tumor necrosis factor (TNF), results in fever. Chemokines, such as IL-8 and granulocyte colony-stimulating factor, stimulate the release of neutrophils and their attraction to the lung, producing both peripheral leukocytosis and increased purulent secretions. Inflammatory mediators released by macrophages and the newly recruited neutrophils create an alveolar capillary leak equivalent to that seen in the acute respiratory distress syndrome (ARDS), although in pneumonia this leak is localized (at least initially). Even erythrocytes can cross the alveolar-capillary membrane, with consequent hemoptysis. The capillary leak results in a radiographic infiltrate and rales detectable on auscultation, and hypoxemia results from alveolar filling. Moreover, some bacterial pathogens appear to interfere with the hypoxemic vasoconstriction that would normally occur with fluid-filled alveoli, and this

interference can result in severe hypoxemia. Increased respiratory drive in the systemic inflammatory response syndrome (SIRS; Chap. 28) leads to respiratory alkalosis. Decreased compliance due to capillary leak, hypoxemia, increased respiratory drive, increased secretions, and occasionally infection-related bronchospasm all lead to dyspnea. If severe enough, the changes in lung mechanics secondary to reductions in lung volume and compliance and the intrapulmonary shunting of blood may cause the patient's death.

PATHOLOGY

Classic pneumonia evolves through a series of pathologic changes. The initial phase is one of *edema*, with the presence of a proteinaceous exudate—and often of bacteria—in the alveoli. This phase is rarely evident in clinical or autopsy specimens because it is so rapidly followed by a *red hepatization* phase. The presence of erythrocytes in the cellular intraalveolar exudate gives this second stage its name, but neutrophil influx is more important from the standpoint of host defense. Bacteria are occasionally seen in pathologic specimens collected during this phase. In the third phase, *gray hepatization*, no new erythrocytes are extravasating, and those already present have been lysed and degraded. The neutrophil is the predominant cell, fibrin deposition is abundant, and bacteria have disappeared. This phase corresponds with successful containment of the infection and improvement in gas exchange. In the final phase, *resolution*, the macrophage reappears as the dominant cell type in the alveolar space, and the debris of neutrophils, bacteria, and fibrin has been cleared, as has the inflammatory response.

This pattern has been described best for lobar pneumococcal pneumonia and may not apply to pneumonias of all etiologies, especially viral or *Pneumocystis* pneumonia. In VAP, respiratory bronchiolitis may precede the development of a radiologically apparent infiltrate. Because of the microaspiration mechanism, a bronchopneumonia pattern is most common in nosocomial pneumonias, whereas a lobar pattern is more common in bacterial CAP. Despite the radiographic appearance, viral and *Pneumocystis* pneumonias represent alveolar rather than interstitial processes.

COMMUNITY-ACQUIRED PNEUMONIA

ETIOLOGY

The extensive list of potential etiologic agents in CAP includes bacteria, fungi, viruses, and protozoa. Newly identified pathogens include hantaviruses, metapneumoviruses, the coronavirus responsible for severe acute respiratory syndrome (SARS), and community-acquired strains of methicillin-resistant *Staphylococcus aureus* (MRSA). Most cases of CAP, however, are caused by relatively few pathogens **(Table 11-2)**. Although *Streptococcus pneumoniae* is most common, other organisms must also be considered in light of the patient's risk factors and severity of illness. In most cases, it is most useful to think of the potential causes as either "typical" bacterial pathogens or "atypical" organisms. The former category includes *S. pneumoniae*, *Haemophilus influenzae*, and (in selected patients) *S. aureus* and gram-negative bacilli such as *Klebsiella pneumoniae* and *Pseudomonas aeruginosa*. The "atypical" organisms include *Mycoplasma pneumoniae* and *Chlamydia pneumoniae* (in outpatients) and *Legionella* spp. (in inpatients) as well as respiratory viruses such as influenza viruses, adenoviruses, and respiratory syncytial viruses. Data suggest that a virus may be responsible for up to 18% of cases of CAP that require admission to the hospital. The atypical organisms cannot be cultured on standard media, nor can they be seen on Gram's stain. The frequency and importance of atypical pathogens have significant implications for therapy. These organisms are intrinsically resistant to all β-lactam agents and must be treated with a macrolide, a fluoroquinolone, or a tetracycline. In the ~10–15% of CAP cases that are polymicrobial, the etiology often includes a combination of typical and atypical pathogens.

TABLE 11-2

MICROBIAL CAUSES OF COMMUNITY-ACQUIRED PNEUMONIA, BY SITE OF CARE

OUTPATIENTS	HOSPITALIZED PATIENTS	
	NON-ICU	ICU
Streptococcus pneumoniae	*S. pneumoniae*	*S. pneumoniae*
Mycoplasma pneumoniae	*M. pneumoniae*	*Staphylococcus aureus*
Haemophilus influenzae	*Chlamydia pneumoniae*	*Legionella* spp.
C. pneumoniae		Gram-negative bacilli
Respiratory viruses[a]	*H. influenzae*	*H. influenzae*
	Legionella spp.	
	Respiratory viruses[a]	

[a]Influenza A and B viruses, adenoviruses, respiratory syncytial viruses, parainfluenza viruses.
Note: Pathogens are listed in descending order of frequency. ICU, intensive care unit.

Anaerobes play a significant role only when an episode of aspiration has occurred days to weeks before presentation for pneumonia. The combination of an unprotected airway (e.g., in patients with alcohol or drug overdose or a seizure disorder) and significant gingivitis constitutes the major risk factor. Anaerobic pneumonias are often complicated by abscess formation and significant empyemas or parapneumonic effusions.

S. aureus pneumonia is well known to complicate influenza infection. However, MRSA has been reported as the primary etiologic agent of CAP. While this entity is still relatively uncommon, clinicians must be aware of its potentially serious consequences such as necrotizing pneumonia. Two important developments have led to this problem: the spread of MRSA from the hospital setting to the community and the emergence of genetically distinct strains of MRSA in the community. The former circumstance is more likely to result in HCAP, whereas the novel community-acquired MRSA (CA-MRSA) strains have infected healthy individuals who have had no association with health care.

Unfortunately, despite a careful history and physical examination as well as routine radiographic studies, the causative pathogen in a case of CAP is difficult to predict with any degree of certainty; in more than one-half of cases, a specific etiology is never determined. Nevertheless, epidemiologic and risk factors may suggest the involvement of certain pathogens **(Table 11-3)**.

TABLE 11-3

EPIDEMIOLOGIC FACTORS SUGGESTING POSSIBLE CAUSES OF COMMUNITY-ACQUIRED PNEUMONIA

FACTOR	POSSIBLE PATHOGEN(S)
Alcoholism	*Streptococcus pneumoniae*, oral anaerobes, *Klebsiella pneumoniae*, *Acinetobacter* spp., *Mycobacterium tuberculosis*
COPD and/or smoking	*Haemophilus influenzae*, *Pseudomonas aeruginosa*, *Legionella* spp., *S. pneumoniae*, *Moraxella catarrhalis*, *Chlamydia pneumoniae*
Structural lung disease (e.g., bronchiectasis)	*P. aeruginosa*, *Burkholderia cepacia*, *Staphylococcus aureus*
Dementia, stroke, decreased level of consciousness	Oral anaerobes, gram-negative enteric bacteria
Lung abscess	CA-MRSA, oral anaerobes, endemic fungi, *M. tuberculosis*, atypical mycobacteria
Travel to Ohio or St. Lawrence river valleys	*Histoplasma capsulatum*
Travel to southwestern United States	Hantavirus, *Coccidioides* spp.
Travel to Southeast Asia	*Burkholderia pseudomallei*, avian influenza virus
Stay in hotel or on cruise ship in previous 2 weeks	*Legionella* spp.
Local influenza activity	Influenza virus, *S. pneumoniae*, *S. aureus*
Exposure to bats or birds	*H. capsulatum*
Exposure to birds	*Chlamydia psittaci*
Exposure to rabbits	*Francisella tularensis*
Exposure to sheep, goats, parturient cats	*Coxiella burnetii*

Abbreviations: CA-MRSA, community-acquired methicillin-resistant *Staphylococcus aureus;* COPD, chronic obstructive pulmonary disease.

EPIDEMIOLOGY

In the United States, ~80% of the 4 million CAP cases that occur annually are treated on an outpatient basis, and ~20% are treated in the hospital. CAP results in more than 600,000 hospitalizations, 64 million days of restricted activity, and 45,000 deaths annually. The overall yearly cost associated with CAP is estimated at $9–10 billion. The incidence rates are highest at the extremes of age. The overall annual rate in the United States is 12 cases per 1000 persons, but the figure increases to 12–18 per 1000 among children <4 years of age and to 20 per 1000 among persons >60 years of age.

The risk factors for CAP in general and for pneumococcal pneumonia in particular have implications for treatment regimens. Risk factors for CAP include alcoholism, asthma, immunosuppression, institutionalization, and an age of ≥70 years versus 60–69 years. Risk factors for pneumococcal pneumonia include dementia, seizure disorders, heart failure, cerebrovascular disease, alcoholism, tobacco smoking, chronic obstructive pulmonary disease (COPD), and HIV infection. CA-MRSA pneumonia is more likely in patients with skin colonization or infection with CA-MRSA. Enterobacteriaceae tend to infect patients who have recently been hospitalized and/or received antibiotic therapy or who have comorbidities such as alcoholism, heart failure, or renal failure. *P. aeruginosa* is a particular problem in patients with severe structural lung disease, such as bronchiectasis, cystic fibrosis, or severe COPD. Risk factors for *Legionella* infection include diabetes, hematologic malignancy, cancer, severe renal disease, HIV infection, smoking, male gender, and a recent hotel stay or ship cruise. (Many of these risk factors would now reclassify as HCAP some cases that were previously designated CAP.)

CLINICAL MANIFESTATIONS

CAP can vary from indolent to fulminant in presentation and from mild to fatal in severity. The various signs and symptoms that depend on the progression and severity of the infection include both constitutional findings and manifestations limited to the lung and associated structures. In light of the pathobiology of the disease, many of the findings are to be expected.

The patient is frequently febrile with tachycardia or may have a history of chills and/or sweats. Cough may be either nonproductive or productive of mucoid, purulent, or blood-tinged sputum. Depending on severity, the patient may be able to speak in full sentences or may be very short of breath. If the pleura is involved, the patient may experience pleuritic chest pain. Up to 20% of patients may have gastrointestinal symptoms such as nausea, vomiting, and/or diarrhea. Other symptoms may include fatigue, headache, myalgias, and arthralgias.

Findings on physical examination vary with the degree of pulmonary consolidation and the presence or absence of a significant pleural effusion. An increased respiratory rate and use of accessory muscles of respiration are common. Palpation may reveal increased or decreased tactile fremitus, and the percussion note can vary from dull to flat, reflecting underlying consolidated lung and pleural fluid, respectively. Crackles, bronchial breath sounds, and possibly a pleural friction rub may be heard on auscultation. The clinical presentation may not be so obvious in the elderly, who may initially display new-onset or worsening confusion and few other manifestations. Severely ill patients may have septic shock and evidence of organ failure.

DIAGNOSIS

When confronted with possible CAP, the physician must ask two questions: Is this pneumonia, and, if so, what is the likely etiology? The former question is typically answered by clinical and radiographic methods, whereas the latter requires the aid of laboratory techniques.

Clinical diagnosis

The differential diagnosis includes both infectious and noninfectious entities such as acute bronchitis, acute exacerbations of chronic bronchitis, heart failure, pulmonary embolism, and radiation pneumonitis. The importance of a careful history cannot be overemphasized. For example, known cardiac disease may suggest worsening pulmonary edema, while underlying carcinoma may suggest lung injury secondary to irradiation. Epidemiologic clues, such as recent travel to areas with known endemic pathogens (e.g., the U.S. southwest), may alert the physician to specific possibilities (Table 11-3).

Unfortunately, the sensitivity and specificity of the findings on physical examination are less than ideal, averaging 58% and 67%, respectively. Therefore, chest radiography is often necessary to differentiate CAP from other conditions. Radiographic findings may include risk factors for increased severity (e.g., cavitation or multilobar involvement). Occasionally, radiographic results suggest an etiologic diagnosis. For example, pneumatoceles suggest infection with *S. aureus*, and an upper-lobe cavitating lesion suggests tuberculosis. CT is rarely necessary but may be of value in a patient with suspected postobstructive pneumonia caused by a tumor or foreign body. For outpatients, the clinical and radiologic assessments are usually all that is done before treatment for CAP is started since most laboratory results are not available soon enough to influence initial management significantly. In certain cases, the availability of rapid point-of-care outpatient diagnostic tests can be very important (e.g., rapid diagnosis of influenza virus infection can prompt specific anti-influenza drug treatment and secondary prevention).

Etiologic diagnosis

The etiology of pneumonia usually cannot be determined solely on the basis of clinical presentation; instead, the physician must rely upon the laboratory for support.

Except for the 2% of CAP patients who are admitted to the intensive care unit (ICU), no data exist to show that treatment directed at a specific pathogen is statistically superior to empirical therapy. The benefit of establishing a microbial etiology can therefore be questioned, particularly in light of the cost of diagnostic testing. However, a number of reasons can be advanced for attempting an etiologic diagnosis. Identification of an unexpected pathogen allows narrowing of the initial empirical regimen that decreases antibiotic selection pressure, lessening the risk of resistance. Pathogens with important public safety implications such as *Mycobacterium tuberculosis* and influenza virus, may be found in some cases. Finally, without culture and susceptibility data, trends in resistance cannot be followed accurately, and appropriate empirical therapeutic regimens are harder to devise.

Gram's stain and culture of sputum

The main purpose of the sputum Gram's stain is to ensure that a sample is suitable for culture. However, Gram's staining may also identify certain pathogens (e.g., *S. pneumoniae*, *S. aureus*, and gram-negative bacteria) by their characteristic appearance. To be adequate for culture, a sputum sample must have >25 neutrophils and <10 squamous epithelial cells per low-power field. The sensitivity and specificity of the sputum Gram's stain and culture are highly variable. Even in cases of proven bacteremic pneumococcal pneumonia, the yield of positive cultures from sputum samples is ≤50%.

Some patients, particularly elderly individuals, may not be able to produce an appropriate expectorated sputum sample. Others may already have started a course of antibiotics that can interfere with culture results at the time a sample is obtained. Inability to produce sputum can be a consequence of dehydration, and the correction of this condition may result in increased sputum production and a more obvious infiltrate on chest radiography. For patients admitted to the ICU and intubated, a deep-suction aspirate or bronchoalveolar lavage sample (obtained either via bronchoscopy or non-bronchoscopically) has a high yield on culture when sent to the microbiology laboratory as soon as possible. Since the etiologies in severe CAP are somewhat different from those in milder disease (Table 11-2), the greatest benefit of staining and culturing respiratory secretions is to alert the physician of unsuspected and/or resistant pathogens and to permit appropriate modification of therapy. Other stains and cultures (e.g., specific stains for *M. tuberculosis* or fungi) may be useful as well.

Blood cultures

The yield from blood cultures, even when samples are collected before antibiotic therapy, is disappointingly low. Only ~5–14% of cultures of blood from patients hospitalized with CAP are positive, and the most frequently isolated pathogen is *S. pneumoniae*. Since recommended empirical regimens all provide pneumococcal coverage, a blood culture positive for this pathogen has little, if any, effect on clinical outcome. However, susceptibility data may allow narrowing of antibiotic therapy in appropriate cases. Because of the low yield and the lack of significant impact on outcome, blood cultures are no longer considered *de rigueur* for all hospitalized CAP patients. Certain high-risk patients—including those with neutropenia secondary to pneumonia, asplenia, or complement deficiencies; chronic liver disease; or severe CAP—should have blood cultured.

Antigen tests

Two commercially available tests detect pneumococcal and certain *Legionella* antigens in urine. The test for *L. pneumophila* detects only serogroup 1, but this serogroup accounts for most community-acquired cases of Legionnaires' disease. The sensitivity and specificity of the *Legionella* urine antigen test are as high as 90% and 99%, respectively. The pneumococcal urine antigen test is also quite sensitive and specific (80% and >90%, respectively). Although false-positive results can be obtained with samples from pneumococcus-colonized children, the test is generally reliable. Both tests can detect antigen even after the initiation of appropriate antibiotic therapy. Other antigen tests include a rapid test for influenza virus and direct fluorescent antibody tests for influenza virus and respiratory syncytial virus; the latter tests are only poorly sensitive.

Polymerase chain reaction

Polymerase chain reaction (PCR) tests, which amplify a microorganism's DNA or RNA, are available for a number of pathogens, including *L. pneumophila* and mycobacteria. In addition, a multiplex PCR can detect the nucleic acid of *Legionella* spp., *M. pneumoniae*, and *C. pneumoniae*. However, the use of these PCR assays is generally limited to research studies. In patients with pneumococcal pneumonia, an increased bacterial load documented by PCR is associated with an increased risk of septic shock, need for mechanical ventilation, and death. Such a test could conceivably help identify patients suitable for ICU admission.

Serology

A fourfold rise in specific IgM antibody titer between acute- and convalescent-phase serum samples is generally considered diagnostic of infection with the pathogen in question. In the past, serologic tests were used to help identify atypical pathogens as well as selected unusual organisms such as *Coxiella burnetii*. Recently, however, they have fallen out of favor because of the time required to obtain a final result for the convalescent-phase sample.

| TREATMENT | Community-Acquired Pneumonia |

SITE OF CARE   The cost of inpatient management exceeds that of outpatient treatment by a factor of 20, and hospitalization accounts for most CAP-related expenditures. Thus the decision to admit a patient with CAP to the hospital has considerable implications. Certain patients clearly can be managed at home, and others clearly require treatment in the hospital, but the choice is sometimes difficult. Tools that objectively assess the risk of adverse outcomes, including severe illness and death, can minimize unnecessary hospital admissions. There are currently two sets of criteria: the Pneumonia Severity Index (PSI), a prognostic model used to identify patients at low risk of dying; and the CURB-65 criteria, a severity-of-illness score.

To determine the PSI, points are given for 20 variables, including age, coexisting illness, and abnormal physical and laboratory findings. On the basis of the resulting score, patients are assigned to one of five classes with the following mortality rates: class 1, 0.1%; class 2, 0.6%; class 3, 2.8%; class 4, 8.2%; and class 5, 29.2%. Clinical trials demonstrate that routine use of the PSI results in lower admission rates for class 1 and class 2 patients. Patients in classes 4 and 5 should be admitted to the hospital, while those in class 3 should ideally be admitted to an observation unit until a further decision can be made.

The CURB-65 criteria include five variables: confusion (C); urea >7 mmol/L (U); respiratory rate ≥30/min (R); blood pressure, systolic ≤90 mmHg or diastolic ≤60 mmHg (B); and age ≥65 years (65). Patients with a score of 0, among whom the 30-day mortality rate is 1.5%, can be treated outside the hospital. With a score of 2, the 30-day mortality rate is 9.2%, and patients should be admitted to the hospital. Among patients with scores of ≥3, mortality rates are 22% overall; these patients may require admission to an ICU.

It is not clear which assessment tool is superior. The PSI is less practical in a busy emergency room setting because of the need to assess 20 variables. While the CURB-65 criteria are easily remembered, they have not been studied as extensively. Whichever system is used, these objective criteria must always be tempered by careful consideration of factors relevant to individual patients, including the ability to comply reliably with an oral antibiotic regimen and the resources available to the patient outside the hospital. In fact, neither the PSI nor CURB-65 is ideal for determining the need for ICU care. The severity criteria proposed by the Infectious Diseases Society of America (IDSA) and the American Thoracic Society (ATS) in their guidelines for the management of CAP are better suited to this purpose.

ANTIBIOTIC RESISTANCE Antimicrobial resistance is a significant problem that threatens to diminish our therapeutic armamentarium. Misuse of antibiotics results in increased antibiotic selection pressure that can affect resistance locally or even globally by clonal dissemination. For CAP, the main resistance issues currently involve *S. pneumoniae* and CA-MRSA.

S. pneumoniae In general, pneumococcal resistance is acquired (1) by direct DNA incorporation and remodeling resulting from contact with closely related oral commensal bacteria, (2) by the process of natural transformation, or (3) by mutation of certain genes.

The cutoff for penicillin susceptibility in pneumonia has recently been raised from a minimal inhibitory concentration (MIC) of ≤0.6 μg/mL to an MIC of ≤2 μg/mL. Cutoffs for intermediate resistance have been raised to 4 μg/mL (from 0.1–1 μg/mL) and ≥8 μg/mL (from ≥2 μg/mL), respectively. These changes in susceptibility thresholds have resulted in a dramatic decrease in the proportion of pneumococcal isolates considered nonsusceptible. For meningitis, MIC thresholds remain at the former levels. Fortunately, resistance to penicillin appeared to plateau even before the change in MIC thresholds. Pneumococcal resistance to β-lactam drugs is due solely to low-affinity penicillin-binding proteins. Risk factors for penicillin-resistant pneumococcal infection include recent antimicrobial therapy, an age of <2 years or >65 years, attendance at day-care centers, recent hospitalization, and HIV infection.

In contrast to penicillin resistance, resistance to macrolides is increasing through several mechanisms. *Target-site modification* is caused by ribosomal methylation in 23S rRNA encoded by the *ermB* gene, resulting in resistance to macrolides, lincosamides, and streptogramin B–type antibiotics. This MLS$_B$ phenotype is associated with high-level resistance, with typical MICs of ≥64 μg/mL. The *efflux mechanism* encoded by the *mef* gene (M phenotype) is usually associated with low-level resistance (MICs, 1–32 μg/mL). These two mechanisms account for ~45% and ~65%, respectively, of resistant pneumococcal isolates in the United States. High-level resistance to macrolides is more common in Europe, whereas lower-level resistance seems to predominate in North America. Although clinical failures with macrolides have been reported, many experts think that these drugs still have a role to play in the management of pneumococcal pneumonia in North America.

Pneumococcal resistance to fluoroquinolones (e.g., ciprofloxacin and levofloxacin) has been reported. Changes can occur in one or both target sites (topoisomerases II and IV); changes in these two sites usually result from mutations in the *gyrA* and *parC* genes, respectively. The increasing number of pneumococcal isolates that, although still testing susceptible to fluoroquinolones, already have a mutation in one target site is of concern. Such organisms may be more likely to undergo a second step mutation that will render them fully resistant to fluoroquinolones. In addition, an efflux pump may play a role in pneumococcal resistance to fluoroquinolones.

Isolates resistant to drugs from three or more antimicrobial classes with different mechanisms of action are considered MDR. The propensity for an association of pneumococcal resistance to penicillin with reduced susceptibility to other drugs such as macrolides, tetracyclines, and trimethoprim-sulfamethoxazole, is also of concern. In the United States, 58.9% of penicillin-resistant pneumococcal isolates from blood are also resistant to macrolides.

The most important risk factor for antibiotic-resistant pneumococcal infection is use of a specific antibiotic within the previous 3 months. Therefore, a patient's history of prior antibiotic treatment is a critical factor in avoiding the use of an inappropriate antibiotic.

CA-MRSA CAP due to MRSA may be caused by infection with the classic hospital-acquired strains or with the more recently identified, genotypically and phenotypically distinct community-acquired strains. Most infections with the former strains have been acquired either directly or indirectly by contact with the health care environment and would now be classified as HCAP. In some hospitals, CA-MRSA strains are displacing the classic hospital-acquired strains—a trend suggesting that the newer strains may be more robust.

Methicillin resistance in *S. aureus* is determined by the *mecA* gene, which encodes for resistance to all β-lactam drugs. At least five *staphylococcal chromosomal cassette mec* (*SCCmec*) types have been described. The typical hospital-acquired strain usually has type II or III, whereas CA-MRSA has a type IV SCC*mec* element. CA-MRSA isolates tend to be less resistant than the older hospital-acquired strains and are often susceptible to trimethoprim-sulfamethoxazole, clindamycin, and tetracycline in addition to vancomycin and linezolid. However, CA-MRSA strains may also carry genes for superantigens, such as enterotoxins B and C and Panton-Valentine leukocidin, a membrane-tropic toxin that can create cytolytic pores in polymorphonuclear neutrophils, monocytes, and macrophages.

Gram-Negative Bacilli A detailed discussion of resistance among gram-negative bacilli is beyond the scope of this chapter. Fluoroquinolone resistance among isolates of *Escherichia coli* from the community appears to be increasing. *Enterobacter* spp. are typically resistant to cephalosporins; the drugs of choice for use against these bacteria are usually fluoroquinolones or carbapenems. Similarly, when infections due to bacteria producing extended-spectrum β-lactamases are documented or suspected, a fluoroquinolone or a carbapenem should be used; these MDR strains are more likely to be involved in HCAP.

INITIAL ANTIBIOTIC MANAGEMENT Since the physician rarely knows the etiology of CAP at the outset of treatment, initial therapy is usually empirical and is designed to cover the most likely pathogens (Table 11-4). In all cases, antibiotic treatment should be initiated as expeditiously as possible. The CAP treatment guidelines in the United States (summarized in Table 11-4) represent joint statements from the IDSA and the ATS; the Canadian guidelines come from the Canadian Infectious Disease Society and the Canadian Thoracic Society. In these guidelines, coverage is always provided for the pneumococcus and the atypical pathogens. In contrast, guidelines from some European countries do not always include atypical coverage based on local epidemiologic data. The U.S.–Canadian approach is supported by retrospective data from several studies of administrative databases including thousands of patients. Atypical pathogen coverage provided by the addition of a macrolide to a cephalosporin or by the use of a fluoroquinolone alone has been consistently associated with a significant reduction in mortality rates compared with those for β-lactam coverage alone.

Therapy with a macrolide or a fluoroquinolone within the previous 3 months is associated with an increased likelihood of infection with a resistant strain of *S. pneumoniae*. For this reason, a fluoroquinolone-based regimen should be used for patients recently given a macrolide, and vice versa (Table 11-4).

TABLE 11-4

EMPIRICAL ANTIBIOTIC TREATMENT OF COMMUNITY-ACQUIRED PNEUMONIA

Outpatients

Previously healthy and no antibiotics in past 3 months
- A macrolide (clarithromycin [500 mg PO bid] or azithromycin [500 mg PO once, then 250 mg qd]) *or*
- Doxycycline (100 mg PO bid)

Comorbidities or antibiotics in past 3 months: select an alternative from a different class
- A respiratory fluoroquinolone (moxifloxacin [400 mg PO qd], gemifloxacin [320 mg PO qd], levofloxacin [750 mg PO qd]) *or*
- A β-lactam (preferred: high-dose amoxicillin [1 g tid] or amoxicillin/clavulanate [2 g bid]; alternatives: ceftriaxone [1–2 g IV qd], cefpodoxime [200 mg PO bid], cefuroxime [500 mg PO bid]) *plus* a macrolide[a]

In regions with a high rate of "high-level" pneumococcal macrolide resistance,[b] consider alternatives listed above for patients with comorbidities.

Inpatients, Non-ICU

- A respiratory fluoroquinolone (moxifloxacin [400 mg PO or IV qd], gemifloxacin [320 mg PO qd], levofloxacin [750 mg PO or IV qd])
- A β-lactam[c] (cefotaxime [1–2 g IV q8h], ceftriaxone [1–2 g IV qd], ampicillin [1–2 g IV q4–6h], ertapenem [1 g IV qd in selected patients]) *plus* a macrolide[d] (oral clarithromycin or azithromycin [as listed above for previously healthy patients] or IV azithromycin [1 g once, then 500 mg qd])

Inpatients, ICU

- A β-lactam[e] (cefotaxime [1–2 g IV q8h], ceftriaxone [2 g IV qd], ampicillin-sulbactam [2 g IV q8h]) *plus*
- Azithromycin or a fluoroquinolone (as listed above for inpatients, non-ICU)

Special Concerns

If *Pseudomonas* is a consideration
- An antipneumococcal, antipseudomonal β-lactam (piperacillin/tazobactam [4.5 g IV q6h], cefepime [1–2 g IV q12h], imipenem [500 mg IV q6h], meropenem [1 g IV q8h]) *plus* either ciprofloxacin (400 mg IV q12h) or levofloxacin (750 mg IV qd)
- The above β-lactams *plus* an aminoglycoside (amikacin [15 mg/kg qd] or tobramycin [1.7 mg/kg qd] and azithromycin)
- The above β-lactams[f] *plus* an aminoglycoside *plus* an antipneumococcal fluoroquinolone

If CA-MRSA is a consideration
- Add linezolid (600 mg IV q12h) or vancomycin (1 g IV q12h).

[a]Doxycycline (100 mg PO bid) is an alternative to the macrolide.
[b]MICs of >16 μg/mL in 25% of isolates.
[c]A respiratory fluoroquinolone should be used for penicillin-allergic patients.
[d]Doxycycline (100 mg IV q12h) is an alternative to the macrolide.
[e]For penicillin-allergic patients, use a respiratory fluoroquinolone and aztreonam (2 g IV q8h).
[f]For penicillin-allergic patients, substitute aztreonam.
Abbreviations: CA-MRSA, community-acquired methicillin-resistant *Staphylococcus aureus;* ICU, intensive care unit.

Once the etiologic agent(s) and susceptibilities are known, therapy may be altered to target the specific pathogen(s). However, this decision is not always straightforward. If blood cultures yield *S. pneumoniae* sensitive to penicillin after 2 days of treatment with a macrolide plus a β-lactam or with a fluoroquinolone alone, should therapy be switched to penicillin alone? The concern here is that a β-lactam alone would not be effective in the potential 15% of cases with atypical co-infection. No standard approach exists. In all cases, the individual patient and the various risk factors must be considered.

Management of bacteremic pneumococcal pneumonia is also controversial. Data from nonrandomized studies suggest that combination therapy (especially with a macrolide and a β-lactam) is associated with a lower mortality rate than monotherapy, particularly in severely ill patients. The exact reason is unknown, but possible explanations include an additive or synergistic antibacterial effect, antimicrobial tolerance, atypical co-infection, or the immunomodulatory effects of the macrolides.

For patients with CAP who are admitted to the ICU, the risk of infection with *P. aeruginosa* or CA-MRSA is increased, and coverage should be considered when a patient has risk factors or a Gram's stain suggestive of these pathogens (Table 11-4). If CA-MRSA infection is suspected, either linezolid or vancomycin should be added to the initial empirical regimen. There is concern about vancomycin's loss of potency against MRSA; in addition, vancomycin does not reach significant concentrations in epithelial lining fluid, whereas concentrations of linezolid at this site exceed the MIC for MRSA during the entire dosing interval.

Although hospitalized patients have traditionally received initial therapy by the IV route, some drugs—particularly the fluoroquinolones—are very well absorbed and can be given orally from the outset to select patients. For patients initially treated IV, a switch to oral treatment is appropriate as long as the patient can ingest and absorb the drugs, is hemodynamically stable, and is showing clinical improvement.

The duration of treatment for CAP has generated considerable interest. Patients were previously treated for 10–14 days, but studies with fluoroquinolones and telithromycin suggest that a 5-day course is sufficient for otherwise uncomplicated CAP. Even a single dose of ceftriaxone has been associated with a significant cure rate. A longer course is required for patients with bacteremia, metastatic infection, or infection with a virulent pathogen such as *P. aeruginosa* or CA-MRSA.

GENERAL CONSIDERATIONS In addition to appropriate antimicrobial therapy, certain general considerations apply in dealing with CAP, HCAP, or HAP/VAP.

Adequate hydration, oxygen therapy for hypoxemia, and assisted ventilation when necessary are critical to the success of therapy. Patients with severe CAP who remain hypotensive despite fluid resuscitation may have adrenal insufficiency and may respond to glucocorticoid treatment. Immunomodulatory therapy in the form of drotrecogin alfa (activated) should be considered for CAP patients with persistent septic shock and APACHE II scores of ≥25, particularly if the infection is caused by *S. pneumoniae*. The value of other forms of adjunctive therapy, including glucocorticoids, statins, and angiotensin-converting enzyme inhibitors, remains unproven in the management of CAP.

Failure to Improve Patients who are slow to respond to therapy should be reevaluated at about day 3 (sooner if their condition is worsening rather than simply not improving), and a number of possible scenarios should be considered. A number of noninfectious conditions can mimic pneumonia, including pulmonary edema, pulmonary embolism, lung carcinoma, radiation and hypersensitivity pneumonitis, and connective tissue disease involving the lungs. If the patient has CAP and treatment is aimed at the correct pathogen, the lack of response may be explained in a number of ways. The pathogen may be resistant to the drug selected, or a sequestered focus (e.g., a lung abscess or empyema) may be blocking access of the antibiotic(s) to the pathogen. The patient may be getting either the wrong drug or the correct drug at the wrong dose or frequency of administration. It is also possible that CAP is the correct diagnosis but that an unsuspected pathogen (e.g., CA-MRSA, *M. tuberculosis*, or a fungus) is the cause. Nosocomial superinfections—both pulmonary and extrapulmonary—are possible explanations for failure to improve or worsening. In all cases of delayed response or deteriorating condition, the patient must be carefully reassessed and appropriate studies initiated. These studies may include such diverse procedures as CT and bronchoscopy.

Complications As in other severe infections, common complications of severe CAP include respiratory failure, shock and multiorgan failure, coagulopathy, and exacerbation of comorbid illnesses. Three particularly noteworthy conditions are metastatic infection, lung abscess, and complicated pleural effusion. Metastatic infection (e.g., brain abscess or endocarditis), although unusual, deserves immediate attention by the physician, with a detailed workup and proper treatment. Lung abscess may occur in association with aspiration or with infection caused by a single CAP pathogen such as CA-MRSA, *P. aeruginosa*, or (rarely) *S. pneumoniae*. Aspiration pneumonia is typically a mixed polymicrobial infection involving both aerobes and anaerobes. In either scenario, drainage should be established, and antibiotics that cover the known or suspected pathogens should be administered. A significant pleural effusion should be tapped for both diagnostic and therapeutic purposes. If the fluid has a pH of <7, a glucose level of <2.2 mmol/L, and a lactate dehydrogenase concentration of >1000 U/L or if bacteria are seen or cultured, then the fluid should be drained; a chest tube is usually required.

Follow-Up Fever and leukocytosis usually resolve within 2–4 days in otherwise healthy patients with CAP, but physical findings may persist longer. Chest radiographic abnormalities are slowest to resolve and may require 4–12 weeks to clear, with the speed of clearance depending on the patient's age and underlying lung disease. Patients may be discharged from the hospital once their clinical conditions are stable, with no active medical problems requiring hospital care. The site of residence after discharge (nursing home, home with family, home alone) is an important consideration, particularly for elderly patients. For a patient whose condition is improving and who (if hospitalized) has been discharged, a follow-up radiograph can be done ~4–6 weeks later. If relapse or recurrence is documented, particularly in the same lung segment, the possibility of an underlying neoplasm must be considered.

PROGNOSIS

The prognosis of CAP depends on the patient's age, comorbidities, and site of treatment (inpatient or outpatient). Young patients without comorbidity do well and usually recover fully after ~2 weeks. Older patients and those with comorbid conditions can take several weeks longer to recover fully. The overall mortality rate for the outpatient group is <1%. For patients requiring hospitalization, the overall mortality rate is estimated at 10%, with ~50% of deaths directly attributable to pneumonia.

PREVENTION

The main preventive measure is vaccination. The recommendations of the Advisory Committee on Immunization Practices should be followed for influenza and pneumococcal vaccines. In the event of an influenza outbreak, unprotected patients at risk from complications should be vaccinated immediately and given chemoprophylaxis with either oseltamivir or zanamivir for 2 weeks—i.e., until vaccine-induced antibody levels are sufficiently high. Because of an increased risk of pneumococcal infection, even among patients without obstructive lung disease, smokers should be strongly encouraged to stop smoking.

An available 7-valent pneumococcal conjugate vaccine produces T cell–dependent antigens that result in long-term immunologic memory. Administration of this vaccine to children has led to an overall decrease in the prevalence of antimicrobial-resistant pneumococci and in the incidence of invasive pneumococcal disease among both children and adults. However, vaccination can be followed by the replacement of vaccine serotypes with nonvaccine serotypes (e.g., 19A and 35B).

HEALTH CARE–ASSOCIATED PNEUMONIA

HCAP represents a transition between classic CAP and typical HAP. The definition of HCAP is still in some degree of flux because of a lack of large-scale studies. Several of the studies that are available have been limited to patients with culture-positive pneumonia. In these studies, the incidence of MDR pathogens in HCAP was as high as or higher than in HAP/VAP. MRSA in particular was more common in HCAP than in traditional HAP/VAP. Conversely, prospective studies in nontertiary-care centers have found a low incidence of MDR pathogens in HCAP.

The patients at greatest risk for HCAP are not well defined. Patients from nursing homes are not always at elevated risk for infection with MDR pathogens. Careful evaluation of nursing home residents with pneumonia suggests that their risk of MDR infection is low if they have not recently received antibiotics and are independent in most activities of daily living. Conversely, nursing home patients are at increased risk of infection with influenza virus and other atypical pneumonia pathogens. Undue concern about MDR pathogens occasionally results in a failure to cover atypical pathogens in treating nursing home patients. In addition, patients receiving home infusion therapy or undergoing chronic dialysis are probably at particular risk for MRSA pneumonia but may not be at greater risk for infection with *Pseudomonas* or *Acinetobacter* than are other patients who develop CAP.

In general, the management of HCAP due to MDR pathogens is similar to that of MDR HAP/VAP. This topic will therefore be covered in subsequent sections on HAP and VAP. The prognosis of HCAP is intermediate between that of CAP and VAP and is closer to that of HAP.

VENTILATOR-ASSOCIATED PNEUMONIA

Most research on VAP has focused on illness in the hospital setting. However, the information and principles based on this research can be applied to non-ICU HAP and HCAP as well. The greatest difference between VAP and HCAP/HAP is the return to dependence on expectorated sputum for a microbiologic diagnosis of VAP (as for that of CAP), which is further complicated by frequent colonization by pathogens in patients with HAP or HCAP.

Etiology

Potential etiologic agents of VAP include both MDR and non-MDR bacterial pathogens (Table 11-5). The non-MDR group is nearly identical to the pathogens found in severe CAP (Table 11-2); it is not surprising that such pathogens predominate if VAP develops in the first 5–7 days of the hospital stay. However, if patients have other risk factors for HCAP, MDR pathogens are a consideration, even early in the hospital course. The relative frequency of individual MDR pathogens can vary significantly from hospital to hospital and even between different critical care units within the same institution. Most hospitals have problems with *P. aeruginosa* and MRSA, but other MDR pathogens are often institution-specific. Less commonly, fungal and viral pathogens cause VAP, usually affecting severely immunocompromised patients. Rarely, community-associated viruses cause mini-epidemics, usually when introduced by ill health care workers.

Epidemiology

Pneumonia is a common complication among patients requiring mechanical ventilation. Prevalence estimates vary between 6 and 52 cases per 100 patients, depending on the population studied. On any given day in the ICU, an average of 10% of patients will have pneumonia—VAP in the overwhelming majority of cases. The frequency of diagnosis is not static but changes with the duration of mechanical ventilation, with the highest hazard ratio in the first 5 days and a plateau in additional cases (1% per day) after ~2 weeks. However, the cumulative rate among patients

TABLE 11-5

MICROBIOLOGIC CAUSES OF VENTILATOR-ASSOCIATED PNEUMONIA

NON-MDR PATHOGENS	MDR PATHOGENS
Streptococcus pneumoniae	*Pseudomonas aeruginosa*
Other *Streptococcus* spp.	MRSA
Haemophilus influenzae	*Acinetobacter* spp.
MSSA	Antibiotic-resistant Enterobacteriaceae
Antibiotic-sensitive Enterobacteriaceae	*Enterobacter* spp.
Escherichia coli	ESBL-positive strains
Klebsiella pneumoniae	*Klebsiella* spp.
Proteus spp.	*Legionella pneumophila*
Enterobacter spp.	*Burkholderia cepacia*
Serratia marcescens	*Aspergillus* spp.

Abbreviations: ESBL, extended-spectrum β-lactamase; MDR, multidrug-resistant; MRSA, methicillin-resistant *Staphylococcus aureus;* MSSA, methicillin-sensitive *S. aureus.*

who remain ventilated for as long as 30 days is as high as 70%. These rates often do not reflect the recurrence of VAP in the same patient. Once a ventilated patient is transferred to a chronic-care facility or to home, the incidence of pneumonia drops significantly, especially in the absence of other risk factors for pneumonia. However, in chronic ventilator units, purulent tracheobronchitis becomes a significant issue, often interfering with efforts to wean patients off mechanical ventilation.

Three factors are critical in the pathogenesis of VAP: colonization of the oropharynx with pathogenic microorganisms, aspiration of these organisms from the oropharynx into the lower respiratory tract, and compromise of the normal host defense mechanisms. Most risk factors and their corresponding prevention strategies pertain to one of these three factors (Table 11-6).

The most obvious risk factor is the endotracheal tube, which bypasses the normal mechanical factors preventing aspiration. While the presence of an endotracheal tube may prevent large-volume aspiration, microaspiration is actually exacerbated by secretions pooling above the cuff. The endotracheal tube and the concomitant need for suctioning can damage the tracheal mucosa, thereby facilitating tracheal colonization. In addition, pathogenic bacteria can form a glycocalyx biofilm on the tube's surface that protects them from both antibiotics and host defenses. The bacteria can also be dislodged during suctioning and can reinoculate the trachea, or tiny fragments of glycocalyx can embolize to distal airways, carrying bacteria with them.

In a high percentage of critically ill patients, the normal oropharyngeal flora is replaced by pathogenic microorganisms. The most important risk factors are antibiotic selection pressure, cross-infection from other infected/colonized patients or contaminated equipment, and malnutrition. Of these factors, antibiotic exposure poses the greatest risk by far. Pathogens such as *P. aeruginosa* almost never cause infection in patients without prior exposure to antibiotics. The recent emphasis on hand hygiene has lowered the cross-infection rate.

How the lower respiratory tract defenses become overwhelmed remains poorly understood. Almost all intubated patients experience microaspiration and are at least transiently colonized with pathogenic bacteria. However, only around one-third of colonized patients develop VAP. Colony counts increase to high levels, sometimes days before the development of clinical pneumonia; these increases suggest that the final step in VAP development, independent of aspiration and oropharyngeal colonization, is the overwhelming of host defenses. Severely ill patients with sepsis and trauma appear to enter a state of immunoparalysis several days after admission to the ICU—a time that corresponds to the greatest risk of developing VAP. The mechanism of this immunosuppression is not clear, although several factors have been suggested.

TABLE 11-6

PATHOGENIC MECHANISMS AND CORRESPONDING PREVENTION STRATEGIES FOR VENTILATOR-ASSOCIATED PNEUMONIA

PATHOGENIC MECHANISM	PREVENTION STRATEGY
Oropharyngeal colonization with pathogenic bacteria	
Elimination of normal flora	Avoidance of prolonged antibiotic courses
Large-volume oropharyngeal aspiration around time of intubation	Short course of prophylactic antibiotics for comatose patients[a]
Gastroesophageal reflux	Postpyloric enteral feeding[b]; avoidance of high gastric residuals, prokinetic agents
Bacterial overgrowth of stomach	Prophylactic agents that raise gastric pH[b]; selective decontamination of digestive tract with nonabsorbable antibiotics[b]
Cross-infection from other colonized patients	Hand washing, especially with alcohol-based hand rub; intensive infection control education[a]; isolation; proper cleaning of reusable equipment
Large-volume aspiration	Endotracheal intubation; avoidance of sedation; decompression of small-bowel obstruction
Microaspiration around endotracheal tube	
Endotracheal intubation	Noninvasive ventilation[a]
Prolonged duration of ventilation	Daily awakening from sedation,[a] weaning protocols[a]
Abnormal swallowing function	Early percutaneous tracheostomy[a]
Secretions pooled above endotracheal tube	Head of bed elevated[a]; continuous aspiration of subglottic secretions with specialized endotracheal tube[a]; avoidance of reintubation; minimization of sedation and patient transport
Altered lower respiratory host defenses	Tight glycemic control[b]; lowering of hemoglobin transfusion threshold; specialized enteral feeding formula

[a]Strategies demonstrated to be effective in at least one randomized controlled trial.
[b]Strategies with negative randomized trials or conflicting results.

Hyperglycemia affects neutrophil function, and trials suggest that keeping the blood sugar close to normal with exogenous insulin may have beneficial effects, including a decreased risk of infection. More frequent transfusions also adversely affect the immune response.

Clinical manifestations

The clinical manifestations are generally the same in VAP as in all other forms of pneumonia: fever, leukocytosis, increase in respiratory secretions, and pulmonary consolidation on physical examination, along with a new or changing radiographic infiltrate. The frequency of abnormal chest radiographs before the onset of pneumonia in intubated patients and the limitations of portable radiographic technique make interpretation of radiographs more difficult than in patients who are not intubated. Other clinical features may include tachypnea, tachycardia, worsening oxygenation, and increased minute ventilation.

Diagnosis

No single set of criteria is reliably diagnostic of pneumonia in a ventilated patient. The inability to identify such patients compromises efforts to prevent and treat VAP and even calls into question estimates of the impact of VAP on mortality rates.

Application of clinical criteria consistently results in overdiagnosis of VAP, largely because of three common findings in at-risk patients: (1) tracheal colonization with pathogenic bacteria in patients with endotracheal tubes, (2) multiple alternative causes of radiographic infiltrates in mechanically ventilated patients, and (3) the high frequency of other sources of fever in critically ill patients. The differential diagnosis of VAP includes a number of entities such as atypical pulmonary edema, pulmonary contusion, alveolar hemorrhage, hypersensitivity pneumonitis, ARDS, and pulmonary embolism. Clinical findings in ventilated patients with fever and/or leukocytosis may have alternative causes, including antibiotic-associated diarrhea, sinusitis, urinary tract infection, pancreatitis, and drug fever. Conditions mimicking pneumonia are often documented in patients in whom VAP has been ruled out by accurate diagnostic techniques. Most of these alternative diagnoses do not require antibiotic treatment; require antibiotics different from those used to treat VAP; or require some additional intervention, such as surgical drainage or catheter removal, for optimal management.

This diagnostic dilemma has led to debate and controversy. The major question is whether a quantitative-culture approach as a means of eliminating false-positive clinical diagnoses is superior to the clinical approach enhanced by principles learned from quantitative-culture studies. The most recent IDSA/ATS guidelines for HCAP suggest that either approach is clinically valid.

Quantitative-culture approach

The essence of the quantitative-culture approach is to discriminate between colonization and true infection by determining the bacterial burden. The more distal in the respiratory tree the diagnostic sampling, the more specific the results and, therefore, the lower the threshold of growth necessary to diagnose pneumonia and exclude colonization. For example, a quantitative endotracheal aspirate yields proximate samples, and the diagnostic threshold is 10^6 cfu/mL. The protected specimen brush method, in contrast, obtains distal samples and has a threshold of 10^3 cfu/mL. Conversely, sensitivity declines as more distal secretions are obtained, especially when they are collected blindly (i.e., by a technique other than bronchoscopy). Additional tests that may increase the diagnostic yield include Gram's stain, differential cell counts, staining for intracellular organisms, and detection of local protein levels elevated in response to infection.

Several studies have compared patient cohorts managed by the various quantitative-culture methods. While these studies documented issues of relative sensitivity and specificity, outcomes were not significantly different for the various groups of patients. The IDSA/ATS guidelines suggest that all these methods are appropriate and that the choice depends on availability and local expertise.

The Achilles heel of the quantitative approach is the effect of antibiotic therapy. With sensitive microorganisms, a single antibiotic dose can reduce colony counts below the diagnostic threshold. Recent changes in antibiotic therapy are the most significant. After 3 days, the operating characteristics of the tests are almost the same as if no antibiotic therapy has been given. Conversely, colony counts above the diagnostic threshold during antibiotic therapy suggest that the current antibiotics are ineffective. Even the normal host response may be sufficient to reduce quantitative-culture counts below the diagnostic threshold if sampling is delayed. In short, expertise in quantitative-culture techniques is critical, with a specimen obtained as soon as pneumonia is suspected and before antibiotic therapy is initiated or changed.

In a study comparing the quantitative with the clinical approach, use of bronchoscopic quantitative cultures resulted in significantly less antibiotic use at 14 days after study entry and lower rates of mortality and severity-adjusted mortality at 28 days. In addition, more alternative sites of infection were found in patients randomized to the quantitative-culture strategy. A critical aspect of this study was that antibiotic treatment was initiated only in patients whose gram-stained respiratory sample was positive or who displayed signs of hemodynamic instability. Fewer than one-half as many patients were treated for pneumonia in the bronchoscopy group, and only one-third as many microorganisms were cultured. Other studies that did not demonstrate a similar beneficial impact of quantitative culture on outcomes did not tightly link antibiotic treatment to the results of quantitative culture and other tests.

Clinical approach

The lack of specificity of a clinical diagnosis of VAP has led to efforts to improve the diagnostic criteria. The Clinical Pulmonary Infection Score (CPIS) was developed by weighting of the various clinical criteria usually used for the diagnosis of VAP (Table 11-7). Use of the CPIS allows the selection of low-risk patients who may need only short-course antibiotic therapy or no treatment at all. Moreover, studies have demonstrated that the absence of bacteria in gram-stained endotracheal aspirates makes pneumonia an unlikely cause of fever or pulmonary infiltrates. These findings, coupled with a heightened awareness of the alternative diagnoses possible in patients with suspected VAP, can prevent inappropriate treatment for this disease. Furthermore, data show that the absence of an MDR pathogen in tracheal aspirate cultures eliminates the need for MDR coverage when empirical antibiotic therapy is narrowed. Since the most likely explanations for the mortality benefit of bronchoscopic quantitative cultures are decreased antibiotic selection pressure (which reduces the risk of subsequent infection with MDR pathogens) and identification of alternative sources of infection, a clinical diagnostic approach that incorporates such principles may result in similar outcomes.

TABLE 11-7

CLINICAL PULMONARY INFECTION SCORE (CPIS)	
CRITERION	**SCORE**
Fever (°C)	
≥38.5 but ≤38.9	1
>39 or <36	2
Leukocytosis	
<4000 or >11,000/µL	1
Bands >50%	1 (additional)
Oxygenation (mmHg)	
Pa_{O_2}/FI_{O_2} <250 and no ARDS	2
Chest radiograph	
Localized infiltrate	2
Patchy or diffuse infiltrate	1
Progression of infiltrate (no ARDS or CHF)	2
Tracheal aspirate	
Moderate or heavy growth	1
Same morphology on Gram's stain	1 (additional)
Maximal score[a]	12

[a]At the time of the original diagnosis, the progression of the infiltrate is not known and tracheal aspirate culture results are often unavailable; thus, the maximal score is initially 8–10.

Abbreviations: ARDS, acute respiratory distress syndrome; CHF, congestive heart failure.

TREATMENT Ventilator-Associated Pneumonia

Many studies have demonstrated higher mortality rates with inappropriate than with appropriate empirical antibiotic therapy. The key to appropriate antibiotic management of VAP is an appreciation of the patterns of resistance of the most likely pathogens in any given patient.

ANTIBIOTIC RESISTANCE If it were not for the risk of infection with MDR pathogens (Table 11-1), VAP could be treated with the same antibiotics used for severe CAP. However, antibiotic selection pressure leads to the frequent involvement of MDR pathogens by selecting either for drug-resistant isolates of common pathogens (MRSA and extended-spectrum β-lactamase–positive Enterobacteriaceae) or for intrinsically resistant pathogens (*P. aeruginosa* and *Acinetobacter* spp.). Frequent use of β-lactam drugs, especially cephalosporins, appears to be the major risk factor for infection with MRSA and extended spectrum β-lactamase–positive strains.

P. aeruginosa has demonstrated the ability to develop resistance to all routinely used antibiotics. Unfortunately, even if initially sensitive, *P. aeruginosa* isolates have also shown a propensity to develop resistance during treatment. Either derepression of resistance genes or selection of resistant clones within the large bacterial inoculum associated with most pneumonias may be the cause. *Acinetobacter* spp., *Stenotrophomonas maltophilia*, and *Burkholderia cepacia* are intrinsically resistant to many of the empirical antibiotic regimens employed (see next). VAP caused by these pathogens emerges during treatment of other infections, and resistance is always evident at initial diagnosis.

EMPIRICAL THERAPY Recommended options for empirical therapy are listed in Table 11-8. Treatment should be started once diagnostic specimens have been obtained. The major factor in the selection of agents is the presence of risk factors for MDR pathogens. Choices among the various options listed depend on local patterns of resistance and the patient's prior antibiotic exposure.

The majority of patients *without* risk factors for MDR infection can be treated with a single agent. The major difference from CAP is the markedly lower incidence of atypical pathogens in VAP; the exception is *Legionella*, which can be a nosocomial pathogen, especially with breakdowns in the treatment of potable water in the hospital.

The standard recommendation for patients *with* risk factors for MDR infection is for three antibiotics: two directed at *P. aeruginosa* and one at MRSA. The choice of a β-lactam agent provides the greatest variability in coverage, yet the use of the broadest-spectrum agent— a carbapenem, even in an antibiotic combination—still represents inappropriate initial therapy in 10–15% of cases.

SPECIFIC TREATMENT Once an etiologic diagnosis is made, broad-spectrum empirical therapy can be modified to address the known pathogen specifically. For patients with MDR risk factors, antibiotic regimens can be reduced to a single agent in more than one-half of cases and to a two-drug combination in more than one-quarter of cases. Only a minority of cases require a complete course with three drugs. A negative tracheal-aspirate culture or growth below the threshold for quantitative cultures, especially if the sample was obtained before any antibiotic change, strongly suggests that antibiotics should be discontinued. Identification of other confirmed or suspected sites of infection may require ongoing antibiotic therapy, but the spectrum of pathogens (and the corresponding antibiotic choices) may be different from those for VAP. If the CPIS decreases over the first 3 days, antibiotics should be stopped after 8 days. An 8-day course of therapy is just as effective as a 2-week course and is associated with less frequent emergence of antibiotic-resistant strains.

The major controversy regarding specific therapy for VAP concerns the need for ongoing combination treatment of *Pseudomonas* infection. No randomized controlled trials have demonstrated a benefit of combination therapy with a β-lactam and an aminoglycoside, nor have subgroup analyses in other trials found a

TABLE 11-8

EMPIRICAL ANTIBIOTIC TREATMENT OF HEALTH CARE–ASSOCIATED PNEUMONIA
Patients without Risk Factors for MDR Pathogens
Ceftriaxone (2 g IV q24h) *or*   Moxifloxacin (400 mg IV q24h), ciprofloxacin (400 mg IV q8h), or levofloxacin (750 mg IV q24h) *or*   Ampicillin/sulbactam (3 g IV q6h) *or*   Ertapenem (1 g IV q24h)
Patients with Risk Factors for MDR Pathogens
1. A β-lactam: Ceftazidime (2 g IV q8h) or cefepime (2 g IV q8–12h) *or*   Piperacillin/tazobactam (4.5 g IV q6h), imipenem (500 mg IV q6h or 1 g IV q8h), or meropenem (1 g IV q8h) *plus*   2. A second agent active against gram-negative bacterial pathogens: Gentamicin or tobramycin (7 mg/kg IV q24h) or amikacin (20 mg/kg IV q24h) *or*   Ciprofloxacin (400 mg IV q8h) or levofloxacin (750 mg IV q24h) *plus*   3. An agent active against gram-positive bacterial pathogens: Linezolid (600 mg IV q12h) *or*   Vancomycin (15 mg/kg, up to 1 g IV, q12h)

Abbreviation: MDR, multidrug-resistant.

survival benefit with such a regimen. The unacceptably high rates of clinical failure and death for VAP caused by *P. aeruginosa* despite combination therapy (see "Failure to Improve," next) indicate that better regimens are needed—including, perhaps, aerosolized antibiotics.

VAP caused by MRSA is associated with a 40% clinical failure rate when treated with standard-dose vancomycin. One proposed solution is the use of high-dose individualized treatment, although the risk of renal toxicity increases with this strategy. In addition, the MIC of vancomycin has been increasing, and a high percentage of clinical failures occur when the MIC is in the upper range of sensitivity (i.e., 1.5–2 μg/mL). Linezolid appears to be more efficacious than the standard dose of vancomycin and may be the preferred agent in patients with renal insufficiency and in those infected with high-MIC isolates of MRSA.

FAILURE TO IMPROVE Treatment failure is not uncommon in VAP, especially in that caused by MDR pathogens. In addition to the 40% failure rate for MRSA infection treated with vancomycin, VAP due to *Pseudomonas* has a 50% failure rate, no matter what the regimen. The causes of clinical failure vary with the pathogen(s) and the antibiotic(s). Inappropriate therapy can usually be minimized by use of the recommended triple-drug regimen (Table 11-8). However, the emergence of β-lactam resistance during therapy is an important problem, especially in infection with *Pseudomonas* and *Enterobacter* spp. Recurrent VAP caused by the same pathogen is possible because the biofilm on endotracheal tubes allows reintroduction of the microorganism. However, studies of VAP caused by *Pseudomonas* show that approximately one-half of recurrent cases are caused by a new strain. Inadequate local levels of vancomycin are the likely cause of treatment failure in VAP due to MRSA.

Treatment failure is very difficult to diagnose. Pneumonia due to a new superinfection, the presence of extrapulmonary infection, and drug toxicity must be considered in the differential diagnosis of treatment failure. Serial CPIS appears to track the clinical response accurately, while repeat quantitative cultures may clarify the microbiologic response. A persistently elevated or rising CPIS value by day 3 of therapy is likely to indicate failure. The most sensitive component of the CPIS is improvement in oxygenation.

COMPLICATIONS Apart from death, the major complication of VAP is prolongation of mechanical ventilation, with corresponding increases in length of stay in the ICU and in the hospital. In most studies, an additional week of mechanical ventilation because of VAP is common. The additional expense of this complication often warrants costly and aggressive efforts at prevention.

In rare cases, some types of necrotizing pneumonia (e.g., that due to *P. aeruginosa*) result in significant pulmonary hemorrhage. More commonly, necrotizing infections result in the long-term complications of bronchiectasis and parenchymal scarring leading to recurrent pneumonias. The long-term complications of pneumonia are underappreciated. Pneumonia results in a catabolic state in a patient already nutritionally at risk. The muscle loss and general debilitation from an episode of VAP often require prolonged rehabilitation and, in the elderly, commonly result in an inability to return to independent function and the need for nursing home placement.

FOLLOW-UP Clinical improvement, if it occurs, is usually evident within 48–72 h of the initiation of antimicrobial treatment. Because findings on chest radiography often worsen initially during treatment, they are less helpful than clinical criteria as an indicator of clinical response in severe pneumonia. Seriously ill patients with pneumonia often undergo follow-up chest radiography daily, at least until they are being weaned off mechanical ventilation. Once a patient has been extubated and is in stable condition, follow-up radiographs may not be necessary for a few weeks.

Prognosis

VAP is associated with significant mortality. Crude mortality rates of 50–70% have been reported, but the real issue is attributable mortality. Many patients with VAP have underlying diseases that would result in death even if VAP did not occur. Attributable mortality exceeded 25% in one matched cohort study. Patients who develop VAP are at least twice as likely to die as those who do not. Some of the variability in VAP mortality rates is clearly related to the type of patient and ICU studied. VAP in trauma patients is not associated with attributable mortality, possibly because many of the patients were otherwise healthy before being injured. However, the causative pathogen also plays a major role. Generally, MDR pathogens are associated with significantly greater attributable mortality than non–MDR pathogens. Pneumonia caused by some pathogens (e.g., *S. maltophilia*) is simply a marker for a patient whose immune system is so compromised that death is almost inevitable.

Prevention

(Table 11-6) Because of the significance of the endotracheal tube as a risk factor for VAP, the most important preventive intervention is to avoid endotracheal intubation or at least to minimize its duration. Successful use of noninvasive ventilation via a nasal or full-face mask avoids many of the problems associated with endotracheal tubes. Strategies that minimize the duration of ventilation through daily holding of sedation and formal weaning protocols have also been highly effective in preventing VAP.

Unfortunately, a tradeoff in risks is sometimes required. Aggressive attempts to extubate early may result in reintubation(s) and increase aspiration, posing a risk of VAP. Heavy continuous sedation increases the risk, but self-extubation because of too little sedation is also a risk. The tradeoffs also apply to antibiotic therapy. Short-course antibiotic prophylaxis can decrease the risk of VAP in comatose patients requiring intubation, and data suggest that antibiotics decrease VAP rates in general. However, the major benefit appears to be a decrease in the incidence of early-onset VAP, which is usually caused by the less pathogenic non-MDR microorganisms. Conversely, prolonged courses of antibiotics consistently increase the risk of VAP caused by the more lethal MDR pathogens. Despite its virulence and associated mortality, VAP caused by *Pseudomonas* is rare among patients who have not recently received antibiotics.

Minimizing the amount of microaspiration around the endotracheal tube cuff is also a strategy for avoidance of VAP. Simply elevating the head of the bed (at least 30° above horizontal but preferably 45°) decreases VAP rates. Specially modified endotracheal tubes that allow removal of the secretions pooled above the cuff may also prevent VAP. The risk-to-benefit ratio of transporting the patient outside the ICU for diagnostic tests or procedures should be carefully considered, since VAP rates are increased among transported patients.

Emphasis on the avoidance of agents that raise gastric pH and on oropharyngeal decontamination has been diminished by the equivocal and conflicting results of more recent clinical trials. The role in the pathogenesis of VAP that is played by the overgrowth of bacterial components of the bowel flora in the stomach has also been downplayed. MRSA and the nonfermenters *P. aeruginosa* and *Acinetobacter* spp. are not normally part of the bowel flora but reside primarily in the nose and on the skin, respectively. Therefore, an emphasis on controlling overgrowth of the bowel flora may be relevant only in certain populations, such as liver transplant recipients and patients who have undergone other major intraabdominal procedures or who have bowel obstruction.

In outbreaks of VAP due to specific pathogens, the possibility of a breakdown in infection control measures (particularly contamination of reusable equipment) should be investigated. Even high rates of pathogens that are already common in a particular ICU may be a result of cross-infection. Education and reminders of the need for consistent hand washing and other infection control practices can minimize this risk.

HOSPITAL-ACQUIRED PNEUMONIA

While significantly less well studied than VAP, HAP in nonintubated patients—both inside and outside the ICU—is similar to VAP. The main differences are in the higher frequency of non-MDR pathogens and the better underlying host immunity in nonintubated patients. The lower frequency of MDR pathogens allows monotherapy in a larger proportion of cases of HAP than of VAP.

The only pathogens that may be more common in the non-VAP population are anaerobes. The greater risk of macroaspiration by nonintubated patients and the lower oxygen tensions in the lower respiratory tract of these patients increase the likelihood of a role for anaerobes. While more common in patients with HAP, anaerobes are usually only contributors to polymicrobial pneumonias except in patients with large-volume aspiration or in the setting of bowel obstruction/ileus. As in the management of CAP, specific therapy targeting anaerobes probably is not indicated (unless gross aspiration is a concern) since many of the recommended antibiotics are active against anaerobes.

Diagnosis is even more difficult for HAP in the nonintubated patient than for VAP. Lower respiratory tract samples appropriate for culture are considerably more difficult to obtain from nonintubated patients. Many of the underlying diseases that predispose a patient to HAP are also associated with an inability to cough adequately. Since blood cultures are infrequently positive (<15% of cases), the majority of patients with HAP do not have culture data on which antibiotic modifications can be based. Therefore, de-escalation of therapy is less likely in patients with risk factors for MDR pathogens. Despite these difficulties, the better host defenses in non-ICU patients result in lower mortality rates than are documented for VAP. In addition, the risk of antibiotic failure is lower in HAP.

CHAPTER 12

TUBERCULOSIS

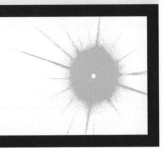

Mario C. Raviglione ■ Richard J. O'Brien

Tuberculosis (TB), which is one of the oldest diseases known to affect humans and is likely to have existed in prehominids, is a major cause of death worldwide. This disease is caused by bacteria of the *Mycobacterium tuberculosis* complex and usually affects the lungs, although other organs are involved in up to one-third of cases. If properly treated, TB caused by drug-susceptible strains is curable in virtually all cases. If untreated, the disease may be fatal within 5 years in 50–65% of cases. Transmission usually takes place through the airborne spread of droplet nuclei produced by patients with infectious pulmonary TB.

ETIOLOGIC AGENT

Mycobacteria belong to the family Mycobacteriaceae and the order Actinomycetales. Of the pathogenic species belonging to the *M. tuberculosis* complex, the most common and important agent of human disease is *M. tuberculosis*. The complex includes *M. bovis* (the bovine tubercle bacillus—characteristically resistant to pyrazinamide, once an important cause of TB transmitted by unpasteurized milk, and currently the cause of a small percentage of cases worldwide), *M. caprae* (related to *M. bovis*), *M. africanum* (isolated from cases in West, Central, and East Africa), *M. microti* (the "vole" bacillus, a less virulent and rarely encountered organism), *M. pinnipedii* (a bacillus infecting seals and sea lions in the Southern Hemisphere and recently isolated from humans), and *M. canetti* (a rare isolate from East African cases that produces unusual smooth colonies on solid media and is considered closely related to a supposed progenitor type).

M. tuberculosis is a rod-shaped, nonspore-forming, thin aerobic bacterium measuring 0.5 μm by 3 μm. Mycobacteria, including *M. tuberculosis*, are often neutral on Gram's staining. However, once stained, the bacilli cannot be decolorized by acid alcohol; this characteristic justifies their classification as acid-fast bacilli (AFB; Fig. 12-1). Acid fastness is due mainly to the organisms' high content of mycolic acids, long-chain cross-linked fatty acids, and other cell-wall lipids. Microorganisms other than mycobacteria that display some acid fastness include species of *Nocardia* and *Rhodococcus*, *Legionella micdadei*, and the protozoa *Isospora* and *Cryptosporidium*. In the mycobacterial cell wall, lipids (e.g., mycolic acids) are linked to underlying arabinogalactan and peptidoglycan. This structure confers very low permeability of the cell wall, thus reducing the effectiveness of most antibiotics. Another molecule in the mycobacterial cell wall, lipoarabinomannan, is involved in the pathogen-host interaction and facilitates the survival of *M. tuberculosis* within macrophages. The complete

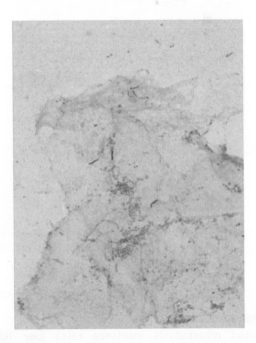

FIGURE 12-1

Acid-fast bacillus smear showing *M. tuberculosis* bacilli. (*Courtesy of the CDC, Atlanta.*)

genome sequence of *M. tuberculosis* comprises 4043 genes encoding 3993 proteins and 50 genes encoding RNAs; its high guanine–plus–cytosine content (65.6%) is indicative of an aerobic "lifestyle." A large proportion of genes are devoted to the production of enzymes involved in cell wall metabolism.

EPIDEMIOLOGY

More than 5.8 million new cases of TB (all forms, both pulmonary and extrapulmonary) were reported to the World Health Organization (WHO) in 2009; 95% of cases were reported from developing countries. However, because of insufficient case detection and incomplete notification, reported cases represent only ~63% (range, 60–67%) of total estimated cases. The WHO estimated that 9.4 million (range, 8.9–9.9 million) new cases of TB occurred worldwide in 2009, 95% of them in developing countries of Asia (5.2 million), Africa (2.8 million), the Middle East (0.7 million), and Latin America (0.3 million). It is further estimated that 1.7 million (range, 1.5–1.9 million) deaths from TB, including 0.4 million among people living with HIV infection, occurred in 2008, 96% of them in developing countries. Estimates of TB incidence rates (per 100,000 population) and numbers of TB-related deaths in 2008 are depicted in **Figs. 12-2** and **12-3**, respectively. During the late 1980s and early 1990s, numbers of reported cases of TB increased in industrialized countries. These increases were related largely to immigration from countries with a high prevalence of TB; infection with HIV; social problems, such as increased urban poverty, homelessness, and drug abuse; and dismantling of TB services. During the past few years, numbers of reported cases have begun to decline again or stabilized in industrialized nations. In the United States, with the implementation of stronger control programs, the decrease resumed in 1993. In 2009, 11,540 cases of TB (3.8 cases per 100,000 population) were reported to the Centers for Disease Control and Prevention (CDC).

In the United States, TB is uncommon among young adults of European descent, who have only rarely been exposed to *M. tuberculosis* infection during recent decades. In contrast, because of a high risk of transmission in the past, the prevalence of *M. tuberculosis* infection is relatively high among elderly whites. Blacks, however, account for the highest proportion of cases (41.4% of 4499) among U.S.-born persons. TB in the United States is also a disease of adult members of the HIV-infected population, the foreign-born population (60% of all cases in 2009), and disadvantaged/marginalized populations. Overall, more TB cases were reported among Hispanics than among other ethnic groups; next in frequency were cases among Asians and blacks, with the highest rates per capita among Asians. Similarly, in Europe, TB has reemerged as an important public health problem, mainly as a result of cases among immigrants from high-prevalence countries and among marginalized populations. In many western European countries, there are currently more cases among foreign-born than native populations.

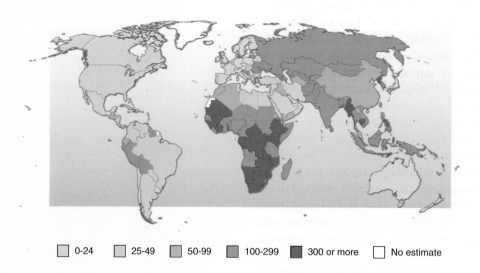

| 0-24 | 25-49 | 50-99 | 100-299 | 300 or more | No estimate |

FIGURE 12-2

Estimated tuberculosis incidence rates (per 100,000 population) in 2008. The designations employed and the presentation of material on this map do not imply the expression of any opinion whatsoever on the part of the WHO concerning the legal status of any country, territory, city, or area or of its authorities or concerning the delimitation of its frontiers or boundaries. White lines on maps represent approximate border lines for which there may not yet be full agreement. (*Courtesy of the Stop TB Department, WHO; with permission.*)

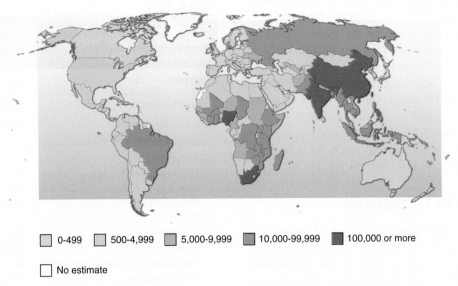

□ 0-499   □ 500-4,999   □ 5,000-9,999   ▨ 10,000-99,999   ■ 100,000 or more

□ No estimate

FIGURE 12-3
Estimated numbers of tuberculosis-related deaths in 2008. (*See disclaimer in Fig. 12-2. Courtesy of the Stop TB Department, WHO; with permission.*)

Recent data on global trends indicate that in 2009 TB incidence was stable or falling in most regions; this trend began in 2004 and appears to continue, with an average annual decline of <1% globally. This global decrease is due largely to a reduction (after a peak in 2004) in sub-Saharan Africa, where incidence had risen steeply since the 1980s as a result of the HIV epidemic and the weakness of health systems and services. In eastern Europe, incidence increased during the 1990s because of deterioration in socioeconomic conditions and the health care infrastructure; however, after peaking in 2001, incidence has since declined slowly.

Of the 9.4 million new cases estimated for 2009, 12% (1.1 million) were associated with HIV, and 80% of these HIV-associated cases occurred in Africa. An estimated 0.4 million deaths due to HIV-associated TB occurred in 2008. Furthermore, an estimated 440,000 cases of multi-drug-resistant TB (MDR-TB), a form of disease caused by bacilli resistant at least to isoniazid and rifampin, may have emerged in 2008. At present, >90% of these cases are not identified because of a lack of culture and drug-susceptibility testing capacity in most settings worldwide. The independent states of the former Soviet Union have reported the highest rates of MDR-TB among new cases (up to 20% or even higher); several provinces of China follow, with peaks of 10%. Overall, 60% of all MDR-TB cases are in India, China, and the Russian Federation. Starting in 2006, 58 countries, including the United States, reported cases of extensively drug-resistant TB (XDR-TB), in which MDR-TB is compounded by additional resistance to the most powerful second-line anti-TB drugs (fluoroquinolones and at least one of the injectable drugs amikacin, kanamycin, and capreomycin). Probably ~10% of the MDR-TB cases worldwide are

XDR-TB, but the vast majority of XDR cases remain undiagnosed.

FROM EXPOSURE TO INFECTION

M. tuberculosis is most commonly transmitted from a person with infectious pulmonary TB to others by droplet nuclei, which are aerosolized by coughing, sneezing, or speaking. The tiny droplets dry rapidly; the smallest (<5–10 μm in diameter) may remain suspended in the air for several hours and may reach the terminal air passages when inhaled. There may be as many as 3000 infectious nuclei per cough. Other routes of transmission of tubercle bacilli (e.g., through the skin or the placenta) are uncommon and of no epidemiologic significance. The probability of contact with a person who has an infectious form of TB, the intimacy and duration of that contact, the degree of infectiousness of the case, and the shared environment in which the contact takes place are all important determinants of the likelihood of transmission. Several studies of close-contact situations have clearly demonstrated that TB patients whose sputum contains AFB visible by microscopy are the most likely to transmit the infection. The most infectious patients have cavitary pulmonary disease or, much less commonly, laryngeal TB and produce sputum containing as many as 10^5–10^7 AFB/mL. Patients with sputum smear–negative/culture-positive TB are less infectious, although they have been responsible for up to 20% of transmission in some studies in the United States, and those with culture-negative pulmonary TB and extrapulmonary TB are essentially noninfectious. Because persons with both HIV infection and TB are less likely to have cavitations, they may be less infectious than persons without HIV co-infection. Crowding in poorly ventilated rooms is one of the most important factors in the transmission of tubercle bacilli, since it increases the intensity of contact with a case.

In short, the risk of acquiring *M. tuberculosis* infection is determined mainly by exogenous factors. Because of delays in seeking care and in making a diagnosis, it is generally believed that, in high-prevalence settings, up to 20 contacts may be infected by each AFB-positive case before the index case is found to have TB.

FROM INFECTION TO DISEASE

Unlike the risk of acquiring infection with *M. tuberculosis*, the risk of developing disease after being infected depends largely on endogenous factors, such as the individual's innate immunologic and nonimmunologic defenses and level of function of cell-mediated immunity (CMI). Clinical illness directly following infection is classified as *primary TB* and is common among children in the first few years of life and among immunocompromised persons. Although primary TB may be severe and disseminated, it is not generally associated with high-level transmissibility. When infection is acquired later in life, the chance is greater that the mature immune system will contain it at least temporarily. Dormant bacilli, however, may persist for years before reactivating to produce *secondary (or postprimary) TB*, which, because of frequent cavitation, is more often infectious than is primary disease. Overall, it is estimated that up to 10% of infected persons will eventually develop active TB in their lifetime, with half of them doing so during the first year after infection. The risk is much higher among HIV-infected persons. Reinfection of a previously infected individual, which is common in areas with high rates of TB transmission, may also favor the development of disease. At the height of the TB resurgence in the United States in the early 1990s, molecular typing and comparison of strains of *M. tuberculosis* suggested that up to one-third of cases of active TB in some inner-city communities were due to recent transmission rather than to reactivation of latent infection. Age is an important determinant of the risk of disease after infection. Among infected persons, the incidence of TB is highest during late adolescence and early adulthood; the reasons are unclear. The incidence among women peaks at 25–34 years of age. In this age group rates among women may be higher than those among men, while at older ages the opposite is true. The risk increases in the elderly, possibly because of waning immunity and comorbidity.

A variety of diseases and conditions favor the development of active TB (Table 12-1). In absolute terms, the most potent risk factor for TB among infected individuals is clearly HIV co-infection, which suppresses cellular immunity. The risk that latent *M. tuberculosis* infection will

TABLE 12-1

RISK FACTORS FOR ACTIVE TUBERCULOSIS AMONG PERSONS WHO HAVE BEEN INFECTED WITH TUBERCLE BACILLI

FACTOR	RELATIVE RISK/ODDS[a]
Recent infection (<1 year)	12.9
Fibrotic lesions (spontaneously healed)	2–20
Comorbidity	
HIV infection	21–>30
Silicosis	30
Chronic renal failure/hemodialysis	10–25
Diabetes	2–4
IV drug use	10–30
Immunosuppressive treatment	10
Gastrectomy	2–5
Jejunoileal bypass	30–60
Posttransplantation period (renal, cardiac)	20–70
Tobacco smoking	2–3
Malnutrition and severe underweight	2

[a]Old infection = 1.

proceed to active disease is directly related to the patient's degree of immunosuppression. In a study of HIV-infected, tuberculin skin test (TST)–positive persons, this risk varied from 2.6 to 13.3 cases per 100 person-years and increased as the CD4+ T cell count decreased.

NATURAL HISTORY OF DISEASE

Studies conducted in various countries before the advent of chemotherapy showed that untreated TB is often fatal. About one-third of patients died within 1 year after diagnosis, and more than 50% died within 5 years. The 5-year mortality rate among sputum smear–positive cases was 65%. Of the survivors at 5 years, ~60% had undergone spontaneous remission, while the remainder were still excreting tubercle bacilli. With effective, timely, and proper chemotherapy, patients have a very high chance of being cured. However, improper use of anti-TB drugs, while reducing mortality rates, may also result in large numbers of chronic infectious cases, often with drug-resistant bacilli.

PATHOGENESIS AND IMMUNITY

INFECTION AND MACROPHAGE INVASION

The interaction of *M. tuberculosis* with the human host begins when droplet nuclei containing microorganisms from infectious patients are inhaled. While the majority of inhaled bacilli are trapped in the upper airways and expelled by ciliated mucosal cells, a fraction (usually <10%) reach the alveoli. There, alveolar macrophages that have not yet been activated phagocytize the bacilli. Adhesion of mycobacteria to macrophages results largely from binding of the bacterial cell wall with a variety of macrophage cell-surface molecules, including complement receptors, the mannose receptor, the immunoglobulin GFcγ receptor, and type A scavenger receptors. Phagocytosis is enhanced by complement activation leading to opsonization of bacilli with C3 activation products such as C3b. After a phagosome forms, the survival of *M. tuberculosis* within it seems to depend on reduced acidification due to lack of accumulation of vesicular proton-adenosine triphosphatase. A complex series of events is probably generated by the bacterial cell-wall glycolipid lipoarabinomannan. This glycolipid inhibits the intracellular increase of Ca^{2+}. Thus, the Ca^{2+}/calmodulin pathway (leading to phagosome-lysosome fusion) is impaired, and the bacilli may survive within the phagosomes. The *M. tuberculosis* phagosome has been found to inhibit the production of phosphatidylinositol 3-phosphate (PI3P). Normally, PI3P earmarks phagosomes for membrane sorting and maturation including phagolysosome formation, which would destroy the bacteria. Bacterial factors have also been found to block the newly identified host defense of autophagy, in which the cell sequesters the phagosome in a double-membrane vesicle (*autophagosome*) that is destined to fuse with lysosomes. If the bacilli are successful in arresting phagosome maturation, then replication begins and the macrophage eventually ruptures and releases its bacillary contents. Other uninfected phagocytic cells are then recruited to continue the infection cycle by ingesting dying macrophages and their bacillary content, thus in turn becoming infected themselves and expanding the infection.

VIRULENCE OF TUBERCLE BACILLI

Since the elucidation of the *M. tuberculosis* genome in 1998, large mutant collections have been generated, and many bacterial genes that contribute to *M. tuberculosis* virulence have been found. Different patterns of virulence defects have been defined in various animal models, predominantly mice but also guinea pigs, rabbits, and nonhuman primates. The *katG* gene encodes for a catalase/peroxidase enzyme that protects against oxidative stress and is required for isoniazid activation and subsequent bactericidal activity. Region of difference 1 (RD1) is a 9.5-kb locus that encodes two key small protein antigens—early secretory antigen-6 (ESAT-6) and culture filtrate protein-10 (CFP-10)—as well as a putative secretion apparatus that may facilitate their egress; the absence of this locus in the vaccine strain *M. bovis* bacille Calmette-Guérin (BCG) has

been shown to be a key attenuating mutation. A recent observation in *Mycobacterium marinum*, the validity of which needs to be confirmed in *M. tuberculosis*, showed that a mutation in the RD1 virulence locus encoding the ESX1 secretion system impairs the capacity of apoptotic macrophages to recruit uninfected cells for further rounds of infection. The results are less replication and fewer new granulomas. Mutants lacking key enzymes of bacterial biosynthesis become auxotrophic for the missing substrate and are often totally unable to proliferate in animals; these include the *leuD* and *panCD* mutants, which require leucine and pantothenic acid, respectively. The isocitrate lyase gene *icl1* encodes a key step in the glyoxylate shunt that facilitates bacterial growth on fatty acid substrates; this gene is required for long-term persistence of *M. tuberculosis* infection in mice with chronic TB. *M. tuberculosis* mutants in regulatory genes such as sigma factor C and sigma factor H (*sigC* and *sigH*) are associated with normal bacterial growth in mice, but they fail to elicit full tissue pathology. Finally, the recently identified mycobacterial protein CarD (expressed by the *carD* gene) seems essential for the control of rRNA transcription that is required for replication and persistence in the host cell. Its loss exposes mycobacteria to oxidative stress, starvation, DNA damage, and ultimately sensitivity to killing by a variety of host mutagens and defensive mechanisms.

INNATE RESISTANCE TO INFECTION

Several observations suggest that genetic factors play a key role in innate nonimmune resistance to infection with *M. tuberculosis* and the development of disease. The existence of this resistance, which is polygenic in nature, is suggested by the differing degrees of susceptibility to TB in different populations. In mice, a gene called *Nramp1* (natural resistance–associated macrophage protein 1) plays a regulatory role in resistance/susceptibility to mycobacteria. The human homologue NRAMP1, which maps to chromosome 2q, may play a role in determining susceptibility to TB, as is suggested by a study among West Africans. Recent studies of mouse genetics identified a novel host resistance gene, *ipr1*, that is encoded within the *sst1* locus; *ipr1* encodes an interferon (IFN)-inducible nuclear protein that interacts with other nuclear proteins in macrophages primed with IFNs or infected by *M. tuberculosis*. In addition, polymorphisms in multiple genes, such as those encoding for various histocompatibility leukocyte antigen (HLA) alleles, IFN-γ, T cell growth factor β, interleukin (IL) 10, mannose-binding protein, IFN-γ receptor, Toll-like receptor 2, vitamin D receptor, and IL-1, have been associated with susceptibility to TB.

THE HOST RESPONSE AND GRANULOMA FORMATION

In the initial stage of host-bacterium interaction, prior to the onset of an acquired CMI response, *M. tuberculosis* undergoes a period of extensive growth within naïve unactivated macrophages, and additional naïve macrophages are recruited to the early granuloma. Studies suggest that *M. tuberculosis* uses a specific virulence mechanism to subvert host cellular signaling and to elicit an early proinflammatory response that promotes granuloma expansion and bacterial growth during this key early phase. A recent study of *M. marinum* infection in zebrafish has delineated the likely molecular mechanism by which mycobacteria induce granuloma formation. The mycobacterial protein ESAT-6 induces secretion of matrix metalloproteinase 9 (MMP9) by nearby epithelial cells that are in contact with infected macrophages. MMP9 in turn stimulates recruitment of naïve macrophages, thus inducing granuloma maturation and bacterial growth. Disruption of MMP9 function results in reduced bacterial growth. Another study has shown that *M. tuberculosis*–derived cyclic AMP is secreted from the phagosome into host macrophages, subverting the cell's signal transduction pathways and stimulating an elevation in the secretion of tumor necrosis factor α (TNF-α) and further proinflammatory cell recruitment. Ultimately, the chemoattractants and bacterial products released during the repeated rounds of cell lysis and infection of newly arriving macrophages enable dendritic cells to access bacilli; these cells migrate to the draining lymph nodes and present mycobacterial antigens to T lymphocytes. At this point, the development of CMI and humoral immunity begins. These initial stages of infection are usually asymptomatic.

About 2–4 weeks after infection, two host responses to *M. tuberculosis* develop: a macrophage-activating CMI response and a tissue-damaging response. The *macrophage-activating response* is a T cell–mediated phenomenon resulting in the activation of macrophages that are capable of killing and digesting tubercle bacilli. The *tissue-damaging response* is the result of a delayed-type hypersensitivity (DTH) reaction to various bacillary antigens; it destroys unactivated macrophages that contain multiplying bacilli but also causes caseous necrosis of the involved tissues (see later). Although both of these responses can inhibit mycobacterial growth, it is the balance between the two that determines the form of TB that will develop subsequently.

With the development of specific immunity and the accumulation of large numbers of activated macrophages at the site of the primary lesion, granulomatous lesions (tubercles) are formed. These lesions consist of accumulations of lymphocytes and activated macrophages that evolve toward epithelioid and giant cell morphologies. Initially, the tissue-damaging response can limit mycobacterial growth within macrophages. As stated earlier, this response, mediated by various bacterial products, not only destroys macrophages but also produces early solid necrosis in the center of the tubercle. Although *M. tuberculosis* can survive, its growth is inhibited within this necrotic environment by low oxygen tension and low pH. At this point, some lesions may heal by fibrosis, with subsequent calcification, whereas inflammation and necrosis occur in other lesions. Some observations have challenged the traditional view that any encounter between mycobacteria and macrophages results in chronic infection. It is possible that an immune response capable of eradicating early infection may sometimes develop as a consequence, for instance, of disabling mutations in mycobacterial genomes rendering their replication ineffective.

MACROPHAGE-ACTIVATING RESPONSE

CMI is critical at this early stage. In the majority of infected individuals, local macrophages are activated when bacillary antigens processed by macrophages stimulate T lymphocytes to release a variety of lymphokines. These activated macrophages aggregate around the lesion's center and effectively neutralize tubercle bacilli without causing further tissue destruction. In the central part of the lesion, the necrotic material resembles soft cheese (*caseous necrosis*)—a phenomenon that may also be observed in other conditions, such as neoplasms. Even when healing takes place, viable bacilli may remain dormant within macrophages or in the necrotic material for many years. These "healed" lesions in the lung parenchyma and hilar lymph nodes may later undergo calcification.

DELAYED-TYPE HYPERSENSITIVITY

In a minority of cases, the macrophage-activating response is weak, and mycobacterial growth can be inhibited only by intensified DTH reactions, which lead to lung tissue destruction. The lesion tends to enlarge further, and the surrounding tissue is progressively damaged. At the center of the lesion, the caseous material liquefies. Bronchial walls as well as blood vessels are invaded and destroyed, and cavities are formed. The liquefied caseous material, containing large numbers of bacilli, is drained through bronchi. Within the cavity, tubercle bacilli multiply, spill into the airways, and are discharged into the environment through expiratory maneuvers such as coughing and talking. In the early stages of infection, bacilli are usually transported by macrophages to regional lymph nodes, from which they gain access to the central venous return; from there they reseed the lungs and may also disseminate beyond the pulmonary vasculature throughout the body via the systemic circulation. The resulting extrapulmonary lesions may undergo the same evolution as those in the lungs, although most tend to heal. In young children with poor natural immunity, hematogenous dissemination may result in fatal miliary TB or tuberculous meningitis.

ROLE OF MACROPHAGES AND MONOCYTES

While CMI confers partial protection against *M. tuberculosis*, humoral immunity plays a less well-defined role in protection (although evidence is accumulating on the existence of antibodies to lipoarabinomannan, which may prevent dissemination of infection in children). In the case of CMI, two types of cells are essential: macrophages, which directly phagocytize tubercle bacilli, and T cells (mainly CD4+ T lymphocytes), which induce protection through the production of cytokines, especially IFN-γ. After infection with *M. tuberculosis*, alveolar macrophages secrete various cytokines responsible for a number of events (e.g., the formation of granulomas) as well as systemic effects (e.g., fever and weight loss). Monocytes and macrophages attracted to the site are key components of the immune response. Their primary mechanism is probably related to production of nitric oxide, which has antimycobacterial activity and increases the synthesis of cytokines such as TNF-α and IL-1, which in turn regulate the release of reactive nitrogen intermediates. In addition, macrophages can undergo apoptosis—a defensive mechanism to prevent release of cytokines and bacilli via their sequestration in the apoptotic cell.

ROLE OF T LYMPHOCYTES

Alveolar macrophages, monocytes, and dendritic cells are also critical in processing and presenting antigens to T lymphocytes, primarily CD4+ and CD8+ T cells; the result is the activation and proliferation of CD4+ T lymphocytes, which are crucial to the host's defense against *M. tuberculosis*. Qualitative and quantitative defects of CD4+ T cells explain the inability of HIV-infected individuals to contain mycobacterial proliferation. Activated CD4+ T lymphocytes can differentiate into cytokine-producing T_H1 or T_H2 cells. T_H1 cells produce IFN-γ—an activator of macrophages and monocytes—and IL-2. T_H2 cells produce IL-4, IL-5, IL-10, and IL-13 and may also promote humoral immunity. The interplay of these various cytokines and their cross-regulation determine the host's response. The role of cytokines in promoting intracellular killing of mycobacteria, however, has not been entirely elucidated. IFN-γ may induce the generation of reactive nitrogen intermediates and regulate genes involved in bactericidal effects. TNF-α also seems to be important. Observations made originally in transgenic knockout mice and more recently in humans suggest that other T cell subsets, especially CD8+ T cells, may play

an important role. CD8+ T cells have been associated with protective activities via cytotoxic responses and lysis of infected cells as well as with production of IFN-γ and TNF-α. Finally, natural killer cells act as co-regulators of CD8+ T cell lytic activities, and γδ T cells are increasingly thought to be involved in protective responses in humans.

MYCOBACTERIAL LIPIDS AND PROTEINS

Lipids have been involved in mycobacterial recognition by the innate immune system, and lipoproteins (such as 19-kDa lipoprotein) have been proven to trigger potent signals through Toll-like receptors present in blood dendritic cells. *M. tuberculosis* possesses various protein antigens. Some are present in the cytoplasm and cell wall; others are secreted. That the latter are more important in eliciting a T lymphocyte response is suggested by experiments documenting the appearance of protective immunity in animals after immunization with live, protein-secreting mycobacteria. Among the antigens that may play a protective role are the 30-kDa (or 85B) and ESAT-6 antigens. Protective immunity is probably the result of reactivity to many different mycobacterial antigens.

SKIN TEST REACTIVITY

Coincident with the appearance of immunity, DTH to *M. tuberculosis* develops. This reactivity is the basis of the TST, which is used primarily for the detection of *M. tuberculosis* infection in persons without symptoms. The cellular mechanisms responsible for TST reactivity are related mainly to previously sensitized CD4+ T lymphocytes, which are attracted to the skin-test site. There, they proliferate and produce cytokines. While DTH is associated with protective immunity (TST-positive persons being less susceptible to a new *M. tuberculosis* infection than TST-negative persons), it by no means guarantees protection against reactivation. In fact, cases of active TB are often accompanied by strongly positive skin-test reactions. There is also evidence of reinfection with a new strain of *M. tuberculosis* in patients previously treated for active disease. This evidence underscores the fact that previous latent or active TB may not confer fully protective immunity.

CLINICAL MANIFESTATIONS

TB is classified as pulmonary, extrapulmonary, or both. Before the advent of HIV infection, ~80% of all new cases of TB were limited to the lungs. However, up to two-thirds of HIV-infected patients with TB may have both pulmonary and extrapulmonary TB or extrapulmonary TB alone.

PULMONARY TB

Pulmonary TB can be conventionally categorized as primary or postprimary (adult-type, secondary). This distinction has been challenged by molecular evidence from TB-endemic areas indicating that a large percentage of cases of adult pulmonary TB result from recent infection (either primary infection or reinfection) and not from reactivation.

Primary disease

Primary pulmonary TB occurs soon after the initial infection with tubercle bacilli. It may be asymptomatic or present with fever and occasionally pleuritic chest pain. In areas of high TB transmission, this form of disease is often seen in children. Because most inspired air is distributed to the middle and lower lung zones, these areas of the lungs are most commonly involved in primary TB. The lesion forming after initial infection (the Ghon focus) is usually peripheral and accompanied by transient hilar or paratracheal lymphadenopathy, which may not be visible on standard chest radiography. Some patients develop erythema nodosum in the legs or phlyctenular conjunctivitis. In the majority of cases, the lesion heals spontaneously and only becomes evident as a small calcified nodule. Pleural reaction overlying a subpleural focus is also common. The Ghon focus, with or without overlying pleural reaction, thickening, and regional lymphadenopathy, is referred to as the *Ghon complex.*

In young children with immature CMI and in persons with impaired immunity (e.g., those with malnutrition or HIV infection), primary pulmonary TB may progress rapidly to clinical illness. The initial lesion increases in size and can evolve in different ways. Pleural effusion, which is found in up to two-thirds of cases, results from the penetration of bacilli into the pleural space from an adjacent subpleural focus. In severe cases, the primary site rapidly enlarges, its central portion undergoes necrosis, and cavitation develops (*progressive primary TB*). TB in young children is almost invariably accompanied by hilar or paratracheal lymphadenopathy due to the spread of bacilli from the lung parenchyma through lymphatic vessels. Enlarged lymph nodes may compress bronchi, causing total obstruction with distal collapse, partial obstruction with large-airway wheezing, or a ball-valve effect with segmental/lobar hyperinflation. Lymph nodes may also rupture into the airway with development of pneumonia, often including areas of necrosis and cavitation, distal to the obstruction. Bronchiectasis may develop in any segment/lobe damaged by progressive caseating pneumonia. Occult hematogenous dissemination commonly follows primary infection. However, in the absence of a sufficient acquired immune response, which usually contains the infection,

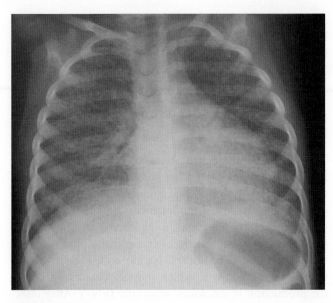

FIGURE 12-4
Chest radiograph showing bilateral miliary (millet-sized) infiltrates in a child. (*Courtesy of Prof. Robert Gie, Department of Paediatrics and Child Health, Stellenbosch University, South Africa; with permission.*)

disseminated or miliary disease may result (**Fig. 12-4**). Small granulomatous lesions develop in multiple organs and may cause locally progressive disease or result in tuberculous meningitis; this is a particular concern in very young children and immunocompromised persons (e.g., patients with HIV infection).

Postprimary (adult-type) disease

Also referred to as *reactivation* or *secondary TB*, postprimary TB is probably most accurately termed *adult-type TB*, since it may result from endogenous reactivation of distant latent infection or recent infection (primary infection or reinfection). It is usually localized to the apical and posterior segments of the upper lobes, where the substantially higher mean oxygen tension (compared with that in the lower zones) favors mycobacterial growth. The superior segments of the lower lobes are also more frequently involved. The extent of lung parenchymal involvement varies greatly, from small infiltrates to extensive cavitary disease. With cavity formation, liquefied necrotic contents are ultimately discharged into the airways and may undergo bronchogenic spread, resulting in satellite lesions within the lungs that may in turn undergo cavitation (**Figs. 12-5 and 12-6**). Massive involvement of pulmonary segments or lobes, with coalescence of lesions, produces caseating pneumonia. While up to one-third of untreated patients reportedly succumb to severe pulmonary TB within a few months after onset (the classic "galloping consumption" of the past), others may undergo a process of spontaneous remission or proceed along a chronic, progressively debilitating course ("consumption" or *phthisis*).

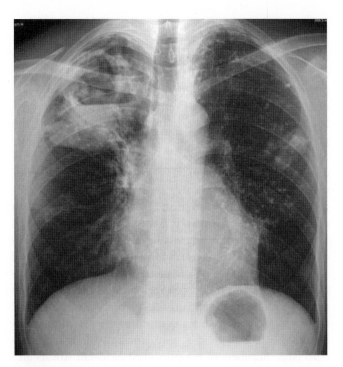

FIGURE 12-5

Chest radiograph showing a right-upper-lobe infiltrate and a cavity with an air-fluid level in a patient with active tuberculosis. (*Courtesy of Dr. Andrea Gori, Department of Infectious Diseases, S. Paolo University Hospital, Milan, Italy; with permission.*)

Under these circumstances, some pulmonary lesions become fibrotic and may later calcify, but cavities persist in other parts of the lungs. Individuals with such chronic disease continue to discharge tubercle bacilli into the environment. Most patients respond to treatment, with defervescence, decreasing cough, weight gain, and a general improvement in well-being within several weeks.

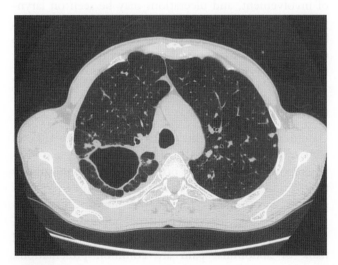

FIGURE 12-6

CT scan showing a large cavity in the right lung of a patient with active tuberculosis. (*Courtesy of Dr. Enrico Girardi, National Institute for Infectious Diseases, Spallanzani Hospital, Rome, Italy; with permission.*)

Early in the course of disease, symptoms and signs are often nonspecific and insidious, consisting mainly of diurnal fever and night sweats due to defervescence, weight loss, anorexia, general malaise, and weakness. However, in up to 90% of cases, cough eventually develops—often initially nonproductive and limited to the morning and subsequently accompanied by the production of purulent sputum, sometimes with blood streaking. Hemoptysis develops in 20–30% of cases, and massive hemoptysis may ensue as a consequence of the erosion of a blood vessel in the wall of a cavity. Hemoptysis, however, may also result from rupture of a dilated vessel in a cavity (*Rasmussen's aneurysm*) or from aspergilloma formation in an old cavity. Pleuritic chest pain sometimes develops in patients with subpleural parenchymal lesions or pleural disease. Extensive disease may produce dyspnea and, in rare instances, adult respiratory distress syndrome. Physical findings are of limited use in pulmonary TB. Many patients have no abnormalities detectable by chest examination, whereas others have detectable rales in the involved areas during inspiration, especially after coughing. Occasionally, rhonchi due to partial bronchial obstruction and classic amphoric breath sounds in areas with large cavities may be heard. Systemic features include fever (often low grade and intermittent) in up to 80% of cases and wasting. Absence of fever, however, does not exclude TB. In some cases, pallor and finger clubbing develop. The most common hematologic findings are mild anemia, leukocytosis, and thrombocytosis with a slightly elevated erythrocyte sedimentation rate and/or C-reactive protein level. None of these findings is consistent or sufficiently accurate for diagnostic purposes. Hyponatremia due to the syndrome of inappropriate secretion of antidiuretic hormone has also been reported.

EXTRAPULMONARY TB

In order of frequency, the extrapulmonary sites most commonly involved in TB are the lymph nodes, pleura, genitourinary tract, bones and joints, meninges, peritoneum, and pericardium. However, virtually all organ systems may be affected. As a result of hematogenous dissemination in HIV-infected individuals, extrapulmonary TB is seen more commonly today than in the past.

Lymph node TB (tuberculous lymphadenitis)

The most common presentation of extrapulmonary TB in both HIV-seronegative and HIV-infected patients (35% in general and >40% of cases in the United States in recent series), lymph node disease is particularly frequent among HIV-infected patients and in children. In the United States, besides children, women (particularly non-Caucasians) seem to be especially susceptible. Once caused mainly by *M. bovis*, tuberculous lymphadenitis is today due largely to *M. tuberculosis*. Lymph node TB presents as painless swelling of the lymph nodes, most commonly at posterior cervical and supraclavicular sites (a condition historically referred to as *scrofula*). Lymph nodes are usually discrete in early disease but develop into a matted nontender mass over time and may result in a fistulous tract draining caseous material. Associated pulmonary disease is present in <50% of cases, and systemic symptoms are uncommon except in HIV-infected patients. The diagnosis is established by fine-needle aspiration biopsy (with a yield of up to 80%) or surgical excision biopsy. Bacteriologic confirmation is achieved in the vast majority of cases, granulomatous lesions with or without visible AFBs are typically seen, and cultures are positive in 70–80% of cases. Among HIV-infected patients, granulomas are less well organized and are frequently absent entirely, but bacterial loads are heavier than in HIV-seronegative patients, with higher yields from microscopy and culture. Differential diagnosis includes a variety of infectious conditions, neoplastic diseases such as lymphomas or metastatic carcinomas, and rare disorders like Kikuchi's disease (necrotizing histiocytic lymphadenitis), Kimura's disease, and Castleman's disease.

Pleural TB

Involvement of the pleura accounts for ~20% of extrapulmonary cases in the United States and elsewhere. Isolated pleural effusion usually reflects recent primary infection, and the collection of fluid in the pleural space represents a hypersensitivity response to mycobacterial antigens. Pleural disease may also result from contiguous parenchymal spread, as in many cases of pleurisy accompanying postprimary disease. Depending on the extent of reactivity, the effusion may be small, remain unnoticed, and resolve spontaneously or may be sufficiently large to cause symptoms such as fever, pleuritic chest pain, and dyspnea. Physical findings are those of pleural effusion: dullness to percussion and absence of breath sounds. A chest radiograph reveals the effusion and, in up to one-third of cases, also shows a parenchymal lesion. Thoracentesis is required to ascertain the nature of the effusion and to differentiate it from manifestations of other etiologies. The fluid is straw colored and at times hemorrhagic; it is an exudate with a protein concentration >50% of that in serum (usually ~4–6 g/dL), a normal to low glucose concentration, a pH of ~7.3 (occasionally <7.2), and detectable white blood cells (usually 500–6000/μL). Neutrophils may predominate in the early stage, but lymphocyte predominance is the typical finding later. Mesothelial cells are generally rare or absent. AFB are seen on direct smear in only 10–25% of cases, but cultures may be positive for *M. tuberculosis* in 25–75% of cases; positive cultures are more common

among postprimary cases. Determination of the pleural concentration of adenosine deaminase (ADA) is a useful screening test: tuberculosis is virtually excluded if the value is very low. Lysozyme is also present in the pleural effusion. Measurement of IFN-γ, either directly or through stimulation of sensitized T cells with mycobacterial antigens, can be helpful. Needle biopsy of the pleura is often required for diagnosis and reveals granulomas and/or yields a positive culture in up to 80% of cases. This form of pleural TB responds rapidly to chemotherapy and may resolve spontaneously. Concurrent glucocorticoid administration may reduce the duration of fever and/or chest pain but is of not proven benefit.

Tuberculous empyema is a less common complication of pulmonary TB. It is usually the result of the rupture of a cavity, with spillage of a large number of organisms into the pleural space. This process may create a bronchopleural fistula with evident air in the pleural space. A chest radiograph shows hydropneumothorax with an air-fluid level. The pleural fluid is purulent and thick and contains large numbers of lymphocytes. Acid-fast smears and mycobacterial cultures are often positive. Surgical drainage is usually required as an adjunct to chemotherapy. Tuberculous empyema may result in severe pleural fibrosis and restrictive lung disease. Removal of the thickened visceral pleura (decortication) is occasionally necessary to improve lung function.

TB of the upper airways

Nearly always a complication of advanced cavitary pulmonary TB, TB of the upper airways may involve the larynx, pharynx, and epiglottis. Symptoms include hoarseness, dysphonia, and dysphagia in addition to chronic productive cough. Findings depend on the site of involvement, and ulcerations may be seen on laryngoscopy. Acid-fast smear of the sputum is often positive, but biopsy may be necessary in some cases to establish the diagnosis. Carcinoma of the larynx may have similar features but is usually painless.

Genitourinary TB

Genitourinary TB, which accounts for ~10–15% of all extrapulmonary cases in the United States and elsewhere, may involve any portion of the genitourinary tract. Local symptoms predominate, and up to 75% of patients have chest radiographic abnormalities suggesting previous or concomitant pulmonary disease. Urinary frequency, dysuria, nocturia, hematuria, and flank or abdominal pain are common presentations. However, patients may be asymptomatic and the disease discovered only after severe destructive lesions of the kidneys have developed. Urinalysis gives abnormal results in 90% of cases, revealing pyuria and hematuria. The documentation of culture-negative pyuria in acidic urine raises the suspicion of TB. IV pyelography, abdominal CT, or MRI (Fig. 12-7) may show deformities and obstructions, and calcifications and ureteral strictures are suggestive findings. Culture of three morning urine specimens yields a definitive diagnosis in nearly 90% of cases. Severe ureteral strictures may lead to hydronephrosis and renal damage. Genital TB is diagnosed more commonly in female than in male patients. In female patients, it affects the fallopian tubes and the endometrium and may cause infertility, pelvic pain, and menstrual abnormalities. Diagnosis requires biopsy or culture of specimens obtained by dilatation and curettage. In male patients, genital TB preferentially affects the epididymis, producing a slightly tender mass that may drain externally through a fistulous tract; orchitis and prostatitis may also develop. In almost half of cases of genitourinary TB, urinary tract disease is also present. Genitourinary TB responds well to chemotherapy.

Skeletal TB

In the United States, TB of the bones and joints is responsible for ~10% of extrapulmonary cases. In bone and joint disease, pathogenesis is related to reactivation of hematogenous foci or to spread from adjacent paravertebral lymph nodes. Weight-bearing joints (the spine in 40% of cases, the hips in 13%, and the knees in 10%) are most commonly affected. Spinal TB (Pott's disease or tuberculous spondylitis; Fig. 12-8) often involves

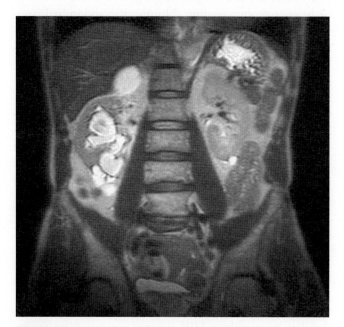

FIGURE 12-7
MRI of culture-confirmed renal tuberculosis. T2-weighted coronary plane: coronal sections showing several renal lesions in both the cortical and the medullary tissues of the right kidney. (*Courtesy of Dr. Alberto Matteelli, Department of Infectious Diseases, University of Brescia, Italy; with permission.*)

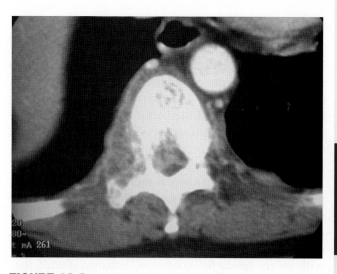

FIGURE 12-8
CT scan demonstrating destruction of the right pedicle of T10 due to Pott's disease. The patient, a 70-year-old Asian woman, presented with back pain and weight loss and had biopsy-proven tuberculosis. (*Courtesy of Charles L. Daley, MD, University of California, San Francisco; with permission.*)

two or more adjacent vertebral bodies. While the upper thoracic spine is the most common site of spinal TB in children, the lower thoracic and upper lumbar vertebrae are usually affected in adults. From the anterior superior or inferior angle of the vertebral body, the lesion slowly reaches the adjacent body, later affecting the intervertebral disk. With advanced disease, collapse of vertebral bodies results in kyphosis (*gibbus*). A paravertebral "cold" abscess may also form. In the upper spine, this abscess may track to and penetrate the chest wall, presenting as a soft tissue mass; in the lower spine, it may reach the inguinal ligaments or present as a psoas abscess. CT or MRI reveals the characteristic lesion and suggests its etiology. The differential diagnosis includes tumors and other infections. Pyogenic bacterial osteomyelitis, in particular, involves the disk very early and produces rapid sclerosis. Aspiration of the abscess or bone biopsy confirms the tuberculous etiology, as cultures are usually positive and histologic findings highly typical. A catastrophic complication of Pott's disease is paraplegia, which is usually due to an abscess or a lesion compressing the spinal cord. Paraparesis due to a large abscess is a medical emergency and requires rapid drainage. TB of the hip joints, usually involving the head of the femur, causes pain; TB of the knee produces pain and swelling. If the disease goes unrecognized, the joints may be destroyed. Diagnosis requires examination of the synovial fluid, which is thick in appearance, with a high protein concentration and a variable cell count. Although synovial fluid culture is positive in a high percentage of cases, synovial biopsy and tissue culture may be necessary to establish the diagnosis. Skeletal TB responds to chemotherapy, but severe cases may require surgery.

Tuberculous meningitis and tuberculoma

TB of the central nervous system accounts for ~5% of extrapulmonary cases in the United States. It is seen most often in young children but also develops in adults, especially those infected with HIV. Tuberculous meningitis results from the hematogenous spread of primary or postprimary pulmonary TB or from the rupture of a subependymal tubercle into the subarachnoid space. In more than half of cases, evidence of old pulmonary lesions or a miliary pattern is found on chest radiography. The disease often presents subtly as headache and slight mental changes after a prodrome of weeks of low-grade fever, malaise, anorexia, and irritability. If not recognized, tuberculous meningitis may evolve acutely with severe headache, confusion, lethargy, altered sensorium, and neck rigidity. Typically, the disease evolves over 1–2 weeks, a course longer than that of bacterial meningitis. Since meningeal involvement is pronounced at the base of the brain, paresis of cranial nerves (ocular nerves in particular) is a frequent finding, and the involvement of cerebral arteries may produce focal ischemia. The ultimate evolution is toward coma, with hydrocephalus and intracranial hypertension.

Lumbar puncture is the cornerstone of diagnosis. In general, examination of cerebrospinal fluid (CSF) reveals a high leukocyte count (up to 1000/μL), usually with a predominance of lymphocytes but sometimes with a predominance of neutrophils in the early stage; a protein content of 1–8 g/L (100–800 mg/dL); and a low glucose concentration. However, any of these three parameters can be within the normal range. AFB are seen on direct smear of CSF sediment in up to one-third of cases, but repeated lumbar punctures increase the yield. Culture of CSF is diagnostic in up to 80% of cases and remains the gold standard. Polymerase chain reaction (PCR) has a sensitivity of up to 80%, but rates of false-positivity reach 10%. Imaging studies (CT and MRI) may show hydrocephalus and abnormal enhancement of basal cisterns or ependyma. If unrecognized, tuberculous meningitis is uniformly fatal. This disease responds to chemotherapy; however, neurologic sequelae are documented in 25% of treated cases, in most of which the diagnosis has been delayed. Clinical trials have demonstrated that patients given adjunctive glucocorticoids may experience faster resolution of CSF abnormalities and elevated CSF pressure. In one study, adjunctive dexamethasone (0.4 mg/kg per day given IV and tapering by 0.1 mg/kg per week until the fourth week, when 0.1 mg/kg per day was administered; followed by 4 mg/d given by mouth and tapering by 1 mg per week until the fourth week, when 1 mg/d was administered) significantly enhanced the chances of survival among persons >14 years of age but did not reduce the frequency of neurologic sequelae.

Tuberculoma, an uncommon manifestation of central nervous system TB, presents as one or more space-occupying lesions and usually causes seizures and focal signs. CT or MRI reveals contrast-enhanced ring lesions, but biopsy is necessary to establish the diagnosis.

Gastrointestinal TB

Gastrointestinal TB is uncommon, making up 3.5% of extrapulmonary cases in the United States. Various pathogenetic mechanisms are involved: swallowing of sputum with direct seeding, hematogenous spread, or (largely in developing areas) ingestion of milk from cows affected by bovine TB. Although any portion of the gastrointestinal tract may be affected, the terminal ileum and the cecum are the sites most commonly involved. Abdominal pain (at times similar to that associated with appendicitis) and swelling, obstruction, hematochezia, and a palpable mass in the abdomen are common findings at presentation. Fever, weight loss, anorexia, and night sweats are also common. With intestinal-wall involvement, ulcerations and fistulae may simulate Crohn's disease; the differential diagnosis with this entity is always difficult. Anal fistulae should prompt an evaluation for rectal TB. As surgery is required in most cases, the diagnosis can be established by histologic examination and culture of specimens obtained intraoperatively.

Tuberculous peritonitis follows either the direct spread of tubercle bacilli from ruptured lymph nodes and intraabdominal organs (e.g., genital TB in women) or hematogenous seeding. Nonspecific abdominal pain, fever, and ascites should raise the suspicion of tuberculous peritonitis. The coexistence of cirrhosis in patients with tuberculous peritonitis complicates the diagnosis. In tuberculous peritonitis, paracentesis reveals an exudative fluid with a high protein content and leukocytosis that is usually lymphocytic (although neutrophils occasionally predominate). The yield of direct smear and culture is relatively low; culture of a large volume of ascitic fluid can increase the yield, but peritoneal biopsy (with a specimen best obtained by laparoscopy) is often needed to establish the diagnosis.

Pericardial TB (tuberculous pericarditis)

Due either to direct extension from adjacent mediastinal or hilar lymph nodes or to hematogenous spread, pericardial TB has often been a disease of the elderly in countries with low TB prevalence. However, it also develops frequently in HIV-infected patients. Case-fatality rates are as high as 40% in some series. The onset may be subacute, although an acute presentation, with dyspnea, fever, dull retrosternal pain, and a pericardial friction rub, is possible. An effusion eventually develops in many cases; cardiovascular symptoms and signs of cardiac tamponade may ultimately appear. In the presence of effusion, TB must be suspected if the patient belongs to a high-risk population (HIV-infected, originating in a high-prevalence country); if there is evidence of previous TB in other organs; or if echocardiography, CT, or MRI shows effusion and thickness across the pericardial space. A definitive diagnosis can be obtained by pericardiocentesis under echocardiographic guidance. The pericardial fluid must be submitted for biochemical, cytologic, and microbiologic study. The effusion is exudative in nature, with a high count of lymphocytes and monocytes. Hemorrhagic effusion is common. Direct smear examination is very rarely positive. Culture of pericardial fluid reveals *M. tuberculosis* in up to two-thirds of cases, while pericardial biopsy has a higher yield. High levels of ADA, lysozyme, and IFN-γ may suggest a tuberculous etiology. PCR may also be useful.

Without treatment, pericardial TB is usually fatal. Even with treatment, complications may develop, including chronic constrictive pericarditis with thickening of the pericardium, fibrosis, and sometimes calcification, which may be visible on a chest radiograph. Systematic reviews and meta-analyses show that adjunctive glucocorticoid treatment remains controversial with no conclusive evidence of benefits for all principal outcomes of pericarditis—i.e., no significant impact on resolution of effusion, no significant difference in functional status after treatment, and no significant reduction in the frequency of development of constriction or death. However, in HIV-infected patients, glucocorticoids do improve functional status after treatment.

Caused by direct extension from the pericardium or through retrograde lymphatic extension from affected mediastinal lymph nodes, tuberculous myocarditis is an extremely rare disease. Usually it is fatal and is diagnosed post-mortem.

Miliary or disseminated TB

Miliary TB is due to hematogenous spread of tubercle bacilli. Although in children it is often the consequence of primary infection, in adults it may be due to either recent infection or reactivation of old disseminated foci. The lesions are usually yellowish granulomas 1–2 mm in diameter that resemble millet seeds (thus the term *miliary*, coined by nineteenth-century pathologists). Clinical manifestations are nonspecific and protean, depending on the predominant site of involvement. Fever, night sweats, anorexia, weakness, and weight loss are presenting symptoms in the majority of cases. At times, patients have a cough and other respiratory symptoms due to pulmonary involvement as well as abdominal symptoms. Physical findings include hepatomegaly, splenomegaly, and lymphadenopathy. Eye examination may reveal choroidal tubercles, which are pathognomonic of miliary TB,

in up to 30% of cases. Meningismus occurs in <10% of cases. A high index of suspicion is required for the diagnosis of miliary TB. Frequently, chest radiography (Fig. 12-4) reveals a miliary reticulonodular pattern (more easily seen on underpenetrated film), although no radiographic abnormality may be evident early in the course and among HIV-infected patients. Other radiologic findings include large infiltrates, interstitial infiltrates (especially in HIV-infected patients), and pleural effusion. Sputum smear microscopy is negative in 80% of cases. Various hematologic abnormalities may be seen, including anemia with leukopenia, lymphopenia, neutrophilic leukocytosis and leukemoid reactions, and polycythemia. Disseminated intravascular coagulation has been reported. Elevation of alkaline phosphatase levels and other abnormal values in liver function tests are detected in patients with severe hepatic involvement. The TST may be negative in up to half of cases, but reactivity may be restored during chemotherapy. Bronchoalveolar lavage and transbronchial biopsy are more likely to provide bacteriologic confirmation, and granulomas are evident in liver or bone-marrow biopsy specimens from many patients. If it goes unrecognized, miliary TB is lethal; with proper early treatment, however, it is amenable to cure. Glucocorticoid therapy has not proved beneficial.

A rare presentation seen in the elderly is *cryptic miliary TB* that has a chronic course characterized by mild intermittent fever, anemia, and—ultimately—meningeal involvement preceding death. An acute septicemic form, *nonreactive miliary TB*, occurs very rarely and is due to massive hematogenous dissemination of tubercle bacilli. Pancytopenia is common in this form of disease, which is rapidly fatal. At postmortem examination, multiple necrotic but nongranulomatous ("nonreactive") lesions are detected.

Less common extrapulmonary forms

TB may cause chorioretinitis, uveitis, panophthalmitis, and painful hypersensitivity-related phlyctenular conjunctivitis. Tuberculous otitis is rare and presents as hearing loss, otorrhea, and tympanic membrane perforation. In the nasopharynx, TB may simulate granulomatosis with polyangiitis (Wegener's). Cutaneous manifestations of TB include primary infection due to direct inoculation, abscesses and chronic ulcers, scrofuloderma, lupus vulgaris (a smoldering disease with nodules, plaques, and fissures), miliary lesions, and erythema nodosum. Tuberculous mastitis results from retrograde lymphatic spread, often from the axillary lymph nodes. Adrenal TB is a manifestation of disseminated disease presenting rarely as adrenal insufficiency. Finally, congenital TB results from transplacental spread of tubercle bacilli to the fetus or from ingestion of contaminated amniotic fluid. This rare disease affects the liver, spleen, lymph nodes, and various other organs.

TB is one of the most common diseases among HIV-infected persons worldwide and a major cause of death. In some African countries, the rate of HIV infection among TB patients reaches 70–80% in certain urban settings. A person with a positive TST who acquires HIV infection has a 3–13% annual risk of developing active TB. A new TB infection acquired by an HIV-infected individual may evolve to active disease in a matter of weeks rather than months or years. TB can appear at any stage of HIV infection, and its presentation varies with the stage. When CMI is only partially compromised, pulmonary TB presents in a typical manner (Figs. 12-4 and 12-5), with upper-lobe infiltrates and cavitation and without significant lymphadenopathy or pleural effusion. In late stages of HIV infection, a primary TB–like pattern, with diffuse interstitial or miliary infiltrates, little or no cavitation, and intrathoracic lymphadenopathy, is more common. However, these forms are becoming less common because of the expanded use of antiretroviral treatment (ART). Overall, sputum smears may be positive less frequently among TB patients with HIV infection than among those without; thus, the diagnosis of TB may be unusually difficult, especially in view of the variety of HIV-related pulmonary conditions mimicking TB. Extrapulmonary TB is common among HIV-infected patients. In various series, extrapulmonary TB—alone or in association with pulmonary disease—has been documented in 40–60% of all cases in HIV-co-infected individuals. The most common forms are lymphatic, disseminated, pleural, and pericardial. Mycobacteremia and meningitis are also frequent, particularly in advanced HIV disease. The diagnosis of TB in HIV-infected patients may be difficult not only because of the increased frequency of sputum-smear negativity (up to 40% in culture-proven pulmonary cases) but also because of atypical radiographic findings, a lack of classic granuloma formation in the late stages, and a negative TST. Delays in treatment may prove fatal.

Exacerbations in systemic or respiratory symptoms, signs, and laboratory or radiographic manifestations of TB—termed the *immune reconstitution inflammatory syndrome* (IRIS)—have been associated with the administration of ART. Usually occurring 1–3 months after initiation of ART, IRIS is more common among patients with advanced immunosuppression and extrapulmonary TB. "Unmasking IRIS" may also develop after the initiation of ART in patients with undiagnosed subclinical TB. The presumed pathogenesis of IRIS is an immune response that is elicited by antigens released as bacilli are killed during effective chemotherapy and that is temporally associated with improving immune function. The first priority in the management of a possible case of IRIS is to ensure that the clinical syndrome does not represent a failure of TB treatment or the development of another infection. Mild paradoxical reactions can be managed with symptom-based treatment. Glucocorticoids have been used for more severe reactions, although their use in this setting has not been formally evaluated in clinical trials.

Recommendations for the prevention and treatment of TB in HIV-infected individuals are provided later.

DIAGNOSIS

The key to the diagnosis of TB is a high index of suspicion. Diagnosis is not difficult with a high-risk patient—e.g., a homeless alcoholic who presents with typical symptoms and a classic chest radiograph showing upper-lobe infiltrates with cavities (Fig. 12-5). On the other hand, the diagnosis can easily be missed in an elderly nursing home resident or a teenager with a focal infiltrate. Often, the diagnosis is first entertained when the chest radiograph of a patient being evaluated for respiratory symptoms is abnormal. If the patient has no complicating medical conditions that cause immunosuppression, the chest radiograph may show typical upper-lobe infiltrates with cavitation (Fig. 12-5). The longer the delay between the onset of symptoms and the diagnosis, the more likely is the finding of cavitary disease. In contrast, immunosuppressed patients, including those with HIV infection, may have "atypical" findings on chest radiography—e.g., lower-zone infiltrates without cavity formation.

AFB MICROSCOPY

A presumptive diagnosis is commonly based on the finding of AFB on microscopic examination of a diagnostic specimen, such as a smear of expectorated sputum or of tissue (e.g., a lymph node biopsy). Although inexpensive, AFB microscopy has relatively low sensitivity (40–60%) in culture-confirmed cases of pulmonary TB. The traditional method—light microscopy of specimens stained with Ziehl-Neelsen basic fuchsin dyes—is nevertheless satisfactory, although time-consuming. Most modern laboratories processing large numbers of diagnostic specimens use auramine-rhodamine staining and fluorescence microscopy. Less expensive light-emitting diode (LED) fluorescence microscopes are now available and should, over time, replace conventional light and fluorescence microscopes, especially facilitating the use of this technology in developing countries. For patients with suspected pulmonary TB, it has been recommended that two or three sputum specimens, preferably collected early in the morning, should be submitted to the laboratory for AFB smear and mycobacterial culture. Recent reviews have emphasized that two specimens collected on the same visit may be as effective as three. If tissue is obtained, it is critical that the portion of the specimen intended for culture not be put in formaldehyde. The use of AFB microscopy on urine or gastric lavage fluid is limited by the presence of commensal mycobacteria that can cause false-positive results.

MYCOBACTERIAL CULTURE

Definitive diagnosis depends on the isolation and identification of *M. tuberculosis* from a clinical specimen or the identification of specific sequences of DNA in a nucleic acid amplification test (see next). Specimens may be inoculated onto egg- or agar-based medium (e.g., Löwenstein-Jensen or Middlebrook 7H10) and incubated at 37°C (under 5% CO_2 for Middlebrook medium). Because most species of mycobacteria, including *M. tuberculosis*, grow slowly, 4–8 weeks may be required before growth is detected. Although *M. tuberculosis* may be identified presumptively on the basis of growth time and colony pigmentation and morphology, a variety of biochemical tests have traditionally been used to speciate mycobacterial isolates. In modern, well-equipped laboratories, the use of liquid culture for isolation and species identification by molecular methods or high-pressure liquid chromatography of mycolic acids has replaced isolation on solid media and identification by biochemical tests. A low-cost, rapid immunochromatographic lateral flow assay based on detection of MTP64 antigen may also be used for species identification of *M. tuberculosis* complex in culture isolates. These new methods, which should be introduced rapidly in developing countries, have decreased the time required for bacteriologic confirmation of TB to 2–3 weeks.

NUCLEIC ACID AMPLIFICATION

Several test systems based on amplification of mycobacterial nucleic acid are available. These systems permit the diagnosis of TB in as little as several hours, with high specificity and sensitivity approaching that of culture. These tests are most useful for the rapid confirmation of TB in persons with AFB-positive specimens but also have utility for the diagnosis of AFB-negative pulmonary and extrapulmonary TB. In settings where these tests are available, nucleic acid amplification testing should be performed on at least one respiratory specimen from patients being evaluated for suspected pulmonary TB.

DRUG SUSCEPTIBILITY TESTING

The initial isolate of *M. tuberculosis* should be tested for susceptibility to isoniazid and rifampin to detect MDR-TB, particularly if one or more risk factors for drug resistance are identified or the patient either fails to respond to initial therapy or has a relapse after the completion of treatment (see "Treatment Failure and Relapse," later). In addition, expanded susceptibility testing for second-line anti-TB drugs (especially the fluoroquinolones and the injectable drugs) is mandatory when MDR-TB is found. Susceptibility testing may be conducted directly (with the clinical specimen) or indirectly (with mycobacterial cultures) on solid or liquid medium. Results are obtained rapidly by direct susceptibility testing on liquid medium, with an average reporting time of 3 weeks. With indirect testing on solid medium, results may be unavailable for ≥8 weeks. Molecular methods for the rapid identification of genetic mutations known to be associated with resistance to rifampin and isoniazid (such as the line probe assays) have been developed and are being widely implemented for screening patients at increased risk of drug-resistant TB. Until the capacity for molecular testing is developed, a few noncommercial culture and drug-susceptibility testing methods (e.g., microscopically observed drug susceptibility, nitrate reductase assays, and colorimetric redox indicator assays) may be useful in resource-limited settings. Their use is limited to national reference laboratories with proven proficiency and adequate external quality control.

RADIOGRAPHIC PROCEDURES

As noted earlier, the initial suspicion of pulmonary TB is often based on abnormal chest radiographic findings in a patient with respiratory symptoms. Although the "classic" picture is that of upper-lobe disease with infiltrates and cavities (Fig. 12-5), virtually any radiographic pattern—from a normal film or a solitary pulmonary nodule to diffuse alveolar infiltrates in a patient with adult respiratory distress syndrome—may be seen. In the era of AIDS, no radiographic pattern can be considered pathognomonic. CT (Fig. 12-6) may be useful in interpreting questionable findings on plain chest radiography and may be helpful in diagnosing some forms of extrapulmonary TB (e.g., Pott's disease; Fig. 12-8). MRI is useful in the diagnosis of intracranial TB.

ADDITIONAL DIAGNOSTIC PROCEDURES

Other diagnostic tests may be used when pulmonary TB is suspected. Sputum induction by ultrasonic nebulization of hypertonic saline may be useful for patients who cannot produce a sputum specimen spontaneously. Frequently, patients with radiographic abnormalities that are consistent with other diagnoses (e.g., bronchogenic carcinoma) undergo fiberoptic bronchoscopy with bronchial brushings and endobronchial or transbronchial biopsy of the lesion. Bronchoalveolar lavage of a lung segment containing an abnormality may also be performed. In all cases, it is essential that specimens be submitted for AFB smear and mycobacterial culture. For the diagnosis of primary pulmonary TB in children, who often do not expectorate sputum, induced sputum specimens and specimens from early-morning gastric lavage may yield positive cultures.

Invasive diagnostic procedures are indicated for patients with suspected extrapulmonary TB. In addition to testing of specimens from involved sites (e.g., CSF for tuberculous meningitis, pleural fluid and biopsy samples for pleural disease), biopsy and culture of bone marrow and liver tissue have a good diagnostic yield in disseminated (miliary) TB, particularly in HIV-infected patients, who also have a high frequency of positive blood cultures. In some cases, cultures are negative but a clinical diagnosis of TB is supported by consistent epidemiologic evidence (e.g., a history of close contact with an infectious patient), a positive TST or IFN-γ release assay (IGRA; see later), and a compatible clinical and radiographic response to treatment. In the United States and other industrialized countries with low rates of TB, some patients with limited abnormalities on chest radiographs and sputum positive for AFB are infected with nontuberculous mycobacteria, most commonly organisms of the *M. avium* complex or *M. kansasii*. Factors favoring the diagnosis of nontuberculous mycobacterial disease over TB include an absence of risk factors for TB, a negative TST or IGRA, and underlying chronic pulmonary disease.

Patients with HIV-associated TB pose several diagnostic problems (see "HIV-associated TB," earlier). Moreover, HIV-infected patients with sputum culture–positive, AFB-positive TB may present with a normal chest radiograph. With the advent of ART, the occurrence of disseminated *M. avium* complex disease that can be confused with TB has become much less common.

SEROLOGIC AND OTHER DIAGNOSTIC TESTS FOR ACTIVE TB

A number of serologic tests based on detection of antibodies to a variety of mycobacterial antigens are marketed in developing countries but not in the United States. Careful independent assessments of these tests suggest that they are not useful as diagnostic aids, especially in persons with a low probability of TB. Various methods aimed at detection of mycobacterial antigens in diagnostic specimens are being investigated but are limited at present by low sensitivity. Determinations of ADA and IFN-γ levels in pleural fluid may be useful as adjunct tests in the diagnosis of pleural TB; the utility of these tests in the diagnosis of other forms of extrapulmonary TB (e.g., pericardial, peritoneal, and meningeal) is less clear.

DIAGNOSIS OF LATENT *M. TUBERCULOSIS* INFECTION

Tuberculin skin testing

In 1891, Robert Koch discovered that components of *M. tuberculosis* in a concentrated liquid culture medium, subsequently named "old tuberculin," were capable of eliciting a skin reaction when injected subcutaneously into patients with TB. In 1932, Seibert and Munday purified this product by ammonium sulfate precipitation to produce an active protein fraction known as *tuberculin purified protein derivative* (PPD). In 1941, PPD-S, developed by Seibert and Glenn, was chosen as the international standard. Later, the WHO and UNICEF sponsored large-scale production of a master batch of PPD (RT23) and made it available for general use. The greatest limitation of PPD is its lack of mycobacterial species specificity, a property due to the large number of proteins in this product that are highly conserved in the various species. In addition, subjectivity of the skin-reaction interpretation, deterioration of the product, and batch-to-batch variations limit the usefulness of PPD.

Skin testing with tuberculin-PPD (TST) is most widely used in screening for latent *M. tuberculosis* infection (LTBI). The test is of limited value in the diagnosis of active TB because of its relatively low sensitivity and specificity and its inability to discriminate between latent infection and active disease. False-negative reactions are common in immunosuppressed patients and in those with overwhelming TB. False-positive reactions may be caused by infections with nontuberculous mycobacteria and by BCG vaccination.

IFN-γ release assays

Two in vitro assays that measure T cell release of IFN-γ in response to stimulation with the highly TB-specific antigens ESAT-6 and CFP-10 are available. The T-SPOT.TB® (Oxford Immunotec, Oxford, UK) is an enzyme-linked immunospot (ELISpot) assay, and the QuantiFERON-TB Gold® (Cellestis Ltd., Carnegie, Australia) is a whole-blood enzyme-linked immunosorbent assay (ELISA) for measurement of IFN-γ. The QuantiFERON-TB Gold In-Tube assay, which facilitates blood collection and initial incubation, also contains another specific antigen, TB7.7.

IGRAs are more specific than the TST as a result of less cross-reactivity due to BCG vaccination and sensitization by nontuberculous mycobacteria. Although diagnostic sensitivity for LTBI cannot be directly estimated because of the lack of a gold standard, these tests have shown better correlation than the TST with exposure to *M. tuberculosis* in contact investigations in low-incidence settings. However, their performance in high TB- and/or HIV-burden settings has been much more varied. Although limited, direct comparative studies of the two assays in routine practice suggest that the ELISpot has a lower rate of indeterminate results and probably has a higher degree of diagnostic sensitivity than whole-blood ELISA. Other potential advantages of IGRAs include logistical convenience, the need for fewer patient visits to complete testing, the avoidance of somewhat subjective measurements such as skin induration, and the ability to perform serial testing without inducing the boosting phenomenon (a spurious TST conversion due to boosting of reactivity on subsequent TSTs among BCG-vaccinated persons and those infected with other mycobacteria). IGRAs require that blood be drawn from patients and delivered to the laboratory in a timely fashion. Because of high specificity and other potential advantages, IGRAs may replace the TST for LTBI diagnosis in low-incidence, high-income settings where cross-reactivity due to BCG might adversely impact the interpretation and utility of the TST.

A number of national guidelines on the use of IGRAs for LTBI testing have been issued. In the United States, an IGRA is preferred over the TST for most persons over the age of 5 years who are being screened for LTBI. However, for those at high risk of progression to active TB (e.g., HIV-infected persons), either test may be used, or both may be used to optimize sensitivity. Because of the paucity of data on IGRA testing in children, the TST is preferred for LTBI testing of children under age 5. In Canada and some European countries, a two-step approach for those with positive TSTs—i.e., initial TST followed by an IGRA—is recommended. However, a TST may boost an IGRA response if the interval between the two tests exceeds 3 days.

TREATMENT   Tuberculosis

The two aims of TB treatment are (1) to interrupt transmission by rendering patients noninfectious and (2) to prevent morbidity and death by curing patients with TB while preventing the emergence of drug resistance. Chemotherapy for TB became possible with the discovery of streptomycin in 1943. Randomized clinical trials clearly indicated that the administration of streptomycin to patients with chronic TB reduced mortality rates and led to cure in the majority of cases. However, monotherapy with streptomycin was frequently associated with the development of resistance to this drug and the attendant failure of treatment. With the introduction into clinical practice of para-aminosalicylic acid (PAS) and isoniazid, it became axiomatic in the early 1950s that cure of TB required the concomitant administration of at least two agents to which the organism was susceptible. Furthermore, early clinical trials demonstrated that a long period of treatment—i.e., 12–24 months—was required to prevent recurrence. The

introduction of rifampin (rifampicin) in the early 1970s heralded the era of effective short-course chemotherapy, with a treatment duration of <12 months. The discovery that pyrazinamide, which was first used in the 1950s, augmented the potency of isoniazid/rifampin regimens led to the use of a 6-month course of this triple-drug regimen as standard therapy.

DRUGS   Four major drugs are considered the first-line agents for the treatment of TB: isoniazid, rifampin, pyrazinamide, and ethambutol (Table 12-2). These drugs are well absorbed after oral administration, with peak serum levels at 2–4 h and nearly complete elimination within 24 h. These agents are recommended on the basis of their bactericidal activity (i.e., their ability to rapidly reduce the number of viable organisms and render patients noninfectious), their sterilizing activity (i.e., their ability to kill all bacilli and thus sterilize the affected tissues, measured in terms of the ability to prevent relapses), and their low rate of induction of drug resistance. Rifapentine and rifabutin, two drugs related to rifampin, are also available in the United States and are useful for selected patients.

TABLE 12-2

RECOMMENDED DOSAGE[a] FOR INITIAL TREATMENT OF TUBERCULOSIS IN ADULTS[b]

	DOSAGE	
DRUG	DAILY DOSE	THRICE-WEEKLY DOSE[c]
Isoniazid	5 mg/kg, max 300 mg	10 mg/kg, max 900 mg
Rifampin	10 mg/kg, max 600 mg	10 mg/kg, max 600 mg
Pyrazinamide	25 mg/kg, max 2 g	35 mg/kg, max 3 g
Ethambutol[d]	15 mg/kg	30 mg/kg

[a]The duration of treatment with individual drugs varies by regimen, as detailed in Table 12-3.
[b]Dosages for children are similar, except that some authorities recommend higher doses of isoniazid (10–15 mg/kg daily; 20–30 mg/kg intermittent) and rifampin (10–20 mg/kg).
[c]Dosages for twice-weekly administration are the same for isoniazid and rifampin but are higher for pyrazinamide (50 mg/kg, with a maximum of 4 g/d) and ethambutol (40–50 mg/d).
[d]In certain settings, streptomycin (15 mg/kg daily, with a maximum dose of 1 g; or 25–30 mg/kg thrice weekly, with a maximum dose of 1.5 g) can replace ethambutol in the initial phase of treatment. However, streptomycin is no longer considered a first-line drug by the ATS, the IDSA, or the CDC.
Source: Based on recommendations of the American Thoracic Society, the Infectious Diseases Society of America, and the Centers for Disease Control and Prevention and of the World Health Organization.

Because of a lower degree of efficacy and a higher degree of intolerability and toxicity, six classes of second-line drugs are generally used only for the treatment of patients with TB resistant to first-line drugs. Included in this group are the injectable aminoglycosides streptomycin (formerly a first-line agent), kanamycin, and amikacin; the injectable polypeptide capreomycin; the oral agents ethionamide, cycloserine, and PAS; and the fluoroquinolone antibiotics. Of the quinolones, third-generation agents are preferred: levofloxacin, gatifloxacin (no longer marketed in the United States because of its severe toxicity), and moxifloxacin. Today amithiozone (thiacetazone) is used very rarely (mainly for MDR-TB) since it is associated with severe and sometimes even fatal skin reactions among HIV-infected patients. Other drugs of unproven efficacy that have been used in the treatment of patients with resistance to most of the first- and second-line agents include clofazimine, amoxicillin/clavulanic acid, clarithromycin, imipenem, and linezolid. Two novel drugs currently under clinical development—OPC-67683, a nitroimidazole; and TMC207, a diarylquinoline—are active against MDR-TB and offer promise in shortening the course of treatment required for drug-susceptible TB as well. Moxifloxacin and gatifloxacin (see earlier) are in late-phase clinical development as 4-month treatment-shortening regimens for drug-susceptible TB.

REGIMENS Standard short-course regimens are divided into an initial, or bactericidal, phase and a continuation, or sterilizing, phase. During the initial phase, the majority of the tubercle bacilli are killed, symptoms resolve, and usually the patient becomes noninfectious. The continuation phase is required to eliminate persisting mycobacteria and prevent relapse. The treatment regimen of choice for virtually all forms of TB in adults consists of a 2-month initial phase of isoniazid, rifampin, pyrazinamide, and ethambutol followed by a 4-month continuation phase of isoniazid and rifampin (Table 12-3). In children, most forms can be safely treated without ethambutol in the intensive phase. Treatment may be given daily throughout the course or intermittently (either three times weekly throughout the course or twice weekly after an initial phase of daily therapy, although the twice-weekly option is not recommended by the WHO). However, HIV-infected patients should receive their initial-phase regimen daily. A continuation phase of once-weekly rifapentine and isoniazid is equally effective for HIV-seronegative patients with noncavitary pulmonary TB who have negative sputum cultures at 2 months. Intermittent treatment is especially useful for patients whose therapy can be directly observed (see later). Patients with cavitary pulmonary TB and delayed sputum-culture conversion (i.e., those who remain culture-positive at 2 months) should have

the continuation phase extended by 3 months, for a total course of 9 months. For patients with sputum culture–negative pulmonary TB, the duration of treatment may be reduced to a total of 4 months. To prevent isoniazid-related neuropathy, pyridoxine (10–25 mg/d) should be added to the regimen given to persons at high risk of vitamin B6 deficiency (e.g., alcoholics; malnourished persons; pregnant and lactating women; and patients with conditions such as chronic renal failure, diabetes, and HIV infection, which are also associated with neuropathy). A full course of therapy (completion of treatment) is defined more accurately by the total number of doses taken than by the duration of treatment. Specific recommendations on the required numbers of doses for each of the various treatment regimens have been published jointly by the American Thoracic Society, the Infectious Diseases Society of America, and the CDC. In some developing countries where the ability to ensure compliance with treatment is limited, a continuation-phase regimen of daily isoniazid and ethambutol for 6 months has been used. However, this regimen is associated with a higher rate of relapse and failure, especially among HIV-infected patients, and is no longer recommended by the WHO.

Lack of adherence to treatment is recognized worldwide as the most important impediment to cure. Moreover, the tubercle bacilli infecting patients who do not adhere to the prescribed regimen are likely to become drug resistant. Both patient- and provider-related factors may affect compliance. Patient-related factors include a lack of belief that the illness is significant and/or that treatment will have a beneficial effect; the existence of concomitant medical conditions (notably substance abuse); lack of social support; and poverty, with attendant joblessness and homelessness. Provider-related factors that may promote compliance include the education and encouragement of patients, the offering of convenient clinic hours, and the provision of incentives and enablers such as meals and travel vouchers. In addition to specific measures addressing noncompliance, two other strategic approaches are used: direct observation of treatment and provision of fixed-drug-combination products. Because it is difficult to predict which patients will adhere to the recommended treatment, all patients should have their therapy directly supervised, especially during the initial phase. In the United States, personnel to supervise therapy are usually available through TB control programs of local public health departments. Supervision increases the proportion of patients completing treatment and greatly lessens the chances of relapse and acquired drug resistance. Fixed-drug-combination products (e.g., isoniazid/rifampin, isoniazid/rifampin/pyrazinamide, and isoniazid/rifampin/pyrazinamide/ethambutol) are available (except, in the United States, for the four-drug fixed

TABLE 12-3

RECOMMENDED ANTITUBERCULOSIS TREATMENT REGIMENS

| INDICATION | INITIAL PHASE | | CONTINUATION PHASE | |
	DURATION, MONTHS	DRUGS	DURATION, MONTHS	DRUGS
New smear- or culture-positive cases	2	HRZE[a,b]	4	HR[a,c,d]
New culture-negative cases	2	HRZE[a]	4	HR[a]
Pregnancy	2	HRE[e]	7	HR
Relapses and treatment default (pending susceptibility testing)	3	HRZES[f]	5	HRE
Failures[g]	—	—	—	—
Resistance (or intolerance) to H	Throughout (6)	RZE[h]		
Resistance (or intolerance) to R	Throughout (12–18)	HZEQ[i]		
Resistance to H + R	Throughout (at least 20 months)	ZEQ + S (or another injectable agent[j])		
Resistance to all first-line drugs	Throughout (at least 20 months)	1 injectable agent[j] + 3 of these 4: ethionamide, cycloserine, Q, PAS		
Intolerance to Z	2	HRE	7	HR

[a]All drugs can be given daily or intermittently (three times weekly throughout). A twice-weekly regimen after 2–8 weeks of daily therapy during the initial phase is sometimes used, although it is not recommended by the WHO.

[b]Streptomycin can be used in place of ethambutol but is no longer considered to be a first-line drug by the ATS/IDSA/CDC.

[c]The continuation phase should be extended to 7 months for patients with cavitary pulmonary tuberculosis who remain sputum culture–positive after the initial phase of treatment.

[d]HIV-negative patients with noncavitary pulmonary tuberculosis who have negative sputum AFB smears after the initial phase of treatment can be given once-weekly rifapentine/isoniazid in the continuation phase.

[e]The 6-month regimen with pyrazinamide can probably be used safely during pregnancy and is recommended by the WHO and the International Union Against Tuberculosis and Lung Disease. If pyrazinamide is not included in the initial treatment regimen, the minimum duration of therapy is 9 months.

[f]Streptomycin should be discontinued after 2 months. Drug susceptibility results will determine the best regimen option.

[g]The regimen is tailored according to the results of drug susceptibility tests. The availability of rapid molecular methods to identify drug resistance allows initiation of a proper regimen at the start of treatment.

[h]A fluoroquinolone may strengthen the regimen for patients with extensive disease.

[i]Streptomycin for the initial 2 months may strengthen the regimen for patients with extensive disease.

[j]Amikacin, kanamycin, or capreomycin. All these agents should be used for at least 6 months and for 4 months after culture conversion. If susceptibility is confirmed, streptomycin could be used as the injectable agent.

Abbreviations: E, ethambutol; H, isoniazid; PAS, para-aminosalicylic acid; Q, a quinolone antibiotic; R, rifampin; S, streptomycin; Z, pyrazinamide.

drug combination) and are strongly recommended as a means of minimizing the likelihood of prescription error and of the development of drug resistance as the result of monotherapy. In some formulations of these combination products, the bioavailability of rifampin has been found to be substandard. In North America and Europe, regulatory authorities ensure that combination products are of good quality; however, this type of quality assurance cannot be assumed to be operative in less affluent countries. Alternative regimens for patients who exhibit drug intolerance or adverse reactions are listed in Table 12-3. However, severe side effects prompting discontinuation of any of the first-line drugs and use of these alternative regimens are uncommon.

MONITORING TREATMENT RESPONSE AND DRUG TOXICITY Bacteriologic evaluation is essential in monitoring the response to treatment for TB. Patients with pulmonary disease should have their sputum examined monthly until cultures become negative. With the recommended regimen, >80% of patients will have negative sputum cultures at the end of the second month of treatment. By the end of the third month, virtually all patients should be culture-negative. In some patients, especially those with extensive cavitary disease and large numbers of organisms, AFB smear conversion may lag behind culture conversion. This phenomenon is presumably due to the expectoration and microscopic visualization of dead bacilli. As noted earlier, patients with cavitary disease in whom sputum culture conversion does not occur by 2 months require extended treatment. When a patient's sputum cultures remain positive at ≥3 months, treatment failure and drug resistance or poor adherence to the regimen should be suspected (see later). A sputum specimen should be collected by the end of treatment to document cure. If mycobacterial cultures are not practical, then monitoring by AFB smear examination should be undertaken at 2, 5, and 6 months. Patients whose smears remain positive at 2 months should undergo a repeat examination at 3 months. Smears that are positive after 3 months of treatment when the patient is known to be adherent are indicative of treatment failure and possible drug resistance. Therefore, drug susceptibility testing should be done. Bacteriologic monitoring of patients with extrapulmonary TB is more difficult and often is not feasible. In these cases, the response to treatment must be assessed clinically and radiographically.

Monitoring of the response during chemotherapy by serial chest radiographs is not recommended, as radiographic changes may lag behind bacteriologic response and are not highly sensitive. After the completion of treatment, neither sputum examination nor chest radiography is recommended for routine follow-up purposes. However, a chest radiograph obtained at the end of treatment may be useful for comparative purposes should the patient develop symptoms of recurrent TB months or years later. Patients should be instructed to report promptly for medical assessment should they develop any such symptoms.

During treatment, patients should be monitored for drug toxicity (Table 12-3). The most common adverse reaction of significance is hepatitis. Patients should be carefully educated about the signs and symptoms of drug-induced hepatitis (e.g., dark urine, loss of appetite) and should be instructed to discontinue treatment promptly and see their health care provider should these symptoms occur. Although biochemical monitoring is not routinely recommended, all adult patients should undergo baseline assessment of liver function (e.g., measurement of serum levels of hepatic aminotransferases and serum bilirubin). Older patients, those with concomitant diseases, those with a history of hepatic disease (especially hepatitis C), and those using

alcohol daily should be monitored especially closely (i.e., monthly), with repeated measurements of aminotransferases, during the initial phase of treatment. Up to 20% of patients have small increases in aspartate aminotransferase (up to three times the upper limit of normal) that are not accompanied by symptoms and are of no consequence. For patients with symptomatic hepatitis and those with marked (five- to sixfold) elevations in serum levels of aspartate aminotransferase, treatment should be stopped and drugs reintroduced one at a time after liver function has returned to normal. Hypersensitivity reactions usually require the discontinuation of all drugs and rechallenge to determine which agent is the culprit. Because of the variety of regimens available, it is usually not necessary—although it is possible—to desensitize patients. Hyperuricemia and arthralgia caused by pyrazinamide can usually be managed by the administration of acetylsalicylic acid; however, pyrazinamide treatment should be stopped if the patient develops gouty arthritis. Individuals who develop autoimmune thrombocytopenia secondary to rifampin therapy should not receive the drug thereafter. Similarly, the occurrence of optic neuritis with ethambutol is an indication for permanent discontinuation of this drug. Other common manifestations of drug intolerance, such as pruritus and gastrointestinal upset, can generally be managed without the interruption of therapy.

TREATMENT FAILURE AND RELAPSE As stated earlier, treatment failure should be suspected when a patient's sputum smears and/or cultures remain positive after 3 months of treatment. In the management of such patients, it is imperative that the current isolate be tested for susceptibility to first- and second-line agents. Initial molecular testing for rifampin resistance should also be done if the technology is available. When the results of susceptibility testing are expected to become available within a few weeks, changes in the regimen can be postponed until that time. However, if the patient's clinical condition is deteriorating, an earlier change in regimen may be indicated. A cardinal rule in the latter situation is always to add more than one drug at a time to a failing regimen: at least two and preferably three drugs that have never been used and to which the bacilli are likely to be susceptible should be added. The patient may continue to take isoniazid and rifampin along with these new agents pending the results of susceptibility tests.

Patients who experience a recurrence after apparently successful treatment (relapses) are less likely to harbor drug-resistant strains (see later) than are patients in whom treatment has failed. However, if the regimen administered initially does not contain rifampin, the probability of isoniazid resistance is high. Acquired resistance is uncommon among strains from patients who relapse after completing a standard short-course regimen. However, it is prudent to begin the treatment of all patients who have relapsed with all four first-line drugs plus streptomycin, pending the results of susceptibility testing. In less affluent countries and other settings where facilities for culture and drug susceptibility testing are not yet routinely available, the WHO recommends that a standard regimen with all four first-line drugs plus streptomycin be used in all instances of relapse and treatment default. Patients with treatment failure should receive an empirical regimen, including second-line agents, based on their history of anti-TB treatment and the drug resistance patterns in the population (Table 12-3). Once drug susceptibility testing results are available, the regimen should be adjusted accordingly.

DRUG-RESISTANT TB Strains of *M. tuberculosis* resistant to individual drugs arise by spontaneous point mutations in the mycobacterial genome that occur at low but predictable rates (10^{-7}–10^{-10} for the key drugs). Because there is no cross-resistance among the commonly used drugs, the probability that a strain will be resistant to two drugs is the product of the probabilities of resistance to each drug and thus is low. The development of drug-resistant TB is invariably the result of monotherapy—i.e., the failure of the health care provider to prescribe at least two drugs to which tubercle bacilli are susceptible or of the patient to take properly prescribed therapy. Drug-resistant TB may be either primary or acquired. Primary drug resistance is that which develops in a strain infecting a patient who has not previously been treated. Acquired resistance develops during treatment with an inappropriate regimen. In North America and western Europe, rates of primary resistance are generally low, and isoniazid resistance is most common. In the United States, while rates of primary isoniazid resistance have been stable at ~7–8%, the rate of primary MDR-TB has declined from 2.5% in 1993 to 1% since 2000. Resistance rates are higher among foreign-born and HIV-infected patients. As described earlier, worldwide, MDR-TB is an increasingly serious problem in some regions, especially in the states of the former Soviet Union and in other parts of Asia (Fig. 12-9). Even more serious is the recently described occurrence of virtually untreatable XDR-TB due to MDR strains that are resistant to all fluoroquinolones and to at least one of three second-line injectable agents (amikacin, kanamycin, and capreomycin). Drug-resistant TB can be prevented by adherence to the principles of sound therapy: the inclusion of at least two bactericidal drugs to which the organism is susceptible, the use of fixed-drug-combination products, and the verification that patients complete the prescribed course.

Although the 6-month regimen described in Table 12-3 is generally effective for patients with initial isoniazid-resistant disease, it is prudent to include at least ethambutol and possibly pyrazinamide for the full 6 months. In such cases, isoniazid probably does not contribute to a successful outcome and could be omitted. For patients with extensive disease, a fluoroquinolone may be added. Patients whose isolates exhibit monoresistance to rifampin should receive a regimen containing isoniazid, pyrazinamide, ethambutol, and a fluoroquinolone for 12–18 months. MDR-TB is more difficult to manage than is disease caused by drug-susceptible organisms, especially because resistance to other first-line drugs besides isoniazid and rifampin is common. For treatment of TB due to strains resistant to isoniazid and rifampin, combinations of a fluoroquinolone, ethambutol, pyrazinamide,

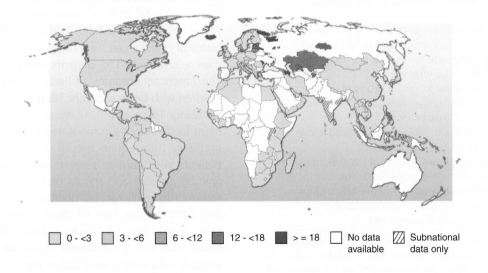

FIGURE 12-9

Percentage of new tuberculosis cases with multidrug resistance in all countries surveyed by the WHO/Union Global Drug Resistance Surveillance Project during 1994–2008. (*See disclaimer in Fig. 12-2. Courtesy of the Stop TB Department, WHO; with permission.*)

and streptomycin or, for strains resistant to streptomycin as well, another injectable agent (amikacin, kanamycin, or capreomycin) should be used. For patients with bacilli resistant to all of the first-line agents, cure may be attained with a combination of four second-line drugs, including one injectable agent (Table 12-3). Although the optimal duration of treatment is not known, a course of at least 20 months, is recommended. Patients with XDR-TB have fewer treatment options and a much poorer prognosis. However, observational studies have shown that aggressive management of cases comprising early drug-susceptibility testing, rational combination of at least five drugs, readjustment of the regimen, strict directly observed therapy, bacteriologic monitoring, and intensive patient support may result in cure rates of up to 60% and may avert deaths. Table 12-4 describes how to manage patients with XDR-TB. For patients with localized disease and sufficient pulmonary reserve, lobectomy or pneumonectomy may be considered. Because the management of patients with MDR- and XDR-TB is complicated by both social and medical factors, care of these patients is ideally provided in specialized centers or, in

TABLE 12-4

MANAGEMENT GUIDELINES FOR PATIENTS WITH DOCUMENTED OR STRONGLY SUSPECTED XDR-TB

1. Use any first-line oral agents that may be effective.
2. Use an injectable agent to which the strain is susceptible, and consider an extended duration of use (12 months or possibly the whole treatment period). If the strain is resistant to all injectable agents, use of an agent that the patient has not previously received is recommended.[a]
3. Use a later-generation fluoroquinolone, such as moxifloxacin.
4. Use all second-line oral agents (para-aminosalicylic acid, cycloserine, ethionamide, or prothionamide) that have not been used extensively in a previous regimen or any that are likely to be effective.
5. Use two or more of the following drugs of unclear role: clofazimine, amoxicillin/clavulanic acid, clarithromycin, imipenem, linezolid, thiacetazone.
6. Consider treatment with high-dose isoniazid if low-level resistance to this drug is documented.
7. Consider adjuvant surgery if there is localized disease.
8. Enforce strong infection-control measures.
9. Implement strict directly observed therapy and full adherence support as well as comprehensive bacteriologic and clinical monitoring.

[a]This recommendation is made because, while the reproducibility and reliability of susceptibility testing with injectable agents are good, there are few data on the correlation of clinical efficacy with test results. Options with XDR-TB are very limited, and some strains may be affected in vivo by an injectable agent even though they test resistant in vitro.
Source: Adapted from the World Health Organization, 2008.

their absence, in the context of programs with adequate resources and capacity.

HIV-ASSOCIATED TB   In general, the standard treatment regimens are equally efficacious in HIV-negative and HIV-positive patients. However, adverse drug effects may be more pronounced in HIV-infected patients. Three important considerations are relevant to TB treatment in HIV-infected patients: an increased frequency of paradoxical reactions, drug interactions between ART and rifamycins, and development of rifampin monoresistance with widely spaced intermittent treatment. IRIS—i.e., the exacerbation of symptoms and signs of TB—has been described earlier. All HIV-infected TB patients are candidates for ART, and the optimal timing for its initiation is as soon as possible and within the first 8 weeks of anti-TB therapy. Rifampin, a potent inducer of enzymes of the cytochrome P450 system, lowers serum levels of many HIV protease inhibitors and some nonnucleoside reverse transcriptase inhibitors—essential drugs used in ART. In such cases, rifabutin, which has much less enzyme-inducing activity, has been recommended in place of rifampin. However, dosage adjustment for rifabutin and/or the antiretroviral drugs may be necessary. Because recommendations are frequently updated, consultation of the CDC website is advised (*www.cdc.gov/tb*). Several clinical trials have found that patients with HIV-associated TB whose immunosuppression is advanced (CD4+ T cell counts of <100/μL) are prone to treatment failure and relapse with rifampin-resistant organisms when treated with "highly intermittent" (i.e., once- or twice-weekly) rifamycin-containing regimens. Consequently, it is recommended that these patients receive daily therapy for at least the initial phase.

SPECIAL CLINICAL SITUATIONS   Although comparative clinical trials of treatment for extrapulmonary TB are limited, the available evidence indicates that most forms of disease can be treated with the 6-month regimen recommended for patients with pulmonary disease. The American Academy of Pediatrics recommends that children with bone and joint TB, tuberculous meningitis, or miliary TB receive 9–12 months of treatment. Treatment for TB may be complicated by underlying medical problems that require special consideration. As a rule, patients with chronic renal failure should not receive aminoglycosides and should receive ethambutol only if serum drug levels can be monitored. Isoniazid, rifampin, and pyrazinamide may be given in the usual doses in cases of mild to moderate renal failure, but the dosages of isoniazid and pyrazinamide should be reduced for all patients with severe renal failure except those undergoing hemodialysis. Patients with hepatic disease pose a special problem because of the hepatotoxicity of isoniazid, rifampin, and pyrazinamide. Patients with severe hepatic disease may be treated with ethambutol, streptomycin, and possibly another drug (e.g., a fluoroquinolone); if required, isoniazid and rifampin may be administered under close supervision. The use of pyrazinamide by patients with liver failure should be avoided. Silicotuberculosis necessitates the extension of therapy by at least 2 months.

The regimen of choice for pregnant women (Table 12-3) is 9 months of treatment with isoniazid and rifampin supplemented by ethambutol for the first 2 months. Although the WHO has recommended routine use of pyrazinamide for pregnant women, this drug has not been recommended in the United States because of insufficient data documenting its safety in pregnancy. Streptomycin is contraindicated because it is known to cause eighth-cranial-nerve damage in the fetus. Treatment for TB is not a contraindication to breast-feeding; most of the drugs administered will be present in small quantities in breast milk, albeit at concentrations far too low to provide any therapeutic or prophylactic benefit to the child.

Medical consultation on difficult-to-manage cases is provided by the CDC Regional Training and Medical Consultation Centers (*www.cdc.gov/tb/education/rtmc/*).

PREVENTION

The best way to prevent TB is to diagnose and isolate infectious cases rapidly and to administer appropriate treatment until patients are rendered noninfectious (usually 2–4 weeks after the start of proper treatment) and the disease is cured. Additional strategies include BCG vaccination and treatment of persons with latent tuberculosis infection who are at high risk of developing active disease.

BCG VACCINATION

BCG was derived from an attenuated strain of *M. bovis* and was first administered to humans in 1921. Many BCG vaccines are available worldwide; all are derived from the original strain, but the vaccines vary in efficacy, ranging from 80% to nil in randomized, placebo-controlled trials. A similar range of efficacy was found in recent observational studies (case-control, historic cohort, and cross-sectional) in areas where infants are vaccinated at birth. These studies also found higher rates of efficacy in the protection of infants and young children from relatively serious forms of TB, such as tuberculous meningitis and miliary TB. BCG vaccine is safe and rarely causes serious complications. The local tissue response begins 2–3 weeks after vaccination, with scar formation and healing within 3 months. Side effects—most commonly, ulceration at the vaccination site and regional lymphadenitis—occur in 1–10% of vaccinated persons.

Some vaccine strains have caused osteomyelitis in ~1 case per million doses administered. Disseminated BCG infection ("BCGitis") and death have occurred in 1–10 cases per 10 million doses administered, although this problem is restricted almost exclusively to persons with impaired immunity, such as children with severe combined immunodeficiency syndrome or adults with HIV infection. BCG vaccination induces TST reactivity, which tends to wane with time. The presence or size of TST reactions after vaccination does not predict the degree of protection afforded.

BCG vaccine is recommended for routine use at birth in countries with high TB prevalence. However, because of the low risk of transmission of TB in the United States, the unreliable protection afforded by BCG, and its impact on the TST, the vaccine has never been recommended for general use in the United States. HIV-infected adults and children should not receive BCG vaccine. Moreover, infants whose HIV status is unknown but who have signs and symptoms consistent with HIV infection or who are born to HIV-infected mothers should not receive BCG.

TREATMENT Latent Tuberculosis Infection

Treatment of selected persons with LTBI aims at preventing active disease. This intervention (also called *preventive chemotherapy* or *chemoprophylaxis*) is based on the results of a large number of randomized, placebo-controlled clinical trials demonstrating that a 6- to 12-month course of isoniazid reduces the risk of active TB in infected people by up to 90%. Analysis of available data indicates that the optimal duration of treatment is 9–10 months. In the absence of reinfection, the protective effect is believed to be lifelong. Clinical trials have shown that isoniazid reduces rates of TB among TST-positive persons with HIV infection. Studies in HIV-infected patients have also demonstrated the effectiveness of shorter courses of rifampin-based treatment.

Candidates for treatment of LTBI (Table 12-5) are identified by TST or IGRA of persons in defined high-risk groups. For skin testing, 5 tuberculin units of polysorbate-stabilized PPD should be injected intradermally into the volar surface of the forearm (Mantoux method). Multipuncture tests are not recommended. Reactions are read at 48–72 h as the transverse diameter (in millimeters) of induration; the diameter of erythema is not considered. In some persons, TST reactivity wanes with time but can be recalled by a second skin test administered ≥1 week after the first (i.e., two-step testing). For persons periodically undergoing the TST, such as health care workers and individuals admitted to long-term-care institutions, initial two-step testing may preclude subsequent misclassification of persons with boosted

TABLE 12-5

TUBERCULIN REACTION SIZE AND TREATMENT OF LATENT *MYCOBACTERIUM TUBERCULOSIS* INFECTION

RISK GROUP	TUBERCULIN REACTION SIZE, mm
HIV-infected persons or persons receiving immuno-suppressive therapy	≥5
Close contacts of tuberculosis patients	≥5[a]
Persons with fibrotic lesions on chest radiography	≥5
Recently infected persons (≤2 years)	≥10
Persons with high-risk medical conditions[b]	≥10
Low-risk persons[c]	≥15

[a]Tuberculin-negative contacts, especially children, should receive prophylaxis for 2–3 months after contact ends and should then undergo repeat TST. Those whose results remain negative should discontinue prophylaxis. HIV-infected contacts should receive a full course of treatment regardless of TST results.
[b]Includes diabetes mellitus, some hematologic and reticuloendothelial diseases, injection drug use (with HIV seronegativity), end-stage renal disease, and clinical situations associated with rapid weight loss.
[c]Except for employment purposes where longitudinal TST screening is anticipated, TST is not indicated for these low-risk persons. A decision to treat should be based on individual risk/benefit considerations.

reactions as TST converters. The cutoff for a positive TST (and thus for treatment) is related both to the probability that the reaction represents true infection and to the likelihood that the individual, if truly infected, will develop TB (Table 12-5). Thus, positive reactions for close contacts of infectious cases, persons with HIV infection, persons receiving drugs that suppress the immune system, and previously untreated persons whose chest radiograph is consistent with healed TB are defined as an area of induration ≥5 mm in diameter. A 10-mm cutoff is used to define positive reactions in most other at-risk persons. For persons with a very low risk of developing TB if infected, a cutoff of 15 mm is used. (Except for employment purposes where longitudinal screening is anticipated, the TST is not indicated for these low-risk persons.) Treatment should be considered for persons from TB-endemic countries who have a history of BCG vaccination. A positive IGRA is based on the manufacturers' recommendations. For the ELISpot assay, there is an uncertainty zone (5–7 spots) for which epidemiologic and clinical factors guide the decision to implement treatment for LTBI. This approach has also been suggested for interpretation of results in the whole-blood assay that are close to the recommended cutoff for a positive test (0.35 IU of IFN-γ). Some TST- and IGRA-negative individuals are also candidates for treatment. Infants and children who have come into contact with infectious cases should be treated and should have a repeat skin test 2 or 3 months after contact ends. Those whose test results remain negative should discontinue treatment. HIV-infected persons who have been exposed to an infectious TB patient should receive treatment regardless of the TST result. Any HIV-infected candidate for LTBI treatment must be screened carefully to exclude active TB, which would necessitate full treatment.

Isoniazid is administered at a daily dose of 5 mg/kg (up to 300 mg/d) for 9 months (Table 12-6). On the basis of cost-benefit analyses, a 6-month period of treatment has been recommended in the past and may be considered for HIV-negative adults with normal chest radiographs when financial considerations are important. When supervised treatment is desirable and feasible, isoniazid may be given at a dose of 15 mg/kg (up to 900 mg) twice weekly. An alternative regimen for adults is 4 months of daily rifampin. A 3-month regimen of isoniazid and rifampin is recommended in the United Kingdom for both adults and children. A previously recommended regimen of 2 months of rifampin and pyrazinamide has been associated with serious and fatal hepatotoxicity and now is generally not recommended. The rifampin regimen should be considered for persons who are likely to have been infected with an isoniazid-resistant strain. Pending the results of a large-scale study of LTBI treatment conducted by the CDC, it is possible that a regimen of isoniazid and rifapentine given once weekly for 12 weeks will also become an option. Furthermore, clinical trials are under way to assess the efficacy of long-term isoniazid administration (i.e., for at least 3 years). Isoniazid should not be given to persons with active liver disease. All persons at increased risk of hepatotoxicity (e.g., those abusing alcohol daily and those with a history of liver disease) should undergo baseline and then monthly assessment of liver function. All patients should be carefully educated about hepatitis and instructed to discontinue use of the drug immediately should any symptoms develop. Moreover, patients should be seen and questioned monthly during therapy about adverse reactions and should be given no more than 1 month's supply of drug at each visit.

It may be more difficult to ensure compliance when treating persons with latent infection than when treating those with active TB. If family members of active cases are being treated, compliance and monitoring may be easier. When feasible, twice-weekly supervised therapy may increase the likelihood of completion. As in active cases, the provision of incentives may also be helpful.

TABLE 12-6

REVISED DRUG REGIMENS FOR TREATMENT OF LATENT TUBERCULOSIS INFECTION (LTBI) IN ADULTS

DRUG	INTERVAL AND DURATION	COMMENTS[a]	RATING[b] (EVIDENCE[c]) HIV-NEGATIVE	RATING[b] (EVIDENCE[c]) HIV-INFECTED
Isoniazid	Daily for 9 months[d,e]	In HIV-infected persons, isoniazid may be administered concurrently with nucleoside reverse transcriptase inhibitors, protease inhibitors, or NNRTIs.	A (II)	A (II)
	Twice weekly for 9 months[d,e]	DOT must be used with twice-weekly dosing.	B (II)	B (II)
	Daily for 6 months[e]	Regimen is not indicated for HIV-infected persons, those with fibrotic lesions on chest radiographs, or children.	B (I)	C (I)
	Twice weekly for 6 months[e]	DOT must be used with twice-weekly dosing.	B (II)	C (I)
Rifampin[f]	Daily for 4 months	Regimen is used for contacts of patients with isoniazid-resistant, rifampin-susceptible tuberculosis. In HIV-infected persons, most protease inhibitors and delavirdine should not be administered concurrently with rifampin. Rifabutin, with appropriate dose adjustments, can be used with protease inhibitors (saquinavir should be augmented with ritonavir) and NNRTIs (except delavirdine). Clinicians should consult web-based updates for the latest specific recommendations.	B (II)	B (III)
Rifampin plus pyrazinamide	Daily for 2 months Twice weekly for 2–3 months	Regimen generally should not be offered for treatment of LTBI in either HIV-infected or HIV-negative persons.	D (II) D (III)	D (II) D (III)

[a]Interactions with HIV-related drugs are updated frequently and are available at *www.aidsinfo.nih.gov/guidelines*.
[b]Strength of the recommendation: A. Both strong evidence of efficacy and substantial clinical benefit support recommendation for use. Should always be offered. B. Moderate evidence for efficacy or strong evidence for efficacy but only limited clinical benefit supports recommendation for use. Should generally be offered. C. Evidence for efficacy is insufficient to support a recommendation for or against use, or evidence for efficacy might not outweigh adverse consequences (e.g., drug toxicity, drug interactions) or cost of the treatment or alternative approaches. Optional. D. Moderate evidence for lack of efficacy or for adverse outcome supports a recommendation against use. Should generally not be offered. E. Good evidence for lack of efficacy or for adverse outcome supports a recommendation against use. Should never be offered.
[c]Quality of evidence supporting the recommendation: I. Evidence from at least one properly randomized controlled trial. II. Evidence from at least one well-designed clinical trial without randomization, from cohort or case-controlled analytic studies (preferably from more than one center), from multiple time-series studies, or from dramatic results in uncontrolled experiments. III. Evidence from opinions of respected authorities based on clinical experience, descriptive studies, or reports of expert committees.
[d]Recommended regimen for persons aged <18 years.
[e]Recommended regimen for pregnant women.
[f]The substitution of rifapentine for rifampin is not recommended because rifapentine's safety and effectiveness have not been established for patients with LTBI.
Abbreviations: DOT, directly observed therapy; NNRTIs, nonnucleoside reverse transcriptase inhibitors.
Source: Adapted from CDC: Targeted tuberculin testing and treatment of latent tuberculosis infection. MMWR Recomm Rep 49:RR-6, 2000.

PRINCIPLES OF TB CONTROL

The highest priority in any TB control program is the prompt detection of cases and the provision of short-course chemotherapy to all TB patients under proper case-management conditions, including directly observed therapy. In addition, in low-prevalence countries with adequate resources (and increasingly in developing countries as well), screening of high-risk groups, such as immigrants from high-prevalence countries, migratory workers, prisoners, homeless individuals, substance abusers, and HIV-seropositive persons, is recommended.

TST-positive high-risk persons should be treated for latent infection. Contact investigation is an important component of efficient TB control. In the United States and other countries worldwide, a great deal of attention has been given to the transmission of TB (particularly in association with HIV infection) in institutional settings such as hospitals, homeless shelters, and prisons. Measures to limit such transmission include respiratory isolation of persons with suspected TB until they are proven to be noninfectious (i.e., at least by sputum AFB smear negativity), proper ventilation in rooms of patients with infectious TB, use of ultraviolet irradiation in areas of increased risk of TB transmission, and periodic screening of personnel who may come into contact with known or unsuspected cases of TB. In the past, radiographic surveys, especially those conducted with portable equipment and miniature films, were advocated for case finding. Today, however, the prevalence of TB in industrialized countries is sufficiently low that "mass miniature radiography" is not cost-effective.

In high-prevalence countries, most TB control programs have made remarkable progress in reducing morbidity and mortality during the past 15 years by adopting and implementing the DOTS strategy promoted by the WHO. Between 1995 and 2008, 36 million TB cases were cured and more than 6 million deaths averted compared with the pre-DOTS period. The DOTS approach consists of: (1) political commitment with increased and sustained financing; (2) case detection through quality-assured bacteriology (starting with microscopic examination of sputum from patients with cough of >2–3 weeks' duration, culture, and possibly drug susceptibility testing); (3) administration of standardized short-course chemotherapy, with direct supervision and patient support; (4) an effective drug supply and management system; and (5) a monitoring and evaluation system, with impact measurement (including assessment of treatment outcomes—e.g., cure, completion of treatment without bacteriologic proof of cure, death, treatment failure, and default—in all cases registered and notified). In 2006, the WHO indicated that, while DOTS remains the essential component of any control strategy, additional steps must be undertaken to reach the 2015 TB control targets set within the United Nations Millennium Development Goals. Thus, a new "Stop TB Strategy" with six components has been promoted: (1) Pursue high-quality DOTS expansion and enhancement. (2) Address HIV-associated TB, MDR-TB, and the needs of poor and vulnerable populations. (3) Contribute to health system strengthening. (4) Engage all care providers. (5) Empower people with TB and [their]

communities. (6) Enable and promote research. As part of the fourth component, evidence-based International Standards for Tuberculosis Care, focused on diagnosis, treatment, and public health responsibilities, have recently been introduced for wide adoption by medical and professional societies, academic institutions, and all practitioners worldwide. Care and control of HIV-associated TB is particularly challenging in developing countries, since existing interventions require collaboration between HIV/AIDS and TB programs as well as standard services. While TB programs must test every patient for HIV in order to provide access to trimethoprim-sulfamethoxazole prophylaxis against common infections and ART, HIV/AIDS programs must regularly screen persons living with HIV/AIDS for active TB and provide treatment for LTBI. Early and active case detection is considered an important intervention not only among persons living with HIV/AIDS but also among other vulnerable populations, as it reduces transmission in a community and provides early effective care. For TB control efforts to succeed, programs must optimize their performance and include additional interventions as described. However, bold public health policies must be enforced to support work on TB control and care. These policies include free access to diagnosis and treatment, at least for the poorest patients; sound regulations to ensure drug quality; rational use of drugs by all care providers; laboratory networks equipped with the latest technology for rapid diagnosis; and airborne infection control in all facilities and congregate settings attended by TB patients, especially where HIV prevalence is high. Finally, elimination of TB will require control and attenuation of the multitude of risk factors (e.g., HIV, smoking, and diabetes) and socioeconomic determinants (e.g., extreme poverty, inadequate living conditions and bad housing, alcoholism, malnutrition, and indoor air pollution) with clear policies within the health sector and other sectors linked to human development and welfare.

CHAPTER 13

INFLUENZA

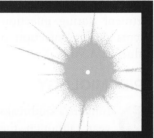

Raphael Dolin

DEFINITION

Influenza is an acute respiratory illness caused by infection with influenza viruses. The illness affects the upper and/or lower respiratory tract and is often accompanied by systemic signs and symptoms such as fever, headache, myalgia, and weakness. Outbreaks of illness of variable extent and severity occur nearly every year. Such outbreaks result in significant morbidity rates in the general population and in increased mortality rates among certain high-risk patients, mainly as a result of pulmonary complications.

ETIOLOGIC AGENT

Influenza viruses are members of the Orthomyxoviridae family, of which influenza A, B, and C viruses constitute three separate genera. The designation of influenza viruses as type A, B, or C is based on antigenic characteristics of the nucleoprotein (NP) and matrix (M) protein antigens. Influenza A viruses are further subdivided (subtyped) on the basis of the surface hemagglutinin (H) and neuraminidase (N) antigens (see later); individual strains are designated according to the site of origin, isolate number, year of isolation, and subtype—for example, influenza A/California/07/2009 (H1N1). Influenza A has 16 distinct H subtypes and 9 distinct N subtypes, of which only H1, H2, H3, N1, and N2 have been associated with epidemics of disease in humans. Influenza B and C viruses are similarly designated, but H and N antigens from these viruses do not receive subtype designations, since intratypic variations in influenza B antigens are less extensive than those in influenza A viruses and may not occur with influenza C virus.

Influenza A and B viruses are major human pathogens and the most extensively studied of the Orthomyxoviridae. Type A and type B viruses are morphologically similar. The virions are irregularly shaped spherical particles, measure 80–120 nm in diameter, and have a lipid envelope from the surface of which the H and N glycoproteins project (Fig. 13-1). The hemagglutinin is the site by which the virus binds to sialic acid cell receptors, whereas the neuraminidase degrades the receptor and plays a role in the release of the virus from infected cells after replication has taken place. Influenza viruses enter cells by receptor-mediated endocytosis, forming a virus-containing endosome. The viral hemagglutinin mediates fusion of the endosomal membrane with the virus envelope, and viral nucleocapsids are subsequently released into the cytoplasm. Immune responses to the H antigen are the major determinants of protection against infection with influenza virus, while those to the N antigen limit viral spread and contribute to reduction of the infection. The lipid envelope of influenza A virus also contains the M proteins M1 and M2, which are involved in stabilization of the lipid envelope and in virus assembly. The virion also contains the NP antigen, which is associated with the viral genome, as well as three polymerase (P) proteins that are essential for transcription and synthesis of viral RNA. Two nonstructural proteins function as an interferon antagonist and posttranscriptional regulator (NS1) and a nuclear export factor (NS2 or NEP).

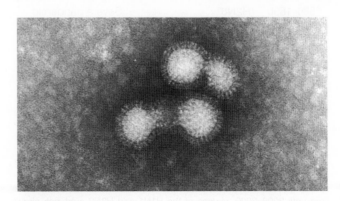

FIGURE 13-1

An electron micrograph of influenza A virus (×40,000).

147

The genomes of influenza A and B viruses consist of eight single-strand RNA segments, which code for the structural and nonstructural proteins. Because the genome is segmented, the opportunity for gene reassortment during infection is high; reassortment often occurs during infection of cells with more than one influenza A virus.

EPIDEMIOLOGY

Influenza outbreaks are recorded virtually every year, although their extent and severity vary widely. Localized outbreaks take place at variable intervals, usually every 1–3 years. Global pandemics have occurred at variable intervals, but much less frequently than interpandemic outbreaks (Table 13-1). The most recent pandemic emerged in March of 2009 and was caused by an influenza A/H1N1 virus that rapidly spread worldwide over the next several months.

Influenza A virus

Antigenic variation and influenza outbreaks and pandemics

The most extensive and severe outbreaks of influenza are caused by influenza A viruses, in part because of the remarkable propensity of the H and N antigens of these viruses to undergo periodic antigenic variation. Major antigenic variations, called *antigenic shifts*, are seen only with influenza A viruses and may be associated with pandemics. Minor variations are called *antigenic drifts*. Antigenic variation may involve the hemagglutinin alone or both the hemagglutinin and the neuraminidase.

TABLE 13-1

EMERGENCE OF ANTIGENIC SUBTYPES OF INFLUENZA A VIRUS ASSOCIATED WITH PANDEMIC OR EPIDEMIC DISEASE

YEARS	SUBTYPE	EXTENT OF OUTBREAK
1889–1890	H2N8[a]	Severe pandemic
1900–1903	H3N8[a]	?Moderate epidemic
1918–1919	H1N1[b] (formerly HswN1)	Severe pandemic
1933–1935	H1N1[b] (formerly H0N1)	Mild epidemic
1946–1947	H1N1	Mild epidemic
1957–1958	H2N2	Severe pandemic
1968–1969	H3N2	Moderate pandemic
1977–1978[c]	H1N1	Mild pandemic
2009–2010[d]	H1N1	Pandemic

[a]As determined by retrospective serologic survey of individuals alive during those years ("seroarchaeology"). [b]Hemagglutinins formerly designated as Hsw and H0 are now classified as variants of H1. [c]From this time until 2008–2009, viruses of the H1N1 and H3N2 subtypes circulated either in alternating years or concurrently. [d]Novel influenza A/H1N1 emerged to cause this pandemic.

An example of an antigenic shift involving both the hemagglutinin and the neuraminidase is that of 1957, when the predominant influenza A virus subtype shifted from H1N1 to H2N2; this shift resulted in a severe pandemic, with an estimated 70,000 excess deaths (i.e., deaths in excess of the number expected without an influenza epidemic) in the United States alone. In 1968, an antigenic shift involving only the hemagglutinin occurred (H2N2 to H3N2); the subsequent pandemic was less severe than that of 1957. In 1977, an H1N1 virus emerged and caused a pandemic that primarily affected younger individuals (i.e., those born after 1957). As can be seen in Table 13-1, H1N1 viruses circulated from 1918 to 1956; thus, individuals born prior to 1957 would be expected to have some degree of immunity to H1N1 viruses. The pandemic of 2009–2010 was caused by an A/H1N1 virus against which little immunity was present in the general population, although approximately one-third of individuals born before 1950 had some apparent immunity to related H1N1 strains.

During most outbreaks of influenza A, a single subtype has circulated at a time. However, since 1977, H1N1 and H3N2 viruses have circulated simultaneously, resulting in outbreaks of varying severity. In some outbreaks, influenza B viruses have also circulated simultaneously with influenza A viruses. In 2009–2010, the pandemic A/H1N1 virus appeared to circulate nearly exclusively.

Avian influenza A viruses

In 1997, human cases of influenza caused by avian influenza viruses (A/H5N1) were detected in Hong Kong during an extensive outbreak of influenza in poultry. Between that time and February 2010, 478 cases of avian influenza in humans were reported in Asia and the Middle East. Nearly all of these cases were associated with contact with infected poultry. Efficient person-to-person transmission has not been observed to date. Mortality rates have been high (60%), and clinical manifestations have differed somewhat from those associated with "typical" outbreaks of influenza (see later). Transmission of avian influenza A/H7N7 viruses from infected poultry to humans has been observed, including outbreaks in the Netherlands, which resulted predominantly in cases of conjunctivitis and some respiratory illnesses. Infection with avian A/H9N2 viruses along with mild respiratory illness has been reported in children in Hong Kong. Because of the absence of widespread immunity to the H5, H7, and H9 viruses, concern persists that avian-to-human transmission might also contribute to the emergence of pandemic strains.

The origin of actual pandemic influenza A virus strains has been partially elucidated with molecular virologic techniques. It appears that the pandemic strains of 1957 and 1968 resulted from a genetic reassortment between human viruses and avian viruses with novel surface glycoproteins (H2N2, H3). The pandemic A/H1N1 virus of 2009–2010 was a quadruple reassortant among swine influenza viruses that circulated in North America and Eurasia, an avian virus, and a human influenza virus. The influenza A/H1N1 virus responsible for the most severe pandemic of modern times (1918–1919) appears to have represented an adaptation of an avian virus to efficient infection of humans.

Features of pandemic and interpandemic influenza A

Pandemics provide the most dramatic evidence of the impact of influenza A. However, illnesses occurring between pandemics (interpandemic disease) also account for extensive mortality and morbidity rates, albeit over a longer period. In the United States, influenza was associated with at least 19,000 excess deaths per season in 1976–1990 and with 36,000 excess deaths per season in 1990–1999. On average, there were 226,000 influenza-associated hospitalizations per year in this country in 1979–2001.

Influenza A viruses that circulate between pandemics demonstrate antigenic drifts in the H antigen. These antigenic drifts result from point mutations involving the RNA segment that codes for the hemagglutinin, which occur most frequently in five hypervariable regions. Epidemiologically significant strains—that is, those with the potential to cause widespread outbreaks—exhibit changes in amino acids in at least two of the major antigenic sites in the hemagglutinin molecule. Since two point mutations are unlikely to occur simultaneously, it is believed that antigenic drifts result from point mutations occurring sequentially during the spread of virus from person to person. Antigenic drifts have been reported nearly annually since 1977 for H1N1 viruses and since 1968 for H3N2 viruses.

Interpandemic influenza A outbreaks usually begin abruptly, peak over a 2- to 3-week period, generally last for 2–3 months, and often subside almost as rapidly as they began. In contrast, pandemic influenza may begin with rapid transmission at multiple locations, have high attack rates, and extend beyond the usual seasonality, with multiple waves of attack before or after the main outbreak. In interpandemic outbreaks, the first indication of influenza activity is an increase in the number of children with febrile respiratory illnesses who present for medical attention. This increase is followed by increases in rates of influenza-like illnesses among adults and eventually by an increase in hospital admissions for patients with pneumonia, worsening of congestive heart failure, and exacerbations of chronic pulmonary disease. Rates of absence from work and school also rise at this time. An increase in the number of deaths caused by pneumonia and influenza is generally a late observation

in an outbreak. Attack rates have been highly variable from outbreak to outbreak in interpandemic influenza but most commonly are in the range of 10–20% of the general population.

While pandemic influenza may occur throughout the year, interpandemic influenza occurs almost exclusively during the winter months in the temperate zones of the Northern and Southern hemispheres. In those locations, it is highly unusual to detect influenza A virus at other times, although rises in serum antibody titer or even outbreaks have been noted rarely during warm-weather months. In contrast, influenza virus infections occur throughout the year in the tropics. Where or how influenza A viruses persist between outbreaks in temperate zones is unknown. It is possible that the viruses are maintained in the human population on a worldwide basis by person-to-person transmission and that large population clusters support a low level of interepidemic transmission. Alternatively, human strains may persist in animal reservoirs. Convincing evidence to support either explanation is not available. In the modern era, rapid transportation may contribute to the transmission of viruses among widespread geographic locales.

The factors that result in the inception and termination of outbreaks of influenza A are incompletely understood. A major determinant of the extent and severity of an outbreak is the level of immunity in the population at risk. With the emergence of an antigenically novel influenza virus to which little or no immunity is present in a community, extensive outbreaks may occur. When the absence of immunity is worldwide, epidemic disease may spread around the globe, resulting in a pandemic. Such pandemic waves can continue for several years, until immunity in the population reaches a high level. In the years following pandemic influenza, antigenic drifts among influenza viruses result in outbreaks of variable severity in populations with high levels of immunity to the pandemic strain that circulated earlier. This situation persists until another antigenically novel pandemic strain emerges. On the other hand, outbreaks sometimes end despite the persistence of a large pool of susceptible individuals in the population. It has been suggested that certain influenza A viruses may be intrinsically less virulent and cause less severe disease than other variants, even in immunologically virgin subjects. If so, then other (undefined) factors besides the level of preexisting immunity must play a role in the epidemiology of influenza.

Influenza B and C viruses

Influenza B virus causes outbreaks that are generally less extensive and are associated with less severe disease than those caused by influenza A virus. The hemagglutinin and neuraminidase of influenza B virus undergo less frequent and less extensive variation than those of influenza A viruses; this characteristic may account, in part, for the lesser extent of disease. Influenza B outbreaks are seen most frequently in schools and military camps, although outbreaks in institutions in which elderly individuals reside have also been noted on occasion. The most serious complication of influenza B virus infection is Reye's syndrome.

In contrast to influenza A and B viruses, influenza C virus appears to be a relatively minor cause of disease in humans. It has been associated with common cold–like symptoms and occasionally with lower respiratory tract illness. The widespread prevalence of serum antibody to this virus indicates that asymptomatic infection may be common.

Influenza-associated morbidity and mortality rates

The morbidity and mortality rates caused by influenza outbreaks continue to be substantial. Most individuals who die in this setting have underlying diseases that place them at high risk for complications of influenza (Table 13-2). Excess annual hospitalizations for groups of adults and children with high-risk medical conditions ranged from 40 to 1900 per 100,000 during outbreaks of influenza in 1973–2004. The most prominent high-risk conditions are chronic cardiac and pulmonary diseases and old age. Mortality rates among individuals with chronic metabolic or renal diseases or certain immunosuppressive diseases have also been elevated, albeit lower than those among patients with chronic cardiopulmonary diseases. In the pandemic of 2009–2010,

TABLE 13-2

PERSONS AT HIGHER RISK FOR COMPLICATIONS OF INFLUENZA
Children from birth to 4 years old
Pregnant women
Persons ≥65 years old
Children and adolescents (6 months to 18 years old) who are receiving long-term aspirin therapy and therefore may be at risk for developing Reye's syndrome after influenza
Adults and children who have chronic disorders of the pulmonary or cardiovascular system, including asthma
Adults and children who have chronic metabolic diseases (including diabetes mellitus), renal dysfunction, hemoglobinopathies, or immunodeficiency (including immunodeficiency caused by medications or by HIV)
Adults and children who have any condition that can compromise respiratory function or compromise the handling of respiratory secretions or can increase the risk of aspiration
Residents of nursing homes and other chronic-care facilities that house persons of any age who have chronic medical conditions

increased risk for severe disease was noted in children from birth to 4 years of age and in pregnant women. The morbidity rate attributable to influenza in the general population is considerable. It is estimated that interpandemic outbreaks of influenza currently incur annual economic costs of more than $87 billion in the United States. For pandemics, it is estimated that annual economic costs would range from $89.7 to $209.4 billion for attack rates of 15–35%.

PATHOGENESIS AND IMMUNITY

The initial event in influenza is infection of the respiratory epithelium with influenza virus acquired from respiratory secretions of acutely infected individuals. In all likelihood, the virus is transmitted via aerosols generated by coughs and sneezes, although hand-to-hand contact, other personal contact, and even fomite transmission may take place. Experimental evidence suggests that infection by a small-particle aerosol (particle diameter, <10 μm) is more efficient than that by larger droplets. Initially, viral infection involves the ciliated columnar epithelial cells, but it may also involve other respiratory tract cells, including alveolar cells, mucous gland cells, and macrophages. In infected cells, virus replicates within 4–6 h, after which infectious virus is released to infect adjacent or nearby cells. In this way, infection spreads from a few foci to a large number of respiratory cells over several hours. In experimentally induced infection, the incubation period of illness has ranged from 18 to 72 h, depending on the size of the viral inoculum. Histopathologic study reveals degenerative changes, including granulation, vacuolization, swelling, and pyknotic nuclei, in infected ciliated cells. The cells eventually become necrotic and desquamate; in some areas, previously columnar epithelium is replaced by flattened and metaplastic epithelial cells. The severity of illness is correlated with the quantity of virus shed in secretions; thus, the degree of viral replication itself may be an important factor in pathogenesis. Despite the frequent development of systemic signs and symptoms such as fever, headache, and myalgias, influenza virus has only rarely been detected in extrapulmonary sites (including the bloodstream). Evidence suggests that the pathogenesis of systemic symptoms in influenza may be related to the induction of certain cytokines, particularly tumor necrosis factor α, interferon α, interleukin 6, and interleukin 8, in respiratory secretions and in the bloodstream.

The host response to influenza infections involves a complex interplay of humoral antibody, local antibody, cell-mediated immunity, interferon, and other host defenses. Serum antibody responses, which can be detected by the second week after primary infection, are measured by a variety of techniques: hemagglutination inhibition (HI), complement fixation (CF), neutralization, enzyme-linked immunosorbent assay (ELISA), and antineuraminidase antibody assay. Antibodies to the hemagglutinin appear to be the most important mediators of immunity; in several studies, HI titers of ≥40 have been associated with protection from infection. Secretory antibodies produced in the respiratory tract are predominantly of the IgA class and also play a major role in protection against infection. Secretory antibody neutralization titers of ≥4 have also been associated with protection. A variety of cell-mediated immune responses, both antigen-specific and antigen-nonspecific, can be detected early after infection and depend on the prior immune status of the host. These responses include T cell proliferative, T cell cytotoxic, and natural killer cell activity. In humans, CD8+ human leukocyte antigen class I–restricted cytotoxic T lymphocytes (CTLs) are directed at conserved regions of internal proteins (NP, M, and P) as well as at the surface proteins H and N. Interferons can be detected in respiratory secretions shortly after the shedding of virus has begun, and rises in interferon titers coincide with decreases in virus shedding.

The host defense factors responsible for cessation of virus shedding and resolution of illness have not been defined specifically. Virus shedding generally stops within 2–5 days after symptoms first appear, at a time when serum and local antibody responses often are not detectable by conventional techniques (although antibody rises may be detected earlier by use of highly sensitive techniques, particularly in individuals with previous immunity to the virus). It has been suggested that interferon, cell-mediated immune responses, and/or nonspecific inflammatory responses all contribute to the resolution of illness. CTL responses may be particularly important in this regard.

CLINICAL MANIFESTATIONS

Influenza has most frequently been described as an illness characterized by the abrupt onset of systemic symptoms, such as headache, feverishness, chills, myalgia, and malaise, as well as accompanying respiratory tract signs, particularly cough and sore throat. In many cases, the onset is so abrupt that patients can recall the precise time they became ill. However, the spectrum of clinical presentations is wide, ranging from a mild, afebrile respiratory illness similar to the common cold (with either a gradual or an abrupt onset) to severe prostration with relatively few respiratory signs and symptoms. In most of the cases that come to a physician's attention, the patient has a fever, with temperatures of 38°–41°C (100.4°–105.8°F). A rapid temperature rise within the first 24 h of illness is generally followed by gradual defervescence over 2–3 days, although, on occasion, fever may last as long as 1 week. Patients report a feverish feeling and chilliness, but true rigors are rare. Headache, either generalized or frontal, is often particularly troublesome. Myalgias may involve any

part of the body but are most common in the legs and lumbosacral area. Arthralgias may also develop.

Respiratory symptoms often become more prominent as systemic symptoms subside. Many patients have a sore throat or persistent cough, which may last for ≥1 week and which is often accompanied by substernal discomfort. Ocular signs and symptoms include pain on motion of the eyes, photophobia, and burning of the eyes.

Physical findings are usually minimal in uncomplicated influenza. Early in the illness, the patient appears flushed and the skin is hot and dry, although diaphoresis and mottled extremities are sometimes evident, particularly in older patients. Examination of the pharynx may yield surprisingly unremarkable results despite a severe sore throat, but injection of the mucous membranes and postnasal discharge are apparent in some cases. Mild cervical lymphadenopathy may be noted, especially in younger individuals. The results of chest examination are largely negative in uncomplicated influenza, although rhonchi, wheezes, and scattered rales have been reported with variable frequency in different outbreaks. Frank dyspnea, hyperpnea, cyanosis, diffuse rales, and signs of consolidation are indicative of pulmonary complications. Patients with apparently uncomplicated influenza have been reported to have a variety of mild ventilatory defects and increased alveolar-capillary diffusion gradients; thus, subclinical pulmonary involvement may be more common than is appreciated.

In uncomplicated influenza, the acute illness generally resolves over 2–5 days, and most patients have largely recovered in 1 week, although cough may persist 1–2 weeks longer. In a significant minority (particularly the elderly), however, symptoms of weakness or lassitude (postinfluenza asthenia) may persist for several weeks and may prove troublesome for persons who wish to resume their full level of activity promptly. The pathogenetic basis for this asthenia is unknown, although pulmonary function abnormalities may persist for several weeks after uncomplicated influenza.

COMPLICATIONS

Complications of influenza (Table 13-2) occur most frequently in patients >65 years old and in those with certain chronic disorders, including cardiac or pulmonary diseases, diabetes mellitus, hemoglobinopathies, renal dysfunction, and immunosuppression. Pregnancy in the second or third trimester predisposes to complications with influenza. Children <5 years old (especially infants) are also at high risk for complications.

Pulmonary complications

Pneumonia

The most significant complication of influenza is pneumonia: "primary" influenza viral pneumonia, secondary bacterial pneumonia, or mixed viral and bacterial pneumonia.

Primary influenza viral pneumonia

Primary influenza viral pneumonia is the least common but most severe of the pneumonic complications. It presents as acute influenza that does not resolve but instead progresses relentlessly, with persistent fever, dyspnea, and eventual cyanosis. Sputum production is generally scanty, but the sputum can contain blood. Few physical signs may be evident early in the illness. In more advanced cases, diffuse rales may be noted, and chest x-ray findings consistent with diffuse interstitial infiltrates and/or acute respiratory distress syndrome may be present. In such cases, arterial blood-gas determinations show marked hypoxia. Viral cultures of respiratory secretions and lung parenchyma, especially if samples are taken early in illness, yield high titers of virus. In fatal cases of primary viral pneumonia, histopathologic examination reveals a marked inflammatory reaction in the alveolar septa, with edema and infiltration by lymphocytes, macrophages, occasional plasma cells, and variable numbers of neutrophils. Fibrin thrombi in alveolar capillaries, along with necrosis and hemorrhage, have also been noted. Eosinophilic hyaline membranes can be found lining alveoli and alveolar ducts.

Primary influenza viral pneumonia has a predilection for individuals with cardiac disease, particularly those with mitral stenosis, but has also been reported in otherwise-healthy young adults as well as in older individuals with chronic pulmonary disorders. In some pandemics of influenza (notably those of 1918 and 1957), pregnancy increased the risk of primary influenza pneumonia. Subsequent epidemics of influenza have been associated with increased rates of hospitalization among pregnant women, which were also noted in the pandemic of 2009–2010.

Secondary bacterial pneumonia

Secondary bacterial pneumonia follows acute influenza. Improvement of the patient's condition over 2–3 days is followed by a reappearance of fever along with clinical signs and symptoms of bacterial pneumonia, including cough, production of purulent sputum, and physical and x-ray signs of consolidation. The most common bacterial pathogens in this setting are *Streptococcus pneumoniae*, *Staphylococcus aureus*, and *Haemophilus influenzae*—organisms that can colonize the nasopharynx and that cause infection in the wake of changes in bronchopulmonary defenses. The etiology can often be determined by Gram's staining and culture of an appropriately obtained sputum specimen. Secondary bacterial pneumonia occurs most frequently in high-risk individuals with chronic pulmonary and cardiac disease and in elderly individuals. Patients with secondary bacterial pneumonia often respond to antibiotic therapy when it is instituted promptly.

Mixed viral and bacterial pneumonia

Perhaps the most common pneumonic complications during outbreaks of influenza have mixed features of viral and bacterial pneumonia. Patients may experience a gradual progression of their acute illness or may show transient improvement followed by clinical exacerbation, with eventual manifestation of the clinical features of bacterial pneumonia. Sputum cultures may contain both influenza A virus and one of the bacterial pathogens described earlier. Patchy infiltrates or areas of consolidation may be detected by physical examination and chest x-ray. Patients with mixed viral and bacterial pneumonia generally have less widespread involvement of the lung than those with primary viral pneumonia, and their bacterial infections may respond to appropriate antibacterial drugs. Mixed viral and bacterial pneumonia occurs primarily in patients with chronic cardiovascular and pulmonary diseases.

Other pulmonary complications

Other pulmonary complications associated with influenza include worsening of chronic obstructive pulmonary disease and exacerbation of chronic bronchitis and asthma. In children, influenza infection may present as croup. Sinusitis as well as otitis media (the latter occurring particularly often in children) may also be associated with influenza.

Extrapulmonary complications

In addition to the pulmonary complications of influenza, a number of extrapulmonary complications may occur. These include *Reye's syndrome*, a serious complication in children that is associated with influenza B and to a lesser extent with influenza A virus infection as well as with varicella-zoster virus infection. An epidemiologic association between Reye's syndrome and aspirin therapy for the antecedent viral infection has been noted, and the syndrome's incidence has decreased markedly with widespread warnings regarding aspirin use by children with acute viral respiratory infections.

Myositis, rhabdomyolysis, and myoglobinuria are occasional complications of influenza infection. Although myalgias are exceedingly common in influenza, true myositis is rare. Patients with acute myositis have exquisite tenderness of the affected muscles, most commonly in the legs, and may not be able to tolerate even the slightest pressure, such as the touch of bedsheets. In the most severe cases, there is frank swelling and bogginess of muscles. Serum levels of creatine phosphokinase and aldolase are markedly elevated, and an occasional patient develops renal failure from myoglobinuria. The pathogenesis of influenza-associated myositis is also unclear, although the presence of influenza virus in affected muscles has been reported.

Myocarditis and pericarditis were reported in association with influenza virus infection during the 1918–1919 pandemic; these reports were based largely on histopathologic findings, and these complications have been reported only infrequently since that time. Electrocardiographic changes during acute influenza are common among patients who have cardiac disease but have been ascribed most often to exacerbations of the underlying cardiac disease rather than to direct involvement of the myocardium with influenza virus.

Central nervous system (CNS) diseases, including encephalitis, transverse myelitis, and Guillain-Barré syndrome, have been reported during influenza. The etiologic relationship of influenza virus to such CNS illnesses remains uncertain. Toxic shock syndrome associated with *S. aureus* or group A streptococcal infection following acute influenza infection has also been reported.

In addition to complications involving the specific organ systems described earlier, influenza outbreaks include a number of cases in which elderly and other high-risk individuals develop influenza and subsequently experience a gradual deterioration of underlying cardiovascular, pulmonary, or renal function—changes that occasionally are irreversible and lead to death. These deaths contribute to the overall excess mortality rate associated with influenza A outbreaks.

Complications of avian influenza

Cases of influenza caused by avian A/H5N1 virus are reportedly associated with high rates of pneumonia (>50%) and extrapulmonary manifestations such as diarrhea and CNS involvement. Deaths have been associated with multisystem dysfunction, including cardiac and renal failure.

LABORATORY FINDINGS AND DIAGNOSIS

During acute influenza, virus may be detected in throat swabs, nasopharyngeal swabs or washes, or sputum. The virus can be isolated by use of tissue culture—or, less commonly, chick embryos—within 48–72 h after inoculation. Most commonly, the laboratory diagnosis is established with rapid tests that detect viral antigens by means of immunologic or enzymatic techniques. The tests are relatively specific but are of variable sensitivity depending on the technique and the virus to be detected. Some rapid tests can distinguish between influenza A and B viruses, but detection of differences in hemagglutinin subtypes requires additional subtype-specific immunologic techniques. The most sensitive and specific in vitro test for influenza virus is reverse-transcriptase polymerase chain reaction; this test proved particularly important in detecting the 2009–2010 pandemic A/H1N1 viruses, for which some rapid antigen detection tests were poorly sensitive. Serologic methods for diagnosis require comparison of antibody titers in sera obtained during the acute illness with those in sera obtained 10–14 days after the onset of illness and are

useful primarily in retrospect. Fourfold or greater titer rises as detected by HI or CF or significant rises as measured by ELISA are diagnostic of acute infection. Other laboratory tests generally are not helpful in the specific diagnosis of influenza virus infection. Leukocyte counts are variable, frequently being low early in illness and normal or slightly elevated later. Severe leukopenia has been described in overwhelming viral or bacterial infection, while leukocytosis with >15,000 cells/μL raises the suspicion of secondary bacterial infection.

DIFFERENTIAL DIAGNOSIS

During a community-wide outbreak, a clinical diagnosis of influenza can be made with a high degree of certainty in patients who present to a physician's office with the typical febrile respiratory illness described earlier. In the absence of an outbreak (i.e., in sporadic or isolated cases), influenza may be difficult to differentiate on clinical grounds alone from an acute respiratory illness caused by any of a variety of respiratory viruses or by *Mycoplasma pneumoniae*. Severe streptococcal pharyngitis or early bacterial pneumonia may mimic acute influenza, although bacterial pneumonias generally do not run a self-limited course. Purulent sputum in which a bacterial pathogen can be detected by Gram's staining is an important diagnostic feature in bacterial pneumonia.

TREATMENT   Influenza

Specific antiviral therapy is available for influenza (Table 13-3): the neuraminidase inhibitors zanamivir, oseltamivir, and peramivir for both influenza A and influenza B and the adamantane agents amantadine and rimantadine for influenza A (Chap. 41). A 5-day course of oseltamivir or zanamivir reduces the duration of signs and symptoms of uncomplicated influenza by 1–1.5 days if treatment is started within 2 days of the onset of illness. Zanamivir may exacerbate bronchospasm in asthmatic patients, and oseltamivir has been associated with nausea and vomiting, whose frequency can be reduced by administration of the drug with food. Oseltamivir has also been associated with neuropsychiatric side effects in children. Peramivir, an investigational neuraminidase inhibitor that can be administered intravenously, is being evaluated in clinical trials, as is an intravenous form of zanamivir. Access to these medications can be sought through the FDA's Emergency Investigational New Drug (E-IND) application procedures.

Amantadine or rimantadine treatment of illness caused by sensitive strains of influenza A virus similarly reduces the duration of symptoms of uncomplicated influenza by ~50% if begun within 48 h of onset of illness. Five to 10% of amantadine recipients experience

TABLE 13-3

ANTIVIRAL MEDICATIONS FOR TREATMENT AND PROPHYLAXIS OF INFLUENZA

	AGE GROUP (YEARS)		
ANTIVIRAL DRUG	CHILDREN (≤12)	13–64	≥65
Oseltamivir			
Treatment, influenza A and B	Age 1–12, dose varies by weight[a]	75 mg PO bid	75 mg PO bid
Prophylaxis, influenza A and B	Age 1–12, dose varies by weight[b]	75 PO qd	75 mg PO qd
Zanamivir			
Treatment, influenza A and B	Age 7–12, 10 mg bid by inhalation	10 mg bid by inhalation	10 mg bid by inhalation
Prophylaxis, influenza A and B	Age 5–12, 10 mg qd by inhalation	10 mg qd by inhalation	10 mg qd by inhalation
Amantadine[c]			
Treatment, influenza A	Age 1–9, 5 mg/kg in 2 divided doses, up to 150 mg/d	Age ≥10, 100 mg PO bid	≤100 mg/d
Prophylaxis, influenza A	Age 1–9, 5 mg/kg in 2 divided doses, up to 150 mg/d	Age ≥10, 100 mg PO bid	≤100 mg/d
Rimantadine[c]			
Treatment, influenza A	Not approved	100 mg PO bid	100–200 mg/d
Prophylaxis, influenza A	Age 1–9, 5 mg/kg in 2 divided doses, up to 150 mg/d	Age ≥10, 100 mg PO bid	100–200 mg/d

[a]<15 kg: 30 mg bid; >15–23 kg: 45 mg bid; >23–40 kg: 60 mg bid; >40 kg: 75 mg bid. For children <1 year of age, see *www.cdc.gov/h1n1flu/recommendations.htm*.

[b]<15 kg: 30 mg qd; >15–23 kg: 45 mg qd; >23–40 kg: 60 mg qd; >40 kg: 75 mg qd. For children <1 year of age, see *www.cdc.gov/h1n1flu/recommendations.htm*.

[c]Amantadine and rimantadine are not currently recommended (2009–2010) because of widespread resistance in influenza A viruses. Their use may be reconsidered if viral susceptibility is reestablished.

mild CNS side effects, primarily jitteriness, anxiety, insomnia, or difficulty concentrating. These side effects disappear promptly upon cessation of therapy. Rimantadine appears to be equally efficacious and is associated with less frequent CNS side effects than is amantadine. In adults, the usual dose of amantadine or rimantadine is 200 mg/d for 3–7 days. Since both drugs are excreted via the kidney, the dose should be reduced to ≤100 mg/d in elderly patients and in patients with renal insufficiency.

The epidemiologic patterns of resistance to the influenza antiviral drugs are crucial elements in agent selection. Since 2005–2006, the vast majority of A/H3N2 viruses, including >90% of U.S. isolates, have been resistant to the adamantanes but have remained sensitive to neuraminidase inhibitors. In contrast, the seasonal A/H1N1 viruses that circulated in 2008–2009 remained sensitive to the adamantanes but were resistant to oseltamivir (although still sensitive to zanamivir). The pandemic A/H1N1 viruses that circulated in 2009–2010 were resistant to the adamantanes but sensitive to zanamivir and usually to oseltamivir; a few oseltamivir-resistant isolates were identified. Up-to-date information on patterns

of resistance to influenza antiviral drugs is available through *www.cdc.gov/flu*.

Ribavirin is a nucleoside analogue with activity against influenza A and B viruses in vitro. It has been reported to be variably effective against influenza when administered as an aerosol but ineffective when administered orally. Its efficacy in the treatment of influenza A or B has not been established.

The therapeutic efficacy of antiviral compounds in influenza has been demonstrated primarily in studies of young adults with uncomplicated disease. The effectiveness of these drugs in the treatment or prevention of complications of influenza is unclear. Pooled analyses of observational investigations and some efficacy studies have suggested that treatment with oseltamivir may reduce the frequency of lower respiratory complications and hospitalization. Therapy for primary influenza pneumonia is directed at maintaining oxygenation and is most appropriately undertaken in an intensive care unit, with aggressive respiratory and hemodynamic support as needed.

Antibacterial drugs should be reserved for the treatment of bacterial complications of acute influenza, such as secondary bacterial pneumonia. The choice of antibiotics should be guided by Gram's staining and culture of appropriate specimens of respiratory secretions, such as sputum. If the etiology of a case of bacterial pneumonia is unclear from an examination of respiratory secretions, empirical antibiotics effective against the most common bacterial pathogens in this setting (*S. pneumoniae*, *S. aureus*, and *H. influenzae*) should be selected.

For uncomplicated influenza in individuals at low risk for complications, symptom-based rather than antiviral therapy may be considered. Acetaminophen or nonsteroidal anti-inflammatory agents can be used for relief of headache, myalgia, and fever, but salicylates should be avoided in children <18 years of age because of the possible association with Reye's syndrome. Since cough is ordinarily self-limited, treatment with cough suppressants generally is not indicated; codeine-containing compounds may be employed if the cough is particularly troublesome. Patients should be advised to rest and maintain hydration during acute illness and to return to full activity only gradually after illness has resolved, especially if it has been severe.

PROPHYLAXIS

The major public health measure for prevention of influenza is vaccination. Both inactivated (killed) and live attenuated vaccines are available and are generated from influenza A and B virus isolates that circulated in the previous influenza seasons and are anticipated to circulate in the upcoming season. For inactivated vaccines, 50–80% protection against influenza is expected if the vaccine virus and the currently circulating viruses are closely related. Available inactivated vaccines have been highly purified and are associated with few reactions. Up to 5% of individuals experience low-grade fever and mild systemic symptoms 8–24 h after vaccination, and up to one-third develop mild redness or tenderness at the vaccination site. Since the vaccine used in the United States and many other countries is produced in eggs, individuals with true hypersensitivity to egg products either should be desensitized or should not be vaccinated. Although the 1976 swine influenza vaccine appears to have been associated with an increased frequency of Guillain-Barré syndrome, influenza vaccines administered since 1976 generally have not been. Possible exceptions were noted during the 1992–1993 and 1993–1994 influenza seasons, when there may have been an excess risk of Guillain-Barré syndrome of slightly more than 1 case per million vaccine recipients. However, the overall health risk following influenza outweighs the potential risk associated with vaccination.

A live attenuated influenza vaccine administered by intranasal spray is available. The vaccine is generated by reassortment between currently circulating strains of influenza A and B virus and a cold-adapted, attenuated master strain. The cold-adapted vaccine is well tolerated and highly efficacious (>90% protective) in young children; in one study, it provided protection against a circulating influenza virus that had drifted antigenically away from the vaccine strain. Live attenuated vaccine is approved for use in healthy nonpregnant persons 2–49 years of age.

Historically, the U.S. Public Health Service has recommended influenza vaccination for certain groups at high risk for complications of influenza on the basis of age or underlying disease or for their close contacts (Table 13-2). While such individuals will continue to be the focus of vaccination programs, the recommendations have been progressively expanded. In 2009–2010, immunization of all children 6 months to 18 years of age was recommended; for 2010–2011, recommendations are for immunization of the entire population above the age of 6 months, including adults. This expanded recommendation reflects increased recognition of previously unappreciated risk factors, including obesity, postpartum conditions, and racial or ethnic influences, as well as an appreciation that more widespread use of vaccine is required for influenza control. Inactivated vaccines may be administered safely to immunocompromised patients. Influenza vaccination is not associated with exacerbations of chronic nervous-system diseases such as multiple sclerosis. Vaccine should be administered early in the autumn before influenza outbreaks occur and should then be given annually to maintain immunity against the most current influenza virus strains.

Although antiviral drugs provide chemoprophylaxis against influenza, their use for that purpose has been limited because of concern about current patterns and further development of resistance. Chemoprophylaxis with oseltamivir or zanamivir has been 84–89% efficacious against influenza A and B (Table 13-3). Chemoprophylaxis with amantadine or rimantadine is no longer recommended because of widespread resistance to these drugs. In earlier studies with sensitive viruses, prophylaxis with amantadine or rimantadine (100–200 mg/d) was 70–100% effective against illness associated with influenza A.

Chemoprophylaxis for healthy persons after community exposure generally is not recommended but may be considered for individuals at high risk of complications who have had close contact with an acutely ill person with influenza. During an outbreak, antiviral chemoprophylaxis can be administered simultaneously with inactivated vaccine, since the drugs do not interfere with an immune response to the vaccine. However, concurrent administration of chemoprophylaxis and live attenuated vaccine may interfere with the immune response to the latter. Antiviral drugs should not be administered until at least 2 weeks after administration of live vaccine, and administration of live vaccine should not begin until at least 48 h after antiviral drug administration

has been stopped. Chemoprophylaxis may also be considered to control nosocomial outbreaks of influenza. For that purpose, prophylaxis should be instituted promptly when influenza activity is detected and must be continued daily for the duration of the outbreak.

CHAPTER 14

COMMON VIRAL RESPIRATORY INFECTIONS

Raphael Dolin

GENERAL CONSIDERATIONS

Acute viral respiratory illnesses are among the most common of human diseases, accounting for one-half or more of all acute illnesses. The incidence of acute respiratory disease in the United States is 3–5.6 cases per person per year. The rates are highest among children <1 year old (6.1–8.3 cases per year) and remain high until age 6, when a progressive decrease begins. Adults have 3–4 cases per person per year. Morbidity from acute respiratory illnesses accounts for 30–50% of time lost from work by adults and for 60–80% of time lost from school by children. The use of antibacterial agents to treat viral respiratory infections represents a major source of abuse of that category of drugs.

It has been estimated that two-thirds to three-fourths of cases of acute respiratory illnesses are caused by viruses. More than 200 antigenically distinct viruses from 10 genera have been reported to cause acute respiratory illness, and it is likely that additional agents will be described in the future. The vast majority of these viral infections involve the upper respiratory tract, but lower respiratory tract disease can also develop, particularly in younger age groups, in the elderly, and in certain epidemiologic settings.

The illnesses caused by respiratory viruses traditionally have been divided into multiple distinct syndromes, such as the "common cold," pharyngitis, croup (laryngotracheobronchitis), tracheitis, bronchiolitis, bronchitis, and pneumonia. Each of these general categories of illness has a certain epidemiologic and clinical profile; for example, croup occurs exclusively in very young children and has a characteristic clinical course. Some types of respiratory illness are more likely to be associated with certain viruses (e.g., the common cold with rhinoviruses), while others occupy characteristic epidemiologic niches (e.g., adenovirus infections in military recruits). The syndromes most commonly associated with infections with the major respiratory virus groups are summarized in Table 14-1. Most respiratory viruses clearly have the potential to cause more than one type of respiratory illness, and features of several types of illness may be found in the same patient. Moreover, the clinical illnesses induced by these viruses are rarely sufficiently distinctive to permit an etiologic diagnosis on clinical grounds alone, although the epidemiologic setting increases the likelihood that one group of viruses rather than another is involved. In general, laboratory methods must be relied on to establish a specific viral diagnosis.

This chapter reviews viral infections caused by six of the major groups of respiratory viruses: rhinoviruses, coronaviruses, respiratory syncytial viruses, metapneumoviruses, parainfluenza viruses, and adenoviruses. The extraordinary outbreaks of lower respiratory tract disease associated with coronaviruses (severe acute respiratory syndrome, or SARS) in 2002–2003 are also discussed. Influenza viruses, which are a major cause of death as well as morbidity, are reviewed in Chap. 13.

RHINOVIRUS INFECTIONS

ETIOLOGIC AGENT

Rhinoviruses are members of the Picornaviridae family, small (15- to 30-nm) nonenveloped viruses that contain a single-stranded RNA genome and have been divided into three genetic species: HRV-A, HRV-B, and HRV-C. In contrast to other members of the picornavirus family, such as enteroviruses, rhinoviruses are acid-labile and are almost completely inactivated at pH ≤ 3. Rhinoviruses grow preferentially at 33°–34°C (the temperature of the human nasal passages) rather than at 37°C (the temperature of the lower respiratory tract). Of the 102 recognized serotypes of rhinovirus, 91 use

TABLE 14-1

ILLNESSES ASSOCIATED WITH RESPIRATORY VIRUSES

	FREQUENCY OF RESPIRATORY SYNDROMES		
VIRUS	MOST FREQUENT	OCCASIONAL	INFREQUENT
Rhinoviruses	Common cold	Exacerbation of chronic bronchitis and asthma	Pneumonia in children
Coronaviruses[a]	Common cold	Exacerbation of chronic bronchitis and asthma	Pneumonia and bronchiolitis
Human respiratory syncytial virus	Pneumonia and bronchiolitis in young children	Common cold in adults	Pneumonia in elderly and immunosuppressed patients
Parainfluenza viruses	Croup and lower respiratory tract disease in young children	Pharyngitis and common cold	Tracheobronchitis in adults; lower respiratory tract disease in immunosuppressed patients
Adenoviruses	Common cold and pharyngitis in children	Outbreaks of acute respiratory disease in military recruits[b]	Pneumonia in children; lower respiratory tract and disseminated disease in immunosuppressed patients
Influenza A viruses	Influenza[c]	Pneumonia and excess mortality in high-risk patients	Pneumonia in healthy individuals
Influenza B viruses	Influenza[c]	Rhinitis or pharyngitis alone	Pneumonia
Enteroviruses	Acute undifferentiated febrile illnesses[d]	Rhinitis or pharyngitis alone	Pneumonia
Herpes simplex viruses	Gingivostomatitis in children; pharyngotonsillitis in adults	Tracheitis and pneumonia in immunocompromised patients	Disseminated infection in immunocompromised patients
Human metapneumoviruses	Upper and lower respiratory tract disease in children	Upper respiratory tract illness in adults	Pneumonia in elderly and immunosuppressed patients

[a]SARS-associated coronavirus (SARS-CoV) caused epidemics of pneumonia from November 2002 to July 2003 (see text).
[b]Serotypes 4 and 7
[c]Fever, cough, myalgia, malaise.
[d]May or may not have a respiratory component.

intercellular adhesion molecule 1 (ICAM-1) as a cellular receptor and constitute the "major" receptor group, 10 use the low-density lipoprotein receptor (LDLR) and constitute the "minor" receptor group, and 1 uses decay-accelerating factor.

EPIDEMIOLOGY

Rhinoviruses are a prominent cause of the common cold and have been detected in up to 50% of common cold–like illnesses by tissue culture and polymerase chain reaction (PCR) techniques. Overall rates of rhinovirus infection are higher among infants and young children and decrease with increasing age. Rhinovirus infections occur throughout the year, with seasonal peaks in early fall and spring in temperate climates. These infections are most often introduced into families

by preschool or grade-school children <6 years old. Of initial illnesses in family settings, 25–70% are followed by secondary cases, with the highest attack rates among the youngest siblings at home. Attack rates also increase with family size.

Rhinoviruses appear to spread through direct contact with infected secretions, usually respiratory droplets. In some studies of volunteers, transmission was most efficient by hand-to-hand contact, with subsequent self-inoculation of the conjunctival or nasal mucosa. Other studies demonstrated transmission by large- or small-particle aerosol. Virus can be recovered from plastic surfaces inoculated 1–3 h previously; this observation suggests that environmental surfaces contribute to transmission. In studies of married couples in which neither partner had detectable serum antibody, transmission was associated with prolonged contact (≥122 h) during a 7-day period. Transmission was infrequent unless (1) virus was recoverable from the donor's hands and nasal mucosa, (2) at least 1000 TCID$_{50}$ of virus was present in nasal washes from the donor, and (3) the donor was at least moderately symptomatic with the "cold." Despite anecdotal observations, exposure to cold temperatures, fatigue, and sleep deprivation have not been associated with increased rates of rhinovirus-induced illness in volunteers, although some studies have suggested that psychologically defined "stress" may contribute to development of symptoms.

Infection with rhinoviruses is worldwide in distribution. By adulthood, nearly all individuals have neutralizing antibodies to multiple serotypes, although the prevalence of antibody to any one serotype varies widely. Multiple serotypes circulate simultaneously, and generally no single serotype or group of serotypes has been more prevalent than the others.

PATHOGENESIS

Rhinoviruses infect cells through attachment to specific cellular receptors; as mentioned earlier, most serotypes attach to ICAM-1, while a few use LDLR. Relatively limited information is available on the histopathology and pathogenesis of acute rhinovirus infections in humans. Examination of biopsy specimens obtained during experimentally induced and naturally occurring illness indicates that the nasal mucosa is edematous, is often hyperemic, and—during acute illness—is covered by a mucoid discharge. There is a mild infiltrate with inflammatory cells, including neutrophils, lymphocytes, plasma cells, and eosinophils. Mucus-secreting glands in the submucosa appear hyperactive; the nasal turbinates are engorged, a condition that may lead to obstruction of nearby openings of sinus cavities. Several mediators—e.g., bradykinin; lysylbradykinin; prostaglandins; histamine; interleukins 1β, 6, and 8; and tumor necrosis factor α—have been linked to the development of signs and symptoms in rhinovirus-induced colds.

The incubation period for rhinovirus illness is short, generally 1–2 days. Virus shedding coincides with the onset of illness or may begin shortly before symptoms develop. The mechanisms of immunity to rhinovirus infection are not well worked out. In some studies, the presence of homotypic antibody has been associated with significantly reduced rates of subsequent infection and illness, but data conflict regarding the relative importance of serum and local antibody in protection from rhinovirus infection.

CLINICAL MANIFESTATIONS

The most common clinical manifestations of rhinovirus infections are those of the common cold. Illness usually begins with rhinorrhea and sneezing accompanied by nasal congestion. The throat is frequently sore, and in some cases sore throat is the initial complaint. Systemic signs and symptoms, such as malaise and headache, are mild or absent, and fever is unusual. Illness generally lasts for 4–9 days and resolves spontaneously without sequelae. In children, bronchitis, bronchiolitis, and bronchopneumonia have been reported; nevertheless, it appears that rhinoviruses are not major causes of lower respiratory tract disease in children. Rhinoviruses may cause exacerbations of asthma and chronic pulmonary disease in adults. The vast majority of rhinovirus infections resolve without sequelae, but complications related to obstruction of the eustachian tubes or sinus ostia, including otitis media or acute sinusitis, can develop. In immunosuppressed patients, particularly bone marrow transplant recipients, severe and even fatal pneumonias have been associated with rhinovirus infections.

DIAGNOSIS

Although rhinoviruses are the most frequently recognized cause of the common cold, similar illnesses are caused by a variety of other viruses, and a specific viral etiologic diagnosis cannot be made on clinical grounds alone. Rather, rhinovirus infection is diagnosed by isolation of the virus from nasal washes or nasal secretions in tissue culture. In practice, this procedure is rarely undertaken because of the benign, self-limited nature of the illness. In most settings, detection of rhinovirus RNA by PCR is more sensitive than that by tissue culture; however, PCR for rhinoviruses is largely a research procedure. Given the many serotypes of rhinovirus, diagnosis by serum antibody tests is currently impractical. Likewise, common laboratory tests, such as white blood cell count and erythrocyte sedimentation rate, are not helpful.

TREATMENT   Rhinovirus Infections

Because rhinovirus infections are generally mild and self-limited, treatment is not usually necessary. Therapy in the form of first-generation antihistamines and nonsteroidal anti-inflammatory drugs may be beneficial in patients with particularly pronounced symptoms, and an oral decongestant may be added if nasal obstruction is particularly troublesome. Reduction of activity is prudent in instances of significant discomfort or fatigability. Antibacterial agents should be used only if bacterial complications such as otitis media or sinusitis develop. Specific antiviral therapy is not available.

PREVENTION

Intranasal application of interferon sprays has been effective in the prophylaxis of rhinovirus infections but is also associated with local irritation of the nasal mucosa. Studies of prevention of rhinovirus infection by blocking of ICAM-1 or by drug binding to parts of the viral capsid (pleconaril) have yielded mixed results. Experimental vaccines to certain rhinovirus serotypes have been generated, but their usefulness is questionable because of the myriad serotypes and the uncertainty about mechanisms of immunity. Thorough hand washing, environmental decontamination, and protection against autoinoculation may help to reduce rates of transmission of infection.

CORONAVIRUS INFECTIONS

ETIOLOGIC AGENT

Coronaviruses are pleomorphic, single-stranded RNA viruses that measure 100–160 nm in diameter. The name derives from the crownlike appearance produced by the club-shaped projections that stud the viral envelope. Coronaviruses infect a wide variety of animal species and have been divided into three antigenic and genetic groups. Before the emergence of the coronavirus associated with SARS (SARS-CoV), coronaviruses recognized as causes of infection in humans fell into groups 1 and 2, which include human isolates HCoV-229E and HCoV-OC43, respectively. SARS-CoV was at first believed to represent a novel group but now is considered to be a distantly related member of group 2. The SARS-CoV strains that have been fully sequenced have shown only minimal variation.

In general, human coronaviruses have been difficult to cultivate in vitro, and some strains grow only in human tracheal organ cultures rather than in tissue culture. SARS-CoV is an exception whose ready growth in African green monkey kidney (Vero E6) cells greatly facilitates its study.

EPIDEMIOLOGY

Generally, human coronavirus infections are present throughout the world. Seroprevalence studies of strains HCoV-229E and HCoV-OC43 have demonstrated that serum antibodies are acquired early in life and increase in prevalence with advancing age, so that >80% of adult populations have antibodies as measured by enzyme-linked immunosorbent assay (ELISA). Overall, coronaviruses account for 10–35% of common colds, depending on the season. Coronavirus infections appear to be particularly prevalent in late fall, winter, and early spring—times when rhinovirus infections are less common.

An extraordinary outbreak of the coronavirus-associated illness known as SARS occurred in 2002–2003. The outbreak apparently began in southern China and eventually resulted in 8096 recognized cases in 28 countries

in Asia, Europe, and North and South America; ~90% of cases occurred in China and Hong Kong. The natural reservoir of SARS-CoV appeared to be the horseshoe bat, and the outbreak may have originated from human contact with infected semidomesticated animals such as the palm civet. In most cases, however, the infection was transmitted from human to human. Case-fatality rates varied among outbreaks, with an overall figure of ~9.5%. The disease appeared to be somewhat milder in cases in the United States and was clearly less severe among children. The outbreak ceased in 2003; 17 cases were detected in 2004, mostly in laboratory-associated settings, and no cases were reported in 2005–2009.

The mechanisms of transmission of SARS are incompletely understood. Clusters of cases suggest that spread may occur by both large and small aerosols and perhaps by the fecal-oral route as well. The outbreak of illness in a large apartment complex in Hong Kong suggested that environmental sources, such as sewage or water, may also play a role in transmission. Some ill individuals ("super-spreaders") appeared to be hyperinfectious and were capable of transmitting infection to 10–40 contacts, although most infections resulted in spread either to no one or to three or fewer individuals.

PATHOGENESIS

Coronaviruses that cause the common cold (e.g., strains HCoV-229E and HCoV-OC43) infect ciliated epithelial cells in the nasopharynx via the aminopeptidase N receptor (group 1) or a sialic acid receptor (group 2). Viral replication leads to damage of ciliated cells and induction of chemokines and interleukins, with consequent common-cold symptoms similar to those induced by rhinoviruses.

SARS-CoV infects cells of the respiratory tract via the angiotensin-converting enzyme 2 receptor. The result is a systemic illness in which virus is also found in the bloodstream, in the urine, and (for up to 2 months) in the stool. Virus persists in the respiratory tract for 2–3 weeks, and titers peak ~10 days after the onset of systemic illness. Pulmonary pathology consists of hyaline membrane formation, desquamation of pneumocytes in alveolar spaces, and an interstitial infiltrate made up of lymphocytes and mononuclear cells. Giant cells are frequently seen, and coronavirus particles have been detected in type II pneumocytes. Elevated levels of proinflammatory cytokines and chemokines have been detected in sera from patients with SARS.

CLINICAL MANIFESTATIONS

After an incubation period that generally lasts 2–7 days (range, 1–14 days), SARS usually begins as a systemic illness marked by the onset of fever, which is often accompanied by malaise, headache, and myalgias and is followed in 1–2 days by a nonproductive cough and dyspnea. Approximately 25% of patients have diarrhea. Chest x-rays can show a variety of infiltrates, including patchy areas of consolidation—most frequently in peripheral and lower lung fields—or interstitial infiltrates, which can progress to diffuse involvement.

In severe cases, respiratory function may worsen during the second week of illness and progress to frank adult respiratory distress syndrome accompanied by multiorgan dysfunction. Risk factors for severe disease include an age of >50 years and comorbidities such as cardiovascular disease, diabetes, or hepatitis. Illness in pregnant women may be particularly severe, but SARS-CoV infection appears to be milder in children than in adults.

The clinical features of common colds caused by human coronaviruses are similar to those of illness caused by rhinoviruses. In studies of volunteers, the mean incubation period of colds induced by coronaviruses (3 days) is somewhat longer than that of illness caused by rhinoviruses, and the duration of illness is somewhat shorter (mean, 6–7 days). In some studies, the amount of nasal discharge was greater in colds induced by coronaviruses than in those induced by rhinoviruses. Coronaviruses other than SARS-CoV have been recovered occasionally from infants with pneumonia and from military recruits with lower respiratory tract disease and have been associated with worsening of chronic bronchitis. Two novel coronaviruses, HCoV-NL63 (group 1) and HCoV-HKU1 (group 2), have been isolated from patients hospitalized with acute respiratory illness. Their overall role as causes of human respiratory disease remains to be determined.

LABORATORY FINDINGS AND DIAGNOSIS

Laboratory abnormalities in SARS include lymphopenia, which is present in ~50% of cases and which mostly affects CD4+ T cells, but also involves CD8+ T cells and natural killer cells. Total white blood cell counts are normal or slightly low, and thrombocytopenia may develop as the illness progresses. Elevated serum levels of aminotransferases, creatine kinase, and lactate dehydrogenase have been reported.

A rapid diagnosis of SARS-CoV infection can be made by reverse-transcription PCR (RT-PCR) of respiratory tract samples and plasma early in illness and of urine and stool later on. SARS-CoV can also be grown from respiratory tract samples by inoculation into Vero E6 tissue culture cells, in which a cytopathic effect is seen within days. RT-PCR appears to be more sensitive than tissue culture, but only around one-third of cases are positive by PCR at initial presentation. Serum antibodies

can be detected by ELISA or immunofluorescence, and nearly all patients develop detectable serum antibodies within 28 days after the onset of illness.

Laboratory diagnosis of coronavirus-induced colds is rarely required. Coronaviruses that cause those illnesses are frequently difficult to cultivate in vitro but can be detected in clinical samples by ELISA or immunofluorescence assays or by RT-PCR for viral RNA. These research procedures can be used to detect coronaviruses in unusual clinical settings.

> **TREATMENT**   Coronavirus Infections
>
> There is no specific therapy of established efficacy for SARS. Although ribavirin has frequently been used, it has little if any activity against SARS-CoV in vitro, and no beneficial effect on the course of illness has been demonstrated. Because of suggestions that immunopathology may contribute to the disease, glucocorticoids have also been widely used, but their benefit, if any, is likewise unestablished. Supportive care to maintain pulmonary and other organ-system functions remains the mainstay of therapy.
>
> The approach to the treatment of common colds caused by coronaviruses is similar to that discussed earlier for rhinovirus-induced illnesses.

PREVENTION

 The recognition of SARS led to a worldwide mobilization of public health resources to apply infection control practices to contain the disease. Case definitions were established, travel advisories were proposed, and quarantines were imposed in certain locales. As of this writing, no additional cases of SARS have been reported since 2004. However, it remains unknown whether the disappearance of cases is a result of control measures, whether it is part of a seasonal or otherwise unexplained epidemiologic pattern of SARS, or when or whether SARS might reemerge. The U.S. Centers for Disease Control and Prevention and the World Health Organization maintain recommendations for surveillance and assessment of potential cases of SARS (*www.cdc.gov/ncidod/sars/*). The frequent transmission of the disease to health care workers makes it mandatory that strict infection-control practices be employed by health care facilities to prevent airborne, droplet, and contact transmission from any suspected cases of SARS. Health care workers who enter areas in which patients with SARS may be present should don gowns, gloves, and eye and respiratory protective equipment (e.g., an N95 filtering facepiece respirator certified by the National Institute for Occupational Safety and Health).

Vaccines have been developed against several animal coronaviruses but not against known human coronaviruses. The emergence of SARS-CoV has stimulated interest in the development of vaccines against such agents.

HUMAN RESPIRATORY SYNCYTIAL VIRUS INFECTIONS

ETIOLOGIC AGENT

Human respiratory syncytial virus (HRSV) is a member of the Paramyxoviridae family (genus *Pneumovirus*). An enveloped virus ~150–350 nm in diameter, HRSV is so named because its replication in vitro leads to the fusion of neighboring cells into large multinucleated syncytia. The single-stranded RNA genome codes for 11 virus-specific proteins. Viral RNA is contained in a helical nucleocapsid surrounded by a lipid envelope bearing two glycoproteins: the G protein, by which the virus attaches to cells, and the F (fusion) protein, which facilitates entry of the virus into the cell by fusing host and viral membranes. HRSV is considered to be of a single antigenic type, but two distinct subgroups (A and B) and multiple subtypes within each subgroup have now been described. Antigenic diversity is reflected by differences in the G protein, while the F protein is highly conserved. Both antigenic groups can circulate simultaneously in outbreaks, although there are typically alternating patterns in which one subgroup predominates over 1- to 2-year periods.

EPIDEMIOLOGY

HRSV is a major respiratory pathogen of young children and the foremost cause of lower respiratory disease in infants. Infection with HRSV is seen throughout the world in annual epidemics that occur in late fall, winter, or spring and last up to 5 months. The virus is rarely encountered during the summer. Rates of illness are highest among infants 1–6 months of age, peaking at 2–3 months of age. The attack rates among susceptible infants and children are extraordinarily high, approaching 100% in settings such as day-care centers where large numbers of susceptible infants are present. By age 2, virtually all children will have been infected with HRSV. HRSV accounts for 20–25% of hospital admissions of young infants and children for pneumonia and for up to 75% of cases of bronchiolitis in this age group. It has been estimated that more than half of infants who are at risk will become infected during an HRSV epidemic.

In older children and adults, reinfection with HRSV is frequent but disease is milder than in infancy. A common cold–like syndrome is the illness most commonly associated with HRSV infection in adults. Severe lower respiratory tract disease with pneumonitis can occur in elderly (often institutionalized) adults and in patients with immunocompromising disorders or treatment, including recipients of stem cell and solid-organ transplants. HRSV is also an important nosocomial pathogen; during an outbreak, it can infect pediatric patients and up to 25–50% of the staff on pediatric wards. The spread of HRSV among families is efficient: up to 40% of siblings may become infected when the virus is introduced into the family setting.

HRSV is transmitted primarily by close contact with contaminated fingers or fomites and by self-inoculation of the conjunctiva or anterior nares. Virus may also be spread by coarse aerosols produced by coughing or sneezing, but it is inefficiently spread by fine-particle aerosols. The incubation period is ~4–6 days, and virus shedding may last for ≥2 weeks in children and for shorter periods in adults. In immunosuppressed patients, shedding can continue for weeks.

PATHOGENESIS

Little is known about the histopathology of minor HRSV infection. Severe bronchiolitis or pneumonia is characterized by necrosis of the bronchiolar epithelium and a peribronchiolar infiltrate of lymphocytes and mononuclear cells. Interalveolar thickening and filling of alveolar spaces with fluid can also be found. The correlates of protective immunity to HRSV are incompletely understood. Because reinfection occurs frequently and is often associated with illness, the immunity that develops after single episodes of infection clearly is not complete or long-lasting. However, the cumulative effect of multiple reinfections is to temper subsequent disease and to provide some temporary measure of protection against infection. Studies of experimentally induced disease in healthy volunteers indicate that the presence of nasal IgA neutralizing antibody correlates more closely with protection than does the presence of serum antibody. Studies in infants, however, suggest that maternally acquired antibody provides some protection from lower respiratory tract disease, although illness can be severe even in infants who have moderate levels of maternally derived serum antibody. The relatively severe disease observed in immunosuppressed patients and experimental animal models indicates that cell-mediated immunity is an important mechanism of host defense against HRSV. Evidence suggests that major histocompatibility class I–restricted cytotoxic T cells may be particularly important in this regard.

CLINICAL MANIFESTATIONS

HRSV infection leads to a wide spectrum of respiratory illnesses. In infants, 25–40% of infections result in lower respiratory tract involvement, including pneumonia, bronchiolitis, and tracheobronchitis. In this age group, illness begins most frequently with rhinorrhea, low-grade fever, and mild systemic symptoms, often accompanied by cough and wheezing. Most patients recover gradually over 1–2 weeks. In more severe illness, tachypnea and dyspnea develop, and eventually frank hypoxia, cyanosis, and apnea can ensue. Physical examination may reveal diffuse wheezing, rhonchi, and rales. Chest radiography shows hyperexpansion, peribronchial thickening, and variable infiltrates ranging from diffuse interstitial infiltrates to segmental or lobar consolidation. Illness may be particularly severe in children born prematurely and in those with congenital cardiac disease, bronchopulmonary dysplasia, nephrotic syndrome, or immunosuppression. One study documented a 37% mortality rate among infants with HRSV pneumonia and congenital cardiac disease.

In adults, the most common symptoms of HRSV infection are those of the common cold, with rhinorrhea, sore throat, and cough. Illness is occasionally associated with moderate systemic symptoms such as malaise, headache, and fever. HRSV has also been reported to cause lower respiratory tract disease with fever in adults, including severe pneumonia in the elderly—particularly in nursing-home residents, among whom its impact can rival that of influenza. HRSV pneumonia can be a significant cause of morbidity and death among patients undergoing stem cell and solid-organ transplantation, in whom case-fatality rates of 20–80% have been reported. Sinusitis, otitis media, and worsening of chronic obstructive and reactive airway disease have also been associated with HRSV infection.

LABORATORY FINDINGS AND DIAGNOSIS

The diagnosis of HRSV infection can be suspected on the basis of a suggestive epidemiologic setting—that is, severe illness among infants during an outbreak of HRSV in the community. Infections in older children and adults cannot be differentiated with certainty from those caused by other respiratory viruses. The specific diagnosis is established by detection of HRSV in respiratory secretions, such as sputum, throat swabs, or nasopharyngeal washes. Virus can be isolated in tissue culture, but this method has been largely supplanted by rapid viral diagnostic techniques consisting of immunofluorescence or ELISA of nasopharyngeal washes, aspirates, and (less satisfactorily) nasopharyngeal swabs. With specimens from children, these techniques have sensitivities and specificities of 80–95%; they are somewhat less sensitive with specimens from adults. RT-PCR detection techniques have shown even higher rates of sensitivity and specificity, particularly in adults. Serologic diagnosis may be made by comparison of acute- and convalescent-phase serum specimens by ELISA or by neutralization or complement-fixation tests. These tests may be useful in older children and adults but are less sensitive in children <4 months of age.

TREATMENT   Human Respiratory Syncytial Virus Infections

Treatment of upper respiratory tract HRSV infection is aimed primarily at the alleviation of symptoms and is similar to that for other viral infections of the upper respiratory tract. For lower respiratory tract infections, respiratory therapy, including hydration, suctioning of secretions, and administration of humidified oxygen and antibronchospastic agents, is given as needed. In severe hypoxia, intubation and ventilatory assistance may be required. Studies of infants with HRSV infection who were given aerosolized ribavirin, a nucleoside analogue active in vitro against HRSV, demonstrated a modest beneficial effect on the resolution of lower respiratory tract illness, including alleviation of blood-gas abnormalities, in some studies. The American Academy of Pediatrics recommends that treatment with aerosolized ribavirin "may be considered" for infants who are severely ill or who are at high risk for complications of HRSV infection; included are premature infants and those with bronchopulmonary dysplasia, congenital heart disease, or immunosuppression. The efficacy of ribavirin against HRSV pneumonia in older children and adults, including those with immunosuppression, has not been established. No benefit has been found in the treatment of HRSV pneumonia with standard immunoglobulin; immunoglobulin with high titers of antibody to HRSV (RSVIg), which is no longer available; or chimeric mouse-human monoclonal IgG antibody to HRSV (palivizumab). Combined therapy with aerosolized ribavirin and palivizumab is being evaluated in immunosuppressed patients with HRSV pneumonia.

PREVENTION

Monthly administration of RSVIg (no longer available) or palivizumab has been approved as prophylaxis against HRSV for children <2 years of age who have bronchopulmonary dysplasia or cyanotic heart disease or who were born prematurely. Considerable interest exists in the development of vaccines against HRSV. Inactivated whole-virus vaccines have been ineffective; in one study, they actually potentiated disease in infants. Other approaches include immunization with purified F and G surface glycoproteins of HRSV or generation of stable, live attenuated virus vaccines. In settings such as pediatric wards where rates of transmission are high, barrier methods for the protection of hands and conjunctivae may be useful in reducing the spread of virus.

HUMAN METAPNEUMOVIRUS INFECTIONS

ETIOLOGIC AGENT

Human metapneumovirus (HMPV) is a viral respiratory pathogen that has been assigned to the Paramyxoviridae family (genus *Metapneumovirus*). Its morphology and genomic organization are similar to those of avian metapneumoviruses, which are recognized respiratory pathogens of turkeys. HMPV particles may be spherical, filamentous, or pleomorphic in shape and measure 150–600 nm in diameter. Particles contain 15-nm projections from the surface that are similar in appearance to those of other Paramyxoviridae. The single-stranded RNA genome codes for nine proteins that, except for the absence of nonstructural proteins, generally correspond to those of HRSV. HMPV is of only one antigenic type; two closely related genotypes (A and B), four subgroups, and two sublineages have been described.

EPIDEMIOLOGY

HMPV infections are worldwide in distribution, are most frequent during the winter, and occur early in life, so that serum antibodies to the virus are present in nearly all children by the age of 5. HMPV infections have been detected in older age groups, including elderly adults, and in both immunocompetent and immunosuppressed hosts. This virus accounts for 1–5% of childhood upper respiratory tract infections and for 10–15% of respiratory tract illnesses requiring hospitalization of children. In addition, HMPV causes 2–4% of acute respiratory illnesses in ambulatory adults and elderly patients. HMPV has been detected in a few cases of SARS, but its role (if any) in these illnesses has not been established.

CLINICAL MANIFESTATIONS

The spectrum of clinical illnesses associated with HMPV is similar to that associated with HRSV and includes both upper and lower respiratory tract illnesses, such as bronchiolitis, croup, and pneumonia. Reinfection with HMPV is common among older children and adults and has manifestations ranging from subclinical infections to common cold syndromes and occasionally pneumonia, which is seen primarily in elderly patients and those with cardiopulmonary diseases. Serious HMPV infections occur in immunocompromised patients, including those with neoplasia and hematopoietic stem cell transplants.

DIAGNOSIS

HMPV can be detected in nasal aspirates and respiratory secretions by immunofluorescence, by PCR, or by growth in rhesus monkey kidney (LLC-MK2) tissue cultures. A serologic diagnosis can be made by ELISA, which uses HMPV-infected tissue culture lysates as sources of antigens.

TREATMENT   Human Metapneumovirus Infections

Treatment for HMPV infections is primarily supportive and symptom-based. Ribavirin is active against HMPV in vitro, but its efficacy in vivo is unknown.

PREVENTION

Vaccines against HMPV are in the early stages of development.

PARAINFLUENZA VIRUS INFECTIONS

ETIOLOGIC AGENT

Parainfluenza viruses belong to the Paramyxoviridae family (genera *Respirovirus* and *Rubulavirus*). They are 150–200 nm in diameter, are enveloped, and contain a single-stranded RNA genome. The envelope is studded with two glycoproteins: one possesses both hemagglutinin and neuraminidase activity, and the other contains fusion activity. The viral RNA genome is enclosed in a helical nucleocapsid and codes for six structural and several accessory proteins. All five serotypes of parainfluenza virus (1, 2, 3, 4A, and 4B) share certain antigens with other members of the Paramyxoviridae family, including mumps and Newcastle disease viruses.

EPIDEMIOLOGY

Parainfluenza viruses are distributed throughout the world; infection with serotypes 4A and 4B has been reported less widely, probably because these types are more difficult than the other three to grow in tissue culture. Infection is acquired in early childhood; by 5 years of age, most children have antibodies to serotypes 1, 2, and 3. Types 1 and 2 cause epidemics during the fall, often occurring in an alternate-year pattern. Type 3 infection has been detected during all seasons of the year, but epidemics have occurred annually in the spring.

The contribution of parainfluenza infections to respiratory disease varies with both the location and the year. In studies conducted in the United States, parainfluenza virus infections have accounted for 4.3–22% of respiratory illnesses in children. In adults, parainfluenza infections are generally mild and account for <10% of respiratory illnesses. The major importance of parainfluenza viruses is as a cause of respiratory illness in young children, in whom they rank second only to HRSV as causes of lower respiratory tract illness. Parainfluenza virus type 1 is the most frequent cause of croup (laryngotracheobronchitis) in children, while serotype 2 causes similar, although generally less severe, disease. Type 3 is an important cause of bronchiolitis and pneumonia in infants, while illnesses associated with types 4A and 4B have generally been mild. Unlike types 1 and 2, type 3 frequently causes illness during the first month of life, when passively acquired maternal antibody is still present. Parainfluenza viruses are spread through infected respiratory secretions, primarily by person-to-person contact and/or by large droplets. The incubation period has varied from 3 to 6 days in experimental infections but may be somewhat shorter for naturally occurring disease in children.

PATHOGENESIS

Immunity to parainfluenza viruses is incompletely understood, but evidence suggests that immunity to infections with serotypes 1 and 2 is mediated by local IgA antibodies in the respiratory tract. Passively acquired serum neutralizing antibodies also confer some protection against infection with types 1, 2, and (to a lesser degree) 3. Studies in experimental animal models and in immunosuppressed patients suggest that T cell–mediated immunity may also be important in parainfluenza virus infections.

CLINICAL MANIFESTATIONS

Parainfluenza virus infections occur most frequently among children, in whom initial infection with serotype 1, 2, or 3 is associated with an acute febrile illness in 50–80% of cases. Children may present with coryza, sore throat, hoarseness, and cough that may or may not be croupy. In severe croup, fever persists, with worsening coryza and sore throat. A brassy or barking cough may progress to frank stridor. Most children recover over the next 1 or 2 days, although progressive airway obstruction and hypoxia ensue occasionally. If bronchiolitis or pneumonia develops, progressive cough accompanied by wheezing, tachypnea, and intercostal retractions may occur. In this setting, sputum production increases modestly. Physical examination shows nasopharyngeal discharge and oropharyngeal injection, along with rhonchi, wheezes, or coarse breath sounds. Chest x-rays can show air trapping and occasionally interstitial infiltrates.

In older children and adults, parainfluenza infections tend to be milder, presenting most frequently as a common cold or as hoarseness, with or without cough. Lower respiratory tract involvement in older children and adults is uncommon, but tracheobronchitis in adults has been reported. Severe, prolonged, and even fatal parainfluenza infection has been reported in children and adults with severe immunosuppression, including hematopoietic stem cell and solid-organ transplant recipients.

LABORATORY FINDINGS AND DIAGNOSIS

The clinical syndromes caused by parainfluenza viruses (with the possible exception of croup in young children) are not sufficiently distinctive to be diagnosed on clinical grounds alone. A specific diagnosis is established by detection of virus in respiratory tract secretions, throat swabs, or nasopharyngeal washings. Viral growth in tissue culture is detected either by hemagglutination or by a cytopathic effect. Rapid viral diagnosis may be made by identification of parainfluenza antigens in exfoliated cells from the respiratory tract with immunofluorescence or ELISA, although these techniques appear to be less sensitive than tissue culture. Highly specific and sensitive PCR assays have also been developed. Serologic diagnosis can be established by hemagglutination inhibition, complement-fixation, or neutralization tests of acute- and convalescent-phase specimens. However, since frequent heterotypic responses occur among the parainfluenza serotypes, the serotype causing illness often cannot be identified by serologic techniques alone.

Acute epiglottitis caused by *Haemophilus influenzae* type b must be differentiated from viral croup. Influenza A virus is also a common cause of croup during epidemic periods.

TREATMENT Parainfluenza Virus Infections

For upper respiratory tract illness, symptoms can be treated as discussed for other viral respiratory tract illnesses. If complications such as sinusitis, otitis, or superimposed bacterial bronchitis develop, appropriate antibacterial antibiotics should be administered. Mild cases of croup should be treated with bed rest and moist air generated by vaporizers. More severe cases require hospitalization and close observation for the development of respiratory distress. If acute respiratory distress develops, humidified oxygen and intermittent racemic epinephrine are usually administered. Aerosolized or systemically administered glucocorticoids are beneficial; the latter have a more profound effect. No specific antiviral therapy is available, although ribavirin is active against parainfluenza viruses in vitro and anecdotal reports describe its use clinically, particularly in immunosuppressed patients.

PREVENTION

Vaccines against parainfluenza viruses are under development.

ADENOVIRUS INFECTIONS

ETIOLOGIC AGENT

Adenoviruses are complex DNA viruses that measure 70–80 nm in diameter. Human adenoviruses belong to the genus *Mastadenovirus*, which includes 51 serotypes. Adenoviruses have a characteristic morphology consisting of an icosahedral shell composed of 20 equilateral triangular faces and 12 vertices. The protein coat (capsid) consists of hexon subunits with group-specific and type-specific antigenic determinants and penton subunits at each vertex primarily containing group-specific antigens. A fiber with a knob at the end projects from each penton; this fiber contains type-specific and some group-specific antigens. Human adenoviruses have been divided into six subgroups (A through F) on the basis of the homology of DNA genomes and other properties. The adenovirus genome is a linear double-stranded DNA that codes for structural and nonstructural polypeptides. The replicative cycle of adenovirus may result either in lytic infection of cells or in the establishment of a latent infection (primarily involving lymphoid cells). Some adenovirus types can induce oncogenic transformation, and tumor formation has been observed in rodents; however, despite intensive investigation, adenoviruses have not been associated with tumors in humans.

EPIDEMIOLOGY

Adenovirus infections most frequently affect infants and children. Infections occur throughout the year but are most common from fall to spring. Adenoviruses account for ~10% of acute respiratory infections in children but for <2% of respiratory illnesses in civilian adults. Nearly 100% of adults have serum antibody to multiple serotypes—a finding indicating that infection is common in childhood. Types 1, 2, 3, and 5 are the most common isolates from children. Certain adenovirus serotypes—particularly 4 and 7 but also 3, 14, and 21—are associated with outbreaks of acute respiratory disease in military recruits in winter and spring. Adenovirus infection can be transmitted by inhalation of aerosolized virus, by inoculation of virus into conjunctival sacs, and probably by the fecal-oral route as well. Type-specific antibody generally develops after infection and is associated with protection, albeit incomplete, against infection with the same serotype.

CLINICAL MANIFESTATIONS

In children, adenoviruses cause a variety of clinical syndromes. The most common is an acute upper respiratory tract infection, with prominent rhinitis. On occasion, lower respiratory tract disease, including bronchiolitis and pneumonia, also develops. Adenoviruses, particularly types 3 and 7, cause pharyngoconjunctival fever, a characteristic acute febrile illness of children that occurs in outbreaks, most often in summer camps. The syndrome is marked by bilateral conjunctivitis in which the bulbar and palpebral conjunctivae have a granular appearance. Low-grade fever is frequently present for the first 3–5 days, and rhinitis, sore throat, and cervical adenopathy develop. The illness generally lasts for 1–2 weeks and resolves spontaneously. Febrile pharyngitis without conjunctivitis has also been associated with adenovirus infection. Adenoviruses have been isolated from cases of whooping cough with or without *Bordetella pertussis*; the significance of adenovirus in that disease is unknown.

In adults, the most frequently reported illness has been acute respiratory disease caused by adenovirus types 4 and 7 in military recruits. This illness is marked by a prominent sore throat and the gradual onset of fever, which often reaches 39°C (102.2°F) on the second or third day of illness. Cough is almost always present, and coryza and regional lymphadenopathy are frequently seen. Physical examination may show pharyngeal edema, injection, and tonsillar enlargement with little or no exudate. If pneumonia has developed, auscultation and x-ray of the chest may indicate areas of patchy infiltration.

Adenoviruses have been associated with a number of non–respiratory tract diseases, including acute diarrheal illness caused by types 40 and 41 in young children and hemorrhagic cystitis caused by types 11 and 21. Epidemic keratoconjunctivitis, caused most frequently by types 8, 19, and 37, has been associated with contaminated common sources such as ophthalmic solutions and roller towels. Adenoviruses have also been implicated in disseminated disease and pneumonia in immunosuppressed patients, including recipients of solid-organ or hematopoietic stem cell transplants. In hematopoietic stem cell transplant recipients, adenovirus infections have been manifested as pneumonia, hepatitis, nephritis, colitis, encephalitis, and hemorrhagic cystitis. In solid-organ transplant recipients, adenovirus infection may involve the organ transplanted (e.g., hepatitis in liver transplants, nephritis in renal transplants) but can disseminate to other organs as well. In patients with AIDS, high-numbered and intermediate adenovirus serotypes have been isolated, usually in the setting of low CD4+ T cell counts, but their isolation often has not been clearly linked to disease manifestations. Adenovirus nucleic acids have been detected in myocardial cells from patients with "idiopathic" myocardiopathies, and adenoviruses have been suggested as causative agents in some cases.

LABORATORY FINDINGS AND DIAGNOSIS

Adenovirus infection should be suspected in the epidemiologic setting of acute respiratory disease in military recruits and in certain of the clinical syndromes (such as pharyngoconjunctival fever or epidemic keratoconjunctivitis) in which outbreaks of characteristic illnesses occur. In most cases, however, illnesses caused by adenovirus infection cannot be differentiated from those caused by a number of other viral respiratory agents and *Mycoplasma pneumoniae*. A definitive diagnosis of adenovirus infection is established by detection of the virus in tissue culture (as evidenced by cytopathic changes) and by specific identification with immunofluorescence or other immunologic techniques. Rapid viral diagnosis can be established by immunofluorescence or ELISA of nasopharyngeal aspirates, conjunctival or respiratory secretions, urine, or stool. Highly sensitive and specific PCR assays and nucleic acid hybridization are also available. Adenovirus types 40 and 41, which have been associated with diarrheal disease in children, require special tissue-culture cells for isolation, and these serotypes are most commonly detected by direct ELISA of stool. Serum antibody rises can be demonstrated by complement-fixation or neutralization tests, ELISA, radioimmunoassay, or (for those adenoviruses that hemagglutinate red cells) hemagglutination inhibition tests.

TREATMENT Adenovirus Infections

Only symptom-based treatment and supportive therapy are available for adenovirus infections, and clinically useful antiviral therapy has not been established. Ribavirin and cidofovir are active in vitro against certain adenoviruses. Retrospective studies and anecdotes describe the use of these agents in disseminated adenovirus infections, but definitive efficacy data from controlled studies are not available.

PREVENTION

Live vaccines have been developed against adenovirus types 4 and 7 and have been used to control illness among military recruits. These vaccines consist of live, unattenuated virus administered in enteric-coated capsules. Infection of the gastrointestinal tract with types 4 and 7 does not cause disease but stimulates local and systemic antibodies that are protective against subsequent acute respiratory disease due to those serotypes. This vaccine has not been produced since 1999, and outbreaks of acute respiratory illness caused by adenovirus types 4 and 7 have again emerged among military recruits. Therefore, a program to redevelop type 4 and 7 vaccines is under way. Adenoviruses are also being studied as live-virus vectors for the delivery of vaccine antigens and for gene therapy.

CHAPTER 15
PNEUMOCYSTIS INFECTIONS

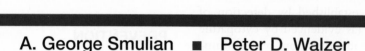

A. George Smulian ■ Peter D. Walzer

DEFINITION AND DESCRIPTION

Pneumocystis is an opportunistic fungal pulmonary pathogen that is an important cause of pneumonia in the immunocompromised host. Although organisms within the *Pneumocystis* genus are morphologically very similar, they are genetically diverse and host-specific. *P. jirovecii* infects humans, whereas *P. carinii*—the original species described in 1909—infects rats. For clarity, only the genus designation *Pneumocystis* will be used in this chapter.

Developmental stages of the organism include the trophic form, the cyst, and the precyst (an intermediate stage). The life cycle of *Pneumocystis* probably involves sexual and asexual reproduction, although definitive proof awaits the development of a reliable culture system. *Pneumocystis* contains several different antigen groups, the most prominent of which are the 95- to 140-kDa major surface glycoprotein (MSG) and kexin (KEX1).

EPIDEMIOLOGY

Serologic surveys have demonstrated that *Pneumocystis* has a worldwide distribution and that most healthy children have been exposed to the organism by 3–4 years of age. Airborne transmission of *Pneumocystis* has been documented in animal studies; person-to-person transmission has been suggested by hospital outbreaks of *Pneumocystis* pneumonia (PcP) and by molecular epidemiologic analysis of isolates. Data suggest that the cyst is the transmissible form.

PATHOGENESIS AND PATHOLOGY

Studies over the past several years have shown that *Pneumocystis* commonly colonizes patients who are immunosuppressed or who have chronic obstructive pulmonary disease. This colonization elicits an inflammatory response and is associated with a decline in lung function.

The host factors that predispose to the development of PcP include defects in cellular and humoral immunity. The risk of PcP among HIV-infected patients rises markedly when circulating CD4+ T cell counts fall below 200/μL. Other persons at risk for PcP are patients receiving immunosuppressive agents (particularly glucocorticoids) for cancer and organ transplantation; those receiving biologic agents such as infliximab and etanercept for rheumatoid arthritis and inflammatory bowel disease; children with primary immunodeficiency diseases; and premature malnourished infants.

The principal host effector cells against *Pneumocystis* are alveolar macrophages, which ingest and kill the organism, releasing a variety of inflammatory mediators. Proliferating organisms remain extracellular within the alveolus, attaching tightly to type I cells. Alveolar damage results in increased alveolar-capillary permeability and surfactant abnormalities, including a fall in phospholipids and an increase in surfactant proteins A and D. The host inflammatory response to lung injury leads to increases in levels of interleukin 8 and in neutrophil counts in bronchoalveolar lavage (BAL) fluid. These changes correlate with disease severity.

On lung sections stained with hematoxylin and eosin, the alveoli are filled with a typical foamy, vacuolated exudate. Severe disease may include interstitial edema, fibrosis, and hyaline membrane formation. The host inflammatory changes usually consist of hypertrophy of alveolar type II cells, a typical reparative response, and a mild mononuclear cell interstitial infiltrate. Malnourished infants display an intense plasma cell infiltrate that gave the disease its early name: interstitial plasma cell pneumonia.

CLINICAL FEATURES

Patients with PcP develop dyspnea, fever, and nonproductive cough. HIV-infected patients are usually ill for several weeks and may have relatively subtle manifestations.

Symptoms in non-HIV-infected patients are of shorter duration and often begin after the glucocorticoid dose has been tapered. A high index of suspicion and a thorough history are key factors in early detection.

Physical findings include tachypnea, tachycardia, and cyanosis, but lung auscultation reveals few abnormalities. Reduced arterial oxygen pressure (Pa_{O2}), increased alveolar-arterial oxygen gradient ($PA_{O2} - Pa_{O2}$), and respiratory alkalosis are evident. Diffusion capacity is reduced, and heightened uptake with nonspecific nuclear imaging techniques (gallium scan) may be noted. Elevated serum concentrations of lactate dehydrogenase, reflecting lung parenchymal damage, and β-D-glucan, a component of the fungal cell wall, have been reported; however, these elevations are not specific for PcP infection.

The classic findings on chest radiography consist of bilateral diffuse infiltrates beginning in the perihilar regions **(Fig. 15-1A)**, but various atypical manifestations (nodular densities, cavitary lesions) have also been reported. Pneumothorax occurs, and its management is often difficult. Early in the course of PcP, the chest radiograph may be normal, although high-resolution CT of the lung may reveal ground-glass opacities at this stage **(Fig. 15-1B)**.

While *Pneumocystis* usually remains confined to the lungs, cases of disseminated infection have occurred in both HIV-infected and non-HIV-infected patients. Common sites of involvement include the lymph nodes, spleen, liver, and bone marrow.

DIAGNOSIS

Because of the nonspecific nature of the clinical picture, the diagnosis must be based on specific identification of the organism. A definitive diagnosis is made by histopathologic staining. Traditional cell wall stains such as methenamine silver selectively stain the wall of *Pneumocystis* cysts, while reagents such as Wright-Giemsa stain the nuclei of all developmental stages. Immunofluorescence with monoclonal antibodies is more sensitive and specific than histologic staining. DNA amplification by PCR may become part of routine diagnostics but may not distinguish colonization from infection.

The successful diagnosis of PcP depends on the collection of proper specimens. In general, the yield from different diagnostic procedures is higher for HIV-infected patients than for non-HIV-infected patients because of the higher organism burden in the former group. Sputum induction and oral washes have gained popularity as simple, noninvasive techniques; however, these procedures require trained and dedicated personnel. Fiberoptic bronchoscopy with BAL, which provides information about the organism burden, the host inflammatory response, and the presence of other opportunistic infections, continues to be the mainstay of *Pneumocystis* diagnosis. Transbronchial biopsy and open lung biopsy, the most invasive procedures, are used only when a diagnosis cannot be made by BAL.

COURSE AND PROGNOSIS

In the typical case of untreated PcP, progressive respiratory embarrassment leads to death. Therapy is most effective when instituted early, before there is extensive alveolar damage. If examination of induced sputum is nondiagnostic and BAL cannot be performed in a timely manner, empirical therapy for PcP is reasonable. However, this practice does not eliminate the need for

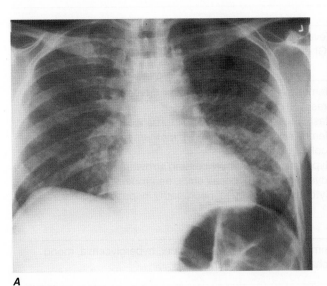

A

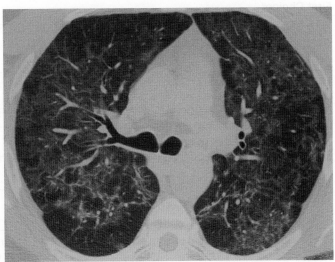

B

FIGURE 15-1
A. Chest radiograph depicting diffuse infiltrates in an HIV-infected patient with PcP. *B*. High-resolution CT of the lung showing ground-glass opacification in an HIV-infected patient with PcP. (*Courtesy of Dr. Cristopher Meyer, with permission.*)

a specific etiologic diagnosis. With improved management of HIV and its complications, mortality rates from PcP among HIV-infected patients are 0–15%. In contrast, rates of early death remain high among patients who require mechanical ventilation (60%) and among non-HIV-infected patients (40%).

TREATMENT   *Pneumocystis* Infections

Trimethoprim-sulfamethoxazole (TMP-SMX), which acts by inhibiting folic acid synthesis, is considered the drug of choice for all forms of PcP (Table 15-1). Therapy is continued for 14 days in non-HIV-infected patients and for 21 days in persons infected with HIV. Since HIV-infected patients respond more slowly than non-HIV-infected patients, it is prudent to wait at least 7 days after the initiation of treatment before concluding that therapy has failed. TMP-SMX is well tolerated by non-HIV-infected patients, whereas more than half of HIV-infected patients experience serious adverse reactions.

Several alternative regimens are available for the treatment of mild to moderate cases of PcP (a Pa_{O_2} of >70 mmHg or a $PA_{O_2} - Pa_{O_2}$ of <35 mmHg while breathing room air). TMP plus dapsone and clindamycin plus primaquine are about as effective as TMP-SMX. Dapsone and primaquine should not be administered to patients with glucose-6-phosphate dehydrogenase

(G6PD) deficiency. Atovaquone is less effective than TMP-SMX but is better tolerated. Since *Pneumocystis* lacks ergosterol, it is not susceptible to antifungal agents that inhibit ergosterol synthesis.

Alternative regimens that are recommended for the treatment of moderate to severe PcP (a Pa_{O_2} of ≤70 mmHg or a $PA_{O_2} - Pa_{O_2}$ of ≥35 mmHg) are parenteral pentamidine, parenteral clindamycin plus primaquine, or trimetrexate plus leucovorin. Parenteral clindamycin plus primaquine may be more efficacious than pentamidine.

Molecular evidence of resistance to sulfonamides and to atovaquone has emerged among clinical *Pneumocystis* isolates. Although prior sulfonamide exposure is a risk factor, this resistance has also occurred in HIV-infected patients who have never received sulfonamides. The outcome of therapy appears to be linked more strongly to traditional measures—e.g., high Acute Physiology, Age, and Chronic Health Evaluation III (APACHE III) scores, need for positive-pressure ventilation, delayed intubation, and development of pneumothorax—than to the presence of molecular markers of sulfonamide resistance.

Early institution of antiretroviral therapy when HIV patients present with PcP has been associated with improved survival rates, but careful attention should be devoted to the possible development of the immune reconstitution inflammatory syndrome. HIV-infected patients frequently experience deterioration of

TABLE 15-1

TREATMENT OF PNEUMOCYSTOSIS

DRUG(S), DOSE, ROUTE	ADVERSE EFFECTS
First Choice[a]	
TMP-SMX (TMP: 5 mg/kg; SMX: 25 mg/kg[b]) q6–8 h PO or IV	Fever, rash, cytopenias, hepatitis, hyperkalemia, GI disturbances
Other Agents[a]	
TMP, 5 mg/kg q6–8h; plus dapsone, 100 mg qd PO	Hemolysis (G6PD deficiency), methemoglobinemia, fever, rash, GI disturbances
Atovaquone, 750 mg bid PO	Rash, fever, GI and hepatic disturbances
Clindamycin, 300–450 mg q6h PO or 600 mg q6–8h IV; plus primaquine, 15–30 mg qd PO	Hemolysis (G6PD deficiency), methemoglobinemia, rash, colitis, neutropenia
Pentamidine, 3–4 mg/kg qd IV	Hypotension, azotemia, cardiac arrhythmias, pancreatitis, dysglycemias, hypocalcemia, neutropenia, hepatitis
Trimetrexate, 45 mg/m² qd IV; plus leucovorin,[c] 20 mg/kg q6h PO or IV	Cytopenias, peripheral neuropathy, hepatic disturbances
Adjunctive Agent	
Prednisone, 40 mg bid × 5 d, 40 mg qd × 5 d, 20 mg qd × 11 d; PO or IV	Immunosuppression, peptic ulcer, hyperglycemia, mood changes, hypertension

[a]Therapy is administered for 14 days to non-HIV-infected patients and for 21 days to HIV-infected patients.
[b]Equivalent of 2 double-strength (DS) tablets. (One DS tablet contains 160 mg of TMP and 800 mg of SMX.)
[c]Leucovorin prevents bone marrow toxicity from trimetrexate.
Abbreviations: GI, gastrointestinal; G6PD, glucose-6-phosphate dehydrogenase; TMP-SMX, trimethoprim-sulfamethoxazole.

TABLE 15-2

PROPHYLAXIS OF PNEUMOCYSTOSIS[a]

DRUG(S), DOSE, ROUTE	COMMENTS
First Choice	
TMP-SMX, 1 DS tablet or 1 SS tablet qd PO[b]	TMP-SMX can be safely reintroduced for treatment of some patients who have had mild to moderate side effects.
Other Agents	
Dapsone, 50 mg bid or 100 mg qd PO	—
Dapsone, 50 mg qd PO; plus pyrimethamine, 50 mg weekly PO; plus leucovorin, 25 mg weekly PO	Leucovorin prevents bone marrow toxicity from pyrimethamine.
Dapsone, 200 mg weekly PO; plus pyrimethamine, 75 mg weekly PO; plus leucovorin, 25 mg weekly PO	Leucovorin prevents bone marrow toxicity from pyrimethamine.
Pentamidine, 300 mg monthly via Respirgard II nebulizer	Adverse reactions include cough and bronchospasm.
Atovaquone, 1500 mg qd PO	—
TMP-SMX, 1 DS tablet three times weekly PO	TMP-SMX can be safely reintroduced for treatment of some patients who have had mild to moderate side effects.

[a]For a list of adverse effects, see Table 15-1.
[b]One DS tablet contains 160 mg of TMP and 800 mg of SMX.
Abbreviations: DS, double-strength; SS, single-strength; TMP-SMX, trimethoprim-sulfamethoxazole.

respiratory function shortly after receiving anti-*Pneumocystis* drugs. The adjunctive administration of tapering doses of glucocorticoids to HIV-infected patients with moderate to severe PcP can prevent this problem and improve the rate of survival (Table 15-1). For maximal benefit, this adjunctive therapy should be started early in the course of the illness. The use of steroids as adjunctive therapy in HIV-infected patients with mild PcP or in non-HIV-infected patients remains to be evaluated.

PREVENTION

Prophylaxis is indicated for HIV-infected patients with CD4+ T cell counts of $<200/\mu L$ or a history of oropharyngeal candidiasis and for both HIV-infected and non-HIV-infected patients who have recovered from PcP. Prophylaxis may be discontinued in HIV-infected patients once CD4+ T cell counts have risen to $>200/\mu L$ and remained at that level for ≥ 3 months. Primary prophylaxis guidelines for immunocompromised hosts not infected with HIV are less clear.

TMP-SMX is the drug of choice for primary and secondary prophylaxis (Table 15-2). This agent also provides protection against toxoplasmosis and some bacterial infections. Alternative regimens are available for individuals intolerant of TMP-SMX (Table 15-2). Although there are no specific recommendations for preventing the spread of *Pneumocystis* in health care facilities, it seems prudent to prevent direct contact between patients with PcP and other susceptible hosts.

CHAPTER 16

BRONCHIECTASIS AND LUNG ABSCESS

Rebecca M. Baron ■ John G. Bartlett

BRONCHIECTASIS

Bronchiectasis refers to an irreversible airway dilation that involves the lung in either a focal or a diffuse manner and that classically has been categorized as cylindrical or tubular (the most common form), varicose, or cystic.

ETIOLOGY

Bronchiectasis can arise from infectious or noninfectious causes (Table 16-1). Clues to the underlying etiology are often provided by the pattern of lung involvement. *Focal bronchiectasis* refers to bronchiectatic changes in a localized area of the lung and can be a consequence of obstruction of the airway—either extrinsic (e.g., due to compression by adjacent lymphadenopathy or parenchymal tumor mass) or intrinsic (e.g., due to an airway tumor or aspirated foreign body, a scarred/stenotic airway, or bronchial atresia from congenital underdevelopment of the airway). *Diffuse bronchiectasis* is characterized by widespread bronchiectatic changes throughout the lung and often arises from an underlying systemic or infectious disease process.

More pronounced involvement of the upper lung fields is most common in cystic fibrosis (CF) and is also observed in postradiation fibrosis, corresponding to the lung region encompassed by the radiation port. Bronchiectasis with predominant involvement of the lower lung fields usually has its source in chronic recurrent aspiration (e.g., due to esophageal motility disorders like those in scleroderma), end-stage fibrotic lung disease (e.g., traction bronchiectasis from idiopathic pulmonary fibrosis), or recurrent immunodeficiency-associated infections (e.g., hypogammaglobulinemia). Bronchiectasis resulting from infection by nontuberculous mycobacteria (NTM; most commonly the *Mycobacterium avium-intracellulare* complex [MAC]) often preferentially affects the midlung fields. Congenital causes of bronchiectasis with predominant midlung field involvement include

the dyskinetic/immotile cilia syndrome. Finally, predominant involvement of the central airways is reported in association with allergic bronchopulmonary aspergillosis (ABPA), in which an immune-mediated reaction to *Aspergillus* damages the bronchial wall. Congenital causes of central airway–predominant bronchiectasis resulting from cartilage deficiency include tracheobronchomegaly (Mounier-Kuhn syndrome) and Williams-Campbell syndrome.

In many cases, the etiology of bronchiectasis is not determined. In case series, as many as 25–50% of patients referred for bronchiectasis have idiopathic disease.

EPIDEMIOLOGY

The epidemiology of bronchiectasis varies greatly with the underlying etiology. For example, patients born with CF often develop significant clinical bronchiectasis in late adolescence or early adulthood, although atypical presentations of CF in adults in their thirties and forties are also possible. In contrast, bronchiectasis resulting from MAC infection classically affects nonsmoking women older than age 50 years. In general, the incidence of bronchiectasis increases with age. Bronchiectasis is more common among women than among men.

In areas where tuberculosis is prevalent, bronchiectasis more frequently occurs as a sequela of granulomatous infection. Focal bronchiectasis can arise from extrinsic compression of the airway by enlarged granulomatous lymph nodes and/or from development of intrinsic obstruction as a result of erosion of a calcified lymph node through the airway wall (e.g., broncholithiasis). Especially in reactivated tuberculosis, parenchymal destruction from infection can result in areas of more diffuse bronchiectasis. Apart from cases associated with tuberculosis, an increased incidence of non-CF bronchiectasis with an unclear underlying mechanism has been reported as a significant problem in

TABLE 16-1

MAJOR ETIOLOGIES OF BRONCHIECTASIS AND PROPOSED WORKUP

PATTERN OF LUNG INVOLVEMENT BY BRONCHIECTASIS	ETIOLOGY BY CATEGORIES (WITH SPECIFIC EXAMPLES)	WORKUP
Focal	Obstruction (e.g., aspirated foreign body, tumor mass)	Chest imaging (chest x-ray and/or chest CT); bronchoscopy
Diffuse	Infection (e.g., bacterial, nontuberculous mycobacterial)	Gram's stain/culture; stains/cultures for acid-fast bacilli and fungi. If no pathogen is identified, consider bronchoscopy with bronchoalveolar lavage (BAL)
	Immunodeficiency (e.g., hypogamma-globulinemia, HIV infection, bronchiolitis obliterans after lung transplantation)	Complete blood count with differential; immunoglobulin measurement; HIV testing
	Genetic causes (e.g., cystic fibrosis, Kartagener's syndrome, α_1 antitrypsin deficiency)	Measurement of chloride levels in sweat (for cystic fibrosis), α_1 antitrypsin levels; nasal or respiratory tract brush/biopsy (for dyskinetic/immotile cilia syndrome); genetic testing
	Autoimmune or rheumatologic causes (e.g., rheumatoid arthritis, Sjögren's syndrome, inflammatory bowel disease); immune-mediated disease (e.g., allergic bronchopulmonary aspergillosis)	Clinical examination with careful joint exam, serologic testing (e.g., for rheumatoid factor). Consider workup for allergic bronchopulmonary aspergillosis, especially in patients with refractory asthma[a]
	Recurrent aspiration	Test of swallowing function and general neuromuscular strength
	Miscellaneous (e.g., yellow nail syndrome; traction bronchiectasis from postradiation fibrosis or idiopathic pulmonary fibrosis)	Guided by clinical condition
	Idiopathic	Exclusion of other causes

[a]Skin testing for *Aspergillus* reactivity; measurement of serum precipitins for *Aspergillus*, serum IgE levels, serum eosinophils, etc.

developing nations. It has been suggested that the high incidence of malnutrition in certain areas may predispose to immune dysfunction and development of bronchiectasis.

PATHOGENESIS AND PATHOLOGY

The most widely cited mechanism of infectious bronchiectasis is the "vicious cycle hypothesis," in which susceptibility to infection and poor mucociliary clearance result in microbial colonization of the bronchial tree. Some organisms, such as *Pseudomonas aeruginosa*, exhibit a particular propensity for colonizing damaged airways and evading host defense mechanisms. Impaired mucociliary clearance can result from inherited conditions such as CF or dyskinetic cilia syndrome, and it has been proposed that a single severe infection (e.g., pneumonia caused by *Bordetella pertussis* or *Mycoplasma pneumoniae*) can result in significant airway damage and poor secretion clearance. The presence of the microbes incites continued chronic inflammation, with consequent damage to the airway wall, continued impairment

of secretion and microbial clearance, and ongoing propagation of the infectious/inflammatory cycle. Moreover, it has been proposed that mediators released directly from bacteria can interfere with mucociliary clearance.

Classic studies of the pathology of bronchiectasis from the 1950s demonstrated significant small-airway wall inflammation and larger-airway wall destruction as well as dilation, with loss of elastin, smooth muscle, and cartilage. It has been proposed that inflammatory cells in the small airways release proteases and other mediators, such as reactive oxygen species and proinflammatory cytokines, that damage the larger-airway walls. Furthermore, the ongoing inflammatory process in the smaller airways results in airflow obstruction. It is believed that antiproteases, such as α_1 antitrypsin, play an important role in neutralizing the damaging effects of neutrophil elastase and in enhancing bacterial killing. In addition to emphysema, bronchiectasis has been observed in patients with α_1 antitrypsin deficiency.

Proposed mechanisms for noninfectious bronchiectasis include immune-mediated reactions that damage the bronchial wall (e.g., those associated with systemic autoimmune conditions such as Sjögren's syndrome and rheumatoid arthritis). *Traction bronchiectasis* refers to dilated airways arising from parenchymal distortion as a result of lung fibrosis (e.g., postradiation fibrosis or idiopathic pulmonary fibrosis).

CLINICAL MANIFESTATIONS

The most common clinical presentation is a persistent productive cough with ongoing production of thick, tenacious sputum. Physical findings often include crackles and wheezing on lung auscultation, and some patients with bronchiectasis exhibit clubbing of the digits. Mild to moderate airflow obstruction is often detected on pulmonary function tests, overlapping with that seen at presentation with other conditions, such as chronic obstructive pulmonary disease (COPD). Acute exacerbations of bronchiectasis are usually characterized by changes in the nature of sputum production, with increased volume and purulence. However, typical signs and symptoms of lung infection, such as fever and new infiltrates, may not be present.

DIAGNOSIS

The diagnosis is usually based on presentation with a persistent chronic cough and sputum production accompanied by consistent radiographic features. While chest radiographs lack sensitivity, the presence of "tram tracks" indicating dilated airways is consistent with bronchiectasis. Chest CT is more specific for bronchiectasis and is the imaging modality of choice for confirming the diagnosis. CT findings include airway dilation (detected as parallel "tram tracks" or as the "signet-ring sign"— a cross-sectional area of the airway with a diameter at least 1.5 times that of the adjacent vessel), lack of bronchial tapering (including the presence of tubular structures within 1 cm from the pleural surface), bronchial wall thickening in dilated airways, inspissated secretions (e.g., the "tree-in-bud" pattern), or cysts emanating from the bronchial wall (especially pronounced in cystic bronchiectasis; **Fig. 16–1**).

APPROACH TO THE PATIENT   Bronchiectasis

The evaluation of a patient with bronchiectasis entails elicitation of a clinical history, chest imaging, and a workup to determine the underlying etiology. Evaluation of focal bronchiectasis almost always requires bronchoscopy to exclude airway obstruction by an underlying mass or foreign body. A workup for diffuse bronchiectasis includes analysis for the major etiologies (Table 16-1). Pulmonary function testing is an important component of a functional assessment of the patient.

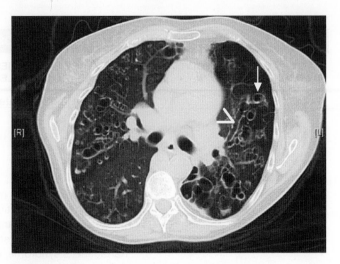

FIGURE 16-1
Representative chest CT image of severe bronchiectasis. This patient's CT demonstrates many severely dilated airways, seen both longitudinally (arrowhead) and in cross-section (arrow).

TREATMENT   Bronchiectasis

Treatment of infectious bronchiectasis is directed at the control of active infection and improvements in secretion clearance and bronchial hygiene so as to decrease the microbial load within the airways and minimize the risk of repeated infections.

ANTIBIOTIC TREATMENT Antibiotics targeting the causative or presumptive pathogen (with *Haemophilus influenzae* and *P. aeruginosa* isolated commonly) should be administered in acute exacerbations, usually for a minimum of 7–10 days. Decisions about treatment of NTM infection can be difficult, given that these organisms can be colonizers as well as pathogens and the prolonged treatment course often is not well tolerated. Consensus guidelines have advised that diagnostic criteria for true clinical infection with NTM should be considered in patients with symptoms and radiographic findings of lung disease who have at least two sputum samples positive on culture; at least one bronchoalveolar lavage (BAL) fluid sample positive on culture; a biopsy sample displaying histopathologic features of NTM infection (e.g., granuloma or a positive stain for acid-fast bacilli) along with one positive sputum culture; or a pleural fluid sample (or a sample from another sterile extrapulmonary site) positive on culture. MAC strains are the most common NTM pathogens, and the recommended regimen for HIV-negative patients includes a macrolide combined with rifampin and ethambutol. Consensus guidelines also recommend macrolide susceptibility testing for clinically significant MAC isolates.

BRONCHIAL HYGIENE The numerous approaches employed to enhance secretion clearance in bronchiectasis include hydration and mucolytic administration, aerosolization of bronchodilators and hyperosmolar agents (e.g., hypertonic saline), and chest physiotherapy (e.g., postural drainage, traditional mechanical chest percussion via hand clapping to the chest, or use of devices such as an oscillatory positive expiratory pressure flutter valve or a high-frequency chest wall oscillation vest). The mucolytic dornase (DNase) is recommended routinely in CF-related bronchiectasis but not in non-CF bronchiectasis, given concerns about lack of efficacy and potential harm in the non-CF population.

ANTI-INFLAMMATORY THERAPY It has been proposed that control of the inflammatory response may be of benefit in bronchiectasis, and relatively small-scale trials have yielded evidence of alleviated dyspnea, decreased need for inhaled β-agonists, and reduced sputum production with inhaled glucocorticoids. However, no significant differences in lung function or bronchiectasis exacerbation rates have been observed. Risks of immunosuppression and adrenal suppression must be carefully considered with use of anti-inflammatory therapy in infectious bronchiectasis. Nevertheless, administration of oral/systemic glucocorticoids may be important in treating bronchiectasis due to certain etiologies, such as ABPA, or non-infectious bronchiectasis due to underlying conditions, especially that in which an autoimmune condition is believed to be active (e.g., rheumatoid arthritis or Sjögren's syndrome). Patients with ABPA may also benefit from a prolonged course of treatment with the oral antifungal agent itraconazole.

REFRACTORY CASES In select cases, surgery can be considered, with resection of a focal area of suppuration. In advanced cases, lung transplantation can be considered.

COMPLICATIONS

In more severe cases of infectious bronchiectasis, recurrent infections and repeated courses of antibiotics can lead to microbial resistance to antibiotics. In certain cases, combinations of antibiotics that have their own independent toxicity profiles may be necessary to treat resistant organisms.

Recurrent infections can result in injury to superficial mucosal vessels, with bleeding and, in severe cases, life-threatening hemoptysis. Management of massive hemoptysis usually requires intubation to stabilize the patient, identifying the source of bleeding, and protecting the nonbleeding lung. Control of bleeding often necessitates bronchial artery embolization and, in severe cases, surgery.

PROGNOSIS

Outcomes of bronchiectasis vary widely with the underlying etiology and may also be influenced by the frequency of exacerbations and (in infectious cases) the specific pathogens involved. In one study, the decline of lung function in patients with non-CF bronchiectasis was similar to that in patients with COPD, with the forced expiratory volume in 1 s (FEV_1) declining by 50–55 mL per year as opposed to 20–30 mL per year for healthy controls.

PREVENTION

Reversal of an underlying immunodeficient state (e.g., by administration of gamma globulin for immunoglobulin-deficient patients) and vaccination of patients with chronic respiratory conditions (e.g., influenza and pneumococcal vaccines) can decrease the risk of recurrent infections. Patients who smoke should be counseled about smoking cessation.

After resolution of an acute infection in patients with recurrences (e.g., ≥3 episodes per year), the use of suppressive antibiotics to minimize the microbial load and reduce the frequency of exacerbations has been proposed, although there is less consensus with regard to this approach in non-CF-associated bronchiectasis than there is in patients with CF-related bronchiectasis. Possible suppressive treatments include (1) administration of an oral antibiotic (e.g., ciprofloxacin) daily for 1–2 weeks per month; (2) use of a rotating schedule of oral antibiotics (to minimize the risk of development of drug resistance); (3) administration of a macrolide antibiotic daily or three times per week (with mechanisms of possible benefit related to non-antimicrobial properties, such as anti-inflammatory effects and reduction of gram-negative bacillary biofilms); (4) inhalation of aerosolized antibiotics (e.g., tobramycin inhalation solution [TOBI]) by select patients on a rotating schedule (e.g., 30 days on, 30 days off) with the goal of decreasing the microbial load without encountering the side effects of systemic drug administration; and (5) intermittent administration of IV antibiotics (e.g., "clean-outs") for patients with more severe bronchiectasis and/or resistant pathogens.

In addition, ongoing, consistent attention to bronchial hygiene can promote secretion clearance and decrease the microbial load in the airways.

LUNG ABSCESS

The term *lung abscess* refers to a microbial infection of the lung that results in necrosis of the pulmonary parenchyma. *Necrotizing pneumonia* or *lung gangrene* refers to multiple small pulmonary abscesses in contiguous areas of the lung, usually resulting from a more virulent infection.

CLASSIFICATION

Lung abscesses are classified by clinical and pathologic features including the tempo of progression, the presence or absence of an associated underlying lesion, and the microbial pathogen responsible. Duration defines the infection as *acute* versus *chronic*, with the dividing line usually at 4–6 weeks. Abscesses occurring in the presence of underlying pulmonary lesions, including tumors or systemic conditions (e.g., HIV infection), are referred to as *secondary*; those that occur in the absence of underlying pulmonary lesions are considered *primary*. The term *nonspecific lung abscess* refers to cases in which no likely pathogen is recovered from expectorated sputum; most such cases are presumed to be due to anaerobic bacteria. *Putrid lung abscess* is a term applied to anaerobic bacterial lung abscesses, which are characterized by distinctive foul-smelling breath, sputum, or empyema fluid.

ETIOLOGY

The likely etiologic agent, appropriate diagnostic testing, and appropriate treatment are frequently indicated by the characteristics of the host and the disease process. A variety of microbial pathogens cause lung abscess (Table 16-2). Most nonspecific lung abscesses are presumed to be due to anaerobic bacteria. Mycobacteria,

TABLE 16-2

MICROBIAL PATHOGENS CAUSING CAVITARY LUNG INFECTION
Aspiration-Prone Host
Anaerobic bacteria plus microaerophilic and/or anaerobic streptococci, *Gemella* spp.
Embolic (endovascular) lesions: usually *Staphylococcus aureus*, *Pseudomonas aeruginosa*, *Fusobacterium necrophorum*[a]
Endemic fungi: *Histoplasma*, *Blastomyces*, *Coccidioides* spp.
Mycobacteria: *M. tuberculosis*, *M. kansasii*, *M. avium*
Immunocompromised Host
M. tuberculosis, *Nocardia asteroides*, *Rhodococcus equi*, *Legionella* spp., *P. aeruginosa*, Enterobacteriaceae (especially *Klebsiella pneumoniae*), *Aspergillus* spp., *Cryptococcus* spp.
Previously Healthy Host
Bacteria: *S. aureus*,[b] *S. milleri*, *K. pneumoniae*, group A *Streptococcus*; *Gemella*, *Legionella*, and *Actinomyces* spp.
Parasites: *Entamoeba histolytica*, *Paragonimus westermani*, *Strongyloides stercoralis*

[a]Lemierre's disease.
[b]Often in a young patient with influenza.

especially *M. tuberculosis*, are a very important cause of pulmonary infections and abscess formation. Fungi and some parasites also cause lung abscess. An acute lung abscess developing in a young, previously healthy patient, especially in conjunction with influenza, is likely to involve *Staphylococcus aureus*; this pathogen generally is seen easily on sputum Gram's stain and culture, and presumptive treatment for methicillin-resistant *S. aureus* is urgent. In an immunocompromised host, suspected pathogens include enteric gram-negative bacilli—especially *Klebsiella pneumoniae* but also agents that are found almost exclusively in patients with defective cell-mediated immunity, such as *Nocardia asteroides* and *Rhodococcus equi*. Lung abscess acquired in other countries may involve *Burkholderia pseudomallei* or *Paragonimus westermani*.

Multiple pulmonary lesions that are not caused by microbes may resemble lung abscess. These include the lesions of pulmonary infarction, bronchiectasis, necrotizing carcinoma, pulmonary sequestration, vasculitides (e.g., periarteritis nodosa, granulomatosis with polyangiitis [Wegener's], Goodpasture syndrome), and cysts or bullae with fluid collections. In some cases, multiple lung abscesses result from septic emboli, most commonly in association with tricuspid valve endocarditis.

CLINICAL FEATURES

The classic presentation of nonspecific lung abscess is an indolent infection that evolves over several days or weeks, usually in a host who has a predisposition to aspiration. A common feature is periodontal infection with pyorrhea or gingivitis. Anaerobes and aerobic or microaerophilic streptococci that colonize the upper airways are implicated in these lesions. The usual symptoms are fatigue, cough, sputum production, and fever. Chills are uncommon. Many patients have evidence of chronic disease, such as weight loss and anemia. Some patients have putrid-smelling sputum indicative of the presence of anaerobes; the foul odor is presumably due to the organisms' production of short-chain fatty acids, such as butyric or succinic acid. Some patients have pleurisy due to pleural involvement by contiguous spread or by a bronchopleural fistula. The pleurisy may be severe and may be the symptom that prompts medical evaluation. Sequential x-rays or CT scans show the evolution of this lesion from pneumonitis to cavitation, a process that generally requires 7–14 days in experimental animals (Fig. 16-2).

DIAGNOSIS

Lung abscess can usually be detected with standard imaging, including chest x-ray and CT (Fig. 16-2). The latter is clearly preferred for precise definition of the lesion and its location and possibly for detection of

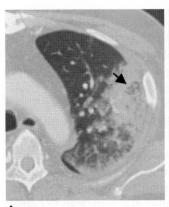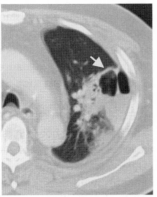

A   **B**

FIGURE 16-2

Representative chest CT demonstrating development of lung abscesses. This patient was immunocompromised due to underlying lymphoma and developed severe *Pseudomonas aeruginosa* pneumonia, as represented by a left lung infiltrate with concern for central regions of necrosis (**panel A**, black arrow). Two weeks later, areas of cavitation with air fluid levels were visible in this region and were consistent with the development of lung abscesses (**panel B**, white arrow). (*Images provided by Dr. Ritu Gill, Division of Chest Radiology, Brigham and Women's Hospital, Boston.*)

underlying lesions. Lymphadenopathy is not associated with bacterial lung abscess; thus this finding suggests an alternative diagnosis.

Microbiologic studies include stains and cultures of expectorated sputum to detect aerobic bacterial pathogens. However, clinical correlations are very important because sputum cultures (especially those that do not satisfy standard cytologic criteria) are unreliable. In appropriate settings, it is important to consider cultures for fungi and mycobacteria. Anaerobic bacteria, the most common causes of primary lung abscess, are not detected in expectorated sputum cultures, and in any case the specimen is subject to anaerobic contamination as it traverses the upper airways. Alternative specimens that may be useful include pleural fluid obtained by thoracentesis in patients who have empyema and quantitative bronchoalveolar lavage (BAL) specimens if they are processed promptly and appropriately for anaerobic bacteria. Many reports describe the use of transtracheal aspiration to bypass the upper airways and obtain a specimen for meaningful anaerobic culture. This procedure, which was used extensively in the 1970s, has largely been abandoned out of concern about adverse consequences and because of a general decline in the pursuit of an etiologic agent in pulmonary infections. Another invasive method for bypassing contamination by the flora of the upper airways is transthoracic needle aspiration under CT guidance; the popularity of this procedure has increased in recent years. In most cases, the etiology of anaerobic lung abscess is clear: the host

is prone to aspiration and has an abscess in a dependent pulmonary segment, with no other likely cause. As stated earlier, putrid breath, sputum, or empyema fluid indicates anaerobic infection.

TREATMENT   Lung Abscess

ANTIBIOTIC SELECTION Treatment depends on the presumed or established etiology. Infections caused by anaerobic bacteria should usually be treated with clindamycin; the initial IV dosage of 600 mg four times daily can be changed to an oral dosage of 300 mg four times daily once the patient becomes afebrile and improves clinically. The duration of therapy is arbitrary, but many experts recommend continuation of oral treatment until imaging shows that chest lesions have cleared or have left a small, stable scar. A shorter course may be effective. An alternative to clindamycin is any β-lactam/β-lactamase inhibitor combination; parenteral treatment may be followed by orally administered amoxicillin/clavulanate. Carbapenems are also effective against anaerobic bacteria as well as streptococci, but the published data with these drugs in the treatment of anaerobic pulmonary infections are sparse. Penicillin was previously regarded as a preferred drug for these infections, but many oral anaerobes produce β-lactamases, and clindamycin proved superior to penicillin G in a randomized clinical trial. Metronidazole is highly active against virtually all anaerobes but not against aerobic microaerophilic streptococci, which play an important role in mixed infections. In therapeutic trials, metronidazole has done poorly unless combined with a β-lactam or another agent active against aerobic and microaerophilic streptococci.

Persistence of fever beyond 5–7 days or progression of the infiltrate suggests failure of therapy and a need to exclude factors such as obstruction, complicating empyema, and involvement of antibiotic-resistant bacteria. Many patients with uncomplicated lung abscesses and all those with atypical presentations or unresponsive abscesses should undergo bronchoscopy and/or CT to detect a possible associated anatomic lesion, such as a tumor, or a foreign body. Quantitative bacteriologic studies using a protected brush catheter or BAL are much less reliable when done after antibiotic therapy. Postural drainage was previously popular for patients with lung abscess, but aggressive attempts to implement this strategy may result in spillage to other pulmonary segments, leading to airway obstruction and clinical deterioration.

Lung abscess due to *S. aureus* is usually treated with vancomycin at a dosage that targets a trough serum level of 15–20 μg/mL. The main alternative is linezolid. Daptomycin should not be used for pulmonary infections. Lung abscesses caused by aerobic gram-negative bacteria need to be treated according to the results of antibiotic sensitivity tests. Most common among the pathogens involved are *K. pneumoniae* (especially the K1 strain in Taiwan) and *P. aeruginosa* in patients with severe chronic lung disease or compromised immune defenses. Pseudomonal lung abscesses usually require prolonged courses of parenteral antibiotics. Carbapenems or β-lactams are frequently combined with aminoglycosides; oral fluoroquinolones are often effective initially, but resistance is common with prolonged use. Aerosolized colistin and aminoglycosides are sometimes used to augment other therapy, but the efficacy of this approach is variable.

Surgery for lung abscesses was developed at the time penicillin became available in the late 1940s. The relative roles of penicillin and resectional surgery were hotly debated at that time, but by the late 1950s penicillin was favored. Initially the standard choice for most lung abscesses, penicillin was subsequently supplanted by the options summarized earlier. Recent large-scale reviews indicate that, in general, surgery is now reserved for ~10–12% of patients. The major indications for surgery are failure to respond to medical management, suspected neoplasm, and hemorrhage. Failure to respond to antibiotics is usually due to an obstructed bronchus and an extremely large abscess (>6 cm in diameter) or to infection involving relatively resistant bacteria, such as *P. aeruginosa*. The usual procedure is lobectomy. An alternative intervention that is becoming popular is percutaneous drainage under CT guidance. Aspirate samples for assay of possible pathogens should be carefully collected.

RESPONSE TO THERAPY Patients with lung abscess usually show clinical improvement, with decreased fever, within 3–5 days of initiation of antibiotic treatment. Defervescence can be expected within 5–10 days. Patients with fevers persisting for 7–14 days should undergo bronchoscopy or other diagnostic tests to better define anatomic changes and microbiologic findings. Cultures of expectorated sputum are not likely to be helpful at this juncture except for detecting pathogens such as mycobacteria and fungi. The response to therapy apparent on serial chest radiographs is delayed in comparison with the clinical course. In fact, infiltrates usually progress during the first 3 days of treatment in approximately one-half of patients. Pleural involvement is relatively common and may develop in dramatic fashion. The most common causes of failures of medical management include a failure to drain pleural collections, an inappropriate choice of antimicrobial therapy, an obstructed bronchus that prevents drainage, a "giant" abscess, a resistant pathogen, or refractory lesions due to immunocompromise.

CHAPTER 17

CYSTIC FIBROSIS

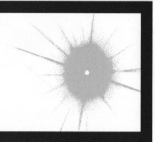

Richard C. Boucher

Cystic fibrosis (CF) is a monogenic disorder that presents as a multisystem disease. The first signs and symptoms typically occur in childhood, but about 5% of patients in the United States are diagnosed as adults. Due to improvements in therapy, >46% of patients are now adults (≥18 years old) and 16.4% are past the age of 30. The median survival is >37.4 years for patients with CF; thus, CF is no longer only a pediatric disease, and internists must be prepared to recognize and treat its many complications. CF is characterized by chronic bacterial infection of the airways that leads to bronchiectasis and bronchiolectasis, exocrine pancreatic insufficiency and intestinal dysfunction, abnormal sweat gland function, and urogenital dysfunction.

PATHOGENESIS

GENETIC CONSIDERATIONS

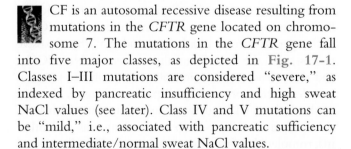 CF is an autosomal recessive disease resulting from mutations in the *CFTR* gene located on chromosome 7. The mutations in the *CFTR* gene fall into five major classes, as depicted in **Fig. 17-1**. Classes I–III mutations are considered "severe," as indexed by pancreatic insufficiency and high sweat NaCl values (see later). Class IV and V mutations can be "mild," i.e., associated with pancreatic sufficiency and intermediate/normal sweat NaCl values.

The prevalence of CF varies with the ethnic origin of a population. CF is detected in approximately 1 in 3000 live births in the Caucasian population of North America and northern Europe, 1 in 17,000 live births of African Americans, and 1 in 90,000 live births of the Asian population of Hawaii. The most common mutation in the *CFTR* gene (~70% of CF chromosomes) is a 3-bp deletion (a class II mutation) that results in an absence of phenylalanine at amino acid position 508 (ΔF_{508})

of the CF gene protein product, known as cystic fibrosis transmembrane conductance regulator (CFTR). The large number (>1500) of relatively uncommon (<2% each) mutations identified in the *CFTR* gene makes genetic testing challenging.

CFTR PROTEIN

The CFTR protein is a single polypeptide chain, containing 1480 amino acids, that functions both as a cyclic AMP–regulated Cl^- channel and a regulator of other ion channels. The fully processed form of CFTR localizes to the plasma membrane in normal epithelia. Biochemical studies indicate that the ΔF_{508} mutation leads to improper maturation and intracellular degradation of the mutant CFTR protein. Thus, absence of CFTR in the plasma membrane is central to the molecular pathophysiology of the ΔF_{508} mutation and other classes I–II mutations. Classes III–IV mutations produce CFTR proteins that are fully processed but are nonfunctional or only partially functional in the plasma membrane. Class V mutations include splicing mutations that produce small amounts of functional CFTR.

EPITHELIAL DYSFUNCTION

The epithelia affected by CF exhibit different functions in their native state, i.e., some are volume-absorbing (airways and distal intestinal epithelia), and some are salt- but not volume-absorbing (sweat duct), whereas others are volume-secretory (proximal intestine and pancreas). Given this diversity of native activities, it is not surprising that CF produces organ-specific effects on electrolyte and water transport. However, the unifying concept is that all affected tissues express abnormal ion transport function.

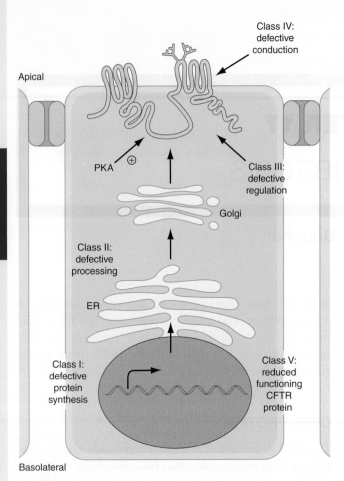

FIGURE 17-1
Schema describing classes of genetic mutations in CFTR gene and effects on CFTR protein/function. Note the ΔF_{508} mutation is a class II mutation and, like class I mutations, would be predicted to produce no mature CFTR protein in the apical membrane. CFTR, cystic fibrosis transmembrane conductance regulator.

ORGAN-SPECIFIC PATHOPHYSIOLOGY

Lung

The diagnostic biophysical hallmark of CF airway epithelia is the raised transepithelial electric potential difference (PD), which reflects both the rate of active ion transport and epithelial resistance to ion flow. CF airway epithelia exhibit abnormalities in both active Cl^- secretion and Na^+ absorption (Fig. 17-2). The Cl^- secretory defect reflects the absence of cyclic AMP–dependent kinase and protein kinase C–regulated Cl^- transport mediated by CFTR itself. An important observation is that there is also a molecularly distinct Ca^{2+}-activated Cl^- channel (CaCC, TMEM16a) expressed in the apical membrane. This channel can substitute for CFTR with regard to Cl^- secretion and is a potential therapeutic target. The abnormal Na^+ transport reflects a second function of CFTR, its function as a tonic

inhibitor of the epithelial Na^+ channel. The molecular mechanisms mediating this action of CFTR remain unknown.

Mucus clearance is the primary innate airways defense mechanism against infection by inhaled bacteria. Normal airways vary the rates of active Na^+ absorption and Cl^- secretion to adjust the volume of liquid (water), i.e., "hydration," on airway surfaces for efficient mucus clearance. The central hypothesis of CF airways pathophysiology is that the faulty regulation of Na^+ absorption and inability to secrete Cl^- via CFTR reduce the volume of liquid on airway surfaces; i.e., they are "dehydrated." Dehydration of both the mucus and the periciliary liquid layers produces adhesion of mucus to the airway surface, which leads to a failure to clear mucus from the airways both by ciliary and cough-dependent mechanisms. The absence of a strict correspondence between gene-mutation class and severity of lung disease suggests important roles for modifier genes and gene-environmental interactions.

The infection that characterizes CF airways involves the mucus layer rather than epithelial or airway wall invasion. The predisposition of CF airways to chronic infection by *Staphylococcus aureus* and *Pseudomonas aeruginosa* is consistent with failure to clear mucus. Recently, it has been demonstrated that the O_2 tension is very low in CF mucus, and adaptations to hypoxemia are important determinants of the physiology of bacteria in the CF lung. Indeed, both mucus stasis and mucus hypoxemia contribute to (1) the propensity for *Pseudomonas* to grow in biofilm colonies within CF airway mucus and (2) the presence of strict anaerobes in CF lungs.

Gastrointestinal tract

The gastrointestinal effects of CF are diverse. In the exocrine pancreas, the absence of the CFTR Cl^- channel in the apical membrane of pancreatic ductal epithelia limits the function of an apical membrane Cl^--HCO_3^- exchanger to secrete bicarbonate and Na^+ (by a passive process) into the duct. The failure to secrete Na^+ HCO_3^- and water leads to retention of enzymes in the pancreas and destruction of virtually all pancreatic tissue. Because of the lack of Cl^- and water secretion, the CF intestinal epithelium fails to flush secreted mucins and other macromolecules from intestinal crypts. The diminished CFTR-mediated liquid secretion may be exacerbated by excessive absorption of liquid, reflecting abnormalities of CFTR-mediated regulation of Na^+ absorption (both mediated by Na^+ channels and possibly other Na^+ transporters, e.g., Na^+-H^+ exchangers). Both dysfunctions lead to dehydrated intraluminal contents and intestinal obstruction. In the hepatobiliary system, defective hepatic ductal salt (Cl^-) and water secretion causes thickened biliary secretions, focal biliary cirrhosis, and bile-duct proliferation in approximately 25–30% of patients with

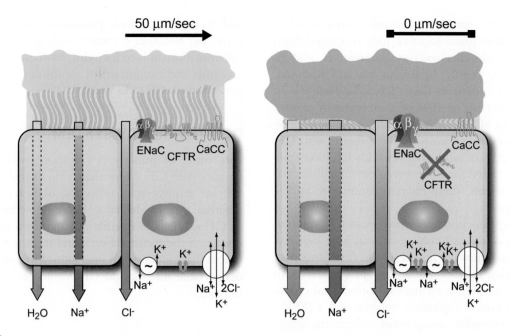

FIGURE 17-2

Comparison of ion transport properties of normal (top) and CF (bottom) airway epithelia. The vectors describe routes and magnitudes of Na⁺ and Cl⁻ transport that is accompanied by osmotically driven water flow. The normal basal pattern for ion transport is absorption of Na⁺ from the lumen via an amiloride-sensitive epithelial Na⁺ channel (ENaC) composed of α, β, and γ ENaC subunits. This process is accelerated in CF. The capacity to initiate cyclic AMP–mediated Cl⁻ secretion is diminished in CF airway epithelia due to abnormal maturation/dysfunction of the CFTR Cl⁻ channel. The accelerated Na⁺ absorption in CF reflects the absence of CFTR inhibitory effects on Na⁺ channels. A Ca^{2+}-activated Cl⁻ channel, likely a product of the TMEM16a gene, is expressed in normal and CF apical membranes and can be activated by extracellular ATP. Horizontal arrows depict velocity of mucociliary clearance (μm/sec).

CF. The inability of the CF gallbladder epithelium to secrete salt and water can lead to both chronic cholecystitis and cholelithiasis.

Sweat gland

CF patients secrete nearly normal volumes of sweat in the sweat acinus, but are not able to absorb NaCl from the sweat duct due to the inability to absorb Cl⁻ via CFTR across ductal epithelial cells. This sweat gland dysfunction is typically measured by measuring Cl⁻ concentrations in sweat collected after iontophoresis of cholinergic agonists.

CLINICAL FEATURES

Most patients with CF present with signs and symptoms of the disease in childhood. Approximately 20% of patients present within the first 24 h of life with gastrointestinal obstruction, termed *meconium ileus.* Other common presentations within the first year or two of life include respiratory tract symptoms, most prominently cough and/or recurrent pulmonary infiltrates, and failure to thrive. A significant proportion of patients (~5%), however, are diagnosed after age 18.

RESPIRATORY TRACT

Upper respiratory tract disease is almost universal in patients with CF. Chronic sinusitis is common in childhood, and the incidence of nasal polyps, which often requires treatment with topical steroids and/or surgery, approaches 25%.

In the lower respiratory tract, the first symptom of CF is cough. With time, the cough becomes persistent and produces viscous, purulent, often greenish-colored sputum. There are protracted periods of clinical stability interrupted by "pulmonary exacerbations," often triggered by viral infections, and defined by increased cough, weight loss, low-grade fever, increased sputum volume, and decrements in pulmonary function. Over the course of years, the exacerbation frequency increases and the recovery of lost lung function becomes incomplete, leading to respiratory failure.

CF patients exhibit a characteristic sputum microbiology. *Haemophilus influenzae* and *S. aureus* are often the first organisms recovered from lung secretions in newly diagnosed CF patients. *P. aeruginosa*, often mucoid and antibiotic-resistant, is typically cultured from lower respiratory tract secretions thereafter. *Burkholderia cepacia* is also recovered from CF sputum and is pathogenic. Patient-to-patient spread of certain strains of these organisms mandates strict infection control in the hospital. Other gram-negative rods recovered from CF sputum include *Alcaligenes xylosoxidans*, *B. gladioli*; and, occasionally, *Proteus*, *Escherichia coli*, and *Klebsiella*. Up to 50% of CF patients have *Aspergillus fumigatus* in their sputum, and up to 10% of these patients exhibit the syndrome of allergic bronchopulmonary aspergillosis. *Mycobacterium tuberculosis* is rare in patients with CF. However, 10–20% of adult patients with CF have sputum cultures positive for nontuberculous mycobacteria, and in some patients, these microorganisms are associated with disease.

The first lung-function abnormalities in CF children, increased ratios of residual volume to total lung capacity, suggest that small-airways disease is the first functional lung abnormality in CF. As disease progresses, both reversible and irreversible changes in forced vital capacity (FVC) and forced expiratory volume in 1 s (FEV_1) develop. The reversible component reflects the accumulation of intraluminal secretions and/or airway reactivity, which occurs in 40–60% of patients with CF. The irreversible component reflects chronic destruction of the airway wall and bronchiolitis.

The earliest chest x-ray change in CF lungs is hyperinflation, reflecting small-airways obstruction. Later, signs of luminal mucus impaction, bronchial cuffing, and finally bronchiectasis, e.g., ring shadows, are noted. For reasons that remain speculative, the right upper lobe displays the earliest and most severe changes.

CF pulmonary disease is associated with many intermittent complications. Pneumothorax is common (>10% of patients). The production of small amounts of blood in sputum is common in CF patients with advanced pulmonary disease. Massive hemoptysis is life-threatening. With advanced lung disease, clubbing of digits appears in virtually all patients with CF. As late events, respiratory failure and cor pulmonale are prominent features of CF.

GASTROINTESTINAL TRACT

Meconium ileus in infants presents with abdominal distention, failure to pass stool, and emesis. The abdominal flat plate can be diagnostic, with small intestinal air-fluid levels, a granular appearance representing meconium, and a small colon. In children and young adults, a syndrome termed *distal intestinal obstruction syndrome* (DIOS) occurs, which presents with right lower quadrant pain, loss of appetite, occasionally emesis, and often a palpable mass. DIOS can be confused with appendicitis, whose frequency is not increased in CF patients.

Exocrine pancreatic insufficiency occurs in >90% of patients with CF. Insufficient pancreatic enzyme secretion yields protein and fat malabsorption, with frequent, bulky, foul-smelling stools. Signs and symptoms of malabsorption of fat-soluble vitamins, including vitamins E

and K, are also noted. Pancreatic beta cells are spared early, but function decreases with age. This effect, plus inflammation-induced insulin resistance, causes hyperglycemia and a requirement for insulin in >29% of older patients with CF (>35 years).

GENITOURINARY SYSTEM

Late onset of puberty is common in both males and females with CF. More than 95% of male patients with CF are azoospermic, reflecting obliteration of the vas deferens due to defective liquid secretion. Some 20% of CF women are infertile due to effects of chronic lung disease on the menstrual cycle and thick, tenacious cervical mucus that blocks sperm migration. Most pregnancies produce viable infants, and CF women breast-feed infants normally.

DIAGNOSIS

The diagnosis of CF rests on the combination of clinical criteria and abnormal CFTR function as documented by sweat tests, nasal PD measurements, and *CFTR* mutation analysis. Elevated sweat Cl^- values are nearly pathognomonic for CF. The sweat concentration values for Cl^- (and Na^+) vary with age, but, typically, a Cl^- concentration of >70 meq/L in adults discriminates between CF and other lung diseases. DNA analysis of the most common mutations identify CF mutations in >90% of affected patients. The nasal PD measurement can document CFTR dysfunction if the sweat Cl^- test is normal or borderline and two CF mutations are not identified. DNA analysis is performed routinely in patients with CF, because pancreatic genotype-phenotype relationships have been identified and mutation class–specific treatments are being developed.

Between 1 and 2% of patients with the clinical syndrome of CF have normal sweat Cl^- values. In most of these patients, the nasal transepithelial PD is raised into the diagnostic range for CF, and sweat acini do not secrete in response to injected β-adrenergic agonists. A single mutation of the *CFTR* gene, 3849 + 10 kb C→T, is associated with most CF patients with normal sweat Cl^- values.

TREATMENT   Cystic Fibrosis

The major objectives of therapy for CF are to promote clearance of secretions and control infection in the lung, provide adequate nutrition, and prevent intestinal obstruction. Ultimately, therapies that restore the processing of misfolded mutant *CFTR* or gene therapy may be the treatments of choice.

LUNG DISEASE More than 95% of CF patients die of complications from lung infection. Theoretically, promoting clearance of adherent mucus should both treat and prevent progression of CF lung disease, whereas antibiotics principally reduce the bacterial burden in the CF lung.

The time-honored techniques for clearing pulmonary secretions are exercise, flutter valves, and chest percussion. Regular use of these maneuvers is effective in preserving lung function. Inhaled hypertonic saline (7%) has demonstrated efficacy in restoring mucus clearance and pulmonary function in short-term studies and in reducing acute exacerbations in a long-term (one-year) study. Hypertonic saline is safe but produces bronchoconstriction in some patients, which can be prevented with coadministered bronchodilators. Inhaled hypertonic saline is becoming a standard of care for all CF patients.

Pharmacologic agents for increasing mucus clearance are in use and in development. An important adjunct to secretion clearance can be recombinant human DNAse, which degrades DNA in CF sputum, increases airflow during short-term administration, and increases the time between pulmonary exacerbations. Most patients receive a therapeutic trial of DNAse for several months to test for efficacy. Clinical trials of experimental drugs aimed at restoring salt and water content of secretions are under way, but these drugs are not yet available for clinical use.

Antibiotics are used to treat lung infection, and their selection is guided by sputum culture results. However, because routine hospital microbiologic cultures are performed under conditions that do not mimic conditions in the CF lung, (e.g., hypoxemia) clinical efficacy often does not correlate with sensitivity testing. Because of increased total-body clearance and volume of distribution of antibiotics in CF patients, the required doses are higher for patients with CF.

Early intervention with antibiotics in infants with infection may eradicate *P. aeruginosa* for extended periods. In older patients with established infection, suppression of bacterial growth is the therapeutic goal. Azithromycin (250 mg/d or 500 mg three times weekly) is often used chronically, although it is unclear whether its actions are antimicrobial or anti-inflammatory. Inhaled aminoglycosides, (e.g., tobramycin 300 mg bid) are also used. "Mild exacerbations," as defined by increased cough and mucus production, are treated with additional oral antibiotics. Oral agents used to treat *Staphylococcus* include a semisynthetic penicillin or a cephalosporin. Oral ciprofloxacin may reduce pseudomonal bacterial counts and control symptoms, but its clinical utility is limited by emergence of resistant organisms. Accordingly, it is often used with an inhaled antibiotic, either tobramycin or colistin (75 mg bid). More severe exacerbations require intravenous antibiotics. Intravenous therapy is given both in hospital and outpatient settings. Usually, two drugs with different mechanisms of action (e.g., a cephalosporin and an aminoglycoside) are used to treat *P. aeruginosa* to minimize emergence of resistant organisms. Drug dosage should be monitored so that levels for gentamicin or tobramycin peak at ranges of ~10 µg/mL and exhibit troughs of <2 µg/mL. Antibiotics directed at *Staphylococcus* and/or *H. influenzae* are added, depending on culture results.

Inhaled β-adrenergic agonists can be useful to control airways constriction, but long-term benefit has not been shown. Oral glucocorticoids may reduce airway inflammation, but their long-term use is limited by adverse side effects; however, they may be useful for treating allergic bronchopulmonary aspergillosis.

The chronic damage to airway walls reflects in part the destructive activities of proteolytic enzymes generated, in part, by inflammatory cells. Specific antiprotease therapies are not available. However, a subset of adolescents with CF may benefit from long-term, high-dose nonsteroidal (ibuprofen) therapy.

Pulmonary complications often require acute interventions. Atelectasis requires treatment with inhaled hypertonic saline, chest physiotherapy, and antibiotics. Pneumothoraxes involving ≤10% of the lung can be observed, but chest tubes are required to expand a collapsed, diseased lung. Small-volume hemoptysis typically requires treatment of lung infection and assessment of coagulation and vitamin K status. For massive hemoptysis, bronchial artery embolization should be performed. The most ominous complications of CF are respiratory failure and cor pulmonale. The most effective conventional therapy for these conditions is vigorous medical management of the lung disease and O_2 supplementation. Ultimately, the only effective treatment for respiratory failure in CF is lung transplantation (Chap. 24). The 2-year survival for lung transplantation exceeds 60%, and transplant-patient deaths result principally from obliterative bronchiolitis.

GASTROINTESTINAL DISEASE Maintenance of adequate nutrition is critical for the health of the CF patient. Most (>90%) CF patients require pancreatic enzyme replacement. Capsules generally contain between 4000 and 20,000 units of lipase. The dose of enzymes (typically no more than 2500 units/kg per meal, to avoid risk of fibrosing colonopathy) is adjusted on the basis of weight, abdominal symptomatology, and stool character. Replacement of fat-soluble vitamins, particularly vitamins E and K, is usually required. Hyperglycemia most often becomes manifest in the adult and typically requires insulin treatment.

For treatment of acute distal intestinal obstruction, megalodiatrizoate or other hypertonic radiocontrast materials delivered by enema to the terminal ileum are used. For control of symptoms, adjustment of pancreatic enzymes and solutions containing osmotically active agents, (e.g., propyleneglycol) is recommended. Persistent symptoms may indicate a gastrointestinal malignancy, which is increased in incidence in patients with CF.

Cholestatic liver disease occurs in about 8% of CF patients. Treatment with urodeoxycholic acid is often initiated, but has not been shown to influence the course of hepatic disease. End-stage liver disease occurs in about 5% of CF patients and is treated by transplantation.

OTHER ORGAN COMPLICATIONS Dehydration due to heat-induced salt loss occurs more readily in CF patients. CF patients also have an increased incidence of osteoarthropathy, renal stones, and osteoporosis, particularly following transplant.

PSYCHOSOCIAL FACTORS CF imposes a tremendous burden on patients, and depression is common. Health insurance, career options, family planning, and life expectancy become major issues. Thus, assisting patients with the psychosocial adjustments required by CF is critical.

CHAPTER 18

CHRONIC OBSTRUCTIVE PULMONARY DISEASE

John J. Reilly, Jr. ■ Edwin K. Silverman ■ Steven D. Shapiro

Chronic obstructive pulmonary disease (COPD) is defined as a disease state characterized by airflow limitation that is not fully reversible (*http://www.goldcopd.com/*). COPD includes *emphysema*, an anatomically defined condition characterized by destruction and enlargement of the lung alveoli; *chronic bronchitis*, a clinically defined condition with chronic cough and phlegm; and *small airways disease*, a condition in which small bronchioles are narrowed. COPD is present only if chronic airflow obstruction occurs; chronic bronchitis *without* chronic airflow obstruction is *not* included within COPD.

COPD is the fourth leading cause of death and affects >10 million persons in the United States. COPD is also a disease of increasing public health importance around the world. Estimates suggest that COPD will rise from the sixth to the third most common cause of death worldwide by 2020.

RISK FACTORS

CIGARETTE SMOKING

By 1964, the Advisory Committee to the Surgeon General of the United States had concluded that cigarette smoking was a major risk factor for mortality from chronic bronchitis and emphysema. Subsequent longitudinal studies have shown accelerated decline in the volume of air exhaled within the first second of the forced expiratory maneuver (FEV_1) in a dose-response relationship to the intensity of cigarette smoking, which is typically expressed as pack-years (average number of packs of cigarettes smoked per day multiplied by the total number of years of smoking). This dose-response relationship between reduced pulmonary function and cigarette smoking intensity accounts for the higher prevalence rates for COPD with increasing age. The historically higher rate of smoking among males is the

likely explanation for the higher prevalence of COPD among males; however, the prevalence of COPD among females is increasing as the gender gap in smoking rates has diminished in the past 50 years.

Although the causal relationship between cigarette smoking and the development of COPD has been absolutely proved, there is considerable variability in the response to smoking. Although pack-years of cigarette smoking is the most highly significant predictor of FEV_1 (Fig. 18-1), only 15% of the variability in FEV_1 is explained by pack-years. This finding suggests that additional environmental and/or genetic factors contribute to the impact of smoking on the development of airflow obstruction.

Although cigar and pipe smoking may also be associated with the development of COPD, the evidence supporting such associations is less compelling, likely related to the lower dose of inhaled tobacco by-products during cigar and pipe smoking.

AIRWAY RESPONSIVENESS AND COPD

A tendency for increased bronchoconstriction in response to a variety of exogenous stimuli, including methacholine and histamine, is one of the defining features of asthma (Chap. 8). However, many patients with COPD also share this feature of airway hyperresponsiveness. The considerable overlap between persons with asthma and those with COPD in airway responsiveness, airflow obstruction, and pulmonary symptoms led to the formulation of the Dutch hypothesis. This suggests that asthma, chronic bronchitis, and emphysema are variations of the same basic disease, which is modulated by environmental and genetic factors to produce these pathologically distinct entities. The alternative British hypothesis contends that asthma and COPD are fundamentally different diseases: Asthma is viewed as largely an allergic phenomenon, while COPD results

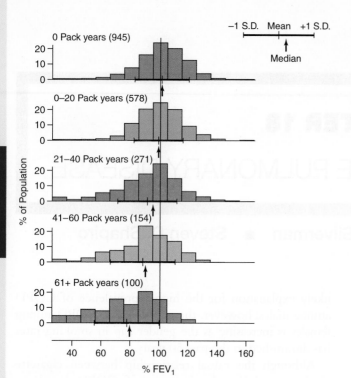

FIGURE 18-1

Distributions of forced expiratory volume in 1 s (FEV$_1$) values in a general population sample, stratified by pack-years of smoking. Means, medians, and ±1 standard deviation of percent predicted FEV$_1$ are shown for each smoking group. Although a dose-response relationship between smoking intensity and FEV$_1$ was found, marked variability in pulmonary function was observed among subjects with similar smoking histories. (*From B Burrows et al: Am Rev Respir Dis 115:95, 1977; with permission.*)

from smoking-related inflammation and damage. Determination of the validity of the Dutch hypothesis vs. the British hypothesis awaits identification of the genetic predisposing factors for asthma and/or COPD, as well as the interactions between these postulated genetic factors and environmental risk factors. Of note, several genes related to the proteinase-antiproteinase hypothesis have been implicated as genetic determinants for both COPD and asthma, including *ADAM33* and macrophage elastase (*MMP12*) as described later.

Longitudinal studies that compared airway responsiveness at the beginning of the study to subsequent decline in pulmonary function have demonstrated that increased airway responsiveness is clearly a significant predictor of subsequent decline in pulmonary function. Thus, airway hyperresponsiveness is a risk factor for COPD.

RESPIRATORY INFECTIONS

The impact of adult respiratory infections on decline in pulmonary function is controversial, but significant long-term reductions in pulmonary function are not typically seen following an episode of bronchitis or pneumonia. The impact of the effects of childhood respiratory illnesses on the subsequent development of COPD has been difficult to assess due to a lack of adequate longitudinal data. Thus, although respiratory infections are important causes of exacerbations of COPD, the association of both adult and childhood respiratory infections to the development and progression of COPD remains to be proven.

OCCUPATIONAL EXPOSURES

Increased respiratory symptoms and airflow obstruction have been suggested to result from general exposure to dust and fumes at work. Several specific occupational exposures, including coal mining, gold mining, and cotton textile dust, have been suggested as risk factors for chronic airflow obstruction. Although nonsmokers in these occupations developed some reductions in FEV$_1$, the importance of dust exposure as a risk factor for COPD, independent of cigarette smoking, is not certain for most of these exposures. However, a recent study found that coal mine dust exposure was a significant risk factor for emphysema in both smokers and nonsmokers. In most cases, the magnitude of these occupational exposures on COPD risk is likely substantially less important than the effect of cigarette smoking.

AMBIENT AIR POLLUTION

Some investigators have reported increased respiratory symptoms in those living in urban compared to rural areas, which may relate to increased pollution in the urban settings. However, the relationship of air pollution to chronic airflow obstruction remains unproved. Prolonged exposure to smoke produced by biomass combustion—a common mode of cooking in some countries—also appears to be a significant risk factor for COPD among women in those countries. However, in most populations, ambient air pollution is a much less important risk factor for COPD than cigarette smoking.

PASSIVE, OR SECOND-HAND, SMOKING EXPOSURE

Exposure of children to maternal smoking results in significantly reduced lung growth. In utero tobacco smoke exposure also contributes to significant reductions in postnatal pulmonary function. Although passive smoke exposure has been associated with reductions in pulmonary function, the importance of this risk factor in the development of the severe pulmonary function reductions in COPD remains uncertain.

GENETIC CONSIDERATIONS

Although cigarette smoking is the major environmental risk factor for the development of COPD, the development of airflow obstruction in smokers is highly variable. Severe α_1 antitrypsin (α_1AT) deficiency is a proven genetic risk factor for COPD; there is increasing evidence that other genetic determinants also exist.

α_1 Antitrypsin deficiency

Many variants of the protease inhibitor (PI or SER-PINA1) locus that encodes α_1AT have been described. The common M allele is associated with normal α_1AT levels. The S allele, associated with slightly reduced α_1AT levels, and the Z allele, associated with markedly reduced α_1AT levels, also occur with frequencies >1% in most white populations. Rare individuals inherit null alleles, which lead to the absence of any α_1AT production through a heterogeneous collection of mutations. Individuals with two Z alleles or one Z and one null allele are referred to as Pi^Z, which is the most common form of severe α_1AT deficiency.

Although only 1–2% of COPD patients are found to have severe α_1AT deficiency as a contributing cause of COPD, these patients demonstrate that genetic factors can have a profound influence on the susceptibility for developing COPD. Pi^Z individuals often develop early-onset COPD, but the ascertainment bias in the published series of Pi^Z individuals—which have usually included many Pi^Z subjects who were tested for α_1AT deficiency because they had COPD—means that the fraction of Pi^Z individuals who will develop COPD and the age-of-onset distribution for the development of COPD in Pi^Z subjects remain unknown. Approximately 1 in 3000 individuals in the United States inherits severe α_1AT deficiency, but only a small minority of these individuals has been recognized. The clinical laboratory test used most frequently to screen for α_1AT deficiency is measurement of the immunologic level of α_1AT in serum (see "Laboratory Findings").

A significant percentage of the variability in pulmonary function among Pi^Z individuals is explained by cigarette smoking; cigarette smokers with severe α_1AT deficiency are more likely to develop COPD at early ages. However, the development of COPD in Pi^Z subjects, even among current or ex-smokers, is not absolute. Among Pi^Z nonsmokers, impressive variability has been noted in the development of airflow obstruction. Asthma and male gender also appear to increase the risk of COPD in Pi^Z subjects. Other genetic and/or environmental factors likely contribute to this variability.

Specific treatment in the form of α_1AT augmentation therapy is available for severe α_1AT deficiency as a weekly IV infusion (see "Treatment," later).

The risk of lung disease in heterozygous Pi^{MZ} individuals, who have intermediate serum levels of α_1AT (~60% of Pi^{MM} levels), is controversial. Although previous general population surveys have not typically shown increased rates of airflow obstruction in Pi^{MZ} compared to Pi^{MM} individuals, case-control studies that compared COPD patients to control subjects have usually found an excess of Pi^{MZ} genotypes in the COPD patient group. Several recent large population studies have suggested that Pi^{MZ} subjects are at slightly increased risk for the development of airflow obstruction, but it remains unclear if all Pi^{MZ} subjects are at slightly increased risk for COPD or if a subset of Pi^{MZ} subjects are at substantially increased risk for COPD due to other genetic or environmental factors.

Other genetic risk factors

Studies of pulmonary function measurements performed in general population samples have suggested that genetic factors other than PI type influence variation in pulmonary function. Familial aggregation of airflow obstruction within families of COPD patients has also been demonstrated.

Association studies have compared the distribution of variants in candidate genes hypothesized to be involved in the development of COPD in COPD patients and control subjects. However, the results have been quite inconsistent, often due to underpowered studies. However, a recent association study comprising 8300 patients and 7 separate cohorts found that a minor allele SNP of *MMP12* (rs2276109) associated with decreased MMP-12 expression has a positive effect on lung function in children with asthma and in adult smokers. Recent genome-wide association studies have identified several COPD loci, including a region near the hedgehog interacting protein (*HHIP*) gene on chromosome 4 and a cluster of genes on chromosome 15 (including components of the nicotinic acetylcholine receptor) that likely contain COPD susceptibility determinants, but the specific genetic determinants in those regions have yet to be definitively identified.

NATURAL HISTORY

The effects of cigarette smoking on pulmonary function appear to depend on the intensity of smoking exposure, the timing of smoking exposure during growth, and the baseline lung function of the individual; other environmental factors may have similar effects. Most individuals follow a steady trajectory of increasing pulmonary function with growth during childhood and adolescence, followed by a gradual decline with aging. Individuals appear to track in their quartile of pulmonary function based upon environmental and genetic factors that put them

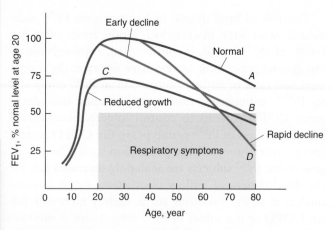

FIGURE 18-2

Hypothetical tracking curves of FEV₁ for individuals throughout their life spans. The normal pattern of growth and decline with age is shown by curve A. Significantly reduced FEV₁ (<65% of predicted value at age 20) can develop from a normal rate of decline after a reduced pulmonary function growth phase (curve C), early initiation of pulmonary function decline after normal growth (curve B), or accelerated decline after normal growth (curve D). (*From B Rijcken: Doctoral dissertation, p 133, University of Groningen, 1991; with permission.*)

on different tracks. The risk of eventual mortality from COPD is closely associated with reduced levels of FEV₁. A graphic depiction of the natural history of COPD is shown as a function of the influences on tracking curves of FEV₁ in **Fig. 18-2**. Death or disability from COPD can result from a normal rate of decline after a reduced growth phase (curve C), an early initiation of pulmonary function decline after normal growth (curve B), or an accelerated decline after normal growth (curve D). The rate of decline in pulmonary function can be modified by changing environmental exposures (i.e., quitting smoking), with smoking cessation at an earlier age providing a more beneficial effect than smoking cessation after marked reductions in pulmonary function have already developed. Genetic factors likely contribute to the level of pulmonary function achieved during growth and to the rate of decline in response to smoking and potentially to other environmental factors as well.

PATHOPHYSIOLOGY

Persistent reduction in forced expiratory flow rates is the most typical finding in COPD. Increases in the residual volume and the residual volume/total lung capacity ratio, nonuniform distribution of ventilation, and ventilation-perfusion mismatching also occur.

AIRFLOW OBSTRUCTION

Airflow limitation, also known as airflow obstruction, is typically determined by spirometry, which involves

forced expiratory maneuvers after the subject has inhaled to total lung capacity. Key parameters obtained from spirometry include FEV₁ and the total volume of air exhaled during the entire spirometric maneuver (forced vital capacity [FVC]). Patients with airflow obstruction related to COPD have a chronically reduced ratio of FEV₁/FVC. In contrast to asthma, the reduced FEV₁ in COPD seldom shows large responses to inhaled bronchodilators, although improvements up to 15% are common. Asthma patients can also develop chronic (not fully reversible) airflow obstruction.

Airflow during forced exhalation is the result of the balance between the elastic recoil of the lungs promoting flow and the resistance of the airways limiting flow. In normal lungs, as well as in lungs affected by COPD, maximal expiratory flow diminishes as the lungs empty because the lung parenchyma provides progressively less elastic recoil and because the cross-sectional area of the airways falls, raising the resistance to airflow. The decrease in flow coincident with decreased lung volume is readily apparent on the expiratory limb of a flow-volume curve. In the early stages of COPD, the abnormality in airflow is only evident at lung volumes at or below the functional residual capacity (closer to residual volume), appearing as a scooped-out lower part of the descending limb of the flow-volume curve. In more advanced disease the entire curve has decreased expiratory flow compared to normal.

HYPERINFLATION

Lung volumes are also routinely assessed in pulmonary function testing. In COPD there is often "air trapping" (increased residual volume and increased ratio of residual volume to total lung capacity) and progressive hyperinflation (increased total lung capacity) late in the disease. Hyperinflation of the thorax during tidal breathing preserves maximum expiratory airflow, because as lung volume increases, elastic recoil pressure increases, and airways enlarge so that airway resistance decreases.

Despite compensating for airway obstruction, hyperinflation can push the diaphragm into a flattened position with a number of adverse effects. First, by decreasing the zone of apposition between the diaphragm and the abdominal wall, positive abdominal pressure during inspiration is not applied as effectively to the chest wall, hindering rib cage movement and impairing inspiration. Second, because the muscle fibers of the flattened diaphragm are shorter than those of a more normally curved diaphragm, they are less capable of generating inspiratory pressures than normal. Third, the flattened diaphragm (with increased radius of curvature, r) must generate greater tension (t) to develop the transpulmonary pressure (p) required to produce tidal breathing. This follows from Laplace's law, $p = 2t/r$. Also, because the thoracic cage is distended beyond its normal resting volume, during tidal breathing the inspiratory muscles must do work to overcome the resistance of the thoracic cage to further inflation instead of gaining the normal assistance from the chest wall recoiling outward toward its resting volume.

GAS EXCHANGE

Although there is considerable variability in the relationships between the FEV_1 and other physiologic abnormalities in COPD, certain generalizations may be made. The Pa_{O_2} usually remains near normal until the FEV_1 is decreased to ~50% of predicted, and even much lower FEV_1 values can be associated with a normal Pa_{O_2}, at least at rest. An elevation of arterial level of carbon dioxide (Pa_{CO_2}) is not expected until the FEV_1 is <25% of predicted and even then may not occur. Pulmonary hypertension severe enough to cause cor pulmonale and right ventricular failure due to COPD typically occurs in individuals who have marked decreases in FEV_1 (<25% of predicted) and chronic hypoxemia (Pa_{O_2} <55 mmHg); however, recent evidence suggests that some patients will develop significant pulmonary hypertension independent of COPD severity.

Nonuniform ventilation and ventilation-perfusion mismatching are characteristic of COPD, reflecting the heterogeneous nature of the disease process within the airways and lung parenchyma. Physiologic studies are consistent with multiple parenchymal compartments having different rates of ventilation due to regional differences in compliance and airway resistance. Ventilation-perfusion mismatching accounts for essentially all of the reduction in Pa_{O_2} that occurs in COPD; shunting is minimal. This finding explains the effectiveness of modest elevations of inspired oxygen in treating hypoxemia due to COPD and therefore the need to consider problems other than COPD when hypoxemia is difficult to correct with modest levels of supplemental oxygen in the patient with COPD.

PATHOLOGY

Cigarette smoke exposure may affect the large airways, small airways (≤2 mm diameter), and alveoli. Changes in large airways cause cough and sputum, while changes in small airways and alveoli are responsible for physiologic alterations. Emphysema and small airway pathology are both present in most persons with COPD; however, they do not appear to be mechanistically related to each other, and their relative contributions to obstruction vary from one person to another.

LARGE AIRWAY

Cigarette smoking often results in mucous gland enlargement and goblet cell hyperplasia leading to

cough and mucus production that define chronic bronchitis, but these abnormalities are not related to airflow limitation. Goblet cells not only increase in number but in extent through the bronchial tree. Bronchi also undergo squamous metaplasia, predisposing to carcinogenesis and disrupting mucociliary clearance. Although not as prominent as in asthma, patients may have smooth-muscle hypertrophy and bronchial hyperreactivity leading to airflow limitation. Neutrophil influx has been associated with purulent sputum of upper respiratory tract infections. Independent of its proteolytic activity, neutrophil elastase is among the most potent secretagogues identified.

SMALL AIRWAYS

The major site of increased resistance in most individuals with COPD is in airways ≤2 mm diameter. Characteristic cellular changes include goblet cell metaplasia, with these mucus-secreting cells replacing surfactant-secreting Clara cells. Infiltration of mononuclear phagocytes is also prominent. Smooth-muscle hypertrophy may also be present. These abnormalities may cause luminal narrowing by fibrosis, excess mucus, edema, and cellular infiltration. Reduced surfactant may increase surface tension at the air-tissue interface, predisposing to airway narrowing or collapse. Respiratory bronchiolitis with mononuclear inflammatory cells collecting in distal airway tissues may cause proteolytic destruction of elastic fibers in the respiratory bronchioles and alveolar ducts where the fibers are concentrated as rings around alveolar entrances.

Because small airway patency is maintained by the surrounding lung parenchyma that provides radial traction on bronchioles at points of attachment to alveolar septa, loss of bronchiolar attachments as a result of extracellular matrix destruction may cause airway distortion and narrowing in COPD.

LUNG PARENCHYMA

Emphysema is characterized by destruction of gas-exchanging air spaces, i.e., the respiratory bronchioles, alveolar ducts, and alveoli. Their walls become perforated and later obliterated with coalescence of small distinct air spaces into abnormal and much larger air spaces. Macrophages accumulate in respiratory bronchioles of essentially all young smokers. Bronchoalveolar lavage fluid from such individuals contains roughly five times as many macrophages as lavage from nonsmokers. In smokers' lavage fluid, macrophages comprise >95% of the total cell count, and neutrophils, nearly absent in nonsmokers' lavage, account for 1–2% of the cells. T lymphocytes, particularly CD8+ cells, are also increased in the alveolar space of smokers.

Emphysema is classified into distinct pathologic types, the most important being centriacinar and panacinar. *Centriacinar emphysema*, the type most frequently associated with cigarette smoking, is characterized by enlarged air spaces found (initially) in association with respiratory bronchioles. Centriacinar emphysema is usually most prominent in the upper lobes and superior segments of lower lobes and is often quite focal. *Panacinar emphysema* refers to abnormally large air spaces evenly distributed within and across acinar units. Panacinar emphysema is usually observed in patients with $\alpha_1 AT$ deficiency, which has a predilection for the lower lobes. Distinctions between centriacinar and panacinar emphysema are interesting and may ultimately be shown to have different mechanisms of pathogenesis. However, garden-variety smoking-related emphysema is usually mixed, particularly in advanced cases, and these pathologic classifications are not helpful in the care of patients with COPD.

PATHOGENESIS

Airflow limitation, the major physiologic change in COPD, can result from both small airway obstruction and emphysema, as discussed earlier. Pathologic findings that can contribute to small airway obstruction are described earlier, but their relative importance is unknown. Fibrosis surrounding the small airways appears to be a significant contributor. Mechanisms leading to collagen accumulation around the airways in the face of increased collagenase activity remain an enigma. Although seemingly counterintuitive, there are several potential mechanisms whereby a proteinase can predispose to fibrosis, including proteolytic activation of transforming growth factor β (TGF-β). Largely due to greater similarity of animal air spaces than airways to humans, we know much more about mechanisms involved in emphysema than small airway obstruction.

The dominant paradigm of the pathogenesis of emphysema comprises four interrelated events **(Fig. 18–3)**: (1) Chronic exposure to cigarette smoke may lead to inflammatory cell recruitment within the terminal air spaces of the lung. (2) These inflammatory cells release elastolytic proteinases that damage the extracellular matrix of the lung. (3) Structural cell death results from oxidant stress and loss of matrix-cell attachment. (4) Ineffective repair of elastin and other extracellular matrix components result in air space enlargement that defines pulmonary emphysema.

THE ELASTASE: ANTIELASTASE HYPOTHESIS

Elastin, the principal component of elastic fibers, is a highly stable component of the extracellular matrix that is

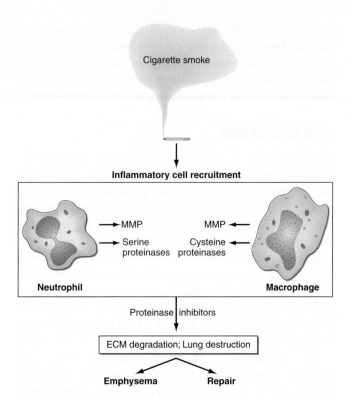

FIGURE 18-3
Pathogenesis of emphysema. Upon long-term exposure to cigarette smoke, inflammatory cells are recruited to the lung; they release proteinases in excess of inhibitors, and if repair is abnormal, this leads to air space destruction and enlargement or emphysema. ECM, extracellular matrix; MMP, matrix metalloproteinase.

critical to the integrity of the lung. The elastase:antielastase hypothesis proposed in the mid-1960s states that the balance of elastin-degrading enzymes and their inhibitors determines the susceptibility of the lung to destruction resulting in air space enlargement. This hypothesis was based on the clinical observation that patients with genetic deficiency in $\alpha_1 AT$, the inhibitor of the serine proteinase neutrophil elastase, were at increased risk of emphysema, and that instillation of elastases, including neutrophil elastase, to experimental animals results in emphysema. The elastase:antielastase hypothesis remains a prevailing mechanism for the development of emphysema. However, a complex network of immune and inflammatory cells and additional proteinases that contribute to emphysema have subsequently been identified.

INFLAMMATION AND EXTRACELLULAR MATRIX PROTEOLYSIS

Macrophages patrol the lower air space under normal conditions. Upon exposure to oxidants from cigarette smoke, macrophages become activated, producing proteinases and chemokines that attract other inflammatory cells. One mechanism of macrophage activation occurs via oxidant-induced inactivation of histone deacetylase-2, shifting the balance toward acetylated or loose chromatin, exposing nuclear factor κB sites and resulting in transcription of matrix metalloproteinases, proinflammatory cytokines such as interleukin 8 (IL-8), and tumor necrosis factor α (TNF-α); this leads to neutrophil recruitment. CD8+ T cells are also recruited in response to cigarette smoke and release interferon inducible protein-10 (IP-10, CXCL-7) that in turn leads to macrophage production of macrophage elastase (matrix metalloproteinase-12 [MMP-12]). Matrix metalloproteinases and serine proteinases, most notably neutrophil elastase, work together by degrading the inhibitor of the other, leading to lung destruction. Proteolytic cleavage products of elastin also serve as a macrophage chemokine, fueling this destructive positive feedback loop.

Autoimmune mechanisms have recently been identified in COPD and may promote the progression of disease. Increased B cells and lymphoid follicles are present in patients, particularly those with advanced disease. Antibodies have been found against elastin fragments, as well; IgG autoantibodies with avidity for pulmonary epithelium and the potential to mediate cytotoxicity have been detected.

Concomitant cigarette smoke–induced loss of cilia in the airway epithelium and impaired macrophage phagocytosis predispose to bacterial infection with neutrophilia. In end-stage lung disease, long after smoking cessation there remains an exuberant inflammatory response, suggesting that mechanisms of cigarette smoke–induced inflammation that initiate the disease differ from mechanisms that sustain inflammation after smoking cessation.

Cell death

Air space enlargement with loss of alveolar units obviously requires disappearance of both extracellular matrix and cells. Cell death can occur from increased oxidant stress both directly from cigarette smoke and from inflammation. Animal models have used endothelial and epithelial cell death as a means to generate transient air space enlargement. Uptake of apoptotic cells by macrophages results in production of growth factors and dampens inflammation, promoting lung repair. Cigarette smoke impairs macrophage uptake of apoptotic cells, limiting repair.

Ineffective repair

The ability of the adult lung to repair damaged alveoli appears limited. It is unlikely that the process of septation that is responsible for alveologenesis during lung development can be reinitiated. The capacity of stem cells to repopulate the lung is under active investigation. It appears difficult for an adult human to completely restore an appropriate extracellular matrix, particularly functional elastic fibers.

CLINICAL PRESENTATION

HISTORY

The three most common symptoms in COPD are cough, sputum production, and exertional dyspnea. Many patients have such symptoms for months or years before seeking medical attention. Although the development of airflow obstruction is a gradual process, many patients date the onset of their disease to an acute illness or exacerbation. A careful history, however, usually reveals the presence of symptoms prior to the acute exacerbation. The development of exertional dyspnea, often described as increased effort to breathe, heaviness, air hunger, or gasping, can be insidious. It is best elicited by a careful history focused on typical physical activities and how the patient's ability to perform them has changed. Activities involving significant arm work, particularly at or above shoulder level, are particularly difficult for patients with COPD. Conversely, activities that allow the patient to brace the arms and use accessory muscles of respiration are better tolerated. Examples of such activities include pushing a shopping cart, walking on a treadmill, or pushing a wheelchair. As COPD advances, the principal feature is worsening dyspnea on exertion with increasing intrusion on the ability to perform vocational or avocational activities. In the most advanced stages, patients are breathless doing simple activities of daily living.

Accompanying worsening airflow obstruction is an increased frequency of exacerbations (described later). Patients may also develop resting hypoxemia and require institution of supplemental oxygen.

PHYSICAL FINDINGS

In the early stages of COPD, patients usually have an entirely normal physical examination. Current smokers may have signs of active smoking, including an odor of smoke or nicotine staining of fingernails. In patients with more severe disease, the physical examination is notable for a prolonged expiratory phase and may include expiratory wheezing. In addition, signs of hyperinflation include a barrel chest and enlarged lung volumes with poor diaphragmatic excursion as assessed by percussion. Patients with severe airflow obstruction may also exhibit use of accessory muscles of respiration, sitting in the characteristic "tripod" position to facilitate the actions of the sternocleidomastoid, scalene, and intercostal muscles. Patients may develop cyanosis, visible in the lips and nail beds.

Although traditional teaching is that patients with predominant emphysema, termed "pink puffers," are thin and noncyanotic at rest and have prominent use of accessory muscles, and patients with chronic bronchitis are more likely to be heavy and cyanotic ("blue bloaters"), current evidence demonstrates that most patients have elements of both bronchitis and emphysema and that the physical examination does not reliably differentiate the two entities.

Advanced disease may be accompanied by systemic wasting, with significant weight loss, bitemporal wasting, and diffuse loss of subcutaneous adipose tissue. This syndrome has been associated with both inadequate oral intake and elevated levels of inflammatory cytokines (TNF-α). Such wasting is an independent poor prognostic factor in COPD. Some patients with advanced disease have paradoxical inward movement of the rib cage with inspiration (Hoover's sign), the result of alteration of the vector of diaphragmatic contraction on the rib cage as a result of chronic hyperinflation.

Signs of overt right heart failure, termed *cor pulmonale*, are relatively infrequent since the advent of supplemental oxygen therapy.

Clubbing of the digits is not a sign of COPD, and its presence should alert the clinician to initiate an investigation for causes of clubbing. In this population, the development of lung cancer is the most likely explanation for newly developed clubbing.

LABORATORY FINDINGS

The hallmark of COPD is airflow obstruction (discussed earlier). Pulmonary function testing shows airflow obstruction with a reduction in FEV_1 and FEV_1/FVC (Chap. 5). With worsening disease severity, lung volumes may increase, resulting in an increase in total lung capacity, functional residual capacity, and residual volume. In patients with emphysema, the diffusing capacity may be reduced, reflecting the lung parenchymal destruction characteristic of the disease. The degree of airflow

obstruction is an important prognostic factor in COPD and is the basis for the Global Initiative for Lung Disease (GOLD) redundant classification (Table 18-1). More recently it has been shown that a multifactorial index incorporating airflow obstruction, exercise performance, dyspnea, and body mass index is a better predictor of mortality rate than pulmonary function alone.

Arterial blood gases and oximetry may demonstrate resting or exertional hypoxemia. Arterial blood gases provide additional information about alveolar ventilation and acid-base status by measuring arterial P_{CO_2} and pH. The change in pH with P_{CO_2} is 0.08 units/10 mmHg acutely and 0.03 units/10 mmHg in the chronic state. Knowledge of the arterial pH therefore allows the classification of ventilatory failure, defined as P_{CO_2} >45 mmHg, into acute or chronic conditions. The arterial blood gas is an important component of the evaluation of patients presenting with symptoms of an exacerbation. An elevated hematocrit suggests the presence of chronic hypoxemia, as does the presence of signs of right ventricular hypertrophy.

Radiographic studies may assist in the classification of the type of COPD. Obvious bullae, paucity of parenchymal markings, or hyperlucency suggests the presence of emphysema. Increased lung volumes and flattening of the diaphragm suggest hyperinflation but do not provide information about chronicity of the changes. Computed tomography (CT) scan is the current definitive test for establishing the presence or absence of emphysema in living subjects (Fig. 18-4). From a practical perspective, the CT scan does little to influence therapy of COPD except in those individuals considering surgical therapy for their disease (described later).

Recent guidelines have suggested testing for α_1AT deficiency in all subjects with COPD or asthma with chronic airflow obstruction. Measurement of the serum α_1AT level is a reasonable initial test. For subjects with

TABLE 18-1

GOLD CRITERIA FOR COPD SEVERITY	
GOLD STAGE	**CHARACTERISTICS**
0: At Risk	Normal spirometry Chronic symptoms (cough, sputum production)
I: Mild COPD	FEV_1/FVC < 70% $FEV_1 \geq$ 80% predicted With or without chronic symptoms (cough, sputum production)
II: Moderate COPD	FEV_1/FVC < 70% 30% $\leq FEV_1$ < 80% predicted (IIA: 50% $\leq FEV_1$ < 80% predicted) (IIB: 30% $\leq FEV_1$ < 50% predicted) With or without chronic symptoms (cough, sputum production, dyspnea)
III: Severe COPD	FEV_1/FVC < 70% FEV_1 < 30% predicted, or the presence of respiratory failure,[a] or clinical signs of right heart failure

[a]Respiratory failure: Pao_2 < 8.0 kPa (60 mmHg) with or without $Paco_2$ > 6.7 kPa (50 mmHg) while breathing air at sea level.
Abbreviation: GOLD, Global Initiative for Lung Disease.
Source: From RA Pauwels et al: Am J Respir Crit Care Med 163:1256, 2001.

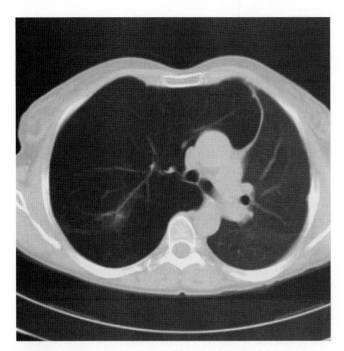

FIGURE 18-4
Chest CT scan of a patient with COPD who underwent a left single-lung transplant. Note the reduced parenchymal markings in the right lung (*left side of figure*) as compared to the left lung, representing emphysematous destruction of the lung, and mediastinal shift to the left, indicative of hyperinflation.

low α_1AT levels, the definitive diagnosis of α_1AT deficiency requires protease inhibitor (PI) type determination. This is typically performed by isoelectric focusing of serum, which reflects the genotype at the PI locus for the common alleles and many of the rare PI alleles as well. Molecular genotyping of DNA can be performed for the common PI alleles (M, S, and Z).

TREATMENT | Chronic Obstructive Pulmonary Disease

STABLE PHASE COPD Only three interventions—smoking cessation, oxygen therapy in chronically hypoxemic patients, and lung volume reduction surgery in selected patients with emphysema—have been demonstrated to influence the natural history of patients with COPD. There is currently suggestive, but not definitive, evidence that the use of inhaled glucocorticoids may alter mortality rate (but not lung function). All other current therapies are directed at improving symptoms and decreasing the frequency and severity of exacerbations. The institution of these therapies should involve an assessment of symptoms, potential risks, costs, and benefits of therapy. This should be followed by an assessment of response to therapy, and a decision should be made whether or not to continue treatment.

PHARMACOTHERAPY

Smoking Cessation It has been shown that middle-aged smokers who were able to successfully stop smoking experienced a significant improvement in the rate of decline in pulmonary function, returning to annual changes similar to that of nonsmoking patients. Thus, all patients with COPD should be strongly urged to quit and educated about the benefits of quitting. An emerging body of evidence demonstrates that combining pharmacotherapy with traditional supportive approaches considerably enhances the chances of successful smoking cessation. There are three principal pharmacologic approaches to the problem: bupropion, originally developed as an antidepressant medication; nicotine replacement therapy available as gum, transdermal patch, inhaler, and nasal spray; and varenicline, a nicotinic acid receptor agonist/antagonist. Current recommendations from the U.S. Surgeon General are that all adult, nonpregnant smokers considering quitting be offered pharmacotherapy, in the absence of any contraindication to treatment.

Bronchodilators In general, bronchodilators are used for symptomatic benefit in patients with COPD. The inhaled route is preferred for medication delivery as the incidence of side effects is lower than that seen with the use of parenteral medication delivery.

Anticholinergic Agents Ipratropium bromide improves symptoms and produces acute improvement in FEV_1. Tiotropium, a long-acting anticholinergic, has been shown to improve symptoms and reduce exacerbations. Studies of both ipratropium and tiotropium have failed to demonstrate that either influences the rate of decline in FEV_1. In a large randomized clinical trial, there was a trend toward reduced mortality rate in the tiotropium-treated patients that approached, but did not reach, statistical significance. Side effects are minor, and a trial of inhaled anticholinergics is recommended in symptomatic patients with COPD.

Beta Agonists These provide symptomatic benefit. The main side effects are tremor and tachycardia. Long-acting inhaled β agonists, such as salmeterol, have benefits comparable to ipratropium bromide. Their use is more convenient than short-acting agents. The addition of a β agonist to inhaled anticholinergic therapy has been demonstrated to provide incremental benefit. A recent report in asthma suggests that those patients, particularly African Americans, using a long-acting β agonist without concomitant inhaled corticosteroids have an increased risk of deaths from respiratory causes. The applicability of these data to patients with COPD is unclear.

Inhaled Glucocorticoids Although a recent trial demonstrated an apparent benefit from the regular use of inhaled glucocorticoids on the rate of decline of lung function, a number of other well-designed randomized trials have not. Patients studied included those with mild to severe airflow obstruction and current and ex-smokers. Patients with significant acute response to inhaled β agonists were excluded from many of these trials, which may impact the generalizability of the findings. Their use has been associated with increased rates of oropharyngeal candidiasis and an increased rate of loss of bone density. Available data suggest that inhaled glucocorticoids reduce exacerbation frequency by ~25%. The impact of inhaled corticosteroids on mortality rates in COPD is controversial. A meta-analysis and several retrospective studies suggest a mortality benefit, but in a recently published randomized trial, differences in mortality rate approached, but did not reach, conventional criteria for statistical significance. A trial of inhaled glucocorticoids should be considered in patients with frequent exacerbations, defined as two or more per year, and in patients who demonstrate a significant amount of acute reversibility in response to inhaled bronchodilators.

Oral Glucocorticoids The chronic use of oral glucocorticoids for treatment of COPD is not recommended because of an unfavorable benefit/risk ratio. The chronic use of oral glucocorticoids is associated with significant side effects, including osteoporosis, weight gain, cataracts, glucose intolerance, and increased risk of infection. A recent study demonstrated that patients tapered off chronic low-dose prednisone (~10 mg/d) did not experience any adverse effect on the frequency of exacerbations, health-related quality of life, or lung function. On average, patients lost ~4.5 kg (~10 lb) when steroids were withdrawn.

Theophylline Theophylline produces modest improvements in expiratory flow rates and vital capacity and a slight improvement in arterial oxygen and carbon dioxide levels in patients with moderate to severe COPD. Nausea is a common side effect; tachycardia and tremor have also been reported. Monitoring of blood theophylline levels is typically required to minimize toxicity.

Oxygen Supplemental O_2 is the only pharmacologic therapy demonstrated to unequivocally decrease mortality rates in patients with COPD. For patients with resting hypoxemia (resting O_2 saturation ≤88% or <90% with signs of pulmonary hypertension or right heart failure), the use of O_2 has been demonstrated to have a significant impact on mortality rate. Patients meeting these criteria should be on continual oxygen supplementation, as the mortality benefit is proportional to the number of hours/day oxygen is used. Various delivery

systems are available, including portable systems that patients may carry to allow mobility outside the home.

Supplemental O_2 is commonly prescribed for patients with exertional hypoxemia or nocturnal hypoxemia. Although the rationale for supplemental O_2 in these settings is physiologically sound, the benefits of such therapy are not well substantiated.

Other Agents N-acetyl cysteine has been used in patients with COPD for both its mucolytic and antioxidant properties. A prospective trial failed to find any benefit with respect to decline in lung function or prevention of exacerbations. Specific treatment in the form of IV $α_1$AT augmentation therapy is available for individuals with severe $α_1$AT deficiency. Despite sterilization procedures for these blood-derived products and the absence of reported cases of viral infection from therapy, some physicians recommend hepatitis B vaccination prior to starting augmentation therapy. Although biochemical efficacy of $α_1$AT augmentation therapy has been shown, a randomized controlled trial of $α_1$AT augmentation therapy has not definitively established the efficacy of augmentation therapy in reducing decline of pulmonary function. Eligibility for $α_1$AT augmentation therapy requires a serum $α_1$AT level <11 $μM$ (approximately 50 mg/dL). Typically, Pi^Z individuals will qualify, although other rare types associated with severe deficiency (e.g., null-null) are also eligible. Since only a fraction of individuals with severe $α_1$AT deficiency will develop COPD, $α_1$AT augmentation therapy is not recommended for severely $α_1$AT-deficient persons with normal pulmonary function and a normal chest CT scan.

NONPHARMACOLOGIC THERAPIES
General Medical Care Patients with COPD should receive the influenza vaccine annually. Polyvalent pneumococcal vaccine is also recommended, although proof of efficacy in this patient population is not definitive.

Pulmonary Rehabilitation This refers to a treatment program that incorporates education and cardiovascular conditioning. In COPD, pulmonary rehabilitation has been demonstrated to improve health-related quality of life, dyspnea, and exercise capacity. It has also been shown to reduce rates of hospitalization over a 6- to 12-month period.

Lung Volume Reduction Surgery (LVRS) Surgery to reduce the volume of lung in patients with emphysema was first introduced with minimal success in the 1950s and was reintroduced in the 1990s. Patients are excluded if they have significant pleural disease, a pulmonary artery systolic pressure >45 mmHg, extreme deconditioning, congestive heart failure, or other severe comorbid conditions. Patients with an FEV_1 <20% of predicted and either diffusely distributed emphysema on

CT scan or diffusing capacity of lung for carbon monoxide (DL_{CO}) <20% of predicted have an increased mortality rate after the procedure and thus are not candidates for LVRS.

The National Emphysema Treatment trial demonstrated that LVRS offers both a mortality benefit and a symptomatic benefit in certain patients with emphysema. The anatomic distribution of emphysema and postrehabilitation exercise capacity are important prognostic characteristics. Patients with upper lobe–predominant emphysema and a low postrehabilitation exercise capacity are most likely to benefit from LVRS.

Lung Transplantation (See also Chap. 24)

COPD is currently the second leading indication for lung transplantation (Fig. 18-4). Current recommendations are that candidates for lung transplantation should be <65 years; have severe disability despite maximal medical therapy; and be free of comorbid conditions such as liver, renal, or cardiac disease. In contrast to LVRS, the anatomic distribution of emphysema and the presence of pulmonary hypertension are not contraindications to lung transplantation. Unresolved issues concerning lung transplantation and COPD include whether single- or double-lung transplant is the preferred procedure.

EXACERBATIONS OF COPD Exacerbations are a prominent feature of the natural history of COPD. Exacerbations are episodes of increased dyspnea and cough and change in the amount and character of sputum. They may or may not be accompanied by other signs of illness, including fever, myalgias, and sore throat. Self-reported health-related quality of life correlates with frequency of exacerbations more closely than it does with the degree of airflow obstruction. Economic analyses have shown that >70% of COPD-related health care expenditures go to emergency department visits and hospital care; this translates to >$10 billion annually in the United States. The frequency of exacerbations increases as airflow obstruction increases; patients with moderate to severe airflow obstruction (GOLD stages III, IV [Table 18-1]) on average have one to three episodes per year. However, some individuals with very severe airflow obstruction do not have frequent exacerbations; the history of prior exacerbations is a strong predictor of future exacerbations.

The approach to the patient experiencing an exacerbation includes an assessment of the severity of the patient's illness, both acute and chronic components; an attempt to identify the precipitant of the exacerbation; and the institution of therapy.

Precipitating Causes and Strategies to Reduce Frequency of Exacerbations

A variety of stimuli may result in the final common pathway of airway inflammation and increased symptoms that are characteristic of COPD exacerbations.

Bacterial infections play a role in many, but by no means all, episodes. Viral respiratory infections are present in approximately one-third of COPD exacerbations. In a significant minority of instances (20–35%), no specific precipitant can be identified.

Despite the frequent implication of bacterial infection, chronic suppressive or "rotating" antibiotics are not beneficial in patients with COPD. This is in contrast to their efficacy in patients with bronchiectasis due to cystic fibrosis, in whom suppressive antibiotics have been shown to reduce frequency of hospital admissions.

The role of pharmacotherapy in reducing exacerbation frequency is less well studied. Chronic oral glucocorticoids are not recommended for this purpose. Inhaled glucocorticoids reduce the frequency of exacerbations by 25–30% in most analyses. The use of inhaled glucocorticoids should be considered in patients with frequent exacerbations or those who have an asthmatic component, i.e., significant reversibility on pulmonary function testing or marked symptomatic improvement after inhaled bronchodilators. Similar magnitudes of reduction have been reported for anticholinergic and long-acting beta-agonist therapy. The influenza vaccine has been shown to reduce exacerbation rates in patients with COPD.

Patient Assessment An attempt should be made to establish the severity of the exacerbation as well as the severity of preexisting COPD. The more severe either of these two components, the more likely that the patient will require hospital admission. The history should include quantification of the degree of dyspnea by asking about breathlessness during activities of daily living and typical activities for the patient. The patient should be asked about fever; change in character of sputum; any ill contacts; and associated symptoms such as nausea, vomiting, diarrhea, myalgias, and chills. Inquiring about the frequency and severity of prior exacerbations can provide important information.

The physical examination should incorporate an assessment of the degree of distress of the patient. Specific attention should be focused on tachycardia, tachypnea, use of accessory muscles, signs of perioral or peripheral cyanosis, the ability to speak in complete sentences, and the patient's mental status. The chest examination should establish the presence or absence of focal findings, degree of air movement, presence or absence of wheezing, asymmetry in the chest examination (suggesting large airway obstruction or pneumothorax mimicking an exacerbation), and the presence or absence of paradoxical motion of the abdominal wall.

Patients with severe underlying COPD, who are in moderate or severe distress or those with focal findings should have a chest x-ray. Approximately 25% of x-rays in this clinical situation will be abnormal, with the most frequent findings being pneumonia and congestive heart failure. Patients with advanced COPD, those with a history of hypercarbia, those with mental status changes (confusion, sleepiness), or those in significant distress should have an arterial blood-gas measurement. The presence of hypercarbia, defined as a P_{CO_2} >45 mmHg, has important implications for treatment (discussed later). In contrast to its utility in the management of exacerbations of asthma, measurement of pulmonary function has not been demonstrated to be helpful in the diagnosis or management of exacerbations of COPD.

There are no definitive guidelines concerning the need for inpatient treatment of exacerbations. Patients with respiratory acidosis and hypercarbia, significant hypoxemia, or severe underlying disease or those whose living situation is not conducive to careful observation and the delivery of prescribed treatment should be admitted to the hospital.

ACUTE EXACERBATIONS

Bronchodilators Typically, patients are treated with an inhaled β agonist, often with the addition of an anticholinergic agent. These may be administered separately or together, and the frequency of administration depends on the severity of the exacerbation. Patients are often treated initially with nebulized therapy, as such treatment is often easier to administer in older patients or to those in respiratory distress. It has been shown, however, that conversion to metered-dose inhalers is effective when accompanied by education and training of patients and staff. This approach has significant economic benefits and also allows an easier transition to outpatient care. The addition of methylxanthines (such as theophylline) to this regimen can be considered, although convincing proof of its efficacy is lacking. If added, serum levels should be monitored in an attempt to minimize toxicity.

Antibiotics Patients with COPD are frequently colonized with potential respiratory pathogens, and it is often difficult to identify conclusively a specific species of bacteria responsible for a particular clinical event. Bacteria frequently implicated in COPD exacerbations include *Streptococcus pneumoniae*, *Haemophilus influenzae*, and *Moraxella catarrhalis*. In addition, *Mycoplasma pneumoniae* or *Chlamydia pneumoniae* are found in 5–10% of exacerbations. The choice of antibiotic should be based on local patterns of antibiotic susceptibility of the above pathogens as well as the patient's clinical condition. Most practitioners treat patients with moderate or severe exacerbations with antibiotics, even in the absence of data implicating a specific pathogen.

Glucocorticoids Among patients admitted to the hospital, the use of glucocorticoids has been demonstrated

to reduce the length of stay, hasten recovery, and reduce the chance of subsequent exacerbation or relapse for a period of up to 6 months. One study demonstrated that 2 weeks of glucocorticoid therapy produced benefit indistinguishable from 8 weeks of therapy. The GOLD guidelines recommend 30–40 mg of oral prednisolone or its equivalent for a period of 10–14 days. Hyperglycemia, particularly in patients with preexisting diagnosis of diabetes, is the most frequently reported acute complication of glucocorticoid treatment.

Oxygen Supplemental O_2 should be supplied to keep arterial saturations ≥90%. Hypoxemic respiratory drive plays a small role in patients with COPD. Studies have demonstrated that in patients with both acute and chronic hypercarbia, the administration of supplemental O_2 does not reduce minute ventilation. It does, in some patients, result in modest increases in arterial P_{CO_2}, chiefly by altering ventilation-perfusion relationships within the lung. This should not deter practitioners from providing the oxygen needed to correct hypoxemia.

Mechanical Ventilatory Support The initiation of noninvasive positive-pressure ventilation (NIPPV) in patients with respiratory failure, defined as Pa_{CO_2} >45 mmHg, results in a significant reduction in mortality rate, need for intubation, complications of therapy, and hospital length of stay. Contraindications to NIPPV include cardiovascular instability, impaired mental status or inability to cooperate, copious secretions or the inability to clear secretions, craniofacial abnormalities or trauma precluding effective fitting of mask, extreme obesity, or significant burns.

Invasive (conventional) mechanical ventilation via an endotracheal tube is indicated for patients with severe respiratory distress despite initial therapy, life-threatening hypoxemia, severe hypercarbia and/or acidosis, markedly impaired mental status, respiratory arrest, hemodynamic instability, or other complications. The goal of mechanical ventilation is to correct the aforementioned conditions. Factors to consider during mechanical ventilatory support include the need to provide sufficient expiratory time in patients with severe airflow obstruction and the presence of auto-PEEP (positive end-expiratory pressure), which can result in patients having to generate significant respiratory effort to trigger a breath during a demand mode of ventilation. The mortality rate of patients requiring mechanical ventilatory support is 17–30% for that particular hospitalization. For patients age >65 admitted to the intensive care unit for treatment, the mortality rate doubles over the next year to 60%, regardless of whether mechanical ventilation was required.

CHAPTER 19
INTERSTITIAL LUNG DISEASES

Talmadge E. King, Jr.

Patients with interstitial lung diseases (ILDs) come to medical attention mainly because of the onset of progressive exertional dyspnea or a persistent nonproductive cough. Hemoptysis, wheezing, and chest pain may be present. Often, the identification of interstitial opacities on chest x-ray focuses the diagnostic approach on one of the ILDs.

ILDs represent a large number of conditions that involve the parenchyma of the lung—the alveoli, the alveolar epithelium, the capillary endothelium, and the spaces between those structures—as well as the perivascular and lymphatic tissues. The disorders in this heterogeneous group are classified together because of similar clinical, roentgenographic, physiologic, or pathologic manifestations. These disorders often are associated with considerable rates of morbidity and mortality, and there is little consensus regarding the best management of most of them.

ILDs have been difficult to classify because >200 known individual diseases are characterized by diffuse parenchymal lung involvement, either as the primary condition or as a significant part of a multiorgan process, as may occur in the connective tissue diseases (CTDs). One useful approach to classification is to separate the ILDs into two groups based on the major underlying histopathology: (1) those associated with predominant inflammation and fibrosis and (2) those with a predominantly granulomatous reaction in interstitial or vascular areas **(Table 19-1)**. Each of these groups can be subdivided further according to whether the cause is known or unknown. For each ILD there may be an acute phase, and there is usually a chronic one as well. Rarely, some are recurrent, with intervals of subclinical disease.

Sarcoidosis, idiopathic pulmonary fibrosis (IPF), and pulmonary fibrosis associated with CTDs are the most common ILDs of unknown etiology. Among the ILDs of known cause, the largest group includes occupational and environmental exposures, especially the inhalation of inorganic dusts, organic dusts, and various fumes or gases (Chaps. 9 and 10) **(Table 19-2)**. A clinical diagnosis is possible for many forms of ILD, especially if an occupational and environmental history is pursued aggressively. High-resolution computed tomography (HRCT) scanning improves the diagnostic accuracy and may eliminate the need for tissue examination in many cases, especially in IPF. For other forms, tissue examination, usually obtained by thoracoscopic lung biopsy, is critical to confirmation of the diagnosis.

PATHOGENESIS

The ILDs are nonmalignant disorders and are not caused by identified infectious agents. The precise pathway(s) leading from injury to fibrosis is not known. Although there are multiple initiating agent(s) of injury, the immunopathogenic responses of lung tissue are limited, and the mechanisms of repair have common features **(Fig. 19-1)**.

As mentioned earlier, the two major histopathologic patterns are a granulomatous pattern and a pattern in which inflammation and fibrosis predominate.

Granulomatous lung disease

This process is characterized by an accumulation of T lymphocytes, macrophages, and epithelioid cells organized into discrete structures (granulomas) in the lung parenchyma. The granulomatous lesions can progress to fibrosis. Many patients with granulomatous lung disease remain free of severe impairment of lung function or, when symptomatic, improve after treatment. The main differential diagnosis is between sarcoidosis and hypersensitivity pneumonitis (Chap. 9).

Inflammation and fibrosis

The initial insult is an injury to the epithelial surface that causes inflammation in the air spaces and alveolar walls

197

TABLE 19-1

MAJOR CATEGORIES OF ALVEOLAR AND INTERSTITIAL INFLAMMATORY LUNG DISEASE

LUNG RESPONSE: ALVEOLITIS, INTERSTITIAL INFLAMMATION, AND FIBROSIS

Known Cause

Asbestos	Residual of acute respiratory distress syndrome
Fumes, gases	Smoking-related
Drugs (antibiotics, amiodarone, gold) and chemotherapy drugs	Desquamative interstitial pneumonia
	Respiratory bronchiolitis–associated interstitial lung disease
Radiation	Langerhans cell granulomatosis (eosinophilic granuloma of
Aspiration pneumonia	the lung)

Unknown Cause

Idiopathic interstitial pneumonias	Pulmonary alveolar proteinosis
Idiopathic pulmonary fibrosis (usual interstitial pneumonia)	Lymphocytic infiltrative disorders (lymphocytic interstitial
Acute interstitial pneumonia (diffuse alveolar damage)	pneumonitis associated with connective tissue disease)
Cryptogenic organizing pneumonia (bronchiolitis obliterans	Eosinophilic pneumonias
with organizing pneumonia)	Lymphangioleiomyomatosis
Nonspecific interstitial pneumonia	Amyloidosis
Connective tissue diseases	Inherited diseases
Systemic lupus erythematosus, rheumatoid arthritis,	Tuberous sclerosis, neurofibromatosis, Niemann-Pick
ankylosing spondylitis, systemic sclerosis, Sjögren's	disease, Gaucher's disease, Hermansky-Pudlak syndrome
syndrome, polymyositis-dermatomyositis	Gastrointestinal or liver diseases (Crohn's disease, primary
Pulmonary hemorrhage syndromes	biliary cirrhosis, chronic active hepatitis, ulcerative colitis)
Goodpasture's syndrome, idiopathic pulmonary	Graft-versus-host disease (bone marrow transplantation;
hemosiderosis, isolated pulmonary capillaritis	solid organ transplantation)

LUNG RESPONSE: GRANULOMATOUS

Known Cause

Hypersensitivity pneumonitis (organic dusts)	Inorganic dusts: beryllium, silica

Unknown Cause

Sarcoidosis	Bronchocentric granulomatosis
Granulomatous vasculitides	Lymphomatoid granulomatosis
Granulomatosis with polyangiitis (Wegener's), allergic granu-	
lomatosis of Churg-Strauss	

(Fig. 19–2). If the disease becomes chronic, inflammation spreads to adjacent portions of the interstitium and vasculature and eventually causes interstitial fibrosis. Important histopathologic patterns found in the ILDs include usual interstitial pneumonia (UIP), nonspecific interstitial pneumonia, respiratory bronchiolitis/desquamative interstitial pneumonia, organizing pneumonia, diffuse alveolar damage (acute or organizing), and lymphocytic interstitial pneumonia. The development of irreversible scarring (fibrosis) of alveolar walls, airways, or vasculature is the most feared outcome in all of these conditions because it is often progressive and leads to significant derangement of ventilatory function and gas exchange.

HISTORY

Duration of illness

Acute presentation (days to weeks), although unusual, occurs with allergy (drugs, fungi, helminths), acute interstitial pneumonia (AIP), eosinophilic pneumonia, and hypersensitivity pneumonitis. These conditions may be confused with atypical pneumonias because of diffuse alveolar opacities on chest x-ray. *Subacute presentation* (weeks to months) may occur in all ILDs but is seen especially in sarcoidosis, drug-induced ILDs, the alveolar hemorrhage syndromes, cryptogenic organizing pneumonia (COP), and the acute immunologic pneumonia that complicates systemic lupus erythematosus (SLE) or polymyositis. In most ILDs the symptoms and signs form a *chronic presentation* (months to years). Examples include IPF, sarcoidosis, pulmonary Langerhans cell histiocytosis (PLCH) (also known as Langerhans cell granulomatosis, eosinophilic granuloma, or histiocytosis X), pneumoconioses, and CTDs. *Episodic presentations* are unusual and include eosinophilic pneumonia, hypersensitivity pneumonitis, COP, vasculitides, pulmonary hemorrhage, and Churg-Strauss syndrome.

TABLE 19-2

ESTIMATED RELATIVE FREQUENCY OF THE INTERSTITIAL LUNG DISEASES

DIAGNOSIS	RELATIVE FREQUENCY, %
Idiopathic interstitial pneumonias	40
Idiopathic pulmonary fibrosis	55
Nonspecific interstitial pneumonia	25
Respiratory bronchiolitis—ILD and desquamative interstitial pneumonia	15
Cryptogenic organizing pneumonia	3
Acute interstitial pneumonia	<1
Occupational and environmental	26
Sarcoidosis	10
Connective tissue diseases	9
Drug and radiation	1
Pulmonary hemorrhage syndromes	<1
Other	13

Source: From DB Coultas, R Hubbard, in JP Lynch III (ed): *Lung Biology in Health and Disease.* New York, Marcel Dekker, 2004; S Garantziotis et al: J Clin Invest 114:319, 2004.

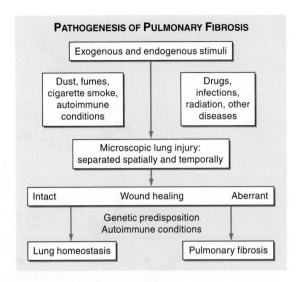

FIGURE 19-1

Proposed mechanism for the pathogenesis of pulmonary fibrosis. The lung is naturally exposed to repetitive injury from a variety of exogenous and endogenous stimuli. Several local and systemic factors (e.g., fibroblasts, circulating fibrocytes, chemokines, growth factors, and clotting factors) contribute to tissue healing and functional recovery. Dysregulation of this intricate network through genetic predisposition, autoimmune conditions, or superimposed diseases can lead to aberrant wound healing, with the result of pulmonary fibrosis. Alternatively, excessive injury to the lung may overwhelm even intact reparative mechanisms and lead to pulmonary fibrosis. (*From S Garantziotis et al: J Clin Invest 114:319, 2004.*)

Age

Most patients with sarcoidosis, ILD associated with CTD, lymphangioleiomyomatosis (LAM), PLCH, and inherited forms of ILD (familial IPF, Gaucher's disease, Hermansky-Pudlak syndrome) present between the ages of 20 and 40 years. Most patients with IPF are older than 60 years.

Gender

LAM and pulmonary involvement in tuberous sclerosis occur exclusively in premenopausal women. In addition, ILD in Hermansky-Pudlak syndrome and in the CTDs is more common in women; an exception is ILD in rheumatoid arthritis (RA), which is more common in men. IPF is more common in men. Because of occupational exposures, pneumoconioses also occur more frequently in men.

Family history

Familial lung fibrosis has been associated with mutations in three genes: the surfactant protein C gene, the surfactant protein A2 gene, and the ATP-binding cassette transporter A3 gene. Familial lung fibrosis is characterized by several patterns of interstitial pneumonia, including nonspecific interstitial pneumonia, desquamative interstitial pneumonia, and UIP. Older age, male sex, and a history of cigarette smoking have been identified as risk factors for familial lung fibrosis. Family associations (with an autosomal dominant pattern) have been identified in tuberous sclerosis and neurofibromatosis. Familial clustering has been identified increasingly in sarcoidosis. The genes responsible for several rare ILDs have been identified, i.e., alveolar microlithiasis, Gaucher's disease, Hermansky-Pudlak syndrome, and Niemann-Pick disease, along with the genes for surfactant homeostasis in pulmonary alveolar proteinosis and for control of cell growth and differentiation in LAM.

Smoking history

Two-thirds to 75% of patients with IPF and familial lung fibrosis have a history of smoking. Patients with PLCH, respiratory bronchiolitis/desquamative interstitial pneumonia (DIP), Goodpasture's syndrome, respiratory bronchiolitis, and pulmonary alveolar proteinosis are usually current or former smokers.

Occupational and environmental history

A strict chronologic listing of the patient's lifelong employment must be sought, including specific duties

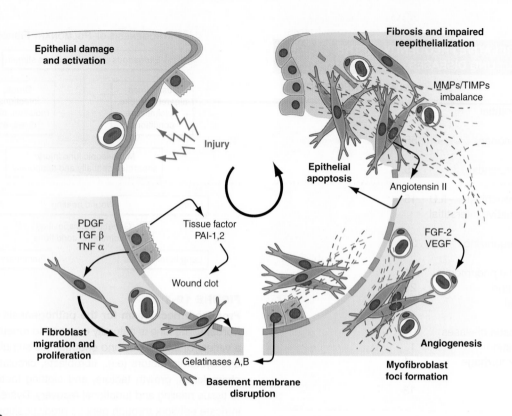

FIGURE 19-2

Cellular basis for the pathogenesis of interstitial lung disease. Multiple microinjuries damage and activate alveolar epithelial cells (*top left*), which in turn induce an antifibrinolytic environment in the alveolar spaces, enhancing wound clot formation. Alveolar epithelial cells secrete growth factors and induce migration and proliferation of fibroblasts and differentiation into myofibroblasts (*bottom left*). Subepithelial myofibroblasts and alveolar epithelial cells produce gelatinases that may increase basement membrane disruption and allow fibroblast–myofibroblast migration (*bottom right*). Angiogenic factors induce neovascularization. Both intraalveolar and interstitial myofibroblasts secrete extracellular matrix proteins, mainly collagens. An imbalance between interstitial collagenases and tissue inhibitors of metalloproteinases provokes the progressive deposit of extracellular matrix (*top right*). Signals responsible for myofibroblast apoptosis seem to be absent or delayed in usual interstitial pneumonia, increasing cell survival. Myofibroblasts produce angiotensinogen that, as angiotensin II, provokes alveolar epithelial cell death, further impairing reepithelialization. Abbreviations: FGF-2, fibroblast growth factor 2; MMPs, metalloproteinases; PAI-1, PAI-2, plasminogen activator inhibitor 1, 2; PDGF, platelet-derived growth factor; TGF-β, transforming growth factor β; TIMPs, tissue inhibitors of metalloproteinases; TNF-α, tumor necrosis factor α; VEGF, vascular endothelial growth factor. (*From M Selman et al: Ann Intern Med 134:136, 2001, with permission.*)

and known exposures. In hypersensitivity pneumonitis (see Fig. 9-1), respiratory symptoms, fever, chills, and an abnormal chest roentgenogram are often temporally related to a hobby (pigeon breeder's disease) or to the workplace (farmer's lung) (Chap. 9). Symptoms may diminish or disappear after the patient leaves the site of exposure for several days; similarly, symptoms may reappear when the patient returns to the exposure site.

Other important past history

Parasitic infections may cause pulmonary eosinophilia, and therefore a travel history should be taken in patients with known or suspected ILD. History of risk factors for HIV infection should be elicited because several processes may occur at the time of initial presentation or during the clinical course, e.g., HIV infection, organizing pneumonia, AIP, lymphocytic interstitial pneumonitis, and diffuse alveolar hemorrhage.

Respiratory symptoms and signs

Dyspnea is a common and prominent complaint in patients with ILD, especially the idiopathic interstitial pneumonias, hypersensitivity pneumonitis, COP, sarcoidosis, eosinophilic pneumonias, and PLCH. Some patients, especially patients with sarcoidosis, silicosis, PLCH, hypersensitivity pneumonitis, lipoid pneumonia, or lymphangitis carcinomatosis, may have extensive parenchymal lung disease on chest x-ray without significant dyspnea, especially early in the course of the illness. Wheezing is an uncommon manifestation of ILD but has been described in patients with chronic eosinophilic pneumonia, Churg-Strauss syndrome, respiratory bronchiolitis, and sarcoidosis. Clinically significant chest pain is uncommon in most ILDs. However, substernal discomfort is common in sarcoidosis. Sudden worsening of dyspnea, especially if associated with acute chest pain, may indicate a spontaneous pneumothorax, which occurs in PLCH, tuberous sclerosis, LAM, and neurofibromatosis. Frank hemoptysis and blood-streaked sputum are rarely presenting manifestations of ILD but can be seen in the diffuse alveolar hemorrhage (DAH) syndromes, LAM, tuberous sclerosis, and the granulomatous vasculitides. Fatigue and weight loss are common in all ILDs.

PHYSICAL EXAMINATION

The findings are usually not specific. Most commonly, physical examination reveals tachypnea and bibasilar end-inspiratory dry crackles, which are common in most forms of ILD associated with inflammation but are less likely to be heard in the granulomatous lung diseases. Crackles may be present in the absence of radiographic abnormalities on the chest radiograph. Scattered late inspiratory high-pitched rhonchi—so-called inspiratory squeaks—are heard in patients with bronchiolitis. The cardiac examination is usually normal except in the middle or late stages of the disease, when findings of pulmonary hypertension and cor pulmonale may become evident. Cyanosis and clubbing of the digits occur in some patients with advanced disease.

LABORATORY

Antinuclear antibodies and anti-immunoglobulin antibodies (rheumatoid factors) are identified in some patients, even in the absence of a defined CTD. A raised lactate dehydrogenase (LDH) level is a nonspecific finding common to ILDs. Elevation of the serum level of angiotensin-converting enzyme is common in sarcoidosis. Serum precipitins confirm exposure when hypersensitivity pneumonitis is suspected, although they are not diagnostic of the process. Antineutrophil cytoplasmic or anti-basement membrane antibodies are useful if vasculitis is suspected. The electrocardiogram is usually normal unless pulmonary hypertension is present; then it demonstrates right-axis deviation, right ventricular hypertrophy, or right atrial enlargement or hypertrophy. Echocardiography also reveals right ventricular dilation and/or hypertrophy in the presence of pulmonary hypertension.

CHEST IMAGING STUDIES

Chest x-ray

ILD may be first suspected on the basis of an abnormal chest radiograph, which most commonly reveals a bibasilar reticular pattern. A nodular or mixed pattern of alveolar filling and increased reticular markings also may be present. A subgroup of ILDs exhibit nodular opacities with a predilection for the upper lung zones (sarcoidosis, PLCH, chronic hypersensitivity pneumonitis, silicosis, berylliosis, RA [necrobiotic nodular form], ankylosing spondylitis). The chest x-ray correlates poorly with the clinical or histopathologic stage of the disease. The radiographic finding of honeycombing correlates with pathologic findings of small cystic spaces and progressive fibrosis; when present, it portends a poor prognosis. In most cases, the chest radiograph is nonspecific and usually does not allow a specific diagnosis.

Computed tomography

High-resolution computed tomography is superior to the plain chest x-ray for early detection and confirmation of suspected ILD **(Fig. 19-3)**. In addition, HRCT allows better assessment of the extent and distribution of disease, and it is especially useful in the investigation of patients with a normal chest radiograph. Coexisting disease is often best recognized on HRCT scanning, e.g., mediastinal adenopathy, carcinoma, or emphysema. In the appropriate clinical setting HRCT may be sufficiently characteristic to preclude the need for lung biopsy in IPF, sarcoidosis, hypersensitivity pneumonitis, asbestosis, lymphangitic carcinoma, and PLCH. When a lung biopsy is required, HRCT scanning is useful for determining the most appropriate area from which biopsy samples should be taken.

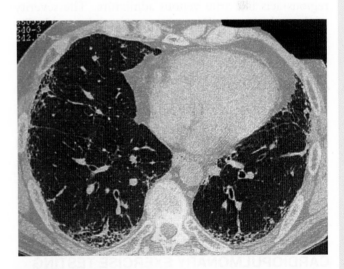

FIGURE 19-3
Idiopathic pulmonary fibrosis. High-resolution CT image shows bibasal, peripheral predominant reticular abnormality with traction bronchiectasis and honeycombing. The lung biopsy showed the typical features of usual interstitial pneumonia.

PULMONARY FUNCTION TESTING

Spirometry and lung volumes

Measurement of lung function is important in assessing the extent of pulmonary involvement in patients with ILD. Most forms of ILD produce a restrictive defect with reduced total lung capacity (TLC), functional residual capacity, and residual volume (Chap. 5). Forced expiratory volume in one second (FEV_1) and forced vital capacity (FVC) are reduced, but these changes are related to the decreased TLC. The FEV_1/FVC ratio is usually normal or increased. Lung volumes decrease as lung stiffness worsens with disease progression. A few disorders produce interstitial opacities on chest x-ray and obstructive airflow limitation on lung function testing (uncommon in sarcoidosis and hypersensitivity pneumonitis but common in tuberous sclerosis and LAM). Pulmonary function studies have been proved to have prognostic value in patients with idiopathic interstitial pneumonias, particularly IPF and nonspecific interstitial pneumonia (NSIP).

Diffusing capacity

A reduction in the diffusing capacity of the lung for carbon monoxide (DL_{CO}) is a common but nonspecific finding in most ILDs. This decrease is due in part to effacement of the alveolar capillary units but, more important, to mismatching of ventilation and perfusion ($\dot{V}/\dot{Q}$). Lung regions with reduced compliance due to either fibrosis or cellular infiltration may be poorly ventilated but may still maintain adequate blood flow, and the ventilation-perfusion mismatch in these regions acts like true venous admixture. The severity of the reduction in DL_{CO} does not correlate with disease stage.

Arterial blood gas

The resting arterial blood gas may be normal or reveal hypoxemia (secondary to a mismatching of ventilation to perfusion) and respiratory alkalosis. A normal arterial O_2 tension (or saturation by oximetry) at rest does not rule out significant hypoxemia during exercise or sleep. Carbon dioxide (CO_2) retention is rare and is usually a manifestation of end-stage disease.

CARDIOPULMONARY EXERCISE TESTING

Because hypoxemia at rest is not always present and because severe exercise-induced hypoxemia may go undetected, it is useful to perform exercise testing with measurement of arterial blood gases to detect abnormalities of gas exchange. Arterial oxygen desaturation, a failure to decrease dead space appropriately with exercise (i.e., a high V_D/V_T [dead space/tidal volume] ratio [Chap. 5]), and an excessive increase in respiratory rate with a lower than expected recruitment of tidal volume provide useful information about physiologic abnormalities and extent of disease. Serial assessment of resting and exercise gas exchange is an excellent method for following disease activity and responsiveness to treatment, especially in patients with IPF. Increasingly, the 6-min walk test is used to obtain a global evaluation of submaximal exercise capacity in patients with ILD. The walk distance and level of oxygen desaturation tend to correlate with the patient's baseline lung function and mirror the patient's clinical course.

FIBEROPTIC BRONCHOSCOPY AND BRONCHOALVEOLAR LAVAGE (BAL)

In selected diseases (e.g., sarcoidosis, hypersensitivity pneumonitis, DAH syndrome, cancer, pulmonary alveolar proteinosis), cellular analysis of BAL fluid may be useful in narrowing the differential diagnostic possibilities among various types of ILD (Table 19-3). The role of BAL in defining the stage of disease and assessment of disease progression or response to therapy remains poorly understood, and the usefulness of BAL in the clinical assessment and management remains to be established.

TISSUE AND CELLULAR EXAMINATION

Lung biopsy is the most effective method for confirming the diagnosis and assessing disease activity. The findings may identify a more treatable process than originally suspected, particularly chronic hypersensitivity pneumonitis, COP, respiratory bronchiolitis–associated ILD, or sarcoidosis. Biopsy should be obtained before the initiation of treatment. A definitive diagnosis avoids confusion and anxiety later in the clinical course if the patient does not respond to therapy or experiences serious side effects from it.

Fiberoptic bronchoscopy with multiple transbronchial lung biopsies (four to eight biopsy samples) is often the initial procedure of choice, especially when sarcoidosis, lymphangitic carcinomatosis, eosinophilic pneumonia, Goodpasture's syndrome, or infection is suspected. If a specific diagnosis is not made by transbronchial biopsy, surgical lung biopsy by video-assisted thoracic surgery or open thoracotomy is indicated. Adequate-sized biopsies from multiple sites, usually from two lobes, should be obtained. Relative contraindications to lung biopsy include serious cardiovascular disease, honeycombing and other roentgenographic evidence of diffuse end-stage disease, severe pulmonary dysfunction, and other major operative risks, especially in the elderly.

TABLE 19-3

DIAGNOSTIC VALUE OF BRONCHOALVEOLAR LAVAGE IN INTERSTITIAL LUNG DISEASE

CONDITION	BRONCHOALVEOLAR LAVAGE FINDING
Sarcoidosis	Lymphocytosis; CD4:CD8 ratio >3.5 most specific of diagnosis
Hypersensitivity pneumonitis	Marked lymphocytosis (>50%)
Organizing pneumonia	Foamy macrophages; mixed pattern of increased cells characteristic; decreased CD4:CD8 ratio
Eosinophilic lung disease	Eosinophils >25%
Diffuse alveolar bleeding	Hemosiderin-laden macrophages, red blood cells
Diffuse alveolar damage, drug toxicity	Atypical hyperplastic type II pneumocytes
Opportunistic infections	*Pneumocystis carinii*, fungi, cytomegalovirus-transformed cells
Lymphangitic carcinomatosis, alveolar cell carcinoma, pulmonary lymphoma	Malignant cells
Alveolar proteinosis	Milky effluent, foamy macrophages and lipoproteinaceous intraalveolar material (periodic acid–Schiff stain–positive)
Lipoid pneumonia	Fat globules in macrophages
Pulmonary Langerhans cell histiocytosis	Increased CD1+ Langerhans cells, electron microscopy demonstrating Birbeck granule in lavaged macrophage (expensive and difficult to perform)
Asbestos-related pulmonary disease	Dust particles, ferruginous bodies
Berylliosis	Positive lymphocyte transformation test to beryllium
Silicosis	Dust particles by polarized light microscopy
Lipoidosis	Accumulation of specific lipopigment in alveolar macrophages

CHAPTER 19 Interstitial Lung Diseases

TREATMENT Interstitial Lung Disease

Although the course of ILD is variable, progression is common and often insidious. All treatable possibilities should be carefully considered. Since therapy does not reverse fibrosis, the major goals of treatment are permanent removal of the offending agent, when known, and early identification and aggressive suppression of the acute and chronic inflammatory process, thereby reducing further lung damage. Hypoxemia (Pao_2 <55 mmHg) at rest and/or with exercise should be managed with supplemental oxygen. Management of cor pulmonale may be required as the disease progresses. Pulmonary rehabilitation has been shown to improve the quality of life in patients with ILD.

DRUG THERAPY Glucocorticoids are the mainstay of therapy for suppression of the alveolitis present in ILD, but the success rate is low. There have been no placebo-controlled trials of glucocorticoids in ILD, and so there is no direct evidence that steroids improve survival in many of the diseases for which they are commonly used. Glucocorticoid therapy is recommended for symptomatic ILD patients with eosinophilic pneumonias, COP, CTD, sarcoidosis, hypersensitivity pneumonitis, acute inorganic dust exposures, acute radiation pneumonitis, DAH, and drug-induced ILD. In organic dust disease, glucocorticoids are recommended for both the acute and chronic stages.

The optimal dose and proper length of therapy with glucocorticoids in the treatment of most ILDs are not known. A common starting dose is prednisone, 0.5–1 mg/kg in a once-daily oral dose (based on the patient's lean body weight). This dose is continued for 4–12 weeks, at which time the patient is reevaluated. If the patient is stable or improved, the dose is tapered to 0.25–0.5 mg/kg and is maintained at this level for an additional 4–12 weeks, depending on the course. Rapid tapering or a shortened course of glucocorticoid treatment can result in recurrence. If the patient's condition continues to decline on glucocorticoids, a second agent (see later) often is added and the prednisone dose is lowered to or maintained at 0.25 mg/kg per d.

Cyclophosphamide and azathioprine (1–2 mg/kg lean body weight per day), with or without glucocorticoids, have been tried with variable success in IPF, vasculitis, progressive systemic sclerosis, and other ILDs. An objective response usually requires at least 8–12 weeks to occur. In situations in which these drugs have failed or could not be tolerated, other agents, including methotrexate, colchicine, penicillamine, and cyclosporine, have been tried. However, their role in the treatment of ILDs remains to be determined.

Many cases of ILD are chronic and irreversible despite the therapy discussed earlier, and lung transplantation may then be considered (Chap. 24).

INDIVIDUAL FORMS OF ILD

IDIOPATHIC PULMONARY FIBROSIS

IPF is the most common form of idiopathic interstitial pneumonia. Separating IPF from other forms of lung fibrosis is an important step in the evaluation of all patients presenting with ILD. IPF has a distinctly poor response to therapy and a bad prognosis.

Clinical manifestations

Exertional dyspnea, a nonproductive cough, and inspiratory crackles with or without digital clubbing may be present on physical examination. HRCT lung scans typically show patchy, predominantly basilar, subpleural reticular opacities, often associated with traction bronchiectasis and honeycombing (Fig. 19-3). Atypical findings that should suggest an alternative diagnosis include extensive ground-glass abnormality, nodular opacities, upper or midzone predominance, and prominent hilar or mediastinal lymphadenopathy. Pulmonary function tests often reveal a restrictive pattern, a reduced DL_{CO}, and arterial hypoxemia that is exaggerated or elicited by exercise.

Histologic findings

Confirmation of the presence of the UIP pattern on histologic examination is essential to confirm this diagnosis. Transbronchial biopsies are not helpful in making the diagnosis of UIP, and surgical biopsy usually is required. The histologic hallmark and chief diagnostic criterion of UIP is a heterogeneous appearance at low magnification with alternating areas of normal lung, interstitial inflammation, foci of proliferating fibroblasts, dense collagen fibrosis, and honeycomb changes. These histologic changes affect the peripheral, subpleural parenchyma most severely. The interstitial inflammation is usually patchy and consists of a lymphoplasmacytic infiltrate in the alveolar septa, associated with hyperplasia of type 2 pneumocytes. The fibrotic zones are composed mainly of dense collagen, although scattered foci of proliferating fibroblasts are a consistent finding. The extent of fibroblastic proliferation is predictive of disease progression. Areas of honeycomb change are composed of cystic fibrotic air spaces that frequently are lined by bronchiolar epithelium and filled with

mucin. Smooth-muscle hyperplasia is commonly seen in areas of fibrosis and honeycomb change. A fibrotic pattern with some features similar to UIP may be found in the chronic stage of several specific disorders, such as pneumoconioses (e.g., asbestosis), radiation injury, certain drug-induced lung diseases (e.g., nitrofurantoin), chronic aspiration, sarcoidosis, chronic hypersensitivity pneumonitis, organized chronic eosinophilic pneumonia, and PLCH. Commonly, other histopathologic features are present in these situations, thus allowing separation of these lesions from the UIP-like pattern. Consequently, the term *usual interstitial pneumonia* is used for patients in whom the lesion is idiopathic and not associated with another condition.

| TREATMENT | Management Issues in Patients with IPF |

Untreated patients with IPF show continued progression of their disease and have a high mortality rate. There is no effective therapy for IPF. Chronic microaspiration secondary to gastroesophageal reflux may play a role in the pathogenesis and natural history of IPF. Patients with IPF and coexisting emphysema (combined pulmonary fibrosis and emphysema [CPFE]) are more likely to require long-term oxygen therapy and develop pulmonary hypertension and may have a more dismal outcome than those without emphysema.

Patients with IPF may have acute deterioration secondary to infections, pulmonary embolism, or pneumothorax. Heart failure and ischemic heart disease are common problems in patients with IPF, accounting for nearly one-third of deaths. These patients also commonly experience an accelerated phase of rapid clinical decline that is associated with a poor prognosis (so-called acute exacerbations of IPF). These acute exacerbations are defined by worsening of dyspnea within a few days to 4 weeks; newly developing diffuse ground-glass abnormality and/or consolidation superimposed on a background reticular or honeycomb pattern consistent with the UIP pattern; worsening hypoxemia; and absence of infectious pneumonia, heart failure, and sepsis. The rate of these acute exacerbations ranges from 10–57%, apparently depending on the length of follow-up. During these episodes, the histopathologic pattern of diffuse alveolar damage is often found on the background of UIP. No therapy has been found to be effective in the management of acute exacerbations of IPF. Often mechanical ventilation is required, but it is usually not successful, with a hospital mortality rate of up to three-fourths of patients. In those who survive, a recurrence of acute exacerbation is common and usually results in death at those times.

Lung transplantation should be considered for patients who experience progressive deterioration despite optimal medical management and who meet the established criteria (Chap. 24).

NONSPECIFIC INTERSTITIAL PNEUMONIA

This condition defines a subgroup of the idiopathic interstitial pneumonias that can be distinguished clinically and pathologically from UIP, DIP, AIP, and idiopathic BOOP. Importantly, many cases with this histopathologic pattern occur in the context of an underlying disorder, such as a connective tissue disease, drug-induced ILD, or chronic hypersensitivity pneumonitis.

Patients with idiopathic NSIP have clinical, serologic, radiographic, and pathologic characteristics highly suggestive of autoimmune disease and meet the criteria for undifferentiated connective tissue disease. Idiopathic NSIP is a subacute restrictive process with a presentation similar to that of IPF but usually at a younger age, most commonly in women who have never smoked. It is often associated with a febrile illness. HRCT shows bilateral, subpleural ground-glass opacities, often associated with lower lobe volume loss (Fig. 19-4). Patchy areas of airspace consolidation and reticular abnormalities may be present, but honeycombing is unusual. The key histopathologic feature of NSIP is the uniformity of interstitial involvement across the biopsy section, and this may be predominantly cellular or fibrosing. There is less temporal and spatial heterogeneity than in UIP, and little or no honeycombing is found. The cellular variant is rare. Unlike patients with IPF (UIP), the majority of patients with NSIP have a good prognosis (5-year mortality rate estimated at <15%), with most showing improvement after treatment with glucocorticoids, often used in combination with azathioprine.

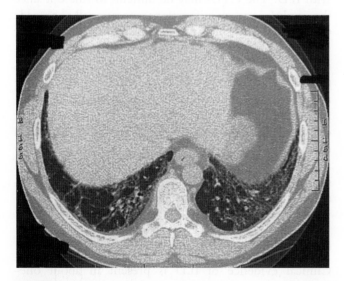

FIGURE 19-4

Nonspecific interstitial pneumonia. High-resolution CT through the lower lung shows volume loss with extensive ground-glass abnormality, reticular abnormality, and traction bronchiectasis. There is sparing on the lung immediately adjacent to the pleura. Histology showed a combination of inflammation and mild fibrosis.

ACUTE INTERSTITIAL PNEUMONIA (HAMMAN-RICH SYNDROME)

AIP is a rare, fulminant form of lung injury characterized histologically by diffuse alveolar damage on lung biopsy. Most patients are older than 40 years. AIP is similar in presentation to the acute respiratory distress syndrome (ARDS) (Chap. 29) and probably corresponds to the subset of cases of idiopathic ARDS. The onset is usually abrupt in a previously healthy individual. A prodromal illness, usually lasting 7–14 days before presentation, is common. Fever, cough, and dyspnea are common manifestations at presentation. Diffuse, bilateral, air-space opacification is present on the chest radiograph. HRCT scans show bilateral, patchy, symmetric areas of ground-glass attenuation. Bilateral areas of air-space consolidation also may be present. A predominantly subpleural distribution may be seen. The diagnosis of AIP requires the presence of a clinical syndrome of idiopathic ARDS and pathologic confirmation of organizing diffuse alveolar damage. Therefore, lung biopsy is required to confirm the diagnosis. Most patients have moderate to severe hypoxemia and develop respiratory failure. Mechanical ventilation is often required. The mortality rate is high (>60%), with most patients dying within 6 months of presentation. Recurrences have been reported. However, those who recover often have substantial improvement in lung function. The main treatment is supportive. It is not clear that glucocorticoid therapy is effective.

CRYPTOGENIC ORGANIZING PNEUMONIA

COP is a clinicopathologic syndrome of unknown etiology. The onset is usually in the fifth and sixth decades. The presentation may be of a flulike illness with cough, fever, malaise, fatigue, and weight loss. Inspiratory crackles are frequently present on examination. Pulmonary function is usually impaired, with a restrictive defect and arterial hypoxemia being most common. The roentgenographic manifestations are distinctive, revealing bilateral, patchy, or diffuse alveolar opacities in the presence of normal lung volume. Recurrent and migratory pulmonary opacities are common. HRCT shows areas of air-space consolidation, ground-glass opacities, small nodular opacities, and bronchial wall thickening and dilation. These changes occur more frequently in the periphery of the lung and in the lower lung zone. Lung biopsy shows granulation tissue within small airways, alveolar ducts, and airspaces, with chronic inflammation in the surrounding alveoli. Glucocorticoid therapy induces clinical recovery in two-thirds of patients. A few patients have rapidly progressive courses with fatal outcomes despite glucocorticoids.

Foci of organizing pneumonia is a nonspecific reaction to lung injury found adjacent to other pathologic processes or as a component of other primary pulmonary disorders (e.g., cryptococcosis, granulomatosis with polyangiitis [Wegener's], lymphoma, hypersensitivity pneumonitis, and eosinophilic pneumonia). Consequently, the clinician must carefully reevaluate any patient found to have this histopathologic lesion to rule out these possibilities.

ILD ASSOCIATED WITH CIGARETTE SMOKING

Desquamative interstitial pneumonia

DIP is a rare but distinct clinical and pathologic entity found almost exclusively in cigarette smokers. The histologic hallmark is the extensive accumulation of macrophages in intraalveolar spaces with minimal interstitial fibrosis. The peak incidence is in the fourth and fifth decades. Most patients present with dyspnea and cough. Lung function testing shows a restrictive pattern with reduced DL_{CO} and arterial hypoxemia. The chest x-ray and HRCT scans usually show diffuse hazy opacities. Clinical recognition of DIP is important because the process is associated with a better prognosis (10-year survival rate is ~70%) in response to smoking cessation. There are no clear data showing that systemic glucocorticoids are effective in DIP.

Respiratory bronchiolitis–associated ILD

Respiratory bronchiolitis–associated ILD (RB-ILD) is considered to be a subset of DIP and is characterized by the accumulation of macrophages in peribronchial alveoli. The clinical presentation is similar to that of DIP. Crackles are often heard on chest examination and occur throughout inspiration; sometimes they continue into expiration. The process is best seen on HRCT lung scanning, which shows bronchial wall thickening, centrilobular nodules, ground-glass opacity, and emphysema with air trapping. RB-ILD appears to resolve in most patients after smoking cessation alone.

Pulmonary Langerhans cell histiocytosis

This is a rare, smoking-related, diffuse lung disease that primarily affects men between the ages of 20 and 40 years. The clinical presentation varies from an asymptomatic state to a rapidly progressive condition. The most common clinical manifestations at presentation are cough, dyspnea, chest pain, weight loss, and fever. Pneumothorax occurs in ~25% of patients. Hemoptysis and diabetes insipidus are rare manifestations. The radiographic features vary with the stage of the disease. The combination of ill-defined or stellate nodules (2–10 mm in diameter), reticular or nodular opacities, bizarre-shaped upper zone cysts, preservation of lung volume, and sparing of the costophrenic angles are characteristics of PLCH. HRCT that reveals a combination of nodules and thin-walled cysts is virtually diagnostic of PLCH. The most common pulmonary function abnormality is a markedly reduced DL_{CO}, although varying degrees of restrictive disease, airflow limitation, and diminished exercise capacity may occur. The characteristic histopathologic finding in PLCH is the presence of nodular sclerosing lesions that contain Langerhans cells accompanied by mixed cellular infiltrates. The nodular lesions are poorly defined and are distributed in a bronchiolocentric fashion with intervening normal lung parenchyma. As the disease advances, fibrosis progresses to involve adjacent lung tissue, leading to pericicatricial air space enlargement, which accounts for the concomitant cystic changes. Discontinuance of smoking is the key treatment, resulting in clinical improvement in one-third of patients. Most patients with PLCH experience persistent or progressive disease. Death due to respiratory failure occurs in ~10% of patients.

ILD ASSOCIATED WITH CONNECTIVE TISSUE DISORDERS

Clinical findings suggestive of a CTD (musculoskeletal pain, weakness, fatigue, fever, joint pain or swelling, photosensitivity, Raynaud's phenomenon, pleuritis, dry eyes, dry mouth) should be sought in any patient with ILD. The CTDs may be difficult to rule out since the pulmonary manifestations occasionally precede the more typical systemic manifestations by months or years. The most common form of pulmonary involvement is the nonspecific interstitial pneumonia histopathologic pattern. However, determining the precise nature of lung involvement in most of the CTDs is difficult due to the high incidence of lung involvement caused by disease-associated complications of esophageal dysfunction (predisposing to aspiration and secondary infections), respiratory muscle weakness (atelectasis and secondary infections), complications of therapy (opportunistic infections), and associated malignancies.

Progressive systemic sclerosis (PSS)

Clinical evidence of ILD is present in about one-half of patients with PSS, and pathologic evidence in three-quarters. Pulmonary function tests show a restrictive pattern and impaired diffusing capacity, often before any clinical or radiographic evidence of lung disease appears. Pulmonary vascular disease alone or in association with pulmonary fibrosis, pleuritis, or recurrent aspiration pneumonitis is strikingly resistant to current modes of therapy.

Rheumatoid arthritis

ILD associated with RA is more common in men. Pulmonary manifestations of RA include pleurisy with or without effusion, ILD in up to 20% of cases, necrobiotic nodules (nonpneumoconiotic intrapulmonary rheumatoid nodules) with or without cavities, Caplan's syndrome (rheumatoid pneumoconiosis), pulmonary hypertension secondary to rheumatoid pulmonary vasculitis, organized pneumonia, and upper airway obstruction due to crico-arytenoid arthritis.

Systemic lupus erythematosus

Lung disease is a common complication in SLE. Pleuritis with or without effusion is the most common pulmonary manifestation. Other lung manifestations include the following: atelectasis, diaphragmatic dysfunction with loss of lung volumes, pulmonary vascular disease, pulmonary hemorrhage, uremic pulmonary edema, infectious pneumonia, and organized pneumonia. Acute lupus pneumonitis characterized by pulmonary capillaritis leading to alveolar hemorrhage is uncommon. Chronic, progressive ILD is uncommon. It is important to exclude pulmonary infection. Although pleuropulmonary involvement may not be evident clinically, pulmonary function testing, particularly $D_{L_{CO}}$, reveals abnormalities in many patients with SLE.

Polymyositis and dermatomyositis (PM/DM)

ILD occurs in ~10% of patients with PM/DM. Diffuse reticular or nodular opacities with or without an alveolar component occur radiographically, with a predilection for the lung bases. ILD occurs more commonly in the subgroup of patients with an anti-Jo-1 antibody that is directed to histidyl tRNA synthetase. Weakness of respiratory muscles contributing to aspiration pneumonia may be present. A rapidly progressive illness characterized by diffuse alveolar damage may cause respiratory failure.

Sjögren's syndrome

General dryness and lack of airway secretion cause the major problems of hoarseness, cough, and bronchitis. Lymphocytic interstitial pneumonitis, lymphoma, pseudolymphoma, bronchiolitis, and bronchiolitis obliterans are associated with this condition. Lung biopsy is frequently required to establish a precise pulmonary diagnosis. Glucocorticoids have been used in the management of ILD associated with Sjögren's syndrome with some degree of clinical success.

DRUG-INDUCED ILD

Many classes of drugs have the potential to induce diffuse ILD, which is manifest most commonly as exertional dyspnea and nonproductive cough. A detailed history of the medications taken by the patient is needed to identify drug-induced disease, including over-the-counter medications, oily nose drops, and petroleum products (mineral oil). In most cases, the pathogenesis is unknown, although a combination of direct toxic effects of the drug (or its metabolite) and indirect inflammatory and immunologic events are likely. The onset of the illness may be abrupt and fulminant, or it may be insidious, extending over weeks to months. The drug may have been taken for several years before a reaction develops (e.g., amiodarone), or the lung disease may occur weeks to years after the drug has been discontinued (e.g., carmustine). The extent and severity of disease are usually dose-related. Treatment consists of discontinuation of any possible offending drug and supportive care.

EOSINOPHILIC PNEUMONIA

(See Chap. 9)

PULMONARY ALVEOLAR PROTEINOSIS (PAP)

Although not strictly an ILD, PAP resembles and is therefore considered with these conditions. It has been proposed that a defect in macrophage function, more specifically an impaired ability to process surfactant, may play a role in the pathogenesis of PAP. This diffuse disease is characterized by the accumulation of an amorphous, periodic acid–Schiff-positive lipoproteinaceous material in the distal air spaces. There is little or no lung inflammation, and the underlying lung architecture is preserved. PAP is an autoimmune disease with a neutralizing antibody of immunoglobulin G isotype against granulocyte-macrophage colony-stimulating factor (GM-CSF). These findings suggest that neutralization of GM-CSF bioactivity by the antibody causes dysfunction of alveolar macrophages, which results in reduced surfactant clearance. There are three distinct classes of PAP: acquired (>90% of all cases), congenital, and secondary. *Congenital PAP* is transmitted in an autosomal recessive manner and is caused by homozygosity for a frameshift mutation (121ins2) in the *SP-B* gene, which leads to an unstable SP-B mRNA, reduced protein levels, and *secondary disturbances of SP-C processing*. *Secondary PAP* is rare among adults and is caused by lysinuric protein intolerance, acute silicosis and other inhalational syndromes, immunodeficiency disorders, and malignancies (almost exclusively of hematopoietic origin) and hematopoietic disorders.

The typical age of presentation is 30–50 years, and males predominate. The clinical presentation is usually insidious and is manifested by progressive exertional dyspnea, fatigue, weight loss, and low-grade fever. A nonproductive cough is common, but occasionally expectoration of "chunky" gelatinous material may occur. Polycythemia, hypergammaglobulinemia, and increased LDH levels are common. Markedly elevated serum levels of lung surfactant proteins A and D have been found in PAP. In the absence of any known secondary cause of PAP, an elevated serum anti-GM-CSF titer is highly sensitive and specific for the diagnosis of acquired PAP. BAL fluid levels of anti-GM-CSF antibodies correlate better with the severity of PAP than do serum titers. Radiographically, bilateral symmetric alveolar opacities located centrally in middle and lower lung zones result in a "bat-wing" distribution. HRCT shows a ground-glass opacification and thickened intralobular structures and interlobular septa. Whole-lung lavage(s) through a double-lumen endotracheal tube provides relief to many patients with dyspnea or progressive hypoxemia and also may provide long-term benefit.

PULMONARY LYMPHANGIOLEIOMYOMATOSIS

Pulmonary LAM is a rare condition that afflicts pre-menopausal women and should be suspected in young women with "emphysema," recurrent pneumothorax, or chylous pleural effusion. It is often misdiagnosed as asthma or chronic obstructive pulmonary disease. Pathologically, LAM is characterized by the proliferation of atypical pulmonary interstitial smooth muscle and cyst formation. The immature-appearing smooth-muscle cells react with monoclonal antibody HMB45, which recognizes a 100-kDa glycoprotein (gp100) originally found in human melanoma cells. Whites are affected much more commonly than are members of other racial groups. The disease accelerates during pregnancy and abates after oophorectomy. Common complaints at presentation are dyspnea, cough, and chest pain. Hemoptysis may be life threatening. Spontaneous pneumothorax occurs in 50% of patients; it may be bilateral and necessitate pleurodesis. Meningioma and renal angiomyolipomas (hamartomas), characteristic findings in the genetic disorder tuberous sclerosis, are also common in patients with LAM. Chylothorax, chyloperitoneum (chylous ascites), chyluria, and chylopericardium are other complications. Pulmonary function testing usually reveals an obstructive or mixed obstructive-restrictive pattern, and gas exchange is often abnormal. HRCT shows thin-walled cysts surrounded by normal lung without zonal predominance. Progression is common, with a median survival of 8–10 years from diagnosis. No therapy is of proven benefit in LAM.

Progesterone (10 mg/d), luteinizing hormone–releasing hormone analogues, and sirolimus have been used. Oophorectomy is no longer recommended, and estrogen-containing drugs should be discontinued. Lung transplantation offers the only hope for cure despite reports of recurrent disease in the transplanted lung.

SYNDROMES OF ILD WITH DIFFUSE ALVEOLAR HEMORRHAGE

Injury to arterioles, venules, and the alveolar septal (alveolar wall or interstitial) capillaries can result in hemoptysis secondary to disruption of the alveolar-capillary basement membrane. This results in bleeding into the alveolar spaces, which characterizes DAH. Pulmonary capillaritis, characterized by a neutrophilic infiltration of the alveolar septae, may lead to necrosis of these structures, loss of capillary structural integrity, and the pouring of red blood cells into the alveolar space. Fibrinoid necrosis of the interstitium and red blood cells within the interstitial space are sometimes seen. Bland pulmonary hemorrhage (i.e., DAH without inflammation of the alveolar structures) also may occur.

The clinical onset is often abrupt, with cough, fever, and dyspnea. Severe respiratory distress requiring ventilatory support may be evident at initial presentation. Although hemoptysis is expected, it can be absent at the time of presentation in one-third of the cases. For patients without hemoptysis, new alveolar opacities, a falling hemoglobin level, and hemorrhagic BAL fluid point to the diagnosis. The chest radiograph is nonspecific and most commonly shows new patchy or diffuse alveolar opacities. Recurrent episodes of DAH may lead to pulmonary fibrosis, resulting in interstitial opacities on the chest radiograph. An elevated white blood cell count and falling hematocrit are common. Evidence for impaired renal function caused by focal segmental necrotizing glomerulonephritis, usually with crescent formation, also may be present.

Varying degrees of hypoxemia may occur and are often severe enough to require ventilatory support. DL_{CO} may be increased, resulting from the increased hemoglobin within the alveoli compartment. Evaluation of either lung or renal tissue by immunofluorescent techniques indicates an absence of immune complexes (pauci-immune) in granulomatosis with polyangiitis (Wegener's), microscopic polyangiitis pauci-immune glomerulonephritis, and isolated pulmonary capillaritis. A granular pattern is found in the CTDs, particularly SLE, and a characteristic linear deposition is found in Goodpasture's syndrome. Granular deposition of IgA-containing immune complexes is present in Henoch-Schönlein purpura.

The mainstay of therapy for the DAH associated with systemic vasculitis, CTD, Goodpasture's syndrome, and isolated pulmonary capillaritis is IV methylprednisolone, 0.5–2 g daily in divided doses for up to 5 days, followed by a gradual tapering, and then maintenance on an oral preparation. Prompt initiation of therapy is important, particularly in the face of renal insufficiency, since early initiation of therapy has the best chance of preserving renal function. The decision to start other immunosuppressive therapy (cyclophosphamide or azathioprine) acutely depends on the severity of illness.

Goodpasture's syndrome

Pulmonary hemorrhage and glomerulonephritis are features in most patients with this disease. Autoantibodies to renal glomerular and lung alveolar basement membranes are present. This syndrome can present and recur as DAH without an associated glomerulonephritis. In such cases, circulating anti-basement membrane antibody is often absent, and the only way to establish the diagnosis is by demonstrating linear immunofluorescence in lung tissue. The underlying histology may be bland hemorrhage or DAH associated with capillaritis. Plasmapheresis has been recommended as adjunctive treatment.

INHERITED DISORDERS ASSOCIATED WITH ILD

Pulmonary opacities and respiratory symptoms typical of ILD can develop in related family members and in several inherited diseases. These diseases include the phakomatoses, tuberous sclerosis and neurofibromatosis, and the lysosomal storage diseases, Niemann-Pick disease and Gaucher disease. The Hermansky-Pudlak syndrome is an autosomal recessive disorder in which granulomatous colitis and ILD may occur. It is characterized by oculocutaneous albinism, bleeding diathesis secondary to platelet dysfunction, and the accumulation of a chromolipid, lipofuscin material in cells of the reticuloendothelial system. A fibrotic pattern is found on lung biopsy, but the alveolar macrophages may contain cytoplasmic ceroid-like inclusions.

ILD WITH A GRANULOMATOUS RESPONSE IN LUNG TISSUE OR VASCULAR STRUCTURES

Inhalation of organic dusts, which cause hypersensitivity pneumonitis, or of inorganic dust, such as silica, which elicits a granulomatous inflammatory reaction leading to ILD, produces diseases of known etiology (Table 19-1) that are discussed in Chaps. 9 and 10. Sarcoidosis is prominent among granulomatous diseases of unknown cause in which ILD is an important feature.

Granulomatous vasculitides

The granulomatous vasculitides are characterized by pulmonary angiitis (i.e., inflammation and necrosis of blood vessels) with associated granuloma formation (i.e., infiltrates of lymphocytes, plasma cells, epithelioid cells, or histiocytes, with or without the presence of multinucleated giant cells, sometimes with tissue necrosis). The lungs are almost always involved, although any organ system may be affected. Granulomatosis with polyangiitis (Wegener's) and allergic angiitis and granulomatosis (Churg-Strauss syndrome) primarily affect the lung but are associated with a systemic vasculitis as well. The granulomatous vasculitides generally limited to the lung include necrotizing sarcoid granulomatosis and benign lymphocytic angiitis and granulomatosis. Granulomatous infection and pulmonary angiitis due to irritating embolic material (e.g., talc) are important known causes of pulmonary vasculitis.

LYMPHOCYTIC INFILTRATIVE DISORDERS

This group of disorders features lymphocyte and plasma cell infiltration of the lung parenchyma. The disorders either are benign or can behave as low-grade lymphomas. Included are angioimmunoblastic lymphadenopathy with dysproteinemia, a rare lymphoproliferative disorder characterized by diffuse lymphadenopathy, fever, hepatosplenomegaly, and hemolytic anemia, with ILD in some cases.

Lymphocytic interstitial pneumonitis

This rare form of ILD occurs in adults, some of whom have an autoimmune disease or dysproteinemia. It has been reported in patients with Sjögren's syndrome and HIV infection.

Lymphomatoid granulomatosis

This multisystem disorder of unknown etiology is an angiocentric malignant (T cell) lymphoma characterized by a polymorphic lymphoid infiltrate, an angiitis, and granulomatosis. Although it may affect virtually any organ, it is most frequently characterized by pulmonary, skin, and central nervous system involvement.

BRONCHOCENTRIC GRANULOMATOSIS

Rather than a specific clinical entity, bronchocentric granulomatosis (BG) is a descriptive histologic term that is applied to an uncommon and nonspecific pathologic response to a variety of airway injuries. There is evidence that BG is caused by a hypersensitivity reaction to *Aspergillus* or other fungi in patients with asthma. About one-half of the patients described have had chronic asthma with severe wheezing and peripheral blood eosinophilia. In patients with asthma, BG probably represents one pathologic manifestation of allergic bronchopulmonary aspergillosis or another allergic mycosis. In patients without asthma, BG has been associated with RA and a variety of infections, including tuberculosis, echinococcosis, histoplasmosis, coccidioidomycosis, and nocardiosis. The chest roentgenogram reveals irregularly shaped nodular or mass lesions with ill-defined margins, which are usually unilateral and solitary, with upper lobe predominance. Glucocorticoids are the treatment of choice, often with an excellent outcome, although recurrences may occur as therapy is tapered or stopped.

GLOBAL CONSIDERATIONS

Limited epidemiologic data exist describing the prevalence or incidence of ILD in the general population. With a few exceptions, e.g., sarcoidosis and certain occupational and environmental exposures, there appear to be no significant differences in the prevalence or incidence of ILD among various populations. For sarcoidosis, there are important environmental, racial, and genetic differences.

CHAPTER 20

DEEP VENOUS THROMBOSIS AND PULMONARY THROMBOEMBOLISM

Samuel Z. Goldhaber

EPIDEMIOLOGY

Venous thromboembolism (VTE), which encompasses deep venous thrombosis (DVT) and pulmonary embolism (PE), is one of the three major cardiovascular causes of death, along with myocardial infarction and stroke. VTE can cause death from PE or, among survivors, chronic thromboembolic pulmonary hypertension and postphlebitic syndrome. The U.S. Surgeon General has declared that PE is the most common preventable cause of death among hospitalized patients. Medicare has labeled PE and DVT occurring after total hip or knee replacement as unacceptable "never events" and no longer reimburses hospitals for the incremental expenses associated with treating this postoperative complication. New nonprofit organizations have begun educating health care professionals and the public on the medical consequences of VTE, along with risk factors and warning signs.

Between 100,000 and 300,000 VTE-related deaths occur annually in the United States. Mortality rates and length of hospital stay are decreasing as charges for hospital care increase. Approximately three of four symptomatic VTE events occur in the community, and the remainder are hospital acquired. Approximately 14 million (M) hospitalized patients are at moderate to high risk for VTE in the United States annually: 6 M major surgery patients and 8 M medical patients with comorbidities such as heart failure, cancer, and stroke. The prophylaxis paradigm has changed from voluntary to mandatory compliance with guidelines to prevent VTE among hospitalized patients. With an estimated 370,000 PE-related deaths annually in Europe, the projected direct cost for VTE-associated care exceeds 3 billion euros per year. In Japan, as the lifestyle becomes more westernized, the rate of VTE appears to be increasing.

The long-term effects of nonfatal VTE lower the quality of life. Chronic thromboembolic pulmonary hypertension is often disabling and causes breathlessness. A late effect of DVT is *postphlebitic syndrome*, which eventually occurs in more than one-half of DVT patients. Postphlebitic syndrome (also known as *postthrombotic syndrome* or *chronic venous insufficiency*) is a delayed complication of DVT that causes the venous valves of the leg to become incompetent and exude interstitial fluid. Patients complain of chronic ankle or calf swelling and leg aching, especially after prolonged standing. In its most severe form, postphlebitic syndrome causes skin ulceration, especially in the medial malleolus of the leg. There is no effective medical therapy for this condition.

Prothrombotic states

Thrombophilia contributes to the risk of venous thrombosis. The two most common autosomal dominant genetic mutations are factor V Leiden, which causes resistance to activated protein C (which inactivates clotting factors V and VIII), and the prothrombin gene mutation, which increases the plasma prothrombin concentration. Antithrombin, protein C, and protein S are naturally occurring coagulation inhibitors. Deficiencies of these inhibitors are associated with VTE but are rare. Hyperhomocysteinemia can increase the risk of VTE, but lowering the homocysteine level with folate, vitamin B_6, or vitamin B_{12} does not reduce the incidence of VTE. Antiphospholipid antibody syndrome is the most common acquired cause of thrombophilia and is associated with venous or arterial thrombosis. Other common predisposing factors include cancer, systemic arterial hypertension, chronic obstructive pulmonary disease, long-haul air travel, air pollution, obesity, cigarette smoking, eating large amounts of red meat, oral contraceptives, pregnancy, postmenopausal hormone replacement, surgery, and trauma.

PATHOPHYSIOLOGY
Embolization

When venous thrombi are dislodged from their site of formation, they embolize to the pulmonary arterial circulation or, paradoxically, to the arterial circulation through a patent foramen ovale or atrial septal defect. About one-half of patients with pelvic vein thrombosis or proximal leg DVT develop PE, which is often asymptomatic. Isolated calf vein thrombi pose a much lower risk of PE but are the most common source of paradoxical embolism. These tiny thrombi can traverse a patent foramen ovale or atrial septal defect, unlike larger, more proximal leg thrombi. With increased use of chronic indwelling central venous catheters for hyperalimentation and chemotherapy, as well as more frequent insertion of permanent pacemakers and internal cardiac defibrillators, upper extremity venous thrombosis is becoming a more common problem. These thrombi rarely embolize and cause PE.

Physiology

The most common gas exchange abnormalities are hypoxemia (decreased arterial P_{O_2}) and an increased alveolar-arterial O_2 tension gradient, which represents the inefficiency of O_2 transfer across the lungs. Anatomic dead space increases because breathed gas does not enter gas exchange units of the lung. Physiologic dead space increases because ventilation to gas exchange units exceeds venous blood flow through the pulmonary capillaries.

Other pathophysiologic abnormalities include the following:

1. *Increased pulmonary vascular resistance* due to vascular obstruction or platelet secretion of vasoconstricting neurohumoral agents such as serotonin. Release of vasoactive mediators can produce ventilation-perfusion mismatching at sites remote from the embolus, thereby accounting for a potential discordance between a small PE and a large alveolar-arterial O_2 gradient.
2. *Impaired gas exchange* due to increased alveolar dead space from vascular obstruction, hypoxemia from alveolar hypoventilation relative to perfusion in the nonobstructed lung, right-to-left shunting, and impaired carbon monoxide transfer due to loss of gas exchange surface.
3. *Alveolar hyperventilation* due to reflex stimulation of irritant receptors.
4. *Increased airway resistance* due to constriction of airways distal to the bronchi.
5. *Decreased pulmonary compliance* due to lung edema, lung hemorrhage, or loss of surfactant.

Right-ventricular (RV) dysfunction

Progressive right heart failure is the usual cause of death from PE. As pulmonary vascular resistance increases, RV wall tension rises and causes further RV dilation and dysfunction. RV contraction continues even after the left ventricle (LV) starts relaxing at end-systole. Consequently, the interventricular septum bulges into and compresses an intrinsically normal left ventricle. Diastolic LV impairment develops, attributable to septal displacement, and results in reduced LV distensibility and impaired LV filling during diastole. Increased RV wall tension also compresses the right coronary artery, diminishes subendocardial perfusion, limits myocardial oxygen supply, and may precipitate myocardial ischemia and RV infarction. Underfilling of the LV may lead to a fall in left-ventricular cardiac output and systemic arterial pressure, thereby provoking myocardial ischemia due to compromised coronary artery perfusion. Eventually, circulatory collapse and death may ensue.

DIAGNOSIS
Clinical evaluation

VTE mimics other illnesses, and PE is known as "the Great Masquerader," making diagnosis difficult. Occult PE is especially hard to detect when it occurs concomitantly with overt heart failure or pneumonia. In such circumstances, clinical improvement often fails to occur despite standard medical treatment of the concomitant illness. This scenario is a clinical clue to the possible coexistence of PE.

For patients who have DVT, the most common history is a cramp in the lower calf that persists for several days and becomes more uncomfortable as time progresses. For patients who have PE, the most common history is unexplained breathlessness.

In evaluating patients with possible VTE, the initial task is to decide on the clinical likelihood of the disorder. Patients with a low likelihood of DVT or a low-to-moderate likelihood of PE can undergo initial diagnostic evaluation with D-dimer testing alone (see "Blood tests") without obligatory imaging tests (Fig. 20-1). If the D-dimer is abnormally elevated, imaging tests are the next step.

Point score methods are useful for estimating the clinical likelihood of DVT and PE (Table 20-1).

Clinical syndromes

The differential diagnosis is critical because not all leg pain is due to DVT and not all dyspnea is due to PE (Table 20-2). Sudden, severe calf discomfort suggests a ruptured Baker's cyst. Fever and chills usually herald cellulitis rather than DVT, though DVT may be present

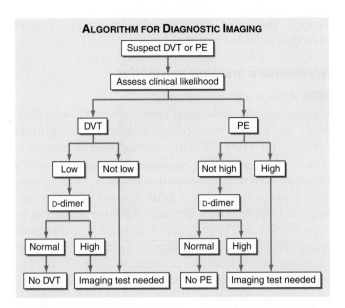

FIGURE 20-1

How to decide whether diagnostic imaging is needed. For assessment of clinical likelihood, see Table 20-1.

TABLE 20-1

CLINICAL DECISION RULES

Low Clinical Likelihood of DVT if Point Score Is Zero or Less; Moderate-Likelihood Score Is 1 to 2; High-Likelihood Score Is 3 or Greater

CLINICAL VARIABLE	SCORE
Active cancer	1
Paralysis, paresis, or recent cast	1
Bedridden for >3 days; major surgery <12 weeks	1
Tenderness along distribution of deep veins	1
Entire leg swelling	1
Unilateral calf swelling >3 cm	1
Pitting edema	1
Collateral superficial nonvaricose veins	1
Alternative diagnosis at least as likely as DVT	–2

High Clinical Likelihood of PE if Point Score Exceeds 4

CLINICAL VARIABLE	SCORE
Signs and symptoms of DVT	3.0
Alternative diagnosis less likely than PE	3.0
Heart rate >100/min	1.5
Immobilization >3 days; surgery within 4 weeks	1.5
Prior PE or DVT	1.5
Hemoptysis	1.0
Cancer	1.0

TABLE 20-2

DIFFERENTIAL DIAGNOSIS

DVT
　Ruptured Baker's cyst
　Cellulitis
　Postphlebitic syndrome/venous insufficiency
PE
　Pneumonia, asthma, chronic obstructive pulmonary disease
　Congestive heart failure
　Pericarditis
　Pleurisy: "viral syndrome," costochondritis, musculoskeletal discomfort
　Rib fracture, pneumothorax
　Acute coronary syndrome
　Anxiety

concomitantly. Physical findings, if present at all, may consist only of mild palpation discomfort in the lower calf. Massive DVT is much easier to recognize. The patient presents with marked thigh swelling and tenderness during palpation of the common femoral vein. In extreme cases, patients are unable to walk or may require a cane, crutches, or a walker.

If the leg is diffusely edematous, DVT is unlikely. More probable is an acute exacerbation of venous insufficiency due to postphlebitic syndrome. Upper extremity venous thrombosis may present with asymmetry in the supraclavicular fossa or in the circumference of the upper arms. A prominent superficial venous pattern may be evident on the anterior chest wall.

Patients with *massive PE* present with systemic arterial hypotension and usually have anatomically widespread thromboembolism. Those with *moderate to large PE* have RV hypokinesis on echocardiography but normal systemic arterial pressure. Patients with *small to moderate PE* have both normal right heart function and normal systemic arterial pressure. They have an excellent prognosis with adequate anticoagulation.

The presence of *pulmonary infarction* usually indicates a small PE but one that is exquisitely painful because it lodges peripherally, near the innervation of pleural nerves. Pleuritic chest pain is more common with small, peripheral emboli. However, larger, more central PEs can occur concomitantly with peripheral pulmonary infarction.

Nonthrombotic PE may be easily overlooked. Possible etiologies include fat embolism after pelvic or long bone fracture, tumor embolism, bone marrow, and air embolism. Cement embolism and bony fragment embolism can occur after total hip or knee replacement. Intravenous drug users may inject themselves with a wide array of substances that can embolize such as hair, talc, and cotton. *Amniotic fluid embolism* occurs when fetal membranes leak or tear at the placental margin. Pulmonary edema in this syndrome probably is due to alveolar capillary leakage.

Dyspnea is the most common symptom of PE, and tachypnea is the most common sign. Dyspnea, syncope, hypotension, or cyanosis indicates a massive PE, whereas pleuritic pain, cough, or hemoptysis often suggests a small embolism situated distally near the pleura. On physical examination, young and previously healthy individuals may appear anxious but otherwise seem well, even with an anatomically large PE. They may have dyspnea only with moderate exertion. They often lack "classic" signs such as tachycardia, low-grade fever, neck vein distention, and an accentuated pulmonic component of the second heart sound. Sometimes paradoxical bradycardia occurs.

Nonimaging diagnostic modalities

Nonimaging tests are best utilized in combination with clinical likelihood assessment of DVT or PE (Fig. 20-1).

Blood tests

The quantitative *plasma D-dimer enzyme-linked immunosorbent assay (ELISA)* rises in the presence of DVT or PE because of the breakdown of fibrin by plasmin. Elevation of D-dimer indicates endogenous although often clinically ineffective thrombolysis. The sensitivity of the D-dimer is >80% for DVT (including isolated calf DVT) and >95% for PE. The D-dimer is less sensitive for DVT than for PE because the DVT thrombus size is smaller. The D-dimer is a useful "rule out" test. More than 95% of patients with a normal (<500 ng/mL) D-dimer do not have PE. The D-dimer assay is not specific. Levels increase in patients with myocardial infarction, pneumonia, sepsis, cancer, and the postoperative state and those in the second or third trimester of pregnancy. Therefore, D-dimer rarely has a useful role among hospitalized patients, because levels are frequently elevated due to systemic illness.

Contrary to classic teaching, *arterial blood gases* lack diagnostic utility for PE, even though both P_{O_2} and Pc_{O_2} often decrease. Among patients suspected of having PE, neither the room air arterial P_{O_2} nor calculation of the alveolar-arterial O_2 gradient can reliably differentiate or triage patients who actually have PE at angiography.

Elevated cardiac biomarkers

Serum troponin and plasma heart-type fatty acid–binding protein levels increase because of RV microinfarction. Myocardial stretch results in elevation of brain natriuretic peptide or NT-pro-brain natriuretic peptide. Elevated cardiac biomarkers predict an increase in major complications and mortality from PE.

Electrocardiogram

The most frequently cited abnormality, in addition to sinus tachycardia, is the S1Q3T3 sign: an S wave in lead I, a Q wave in lead III, and an inverted T wave in lead III. This finding is relatively specific but insensitive. Perhaps the most common abnormality is T-wave inversion in leads V_1 to V_4.

Noninvasive imaging modalities

Venous ultrasonography

Ultrasonography of the deep venous system (Table 20-3) relies on loss of vein compressibility as the primary criterion for DVT. When a normal vein is imaged in cross-section, it readily collapses with gentle manual pressure from the ultrasound transducer. This creates the illusion of a "wink." With acute DVT, the vein loses its compressibility because of passive distention by acute thrombus. The diagnosis of acute DVT is even more secure when thrombus is directly visualized. It appears homogeneous and has low echogenicity (Fig. 20-2). The vein itself often appears mildly dilated, and collateral channels may be absent.

Venous flow dynamics can be examined with Doppler imaging. Normally, manual calf compression causes augmentation of the Doppler flow pattern. Loss of normal respiratory variation is caused by an obstructing DVT or by any obstructive process within the pelvis. Because DVT and PE are so closely related and are both treated with anticoagulation (see "Treatment Deep Venous Thrombosis") confirmed DVT is usually an adequate surrogate for PE. In contrast, a normal venous ultrasound does not exclude PE. About one-half of patients with PE have no imaging evidence of DVT, probably because the clot already has embolized to the lung or is in the pelvic veins, where ultrasonography is usually inadequate. In patients without DVT, the ultrasound examination may identify other reasons for leg discomfort, such as a Baker's cyst (also known as a popliteal or synovial cyst) or a hematoma. For patients with a technically poor or nondiagnostic venous ultrasound, one should consider alternative imaging modalities for DVT, such as computed tomography (CT) and magnetic resonance imaging.

TABLE 20-3

ULTRASONOGRAPHY OF THE DEEP LEG VEINS
Criteria for Establishing the Diagnosis of Acute DVT
Lack of vein compressibility (principal criterion)   Vein does not "wink" when gently compressed in cross-section   Failure to appose walls of vein due to passive distention
Direct Visualization of Thrombus
Homogeneous   Low echogenicity
Abnormal Doppler Flow Dynamics
Normal response: calf compression augments Doppler flow signal and confirms vein patency proximal and distal to Doppler   Abnormal response: flow blunted rather than augmented with calf compression

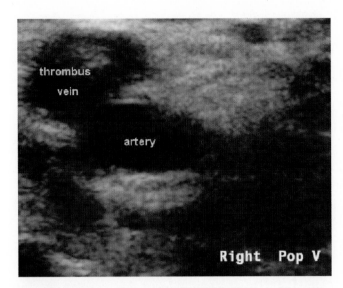

FIGURE 20-2
Acute popliteal DVT on venous ultrasound in a 56-year-old man receiving chemotherapy for lung cancer.

Chest roentgenography

A normal or nearly normal chest x-ray often occurs in PE. Well-established abnormalities include focal oligemia (Westermark's sign), a peripheral wedged-shaped density above the diaphragm (Hampton's hump), and an enlarged right descending pulmonary artery (Palla's sign).

Chest CT

Computed tomography of the chest with intravenous contrast is the principal imaging test for the diagnosis of PE (Fig. 20–3). Multidetector-row spiral CT acquires all chest images with ≤1 mm of resolution during a short breath hold. This generation of CT scanners can image small peripheral emboli. Sixth-order branches can be visualized with resolution superior to that of conventional invasive contrast pulmonary angiography. The CT scan also obtains excellent images of the RV and LV and can be used for risk stratification along with its use as a diagnostic tool. In patients with PE, RV enlargement on chest CT indicates an increased likelihood of death within the next 30 days compared with PE patients who have normal RV size on chest CT. When imaging is continued below the chest to the knee, pelvic and proximal leg DVT also can be diagnosed by CT scanning. In patients without PE, the lung parenchymal images may establish alternative diagnoses not apparent on chest x-ray that explain the presenting symptoms and signs such as pneumonia, emphysema, pulmonary fibrosis, pulmonary mass, and aortic pathology. Sometimes asymptomatic early-stage lung cancer is diagnosed incidentally.

Lung scanning

Lung scanning has become a second-line diagnostic test for PE, used mostly for patients who cannot tolerate

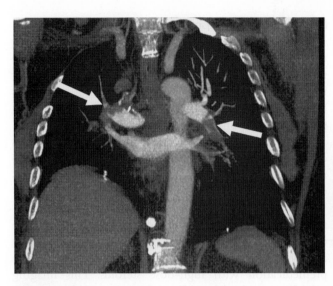

FIGURE 20-3
Large bilateral proximal PE on a coronal chest CT image in a 54-year-old man with lung cancer and brain metastases. He had developed sudden onset of chest heaviness and shortness of breath while at home. There are filling defects in the main and segmental pulmonary arteries bilaterally (*white arrows*). Only the left upper lobe segmental artery is free of thrombus.

intravenous contrast. Small particulate aggregates of albumin labeled with a gamma-emitting radionuclide are injected intravenously and are trapped in the pulmonary capillary bed. The perfusion scan defect indicates absent or decreased blood flow, possibly due to PE. Ventilation scans, obtained with a radiolabeled inhaled gas such as xenon or krypton, improve the specificity of the perfusion scan. Abnormal ventilation scans indicate abnormal nonventilated lung, thereby providing possible explanations for perfusion defects other than acute PE, such as asthma and chronic obstructive pulmonary disease. A high-probability scan for PE is defined as one that indicates two or more segmental perfusion defects in the presence of normal ventilation.

The diagnosis of PE is very unlikely in patients with normal and nearly normal scans but is about 90% certain in patients with high-probability scans. Unfortunately, most patients have nondiagnostic scans, and fewer than one-half of patients with angiographically confirmed PE have a high probability scan. As many as 40% of patients with high clinical suspicion for PE and "low-probability" scans do, in fact, have PE at angiography.

Magnetic resonance (MR) (contrast-enhanced)

When ultrasound is equivocal, MR venography with gadolinium contrast is an excellent imaging modality to diagnose DVT. MR imaging should be considered for suspected VTE patients with renal insufficiency or contrast dye allergy. MR pulmonary angiography may detect large proximal PE but is not reliable for smaller segmental and subsegmental PE.

Echocardiography

Echocardiography is *not* a reliable diagnostic imaging tool for acute PE because most patients with PE have normal echocardiograms. However, echocardiography is a very useful diagnostic tool for detecting conditions that may mimic PE, such as acute myocardial infarction, pericardial tamponade, and aortic dissection.

Transthoracic echocardiography rarely images thrombus directly. The best-known indirect sign of PE on transthoracic echocardiography is McConnell's sign: hypokinesis of the RV free wall with normal motion of the RV apex.

One should consider transesophageal echocardiography when CT scanning facilities are not available or when a patient has renal failure or severe contrast allergy that precludes administration of contrast despite premedication with high-dose steroids. This imaging modality can identify saddle, right main, or left main PE.

Invasive diagnostic modalities

Pulmonary angiography

Chest CT with contrast (see earlier) has virtually replaced invasive pulmonary angiography as a diagnostic test. Invasive catheter-based diagnostic testing is reserved for patients with technically unsatisfactory chest CTs and those in whom an interventional procedure such as catheter-directed thrombolysis or embolectomy is planned. A definitive diagnosis of PE depends on visualization of an intraluminal filling defect in more than one projection. Secondary signs of PE include abrupt occlusion ("cut-off") of vessels, segmental oligemia or avascularity, a prolonged arterial phase with slow filling, and tortuous, tapering peripheral vessels.

Contrast phlebography

Venous ultrasonography has virtually replaced contrast phlebography as the diagnostic test for suspected DVT.

Integrated diagnostic approach

An integrated diagnostic approach (Fig. 20-1) streamlines the workup of suspected DVT and PE (Fig. 20-4).

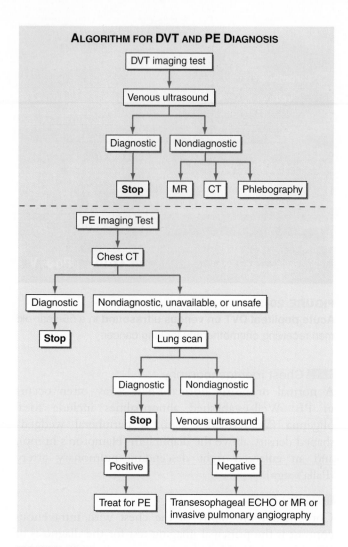

ALGORITHM FOR DVT AND PE DIAGNOSIS

FIGURE 20-4
Imaging tests to diagnose DVT and PE.

strategy. The presence of hemodynamic instability, RV dysfunction, RV enlargement, or elevation of the troponin level due to RV microinfarction can identify high-risk patients. RV hypokinesis on echocardiography, RV enlargement on chest CT, and troponin elevation predict an increased mortality rate from PE.

Primary therapy should be reserved for patients at high risk of an adverse clinical outcome. When RV function remains normal in a hemodynamically stable patient, a good clinical outcome is highly likely with anticoagulation alone (Fig. 20-5).

TREATMENT   Pulmonary Embolism

PRIMARY THERAPY VERSUS SECONDARY PREVENTION *Primary therapy* consists of clot dissolution with thrombolysis or removal of PE by embolectomy. Anticoagulation with heparin and warfarin or placement of an inferior vena caval filter constitutes *secondary prevention* of recurrent PE rather than primary therapy.

RISK STRATIFICATION Rapid and accurate risk stratification is critical in determining the optimal treatment

---

TREATMENT   Massive Pulmonary Embolism

ANTICOAGULATION Anticoagulation is the foundation for successful treatment of DVT and PE (Table 20-4). Immediately effective anticoagulation is initiated with a parenteral drug: unfractionated heparin (UFH), low-molecular-weight heparin (LMWH), or fondaparinux.

ALGORITHM FOR PE MANAGEMENT

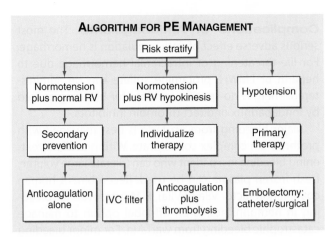

FIGURE 20-5

Acute management of pulmonary thromboembolism. RV, right ventricular; IVC, inferior vena cava.

One should use a direct thrombin inhibitor—argatroban, lepirudin, or bivalirudin—in patients with proven or suspected heparin-induced thrombocytopenia. Parenteral agents are continued as a transition or "bridge" to stable, long-term anticoagulation with a vitamin K antagonist (exclusively warfarin in the United States). Warfarin requires 5–7 days to achieve a therapeutic effect. During that period, one should overlap the parenteral and oral agents. After 5–7 days of anticoagulation, residual thrombus begins to endothelialize in the vein or pulmonary artery. However, anticoagulants do *not* directly dissolve thrombus that already exists.

Unfractionated Heparin Unfractionated heparin anticoagulates by binding to and accelerating the activity of antithrombin, thus preventing additional thrombus formation and permitting endogenous fibrinolytic mechanisms to lyse clot that already has formed. UFH is dosed

TABLE 20-4

ANTICOAGULATION OF VTE

Immediate Parenteral Anticoagulation

Unfractionated heparin, bolus and continuous infusion, to achieve aPTT two to three times the upper limit of the laboratory normal, *or*
Enoxaparin 1 mg/kg twice daily with normal renal function, *or*
Dalteparin 200 U/kg once daily or 100 U/kg twice daily, with normal renal function, *or*
Tinzaparin 175 U/kg once daily with normal renal function, *or*
Fondaparinux weight-based once daily; adjust for impaired renal function

Warfarin Anticoagulation

Usual start dose is 5 mg
Titrate to INR, target 2.0–3.0
Continue parenteral anticoagulation for a minimum of 5 days and until two sequential INR values, at least 1 day apart, achieve the target INR range.

to achieve a target activated partial thromboplastin time (aPTT) that is 2–3 times the upper limit of the laboratory normal. This is usually equivalent to an aPTT of 60–80 s. For UFH, a typical intravenous bolus is 5000–10,000 units followed by a continuous infusion of 1000–1500 U/h. Nomograms based on a patient's weight may assist in adjusting the dose of heparin. The most popular nomogram utilizes an initial bolus of 80 U/kg, followed by an initial infusion rate of 18/kg per h.

The major advantage of UFH is its short half-life. This is especially useful if the patient may undergo an invasive procedure such as embolectomy. The major disadvantage of UFH is that achieving the target aPTT is empirical and may require repeated blood sampling and heparin dose adjustment every 4–6 h. Furthermore, patients are at risk of developing heparin-induced thrombocytopenia.

Low-Molecular-Weight Heparins These fragments of UFH exhibit less binding to plasma proteins and endothelial cells and consequently have greater bioavailability, a more predictable dose response, and a longer half-life than does UFH. No monitoring or dose adjustment is needed unless the patient is markedly obese or has chronic kidney disease.

There are two commonly used LMWH preparations in the United States: enoxaparin and dalteparin. *Enoxaparin* is approved as a bridge to warfarin for VTE. *Dalteparin* is also approved as monotherapy without warfarin for symptomatic VTE patients with cancer in a dose of 200 U/kg once daily for 30 days, followed by 150 U/kg once daily for months 2–6. These weight-adjusted LMWH doses must be reduced in patients with chronic kidney disease because the kidneys metabolize LMWH.

Fondaparinux Fondaparinux, an anti-Xa pentasaccharide, is administered as a once-daily subcutaneous injection in a prefilled syringe to treat DVT and PE as a "bridge" to warfarin. No laboratory monitoring is required. Patients weighing <50 kg receive 5 mg, patients weighing 50–100 kg receive 7.5 mg, and patients weighing >100 kg receive 10 mg. Fondaparinux is synthesized in a laboratory and, unlike LMWH or UFH, is not derived from animal products. It does not cause heparin-induced thrombocytopenia. The dose must be adjusted downward for patients with renal dysfunction because the kidneys metabolize the drug.

Warfarin This vitamin K antagonist prevents carboxylation activation of coagulation factors II, VII, IX, and X. The full effect of warfarin requires at least 5 days even if the prothrombin time, used for monitoring, becomes elevated more rapidly. If warfarin is initiated as monotherapy during an acute thrombotic illness, a paradoxical exacerbation of hypercoagulability can increase the likelihood of thrombosis rather than prevent it. Overlapping UFH, LMWH, or fondaparinux with warfarin for at least 5 days can counteract the early procoagulant effect of unopposed warfarin.

Warfarin Dosing In an average-size adult, warfarin usually is initiated in a dose of 5 mg. Doses of 7.5 or 10 mg can be used in obese or large-framed young patients who are otherwise healthy. Patients who are malnourished or who have received prolonged courses of antibiotics are probably deficient in vitamin K and should receive smaller initial doses of warfarin, such as 2.5 mg. The prothrombin time is standardized by calculating the international normalized ratio (INR), which assesses the anticoagulant effect of warfarin. The target INR is usually 2.5, with a range of 2.0–3.0.

The warfarin dose is titrated to achieve the target INR. Proper dosing is difficult because hundreds of drug-drug and drug-food interactions affect warfarin metabolism. Variables such as increasing age and comorbidities such as systemic illness reduce the required warfarin dose. Pharmacogenomics may provide more precise initial dosing of warfarin, especially for patients who require unusually large or small doses. *CYP2C9* variant alleles impair the hydroxylation of S-warfarin, thereby lowering the dose requirement. Variants in the gene encoding the vitamin K epoxide reductase complex 1 (*VKORC1*) can predict whether patients require low, moderate, or high warfarin doses. Nevertheless, more than half of warfarin dosing variability is caused by clinical factors such as age, sex, weight, concomitant drugs, and comorbid illnesses.

Nomograms have been developed (*www.warfarindosing.org*) to help clinicians initiate warfarin dosing based on clinical information and, if available, pharmacogenetic data. However, most practitioners utilize empirical dosing with an "educated guess." Centralized anticoagulation clinics have improved the efficacy and safety of warfarin dosing. Patients maintain a therapeutic INR more often if they self-monitor their INR with a home point-of-care fingerstick machine rather than obtaining a coagulation laboratory INR. The patient subgroup with the best results self-adjusts warfarin doses as well as self-tests INRs.

Novel Anticoagulants Novel oral anticoagulants are administered in a fixed dose, establish effective anticoagulation within hours of administration, require no laboratory coagulation monitoring, and have few of the drug-drug or drug-food interactions that make warfarin so difficult to dose. Rivaroxaban, a factor Xa inhibitor, and dabigatran, a direct thrombin inhibitor, are approved in Canada and Europe for prevention of VTE after total hip and total knee replacement. In a large-scale trial of acute VTE treatment, dabigatran was as effective as warfarin and had less nonmajor bleeding. Because of these drugs' rapid onset of action and relatively short half-life compared with warfarin, "bridging" with a parenteral anticoagulant is not required.

Complications of Anticoagulants The most serious adverse effect of anticoagulation is hemorrhage. For life-threatening or intracranial hemorrhage due to heparin or LMWH, protamine sulfate can be administered. There is no specific antidote for bleeding caused by fondaparinux or direct thrombin inhibitors.

Major bleeding from warfarin is best managed with prothrombin complex concentrate. With non-life threatening bleeding in a patient who can tolerate large volume, fresh-frozen plasma can be used. Recombinant human coagulation factor VIIa (rFVIIa), FDA-approved for bleeding in hemophiliacs, is an off-label option to manage catastrophic bleeding from warfarin. For minor bleeding or to manage an excessively high INR in the absence of bleeding, oral vitamin K may be administered.

Heparin-induced thrombocytopenia (HIT) and osteopenia are far less common with LMWH than with UFH. Thrombosis due to HIT should be managed with a direct thrombin inhibitor: argatroban for patients with renal insufficiency and lepirudin for patients with hepatic failure. In the setting of percutaneous coronary intervention, one should administer bivalirudin.

During pregnancy, warfarin should be avoided if possible because of warfarin embryopathy, which is most common with exposure during the sixth through twelfth week of gestation. However, women can take warfarin postpartum and breast-feed safely. Warfarin can also be administered safely during the second trimester.

Duration of Hospital Stay Acute DVT patients with good family and social support, permanent residence, telephone service, and no hearing or language impairment often can be managed as outpatients. They, a family member, or a visiting nurse must administer a parenteral anticoagulant. Warfarin dosing can be titrated to the INR and adjusted on an outpatient basis.

Acute PE patients, who traditionally have required hospital stays of 5–7 days for intravenous heparin as a "bridge" to warfarin, can be considered for abbreviated hospitalization if they have a reliable support system at home and an excellent prognosis. Criteria include clinical stability, absence of chest pain or shortness of breath, normal RV size and function, and normal levels of cardiac biomarkers.

Duration of Anticoagulation Patients with PE after surgery, trauma, or estrogen exposure (from oral contraceptives, pregnancy, or postmenopausal therapy) ordinarily have a low rate of recurrence after 3–6 months of anticoagulation. For DVT isolated to an upper extremity or calf that has been provoked by surgery, trauma, estrogen, or an indwelling central venous catheter or pacemaker, 3 months of anticoagulation suffices. For provoked proximal leg DVT or PE, 3 to 6 months of anticoagulation is sufficient. For patients with cancer and

VTE, the consensus is to prescribe 3–6 months of LMWH as monotherapy without warfarin and to continue anticoagulation indefinitely unless the patient is rendered cancer-free. However, there is uncertainty whether subsequent anticoagulation should continue with LMWH or whether the patient should be placed on warfarin.

Among patients with idiopathic, unprovoked VTE, the recurrence rate is high after cessation of anticoagulation. VTE that occurs during long-haul air travel is considered unprovoked. It appears that unprovoked VTE is often a chronic illness, with latent periods between flares of recurrent episodes. American College of Chest Physicians (ACCP) guidelines recommend considering anticoagulation for an indefinite duration with a target INR between 2 and 3 for patients with idiopathic VTE. An alternative approach after the first 6 months of anticoagulation is to reduce the intensity of anticoagulation and to lower the target INR range to between 1.5 and 2.

Counterintuitively, the presence of genetic mutations such as heterozygous factor V Leiden and prothrombin gene mutation do not appear to increase the risk of recurrent VTE. However, patients with moderate or high levels of anticardiolipin antibodies probably warrant indefinite-duration anticoagulation even if the initial VTE was provoked by trauma or surgery.

INFERIOR VENA CAVAL (IVC) FILTERS

The two principal indications for insertion of an IVC filter are (1) active bleeding that precludes anticoagulation and (2) recurrent venous thrombosis despite intensive anticoagulation. Prevention of recurrent PE in patients with right heart failure who are not candidates for fibrinolysis and prophylaxis of extremely high-risk patients are "softer" indications for filter placement. The filter itself may fail by permitting the passage of small- to medium-size clots. Large thrombi may embolize to the pulmonary arteries via collateral veins that develop. A more common complication is caval thrombosis with marked bilateral leg swelling.

Paradoxically, by providing a nidus for clot formation, filters double the DVT rate over the ensuing 2 years after placement. Retrievable filters can now be placed for patients with an anticipated temporary bleeding disorder or for patients at temporary high risk of PE, such as individuals undergoing bariatric surgery who have a prior history of perioperative PE. The filters can be retrieved up to several months after insertion unless thrombus forms and is trapped within the filter. The retrievable filter becomes permanent if it remains in place or if, for technical reasons such as rapid endothelialization, it cannot be removed.

MAINTAINING ADEQUATE CIRCULATION

For patients with massive PE and hypotension, one should administer 500 mL of normal saline. Additional fluid should be infused with extreme caution because excessive fluid administration exacerbates RV wall stress, causes more profound RV ischemia, and worsens LV compliance and filling by causing further interventricular septal shift toward the LV. Dopamine and dobutamine are first-line inotropic agents for treatment of PE-related shock. There should be a low threshold for initiating these pressors. Often, a "trial-and-error" approach works best; one should consider norepinephrine, vasopressin, or phenylephrine.

FIBRINOLYSIS Successful fibrinolytic therapy rapidly reverses right heart failure and may result in a lower rate of death and recurrent PE by (1) dissolving much of the anatomically obstructing pulmonary arterial thrombus, (2) preventing the continued release of serotonin and other neurohumoral factors that exacerbate pulmonary hypertension, and (3) lysing much of the source of the thrombus in the pelvic or deep leg veins, thereby decreasing the likelihood of recurrent PE.

The preferred fibrinolytic regimen is 100 mg of recombinant tissue plasminogen activator (tPA) administered as a continuous peripheral intravenous infusion over 2 h. Patients appear to respond to fibrinolysis for up to 14 days after the PE has occurred.

Contraindications to fibrinolysis include intracranial disease, recent surgery, and trauma. The overall major bleeding rate is about 10%, including a 1–3% risk of intracranial hemorrhage. Careful screening of patients for contraindications to fibrinolytic therapy (Chap. 33) is the best way to minimize bleeding risk.

The only FDA-approved indication for PE fibrinolysis is massive PE. For patients with preserved systolic blood pressure and submassive PE with moderate or severe RV dysfunction, ACCP guidelines for fibrinolysis recommend individual patient risk assessment of the thrombotic burden versus the bleeding risk.

PULMONARY EMBOLECTOMY The risk of intracranial hemorrhage with fibrinolysis has prompted a renaissance of surgical embolectomy. More prompt referral before the onset of irreversible cardiogenic shock and multisystem organ failure and improved surgical technique have resulted in a high survival rate. A possible alternative to open surgical embolectomy is catheter embolectomy. New-generation catheters are under development.

PULMONARY THROMBOENDARTERECTOMY Chronic thromboembolic pulmonary hypertension occurs in 2–4% of acute PE patients. Therefore, PE patients who have initial pulmonary hypertension (usually diagnosed with Doppler echocardiography) should be followed up at about 6 weeks with a repeat echocardiogram to determine whether pulmonary arterial pressure has normalized. Patients impaired by dyspnea due to chronic thromboembolic pulmonary hypertension should be considered for pulmonary thromboendarterectomy, which, if successful, can markedly reduce, and at times even cure, pulmonary hypertension. The operation requires median sternotomy, cardiopulmonary bypass, deep hypothermia, and periods of hypothermic circulatory arrest. The mortality rate at experienced centers is approximately 5%.

EMOTIONAL SUPPORT Patients with VTE may feel overwhelmed when they learn that they are susceptible to recurrent PE or DVT. They worry about the health of their families and the genetic implications of their illness. Those who are advised to discontinue warfarin after 3–6 months of therapy may feel especially vulnerable. At Brigham and Woman's Hospital a physican-nurse–facilitated PE support group has been maintained for patients and has met monthly for more than 15 years.

PREVENTION OF POSTPHLEBITIC SYN-DROME Daily use of below-knee 30- to 40-mmHg vascular compression stockings will halve the rate of developing postphlebitic syndrome. These stockings should be prescribed as soon as DVT is diagnosed and should be fitted carefully to maximize their benefit. When patients are in bed, the stockings need not be worn.

PREVENTION OF VTE

Prophylaxis (Table 20-5) is of paramount importance because VTE is difficult to detect and poses a profound medical and economic burden. Computerized reminder systems can increase the use of preventive measures and at Brigham and Women's Hospital have reduced the symptomatic VTE rate by more than 40%. Patients who have undergone total hip or knee replacement or cancer surgery will benefit from extended pharmacologic prophylaxis for a total of 4–5 weeks.

TABLE 20-5

PREVENTION OF VENOUS THROMBOEMBOLISM	
CONDITION	PROPHYLAXIS STRATEGY
High-risk general surgery	Mini-UFH or LMWH
Thoracic surgery	Mini-UFH + IPC
Cancer surgery, including gynecologic cancer surgery	LMWH, consider 1 month of prophylaxis
Total hip replacement, total knee replacement, hip fracture surgery	LMWH, fondaparinux (a pentasaccharide) 2.5 mg SC, once daily, or (except for total knee replacement) warfarin (target INR 2.5); rivaroxaban or dalteparin in countries where it is approved
Neurosurgery	IPC
Neurosurgery for brain tumor	Mini-UFH or LMWH, + IPC + predischarge venous ultrasonography
Benign gynecologic surgery	Mini-UFH
Medically ill patients	Mini-UFH or LMWH
Anticoagulation contraindicated	IPC
Long-haul air travel	Consider LMWH for very high-risk patients

Note: Mini-UFH, mini-dose unfractionated heparin, 5000 units subcutaneously twice (less effective) or three times daily (more effective); LMWH, low-molecular-weight heparin, typically in the United States enoxaparin, 40 mg once daily, or dalteparin, 2500 or 5000 units once daily; IPC, intermittent pneumatic compression devices.

CHAPTER 21

DISORDERS OF THE PLEURA AND MEDIASTINUM

Richard W. Light

DISORDERS OF THE PLEURA

PLEURAL EFFUSION

The pleural space lies between the lung and the chest wall and normally contains a very thin layer of fluid, which serves as a coupling system. A pleural effusion is present when there is an excess quantity of fluid in the pleural space.

Etiology

Pleural fluid accumulates when pleural fluid formation exceeds pleural fluid absorption. Normally, fluid enters the pleural space from the capillaries in the parietal pleura and is removed via the lymphatics in the parietal pleura. Fluid also can enter the pleural space from the interstitial spaces of the lung via the visceral pleura or from the peritoneal cavity via small holes in the diaphragm. The lymphatics have the capacity to absorb 20 times more fluid than is formed normally. Accordingly, a pleural effusion may develop when there is excess pleural fluid formation (from the interstitial spaces of the lung, the parietal pleura, or the peritoneal cavity) or when there is decreased fluid removal by the lymphatics.

Diagnostic approach

When a patient is found to have a pleural effusion, an effort should be made to determine the cause (Fig. 21-1). The first step is to determine whether the effusion is a transudate or an exudate. A *transudative pleural effusion* occurs when *systemic factors* that influence the formation and absorption of pleural fluid are altered. The leading causes of transudative pleural effusions in the United States are left-ventricular failure and cirrhosis. An *exudative pleural effusion* occurs when *local factors* that influence the formation and absorption of pleural fluid

are altered. The leading causes of exudative pleural effusions are bacterial pneumonia, malignancy, viral infection, and pulmonary embolism. The primary reason for making this differentiation is that additional diagnostic procedures are indicated with exudative effusions to define the cause of the local disease.

Transudative and exudative pleural effusions are distinguished by measuring the lactate dehydrogenase (LDH) and protein levels in the pleural fluid. Exudative pleural effusions meet at least one of the following criteria, whereas transudative pleural effusions meet none:

1. Pleural fluid protein/serum protein >0.5
2. Pleural fluid LDH/serum LDH >0.6
3. Pleural fluid LDH more than two-thirds normal upper limit for serum

These criteria misidentify ~25% of transudates as exudates. If one or more of the exudative criteria are met and the patient is clinically thought to have a condition producing a transudative effusion, the difference between the protein levels in the serum and the pleural fluid should be measured. If this gradient is >31 g/L (3.1 g/dL), the exudative categorization by these criteria can be ignored because almost all such patients have a transudative pleural effusion.

If a patient has an exudative pleural effusion, the following tests on the pleural fluid should be obtained: description of the appearance of the fluid, glucose level, differential cell count, microbiologic studies, and cytology.

Effusion due to heart failure

The most common cause of pleural effusion is left-ventricular failure. The effusion occurs because the increased amounts of fluid in the lung interstitial spaces exit in part across the visceral pleura; this overwhelms

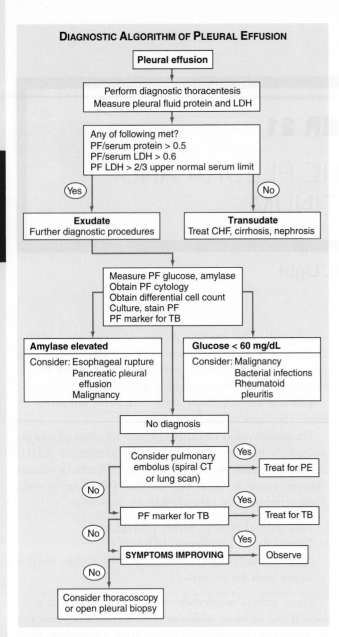

FIGURE 21-1
Approach to the diagnosis of pleural effusions. CHF, congestive heart failure; CT, computed tomography; LDH, lactate dehydrogenase; PE, pulmonary embolism; TB, tuberculosis; PF, pleural fluid.

the capacity of the lymphatics in the parietal pleura to remove fluid. In patients with heart failure, a diagnostic thoracentesis should be performed if the effusions are not bilateral and comparable in size, if the patient is febrile, or if the patient has pleuritic chest pain to verify that the patient has a transudative effusion. Otherwise the patient's heart failure is treated. If the effusion persists despite therapy, a diagnostic thoracentesis should be performed. A pleural fluid N-terminal pro-brain natriuretic peptide (NT-proBNP) >1500 pg/mL is virtually diagnostic of an effusion secondary to congestive heart failure.

Hepatic hydrothorax

Pleural effusions occur in ~5% of patients with cirrhosis and ascites. The predominant mechanism is the direct movement of peritoneal fluid through small openings in the diaphragm into the pleural space. The effusion is usually right-sided and frequently is large enough to produce severe dyspnea.

Parapneumonic effusion

Parapneumonic effusions are associated with bacterial pneumonia, lung abscess, or bronchiectasis and are probably the most common cause of exudative pleural effusion in the United States. *Empyema* refers to a grossly purulent effusion.

Patients with aerobic bacterial pneumonia and pleural effusion present with an acute febrile illness consisting of chest pain, sputum production, and leukocytosis. Patients with anaerobic infections present with a subacute illness with weight loss, a brisk leukocytosis, mild anemia, and a history of some factor that predisposes them to aspiration.

The possibility of a parapneumonic effusion should be considered whenever a patient with bacterial pneumonia is initially evaluated. The presence of free pleural fluid can be demonstrated with a lateral decubitus radiograph, computed tomography (CT) of the chest, or ultrasound. If the free fluid separates the lung from the chest wall by >10 mm, a therapeutic thoracentesis should be performed. Factors indicating the likely need for a procedure more invasive than a thoracentesis (in increasing order of importance) include the following:

1. Loculated pleural fluid
2. Pleural fluid pH <7.20
3. Pleural fluid glucose <3.3 mmol/L (<60 mg/dL)
4. Positive Gram stain or culture of the pleural fluid
5. Presence of gross pus in the pleural space

If the fluid recurs after the initial therapeutic thoracentesis and if any of these characteristics are present, a repeat thoracentesis should be performed. If the fluid cannot be completely removed with the therapeutic thoracentesis, consideration should be given to inserting a chest tube and instilling a fibrinolytic agent (e.g., tissue plasminogen activator, 10 mg) or performing a thoracoscopy with the breakdown of adhesions. Decortication should be considered when these measures are ineffective.

Effusion secondary to malignancy

Malignant pleural effusions secondary to metastatic disease are the second most common type of exudative pleural effusion. The three tumors that cause ~75% of all malignant pleural effusions are lung carcinoma, breast carcinoma, and lymphoma. Most patients complain of dyspnea, which is frequently out of proportion to the size of the effusion. The pleural fluid is an exudate, and its glucose level may be reduced if the tumor burden in the pleural space is high.

The diagnosis usually is made via cytology of the pleural fluid. If the initial cytologic examination is negative, thoracoscopy is the best next procedure if malignancy is strongly suspected. At the time of thoracoscopy, a procedure such as pleural abrasion should be performed to effect a pleurodesis. An alternative to thoracoscopy is CT- or ultrasound-guided needle biopsy of pleural thickening or nodules. Patients with a malignant pleural effusion are treated symptomatically for the most part, since the presence of the effusion indicates disseminated disease and most malignancies associated with pleural effusion are not curable with chemotherapy. The only symptom that can be attributed to the effusion itself is dyspnea. If the patient's lifestyle is compromised by dyspnea and if the dyspnea is relieved with a therapeutic thoracentesis, one of the following procedures should be considered: (1) insertion of a small indwelling catheter or (2) tube thoracostomy with the instillation of a sclerosing agent such as doxycycline, 500 mg.

Mesothelioma

Malignant mesotheliomas are primary tumors that arise from the mesothelial cells that line the pleural cavities; most are related to asbestos exposure. Patients with mesothelioma present with chest pain and shortness of breath. The chest radiograph reveals a pleural effusion, generalized pleural thickening, and a shrunken hemithorax. Thoracoscopy or open pleural biopsy is usually necessary to establish the diagnosis. Chest pain should be treated with opiates, and shortness of breath with oxygen and/or opiates.

Effusion secondary to pulmonary embolization

The diagnosis most commonly overlooked in the differential diagnosis of a patient with an undiagnosed pleural effusion is pulmonary embolism. Dyspnea is the most common symptom. The pleural fluid is almost always an exudate. The diagnosis is established by spiral CT scan or pulmonary arteriography (Chap. 20). Treatment of a patient with a pleural effusion secondary to pulmonary embolism is the same as it is for any patient with pulmonary emboli. If the pleural effusion increases in size after anticoagulation, the patient probably has recurrent emboli or another complication, such as a hemothorax or a pleural infection.

Tuberculous pleuritis

(See also Chap. 12) In many parts of the world, the most common cause of an exudative pleural effusion is tuberculosis (TB), but tuberculous effusions are relatively uncommon in the United States. Tuberculous pleural effusions usually are associated with primary TB and are thought to be due primarily to a hypersensitivity reaction to tuberculous protein in the pleural space. Patients with tuberculous pleuritis present with fever, weight loss, dyspnea, and/or pleuritic chest pain. The pleural fluid is an exudate with predominantly small lymphocytes. The diagnosis is established by demonstrating high levels of TB markers in the pleural fluid (adenosine deaminase >40 IU/L or interferon γ >140 pg/mL). Alternatively, the diagnosis can be established by culture of the pleural fluid, needle biopsy of the pleura, or thoracoscopy. The recommended treatments of pleural and pulmonary TB are identical (Chap. 12).

Effusion secondary to viral infection

Viral infections are probably responsible for a sizable percentage of undiagnosed exudative pleural effusions. In many series, no diagnosis is established for ~20% of exudative effusions, and these effusions resolve spontaneously with no long-term residua. The importance of these effusions is that one should not be too aggressive in trying to establish a diagnosis for the undiagnosed effusion, particularly if the patient is improving clinically.

Chylothorax

A chylothorax occurs when the thoracic duct is disrupted and chyle accumulates in the pleural space. The most common cause of chylothorax is trauma (most frequently thoracic surgery), but it also may result from tumors in the mediastinum. Patients with chylothorax present with dyspnea, and a large pleural effusion is present on the chest radiograph. Thoracentesis reveals milky fluid, and biochemical analysis reveals a triglyceride level that exceeds 1.2 mmol/L (110 mg/dL). Patients with chylothorax and no obvious trauma should have a lymphangiogram and a mediastinal CT scan to assess the mediastinum for lymph nodes. The treatment of choice for most chylothoraxes is insertion of a chest tube plus the administration of octreotide. If these modalities fail, a pleuroperitoneal shunt should be placed unless the patient has chylous ascites. An alternative treatment is ligation of the thoracic duct. Patients with chylothoraxes should not undergo prolonged tube thoracostomy with chest tube drainage because this will lead to malnutrition and immunologic incompetence.

Hemothorax

When a diagnostic thoracentesis reveals bloody pleural fluid, a hematocrit should be obtained on the pleural fluid. If the hematocrit is more than one-half of that in the peripheral blood, the patient is considered to have a hemothorax. Most hemothoraxes are the result of trauma; other causes include rupture of a blood vessel or tumor. Most patients with hemothorax should be treated with tube thoracostomy, which allows continuous quantification of bleeding. If the bleeding emanates from a laceration of the pleura, apposition of the two pleural surfaces is likely to stop the bleeding. If the pleural hemorrhage exceeds 200 mL/h, consideration should be given to thoracoscopy or thoracotomy.

Miscellaneous causes of pleural effusion

There are many other causes of pleural effusion (Table 21-1). Key features of some of these conditions are as follows: If the pleural fluid amylase level is elevated, the diagnosis of esophageal rupture or pancreatic disease is likely. If the patient is febrile, has predominantly polymorphonuclear cells in the pleural fluid, and has no pulmonary parenchymal abnormalities, an intraabdominal abscess should be considered.

The diagnosis of an asbestos pleural effusion is one of exclusion. Benign ovarian tumors can produce ascites and a pleural effusion (Meigs' syndrome), as can the ovarian hyperstimulation syndrome. Several drugs can cause pleural effusion; the associated fluid is usually eosinophilic. Pleural effusions commonly occur after coronary artery bypass surgery. Effusions occurring within the first weeks are typically left-sided and bloody, with large numbers of eosinophils, and respond to one or two therapeutic thoracenteses. Effusions occurring after the first few weeks are typically left-sided and clear yellow, with predominantly small lymphocytes, and tend to recur. Other medical manipulations that induce pleural effusions include abdominal surgery; radiation therapy; liver, lung, or heart transplantation; and the intravascular insertion of central lines.

PNEUMOTHORAX

Pneumothorax is the presence of gas in the pleural space. A *spontaneous pneumothorax* is one that occurs without antecedent trauma to the thorax. A *primary spontaneous pneumothorax* occurs in the absence of underlying lung disease, whereas a *secondary pneumothorax* occurs in its presence. A *traumatic pneumothorax* results from penetrating or nonpenetrating chest injuries. A *tension pneumothorax* is a pneumothorax in which the pressure in the pleural space is positive throughout the respiratory cycle.

Primary spontaneous pneumothorax

Primary spontaneous pneumothoraxes are usually due to rupture of apical pleural blebs, small cystic spaces that lie within or immediately under the visceral pleura. Primary spontaneous pneumothoraxes occur almost exclusively in smokers; this suggests that these patients have subclinical lung disease. Approximately one-half of patients with

TABLE 21-1

DIFFERENTIAL DIAGNOSES OF PLEURAL EFFUSIONS

Transudative Pleural Effusions

1. Congestive heart failure	5. Peritoneal dialysis
2. Cirrhosis	6. Superior vena cava
3. Pulmonary embolization	obstruction
4. Nephrotic syndrome	7. Myxedema
	8. Urinothorax

Exudative Pleural Effusions

1. Neoplastic diseases	6. Post-coronary artery
a. Metastatic disease	bypass surgery
b. Mesothelioma	7. Asbestos exposure
2. Infectious diseases	8. Sarcoidosis
a. Bacterial infections	9. Uremia
b. Tuberculosis	10. Meigs' syndrome
c. Fungal infections	11. Yellow nail syndrome
d. Viral infections	12. Drug-induced pleural
e. Parasitic infections	disease
3. Pulmonary embolization	a. Nitrofurantoin
4. Gastrointestinal disease	b. Dantrolene
a. Esophageal perforation	c. Methysergide
b. Pancreatic disease	d. Bromocriptine
c. Intraabdominal	e. Procarbazine
abscesses	f. Amiodarone
d. Diaphragmatic hernia	g. Dasatinib
e. After abdominal	13. Trapped lung
surgery	14. Radiation therapy
f. Endoscopic variceal	15. Post-cardiac injury
sclerotherapy	syndrome
g. After liver transplant	16. Hemothorax
5. Collagen vascular	17. Iatrogenic injury
diseases	18. Ovarian hyperstimulation
a. Rheumatoid pleuritis	syndrome
b. Systemic lupus	19. Pericardial disease
erythematosus	20. Chylothorax
c. Drug-induced lupus	
d. Immunoblastic	
lymphadenopathy	
e. Sjögren's syndrome	
f. Granulomatosis with	
polyangiitis (Wegener's)	
g. Churg-Strauss	
syndrome	

an initial primary spontaneous pneumothorax will have a recurrence. The initial recommended treatment for primary spontaneous pneumothorax is simple aspiration. If the lung does not expand with aspiration or if the patient has a recurrent pneumothorax, thoracoscopy with stapling of blebs and pleural abrasion is indicated. Thoracoscopy or thoracotomy with pleural abrasion is almost 100% successful in preventing recurrences.

Secondary pneumothorax

Most secondary pneumothoraxes are due to chronic obstructive pulmonary disease, but pneumothoraxes have been reported with virtually every lung disease.

Pneumothorax in patients with lung disease is more life-threatening than it is in normal individuals because of the lack of pulmonary reserve in these patients. Nearly all patients with secondary pneumothorax should be treated with tube thoracostomy. Most should also be treated with thoracoscopy or thoracotomy with the stapling of blebs and pleural abrasion. If the patient is not a good operative candidate or refuses surgery, pleurodesis should be attempted by the intrapleural injection of a sclerosing agent such as doxycycline.

Traumatic pneumothorax

Traumatic pneumothoraxes can result from both penetrating and nonpenetrating chest trauma. Traumatic pneumothoraxes should be treated with tube thoracostomy unless they are very small. If a hemopneumothorax is present, one chest tube should be placed in the superior part of the hemithorax to evacuate the air and another should be placed in the inferior part of the hemithorax to remove the blood. Iatrogenic pneumothorax is a type of traumatic pneumothorax that is becoming more common. The leading causes are transthoracic needle aspiration, thoracentesis, and the insertion of central intravenous catheters. Most can be managed with supplemental oxygen or aspiration, but if these measures are unsuccessful, a tube thoracostomy should be performed.

Tension pneumothorax

This condition usually occurs during mechanical ventilation or resuscitative efforts. The positive pleural pressure is life-threatening both because ventilation is severely compromised and because the positive pressure is transmitted to the mediastinum, resulting in decreased venous return to the heart and reduced cardiac output.

Difficulty in ventilation during resuscitation or high peak inspiratory pressures during mechanical ventilation strongly suggest the diagnosis. The diagnosis is made by physical examination showing an enlarged hemithorax with no breath sounds, hyperresonance to percussion, and shift of the mediastinum to the contralateral side. Tension pneumothorax must be treated as a medical emergency. If the tension in the pleural space is not relieved, the patient is likely to die from inadequate cardiac output or marked hypoxemia. A large-bore needle should be inserted into the pleural space through the second anterior intercostal space. If large amounts of gas escape from the needle after insertion, the diagnosis is confirmed. The needle should be left in place until a thoracostomy tube can be inserted.

DISORDERS OF THE MEDIASTINUM

The mediastinum is the region between the pleural sacs. It is separated into three compartments. The *anterior mediastinum* extends from the sternum anteriorly to the pericardium and brachiocephalic vessels posteriorly. It contains the thymus gland, the anterior mediastinal lymph nodes, and the internal mammary arteries and veins. The *middle mediastinum* lies between the anterior and posterior mediastina and contains the heart; the ascending and transverse arches of the aorta; the venae cavae; the brachiocephalic arteries and veins; the phrenic nerves; the trachea, the main bronchi, and their contiguous lymph nodes; and the pulmonary arteries and veins. The *posterior mediastinum* is bounded by the pericardium and trachea anteriorly and the vertebral column posteriorly. It contains the descending thoracic aorta, the esophagus, the thoracic duct, the azygos and hemiazygos veins, and the posterior group of mediastinal lymph nodes.

MEDIASTINAL MASSES

The first step in evaluating a mediastinal mass is to place it in one of the three mediastinal compartments, since each has different characteristic lesions. The most common lesions in the anterior mediastinum are thymomas, lymphomas, teratomatous neoplasms, and thyroid masses. The most common masses in the middle mediastinum are vascular masses, lymph node enlargement from metastases or granulomatous disease, and pleuropericardial and bronchogenic cysts. In the posterior mediastinum, neurogenic tumors, meningoceles, meningomyeloceles, gastroenteric cysts, and esophageal diverticula are commonly found.

CT scanning is the most valuable imaging technique for evaluating mediastinal masses and is the only imaging technique that should be done in most instances. Barium studies of the gastrointestinal tract are indicated in many patients with posterior mediastinal lesions, since hernias, diverticula, and achalasia are readily diagnosed in this manner. An ^{131}I scan can efficiently establish the diagnosis of intrathoracic goiter.

A definite diagnosis can be obtained with mediastinoscopy or anterior mediastinotomy in many patients with masses in the anterior or middle mediastinal compartments. A diagnosis can be established without thoracotomy via percutaneous fine-needle aspiration biopsy or endoscopic transesophageal or endobronchial ultrasound-guided biopsy of mediastinal masses in most cases. Alternative ways to establish the diagnosis are video-assisted thoracoscopy, mediastinoscopy, and mediastinotomy. In many cases the diagnosis can be established and the mediastinal mass removed with video-assisted thoracoscopy.

ACUTE MEDIASTINITIS

Most cases of acute mediastinitis either are due to esophageal perforation or occur after median sternotomy for cardiac surgery. Patients with esophageal rupture are acutely ill with chest pain and dyspnea due to the mediastinal infection. The esophageal rupture can occur spontaneously or as a complication of esophagoscopy or the insertion of a Blakemore tube. Appropriate treatment consists of exploration of the mediastinum with primary repair of the esophageal tear and drainage of the pleural space and the mediastinum.

The incidence of mediastinitis after median sternotomy is 0.4–5.0%. Patients most commonly present with wound drainage. Other presentations include sepsis and a widened mediastinum. The diagnosis usually is established with mediastinal needle aspiration. Treatment includes immediate drainage, debridement, and parenteral antibiotic therapy, but the mortality rate still exceeds 20%.

CHRONIC MEDIASTINITIS

The spectrum of chronic mediastinitis ranges from granulomatous inflammation of the lymph nodes in the mediastinum to fibrosing mediastinitis. Most cases are due to histoplasmosis or TB, but sarcoidosis, silicosis, and other fungal diseases are at times causative. Patients with granulomatous mediastinitis are usually asymptomatic. Those with fibrosing mediastinitis usually have signs of compression of a mediastinal structure such as the superior vena cava or large airways, phrenic or recurrent laryngeal nerve paralysis, or obstruction of the

pulmonary artery or proximal pulmonary veins. Other than antituberculous therapy for tuberculous mediastinitis, no medical or surgical therapy has been demonstrated to be effective for mediastinal fibrosis.

PNEUMOMEDIASTINUM

In this condition, there is gas in the interstices of the mediastinum. The three main causes are (1) alveolar rupture with dissection of air into the mediastinum, (2) perforation or rupture of the esophagus, trachea, or main bronchi, and (3) dissection of air from the neck or the abdomen into the mediastinum. Typically, there is severe substernal chest pain with or without radiation into the neck and arms. The physical examination usually reveals subcutaneous emphysema in the suprasternal notch and *Hamman's sign*, which is a crunching or clicking noise synchronous with the heartbeat and is best heard in the left lateral decubitus position. The diagnosis is confirmed with the chest radiograph. Usually no treatment is required, but the mediastinal air will be absorbed faster if the patient inspires high concentrations of oxygen. If mediastinal structures are compressed, the compression can be relieved with needle aspiration.

CHAPTER 22

DISORDERS OF VENTILATION

John F. McConville ■ Julian Solway

DEFINITION AND PHYSIOLOGY

In health the arterial level of carbon dioxide (Pa_{CO_2}) is maintained between 37 and 43 mmHg at sea level. All disorders of ventilation result in abnormal measurements of Pa_{CO_2}. This chapter reviews chronic ventilatory disorders that are reflected in abnormal Pa_{CO_2}.

The continuous production of CO_2 by cellular metabolism necessitates its efficient elimination by the respiratory system. The relationship between CO_2 production and Pa_{CO_2} is described by the equation, $Pa_{CO_2} = (k)(\dot{V}_{CO_2})/\dot{V}A$, where $\dot{V}_{CO_2}$ represents the carbon dioxide production, k is a constant and $\dot{V}A$ is fresh gas alveolar ventilation (Chap. 5). $\dot{V}A$ can be calculated as minute ventilation x(1-Vd/Vt), where the dead space fraction Vd/Vt represents the portion of a tidal breath that remains within the conducting airways at the conclusion of inspiration and does not, therefore, contribute to alveolar ventilation. As such, all disturbances of Pa_{CO_2} must reflect altered CO_2 production, minute ventilation, or dead space fraction.

Diseases that alter $\dot{V}_{CO_2}$ are often acute (sepsis, burns, or pyrexia, for example), and their contribution to ventilatory abnormalities and/or respiratory failure is reviewed elsewhere. Chronic ventilatory disorders typically involve inappropriate levels of minute ventilation or increased dead space fraction. Characterization of these disorders requires a review of the normal respiratory cycle.

The spontaneous cycle of inspiration and expiration is automatically generated in the brainstem. Two groups of neurons located within the medulla are particularly important: the dorsal respiratory group (DRG) and the ventral respiratory column (VRC). These neurons have widespread projections, including the descending projections into the contralateral spinal cord, where they perform many functions. They initiate activity in the phrenic nerve/diaphragm, project to the upper airway muscle groups and spinal respiratory neurons, and innervate the intercostal and abdominal muscles that participate in normal respiration. The DRG acts as the initial integration site for many of the afferent nerves relaying information about the partial pressure of arterial oxygen (Pa_{O_2}), Pa_{CO_2}, pH, and blood pressure from the carotid and aortic chemoreceptors and baroreceptors to the central nervous system (CNS). In addition, the vagus nerve relays information from stretch receptors and juxtapulmonary-capillary receptors in the lung parenchyma and chest wall to the DRG. The respiratory rhythm is generated within the VRC, as well as the more rostrally located parafacial respiratory group (pFRG), which is particularly important for the generation of active expiration. One particularly important area within the VRC is the so-called pre-Bötzinger complex. This area is responsible for the generation of various forms of inspiratory activity, and lesioning of the pre-Bötzinger complex leads to the complete cessation of breathing. The neural output of these medullary respiratory networks can be voluntarily suppressed or augmented by input from higher brain centers and the autonomic nervous system. During normal sleep there is an attenuated response to hypercapnia and hypoxemia resulting in mild nocturnal hypoventilation that corrects upon awakening.

Once neural input has been delivered to the respiratory pump muscles, normal gas exchange requires an adequate amount of respiratory muscle strength to overcome the elastic and resistive loads of the respiratory system (Fig. 22-1A, Chap. 5). In health, the strength of the respiratory muscles readily accomplishes this, and normal respiration continues indefinitely. Reduction in respiratory drive or neuromuscular competence or substantial increase in respiratory load can diminish minute ventilation, resulting in hypercapnia (Fig. 22-1B). Alternatively, if normal respiratory muscle strength is coupled with excessive respiratory drive, then alveolar hyperventilation ensues and leads to hypocapnia (Fig. 22-1C).

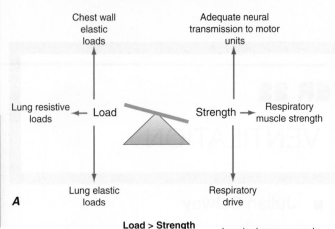

Excess respiratory muscle strength in health

A

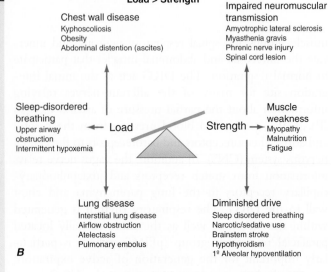

Load > Strength

B

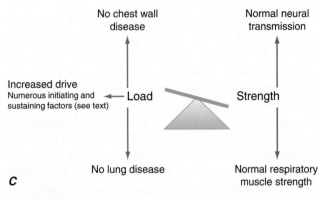

Increased drive with acceptable strength

C

FIGURE 22-1

Examples of balance between respiratory system strength and load. *A.* Excess respiratory muscle strength in health. *B.* Load greater than strength. *C.* Increased drive with acceptable strength.

HYPOVENTILATION

CLINICAL FEATURES

Diseases that reduce minute ventilation or increase dead space fall into four major categories: parenchymal lung and chest wall disease, sleep disordered

TABLE 22-1

SIGNS AND SYMPTOMS OF HYPOVENTILATION

Dyspnea during activities of daily living
Orthopnea in diseases affecting diaphragm function
Poor quality sleep
Daytime hypersomnolence
Early morning headaches
Anxiety
Impaired cough in neuromuscular diseases

breathing, neuromuscular disease, and respiratory drive disorders (Fig. 22-1B). The clinical manifestations of hypoventilation syndromes are nonspecific (Table 22-1) and vary depending on the severity of hypoventilation, the rate at which hypercapnia develops, the degree of compensation for respiratory acidosis, and the underlying disorder. Patients with parenchymal lung or chest wall disease typically present with shortness of breath and diminished exercise tolerance. Episodes of increased dyspnea and sputum production are hallmarks of obstructive lung diseases, such as chronic obstructive pulmonary disease (COPD), whereas progressive dyspnea and cough are common in interstitial lung diseases. Excessive daytime somnolence, poor quality sleep, and snoring are common among patients with sleep-disordered breathing. Sleep disturbance and orthopnea are also described in neuromuscular disorders. As neuromuscular weakness progresses, the respiratory muscles, including the diaphragm, are placed at a mechanical disadvantage in the supine position due to the upward movement of the abdominal contents. New-onset orthopnea is frequently a sign of reduced respiratory muscle force generation. More commonly, however, extremity weakness or bulbar symptoms develop prior to sleep disturbance in neuromuscular diseases, such as amyotrophic lateral sclerosis (ALS) or muscular dystrophy. Patients with respiratory drive disorders do not have symptoms distinguishable from other causes of chronic hypoventilation.

The clinical course of patients with chronic hypoventilation from neuromuscular or chest wall disease follows a characteristic sequence: An asymptomatic stage where daytime Pa_{O_2} and Pa_{CO_2} are normal, followed by nocturnal hypoventilation, initially during rapid eye movement (REM) sleep and later in non-REM sleep. Finally, if vital capacity drops further, daytime hypercapnia develops. Symptoms can develop at any point along this time course and often depend on the pace of respiratory muscle functional decline. Regardless of cause, the hallmark of all alveolar hypoventilation syndromes is an increase in alveolar P_{CO_2} (PA_{CO_2}) and, therefore, in Pa_{CO_2}. The resulting respiratory acidosis eventually leads to a compensatory increase in plasma bicarbonate concentration. The increase in PA_{CO_2} results in an obligatory decrease in PA_{O_2}, often resulting in hypoxemia. If severe, the hypoxemia manifests clinically as cyanosis and can stimulate erythropoiesis, thereby inducing secondary erythrocytosis. The combination of chronic hypoxemia and hypercapnia may also induce pulmonary vasoconstriction, leading eventually to pulmonary hypertension, right-ventricular hypertrophy, and right heart failure.

DIAGNOSIS

Elevated plasma bicarbonate in the absence of volume depletion is suggestive of hypoventilation. An arterial blood gas demonstrating elevated Pa_{CO_2} with a normal pH confirms chronic alveolar hypoventilation. The subsequent evaluation to identify an etiology should initially focus on whether the patient has lung disease or chest wall abnormalities. Physical examination, imaging studies (chest x-ray and/or CT scan), and pulmonary function tests are sufficient to identify most lung/chest wall disorders leading to hypercapnia. If these evaluations are unrevealing, then the clinician should screen for obstructive sleep apnea (OSA), the most frequent sleep disorder leading to chronic hypoventilation. Several screening tools have been developed to identify patients at risk for OSA. The Berlin Questionnaire has been validated in a primary care setting and identifies patients likely to have OSA. The Epworth Sleepiness Scale (ESS) and the STOP-Bang questionnaire have not been validated in outpatient primary care settings but are quick and easy to use. The ESS measures daytime sleepiness, with a score of ≥10 identifying individuals who warrant additional investigation. The STOP-Bang survey has been used in preoperative clinics to identify patients at risk of having OSA. In this population, it has 93% sensitivity and 90% negative predictive value.

If the ventilatory apparatus (lung, airways, chest wall) is not responsible for chronic hypercapnia, then the focus should shift to respiratory drive and neuromuscular disorders. There is an attenuated increase in minute ventilation in response to elevated CO_2 and/or low O_2 in respiratory drive disorders. These diseases are difficult to diagnose and should be suspected when patients with hypercapnia are found to have normal respiratory muscle strength, normal pulmonary function, and normal alveolar-arterial P_{O_2} difference. Hypoventilation is more marked during sleep in patients with respiratory drive defects, and polysomnography often reveals central apneas, hypopneas, or hypoventilation. Brain imaging (CT scan or MRI) can sometimes identify structural abnormalities in the pons or medulla that result in hypoventilation. Chronic narcotic use or significant hypothyroidism can depress the central respiratory drive and lead to chronic hypercapnia, as well.

Respiratory muscle weakness has to be profound before lung volumes are compromised and hypercapnia develops. Typically, physical examination reveals decreased strength in major muscle groups prior to the development of hypercapnia. Measurement of maximum inspiratory and expiratory pressures or forced vital capacity (FVC) can be used to monitor for respiratory muscle involvement in diseases with progressive muscle weakness. These patients also have increased risk for sleep-disordered breathing, including hypopneas, central and obstructive apneas, and hypoxemia. Nighttime oximetry and polysomnography are helpful in better characterizing sleep disturbances in this patient population.

| TREATMENT | Hypoventilation |

Nocturnal noninvasive positive-pressure ventilation (NIPPV) has been used successfully in the treatment of hypoventilation and apneas, both central and obstructive, in patients with neuromuscular and chest wall disorders. Nocturnal NIPPV has been shown to improve daytime hypercapnia, prolong survival, and improve health-related quality of life when daytime hypercapnia is documented. ALS guidelines recommend nocturnal NIPPV if symptoms of hypoventilation exist AND one of the following criteria is present: Pa_{CO_2} ≥45 mmHg; nocturnal oximetry demonstrates oxygen saturation ≤88% for 5 consecutive minutes; maximal inspiratory pressure <60 cm H_2O; and FVC <50% predicted. However, at present there is inconclusive evidence to support preemptive nocturnal NIPPV use in all patients with neuromuscular and chest wall disorders who demonstrate nocturnal, but not daytime, hypercapnia. Nevertheless, at some point the institution of full-time ventilatory support with either pressure or volume-preset modes is required in progressive neuromuscular disorders. There is less evidence to direct the timing of this decision, but ventilatory failure requiring mechanical ventilation and chest infections related to ineffective cough are frequent triggers for the institution of full-time ventilatory support.

Treatment of chronic hypoventilation from lung or neuromuscular diseases should be directed at the underlying disorder. Pharmacologic agents that stimulate respiration, such as medroxyprogesterone and acetazolamide, have been poorly studied in chronic hypoventilation and should not replace treatment of the underlying disease process. Regardless of the cause, excessive metabolic alkalosis should be corrected, as plasma bicarbonate levels elevated out of proportion to the degree of chronic respiratory acidosis can result in additional hypoventilation. When indicated, administration of supplemental oxygen is effective in attenuating hypoxemia, polycythemia, and pulmonary hypertension.

Phrenic nerve or diaphragm pacing is a potential therapy for patients with hypoventilation from high cervical spinal cord lesions or respiratory drive disorders. Prior to surgical implantation, patients should have nerve conduction studies to ensure normal bilateral phrenic nerve function. Small case series suggest that effective diaphragmatic pacing can improve quality of life in these patients.

HYPOVENTILATION SYNDROMES

OBESITY HYPOVENTILATION SYNDROME

The diagnosis of obesity hypoventilation syndrome (OHS) requires: body mass index (BMI) ≥ 30 kg/m^2, sleep-disordered breathing and chronic daytime alveolar hypoventilation, defined as $Pa_{CO_2} \geq 45$ mmHg, and $Pa_{O_2} < 70$ mmHg in the absence of other known causes of hypercapnia. In almost 90% of cases, the sleep-disordered breathing is in the form of OSA. Several international studies in different populations confirm that the overall prevalence of obstructive sleep apnea syndrome, defined by an apnea hypopnea index ≥ 5 AND daytime sleepiness, is approximately 3–4% in middle-aged men and 2% in middle-aged women. Thus, the population at risk for the development of OHS continues to rise as the worldwide obesity epidemic persists. Although no population-based prevalence studies of OHS have been performed, some estimates suggest there may be as many as 500,000 individuals with OHS in the United States.

Several studies suggest that severe obesity (BMI >40 kg/m^2) and severe OSA apnea-hypopnea index ([AHI] >30 events per hour) are risk factors for the development of OHS. The pathogenesis of hypoventilation in these patients is multifactorial and incompletely understood. Defects in central respiratory drive have been demonstrated in OHS patients but often improve with treatment. This suggests central defects may not be the primary disturbance that leads to chronic hypercapnia. The treatment of OHS is similar to that for OSA: weight reduction and continuous positive airway pressure (CPAP) therapy during sleep. CPAP improves daytime hypercapnia and hypoxemia in the majority of patients with OHS. There is not conclusive evidence to suggest that bilevel positive airway pressure (BiPAP) is superior to CPAP. Bilevel positive airway pressure should be reserved for patients not able to tolerate high levels of CPAP support or patients that remain hypoxemic despite resolution of obstructive respiratory events.

CENTRAL HYPOVENTILATION SYNDROME

This syndrome can present later in life or in the neonatal period where it is often called Ondine's curse or congenital central hypoventilation syndrome (CCHS). Abnormalities in the gene encoding PHOX2b, a transcription factor with a role in neuronal development, have been implicated in the pathogenesis of congenital central hypoventilation syndrome. Regardless of the age of onset, these patients have absent respiratory response to hypoxia or hypercapnia, mildly elevated Pa_{CO_2} while awake, and markedly elevated Pa_{CO_2} during non-REM sleep. Interestingly, these patients are able to augment their ventilation and "normalize" Pa_{CO_2} during exercise. These patients typically require NIPPV or mechanical ventilation as therapy and should be considered for phrenic nerve or diaphragmatic pacing at centers with experience performing these procedures.

HYPERVENTILATION

CLINICAL FEATURES

Hyperventilation is defined as ventilation in excess of metabolic requirements (CO_2 production) leading to a reduction in Pa_{CO_2}. The physiology of patients with chronic hyperventilation is poorly understood, and there is no typical clinical presentation. Symptoms can include dyspnea, paresthesias, tetany, headache, dizziness, visual disturbances, and atypical chest pain. Because symptoms can be so diverse, patients with chronic hyperventilation present to a variety of health care providers, including internists, neurologists, psychologists, psychiatrists, and pulmonologists.

It is helpful to think of hyperventilation as having initiating and sustaining factors. Some investigators believe that an initial event leads to increased alveolar ventilation and a drop in Pa_{CO_2} to ~20 mmHg. The ensuing onset of chest pain, breathlessness, paresthesia, or altered consciousness can be alarming. The resultant increase in minute volume to relieve these acute symptoms only serves to exacerbate symptoms that are often misattributed by the patient and health care workers to cardiopulmonary disorders. An unrevealing evaluation for causes of these symptoms often results in patients being anxious and fearful of additional attacks. It is important to note that *anxiety disorders and panic attacks are NOT synonymous with hyperventilation*. Anxiety can be both an initiating and sustaining factor in the pathogenesis of chronic hyperventilation, but these are not necessary for the development of chronic hypocapnia.

DIAGNOSIS

Respiratory symptoms associated with acute hyperventilation can be the initial manifestation of systemic illnesses such as diabetic ketoacidosis. Causes of acute hyperventilation need to be excluded before a diagnosis of chronic hyperventilation is considered. Arterial blood gas sampling that demonstrates a compensated respiratory alkalosis with a near-normal pH, low Pa_{CO_2} and low calculated bicarbonate are necessary to confirm chronic hyperventilation. Other causes of respiratory alkalosis, such as mild asthma, need to be diagnosed and treated before chronic hyperventilation can be considered. A high index of suspicion is required as increased minute ventilation can be difficult to detect on physical examination. Once chronic hyperventilation is established, a sustained 10% increase in alveolar ventilation is enough to perpetuate hypocapnia. This increase can be accomplished with subtle changes in the respiratory pattern, such as occasional sigh breaths or yawning two to three times per minute.

TREATMENT	Hyperventilation

There are few well-controlled treatment studies of chronic hyperventilation because of its diverse features and the lack of a universally accepted diagnostic process. Clinicians often spend considerable time identifying initiating factors, excluding alternative diagnoses and discussing the patient's concerns and fears. In some patients, reassurance and frank discussion about hyperventilation can be liberating. Identifying and eliminating habits that perpetuate hypocapnia, such as frequent yawning or sigh breathing, can be helpful. Some evidence suggests that breathing exercises and diaphragmatic retraining may be beneficial for some patients. The evidence for using medications to treat hyperventilation is scant. Beta-blockers may be helpful in patients with sympathetically mediated symptoms, such as palpitations and tremors.

ACKNOWLEDGMENTS

We would like to acknowledge Eliot A. Phillipson for earlier versions of this chapter and Jan-Marino Ramirez for his careful critique and helpful suggestions.

CHAPTER 23
SLEEP APNEA

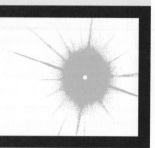

Neil J. Douglas

OBSTRUCTIVE SLEEP APNEA

Obstructive sleep apnea/hypopnea syndrome (OSAHS) is one of the most important medical conditions identified in the last 50 years. It is a major cause of morbidity, a significant cause of mortality, and the most common medical cause of daytime sleepiness. Central sleep apnea is a rare clinical problem.

DEFINITION

OSAHS is defined as the coexistence of unexplained excessive daytime sleepiness with at least five obstructed breathing events (apnea or hypopnea) per hour of sleep (Table 23-1). This event threshold may have to be increased in the elderly. *Apneas* are defined in adults as breathing pauses lasting ≥10 s and hypopneas as events ≥10 s in which there is continued breathing but ventilation is reduced by at least 50% from the previous baseline during sleep. As a syndrome, OSAHS is the association

of a clinical picture with specific abnormalities on testing; asymptomatic individuals with abnormal breathing during sleep should not be labeled as having OSAHS.

MECHANISM OF OBSTRUCTION

Apneas and hypopneas are caused by the airway being sucked closed on inspiration during sleep. This occurs as the upper-airway dilating muscles—like all striated muscles—relax during sleep. In patients with OSAHS, the dilating muscles fail to oppose negative pressure within the airway during inspiration. The primary defect is not in the upper-airway muscles, which function normally in OSAHS patients when awake. These patients have narrow upper airways already during wakefulness, but when they are awake, their airway dilating muscles have increased activity, which ensures airway patency. However, during sleep, muscle tone falls and the airway narrows; snoring may commence before the airway occludes, and apnea results. Apneas and hypopneas terminate when the subject arouses,

TABLE 23-1

CLINICAL INDICATORS IN THE SLEEPY PATIENT			
	OSAHS	**NARCOLEPSY**	**IHS**
Age of onset (years)	35–60	10–30	10–30
Cataplexy	No	Yes	No
Night sleep			
Duration	Normal	Normal	Long
Awakenings	Occasional	Frequent	Rare
Snoring	Yes, loud	Occasional	Occasional
Morning drunkenness	Occasional	Occasional	Common
Daytime naps			
Frequency	Usually few	Many	Few
Time of day	Afternoon/evening	Afternoon/evening	Morning
Duration	<1 h	<1 h	>1 h

Note: Features suggesting obstructive sleep apnea/hypopnea syndrome (OSAHS), narcolepsy, or idiopathic hypersomnolence (IHS).

i.e., wakens briefly, from sleep. This arousal is sometimes too subtle to be seen on the electroencephalogram but may be detected by cardiac acceleration, blood pressure elevation, or increase in sympathetic tone. The arousal results in return of upper-airway dilating muscle tone, and thus airway patency is resumed.

Factors predisposing to OSAHS by narrowing the pharynx include obesity—in Western populations around 50% of OSAHS patients have a body mass index (BMI) >30 kg/m^2—and shortening of the mandible and/or maxilla. This change in jaw shape may be subtle and can be familial. Hypothyroidism and acromegaly predispose to OSAHS by narrowing the upper airway with tissue infiltration. Other predisposing factors for OSAHS include male sex and middle age (40–65 years), myotonic dystrophy, Ehlers-Danlos syndrome, and, perhaps, smoking.

EPIDEMIOLOGY

OSAHS occurs in around 1–4% of middle-aged males and is about half as common in women. The syndrome also occurs in childhood—usually associated with tonsil or adenoid enlargement—and in the elderly, although the frequency is slightly lower in old age. Irregular breathing during sleep *without* daytime sleepiness is much more common, occurring in perhaps a quarter of the middle-aged male population. As these individuals are asymptomatic, they do not have OSAHS, but there is increasing epidemiologic evidence of an association of irregular breathing during sleep with increased vascular risk even in the nonsleepy.

CLINICAL FEATURES

Randomized controlled treatment trials have shown that OSAHS causes daytime sleepiness; impaired vigilance, cognitive performance and driving; depression; disturbed sleep; and hypertension. Daytime sleepiness may range from mild to irresistible and can be indistinguishable from that in narcolepsy. The sleepiness may cause inability to work effectively, damage interpersonal relationships, and prevent socializing. The somnolence is dangerous, with a three- to sixfold risk of road accidents. Experiments with normal subjects repeatedly aroused from sleep indicate that the sleepiness results, at least in part, from the repetitive sleep disruption associated with the breathing abnormality. Other symptoms include difficulty concentrating, unrefreshing nocturnal sleep, nocturnal choking, nocturia, and decreased libido. Partners report nightly loud snoring in all postures, which may be punctuated by the silence of apneas.

Cardiovascular and cerebrovascular events

OSAHS raises 24-h mean blood pressure. The increase is greater in those with recurrent nocturnal hypoxemia, is at least 4–5 mmHg, and may be as great as 10 mmHg in those with >20% arterial oxygen desaturations per hour of sleep. This rise probably results from a combination of surges in blood pressure accompanying each arousal at apnea/hypopnea termination and from the associated 24-h increases in sympathetic tone.

Epidemiologic data in normal populations indicate that this rise in blood pressure would increase the risk of myocardial infarction by around 20% and that of stroke by about 40%. Although there are no long-term randomized controlled trials to indicate whether this is true in OSAHS patients—such studies would be unethical—observational studies suggest an increase in cardiovascular and stroke risk in patients with untreated OSAHS. Furthermore, epidemiologic studies suggest increased vascular risk in normal subjects with raised apneas and hypopneas during sleep. Patients with recent stroke have a high frequency of apneas and hypopneas during sleep. These seem largely to be a consequence, not a cause, of the stroke and to decline over the weeks after the vascular event. There is no evidence that treating the apneas and hypopneas improves stroke outcome.

Diabetes mellitus

The association of OSAHS with diabetes mellitus is not due only to the fact that obesity is common in both conditions. Increased apneas and hypopneas during sleep are associated with insulin resistance independent of obesity. In addition, uncontrolled trials suggest OSAHS can aggravate diabetes and that treating OSAHS in patients who also have diabetes decreases their insulin requirements.

Liver

Hepatic dysfunction also has been associated with irregular breathing during sleep. Non-alcohol-drinking subjects with apneas and hypopneas during sleep were found to have raised liver enzymes and more steatosis and fibrosis on liver biopsy, independent of body weight.

Anesthestic risk

Patients with OSAHS are at increased risk perioperatively as their upper airways may obstruct during the recovery period or as a consequence of sedation. Patients whom anesthesiologists have difficulty intubating are much more likely to have irregular breathing during sleep. Anesthesiologists should thus take preoperative sleep histories and take the appropriate precautions with patients who might have OSAHS.

Differential diagnosis

Causes of sleepiness that may need to be distinguished include (Table 23-1) the following:

- *Insufficient sleep*: this usually can be diagnosed by history.
- *Shift work*: a major cause of sleepiness, especially in those >40 years old.
- *Psychological psychiatric causes:* depression is a major cause of sleepiness.
- *Drugs*: both stimulant and sedative drugs can produce sleepiness.
- *Narcolepsy*: around 50 times less common than OSAHS, narcolepsy is usually evident from childhood or the teens and is associated with cataplexy.
- *Idiopathic hypersomnolence*: this is an ill–defined condition typified by long sleep duration and sleepiness.
- *Phase alteration syndromes*: both the phase delay and the less common phase advancement syndromes are characterized by sleepiness at the appropriate time of day.

Who to refer for diagnosis

Anyone whose troublesome sleepiness is not readily explained and rectified by considering the differential diagnosis earlier should be referred to a sleep specialist. The guideline the author uses for patients with troublesome sleepiness includes those with an Epworth Sleepiness Score >11 (Table 23-2) and also those whose sleepiness during work or driving poses problems. The Epworth Score is not a perfect measure for detecting sleepiness, as many whose lives are troubled by frequently fighting sleepiness but who never doze will correctly give themselves a low Epworth Score. The patient and his or her partner often give divergent scores for the patient's sleepiness, and in such cases the higher of the two scores should be used.

Diagnosis

OSAHS requires lifelong treatment, and the diagnosis has to be made or excluded with certainty. This will hinge on obtaining a good sleep history from the patient and partner, with both completing sleep questionnaires, including the Epworth Sleepiness Score (Table 23-2). Physical examination must include assessment of obesity, jaw structure, the upper airway, blood pressure, and possible predisposing causes, including hypothyroidism and acromegaly (see earlier).

In those with appropriate clinical features, the diagnostic test must demonstrate recurrent breathing pauses during sleep. This may be full polysomnography with recording of multiple respiratory and neurophysiologic

TABLE 23-2

EPWORTH SLEEPINESS SCORE

How often are you likely to doze off or fall asleep in the following situations, in contrast to feeling just tired? This refers to your usual way of life in recent times. Even if you have not done some of these things recently, try to work out how they would have affected you. Use the following scale to choose the *most appropriate number* for each situation:

0 = would *never* doze

1 = *slight* chance of dozing

2 = *moderate* chance of dozing

3 = *high* chance of dozing

Sitting and reading	....
Watching TV	....
Sitting, inactive in a public place (e.g., a theater or a meeting)	....
As a passenger in a car for an hour without a break	....
Lying down to rest in the afternoon when circumstances permit	....
Sitting and talking to someone	....
Sitting quietly after lunch without alcohol	....
In a car, while stopped for a few minutes in traffic	....
TOTAL	....

Source: From MW Johns: Sleep 14:540, 1991.

signals during sleep. Increasingly, especially outside the United States, most diagnostic tests are "limited studies"—recording respiratory and oxygenation patterns overnight without neurophysiologic recording. Such approaches in expert hands produce good patient outcomes and are cost-effective. It is sensible to use such limited sleep studies as the first-line diagnostic test and then allow positively diagnosed patients to proceed to treatment. A reasonable approach at present is for patients with troublesome sleepiness but negative limited studies to have polysomnography to exclude or confirm OSAHS.

TREATMENT ▸ **Obstructive Sleep Apnea**

WHOM TO TREAT There is evidence from robust randomized controlled trials (RCTs) that treatment improves symptoms, sleepiness, driving, cognition, mood, quality of life, and blood pressure in patients who have an Epworth Score >11, troublesome sleepiness while driving or working, and >15 apneas + hypopneas per hour of sleep. For those with similar degrees of sleepiness and 5–15 events per hour of sleep, RCTs indicate improvements in symptoms, including subjective sleepiness, with less strong evidence indicating gains in cognition and quality of life. There is no evidence of blood pressure improvements in this group. There is no robust evidence that treating nonsleepy subjects improves their symptoms, function, or blood pressure, and so treatment cannot be advocated for this large group, although this may change with further RCTs or less obtrusive therapy.

HOW TO TREAT All patients diagnosed with OSAHS should have the condition and its significance explained to them and their partners. This should be accompanied by written and/or Web-based information and a discussion of the implications of the local driving regulations. Rectifiable predispositions should be discussed; this often includes weight loss and alcohol reduction both to reduce weight and because alcohol acutely decreases upper-airway dilating muscle tone, thus predisposing to obstructed breathing. Sedative drugs, which also impair airway tone, should be carefully withdrawn.

Continuous Positive Airway Pressure (CPAP) CPAP therapy works by blowing the airway open during sleep, usually with pressures of 5–20 mmHg. CPAP has been shown in randomized placebo-controlled trials to improve breathing during sleep, sleep quality, sleepiness, blood pressure, vigilance, cognition, and driving ability as well as mood and quality of life in patients with OSAHS. However, this is obtrusive therapy, and care must be taken to explain the need for the treatment to patients and their partners and to intensively support patients on CPAP with telephone or Web support and regular follow-up. Initiation should include finding the most comfortable mask from the ranges of several manufacturers and trying the system for at least 30 min during the day to prepare for the overnight trial. An overnight monitored trial of CPAP is used to identify the pressure required to keep the patient's airway patent. The development of pressure-varying CPAP machines has made an in-lab CPAP night trial unnecessary, but treatment must be initiated in a supportive environment. Thereafter, patients can be treated with fixed-pressure CPAP machines set at the determined pressure or with a self-adjusting intelligent CPAP device. The main side effect of CPAP is airway drying, which can be countered by using an integral heated humidifier. CPAP use is imperfect, but around 94% of patients with severe OSAHS are still using their therapy after 5 years on objective monitoring.

Mandibular Repositioning Splint (MRS) Also called oral devices, MRSs work by holding the lower jaw and the tongue forward, thereby widening the pharyngeal airway. MRSs have been shown in RCTs to improve OSAHS patients' breathing during sleep, daytime somnolence, and blood pressure. As there are many devices with differing designs with unknown relative efficacy, these results cannot be generalized to all MRSs. Self-reports of the use of devices long-term suggest high dropout rates.

Surgery Four forms of surgery have a role in OSAHS, although it must be remembered that these patients have a raised perioperative risk. Bariatric surgery can be curative in the morbidly obese. Tonsillectomy can be highly effective in children but rarely in adults. Tracheostomy is curative but rarely used because of the associated morbidity rate but should not be overlooked in severe cases. Jaw advancement surgery—particularly maxillomandibular osteotomy—is effective in those with retrognathia (posterior displacement of the mandible) and should be considered particularly in young and thin patients. There is no robust evidence that pharyngeal surgery, including uvulopalatopharyngoplasty (whether by scalpel, laser, or thermal techniques) helps OSAHS patients.

Drugs Unfortunately, no drugs are clinically useful in the prevention or reduction of apneas and hypopneas. A marginal improvement in sleepiness in patients who remain sleepy despite CPAP can be produced by modafinil, but the clinical value is debatable and the financial cost is significant.

CHOICE OF TREATMENT CPAP and MRS are the two most widely used and best evidence-based therapies. Direct comparisons in RCTs indicate better outcomes with CPAP in terms of apneas and hypopneas, nocturnal oxygenation, symptoms, quality of life, mood, and vigilance. Adherence to CPAP is generally better than that to an MRS, and there is evidence that CPAP improves driving, whereas there are no such data on MRSs. Thus, CPAP is the current treatment of choice. However, MRSs are evidence-based second-line therapy in those who fail CPAP. In younger, thinner patients, maxillomandibular advancement should be considered.

HEALTH RESOURCES Untreated OSAHS patients are heavy users of health care and dangerous drivers; they also work beneath their potential. Treatment of OSAHS with CPAP is cost-effective in terms of reducing the health care costs of associated illness and associated accidents.

CENTRAL SLEEP APNEA

Central sleep apneas (CSAs) are respiratory pauses caused by lack of respiratory effort. They occur occasionally in normal subjects, particularly at sleep onset and in rapid eye movement (REM) sleep, and are transiently increased after ascent to altitude. Recurrent CSA is most commonly found in the presence of cardiac failure or neurologic disease, especially stroke. Spontaneous central sleep syndrome is rare and can be classified on the basis of the arterial P_{CO_2}.

Hypercapnic CSA occurs in conjunction with diminished ventilatory drive in Ondine's curse (central alveolar hypoventilation). Patients with normocapnic spontaneous CSA have a normal or low arterial P_{CO_2} when awake, with brisk ventilatory responses to hypercapnia. This combination results in unstable ventilatory control, with subjects breathing close to or below their apneic threshold for P_{CO_2} during sleep; this apneic tendency is compounded by cycles of arousal-induced hyperventilation, inducing further hypocapnia.

CLINICAL FEATURES

Patients may present with sleep maintenance insomnia, which is relatively unusual in OSAHS. Daytime sleepiness may occur.

INVESTIGATION

Many apneas previously labeled central because of absent thoracoabdominal movement are actually obstructive, identification of movement being particularly difficult in the very obese. CSA can be identified with certainty only if either esophageal pressure or respiratory muscle electromyography is recorded and shown to be absent during the events.

TREATMENT Central Sleep Apnea

Patients with underlying cardiac failure should have their failure treated appropriately. CPAP may improve outcome but is difficult to initiate and has not been shown to improve survival. Patients with spontaneous normocapnic CSA may be treated with acetazolamide. In a minority of patients, CPAP is effective, perhaps because in some patients with OSAHS, pharyngeal collapse initiates reflex inhibition of respiration, and this is prevented by CPAP. Oxygen and nocturnal nasal positive-pressure ventilation also may be tried.

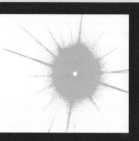

CHAPTER 24
LUNG TRANSPLANTATION

Elbert P. Trulock

Lung transplantation is a therapeutic consideration for many patients with nonmalignant end-stage lung disease, and it prolongs survival and improves quality of life in appropriately selected recipients. Since 1985 more than 25,000 procedures have been recorded worldwide, and ~2200 transplants have been reported annually in recent years.

INDICATIONS

The indications span the gamut of lung diseases. The most common indications in the last few years have been chronic obstructive pulmonary disease (COPD), ~30%; idiopathic pulmonary fibrosis (IPF), ~30%; cystic fibrosis (CF), ~15%; α_1-antitrypsin deficiency emphysema, ~3%; and idiopathic pulmonary arterial hypertension (IPAH), ~2%. Other diseases have accounted for the balance of primary indications, and retransplantation has accounted for ~4% of procedures.

RECIPIENT SELECTION

Transplantation should be considered when other therapeutic options have been exhausted and when the patient's prognosis is expected to improve as a result of the procedure. Survival rates after transplantation can be compared with predictive indices for the patient's disease, but each patient's clinical course must be integrated into the assessment, too. Moreover, quality of life is a primary motive for transplantation for many patients, and the prospect of improved quality-adjusted survival is often attractive even if the survival advantage itself may be marginal.

Disease-specific consensus guidelines for referring patients for evaluation and for proceeding with transplantation are summarized in Table 24-1 and are linked to clinical, physiologic, radiographic, and pathologic features that influence the prognosis of the respective diseases. Candidates for lung transplantation are also thoroughly screened for comorbidities that might affect the outcome adversely. Conditions such as systemic hypertension, diabetes mellitus, gastroesophageal reflux, and osteoporosis are not unusual, but if uncomplicated and adequately managed, they do not disqualify patients from transplantation. The upper age limit is ~65–70 years at most centers.

Standard exclusions include HIV infection, chronic active hepatitis B or C infection, uncontrolled or untreatable pulmonary or extrapulmonary infection, uncured malignancy, active cigarette smoking, drug or alcohol dependency, irreversible physical deconditioning, chronic nonadherence with medical care, significant disease of another vital organ (e.g., heart, liver, or kidney), and psychiatric or psychosocial situations that could substantially interfere with posttransplantation management. Other problems that may compromise the outcome constitute relative contraindications. Some typical issues are ventilator-dependent respiratory failure, previous thoracic surgical procedures, obesity, and coronary artery disease. Chronic infection with antibiotic-resistant *Pseudomonas* species, *Burkholderia* species, *Aspergillus* species, or nontuberculous mycobacteria is a unique concern in some patients with CF. The potential impact of these and other factors has to be judged in clinical context to determine an individual candidate's suitability for transplantation.

WAITING LIST AND ORGAN ALLOCATION

Organ allocation policies are influenced by medical, ethical, geographic, and political factors, with systems varying from country to country. Regardless of the system, potential recipients are placed on a waiting list and must be matched for blood group compatibility and, with some latitude, for lung size with an acceptable donor. Most lungs are procured from deceased donors after brain death, but only ~15–17% of brain-death organ donors yield either one or two lungs suitable for transplantation. Lungs from donors after cardiac death have been utilized to a limited extent.

TABLE 24-1

DISEASE-SPECIFIC GUIDELINES FOR REFERRAL AND TRANSPLANTATION

Chronic Obstructive Pulmonary Disease

Referral
    BODE index >5
Transplantation
    BODE index 7–10
    or
    any of the following criteria:
        Hospitalization for exacerbation, with Pa_{CO_2} >50 mmHg
        Pulmonary hypertension or cor pulmonale despite oxygen therapy
        FEV_1<20% with either DL_{CO} <20% or diffuse emphysema

Cystic Fibrosis/Bronchiectasis

Referral
    FEV_1<30% or rapidly declining FEV_1
    Hospitalization in ICU for exacerbation
    Increasing frequency of exacerbations
    Refractory or recurrent pneumothorax
    Recurrent hemoptysis not controlled by bronchial artery embolization
Transplantation
    Oxygen-dependent respiratory failure
    Hypercapnia
    Pulmonary hypertension

Idiopathic Pulmonary Fibrosis

Referral
    Pathologic or radiographic evidence of UIP regardless of vital capacity
Transplantation
    Pathologic or radiographic evidence of UIP
    and
    any of the following criteria
        DL_{CO} <39%
        Decrement in FVC ≥10% during 6 months of follow-up
        Decrease in Sp_{O_2} below 88% during a 6-min walk test
        Honeycombing on HRCT (fibrosis score >2)

Idiopathic Pulmonary Arterial Hypertension

Referral
    NYHA functional class III or IV regardless of therapy
    Rapidly progressive disease
Transplantation
    Failing therapy with intravenous epoprostenol (or equivalent drug)
    Persistent NYHA functional class III or IV on maximal medical therapy
    Low (<350 m) or declining 6-min walk test
    Cardiac index <2 L/min/m²
    Right atrial pressure >15 mmHg

Abbreviations: BODE, body-mass index (B), airflow obstruction (O), dyspnea (D), exercise capacity (E); FVC, forced vital capacity; FEV_1, forced expiratory volume in 1 s; DL_{CO}, diffusing capacity for carbon monoxide; Pa_{CO_2}, partial pressure of carbon dioxide in arterial blood; Sp_{O_2}, arterial oxygen saturation by pulse oximetry; ICU, intensive care unit; UIP, usual interstitial pneumonitis; HRCT, high-resolution computed tomography; NYHA, New York Heart Association.
Source: Summarized from Orens et al. For BODE index, BR Celli et al: N Engl J Med 350:1005, 2004.

A priority algorithm for allocating donor lungs was implemented in the United States in 2005. A lung allocation score that is based on the patient's risk of death on the waiting list and likelihood of survival after transplantation determines priority. The score can range from zero to 100, and precedence for transplantation is ranked from highest to lowest scores. Both the lung disease and its severity affect a patient's score; parameters in the score must be updated biannually but can be submitted for calculation of a new score whenever the patient's condition changes. The median score for all candidates on the waiting list is usually ~34–35, but the distribution of scores tends to be higher among patients with IPF and CF than among patients with COPD and IPAH. Under this priority system, the median waiting time for transplantation has fallen to <6 months, and the annual number of deaths on the waiting list has dropped by ~50%. The main indication for transplantation has also shifted from COPD to IPF. Overall survival rates in the first two years after transplantation have not changed substantially under this system; however, recipients with lung allocation scores >60 have had lower survival rates in the first two years compared with recipients with lower scores.

TRANSPLANT PROCEDURE

Bilateral transplantation is mandatory for CF and other forms of bronchiectasis because the risk of spillover infection from a remaining native lung precludes single-lung transplantation. Heart-lung transplantation is obligatory for Eisenmenger syndrome with complex anomalies that cannot be readily repaired in conjunction with lung transplantation and for concomitant end-stage lung and heart disease. However, cardiac replacement is not necessary for cor pulmonale because right ventricular function will recover when pulmonary vascular afterload is normalized by lung transplantation.

Either bilateral or single-lung transplantation is an option for other diseases unless there is a special consideration, but bilateral transplantation has been utilized increasingly for most indications. Recently, ~65% of procedures in the United States have been bilateral, and in the international registry, ~55% of transplants for COPD, ~50% for IPF, and ~90% for IPAH have been bilateral.

Living donor lobar transplantation has a limited role in adult lung transplantation. It has been performed predominantly in teenagers or young adults with CF, and it usually has been reserved for patients who were unlikely to survive the wait for a deceased organ donor.

POSTTRANSPLANTATION MANAGEMENT

Induction therapy with an antilymphocyte globulin or an interleukin 2 receptor antagonist is utilized by ~50%

of centers, and a three-drug maintenance immunosuppressive regimen that includes a calcineurin inhibitor (cyclosporine or tacrolimus), a purine synthesis antagonist (azathioprine or a mycophenolic acid precursor), and prednisone is traditional. Subsequently, other drugs, such as sirolimus, may be substituted into the regimen for various reasons. Prophylaxis for *Pneumocystis jiroveci* pneumonia is standard, and prophylaxis against cytomegalovirus (CMV) infection and fungal infection is part of many protocols. The dose of cyclosporine, tacrolimus, and sirolimus is adjusted by blood-level monitoring. All these agents are metabolized by the hepatic cytochrome P450 system, and interactions with medications that affect this pathway can significantly alter the clearance and blood level of these drugs.

Routine management focuses on monitoring the allograft, regulating immunosuppressive therapy, and detecting problems or complications expeditiously. Regular contact with a nurse coordinator, physician follow-up, chest radiographs, blood tests, and spirometry are customary, and periodic surveillance bronchoscopies are employed in some programs. If recovery is uncomplicated, lung function rapidly improves and then stabilizes by 3–6 months after transplantation. Subsequently, the variation in spirometric measurements is small, and a sustained decline of ≥10–15% signals a potentially significant problem.

OUTCOMES

Survival

Major registries publish survival (Table 24-2) and other outcomes annually (*www.ishlt.org; www.ustransplant.org*).

In the international registry, survival half-life for the main indications is in the range of 4–6 years; however, age and transplant procedure have a significant impact on outcome. For recipients 18–59 years of age, the survival half-life is 5–6 years, but it decreases to 4 years for those 60–65 years old and to 3 years for those >65 years old. Survival over 10 years has been significantly better after bilateral transplantation than after unilateral transplantation for COPD, α_1-antitrypsin deficiency emphysema, IPF, and IPAH.

The main sources of perioperative mortality include technical complications of the operation, primary graft dysfunction, and infections. Acute rejection and CMV infection are common problems in the first year, but neither is usually fatal. Beyond the first year, chronic rejection and non-CMV infections cause the majority of deaths.

Function

Regardless of the disease, successful transplantation impressively restores cardiopulmonary function. After bilateral transplantation, pulmonary function tests are typically normal; after unilateral transplantation, a mild abnormality characteristic of the remaining diseased lung is still apparent. Formal exercise testing usually demonstrates some impairment in maximum work rate and maximum oxygen uptake, but few recipients report any limitation to activities of daily living.

Quality of life

Both overall and health-related quality of life are enhanced. With multidimensional profiles, improvements extend across most domains and are sustained longitudinally unless

TABLE 24-2

RECIPIENT SURVIVAL, BY PRETRANSPLANTATION DIAGNOSIS (1990–2006)

DIAGNOSIS	n	SURVIVAL RATE, %				
		3 MONTHS	1 YEAR	3 YEARS	5 YEARS	10 YEARS
Chronic obstructive pulmonary disease						
Bilateral	2444	93	85	69	57	31
Single	5316	90	81	63	47	19
α_1-Antitrypsin deficiency emphysema						
Bilateral	956	88	79	67	58	36
Single	969	87	77	61	51	28
Cystic fibrosis	3275	90	82	66	56	39
Idiopathic pulmonary fibrosis						
Bilateral	1290	81	72	59	48	28
Single	2641	85	73	56	43	19
Idiopathic pulmonary arterial hypertension						
Bilateral	710	75	69	59	51	33
Single	260	71	61	51	41	24
Sarcoidosis	506	83	70	56	51	31

Source: Data from *www.ishlt.org/registries/slides.asp?slides=heartLungRegistry*.

chronic rejection or another complication develops. Other problems that detract from quality of life include renal dysfunction and drug side effects.

Cost

The cost of transplantation depends on the health care system, other health care policies, and economic factors that vary from country to country. In the United States in 2008 the average billed charge per transplant for the period 30 days before transplantation through 180 days after the transplant admission was $450,400 for single-lung transplantation and $657,800 for bilateral lung transplantation. For bilateral transplantation, the total cost included the following charges: all care during 30 days before transplantation, $20,700; donor organ procurement, $96,500; hospital transplant admission, $344,700; physician fees during transplant admission, $59,300; all inpatient and outpatient care during 180 days after transplant admission, $113,800; and all outpatient drugs, including immunosuppressants, from discharge for the transplant to 180 days after transplant admission, $22,800.

Complications

Lung transplantation can be complicated by a variety of problems (Table 24-3). Aside from predicaments that are unique to transplantation, side effects and toxicities of the immunosuppressive medications can cause new medical problems or aggravate preexisting conditions.

Graft dysfunction

Primary graft dysfunction (PGD) is an acute lung injury that is a manifestation of multiple potential insults to the donor organ inherent in the transplantation process. The principal clinical features are diffuse pulmonary infiltrates and hypoxemia within 72 h of transplantation; however, the presentation can be mimicked by pulmonary venous obstruction, hyperacute rejection, pulmonary edema, and pneumonia.

The severity is variable, and a standardized grading system has been established. Up to 50% of recipients may have some degree of PGD, and ~10–20% have severe PGD. The treatment follows the conventional, supportive paradigm for acute lung injury. Inhaled nitric oxide and extracorporeal membrane oxygenation have been used in severe cases; retransplantation also has been performed, but retransplantation in the first 30 days has a poor survival rate (~30% at 1 year). Most recipients with mild PGD recover, but the mortality rate for severe PGD has been ~40–60%. PGD also is associated with longer postoperative ventilator support, longer intensive care unit and hospital stays, higher costs, and excess morbidity rates and severe PGD is probably a risk factor for the later development of chronic rejection.

Airway complications

The bronchial blood supply to the donor lung is disrupted during procurement. Bronchial revascularization during transplantation is technically feasible in some cases, but it is not widely practiced. Consequently, after

TABLE 24-3

MAJOR POTENTIAL COMPLICATIONS OF LUNG TRANSPLANTATION AND IMMUNOSUPPRESSION	
CATEGORY	**COMPLICATION**
Allograft	Primary graft dysfunction; anastomotic dehiscence or stenosis; ischemic airway injury with bronchostenosis or bronchomalacia; rejection; infection; recurrence of primary disease (sarcoidosis, lymphangioleiomyomatosis, giant cell interstitial pneumonitis, diffuse panbronchiolitis, pulmonary alveolar proteinosis, Langerhans cell histiocytosis)
Thoracic	Phrenic nerve injury—diaphragmatic dysfunction; recurrent laryngeal nerve injury—vocal cord dysfunction; cervical ganglia injury—Horner's syndrome; pneumothorax; pleural effusion; chylothorax; empyema
Cardiovascular	Intraoperative or perioperative air embolism; postoperative pericarditis; perioperative myocardial injury/infarction; venous thromboembolism; supraventricular dysrhythmias; systemic hypertension
Gastrointestinal	Esophagitis (especially *Candida*, herpes, or cytomegalovirus [CMV]); gastroparesis; gastroesophageal reflux; diarrhea (*Clostridium difficile*; medications, especially mycophenolate mofetil and sirolimus); colitis (*C. difficile*; CMV)
Hepatobiliary	Hepatitis (especially CMV or medications); acalculous cholecystitis
Renal	Calcineurin inhibitor nephropathy; hemolytic-uremic syndrome (thrombotic microangiopathy)
Neurologic	Tremors; seizures; reversible posterior leukoencephalopathy; headaches
Musculoskeletal	Steroid myopathy; rhabdomyolysis (cyclosporine + HMG-CoA reductase inhibitor treatment); osteoporosis; avascular necrosis
Metabolic	Obesity; diabetes mellitus; hyperlipidemia; idiopathic hyperammonemia
Hematologic	Anemia; leukopenia; thrombocytopenia; thrombotic microangiopathy
Oncologic	Lymphoproliferative disease and lymphoma; skin cancers; other malignancies

implantation the donor bronchus is dependent on retrograde bronchial blood flow from the pulmonary circulation and is vulnerable to ischemia.

The spectrum of airway problems includes anastomotic necrosis and dehiscence, occlusive granulation tissue, anastomotic or bronchial stenosis, and bronchomalacia. The incidence has been in the range of 7–18%, but the associated mortality rate has been low. These problems usually can be managed bronchoscopically with techniques such as simple endoscopic debridement, laser photoresection, balloon dilatation, and bronchial stenting.

Rejection

Rejection is the main limitation to better medium- and long-term survival. It is an immunologic response to alloantigen recognition, and both cell-mediated and antibody-mediated (humoral) cascades can play a role. Cellular rejection is effected by T lymphocyte interactions with donor alloantigens, mainly in the major histocompatibility complex (MHC), whereas humoral rejection is driven by antibodies to donor MHC alloantigens or possibly to non-MHC antigens on epithelial or endothelial cells.

Rejection often is categorized as acute or chronic without mention of the mechanism. Acute rejection is cell-mediated, and its incidence is highest in the first 6–12 months after transplantation. In contrast, chronic rejection generally emerges later, and both alloimmune and nonalloimmune fibroproliferative reactions may contribute to its pathogenesis.

Acute cellular rejection

With current immunosuppressive regimens, ~25–40% of recipients have acute rejection in the first year. Acute cellular rejection (ACR) can be clinically silent, or it can be manifested by nonspecific symptoms or signs that may include cough, low-grade fever, dyspnea, hypoxemia, inspiratory crackles, interstitial infiltrates, and declining lung function; however, clinical impression is not reliable. The diagnosis is confirmed by transbronchial biopsies showing the characteristic lymphocytic infiltrates around arterioles or bronchioles, and a standardized pathologic scheme is used to grade the biopsies.

Minimal ACR on a surveillance biopsy in a clinically stable recipient often is left untreated, but higher grades generally are treated regardless of the clinical situation. Treatment usually includes a short course of high-dose steroid therapy and adjustment of the maintenance immunosuppressive regimen. Most episodes respond to this approach; however, more intensive therapy is sometimes necessary for persistent or recurrent episodes.

Chronic rejection

This complication is the main impediment to better long-term survival rates, and it is the source of substantial morbidity rates because of its impact on lung function and quality of life. Clinically, it is characterized physiologically by airflow limitation and pathologically by bronchiolitis obliterans; the process is denoted bronchiolitis obliterans syndrome (BOS). Transbronchial biopsies are relatively insensitive for detecting bronchiolitis obliterans, and pathologic confirmation is not required for diagnosis. Thus, after other causes of graft dysfunction have been excluded, the diagnosis of BOS is based primarily on a sustained decrement ($\geq$20%) in forced expiratory volume in 1s (FEV_1), although smaller declines in FEV_1 ($\geq$10%) or in forced expiratory flow FEF_{25-75}% may presage BOS. Spirometric criteria for diagnosis and staging of BOS have been standardized.

The prevalence of BOS approaches 50% by 5 years after transplantation. Antecedent ACR is the main risk factor, but PGD, CMV pneumonitis, other community-acquired respiratory viral infections, and gastroesophageal reflux have been implicated as well. BOS can present acutely and imitate infectious bronchitis, or it can manifest as an insidious decline in lung function. The chest radiograph is typically unchanged; computed tomography may reveal mosaic perfusion, air trapping, ground-glass opacities, or bronchiolectasis. Bronchoscopy is indicated to eliminate other processes, but transbronchial biopsies identify bronchiolitis obliterans in a minority of cases.

BOS usually is treated with augmented immunosuppression, but there is no consensus about therapy. Strategies include changes in the maintenance drug regimen, including the addition of azithromycin, antilymphocyte globulin, photopheresis, and total lymphoid irradiation. Although therapy may stabilize lung function, the overall results of treatment have been disappointing; median survival after onset has been ~3–4 years. Retransplantation is a consideration if clinical circumstances and other comorbidities are not prohibitive, but survival has been inferior to that with primary transplantation.

Humoral rejection

The role of antibody-mediated rejection is still evolving. Hyperacute rejection is caused by preformed human leukocyte (HLA) antibodies in the recipient, but it is minimized by pretransplantation antibody screening coupled with virtual or direct cross-matching with any potential donor. Donor-specific HLA antibodies develop after transplantation in up to 50% of recipients, and their presence has been associated with an increased risk of both ACR and BOS and with poorer overall survival. However, the mechanisms by which these antibodies could contribute to ACR or BOS or could otherwise be detrimental have not been unraveled. Formal criteria for antibody-mediated rejection have been defined for renal transplantation, but few cases in lung transplantation fulfill them. Nonetheless, episodes of acute lung allograft dysfunction occasionally have been attributed directly to antibody-mediated injury. If treatment is indicated, therapies that may deplete antibodies include plasmapheresis, intravenous immune globulin, and rituximab.

Infection

The lung allograft is especially susceptible to infection, which has been one of the leading causes of death. In addition to a blunted immune response from the immunosuppressive drugs, other normal defenses are compromised: the cough reflex is diminished, and mucociliary clearance is impaired in the transplanted lung. The spectrum of infections includes both opportunistic and nonopportunistic pathogens.

Bacterial bronchitis or pneumonia can occur at any time, but it is very common in the perioperative period. Later, bronchitis occurs frequently in recipients with BOS, and *Pseudomonas aeruginosa* or methicillin–resistant *Staphylococcus aureus* is often the culprit.

CMV is the most common viral infection. Although gastroenteritis, colitis, and hepatitis can occur, CMV viremia and CMV pneumonia are the main illnesses. Most episodes occur in the first 6 months, and treatment with ganciclovir is effective unless resistance develops. Other community-acquired viruses such as influenza, parainfluenza, and respiratory syncytial virus also contribute to respiratory complications. The most problematic fungal infections are caused by *Aspergillus* species. The spectrum encompasses simple pulmonary colonization, tracheobronchitis, invasive pulmonary aspergillosis, and disseminated aspergillosis, and the clinical scenario dictates treatment.

Other complications

Other potential complications are listed in Table 24-3. Many of them are related to side effects or toxicities of the immunosuppressive drugs. Management of these general medical problems is guided by standard practices, but the complex milieu of transplantation requires close collaboration and good communication among health care providers.

SECTION III

GENERAL APPROACH TO THE CRITICALLY ILL PATIENT

CHAPTER 25

APPROACH TO THE PATIENT WITH CRITICAL ILLNESS

John P. Kress ■ Jesse B. Hall

The care of critically ill patients requires a thorough understanding of pathophysiology and is centered initially on resuscitation of patients at extremes of physiologic deterioration. This resuscitation is often fast-paced and occurs early without a detailed awareness of the patients' chronic medical problems. While physiologic stabilization is taking place, intensivists attempt to gather important background medical information to supplement the real-time assessment of the patients' current physiologic conditions. Numerous tools are available to assist intensivists in the accurateassessment of pathophysiology and management to incipient organ failure, offering a window of opportunity for diagnosing and treating underlying disease(s) in a stabilized patient. Indeed, the use of invasive interventions such as mechanical ventilation and renal replacement therapy is commonplace in the intensive care unit. An appreciation of the risks and benefits of such aggressive and often invasive interventions is vital to assure an optimal patient outcome. Nonetheless, intensivists must recognize when patients' chances for recovery are remote or impossible and counsel and comfort dying patients and their significant others. Critical care physicians often must redirect the goals of care from resuscitation and cure to comfort when the resolution of an underlying illness is not possible.

ASSESSMENT OF SEVERITY OF ILLNESS

Categorization of a patient's illness into grades of severity occurs frequently in the intensive care unit (ICU). Numerous severity-of-illness (SOI) scoring systems have been developed and validated over the last two decades. Although these scoring systems have been validated as tools to assess populations of critically ill patients, their utility in predicting individual patient outcomes is not clear.

SOI scoring systems are important for defining populations of critically ill patients. This allows effective comparison of groups of patients enrolled in clinical trials. To be assured that a purported benefit of a therapy is real, investigators must be assured that different groups involved in a clinical trial have similar illness severities. SOI scores are also useful in guiding hospital administrative policies. Allocation of resources such as nursing and ancillary care can be directed by such scoring systems. SOI scoring systems also can assist in the assessment of quality of ICU care over time. Scoring system validations are based on the premise that increasing age, the presence of chronic medical illnesses, and increasingly severe derangements from normal physiology are associated with increased mortality rates. All currently existing SOI scoring systems are derived from patients who already have been admitted to the ICU. There are no established scoring systems available that purport to direct clinicians' decision-making regarding criteria for admission to an ICU.

Currently, the most commonly utilized scoring systems are the APACHE (acute physiology and chronic health evaluation) system and the SAPS (simplified acute physiology score) system. These systems were designed to predict outcomes in critical illness and use common variables that include age; vital signs; assessments of respiratory, renal, and neurologic function; and an evaluation of chronic medical illnesses.

APACHE II SCORING SYSTEM

The APACHE II system is the most commonly used SOI scoring system in North America. Age, type of ICU admission (after elective surgery vs. nonsurgical or after emergency surgery), a chronic health problem score, and 12 physiologic variables (the most severely abnormal of each in the first 24 h of ICU admission) are used to derive a score. The predicted hospital mortality is derived from a formula that takes into account the APACHE II score, the need for emergency surgery, and a weighted, disease-specific diagnostic category (Table 25-1). The relationship between APACHE II score and mortality is illustrated in Fig. 25-1. Updated versions of the APACHE scoring system (APACHE III and APACHE IV) have been published. APACHE III is derived from a larger database than APACHE II and utilizes a daily clinical update protocol to provide daily modification of predicted mortality. APACHE IV uses a

TABLE 25-1

CALCULATION OF ACUTE PHYSIOLOGY AND CHRONIC HEALTH EVALUATION II (APACHE II)[a]

Acute Physiology Score

SCORE	4	3	2	1	0	1	2	3	4
Rectal temperature, °C	≥41	39.0–40.9		38.5–38.9	36.0–38.4	34.0–35.9	32.0–33.9	30.0–31.9	≤29.9
Mean blood pressure, mmHg	≥160	130–159	110–129		70–109		50–69		≤49
Heart rate	≥180	140–179	110–139		70–109		55–69	40–54	≤39
Respiratory rate	≥50	35–49		25–34	12–24	10–11	6–9		≤5
Arterial pH	≥7.70	7.60–7.69		7.50–7.59	7.33–7.49		7.25–7.32	7.15–7.24	<7.15
Oxygenation									
If $FI_{O_2} > 0.5$, use $(A-a) D_{O_2}$	≥500	350–499	200–349	<200					
If $FI_{O_2} \leq 0.5$, use Pa_{O_2}					≥70	61–70		55–60	<55
Serum sodium, meq/L	≥180	160–179	155–159	150–154	130–149		120–129	111–119	≤110
Serum potassium, meq/L	≥7.0	6.0–6.9		5.5–5.9	3.5–5.4	3.0–3.4	2.5–2.9		<2.5
Serum creatinine, mg/dL	≥3.5	2.0–3.4	1.5–1.9		0.6–1.4		<0.6		
Hematocrit	≥60		50–59.9	46–49.9	30–45.9		20–29.9		<20
WBC count, 10^3/mL	≥40		20–39.9	15–19.9	3–14.9		1–2.9		<1

Glasgow Coma Score[b,c]

EYE OPENING	VERBAL (NONINTUBATED)	VERBAL (INTUBATED)	MOTOR ACTIVITY
4—Spontaneous	5—Oriented and talks	5—Seems able to talk	6—Verbal command
3—Verbal stimuli	4—Disoriented and talks	3—Questionable ability to talk	5—Localizes to pain
2—Painful stimuli	3—Inappropriate words	1—Generally unresponsive	4—Withdraws to pain
1—No response	2—Incomprehensible sounds		3—Decorticate
	1—No response		2—Decerebrate
			1—No response

Points Assigned to Age and Chronic Disease as Part of the APACHE II Score

AGE, YEARS	SCORE
<45	0
45–54	2
55–64	3
65–74	5
≥75	6

CHRONIC HEALTH (HISTORY OF CHRONIC CONDITIONS)[d]	SCORE
None	0
If patient is admitted after elective surgery	2
If patient is admitted after emergency surgery or for reason other than after elective surgery	5

[a]APACHE II score is the sum of the acute physiology score (vital signs, oxygenation, laboratory values), Glasgow coma score, age, and chronic health points. Worst values during first 24 h in the ICU should be used.

[b]Glasgow coma score (GCS) = eye-opening score + verbal (intubated or nonintubated) score + motor score.

[c]For GCS component of acute physiology score, subtract GCS from 15 to obtain points assigned.

[d]Chronic health conditions: liver, cirrhosis with portal hypertension or encephalopathy; cardiovascular, class IV angina (at rest or with minimal self-care activities); pulmonary, chronic hypoxemia or hypercapnia, polycythemia, ventilator dependent; kidney, chronic peritoneal or hemodialysis; immune, immunocompromised host.

Note: $(A-a) D_{O_2}$, alveolar-arterial oxygen difference; WBC, white blood (cell) count.

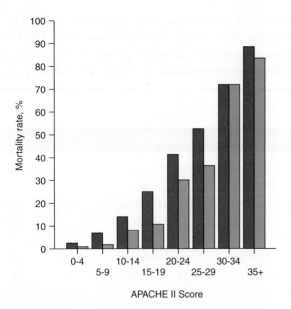

FIGURE 25-1
APACHE II survival curve. Blue, nonoperative; green, post-operative.

modified statistical model of logistic regression; it is the most recently released version of this scoring system.

THE SAPS SCORING SYSTEM

The SAPS II score, used more frequently in Europe, was derived in a manner similar to the APACHE scores. This score is not disease-specific but, rather, incorporates three underlying disease variables (AIDS, metastatic cancer, and hematologic malignancy).

Severity of illness scoring systems cannot be used to predict survival in individual patients. Accordingly, the use of these scoring systems to direct therapy and clinical decision-making cannot be recommended at present. Instead, these tools should be used as important data to complement clinical bedside decision-making.

SHOCK

(See also Chap. 27)

INITIAL EVALUATION

Shock is a common condition necessitating admission to the ICU or occurring in the course of critical care. Shock is defined by the presence of multisystem end organ hypoperfusion. Clinical indicators include reduced mean arterial pressure (MAP), tachycardia, tachypnea, cool skin and extremities, acute altered mental status, and oliguria. Hypotension is usually, though not always, present. The end result of multiorgan hypoperfusion is tissue hypoxia, often clinically manifested by lactic acidosis. Since the MAP is the product of cardiac output and

systemic vascular resistance (SVR), reductions in blood pressure can be caused by decreased cardiac output and/or decreased SVR. Accordingly, the initial evaluation of a hypotensive patient should include an assessment of the adequacy of cardiac output; this should be part of the earliest assessment of the patient by the clinician at the bedside once shock is contemplated (Fig. 25-2). Clinical evidence of *diminished* cardiac output includes a narrow pulse pressure—a marker that correlates with stroke volume—and cool extremities with delayed capillary refill. Signs of *increased* cardiac output include a widened pulse pressure (particularly with a reduced diastolic pressure), warm extremities with bounding pulses, and rapid capillary refill. If a hypotensive patient has clinical signs of increased cardiac output, one can infer that the reduced blood pressure is a result of decreased SVR.

In hypotensive patients with signs of a reduced cardiac output, an assessment of intravascular and cardiac volume status is appropriate. A hypotensive patient with decreased intravascular volume status may have a history suggesting hemorrhage or other volume losses (e.g., vomiting, diarrhea, polyuria). The jugular venous pressure (JVP) may be reduced in such a patient, although the change in right

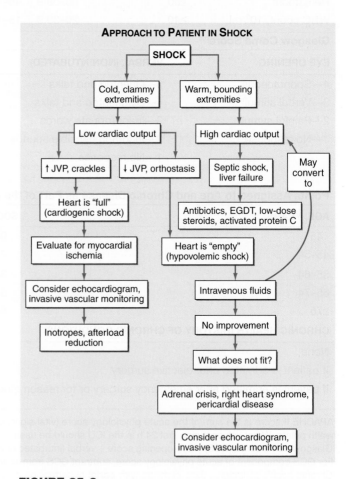

FIGURE 25-2
Approach to patient in shock. EGDT, early goal-directed therapy; JVP, jugular venous pulse.

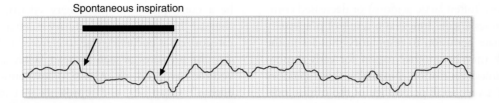

FIGURE 25-3
Right atrial pressure change during spontaneous respiration in a patient with shock who will increase cardiac output in response to intravenous fluid administration. The right atrial pressure decreases from 7 mmHg to 4 mmHg. The horizontal bar marks the time of spontaneous inspiration.

Spontaneous inspiration

atrial pressure as a function of spontaneous respiration is a better predictor of fluid responsiveness (**Fig. 25-3**). Patients with fluid-responsive (i.e., hypovolemic) shock also may manifest large changes in pulse pressure as a function of respiration during positive-pressure mechanical ventilation (**Fig. 25-4**). A hypotensive patient with increased intravascular volume status and cardiac dysfunction may have S_3 and/or S_4 gallops on examination, increased JVP, extremity edema, and crackles on lung auscultation. The chest x-ray may show cardiomegaly, widening of the vascular pedicle, Kerley B lines, and pulmonary edema. Chest pain and electrocardiographic changes consistent with ischemia may be noted (Chap. 30).

In hypotensive patients with clinical evidence of increased cardiac output, a search for causes of decreased SVR is appropriate. The most common cause of high cardiac output hypotension is sepsis (Chap. 28). Other causes of high cardiac output hypotension include liver failure, severe pancreatitis, burns and other trauma that elicit the systemic inflammatory response syndrome (SIRS), anaphylaxis, thyrotoxicosis, and peripheral arteriovenous shunts.

In summary, the most common categories of shock are hypovolemic, cardiogenic, and high cardiac output with decreased SVR (high-output hypotension). Certainly these categories may overlap and occur simultaneously (e.g., hypovolemic and septic shock).

The initial assessment of a patient in shock as outlined above should take only a few minutes. It is important that

aggressive, early resuscitation is instituted based on the initial assessment, particularly since early resuscitation of septic and cardiogenic shock may improve survival (see below). If the initial bedside assessment yields equivocal or confounding data, more objective assessments such as echocardiography and/or invasive vascular monitoring may be useful. The goal of early resuscitation is to reestablish adequate tissue perfusion to prevent or minimize end organ injury.

MECHANICAL VENTILATORY SUPPORT

(See also Chap. 26) During the initial resuscitation of patients in shock, principles of advanced cardiac life support should be followed. Since patients in shock may be obtunded and unable to protect the airway, an early assessment of the patient's airway is mandatory during resuscitation from shock. Early intubation and mechanical ventilation often are required. Reasons for the institution of endotracheal intubation and mechanical ventilation include acute hypoxemic respiratory failure and ventilatory failure, which frequently accompany shock. Acute hypoxemic respiratory failure may occur in patients with cardiogenic shock and pulmonary edema (Chap. 30) as well as in those in septic shock with pneumonia or acute respiratory distress syndrome (ARDS) (Chaps. 28 and 29). Ventilatory failure often occurs as a result of an increased load on the respiratory system. This load may present in the form of acute

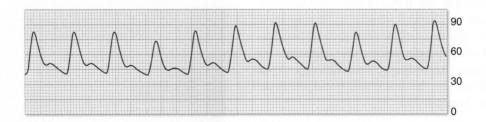

FIGURE 25-4
Pulse pressure change during mechanical ventilation in a patient with shock who will increase cardiac output in response to intravenous fluid administration. The pulse pressure (systolic minus diastolic blood pressure) changes during mechanical ventilation in a patient with septic shock.

metabolic acidosis (often lactic acidosis) or decreased compliance of the lungs ("stiff" lungs) as a result of pulmonary edema. Inadequate perfusion to respiratory muscles in the setting of shock may be another reason for early intubation and mechanical ventilation. Normally, the respiratory muscles receive a very small percentage of the cardiac output. However, in patients who are in shock with respiratory distress for the reasons listed above, the percentage of cardiac output dedicated to respiratory muscles may increase tenfold or more. Lactic acid production from inefficient respiratory muscle activity presents an additional ventilatory load.

Mechanical ventilation may relieve the patient of the work of breathing and allow redistribution of a limited cardiac output to other vital organs, often with an improvement in lactic acidosis. Patients demonstrate signs of respiratory distress with a number of clinical signs, including inability to speak full sentences, accessory use of respiratory muscles, paradoxical abdominal muscle activity, extreme tachypnea (>40 breaths/min), and decreasing respiratory rate despite an increasing drive to breathe. When patients with shock are treated with mechanical ventilation, a major goal of ventilator settings is to assume all or the majority of work of breathing, facilitating a state of minimal respiratory muscle work. With the institution of mechanical ventilation for shock, further declines in MAP are frequently seen. The reasons for this include impeded venous return with positive-pressure ventilation, reduced endogenous catecholamine secretion once the stress associated with respiratory failure abates, and the actions of drugs used to facilitate endotracheal intubation (e.g., barbiturates, benzodiazepines, opiates), all of which may result in hypotension. Accordingly, hypotension should be anticipated after endotracheal intubation and positive-pressure ventilation. Many of these patients have a component of hypovolemia, which may respond to IV volume administration. Fig. 25-2 summarizes the diagnosis and treatment of different types of shock. For further discussion of individual forms of shock, see Chaps. 27, 28, and 30.

RESPIRATORY FAILURE

Respiratory failure is one of the most common reasons patients are admitted to the ICU. In some ICUs, ≥75% of patients require mechanical ventilation during their stay. Respiratory failure can be categorized mechanistically, based on pathophysiologic derangements in respiratory function. Accordingly, four different types of respiratory failure can be described, based on these pathophysiologic derangements.

Type I, acute hypoxemic respiratory failure

This occurs when alveolar flooding and subsequent intrapulmonary shunt physiology occur. Alveolar flooding may

be a consequence of pulmonary edema, pneumonia, or alveolar hemorrhage. Pulmonary edema can be further categorized as occurring due to elevated pulmonary microvascular pressures as seen in heart failure and intravascular volume overload or ARDS ("low-pressure pulmonary edema"; Chap. 29) and represents an extreme degree of lung injury. This syndrome is defined by diffuse bilateral airspace edema seen on chest radiography, the absence of left atrial hypertension, and profound shunt physiology (Fig. 25-5) in a clinical setting in which this syndrome is known to occur, including sepsis, gastric aspiration, pneumonia, near-drowning, multiple blood transfusions, and pancreatitis. The mortality rate of patients with ARDS was traditionally very high (50–70%), although recent changes in ventilator management strategy have led to reports of mortality rates closer to 30% (see later).

For many years, physicians have suspected that mechanical ventilation of patients with acute lung injury and ARDS may propagate lung injury. Cyclical collapse and reopening of alveoli may be partly responsible for this. As seen in Fig. 25-6, the pressure-volume relationship of the lung in ARDS is not linear. Alveoli may collapse at very low lung volumes. Animal studies have suggested that stretching and overdistention of injured alveoli during mechanical ventilation can further injure the lung. Concern over this alveolar overdistention, termed *ventilator-induced "volutrauma,"*

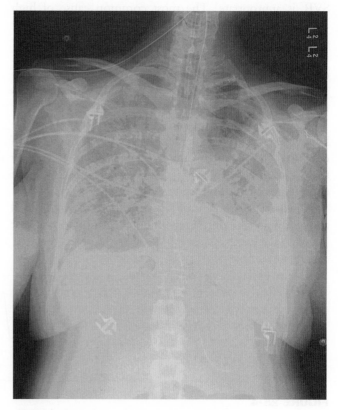

FIGURE 25-5

Chest radiograph of a patient with ARDS. ARDS, acute respiratory distress syndrome.

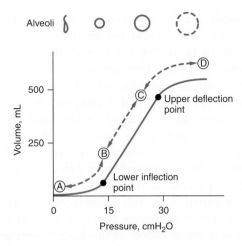

FIGURE 25-6
Pressure-volume relationship of the lungs of a patient with ARDS. At the lower inflection point, collapsed alveoli begin to open, and the lung compliance changes. At the upper deflection point, alveoli become overdistended. The shape and size of alveoli are illustrated at the top. ARDS, acute respiratory distress syndrome.

led to a multicenter, randomized, prospective trial to compare traditional ventilator strategies for acute lung injury and ARDS (large tidal volume—12 mL/kg ideal body weight) to a low tidal volume (6 mL/kg ideal body weight). This study showed a dramatic reduction in mortality rate in the low tidal volume group (large tidal volume—39.8% mortality rate versus low tidal volume—31% mortality rate) and confirmed that ventilator management could affect outcomes in these patients. In addition, a "fluid conservative" management strategy (maintaining a relatively low central venous pressure [CVP] or pulmonary capillary wedge pressure [PCWP]) is associated with the need for fewer days of mechanical ventilation compared with a "fluid liberal" management strategy (maintaining a relatively high CVP or PCWP) in acute lung injury and ARDS.

Type II respiratory failure

This type of respiratory failure occurs as a result of alveolar hypoventilation and results in the inability to eliminate carbon dioxide effectively. Mechanisms by which this occurs are categorized by impaired central nervous system (CNS) drive to breathe, impaired strength with failure of neuromuscular function in the respiratory system, and increased load(s) on the respiratory system. Reasons for diminished CNS drive to breathe include drug overdose, brainstem injury, sleep-disordered breathing, and hypothyroidism. Reduced strength can be due to impaired neuromuscular transmission (e.g., myasthenia gravis, Guillain-Barré syndrome, amyotrophic lateral sclerosis, phrenic nerve injury) or respiratory muscle weakness (e.g., myopathy, electrolyte derangements, fatigue).

The overall load on the respiratory system can be sub-classified into increased resistive loads (e.g., bronchospasm), loads due to reduced lung compliance (e.g., alveolar edema, atelectasis, intrinsic positive end-expiratory pressure [autoPEEP]—see later), loads due to reduced chest wall compliance (e.g., pneumothorax, pleural effusion, abdominal distention), and loads due to increased minute ventilation requirements (e.g., pulmonary embolus with increased dead space fraction, sepsis).

The mainstays of therapy for type II respiratory failure are treatments directed at reversing the underlying cause(s) of ventilatory failure. Noninvasive positive-pressure ventilation using a mechanical ventilator with a tight-fitting face or nasal mask that avoids endotracheal intubation often can stabilize these patients. This approach has been shown to be beneficial in treating patients with exacerbations of chronic obstructive pulmonary disease. Noninvasive ventilation has been tested less extensively in other types of type II respiratory failure, but may be attempted nonetheless in the absence of contraindications (hemodynamic instability, inability to protect airway, respiratory arrest).

Type III respiratory failure

This form of respiratory failure occurs as a result of lung atelectasis. Because atelectasis occurs so commonly in the perioperative period, this is also called perioperative respiratory failure. After general anesthesia, decreases in functional residual capacity lead to collapse of dependent lung units. Such atelectasis can be treated by frequent changes in position, chest physiotherapy, upright positioning, and aggressive control of incisional and/or abdominal pain. Noninvasive positive-pressure ventilation may also be used to reverse regional atelectasis.

Type IV respiratory failure

This form results from hypoperfusion of respiratory muscles in patients in shock. Normally, respiratory muscles consume <5% of the total cardiac output and O_2 delivery. Patients in shock often experience respiratory distress due to pulmonary edema (e.g., patients in cardiogenic shock), lactic acidosis, and anemia. In this setting, up to 40% of the cardiac output may be distributed to the respiratory muscles. Intubation and mechanical ventilation can allow redistribution of the cardiac output away from the respiratory muscles and back to vital organs while the shock is treated.

CARE OF THE MECHANICALLY VENTILATED PATIENT

(See also Chap. 26) Whereas a thorough understanding of the pathophysiology of respiratory failure is essential to optimize patient care, recognition of a patient's readiness to be liberated from mechanical ventilation is similarly important. Several studies have shown that subjecting patients to daily spontaneous breathing trials can identify those ready for extubation. Accordingly, all intubated, mechanically ventilated patients should undergo a daily screening of respiratory function. If oxygenation is stable (i.e., $Pa_{O_2}/Fi_{O_2} >200$ and PEEP ≤ 5 cmH$_2$O), cough and airway reflexes are intact, and no vasopressor agents or sedatives are being administered, the patient has passed the screening test and should undergo a spontaneous breathing trial. This trial consists of a period of breathing through the endotracheal tube without ventilator support (both continuous positive airway pressure [CPAP] of 5 cmH$_2$O and an open T-piece breathing system can be used) for 30–120 min. The spontaneous breathing trial is declared a failure and stopped if *any* of the following occur: (1) respiratory rate >35/min for >5 min, (2) O$_2$ saturation <90%, (3) heart rate >140/min or a 20% increase or decrease from baseline, (4) systolic blood pressure <90 mmHg or >180 mmHg, (5) increased anxiety or diaphoresis. If, at the end of the spontaneous breathing trial, the ratio of the respiratory rate and tidal volume in liters (f/V$_T$) is <105, the patient can be extubated. Such protocol-driven approaches to patient care can have an important impact on the duration of mechanical ventilation and length of stay in the ICU. In spite of such a careful approach to liberation from mechanical ventilation, up to 10% of patients will develop respiratory distress after extubation and may require resumption of mechanical ventilation. Many of these patients will require reintubation. The use of noninvasive ventilation in patients who fail extubation may be associated with worse outcomes compared with immediate reintubation.

Mechanically ventilated patients frequently require sedatives and analgesics. Most patients undergoing mechanical ventilation experience pain, which can be elicited by the presence of the endotracheal tube and endotracheal suctioning. Accordingly, early attention to pain control is extremely important. Opiates are the mainstay of therapy for pain control in mechanically ventilated patients. After adequate pain control has been assured, additional indications for sedation for mechanically ventilated patients include anxiolysis; treatment of subjective dyspnea; psychosis; facilitation of nursing care; reduction of autonomic hyperactivity, which may precipitate myocardial ischemia; and reduction of total O$_2$ consumption (V$_{O_2}$).

Neuromuscular blocking agents are occasionally needed to facilitate mechanical ventilation in patients with profound dyssynchrony with the ventilator despite optimal sedation. The use of neuromuscular blocking agents may result in prolonged weakness—a myopathy known as the *postparalytic syndrome*. For this reason, these agents typically are used as a last resort when aggressive sedation fails to achieve patient-ventilator synchrony. Because neuromuscular blocking agents result in pharmacologic paralysis without altering mental status, sedative-induced amnesia is mandatory when these agents are administered.

Amnesia can be achieved reliably with benzodiazepines such as lorazepam and midazolam as well as the IV anesthetic agent propofol. Outside the setting of pharmacologic paralysis, there are few data supporting the idea that amnesia is mandatory in all patients who require intubation and mechanical ventilation. Since many of these patients have impaired hepatic and renal function, sedatives and opiates may accumulate in critically ill patients when they are given for prolonged periods. A protocol-driven approach to sedation of mechanically ventilated patients with daily interruption of sedative infusions paired with daily spontaneous breathing trials has been shown to prevent excessive drug accumulation and shorten the duration of mechanical ventilation and length of stay in the ICU.

MULTIORGAN SYSTEM FAILURE

The syndrome of multiorgan system failure is a common problem associated with critical illness. This syndrome is defined by the simultaneous presence of physiologic dysfunction and/or failure of two or more organs. Typically, this occurs in the setting of severe sepsis, shock of any kind, severe inflammatory conditions such as pancreatitis, and trauma. The fact that multiorgan system failure occurs commonly in the ICU is a testament to our current ability to stabilize and support single-organ failure. The ability to support single-organ failure aggressively (e.g., mechanical ventilation for respiratory failure, renal replacement therapy for acute renal failure) has affected rates of early mortality in critical illness greatly. As a result, it is uncommon for critically ill patients to die in the initial stages of resuscitation. Instead, many patients succumb to critical illness later in the ICU stay, after the initial presenting problem has been stabilized.

Although there is debate regarding specific definitions of organ failure, several general principles governing the syndrome of multiorgan system failure apply. First, organ failure, no matter how defined, must persist beyond 24 h. Second, mortality risk increases as patients accrue additional failing. Third, prognosis is worsened by increased duration of organ failure. These observations remain true across various critical care settings (e.g., medical versus surgical). SIRS is a common basis for multiorgan system failure. Although infection is a common cause of SIRS, "sterile" triggers such as pancreatitis, trauma, and burns often are invoked to explain multiorgan system failure.

MONITORING IN THE ICU

Because respiratory and circulatory failure occurs commonly in critically ill patients, monitoring of the respiratory and cardiovascular systems is undertaken frequently in the ICU. Evaluation of respiratory gas exchange is routine in critical illness. The "gold standard" remains arterial blood-gas analysis, in which pH, partial pressures of O_2 and CO_2, and O_2 saturation are measured directly. With arterial blood-gas analysis, the two main functions of the lung—oxygenation of arterial blood and elimination of CO_2—can be assessed directly. Importantly, the blood pH, which has a profound effect on the drive to breathe, can be assessed only by sampling arterial blood. Though sampling of arterial blood is generally safe, it may be painful and cannot provide continuous information for clinicians routinely. In light of these limitations, noninvasive monitoring of respiratory function is often employed in the critical care setting.

PULSE OXIMETRY

This is the most commonly utilized noninvasive monitor of respiratory function. This technique takes advantage of differences in the absorptive properties of oxygenated and deoxygenated hemoglobin. At wavelengths of 660 nm, oxyhemoglobin reflects light more effectively than does deoxyhemoglobin, whereas the reverse is true in the infrared spectrum (940 nm). A pulse oximeter passes both wavelengths of light through a perfused digit such as a finger, and the relative intensity of light transmission at these two wavelengths is recorded. This allows the derivation of the relative percentage of oxyhemoglobin. Since arterial pulsations produce phasic changes in the intensity of transmitted light, the pulse oximeter is designed to detect only light of alternating intensity. This allows distinction of arterial and venous blood O_2 saturations.

Respiratory system mechanics

These can be measured in patients during mechanical ventilation (Chap. 26). When volume-controlled modes of mechanical ventilation are used, accompanying airway pressures can be easily measured, assuming the patient is passive. The peak airway pressure is determined by two variables: airway resistance and respiratory system compliance. At the end of inspiration, inspiratory flow can be stopped transiently. This end-inspiratory pause (*plateau pressure*) is a static measurement, affected only by respiratory system compliance, not airway resistance. Therefore, during volume-controlled ventilation, the difference between the peak (airway resistance + respiratory system compliance) and plateau (respiratory system compliance only) airway pressures provides a quantitative assessment of airway resistance. Accordingly, during volume-controlled ventilation, patients with increases in airway resistance typically have increased peak airway pressures as well as abnormally high gradients between peak and plateau airway pressures (typically >15 cmH_2O).

The compliance of the respiratory system is defined by the change in pressure of the respiratory system per unit change in volume.

The respiratory system can be divided further into two components: the lungs and the chest wall. Normally, respiratory system compliance is ~100 mL per cmH_2O. Pathophysiologic processes such as pleural effusions, pneumothorax, and increased abdominal girth from ascites all reduce chest wall compliance. Lung compliance may be reduced by pneumonia, pulmonary edema from any cause, or autoPEEP. Accordingly, patients with abnormalities in compliance of the respiratory system (lungs and/or chest wall) typically have elevated peak *and* plateau airway pressures but a normal gradient between peak and plateau airway pressures. AutoPEEP occurs when there is insufficient time for emptying of alveoli before the next inspiratory cycle. Since the alveoli have not decompressed completely, alveolar pressure remains positive at end exhalation (functional residual capacity). This phenomenon results most commonly from critical narrowing of distal airways in disease processes such as asthma and chronic obstructive pulmonary disease. AutoPEEP with resulting alveolar overdistention may result in diminished lung compliance, reflected by abnormally increased plateau airway pressures. Modern mechanical ventilators allow breath-to-breath display of pressure and flow, which may allow detection of problems such as patient-ventilator dyssynchrony, airflow obstruction, and autoPEEP (**Fig. 25-7**).

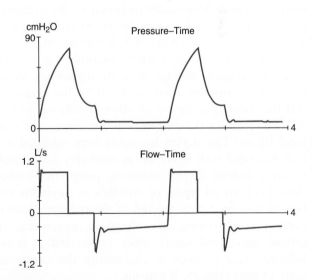

FIGURE 25-7

Increased airway resistance with autoPEEP. The top waveform (airway pressure vs. time) shows a large difference between the peak airway pressure (80 cmH_2O) and the plateau airway pressure (20 cmH_2O). The bottom waveform (flow vs. time) demonstrates airflow throughout expiration (reflected by the flow tracing on the negative portion of the abscissa) that persists up to the next inspiratory effort.

CIRCULATORY STATUS

Oxygen delivery (Q_{O_2}) is a function of cardiac output and the content of O_2 in the arterial blood (Ca_{O_2}). The Ca_{O_2} is determined by the hemoglobin concentration, the arterial hemoglobin saturation, and dissolved O_2 not bound to hemoglobin. For normal adults:

$$Q_{O_2} = 50 \text{ dL/min} \times (1.39 \times 15 \text{ g/dL [hemoglobin}$$
$$\text{concentration]} \times 1.0 \text{ [hemoglobin \% satura-}$$
$$\text{tion]} + 0.0031 \times 100 \text{ [Pa}_{O_2}])$$

$$= 50 \text{ dL/min (cardiac output)} \times 21.16 \text{ mL } O_2 \text{ per}$$
$$\text{dL blood (Ca}_{O_2})$$

$$= 1058 \text{ mL } O_2 \text{ per min}$$

It is apparent that the vast majority of O_2 delivered to tissues is bound to hemoglobin and that the dissolved O_2 (Pa_{O_2}) contributes very little to O_2 content in arterial blood or O_2 delivery. Normally, the content of O_2 in mixed venous blood ($C\bar{v}_{O_2}$) is 15.76 mL O_2 per dL blood, since the mixed venous blood is 75% saturated. Therefore, the normal tissue extraction ratio for O_2 is $Ca_{O_2} \times C\bar{v}_{O_2}/Ca_{O_2}$ ([21.16–15.76]/21.16) or ~25%. A pulmonary artery catheter allows measurements of O_2 delivery and O_2 extraction ratio.

The mixed venous O_2 saturation allows assessment of global tissue perfusion. A reduced mixed venous O_2 saturation may be caused by inadequate cardiac output, reduced hemoglobin concentration, and/or reduced arterial O_2 saturation. An abnormally high O_2 consumption (V_{O_2}) may also lead to a reduced mixed venous O_2 saturation if O_2 delivery is not concomitantly increased. Abnormally increased V_{O_2} by peripheral tissues may be caused by a multitude of problems, such as fever, agitation, shivering, and thyrotoxicosis.

The pulmonary artery catheter originally was designed as a tool to guide therapy in acute myocardial infarction but is currently used in the ICU for evaluation and treatment of a variety of other conditions, such as ARDS, septic shock, congestive heart failure, and acute renal failure. This device has never been validated as a tool associated with reduction in morbidity and mortality rates. Indeed, despite numerous prospective studies, there has been no report of mortality or morbidity rate benefit associated with the use of the pulmonary artery catheter in any setting. Accordingly, it appears that the routine use of pulmonary artery catheterization is not indicated as a monitor to characterize the circulatory status in most critically ill patients.

Recent data suggest that static measurements of circulatory parameters (e.g., CVP, PCWP) do not provide reliable information on the circulatory status of critically ill patients. In contrast, dynamic assessments measuring the impact of breathing on the circulation are more reliable predictors of responsiveness to IV fluid administration. A decrease in CVP of >1 mmHg during inspiration in a spontaneously breathing patient has been shown to predict an increase in cardiac output after IV fluid administration. Similarly, a changing pulse pressure during mechanical ventilation has been shown to predict an increase in cardiac output after IV fluid administration in patients with septic shock.

PREVENTION OF COMPLICATIONS OF CRITICAL ILLNESS

Sepsis in the critical care unit

(See also Chap. 28) Sepsis is a significant problem in the care of critically ill patients. It is the leading cause of death in noncoronary ICUs in the United States, with case rates expected to increase as the population ages with a greater percentage of people vulnerable to infection.

Many therapeutic interventions in the ICU are invasive and predispose patients to infectious complications. These interventions include endotracheal intubation, indwelling vascular catheters, nasally placed enteral feeding tubes, transurethral bladder catheters, and other catheters placed into sterile body cavities (e.g., tube thoracostomy, percutaneous intraabdominal drainage catheters). The longer such devices remain in place, the more prone to these infections patients become. For example, ventilator-associated pneumonia (VAP) correlates strongly with the duration of intubation and mechanical ventilation. Therefore, an important aspect of preventive care is the timely removal of invasive devices as soon as they are no longer needed. Multidrug-resistant organisms are commonplace in the ICU.

An important aspect of critical care is infection control in the ICU. Simple measures such as frequent hand washing are effective but underutilized strategies. Protective isolation of patients with colonization or infection by drug-resistant organisms is another frequently used strategy in the critical care setting. A recent study utilizing silver-coated endotracheal tubes reported a significant reduction in VAP incidence. Studies evaluating multifaceted, evidence-based strategies to decrease catheter-related bloodstream infections have shown improved outcomes from using measures such as hand washing, full-barrier precautions during insertion, chlorhexidine skin preparation, avoidance of the femoral site, and timely catheter removal.

Deep venous thromboses (DVTs)

All ICU patients are at high risk for this complication because of their predilection for being immobile. Therefore, all should receive some form of prophylaxis against DVT. The most commonly employed forms of prophylaxis are subcutaneous low-dose heparin injections and sequential compression devices for the lower extremities. Observational studies report an alarming incidence of the occurrence of DVTs despite the use of these standard prophylactic regimens. Heparin prophylaxis may result in heparin-induced thrombocytopenia (HIT), another relatively common nosocomial complication in critically ill patients.

Low-molecular-weight heparins such as enoxaparin are more effective than unfractionated heparin for DVT prophylaxis in high-risk patients, such as those undergoing orthopedic surgery, and they have a lower incidence of HIT. Fondaparinux, a selective factor Xa inhibitor, is even more effective than enoxaparin in high-risk orthopedic patients.

Stress ulcers

Prophylaxis against stress ulcers is frequently administered in most ICUs; typically, histamine-2 antagonists are given. Currently available data suggest that high-risk patients, such as those with coagulopathy, shock, or respiratory failure requiring mechanical ventilation, benefit from such prophylactic treatment.

Nutrition and glycemic control

These are important issues in critically ill patients that may be associated with respiratory failure, impaired wound healing, and dysfunctional immune response. Early enteral feeding is reasonable, though no data are available to suggest that this improves patient outcome per se. Certainly, enteral feeding, if possible, is preferred over parenteral nutrition, which is associated with numerous complications, including hyperglycemia, fatty liver, cholestasis, and sepsis. In addition, enteral feeding may prevent bacterial translocation across the gut mucosa. Tight glucose control is another area of controversy in critical care. Although one study showed a significant mortality benefit when glucose levels were aggressively normalized in a large group of surgical ICU patients, more recent data suggest that tight glucose control in a large population of both medical and surgical ICU patients resulted in increased rates of mortality.

ICU-acquired weakness

This occurs frequently in patients who survive critical illness. It is particularly common in those with SIRS and/or sepsis. Neuropathies and myopathies both have been described, most commonly after ~1 week in the ICU. The mechanisms behind ICU-acquired weakness syndromes are poorly understood. Intensive insulin therapy may reduce polyneuropathy of critical illness. A recent study of very early physical and occupational therapy in mechanically ventilated critically ill patients reported significant improvements in functional independence at hospital discharge, as well as reduced duration of mechanical ventilation and delirium.

Anemia

This is a common problem in critically ill patients. Studies have shown that the vast majority of ICU patients are anemic. Furthermore, most have anemia of chronic inflammation. Phlebotomy contributes significantly to anemia in ICU patients. Studies have demonstrated that erythropoietin levels are inappropriately reduced in most ICU patients and that exogenous erythropoietin administration may reduce transfusion requirements in the ICU. The hemoglobin level that merits transfusion in critically ill patients has been a long-standing area of controversy. A large, multicenter study involving patients in many different ICU settings challenged the conventional notion that a hemoglobin level of 100 g/L (10 g/dL) is needed in critically ill patients. Red blood cell transfusion is associated with impairment of immune function and increased risk of infections as well as acute lung injury and volume overload, all of which may explain the findings in this study. A conservative transfusion strategy should be the rule in managing critically ill patients who are not actively hemorrhaging.

Acute renal failure

This occurs in a significant percentage of critically ill patients. The most common underlying etiology is acute tubular necrosis, usually precipitated by hypoperfusion and/or nephrotoxic agents. Currently, there are no pharmacologic agents available for prevention of renal injury in critical illness. A recent study showed convincingly that low-dose dopamine is *not* effective in protecting the kidneys from acute injury.

NEUROLOGIC DYSFUNCTION IN CRITICALLY ILL PATIENTS

Delirium

(See also Chap. 35) This state is defined by (1) an acute onset of changes or fluctuations in the course of mental status, (2) inattention, (3) disorganized thinking, and (4) an altered level of consciousness (i.e., other than alert). Delirium is reported to occur in over 80% of mechanically ventilated ICU patients and can be detected by the Confusion Assessment Method (CAM)-ICU. This assessment asks patients to answer simple questions and perform simple tasks and can be completed by the bedside nurse in ~2 min. The differential diagnosis of delirium in ICU patients is broad and includes infectious etiologies (including sepsis), medications (particularly sedatives and analgesics), drug withdrawal, metabolic/electrolyte derangements, intracranial pathology (e.g., stroke, intracranial hemorrhage), seizures, hypoxia, hypertensive crisis, shock, and vitamin deficiencies (particularly thiamine). Patients with ICU delirium have increases in hospital length of stay, time on mechanical ventilation, cognitive impairment at hospital discharge, and 6-month mortality rate. Interventions to reduce ICU delirium have been described recently. The use of the novel sedative dexmedetomidine was associated with reduced ICU delirium compared with midazolam. In addition, as mentioned earlier in the section "ICU-Acquired Weakness," very early physical and occupational therapy in mechanically ventilated patients also has been demonstrated to reduce delirium.

Anoxic cerebral injury

(See also Chap. 35) This condition is common after cardiac arrest and often results in severe and permanent brain injury in patients whose cardiac arrest is resuscitated. Active cooling of patients after cardiac arrest has been shown to improve neurologic outcomes. Therefore, patients who present to the ICU after circulatory arrest from ventricular fibrillation or pulseless ventricular tachycardia should be actively cooled with cooling blankets and ice packs if necessary to achieve a core body temperature of 32–34°C.

Stroke

This is a common cause of neurologic critical illness. Hypertension must be managed carefully, since abrupt reductions in blood pressure may be associated with further brain ischemia and injury. Acute ischemic stroke treated with tissue plasminogen activator (tPA) has an improved neurologic outcome when treatment is given within 3 h of onset of symptoms. The mortality rate is not improved when tPA is compared with placebo, despite the improved neurologic outcome. Cerebral hemorrhage is significantly higher in patients given tPA. A treatment benefit is not seen when tPA therapy is given beyond 3 h. Heparin has not been shown to demonstrate improved outcomes convincingly in patients with acute ischemic stroke.

Subarachnoid hemorrhage

This may occur secondary to aneurysm rupture and is often complicated by cerebral vasospasm, rebleeding, and hydrocephalus. Vasospasm can be detected by either transcranial Doppler assessment or cerebral angiography; it is typically treated with the calcium channel blocker nimodipine, aggressive IV fluid administration, and therapy aimed at increasing blood pressure, typically with vasoactive drugs such as phenylephrine. The IV fluids and vasoactive drugs (hypertensive hypervolemic therapy) are used to overcome the cerebral vasospasm. Early surgical clipping of aneurysms is advocated by most authorities to prevent complications related to rebleeding. Hydrocephalus,

typically heralded by a decreased level of consciousness, may require ventriculostomy drainage.

Status epilepticus

Recurrent or relentless seizure activity is a medical emergency. Cessation of seizure activity is required to prevent irreversible neurologic injury. Lorazepam is the most effective benzodiazepine for treating status epilepticus and is the treatment of choice for controlling seizures acutely. Phenytoin or fosphenytoin should be given concomitantly since lorazepam has a short half-life. Other drugs, such as gabapentin, carbamazepine, and phenobarbital, should be reserved for patients with contraindications to phenytoin (e.g., allergy or pregnancy) or ongoing seizures despite phenytoin.

Brain death

(See also Chap. 35) Though critically ill patients usually die from irreversible cessation of circulatory and respiratory function, a diagnosis of death also may be established by irreversible cessation of all functions of the entire brain, including the brainstem, even if circulatory and respiratory function remains intact on artificial life support. Patients must demonstrate absence of cerebral function (unresponsive to all external stimuli) and brainstem functions (e.g., unreactive pupils, absent ocular movement to head turning or ice water irrigation of ear canals, positive apnea test [no drive to breathe]). Absence of brain function must have an established cause and be permanent without possibility of recovery (e.g., must confirm the absence of sedative effect, hypothermia, hypoxemia, neuromuscular paralysis, or severe hypotension). If there is uncertainty about the cause of coma, studies of cerebral blood flow and electroencephalography should be performed.

WITHHOLDING AND WITHDRAWING CARE

Withholding and withdrawing of care occurs commonly in the ICU setting. The Task Force on Ethics of the Society of Critical Care Medicine reported that it is ethically sound to withhold or withdraw care if a patient or surrogate makes such a request or if the goals of therapy are not achievable according to the physician. Since all medical treatments are justified by their expected benefits, the loss of such an expectation justifies the act of withdrawing or withholding such treatment. Thus, the act of withdrawing care is fundamentally similar to the act of withholding care. An underlying stipulation derived from this report is that an informed patient should have his or her wishes respected with regard to life-sustaining therapy. Implicit in this stipulation is the need to ensure that patients are thoroughly and accurately informed regarding the plausibility and expected results of various therapies.

The act of informing patients and/or surrogate decision makers is the responsibility of the physician and other health care providers. If a patient or surrogate desires therapy deemed futile by the treating physician, the physician is not obligated ethically to provide such treatment. Rather, arrangements may be made to transfer the patient's care to another care provider. Whether the decision to withdraw life support should be initiated by the physician or left to surrogate decision makers is not clear. A recent study reported that slightly more than half of surrogate decision makers preferred to receive such a recommendation, whereas the rest did not. Critical care providers should meet regularly with patients and/or surrogates to discuss prognosis when the withholding or withdrawal of care is being considered. After a consensus among caregivers has been reached regarding withholding or withdrawal of care, this should be relayed to the patient and/or surrogate decision maker. If a decision to withhold or withdraw life-sustaining care for a patient has been reached, aggressive attention to analgesia and anxiolysis is needed. Opiates and benzodiazepines are typically used to achieve these goals.

CHAPTER 26
MECHANICAL VENTILATORY SUPPORT

Bartolome R. Celli

MECHANICAL VENTILATORY SUPPORT

Mechanical ventilation is a therapeutic method that is used to assist or replace spontaneous breathing. The primary indication for initiation of mechanical ventilation is respiratory failure, of which there are two basic types: *hypoxemic* respiratory failure, which is present when arterial O_2 saturation (SaO_2) <90% occurs despite an increased inspired O_2 fraction, and *hypercarbic* respiratory failure, which is characterized by arterial PCO_2 values >50 mmHg. When it is chronic, neither of the two types is obligatorily treated with mechanical ventilation, but when acute, mechanical ventilation may be lifesaving.

INDICATIONS

The most common reasons for instituting mechanical ventilation are acute respiratory failure with hypoxemia (acute respiratory distress syndrome, heart failure with pulmonary edema, pneumonia, sepsis, complications of surgery and trauma), which accounts for ~65% of all ventilated cases, followed by causes of hypercarbic ventilatory failure such as coma (15%), exacerbations of chronic obstructive pulmonary disease (13%), and neuromuscular diseases (5%). The primary objectives of mechanical ventilation are to decrease the work of breathing, thus avoiding respiratory muscle fatigue, and to reverse life-threatening hypoxemia and progressive respiratory acidosis.

In some cases, mechanical ventilation is used as an adjunct to other forms of therapy, such as its use in reducing cerebral blood flow in patients with increased intracranial pressure. Mechanical ventilation also is used frequently in conjunction with endotracheal intubation to prevent aspiration of gastric contents in otherwise unstable patients during gastric lavage for suspected drug overdose or during gastrointestinal endoscopy. In critically ill patients, intubation and mechanical ventilation may be indicated before essential diagnostic or therapeutic studies if it appears that respiratory failure may occur during those maneuvers.

TYPES OF MECHANICAL VENTILATION

In its broadest sense, there are two distinct methods for ventilating patients: noninvasive ventilation (NIV) and invasive ventilation or conventional mechanical ventilation (MV).

Noninvasive ventilation

Noninvasive ventilation has been gaining more acceptance because it is effective in certain conditions, such as acute or chronic respiratory failure, and is associated with fewer complications, namely, pneumonia and tracheolaryngeal trauma. Noninvasive ventilation usually is provided by using a tight-fitting face mask or nasal mask similar to the masks traditionally used for treatment of sleep apnea. Noninvasive ventilation has proved highly effective in patients with respiratory failure from acute exacerbations of chronic obstructive pulmonary disease and is most frequently implemented by using bilevel positive airway pressure ventilation or pressure support ventilation. In both of these modes, a preset positive pressure is applied during inspiration and a lower pressure is applied during expiration at the mask. Both modes are well tolerated by a conscious patient and optimize patient-ventilator synchrony. The major limitation to its widespread application has been patient intolerance because the tight-fitting mask required for NIV can cause both physical and emotional discomfort. In addition, NIV has had limited success in patients with acute hypoxemic respiratory failure, for whom endotracheal intubation and conventional MV remain the ventilatory method of choice.

The most important group of patients who benefit from a trial of NIV are those with acute exacerbations of chronic obstructive pulmonary disease (COPD) leading to respiratory acidosis (pH <7.35). Experience from several well-conducted randomized trials has shown that in patients with ventilatory failure characterized by blood pH levels between 7.25 and 7.35, NIV is associated with low failure rates (15–20%) and good outcomes (intubation rate, length of stay in intensive care, and in some series mortality rates). In more severely ill patients with pH <7.25, the rate of NIV failure is inversely related to the severity of respiratory acidosis, with greater failure as the pH decreases. In patients with milder acidosis (pH >7.35), NIV is not better than conventional therapy that includes controlled oxygen delivery and pharmacotherapy for exacerbations of COPD (systemic corticosteroids, bronchodilators, and, if needed, antibiotics).

Despite its benign outcomes, NIV is not useful in the majority of cases of respiratory failure and is contraindicated in patients with the conditions listed in Table 26-1. Experience shows that NIV can delay lifesaving ventilatory support in those cases and actually results in aspiration or hypoventilation. Once NIV is initiated, patients should be monitored; a reduction in respiratory frequency and a decrease in the use of accessory muscles (scalene, sternomastoid, and intercostals) are good clinical indicators of adequate therapeutic benefit. Arterial blood gases should be obtained at least within hours of the initiation of therapy to ensure that NIV is having the desired effect and that it is safe to continue its application. Lack of benefit within that time frame should alert one to the possible need for conventional MV.

Conventional mechanical ventilation

Conventional mechanical ventilation is implemented once a cuffed tube is inserted into the trachea to allow conditioned gas (warmed, oxygenated, and humidified) to be delivered to the airways and lungs at pressures above atmospheric pressure. Great care has to be taken during the act of intubation to avoid brain-damaging hypoxia. In some patients, intubation can be achieved without added sedation. In most patients, the administration of mild sedation may help facilitate the procedure.

TABLE 26-1

CONTRAINDICATIONS FOR NONINVASIVE VENTILATION
Cardiac or respiratory arrest
Severe encephalopathy
Severe gastrointestinal bleed
Hemodynamic instability
Unstable angina and myocardial infarction
Facial surgery or trauma
Upper airway obstruction
High-risk aspiration and/or inability to protect airways
Inability to clear secretions

Opiates and benzodiazepines are good choices but can have a deleterious effect on hemodynamics in patients with depressed cardiac function or low systemic vascular resistance. Morphine can promote histamine release from tissue mast cells and may worsen bronchospasm in patients with asthma; fentanyl, sufentanil, and alfentanil are acceptable alternatives. Ketamine may increase systemic arterial pressure and has been associated with hallucinatory responses; it should be used with caution in patients with hypertensive crisis or a history of psychiatric disorders. Newer agents such as etomidate and propofol have been used for both induction and maintenance of anesthesia in ventilated patients. They are shorter-acting, and etomidate has fewer adverse hemodynamic effects, but both agents are significantly more expensive than older agents. Great care must be taken to avoid the use of neuromuscular paralysis during intubation; in particular, the use of agents whose mechanism of action includes depolarization at the neuromuscular junction, such as succinylcholine chloride, should be avoided in patients with renal failure, tumor lysis syndrome, crush injuries, medical conditions associated with elevated serum potassium levels, and muscular dystrophy syndromes.

PRINCIPLES OF MECHANICAL VENTILATION

Once the patient has been intubated, the basic principles of applying MV are *to optimize oxygenation while avoiding overstretch and collapse/rerecruitment ventilator-induced lung injury (VILI)*. This concept, which is illustrated in **Fig. 26-1**, has gained acceptance because of important empirical and experimental evidence linking high airway pressures and volumes and overstretching the lung with collapse/rerecruitment with poor outcomes. Although normalization of pH through elimination of CO_2 is desirable, the risk of lung damage associated with the large volume and high pressures needed to achieve this goal has led to the acceptance of permissive hypercapnia. This approach has been found to be well tolerated when care is taken to avoid excess acidosis by pH buffering.

MODES OF VENTILATION

Mode refers to the manner in which ventilator breaths are triggered, cycled, and limited. The *trigger*, either an inspiratory effort or a time-based signal, defines what the ventilator senses to initiate an assisted breath. *Cycle* refers to the factors that determine the end of inspiration. For example, in volume-cycled ventilation, inspiration ends when a specific tidal volume is delivered. Other types of cycling include pressure cycling and time cycling. The *limiting factors* are operator-specified values, such as airway pressure, that are monitored by transducers internal

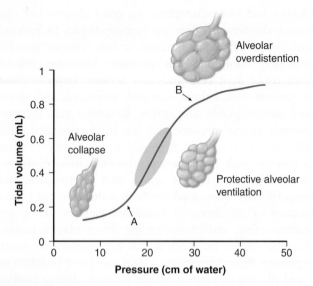

FIGURE 26-1

Hypothetical pressure-volume curve of the lung in a patient on MV. Alveoli tend to close if the distending pressure falls below the lower inflection point (A), whereas they overstretch if the pressure within them is higher than that of the upper inflection point (B). Collapse and opening of ventilated alveoli are associated with poor outcomes in patients with acute respiratory failure. Protective ventilation (*hatched lines*), using lower tidal volume (6 mL/kg of ideal body weight) and maintaining positive end-expiratory pressure to prevent overstretching and collapse/opening of alveoli, has resulted in improved survival in patients on MV.

to the ventilator circuit throughout the respiratory cycle; if the specified values are exceeded, inspiratory flow is terminated, and the ventilator circuit is vented to atmospheric pressure or the specified pressure at the end of expiration (positive end-expiratory pressure [PEEP]). Most patients are ventilated with assist control ventilation, intermittent mandatory ventilation, or pressure-support ventilation, with the latter two modes often used simultaneously (**Table 26-2**).

Assist control ventilation (ACMV)

This is the most widely used mode of ventilation. In this mode, an inspiratory cycle is initiated either by the patient's inspiratory effort or, if none is detected within a specified time window, by a timer signal within the ventilator. Every breath delivered, whether patient- or timer-triggered, consists of the operator-specified tidal volume. Ventilatory rate is determined either by the patient or by the operator-specified backup rate, whichever is of higher frequency. ACMV commonly is used for initiation of mechanical ventilation because it ensures a backup minute ventilation in the absence of an intact respiratory drive and allows for synchronization of the ventilator cycle with the patient's inspiratory effort.

Problems can arise when ACMV is used in patients with tachypnea due to nonrespiratory or nonmetabolic

factors, such as anxiety, pain, and airway irritation. Respiratory alkalemia may develop and trigger myoclonus or seizures. Dynamic hyperinflation leading to increased intrathoracic pressures (so-called auto-PEEP) may occur if the patient's respiratory mechanics are such that inadequate time is available for complete exhalation between inspiratory cycles. Auto-PEEP can limit venous return, decrease cardiac output, and increase airway pressures, predisposing to barotrauma.

Intermittent mandatory ventilation (IMV)

With this mode, the operator sets the number of mandatory breaths of fixed volume to be delivered by the ventilator; between those breaths, the patient can breathe spontaneously. In the most frequently used synchronized mode (SIMV), mandatory breaths are delivered in synchrony with the patient's inspiratory efforts at a frequency determined by the operator. If the patient fails to initiate a breath, the ventilator delivers a fixed-tidal-volume breath and resets the internal timer for the next inspiratory cycle. SIMV differs from ACMV in that only the preset number of breaths is ventilator-assisted.

SIMV allows patients with an intact respiratory drive to exercise inspiratory muscles between assisted breaths, making it useful for both supporting and weaning intubated patients. SIMV may be difficult to use in patients with tachypnea because they may attempt to exhale during the ventilator-programmed inspiratory cycle. When this occurs, the airway pressure may exceed the inspiratory pressure limit, the ventilator-assisted breath will be aborted, and minute volume may drop below that programmed by the operator. In this setting, if the tachypnea is in response to respiratory or metabolic acidosis, a change in ACMV will increase minute ventilation and help normalize the pH while the underlying process is further evaluated and treated.

Pressure-support ventilation (PSV)

This form of ventilation is patient-triggered, flow-cycled, and pressure-limited. It provides graded assistance and differs from the other two modes in that the operator sets the pressure level (rather than the volume) to augment every spontaneous respiratory effort. The level of pressure is adjusted by observing the patient's respiratory frequency. During PSV, the inspiration is terminated when inspiratory airflow falls below a certain level; in most ventilators, this flow rate cannot be adjusted by the operator. When PSV is used, patients receive ventilator assistance only when the ventilator detects an inspiratory effort. PSV frequently is used in combination with SIMV to ensure volume-cycled backup for patients whose respiratory drive is depressed. PSV frequently is well tolerated by most patients who are being weaned;

TABLE 26-2   259

CHARACTERISTICS OF THE MOST COMMONLY USED FORMS OF MECHANICAL VENTILATION

VENTILATORY MODE	VARIABLES SET BY USER (INDEPENDENT)	VARIABLES MONITORED BY USER (DEPENDENT)	TRIGGER CYCLE LIMIT	ADVANTAGES	DISADVANTAGES
ACMV (assist control ventilation)	Tidal volume Ventilator rate Fio$_2$ PEEP level Pressure limit	Peak, mean, and plateau airway pressures VE ABG I/E ratio	Patient effort Timer Pressure limit	Patient control Guaranteed ventilation	Potential to hyperventilate, Barotrauma and volume trauma Every effective breath generates a ventilator volume
IMV (intermittent mandatory ventilation)	Tidal volume Mandatory Ventilator Rate Fio$_2$ PEEP level Pressure limit Between breaths patients can breathe spontaneously	Peak, mean, and plateau airway pressures VE ABG I/E ratio	Patient effort Timer Pressure limit	Patient control Comfort from spontaneous breaths Guaranteed ventilation	Potential dysynchrony May result in hypoventilation
PSV (pressure support ventilation)	Inspiratory pressure level Fio$_2$ PEEP Pressure limit	Tidal volume Respiratory rate VE ABG	Pressure limit Inspiratory flow	Patient control Comfort Assures synchrony	No timer backup May result in hypoventilation
NIV (noninvasive ventilation)	Inspiratory and expiratory pressure level Fio$_2$	Tidal volume Respiratory rate VE ABG	Pressure limit Inspiratory flow	Patient control	Mask interface may cause discomfort and facial bruising Leaks are common Hypoventilation

Abbreviations: ABG, arterial blood gases; Fio$_2$, fraction of inspired oxygen; PEEP, positive end-expiratory pressure; I/E, inspiratory to expiratory time ratio; VE, minute ventilation.

PSV parameters can be set to provide full or nearly full ventilatory support and can be withdrawn to load the respiratory muscles gradually.

There are other modes of ventilation, and each has its own acronym, making it very difficult to understand for those unfamiliar with the terms. All these modes are modifications of the manner and duration in which pressure is applied to the airway and lungs and of the interaction between the mechanical assistance provided by the ventilator and the patient's respiratory effort. Although their use in acute respiratory failure is limited, the following have been used with varying levels of enthusiasm and adoption.

Pressure-control ventilation (PCV)

This form of ventilation is time-triggered, time-cycled, and pressure-limited. During the inspiratory phase, a specified pressure is imposed at the airway opening throughout inspiration. Since the inspiratory airway pressure is specified by the operator, tidal volume and inspiratory flow rate are *dependent*, rather than *independent*, variables and are not operator-specified. PCV is the preferred mode of ventilation for patients in whom it is desirable to regulate peak airway pressures, such as those with preexisting barotrauma, and postoperative thoracic surgical patients, in whom the shear forces across a fresh suture line should be limited. When PCV is used, minute ventilation and tidal volume must be monitored closely; minute ventilation is altered through changes in rate or in the pressure-control value, which changes tidal volume.

Inverse ratio ventilation (IRV)

This mode of ventilation is a variant of PCV that incorporates the use of a prolonged inspiratory time with the appropriate shortening of the expiratory time. It has been used in patients with severe hypoxemic respiratory failure. This approach increases mean distending pressures without increasing peak airway pressures. It is thought to work in conjunction with PEEP to open collapsed alveoli and improve oxygenation, although there are no conclusive data showing that IRV improves outcomes in clinical trials.

■■■ Continuous positive airway pressure (CPAP)

This is not a true support mode of ventilation because all ventilation occurs through the patient's spontaneous efforts. The ventilator provides fresh gas to the breathing circuit with each inspiration and sets the circuit to a constant, operator-specified pressure. CPAP is used to assess extubation potential in patients who have been effectively weaned and require little ventilator support and patients with intact respiratory system function who require an endotracheal tube for airway protection.

NONCONVENTIONAL VENTILATORY STRATEGIES

Several nonconventional ventilator strategies have been evaluated for their ability to improve oxygenation and reduce mortality rates in patients with advanced hypoxemic respiratory failure. These strategies include high-frequency oscillatory ventilation (HFOV), airway pressure release ventilation (APRV), extracorporeal membrane oxygenation (BCMO), and partial liquid ventilation (PLV) using perfluorocarbons. Although case reports and small uncontrolled cohort studies have shown benefit, randomized controlled trials have failed to demonstrate consistent improvements in outcome with any of these strategies. Currently, these approaches should be considered "salvage" techniques and considered for patients with hypoxemia refractory to conventional therapy. Prone positioning of patients with refractory hypoxemia has been explored because in theory it would tend to improve ventilation-perfusion matching. Although this is conceptually appealing and simple to implement, several randomized trial in patients with acute lung injury did not demonstrate a survival advantage with prone positioning despite demonstration of a transient physiologic benefit. The administration of nitric oxide (NO) gas, which has bronchodilator and pulmonary vasodilator effects when delivered through the airways and has been shown to improve arterial oxygenation in many patients with advanced hypoxemic respiratory failure, also failed to improve outcomes in patients with advanced hypoxemic respiratory failure.

Newer, promising strategies are intended to improve patient-ventilator synchrony, a major practical problem during MV. Currently, the more advanced new ventilators allow patients to trigger the ventilator with their own effort while also incorporating flow algorithms that allow termination of cycles once certain preset criteria are reached; this approach has greatly improved patient-ventilator synchrony and comfort. More recently, new modes of ventilation that synchronize not only the timing but also the levels

of assistance to match the patient's effort have been developed. Proportional assist ventilation (PAV) and neurally adjusted ventilatory assist ventilation (NAV) are two modes that are designed to deliver assisted breaths through algorithms incorporating not only pressure, volume, and time but also overall respiratory resistance and compliance in the case of PAV and neural activation of the diaphragm in the case of NAV. Although these modes result in better patient-ventilator synchrony, their practical use in the everyday management of patients on MV needs further study.

PROTECTIVE VENTILATORY STRATEGY

Whichever mode of MV is used, in acute respiratory failure the evidence from several important controlled trials indicates that the use of a protective ventilation approach guided by the principles outlined later and summarized in Fig. 26-1 is safe and offers the best chance of a good outcome:

1. Set a target tidal volume close to 6 mL/kg of ideal body weight.
2. Prevent plateau pressure (static pressure in the airway at the end of inspiration) over 30 cmH_2O.
3. Use the lowest possible fraction of inspired oxygen (FiO_2) to keep $SaO_2 \geq 90\%$.
4. Adjust the PEEP to maintain alveolar patency while preventing overdistention and closure/reopening.

With the application of these techniques, the mortality rate among patients with acute hypoxemic respiratory failure has decreased to ~30% from close to 50% a decade ago.

PATIENT MANAGEMENT

Once the patient has been stabilized with respect to gas exchange, definitive therapy for the underlying process responsible for respiratory failure is initiated. Subsequent modifications in ventilator therapy must be provided in parallel with changes in the patient's clinical status. As improvement in respiratory function is noted, the first priority is to reduce the level of mechanical ventilator support. Patients on full ventilator support should be monitored frequently with the goal of switching to a mode that allows for weaning as soon as possible. Protocols and guidelines that can be applied by paramedical personnel when physicians are not readily available have proved to be of value in shortening ventilator and intensive care unit (ICU) time, with very good outcomes. Patients whose condition continues to deteriorate after ventilator support is initiated may require increased O_2, PEEP, or one of the alternative modes of ventilation.

GENERAL SUPPORT DURING VENTILATION

Patients started on mechanical ventilation usually require sedation and analgesia to maintain an acceptable level of comfort. Often, this consists of a combination of a benzodiazepine and an opiate administered intravenously. Medications commonly used for this purpose include lorazepam, midazolam, diazepam, morphine, and fentanyl. The use of oversedation must be avoided in the ICU. Indeed, recent trials evaluating the effect of daily interruption of sedation in patients with improved ventilatory status show that this results in shorter time on the ventilator and shorter ICU stay.

Immobilized patients in the ICU who are on mechanical ventilator support are at increased risk for deep venous thrombosis and decubitus ulcers. To prevent venous thrombosis, prophylaxis in the form of subcutaneous heparin and/or pneumatic compression boots is prescribed frequently. Fractionated low-molecular-weight heparin appears to be equally effective for this purpose. To help prevent decubitus ulcers, frequent changes in body position and the use of soft mattress overlays and air mattresses are employed. Prophylaxis against diffuse gastrointestinal mucosal injury is indicated for patients on MV. Histamine-receptor antagonists (H_2-receptor antagonists), antacids, and cytoprotective agents such as Carafate (sucralfate) have all been used for this purpose and appear to be effective. Nutrition support by enteral feeding through either a nasogastric or an orogastric tube should be initiated and maintained whenever possible. Delayed gastric emptying is common in critically ill patients on sedative medications but often responds to promotility agents such as metoclopramide. Parenteral nutrition is an alternative to enteral nutrition in patients with severe gastrointestinal pathology who need prolonged MV.

COMPLICATIONS OF MECHANICAL VENTILATION

Endotracheal intubation and mechanical ventilation have direct and indirect effects on the lung and upper airways, the cardiovascular system, and the gastrointestinal system. Pulmonary complications include barotrauma, nosocomial pneumonia, oxygen toxicity, tracheal stenosis, and deconditioning of respiratory muscles. Barotrauma and volutrauma overdistend and disrupt lung tissue; may be clinically manifest by interstitial emphysema, pneumomediastinum, subcutaneous emphysema, or pneumothorax; and can result in the liberation of cytokines from overdistended tissues, further promoting tissue injury. Clinically significant pneumothorax requires tube thoracostomy. Intubated patients are at high risk for ventilator-associated pneumonia (VAP) as a result of aspiration from the upper airways through small leaks around the endotracheal tube cuff; the most common organisms responsible for this condition are *Pseudomonas aeruginosa*, enteric gram-negative rods, and *Staphylococcus aureus*. Because this condition is associated with high mortality rates, early initiation of empirical antibiotics directed against likely pathogens is recommended. *Hypotension* resulting from elevated intrathoracic pressures with decreased venous return is almost always responsive to intravascular volume repletion. In patients who are judged to have respiratory failure on the basis of alveolar edema but in whom the cardiac or pulmonary origin of the edema is unclear, hemodynamic monitoring with a pulmonary arterial catheter may be of value in helping to clarify the cause of the edema.

Gastrointestinal effects of positive-pressure ventilation include stress ulceration and mild to moderate cholestasis.

WEANING FROM MECHANICAL VENTILATION

It is important to consider discontinuation of mechanical ventilation once the underlying respiratory disease begins to reverse. Although the predictive capacities of multiple clinical and physiologic variables have been explored, the consensus from a weaning task force includes the following recommendations: (1) lung injury is stable/resolving, (2) gas exchange is adequate with low PEEP/F_{IO_2} (<8 cmH$_2$O and F$_{IO}$ <0.5), (3) hemodynamic variables are stable (patient off vasopressors), and (4) patient is capable of initiating spontaneous breaths. This "screen" should be done at least daily. If the patient is deemed capable of beginning weaning, the recommendation of the task force is to perform a spontaneous breathing trial (SBT) because several randomized trials support the value of this approach (**Fig. 26-2**). The SBT involves an integrated patient assessment during spontaneous breathing with little or no ventilator support. The SBT is usually implemented with a T-piece using 1–5 cmH$_2$O CPAP or a T-piece with 5–7 cmH$_2$O or PSV from the ventilator to offset the resistance from the endotracheal tube. Once it is determined that the patient can breath spontaneously, a decision must be made about the removal of the artificial airway; this should be done only when it is concluded that the patient has the ability to protect the airway, is able to cough and clear secretions, and is alert enough to follow commands. In addition, other factors must be taken into account, such as the possible difficulty in replacing the tube if that is anticipated. If upper airway difficulty is suspected, an evaluation using a "cuff leak" test (assessing the presence of air movement around a deflated endotracheal tube cuff) is supported by some internists. Despite the application of all of these methods, ~10–15% of extubated patients require reintubation. Several studies suggest that NIV can be used to avert reintubation; this has been particularly useful in patients

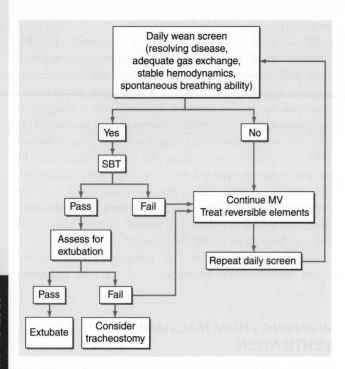

FIGURE 26-2
Flow chart to guide daily approach to managing patients considered for weaning. If the patient fails attempts at extubation, a tracheostomy should be considered.

with ventilatory failure secondary to COPD exacerbation. In this group, earlier extubation with the use of prophylactic NIV has shown good results. The use of NIV to facilitate weaning in other causes of respiratory failure is not currently indicated.

Prolonged mechanical ventilation and tracheostomy

From 5 to 13% of patients on MV will go on to require prolonged MV (>21 days). In these patients, critical care personnel have to make a decision about whether and when to perform a tracheostomy. This decision is individually based on the risk and benefits of tracheostomy and prolonged intubation and the patient's preferences and expected clinical outcomes. A tracheostomy is thought to be more comfortable, require less sedation, and provide a more secure airway, and it seems to reduce weaning time. However, tracheostomy carries the risk of complications, which occur in 5–40% of the procedures and include bleeding, cardiopulmonary arrest, hypoxia due to airway loss, structural damage, postoperative pneumothorax, pneumomediastinum, and wound infection. In patients with long-term tracheostomy, tracheal stenosis, granulation, and the erosion of the innominate artery are complex complications. It is generally agreed that if a patient is in need of MV for more than 10–14 days, a tracheostomy is indicated and should be planned under optimal conditions. Whether it is completed at the bedside or as an operative procedure depends on the local resources and experience. Some 5–10% of patients are deemed unable to wean in the ICU. These patients may benefit from transfer to special units where a multidisciplinary approach, including nutrition optimization, physical therapy with rehabilitation, and slower weaning methods, including SIMV with PSV, results in up to 30% successful weaning. Unfortunately, close to 2% of ventilated patients may ultimately remain unable to wean and become dependent on ventilatory support to maintain life. Most of these patients remain in chronic care institutions, although some who have strong social, economical, and family support may achieve a fulfilling life with home mechanical ventilation.

ACKNOWLEDGMENT

Portions of this chapter were retained from the work of the previous author, Edward Ingenito, MD.

CHAPTER 27

APPROACH TO THE PATIENT WITH SHOCK

Ronald V. Maier

Shock is the clinical syndrome that results from inadequate tissue perfusion. Irrespective of cause, the hypoperfusion-induced imbalance between the delivery of and requirements for oxygen and substrate leads to cellular dysfunction. The cellular injury created by the inadequate delivery of oxygen and substrates also induces the production and release of damage-associated molecular patterns (DAMPs or "danger signals") and inflammatory mediators that further compromise perfusion through functional and structural changes within the microvasculature. This leads to a vicious cycle in which impaired perfusion is responsible for cellular injury that causes maldistribution of blood flow, further compromising cellular perfusion; the latter ultimately causes multiple organ failure (MOF) and, if the process is not interrupted, leads to death. The clinical manifestations of shock are also the result, in part, of autonomic neuroendocrine responses to hypoperfusion as well as the breakdown in organ function induced by severe cellular dysfunction (**Fig. 27-1**).

When very severe and/or persistent, inadequate oxygen delivery leads to irreversible cell injury; only rapid restoration of oxygen delivery can reverse the progression of the shock state. The fundamental approach to management, therefore, is to recognize overt and impending shock in a timely fashion and to intervene emergently to restore perfusion. This often requires the expansion or reexpansion of intravascular blood volume. Control of any inciting pathologic process (e.g., continued hemorrhage, impairment of cardiac function, or infection), must occur simultaneously.

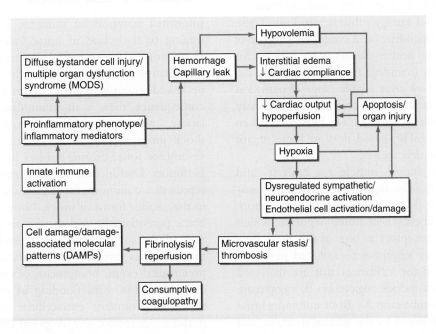

FIGURE 27-1
Shock-induced vicious cycle.

TABLE 27-1

CLASSIFICATION OF SHOCK	
Hypovolemic	Septic
Traumatic	Hyperdynamic (early)
Cardiogenic	Hypodynamic (late)
Intrinsic	Neurogenic
Compressive	Hypoadrenal

Clinical shock is usually accompanied by hypotension (i.e., a mean arterial pressure (MAP) <60 mmHg in previously normotensive persons). Multiple classification schemes have been developed in an attempt to synthesize the seemingly dissimilar processes leading to shock. Strict adherence to a classification scheme may be difficult from a clinical standpoint because of the frequent combination of two or more causes of shock in any individual patient, but the classification shown in Table 27-1 provides a useful reference point from which to discuss and further delineate the underlying processes.

PATHOGENESIS AND ORGAN RESPONSE

MICROCIRCULATION

Normally when cardiac output falls, systemic vascular resistance rises to maintain a level of systemic pressure that is adequate for perfusion of the heart and brain at the expense of other tissues such as muscle, skin, and especially the gastrointestinal (GI) tract. Systemic vascular resistance is determined primarily by the luminal diameter of arterioles. The metabolic rates of the heart and brain are high, and their stores of energy substrate are low. These organs are critically dependent on a continuous supply of oxygen and nutrients, and neither tolerates severe ischemia for more than brief periods (minutes). Autoregulation (i.e., the maintenance of blood flow over a wide range of perfusion pressures), is critical in sustaining cerebral and coronary perfusion despite significant hypotension. However, when MAP drops to ≤60 mmHg, blood flow to these organs falls, and their function deteriorates.

Arteriolar vascular smooth muscle has both α- and β-adrenergic receptors. The α_1 receptors mediate vasoconstriction, while the β_2 receptors mediate vasodilation. Efferent sympathetic fibers release norepinephrine, which acts primarily on α_1 receptors as one of the most fundamental compensatory responses to reduced perfusion pressure. Other constrictor substances that are increased in most forms of shock include angiotensin II, vasopressin, endothelin 1, and thromboxane A_2. Both norepinephrine and epinephrine are released by the adrenal medulla, and the concentrations of these catecholamines in the bloodstream rise. Circulating vasodilators in shock include prostacyclin (prostaglandin [PG] I_2), nitric oxide (NO), and, importantly, products of local metabolism such as adenosine that match flow to the tissue's metabolic needs. The balance between these various vasoconstrictors and vasodilators influences acting upon the microcirculation determines local perfusion.

Transport to cells depends on microcirculatory flow; capillary permeability; the diffusion of oxygen, carbon dioxide, nutrients, and products of metabolism through the interstitium; and the exchange of these products across cell membranes. Impairment of the microcirculation that is central to the pathophysiologic responses in the late stages of all forms of shock, results in the derangement of cellular metabolism that is ultimately responsible for organ failure.

The endogenous response to mild or moderate hypovolemia is an attempt at restitution of intravascular volume through alterations in hydrostatic pressure and osmolarity. Constriction of arterioles leads to reductions in both the capillary hydrostatic pressure and the number of capillary beds perfused, thereby limiting the capillary surface area across which filtration occurs. When filtration is reduced while intravascular oncotic pressure remains constant or rises, there is net reabsorption of fluid into the vascular bed, in accord with Starling's law of capillary interstitial liquid exchange. Metabolic changes (including hyperglycemia and elevations in the products of glycolysis, lipolysis, and proteolysis) raise extracellular osmolarity, leading to an osmotic gradient that increases interstitial and intravascular volume at the expense of intracellular volume.

CELLULAR RESPONSES

Interstitial transport of nutrients is impaired in shock, leading to a decline in intracellular high-energy phosphate stores. Mitochondrial dysfunction and uncoupling of oxidative phosphorylation are the most likely causes for decreased amounts of adenosine triphosphate (ATP). As a consequence, there is an accumulation of hydrogen ions, lactate, and other products of anaerobic metabolism. As shock progresses, these vasodilator metabolites override vasomotor tone, causing further hypotension and hypoperfusion. Dysfunction of cell membranes is thought to represent a common end-stage pathophysiologic pathway in the various forms of shock. Normal cellular transmembrane potential falls, and there is an associated increase in intracellular sodium and water, leading to cell swelling that interferes further with microvascular perfusion. In a preterminal event, homeostasis of calcium via membrane channels is lost with flooding of calcium intracellularly and a concomitant extracellular hypocalcemia. There is also evidence for a widespread but selective apoptotic (programmed cell-death) loss of cells, contributing to organ and immune failure.

NEUROENDOCRINE RESPONSE

Hypovolemia, hypotension, and hypoxia are sensed by baroreceptors and chemoreceptors that contribute to an autonomic response that attempts to restore blood volume, maintain central perfusion, and mobilize metabolic substrates. Hypotension disinhibits the vasomotor center, resulting in increased adrenergic output and reduced vagal activity. Release of norepinephrine from adrenergic neurons induces significant peripheral and splanchnic vasoconstriction, a major contributor to the maintenance of central organ perfusion, while reduced vagal activity increases the heart rate and cardiac output. Loss of vagal activity is also recognized to upregulate the innate immunity inflammatory response. The effects of circulating epinephrine released by the adrenal medulla in shock are largely metabolic, causing increased glycogenolysis and gluconeogenesis and reduced pancreatic insulin release. However, epinephrine also inhibits production and release of inflammatory mediators through stimulation of β-adrenergic receptors on innate immune cells.

Severe pain or other stresses cause the hypothalamic release of adrenocorticotropic hormone (ACTH). This stimulates cortisol secretion that contributes to decreased peripheral uptake of glucose and amino acids, enhances lipolysis, and increases gluconeogenesis. Increased pancreatic secretion of glucagon during stress accelerates hepatic gluconeogenesis and further elevates blood glucose concentration. These hormonal actions act synergistically to increase blood glucose for both selective tissue metabolism and the maintenance of blood volume. Many critically ill patients have recently been shown to exhibit low plasma cortisol levels and an impaired response to ACTH stimulation, which is linked to a decrease in survival. The importance of the cortisol response to stress is illustrated by the profound circulatory collapse that occurs in patients with adrenal cortical insufficiency.

Renin release is increased in response to adrenergic discharge and reduced perfusion of the juxtaglomerular apparatus in the kidney. Renin induces the formation of angiotensin I that is then converted to angiotensin II, an extremely potent vasoconstrictor and stimulator of aldosterone release by the adrenal cortex and of vasopressin by the posterior pituitary. Aldosterone contributes to the maintenance of intravascular volume by enhancing renal tubular reabsorption of sodium, resulting in the excretion of a low-volume, concentrated, sodium-free urine. Vasopressin has a direct action on vascular smooth muscle, contributing to vasoconstriction, and acts on the distal renal tubules to enhance water reabsorption.

CARDIOVASCULAR RESPONSE

Three variables—ventricular filling (preload), the resistance to ventricular ejection (afterload), and myocardial contractility—are paramount in controlling stroke volume. Cardiac output, the major determinant of tissue perfusion, is the product of stroke volume and heart rate. Hypovolemia leads to decreased ventricular preload that in turn reduces the stroke volume. An increase in heart rate is a useful but limited compensatory mechanism to maintain cardiac output. A shock-induced reduction in myocardial compliance is frequent, reducing ventricular end-diastolic volume and hence stroke volume at any given ventricular filling pressure. Restoration of intravascular volume may return stroke volume to normal but only at elevated filling pressures. Increased filling pressures stimulate release of brain natriuretic peptide (BNP) to secrete sodium and volume to relieve the pressure on the heart. Levels of BNP correlate with outcome following severe stress. In addition, sepsis, ischemia, myocardial infarction (MI), severe tissue trauma, hypothermia, general anesthesia, prolonged hypotension, and acidemia may all also impair myocardial contractility and reduce the stroke volume at any given ventricular end-diastolic volume. The resistance to ventricular ejection is significantly influenced by the systemic vascular resistance, which is elevated in most forms of shock. However, resistance is depressed in the early hyperdynamic stage of septic shock (Chap. 28) or neurogenic shock, thereby initially allowing the cardiac output to be maintained or elevated.

The venous system contains nearly two-thirds of the total circulating blood volume, most in the small veins, and serves as a dynamic reservoir for autoinfusion of blood. Active venoconstriction as a consequence of α-adrenergic activity is an important compensatory mechanism for the maintenance of venous return and therefore of ventricular filling during shock. On the other hand, venous dilation, as occurs in neurogenic shock, reduces ventricular filling and hence stroke volume and potentially cardiac output.

PULMONARY RESPONSE

The response of the pulmonary vascular bed to shock parallels that of the systemic vascular bed, and the relative increase in pulmonary vascular resistance, particularly in septic shock, may exceed that of the systemic vascular resistance, leading to right heart failure. Shock-induced tachypnea reduces tidal volume and increases both dead space and minute ventilation. Relative hypoxia and the subsequent tachypnea induce a respiratory alkalosis. Recumbency and involuntary restriction of ventilation secondary to pain reduce functional residual capacity and may lead to atelectasis. Shock and, in particular, resuscitation-induced oxidant radical generation, is recognized as a major cause of acute lung injury and subsequent acute respiratory distress syndrome (ARDS; Chap. 29). These disorders are characterized by noncardiogenic pulmonary edema secondary to diffuse pulmonary capillary endothelial and alveolar epithelial injury, hypoxemia, and bilateral diffuse pulmonary infiltrates. Hypoxemia results from perfusion of underventilated and nonventilated alveoli. Loss of surfactant and lung volume in combination with increased interstitial and alveolar edema reduces lung compliance. The work of breathing and the oxygen requirements of respiratory muscles increase.

RENAL RESPONSE

Acute kidney injury, a serious complication of shock and hypoperfusion, occurs less frequently than heretofore because of early aggressive volume repletion. Acute tubular necrosis is now more frequently seen as a result of the interactions of shock, sepsis, the administration of nephrotoxic agents (such as aminoglycosides and angiographic contrast media), and rhabdomyolysis; the latter may be particularly severe in skeletal muscle trauma. The physiologic response of the kidney to hypoperfusion is to conserve salt and water. In addition to decreased renal blood flow, increased afferent arteriolar resistance accounts for diminished glomerular filtration rate (GFR) that together with increased aldosterone and vasopressin is responsible for reduced urine formation. Toxic injury causes necrosis of tubular epithelium and tubular obstruction by cellular debris with back leak of filtrate. The depletion of renal ATP stores that occurs with prolonged renal hypoperfusion contributes to subsequent impairment of renal function.

METABOLIC DERANGEMENTS

During shock, there is disruption of the normal cycles of carbohydrate, lipid, and protein metabolism. Through the citric acid cycle, alanine in conjunction with lactate, which is converted from pyruvate in the periphery in the presence of oxygen deprivation enhances the hepatic production of glucose. With reduced availability of oxygen, the breakdown of glucose to pyruvate, and ultimately lactate, represents an inefficient cycling of substrate with minimal net energy production. An elevated plasma lactate/pyruvate ratio is preferable to lactate alone as a measure of anaerobic metabolism and reflects inadequate tissue perfusion. Decreased clearance of exogenous triglycerides coupled with increased hepatic lipogenesis causes a significant rise in serum triglyceride concentrations. There is increased protein catabolism as energy substrate, a negative nitrogen balance, and, if the process is prolonged, severe muscle wasting.

INFLAMMATORY RESPONSES

Activation of an extensive network of proinflammatory mediator systems by the innate immune system plays a significant role in the progression of shock and contributes importantly to the development of multiple organ injury, dysfunction (MOD), and failure (MOF) (Fig. 27-2). In those surviving the acute insult, there

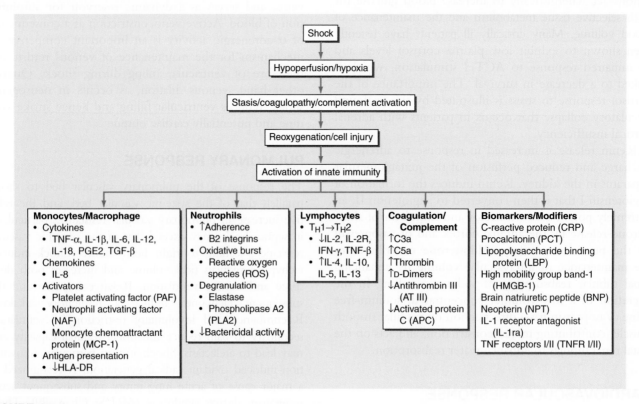

FIGURE 27-2
A schematic of the host immunoinflammatory response to shock.

is a prolonged endogenous counterregulatory response to "turn off" or balance the excessive proinflammatory response. If balance is restored, the patient does well. If the response is excessive, adaptive immunity is suppressed and the patient is highly susceptible to secondary nosocomial infections, which may then drive the inflammatory response and lead to delayed MOF.

Multiple humoral mediators are activated during shock and tissue injury. The complement cascade, activated through both the classic and alternate pathways, generates the anaphylatoxins C3a and C5a. Direct complement fixation to injured tissues can progress to the C5-C9 attack complex, causing further cell damage. Activation of the coagulation cascade (Chap. 39) causes microvascular thrombosis, with subsequent fibrinolysis leading to repeated episodes of ischemia and reperfusion. Components of the coagulation system (e.g., thrombin), are potent proinflammatory mediators that cause expression of adhesion molecules on endothelial cells and activation of neutrophils, leading to microvascular injury. Coagulation also activates the kallikrein-kininogen cascade, contributing to hypotension.

Eicosanoids are vasoactive and immunomodulatory products of arachidonic acid metabolism that include cyclooxygenase-derived prostaglandins (PGs) and thromboxane A_2, as well as lipoxygenase-derived leukotrienes and lipoxins. Thromboxane A_2 is a potent vasoconstrictor that contributes to the pulmonary hypertension and acute tubular necrosis of shock. PGI_2 and PGE_2 are potent vasodilators that enhance capillary permeability and edema formation. The cysteinyl leukotrienes LTC_4 and LTD_4 are pivotal mediators of the vascular sequelae of anaphylaxis, as well as of shock states resulting from sepsis or tissue injury. LTB_4 is a potent neutrophil chemoattractant and secretagogue that stimulates the formation of reactive oxygen species. Platelet-activating factor, an ether-linked, arachidonyl-containing phospholipid mediator, causes pulmonary vasoconstriction, bronchoconstriction, systemic vasodilation, increased capillary permeability, and the priming of macrophages and neutrophils to produce enhanced levels of inflammatory mediators.

Tumor necrosis factor α (TNF-α), produced by activated macrophages, reproduces many components of the shock state, including hypotension, lactic acidosis, and respiratory failure. Interleukin 1β (IL-1β), originally defined as "endogenous pyrogen" and produced by tissue-fixed macrophages, is critical to the inflammatory response. Both are significantly elevated immediately following trauma and shock. IL-6, also produced predominantly by the macrophage, has a slightly delayed peak response but is the best single predictor of prolonged recovery and development of MOF following shock. Chemokines such as IL-8 are potent neutrophil chemoattractants and activators that upregulate adhesion molecules on the neutrophil to enhance aggregation, adherence, and damage to the vascular endothelium. While the endothelium normally produces low levels of NO, the inflammatory response stimulates the inducible isoform of NO synthase (iNOS), which is overexpressed and produces toxic nitrosyl- and oxygen-derived free radicals that contribute to the hyperdynamic cardiovascular response and tissue injury in sepsis.

Multiple inflammatory cells, including neutrophils, macrophages, and platelets, are major contributors to inflammation-induced injury. Margination of activated neutrophils in the microcirculation is a common pathologic finding in shock, causing secondary injury due to the release of toxic oxygen radicals, lipases, primarily PLA2, and proteases. Release of high levels of reactive oxygen intermediates/species (ROI/ROS) rapidly consumes endogenous essential antioxidants and generates diffuse oxygen radical damage. Newer efforts to control ischemia/reperfusion injury include treatment with carbon monoxide, hydrogen sulfide, or other agents to reduce oxidant stress. Tissue-fixed macrophages produce virtually all major mediators of the inflammatory response and orchestrate the progression and duration of the inflammatory response. A major source of activation of the monocyte/macrophage is through the highly conserved membrane toll-like receptors (TLRs) that recognize DAMPs such as HMGB-1, and pathogen-associated molecular patterns (PAMPs) such as endotoxins released following tissue injury, and by pathogenic microbial organisms, respectively. Toll-like receptors also appear important for the chronic inflammation seen in Crohn's disease, ulcerative colitis, and transplant rejection. The variability in individual responses is a genetic predisposition that, in part, is due to single nucleotide polymorphisms (SNPs) in genetic sequences affecting the function and production of various inflammatory mediators.

TREATMENT Shock

MONITORING Patients in shock require care in an ICU. Careful and continuous assessment of the physiologic status is necessary. Arterial pressure through an indwelling line, pulse, and respiratory rate should be monitored continuously; a Foley catheter should be inserted to follow urine flow; and mental status should be assessed frequently. Sedated patients should be allowed to awaken ("drug holiday") daily to assess their neurologic status and to shorten duration of ventilator support.

There is ongoing debate as to the indications for using the flow-directed pulmonary artery catheter (PAC, Swan-Ganz catheter). Most patients in the ICU can be safely managed without the use of a PAC. However, in shock with significant ongoing blood loss, fluid shifts, and underlying cardiac dysfunction, a PAC may be useful. The PAC is placed percutaneously via the subclavian or jugular vein through the central venous circulation and right heart into the pulmonary artery. There are ports both proximal in the right atrium and distal in the pulmonary artery to provide access for infusions and for cardiac output measurements. Right atrial and pulmonary artery pressures (PAPs) are measured, and the pulmonary capillary wedge pressure (PCWP) serves as an approximation of the left atrial pressure. Normal hemodynamic parameters are shown in Table 27-2.

Cardiac output is determined by the thermodilution technique, and high-resolution thermistors can also be used to determine right ventricular end-diastolic volume to monitor further the response of the right heart to fluid resuscitation. A PAC with an oximeter port offers the additional advantage of on-line monitoring of the mixed venous oxygen saturation, an important index of overall tissue perfusion. Systemic and pulmonary vascular resistances are calculated as the ratio of the pressure drop across these vascular beds to the cardiac output. Determinations of oxygen content in arterial and venous blood, together with cardiac output and hemoglobin concentration, allow calculation of oxygen delivery, oxygen consumption, and oxygen-extraction ratio (Table 27-3). The hemodynamic patterns associated with the various forms of shock are shown in Table 27-4.

In resuscitation from shock, it is critical to restore tissue perfusion and optimize oxygen delivery, hemodynamics, and cardiac function rapidly. A reasonable goal of therapy

TABLE 27-2

NORMAL HEMODYNAMIC PARAMETERS

PARAMETER	CALCULATION	NORMAL VALUES
Cardiac output (CO)	$SV \times HR$	4–8 L/min
Cardiac index (CI)	CO/BSA	2.6–4.2 (L/min)/m²
Stroke volume (SV)	CO/HR	50–100 mL/beat
Systemic vascular resistance (SVR)	$([MAP - RAP]/CO) \times 80$	700–1600 dynes · s/cm⁵
Pulmonary vascular resistance (PVR)	$([PAP_m - PCWP]/CO) \times 80$	20–130 dynes · s/cm⁵
Left ventricular stroke work (LVSW)	$SV(MAP - PCWP) \times 0.0136$	60–80 g-m/beat
Right ventricular stroke work (RVSW)	$SV(PAP_m - RAP)$	10–15 g-m/beat

Abbreviations: BSA, body surface area; HR, heart rate; MAP, mean arterial pressure; PAP$_m$, pulmonary artery pressure—mean; PCWP, pulmonary capillary wedge pressure; RAP, right atrial pressure.

TABLE 27-3

OXYGEN TRANSPORT CALCULATIONS

PARAMETER	CALCULATION	NORMAL VALUES
Oxygen-carrying capacity of hemoglobin		1.39 mL/g
Plasma O_2 concentration	$P_{O_2} \times 0.0031$	
Arterial O_2 concentration (Ca_{O_2})	$1.39\ Sa_{O_2} + 0.0031\ Pa_{O_2}$	20 vol%
Venous O_2 concentration (Cv_{O_2})	$1.39\ Sv_{O_2} + 0.0031\ Pv_{O_2}$	15.5 vol%
Arteriovenous O_2 difference ($Ca_{O_2} - Cv_{O_2}$)	$1.39\ (Sa_{O_2} - Sv_{O_2})$ $0.0031\ (Pa_{O_2} - Pv_{O_2})$	3.5 vol%
Oxygen delivery (D_{O_2})	$Ca_{O_2} \times CO$ (L/min) $\times 10$ (dL/L) 1.39 $Sa_{O_2} \times CO \times 10$	800–1600 mL/min
Oxygen uptake (V_{O_2})	$(Ca_{O_2} - Cv_{O_2}) \times CO \times 10$ $1.39\ (Sa_{O_2} - Sv_{O_2}) \times CO \times 10$	150–400 mL/min
Oxygen delivery index (D_{O_2} I)	D_{O_2}/BSA	520–720 (mL/min)/m²
Oxygen uptake index (V_{O_2}I)	V_{O_2}/BSA	115–165 (mL/min)/m²
Oxygen extraction ratio (O_2ER)	$(1 - [V_{O_2}/D_{O_2}]) \times 100$	22–32%

Abbreviations: BSA, body surface area; CO, cardiac output; P$_{O_2}$, partial pressure of oxygen; Pa$_{O_2}$, partial pressure of O_2 in arterial blood; Pv$_{O_2}$, partial pressure of O_2 in venous blood; Sa$_{O_2}$, saturation of hemoglobin with O_2 in arterial blood; Sv$_{O_2}$, saturation of hemoglobin with O_2 in venous blood.

is to achieve a normal mixed venous oxygen-saturation and arteriovenous oxygen-extraction ratio. To enhance oxygen delivery, red cell mass, arterial oxygen saturation, and cardiac output may be augmented singly or simultaneously. An increase in oxygen delivery not accompanied by an increase in oxygen consumption implies that oxygen availability is adequate and that oxygen consumption is not flow dependent. Conversely, an elevation of oxygen consumption with increased delivery implies that the oxygen supply was inadequate. However, cautious interpretation is required due to the link among increased oxygen delivery, cardiac work, and oxygen consumption. A reduction in systemic vascular resistance accompanying an increase in cardiac output indicates that compensatory vasoconstriction is reversing due to improved tissue perfusion. The determination of stepwise expansion of blood volume on cardiac performance allows identification of the optimum preload (Starling's law). An algorithm for the resuscitation of the patient in shock is shown in Fig. 27-3.

TABLE 27-4

PHYSIOLOGIC CHARACTERISTICS OF THE VARIOUS FORMS OF SHOCK

TYPE OF SHOCK	CVP AND PCWP	CARDIAC OUTPUT	SYSTEMIC VASCULAR RESISTANCE	VENOUS O₂ SATURATION
Hypovolemic	↓	↓	↑	↓
Cardiogenic	↑	↓	↑	↓
Septic				
Hyperdynamic	↓↑	↑	↓	↑
Hypodynamic	↓↑	↓	↑	↑↓
Traumatic	↓	↓↑	↑↓	↓
Neurogenic	↓	↓	↓	↓
Hypoadrenal	↓↑	↓	=↓	↓

Abbreviations: CVP, central venous pressure; PCWP, pulmonary capillary wedge pressure.

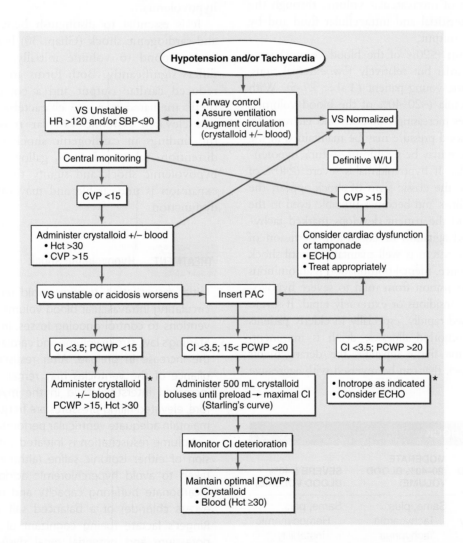

FIGURE 27-3

An algorithm for the resuscitation of the patient in shock.
*Monitor SV$_{O_2}$, SVRI, and RVEDVI as additional markers of correction for perfusion and hypovolemia. Consider age-adjusted CI. SV$_{O_2}$, saturation of hemoglobin with O$_2$ in venous blood; SVRI, systemic vascular resistance index; RVEDVI, right-ventricular end-diastolic volume index. CI, cardiac index in (L/min) per m^2; CVP, central venous pressure; ECHO, echocardiogram; Hct, hematocrit; HR, heart rate; PAC, pulmonary artery catheter; PCWP, pulmonary capillary wedge pressure in mmHg; SBP, systolic blood pressure; VS, vital signs; W/U, work up.

SPECIFIC FORMS OF SHOCK

HYPOVOLEMIC SHOCK

This most common form of shock results either from the loss of red blood cell mass and plasma from hemorrhage or from the loss of plasma volume alone due to extravascular fluid sequestration or GI, urinary, and insensible losses. The signs and symptoms of nonhemorrhagic hypovolemic shock are the same as those of hemorrhagic shock, although they may have a more insidious onset. The normal physiologic response to hypovolemia is to maintain perfusion of the brain and heart while attempting to restore an effective circulating blood volume. There is an increase in sympathetic activity, hyperventilation, collapse of venous capacitance vessels, release of stress hormones, and an attempt to replace the loss of intravascular volume through the recruitment of interstitial and intracellular fluid and by reduction of urine output.

Mild hypovolemia (≤20% of the blood volume) generates mild tachycardia but relatively few external signs, especially in a supine young patient (Table 27-5). With moderate hypovolemia (~20–40% of the blood volume), the patient becomes increasingly anxious and tachycardic; although normal blood pressure may be maintained in the supine position, there may be significant postural hypotension and tachycardia. If hypovolemia is severe (≥40% of the blood volume), the classic signs of shock appear; the blood pressure declines and becomes unstable even in the supine position, and the patient develops marked tachycardia, oliguria, and agitation or confusion. Perfusion of the central nervous system is well maintained until shock becomes severe. Hence, mental obtundation is an ominous clinical sign. The transition from mild to severe hypovolemic shock can be insidious or extremely rapid. If severe shock is not reversed rapidly, especially in elderly patients and those with comorbid illnesses, death is imminent. A very narrow time frame separates the derangements found in severe shock that can be reversed with aggressive resuscitation from those of progressive decompensation and irreversible cell injury.

Diagnosis

Hypovolemic shock is readily diagnosed when there are signs of hemodynamic instability and the source of volume loss is obvious. The diagnosis is more difficult when the source of blood loss is occult, as into the GI tract, or when plasma volume alone is depleted. Even after acute hemorrhage, hemoglobin and hematocrit values do not change until compensatory fluid shifts have occurred or exogenous fluid is administered. Thus, an initial normal hematocrit does not disprove the presence of significant blood loss. Plasma losses cause hemoconcentration, and free water loss leads to hypernatremia. These findings should suggest the presence of hypovolemia.

It is essential to distinguish between hypovolemic and cardiogenic shock (Chap. 30) because, while both may respond to volume initially, definitive therapy differs significantly. Both forms are associated with a reduced cardiac output and a compensatory sympathetic mediated response characterized by tachycardia and elevated systemic vascular resistance. However, the findings in cardiogenic shock of jugular venous distention, rales, and an S_3 gallop distinguish it from hypovolemic shock and signify that ongoing volume expansion is undesirable and may cause further organ dysfunction.

TREATMENT   Hypovolemic Shock

Initial resuscitation requires rapid reexpansion of the circulating intravascular blood volume along with interventions to control ongoing losses. In accordance with Starling's law, stroke volume and cardiac output rise with the increase in preload. After resuscitation, the compliance of the ventricles may remain reduced due to increased interstitial fluid in the myocardium. Therefore, elevated filling pressures are frequently required to maintain adequate ventricular performance.

Volume resuscitation is initiated with the rapid infusion of either isotonic saline (although care must be taken to avoid hyperchloremic acidosis from loss of bicarbonate buffering capacity and replacement with excess chloride) or a balanced salt solution such as Ringer's lactate (being cognizant of the presence of potassium and potential renal dysfunction) through large-bore intravenous lines. Data, particularly on severe traumatic brain injury (TBI), regarding benefits of small volumes of hypertonic saline that more rapidly restore blood pressure are variable, but tend to show improved survival thought to be linked to immunomodulation.

TABLE 27-5

HYPOVOLEMIC SHOCK

MILD (<20% BLOOD VOLUME)	MODERATE (20–40% BLOOD VOLUME)	SEVERE (>40% BLOOD VOLUME)
Cool extremities	Same, plus:	Same, plus:
Increased capillary refill time	Tachycardia	Hemodynamic instability
	Tachypnea	Marked tachycardia
Diaphoresis	Oliguria	Hypotension
Collapsed veins	Postural	Mental status
Anxiety	changes	deterioration (coma)

No distinct benefit from the use of colloid has been demonstrated, and in trauma patients it is associated with a higher mortality, particularly in patients with TBI. The infusion of 2–3 L of salt solution over 20–30 min should restore normal hemodynamic parameters. Continued hemodynamic instability implies that shock has not been reversed and/or there are significant ongoing blood or other volume losses. Continuing acute blood loss, with hemoglobin concentrations declining to ≤100 g/L (10 g/dL), should initiate blood transfusion, preferably as fully cross-matched recently banked (<14 days old) blood. Resuscitated patients are often coagulopathic due to deficient clotting factors in crystalloids and banked packed red blood cells (PRBCs). Early administration of component therapy during massive transfusion (fresh-frozen plasma [FFP] and platelets) approaching a 1:1 ratio of PRBC/FFP appears to improve survival. In extreme emergencies, type-specific or O-negative packed red cells may be transfused. Following severe and/or prolonged hypovolemia, inotropic support with norepinephrine, vasopressin, or dopamine may be required to maintain adequate ventricular performance *but only after* blood volume has been restored. Increases in peripheral vasoconstriction with inadequate resuscitation leads to tissue loss and organ failure. Once hemorrhage is controlled and the patient has stabilized, blood transfusions should not be continued unless the hemoglobin is <~7g/dL. Studies have demonstrated an increased survival in patients treated with this restrictive blood transfusion protocol.

Successful resuscitation also requires support of respiratory function. Supplemental oxygen should always be provided, and endotracheal intubation may be necessary to maintain arterial oxygenation. Following resuscitation from isolated hemorrhagic shock, end-organ damage is frequently less than following septic or traumatic shock. This may be due to the absence of massive activation of the inflammatory innate immune response and consequent nonspecific organ injury and failure.

TRAUMATIC SHOCK

Shock following trauma is, in large measure, due to hemorrhage. However, even when hemorrhage has been controlled, patients can continue to suffer loss of plasma volume into the interstitium of injured tissues. These fluid losses are compounded by injury-induced inflammatory responses that which contribute to the secondary microcirculatory injury. Proinflammatory mediators are induced by DAMPs released from injured tissue and are recognized by the highly conserved membrane receptors of the TLR family (see "Inflammatory Responses"). These receptors on cells of the innate immune system, particularly the circulating monocyte, tissue-fixed macrophage, and dendritic cell, are potent activators of an excessive proinflammatory phenotype in response to cellular injury. This causes secondary tissue injury and maldistribution of blood flow, intensifying tissue ischemia and leading to multiple organ system failure. In addition, direct structural injury to the heart, chest, or head can also contribute to shock. For example, pericardial tamponade or tension pneumothorax impairs ventricular filling, while myocardial contusion depresses myocardial contractility.

TREATMENT Traumatic Shock

Inability of the patient to maintain a systolic blood pressure ≥90 mmHg after trauma-induced hypovolemia is associated with a mortality rate up to ~50%. To prevent this decompensation of homeostatic mechanisms, therapy must be promptly administered.

The initial management of the seriously injured patient requires attention to the "ABCs" of resuscitation: assurance of an *airway* (A), adequate ventilation (*breathing*, B), and establishment of an adequate blood volume to support the *circulation* (C). Control of ongoing hemorrhage requires immediate attention. Early stabilization of fractures, debridement of devitalized or contaminated tissues, and evacuation of hematomata all reduce the subsequent inflammatory response to the initial insult and minimize damaged-tissue release of DAMPs and subsequent diffuse organ injury. Supplementation of depleted endogenous antioxidants also reduces subsequent organ failure and mortality.

CARDIOGENIC SHOCK

See Chap. 30.

COMPRESSIVE CARDIOGENIC SHOCK

With extrinsic compression, the heart and surrounding structures are less compliant, and therefore normal filling pressures generate inadequate diastolic filling and stroke volume. Blood or fluid within the poorly distensible pericardial sac may cause tamponade. Any cause of increased intrathoracic pressure such as tension pneumothorax, herniation of abdominal viscera through a diaphragmatic hernia, or excessive positive-pressure ventilation to support pulmonary function, can also cause compressive cardiogenic shock while simultaneously impeding venous return and preload. Although initially responsive to increased filling pressures produced by volume expansion, as compression increases, cardiogenic shock recurs. The window of opportunity gained by volume loading may be very brief until irreversible shock recurs. Diagnosis and intervention must occur urgently.

The diagnosis of compressive cardiogenic shock is most frequently based on clinical findings, the chest radiograph, and an echocardiogram. The diagnosis of compressive cardiac shock may be more difficult to establish in the setting of trauma when hypovolemia and cardiac compression are present simultaneously. The classic findings of pericardial tamponade include the triad of hypotension, neck vein distention, and muffled heart sounds. Pulsus paradoxus (i.e., an inspiratory reduction in systolic pressure >10 mmHg), may also be noted. The diagnosis is confirmed by echocardiography, and treatment consists of immediate pericardiocentesis or open subxiphoid pericardial window. A tension pneumothorax produces ipsilateral decreased breath sounds, tracheal deviation away from the affected thorax, and jugular venous distention. Radiographic findings include increased intrathoracic volume, depression of the diaphragm of the affected hemithorax, and shifting of the mediastinum to the contralateral side. Chest decompression must be carried out immediately, and, ideally, should occur based on clinical findings rather than awaiting a chest radiograph. Release of air and restoration of normal cardiovascular dynamics are both diagnostic and therapeutic.

SEPTIC SHOCK

See Chap. 28.

NEUROGENIC SHOCK

Interruption of sympathetic vasomotor input after a high cervical spinal cord injury, inadvertent cephalad migration of spinal anesthesia, or devastating head injury may result in neurogenic shock. In addition to arteriolar dilation, venodilation causes pooling in the venous system, which decreases venous return and cardiac output. The extremities are often warm, in contrast to the usual sympathetic vasoconstriction-induced coolness in hypovolemic or cardiogenic shock. Treatment involves a simultaneous approach to the relative hypovolemia and to the loss of vasomotor tone. Excessive volumes of fluid may be required to restore normal hemodynamics if given alone. Once hemorrhage has been ruled out, norepinephrine or a pure α-adrenergic agent (phenylephrine) may be necessary to augment vascular resistance and maintain an adequate mean arterial pressure.

HYPOADRENAL SHOCK

The normal host response to the stress of illness, operation, or trauma requires that the adrenal glands hypersecrete cortisol in excess of that normally required. Hypoadrenal shock occurs in settings in which unrecognized adrenal insufficiency complicates the host response to the stress induced by acute illness or major surgery. Adrenocortical insufficiency may occur as a consequence of the chronic administration of high doses of exogenous glucocorticoids. In addition, recent studies have shown that critical illness, including trauma and sepsis, may also induce a relative hypoadrenal state. Other, less common causes include adrenal insufficiency secondary to idiopathic atrophy, use of etomidate for intubation, tuberculosis, metastatic disease, bilateral hemorrhage, and amyloidosis. The shock produced by adrenal insufficiency is characterized by loss of homeostasis with reductions in systemic vascular resistance, hypovolemia, and reduced cardiac output. The diagnosis of adrenal insufficiency may be established by means of an ACTH stimulation test but is inconsistent.

TREATMENT   Hypoadrenal Shock

In the persistently hemodynamically unstable patient, dexamethasone sodium phosphate, 4 mg, should be given intravenously. This agent is preferred if empiric therapy is required because, unlike hydrocortisone, it does not interfere with the ACTH stimulation test. If the diagnosis of absolute or relative adrenal insufficiency is established as shown by nonresponse to corticotropin stimulation (cortisol ≤9 μg/dL change poststimulation), the patient has a reduced risk of death if treated with hydrocortisone, 100 mg every 6–8 h, and tapered as the patient achieves hemodynamic stability. Simultaneous volume resuscitation and pressor support are required. The need for simultaneous mineralocoid is unclear.

ADJUNCTIVE THERAPIES

The sympathomimetic amines dobutamine, dopamine, and norepinephrine are widely used in the treatment of all forms of shock. Dobutamine is inotropic with simultaneous afterload reduction, thus minimizing cardiac-oxygen consumption increases as cardiac output increases. Dopamine is an inotropic and chronotropic agent that also supports vascular resistance in those whose blood pressure will not tolerate peripheral vascular dilation. Norepinephrine primarily supports blood pressure through vasoconstriction and increases myocardial oxygen consumption while placing marginally perfused tissues such as extremities and splanchnic organs, at risk for ischemia or necrosis, but it is also inotropic without chronotropy. Arginine-vasopressin (antidiuretic hormone) is being used increasingly to increase afterload and may better protect vital organ blood flow and prevent pathologic vasodilation.

REWARMING

Hypothermia is a frequent adverse consequence of massive volume resuscitation. The infusion of large volumes of refrigerated blood products and room temperature crystalloid solutions can rapidly drop core temperatures if fluid is not run through warming devices. Hypothermia may depress cardiac contractility and thereby further impair cardiac output and oxygen delivery/utilization. Hypothermia, particularly temperatures <35°C (<95°F), directly impairs the coagulation pathway, sometimes causing a significant coagulopathy. Rapid rewarming to >35°C (>95°F) significantly decreases the requirement for blood products and produces an improvement in cardiac function. The most effective method for rewarming is endovascular countercurrent warmers through femoral vein cannulation. This process does not require a pump and can rewarm from 30° to 35°C (86° to 95°F) in 30–60 min.

SECTION IV

COMMON CRITICAL ILLNESSES AND SYNDROMES

CHAPTER 28

SEVERE SEPSIS AND SEPTIC SHOCK

Robert S. Munford

DEFINITIONS

(See Table 28-1) Animals mount both local and systemic responses to microbes that traverse their epithelial barriers and enter underlying tissues. Fever or hypothermia, leukocytosis or leukopenia, tachypnea, and tachycardia are the cardinal signs of the systemic response, that is often called the *systemic inflammatory response syndrome* (SIRS). SIRS may have an infectious or a noninfectious etiology. If infection is suspected or proven, a patient with SIRS is said to have *sepsis*. When sepsis is associated with dysfunction of organs distant from the site of infection, the patient has *severe sepsis*. Severe sepsis may be accompanied by hypotension or evidence of hypoperfusion. When hypotension cannot be corrected by infusing fluids, the diagnosis is *septic shock*. These definitions were developed by consensus conference committees in 1992 and 2001 and have been widely used; there is evidence that the different stages may form a continuum.

ETIOLOGY

Sepsis can be a response to any class of microorganism. Microbial invasion of the bloodstream is not essential, since local inflammation can also elicit distant organ dysfunction and hypotension. In fact, blood cultures yield bacteria or fungi in only ~20–40% of cases of severe sepsis and 40–70% of cases of septic shock. Individual gram-negative or gram-positive bacteria account for ~70% of these isolates; the remainder are fungi or a mixture of microorganisms (Table 28-2). In patients whose blood cultures are negative, the etiologic agent is often established by culture or microscopic examination of infected material from a local site; specific identification of microbial DNA or RNA in blood or tissue samples is also used. In some case series, a majority of patients with a clinical picture of severe sepsis or septic shock have had negative microbiologic data.

EPIDEMIOLOGY

Severe sepsis is a contributing factor in >200,000 deaths per year in the United States. The incidence of severe sepsis and septic shock has increased over the past 30 years, and the annual number of cases is now >700,000 (~3 per 1000 population). Approximately two-thirds of the cases occur in patients with significant underlying illness. Sepsis-related incidence and mortality rates increase with age and preexisting comorbidity. The rising incidence of severe sepsis in the United States is attributable to the aging of the population, the increasing longevity of patients with chronic diseases, and the relatively high frequency with which sepsis develops in patients with AIDS. The widespread use of immunosuppressive drugs, indwelling catheters, and mechanical devices also plays a role.

Invasive bacterial infections are prominent causes of death around the world, particularly among young children. In sub-Saharan Africa, for example, careful screening for positive blood cultures found that community-acquired bacteremia accounted for at least one-fourth of deaths of children >1 year of age. Nontyphoidal *Salmonella* species, *Streptococcus pneumoniae*, *Haemophilus influenzae*, and *Escherichia coli* were the most commonly isolated bacteria. Bacteremic children often had HIV infection or were severely malnourished.

PATHOPHYSIOLOGY

Most cases of severe sepsis are triggered by bacteria or fungi that do not ordinarily cause systemic disease in immunocompetent hosts (Table 28-2). To survive within the human body, these microbes often exploit deficiencies in host defenses, indwelling catheters or other foreign matter, or obstructed fluid drainage conduits. Microbial pathogens, in contrast, can circumvent innate defenses because they (1) lack molecules that can be recognized by host receptors (see later) or (2) elaborate toxins or other virulence factors. In both

TABLE 28-1

DEFINITIONS USED TO DESCRIBE THE CONDITION OF SEPTIC PATIENTS

Bacteremia	Presence of bacteria in blood, as evidenced by positive blood cultures
Septicemia	Presence of microbes or their toxins in blood
Systemic inflammatory response syndrome (SIRS)	Two or more of the following conditions: (1) fever (oral temperature >38°C) or hypothermia (<36°C); (2) tachypnea (>24 breaths/min); (3) tachycardia (heart rate >90 beats/min); (4) leukocytosis (>12,000/μL), leucopenia (<4,000/μL), or >10% bands; may have a noninfectious etiology
Sepsis	SIRS that has a proven or suspected microbial etiology
Severe sepsis (similar to "sepsis syndrome")	Sepsis with one or more signs of organ dysfunction—for example: 1. *Cardiovascular:* Arterial systolic blood pressure ≤90 mmHg or mean arterial pressure ≤70 mmHg that responds to administration of intravenous fluid 2. *Renal:* Urine output <0.5 mL/kg per hour for 1 h despite adequate fluid resuscitation 3. *Respiratory:* Pa_{O_2}/Fi_{O_2} ≤250 or, if the lung is the only dysfunctional organ, ≤200 4. *Hematologic:* Platelet count <80,000/μL or 50% decrease in platelet count from highest value recorded over previous 3 days 5. *Unexplained metabolic acidosis:* A pH ≤7.30 or a base deficit ≥5.0 mEq/L and a plasma lactate level >1.5 times upper limit of normal for reporting lab 6. *Adequate fluid resuscitation:* Pulmonary artery wedge pressure ≥12 mmHg or central venous pressure ≥8 mmHg
Septic shock	Sepsis with hypotension (arterial blood pressure <90 mmHg systolic, or 40 mmHg less than patient's normal blood pressure) for at least 1 h despite adequate fluid resuscitation; *or* Need for vasopressors to maintain systolic blood pressure ≥90 mmHg *or* mean arterial pressure ≥70 mmHg
Refractory septic shock	Septic shock that lasts for >1 h and does not respond to fluid or pressor administration
Multiple-organ dysfunction syndrome (MODS)	Dysfunction of more than one organ, requiring intervention to maintain homeostasis
Predisposition–infection–response–organ dysfunction (PIRO)	A grading system that stratifies patients according to four key aspects of illness; attempts to define subgroups of patients, reducing heterogeneity in clinical trials
Critical illness–related corticosteroid insufficiency (CIRCI)	Inadequate corticosteroid activity for the patient's severity of illness; should be suspected when hypotension is not relieved by fluid administration

Source: Adapted from the American College of Chest Physicians/Society of Critical Care Medicine Consensus Conference Committee.

TABLE 28-2

MICROORGANISMS INVOLVED IN EPISODES OF SEVERE SEPSIS AT EIGHT ACADEMIC MEDICAL CENTERS

MICROORGANISM	EPISODES WITH BLOODSTREAM INFECTION, % (n = 436)	EPISODES WITH DOCUMENTED INFECTION BUT NO BLOODSTREAM INFECTION, % (n = 430)	TOTAL EPISODES, % (n = 866)
Gram-negative bacteria[a]	35	44	40
Gram-positive bacteria[b]	40	24	31
Fungi	7	5	6
Polymicrobial	11	21	16
Classic pathogens[c]	<5	<5	<5

[a]Enterobacteriaceae, pseudomonads, *Haemophilus* spp., other gram-negative bacteria.
[b]*Staphylococcus aureus*, coagulase-negative staphylococci, enterococci, *Streptococcus pneumoniae*, other streptococci, other gram-positive bacteria.
[c]Such as *Neisseria meningitidis*, *S. pneumoniae*, *Haemophilus influenzae*, and *Streptococcus pyogenes*.
Source: Adapted from KE Sands et al: JAMA 278:234, 1997.

cases, the body can mount a vigorous inflammatory reaction that results in severe sepsis yet fails to kill the invaders. The septic response may also be induced by microbial exotoxins that act as superantigens (e.g., toxic shock syndrome toxin 1) as well as by many pathogenic viruses.

Host mechanisms for sensing microbes

Animals have exquisitely sensitive mechanisms for recognizing and responding to certain highly conserved microbial molecules. Recognition of the lipid A moiety of lipopolysaccharide (LPS, also called *endotoxin*) is the best-studied example. A host protein (LPS-binding protein) binds lipid A and transfers the LPS to CD14 on the surfaces of monocytes, macrophages, and neutrophils. LPS then is passed to MD-2, that is bound to toll-like receptor (TLR) 4 to form a molecular complex that transduces the LPS recognition signal to the interior of the cell. This signal rapidly triggers the production and release of mediators, such as tumor necrosis factor (TNF; see later), that amplify the LPS signal and transmit it to other cells and tissues. Bacterial peptidoglycan and lipopeptides elicit responses in animals that are generally similar to those induced by LPS; whereas these molecules also may be transferred by CD14, they interact with different TLRs. Having numerous TLR-based receptor complexes (11 different TLRs have been identified so far in humans) allows animals to recognize many conserved microbial molecules; others include lipopeptides (TLR2/1, TLR2/6), flagellin (TLR5), undermethylated DNA sequences (TLR9), and double-stranded RNA (TLR3, TLR7). The ability of some TLRs to serve as receptors for host ligands (e.g., hyaluronans, heparan sulfate, saturated fatty acids) raises the possibility that they also play a role in producing noninfectious sepsis-like states. Other host pattern-recognition proteins that are important for sensing microbial invasion include the intracellular NOD1 and NOD2 proteins, which recognize discrete fragments of bacterial peptidoglycan; early complement components (principally in the alternative pathway); and mannose-binding lectin and C-reactive protein, which activate the classic complement pathway.

A host's ability to recognize certain microbial molecules may influence both the potency of its own defenses and the pathogenesis of severe sepsis. For example, MD-2–TLR4 best senses LPS that has a hexaacyl lipid A moiety (i.e., one with six fatty acyl chains). Most of the commensal aerobic and facultatively anaerobic gram-negative bacteria that trigger severe sepsis and shock (including *E. coli*, *Klebsiella*, and *Enterobacter*) make this lipid A structure. When they invade human hosts, often through breaks in an epithelial barrier, they are typically confined to the subepithelial tissue by a localized inflammatory response. Bacteremia, if it occurs, is intermittent and low-grade, as these bacteria are efficiently cleared from the bloodstream by TLR4-expressing Kupffer cells and splenic macrophages. These mucosal commensals

seem to induce severe sepsis most often by triggering severe local tissue inflammation rather than by circulating within the bloodstream. One exception is *Neisseria meningitidis*. Its hexaacyl LPS seems to be shielded from host recognition by its polysaccharide capsule. This protection may allow meningococci to transit undetected from the nasopharyngeal mucosa into the bloodstream, where they can infect vascular endothelial cells and release large amounts of endotoxin. Host recognition of lipid A may nonetheless influence pathogenesis, as meningococci that produce pentaacyl LPS were isolated from the blood of patients with less severe coagulopathy than was found in patients whose isolates produced hexaacyl lipid A. In contrast, gram-negative bacteria that make lipid A with fewer than six acyl chains (*Yersinia pestis*, *Francisella tularensis*, *Vibrio vulnificus*, *Pseudomonas aeruginosa*, and *Burkholderia pseudomallei*, among others) are poorly recognized by MD-2–TLR4. When these bacteria enter the body, they may initially induce relatively little inflammation. When they do trigger severe sepsis, it is often after they have multiplied to high density in tissues and blood. The importance of LPS recognition in disease pathogenesis has been shown by engineering a virulent strain of *Y. pestis*, which makes tetraacyl LPS at 37°C, to produce hexaacyl LPS; unlike its virulent parent, the mutant strain stimulates local inflammation and is rapidly cleared from tissues. For at least one large class of microbes—gram-negative aerobic bacteria—the pathogenesis of sepsis thus depends, at least in part, upon whether the bacterium's major signal molecule, LPS, can be sensed by the host.

Local and systemic host responses to invading microbes

Recognition of microbial molecules by tissue phagocytes triggers the production and/or release of numerous host molecules (cytokines, chemokines, prostanoids, leukotrienes, and others) that increase blood flow to the infected tissue, enhance the permeability of local blood vessels, recruit neutrophils to the site of infection, and elicit pain. These reactions are familiar elements of local inflammation, the body's frontline innate immune mechanism for eliminating microbial invaders. Systemic responses are activated by neural and/or humoral communication with the hypothalamus and brainstem; these responses enhance local defenses by increasing blood flow to the infected area, augmenting the number of circulating neutrophils, and elevating blood levels of numerous molecules (such as the microbial recognition proteins discussed earlier) that have anti-infective functions.

Cytokines and other mediators

Cytokines can exert endocrine, paracrine, and autocrine effects. TNF-α stimulates leukocytes and vascular endothelial cells to release other cytokines (as well as additional TNF-α), to express cell-surface molecules that enhance neutrophil-endothelial adhesion at sites of infection, and to increase prostaglandin and leukotriene production. Whereas blood levels of TNF-α are not elevated in individuals with localized infections, they increase in most patients with severe sepsis or septic shock. Moreover, IV infusion of TNF-α can elicit the characteristic abnormalities of SIRS. In animals, larger doses of TNF-α induce shock and death.

Although TNF-α is a central mediator, it is only one of many proinflammatory molecules that contribute to innate host defense. Chemokines, most prominently interleukin (IL)-8 and IL-17, attract circulating neutrophils to the infection site. IL-1β exhibits many of the same activities as TNF-α. TNF-α, IL-1β, interferon (IFN) γ, IL-12, IL-17, and other proinflammatory cytokines probably interact synergistically with one another and with additional mediators. The nonlinearity and multiplicity of these interactions have made it difficult to interpret the roles played by individual mediators in both tissues and blood.

Coagulation factors

Intravascular thrombosis, a hallmark of the local inflammatory response, may help wall off invading microbes and prevent infection and inflammation from spreading to other tissues. IL-6 and other mediators promote intravascular coagulation initially by inducing blood monocytes and vascular endothelial cells to express tissue factor. When tissue factor is expressed on cell surfaces, it binds to factor VIIa to form an active complex that can convert factors X and IX to their enzymatically active forms. The result is activation of both extrinsic and intrinsic clotting pathways, culminating in the generation of fibrin. Clotting is also favored by impaired function of the protein C–protein S inhibitory pathway and depletion of antithrombin and proteins C and S, while fibrinolysis is prevented by increased plasma levels of plasminogen activator inhibitor 1. Thus, there may be a striking propensity toward intravascular fibrin deposition, thrombosis, and bleeding; this propensity has been most apparent in patients with intravascular endothelial infections such as meningococcemia. Evidence points to tissue factor–expressing microparticles derived from leukocytes as a potential trigger for intravascular coagulation. Contact-system activation occurs during sepsis but contributes more to the development of hypotension than to disseminated intravascular coagulation (DIC).

Control mechanisms

Elaborate control mechanisms operate within both local sites of inflammation and the systemic compartment.

Local control mechanisms

Host recognition of invading microbes within subepithelial tissues typically ignites immune responses that rapidly kill the invader and then subside to allow tissue recovery. The anti-inflammatory forces that put out the fire and clean up the battleground include molecules that neutralize or inactivate microbial signals. Among these molecules are intracellular factors (e.g., suppressor of cytokine signaling 3 and IL-1 receptor–associated kinase 3) that diminish the production of proinflammatory mediators by neutrophils and macrophages; anti-inflammatory cytokines (IL-10, IL-4); and molecules derived from essential polyunsaturated fatty acids (lipoxins, resolvins, and protectins) that promote tissue restoration. Enzymatic inactivation of microbial signal molecules (e.g., LPS) may be required to restore homeostasis; a leukocyte enzyme, acyloxyacyl hydrolase, has been shown to prevent prolonged inflammation by inactivating LPS in mice.

Systemic control mechanisms

The signaling apparatus that links microbial recognition to cellular responses in tissues is less active in the blood. For example, whereas LPS-binding protein plays a role in recognizing the presence of LPS, in plasma it also prevents LPS signaling by transferring LPS molecules into plasma lipoprotein particles that sequester the lipid A moiety so that it cannot interact with cells. At the high concentrations found in blood, LPS-binding protein also inhibits monocyte responses to LPS, and the soluble (circulating) form of CD14 strips off LPS that has bound to monocyte surfaces.

Systemic responses to infection also diminish cellular responses to microbial molecules. Circulating levels of anti-inflammatory cytokines (e.g., IL-10) increase even in patients with mild infections. Glucocorticoids inhibit cytokine synthesis by monocytes in vitro; the increase in blood cortisol levels early in the systemic response presumably plays a similarly inhibitory role. Epinephrine inhibits the TNF-α response to endotoxin infusion in humans while augmenting and accelerating the release of IL-10; prostaglandin E$_2$ has a similar "reprogramming" effect on the responses of circulating monocytes to LPS and other bacterial agonists. Cortisol, epinephrine, IL-10, and C-reactive protein reduce the ability of neutrophils to attach to vascular endothelium, favoring their demargination and thus contributing to leukocytosis while preventing neutrophil-endothelial adhesion in uninflamed organs. The available evidence thus suggests that the body's systemic responses to injury and infection normally prevent inflammation within organs distant from a site of infection. There is also evidence that these responses may be immunosuppressive.

The acute-phase response increases the blood concentrations of numerous molecules that have anti-inflammatory actions. Blood levels of IL-1 receptor antagonist often greatly exceed those of circulating IL-1β, for example, and this excess may inhibit the binding of IL-1β to its receptors. High levels of soluble TNF receptors neutralize TNF-α that enters the circulation. Other acute-phase proteins are protease inhibitors or antioxidants; these may neutralize potentially harmful molecules released from neutrophils and other inflammatory cells. Increased hepatic production of hepcidin promotes the sequestration of iron in hepatocytes, intestinal epithelial cells, and erythrocytes; this effect reduces iron acquisition by invading microbes while contributing to the normocytic, normochromic anemia associated with inflammation.

It can thus be concluded that both local and systemic responses to infectious agents benefit the host in important ways. Most of these responses and the molecules responsible for them have been highly conserved during animal evolution and therefore may be adaptive. Elucidating how they contribute to lethality—i.e., become maladaptive—remains a major challenge for sepsis research.

Organ dysfunction and shock

As the body's responses to infection intensify, the mixture of circulating cytokines and other molecules becomes very complex: elevated blood levels of more than 50 molecules have been found in patients with septic shock. Although high concentrations of both pro- and anti-inflammatory molecules are found, the net mediator balance in the plasma of these extremely sick patients seems to be anti-inflammatory. For example, blood leukocytes from patients with severe sepsis are often hyporesponsive to agonists such as LPS. In patients with severe sepsis, persistence of leukocyte hyporesponsiveness has been associated with an increased risk of dying. Apoptotic death of B cells, follicular dendritic cells, and CD4+ T lymphocytes also may contribute significantly to the immunosuppressive state.

Endothelial injury
Many investigators have favored widespread vascular endothelial injury as the major mechanism for multiorgan dysfunction. In keeping with this idea, one study found high numbers of vascular endothelial cells in the peripheral blood of septic patients. Leukocyte-derived mediators and platelet-leukocyte-fibrin thrombi may contribute to vascular injury, but the vascular endothelium also seems to play an active role. Stimuli such as TNF-α induce vascular endothelial cells to produce and release cytokines, procoagulant molecules, platelet-activating factor, nitric oxide, and other mediators. In addition, regulated cell-adhesion molecules promote the adherence of neutrophils to endothelial cells. While these responses can attract phagocytes to infected sites and activate their antimicrobial arsenals, endothelial cell activation can also promote increased vascular permeability, microvascular thrombosis, DIC, and hypotension.

Tissue oxygenation may decrease as the number of functional capillaries is reduced by luminal obstruction due to swollen endothelial cells, decreased deformability of circulating erythrocytes, leukocyte-platelet-fibrin thrombi, or compression by edema fluid. On the other hand, studies using orthogonal polarization spectral imaging of the microcirculation in the tongue found that sepsis-associated derangements in capillary flow could be reversed by applying acetylcholine to the surface of the tongue or by giving nitroprusside intravenously; these observations suggest a neuroendocrine basis for the loss of capillary filling. Oxygen utilization by tissues may also be impaired by a state of "hibernation" in which ATP production is diminished as oxidative phosphorylation decreases; nitric oxide may be responsible for inducing this response.

Remarkably, poorly functioning "septic" organs usually appear normal at autopsy. There is typically very little necrosis or thrombosis, and apoptosis is largely confined to lymphoid organs and the gastrointestinal tract. Moreover, organ function usually returns to normal if patients recover. These points suggest that organ dysfunction during severe sepsis has a basis that is principally biochemical, not structural.

Septic shock
The hallmark of septic shock is a decrease in peripheral vascular resistance that occurs despite increased levels of vasopressor catecholamines. Before this vasodilatory phase, many patients experience a period during which oxygen delivery to tissues is compromised by myocardial depression, hypovolemia, and other factors. During this "hypodynamic" period, the blood lactate concentration is elevated and central venous oxygen saturation is low. Fluid administration is usually followed by the hyperdynamic, vasodilatory phase during which cardiac output is normal (or even high) and oxygen consumption declines despite adequate oxygen delivery. The blood lactate level may be normal or increased, and normalization of central venous oxygen saturation may reflect either improved oxygen delivery or left-to-right shunting.

Prominent hypotensive molecules include nitric oxide, β-endorphin, bradykinin, platelet-activating factor, and prostacyclin. Agents that inhibit the synthesis or action of each of these mediators can prevent or reverse endotoxic shock in animals. However, in clinical trials, neither a platelet-activating factor receptor antagonist nor a bradykinin antagonist improved survival rates among patients with septic shock, and a nitric oxide synthase inhibitor, L-N^G-methylarginine HCl, actually increased the mortality rate. Remarkably, recent findings indicate that exogenous nitrite can protect mice from challenge with TNF or LPS. Nitrite provides a storage pool from which nitric oxide can be generated in hypoxic and/or acidic conditions. These findings should renew interest in the possibility of exploiting nitric oxide metabolism to improve survival rates among septic patients.

Severe sepsis: A single pathogenesis?

In some cases, circulating bacteria and their products almost certainly elicit multiorgan dysfunction and hypotension by directly stimulating inflammatory responses within the vasculature. In patients with fulminant meningococcemia, for example, mortality rates have correlated directly with blood levels of endotoxin and bacterial DNA and with the occurrence of DIC. In most patients infected with other gram-negative bacteria, in contrast, circulating bacteria or bacterial molecules may reflect uncontrolled infection at a local tissue site and have little or no direct impact on distant organs; in these patients, inflammatory mediators or neural signals arising from the local site seem to be the key triggers for severe sepsis and septic shock. In a large series of patients with positive blood cultures, the risk of developing severe sepsis was strongly related to the site of primary infection: bacteremia arising from a pulmonary or abdominal source was eightfold more likely to be associated with severe sepsis than was bacteremic urinary tract infection, even after the investigators controlled for age, the kind of bacteria isolated from the blood, and other factors. A third pathogenesis may be represented by severe sepsis due to superantigen-producing *Staphylococcus aureus* or *Streptococcus pyogenes*; the T cell activation induced by these toxins produces a cytokine profile that differs substantially from that elicited by gram-negative bacterial infection. Further evidence for different pathogenetic pathways has come from observations that the pattern of mRNA expression in peripheral-blood leukocytes from children with sepsis is different for gram-positive, gram-negative, and viral pathogens.

The pathogenesis of severe sepsis thus may differ according to the infecting microbe, the ability of the host's innate defense mechanisms to sense it, the site of the primary infection, the presence or absence of immune defects, and the prior physiologic status of the host. Genetic factors are probably important as well, yet despite much study only a few allelic polymorphisms (e.g., in the IL-1β gene) have been associated with sepsis severity in more than one or two analyses. Further studies in this area are needed.

CLINICAL MANIFESTATIONS

The manifestations of the septic response are superimposed on the symptoms and signs of the patient's underlying illness and primary infection. The rate at which severe sepsis develops may differ from patient to patient, and there are striking individual variations in presentation. For example, some patients with sepsis are normo- or hypothermic; the absence of fever is most common in neonates, in elderly patients, and in persons with uremia or alcoholism.

Hyperventilation is often an early sign of the septic response. Disorientation, confusion, and other manifestations of encephalopathy may also develop early on, particularly in the elderly and in individuals with preexisting neurologic impairment. Focal neurologic signs are uncommon, although preexisting focal deficits may become more prominent.

Hypotension and DIC predispose to acrocyanosis and ischemic necrosis of peripheral tissues, most commonly the digits. Cellulitis, pustules, bullae, or hemorrhagic lesions may develop when hematogenous bacteria or fungi seed the skin or underlying soft tissue. Bacterial toxins may also be distributed hematogenously and elicit diffuse cutaneous reactions. On occasion, skin lesions may suggest specific pathogens. When sepsis is accompanied by cutaneous petechiae or purpura, infection with *N. meningitidis* (or, less commonly, *H. influenzae*) should be suspected; in a patient who has been bitten by a tick while in an endemic area, petechial lesions also suggest Rocky Mountain spotted fever. A cutaneous lesion seen almost exclusively in neutropenic patients is ecthyma gangrenosum, usually caused by *P. aeruginosa*. It is a bullous lesion, surrounded by edema, that undergoes central hemorrhage and necrosis. Histopathologic examination shows bacteria in and around the wall of a small vessel, with little or no neutrophilic response. Hemorrhagic or bullous lesions in a septic patient who has recently eaten raw oysters suggest *V. vulnificus* bacteremia, while such lesions in a patient who has recently suffered a dog bite may indicate bloodstream infection due to *Capnocytophaga canimorsus* or *C. cynodegmi*. Generalized erythroderma in a septic patient suggests the toxic shock syndrome due to *S. aureus* or *S. pyogenes*.

Gastrointestinal manifestations such as nausea, vomiting, diarrhea, and ileus may suggest acute gastroenteritis. Stress ulceration can lead to upper gastrointestinal bleeding. Cholestatic jaundice, with elevated levels of serum bilirubin (mostly conjugated) and alkaline phosphatase, may precede other signs of sepsis. Hepatocellular or canalicular dysfunction appears to underlie most cases, and the results of hepatic function tests return to normal with resolution of the infection. Prolonged or severe hypotension may induce acute hepatic injury or ischemic bowel necrosis.

Many tissues may be unable to extract oxygen normally from the blood, so that anaerobic metabolism occurs despite near-normal mixed venous oxygen saturation. Blood lactate levels rise early because of increased glycolysis as well as impaired clearance of the resulting lactate and pyruvate by the liver and kidneys. The blood glucose concentration often increases, particularly in patients with diabetes, although impaired gluconeogenesis and excessive insulin release on occasion produce hypoglycemia. The cytokine-driven acute-phase response inhibits the synthesis of transthyretin while enhancing the production of C-reactive protein, fibrinogen, and complement components. Protein catabolism is often markedly accelerated. Serum albumin levels decline as a result of decreased hepatic synthesis and the movement of albumin into interstitial spaces.

MAJOR COMPLICATIONS

Cardiopulmonary complications

Ventilation-perfusion mismatching produces a fall in arterial P_{O_2} early in the course. Increasing alveolar epithelial injury and capillary permeability result in increased pulmonary water content, which decreases pulmonary compliance and interferes with oxygen exchange. In the absence of pneumonia or heart failure, progressive diffuse pulmonary infiltrates and arterial hypoxemia (Pa_{O_2}/Fi_{O_2}, <300) indicate the development of acute lung injury; more severe hypoxemia (Pa_{O_2}/Fi_{O_2}, <200) denotes the acute respiratory distress syndrome (ARDS). Acute lung injury or ARDS develops in ~50% of patients with severe sepsis or septic shock. Respiratory muscle fatigue can exacerbate hypoxemia and hypercapnia. An elevated pulmonary capillary wedge pressure (>18 mmHg) suggests fluid volume overload or cardiac failure rather than ARDS. Pneumonia caused by viruses or by *Pneumocystis* may be clinically indistinguishable from ARDS.

Sepsis-induced hypotension (see "Septic Shock," earlier) usually results initially from a generalized maldistribution of blood flow and blood volume and from hypovolemia that is due, at least in part, to diffuse capillary leakage of intravascular fluid. Other factors that may decrease effective intravascular volume include dehydration from antecedent disease or insensible fluid losses, vomiting or diarrhea, and polyuria. During early septic shock, systemic vascular resistance is usually elevated and cardiac output may be low. After fluid repletion, in contrast, cardiac output typically increases and systemic vascular resistance falls. Indeed, normal or increased cardiac output and decreased systemic vascular resistance distinguish septic shock from cardiogenic, extracardiac obstructive, and hypovolemic shock; other processes that can produce this combination include anaphylaxis, beriberi, cirrhosis, and overdoses of nitroprusside or narcotics.

Depression of myocardial function, manifested as increased end-diastolic and systolic ventricular volumes with a decreased ejection fraction, develops within 24 h in most patients with severe sepsis. Cardiac output is maintained despite the low ejection fraction because ventricular dilatation permits a normal stroke volume. In survivors, myocardial function returns to normal over several days. Although myocardial dysfunction may contribute to hypotension, refractory hypotension is usually due to low systemic vascular resistance, and death results from refractory shock or the failure of multiple organs rather than from cardiac dysfunction per se.

Adrenal insufficiency

The diagnosis of adrenal insufficiency may be very difficult in critically ill patients. Whereas a plasma cortisol level of ≤15 µg/mL (≤10 µg/mL if the serum albumin concentration is <2.5 mg/dL) indicates adrenal insufficiency (inadequate production of cortisol), many experts now feel that the ACTH (CoSyntropin®) stimulation test is not useful for detecting less profound degrees of corticosteroid deficiency in patients who are critically ill. The concept of critical illness–related corticosteroid insufficiency (CIRCI; Table 28-1) was proposed to encompass the different mechanisms that may produce corticosteroid activity that is inadequate for the severity of a patient's illness. Although CIRCI may result from structural damage to the adrenal gland, it is more commonly due to reversible dysfunction of the hypothalamic-pituitary axis or to tissue corticosteroid resistance resulting from abnormalities of the glucocorticoid receptor or increased conversion of cortisol to cortisone. The major clinical manifestation of CIRCI is hypotension that is refractory to fluid replacement and requires pressor therapy. Some classic features of adrenal insufficiency, such as hyponatremia and hyperkalemia, are usually absent; others, such as eosinophilia and modest hypoglycemia, may sometimes be found. Specific etiologies include fulminant *N. meningitidis* bacteremia, disseminated tuberculosis, AIDS (with cytomegalovirus, *Mycobacterium avium-intracellulare*, or *Histoplasma capsulatum* disease), or the prior use of drugs that diminish glucocorticoid production, such as glucocorticoids, megestrol, etomidate, or ketoconazole.

Renal complications

Oliguria, azotemia, proteinuria, and nonspecific urinary casts are frequently found. Many patients are inappropriately polyuric; hyperglycemia may exacerbate this tendency. Most renal failure is due to acute tubular necrosis induced by hypotension or capillary injury, although some patients also have glomerulonephritis, renal cortical necrosis, or interstitial nephritis. Drug-induced renal damage may complicate therapy, particularly when hypotensive patients are given aminoglycoside antibiotics.

Coagulopathy

Although thrombocytopenia occurs in 10–30% of patients, the underlying mechanisms are not understood. Platelet counts are usually very low (<50,000/µL) in patients with DIC; these low counts may reflect diffuse endothelial injury or microvascular thrombosis, yet thrombi have only infrequently been found upon biopsy of septic organs.

Neurologic complications

When the septic illness lasts for weeks or months, "critical illness" polyneuropathy may prevent weaning from ventilatory support and produce distal motor weakness. Electrophysiologic studies are diagnostic. Guillain-Barré syndrome, metabolic disturbances, and toxin activity must be ruled out.

IMMUNOSUPPRESSION

Patients with severe sepsis are often profoundly immunosuppressed. Manifestations include loss of delayed-type hypersensitivity reactions to common antigens, failure to control the primary infection, and increased risk for secondary infections (e.g., by opportunists such as *Stenotrophomonas maltophilia*, *Acinetobacter calcoaceticus-baumannii*, and *Candida albicans*). Approximately one-third of patients experience reactivation of herpes simplex virus, varicella-zoster virus, or cytomegalovirus infections; the latter are thought to contribute to adverse outcomes in some instances.

LABORATORY FINDINGS

Abnormalities that occur early in the septic response may include leukocytosis with a left shift, thrombocytopenia, hyperbilirubinemia, and proteinuria. Leukopenia may develop. The neutrophils may contain toxic granulations, Döhle bodies, or cytoplasmic vacuoles. As the septic response becomes more severe, thrombocytopenia worsens (often with prolongation of the thrombin time, decreased fibrinogen, and the presence of D-dimers, suggesting DIC), azotemia and hyperbilirubinemia become more prominent, and levels of aminotransferases rise. Active hemolysis suggests clostridial bacteremia, malaria, a drug reaction, or DIC; in the case of DIC, microangiopathic changes may be seen on a blood smear.

During early sepsis, hyperventilation induces respiratory alkalosis. With respiratory muscle fatigue and the accumulation of lactate, metabolic acidosis (with increased anion gap) typically supervenes. Evaluation of arterial blood gases reveals hypoxemia that is initially correctable with supplemental oxygen but whose later refractoriness to 100% oxygen inhalation indicates right-to-left shunting. The chest radiograph may be normal or may show evidence of underlying pneumonia, volume overload, or the diffuse infiltrates of ARDS. The electrocardiogram may show only sinus tachycardia or nonspecific ST–T-wave abnormalities.

Most diabetic patients with sepsis develop hyperglycemia. Severe infection may precipitate diabetic ketoacidosis that may exacerbate hypotension. Hypoglycemia occurs rarely. The serum albumin level declines as sepsis continues. Hypocalcemia is rare.

DIAGNOSIS

There is no specific diagnostic test for the septic response. Diagnostically sensitive findings in a patient with suspected or proven infection include fever or hypothermia, tachypnea, tachycardia, and leukocytosis or leukopenia (Table 28-1); acutely altered mental status, thrombocytopenia, an elevated blood lactate level, or hypotension

also should suggest the diagnosis. The septic response can be quite variable, however. In one study, 36% of patients with severe sepsis had a normal temperature, 40% had a normal respiratory rate, 10% had a normal pulse rate, and 33% had normal white blood cell counts. Moreover, the systemic responses of uninfected patients with other conditions may be similar to those characteristic of sepsis. Noninfectious etiologies of SIRS (Table 28-1) include pancreatitis, burns, trauma, adrenal insufficiency, pulmonary embolism, dissecting or ruptured aortic aneurysm, myocardial infarction, occult hemorrhage, cardiac tamponade, postcardiopulmonary bypass syndrome, anaphylaxis, tumor-associated lactic acidosis, and drug overdose.

Definitive etiologic diagnosis requires isolation of the microorganism from blood or a local site of infection. At least two blood samples should be obtained (from two different venipuncture sites) for culture; in a patient with an indwelling catheter, one sample should be collected from each lumen of the catheter and another via venipuncture. In many cases, blood cultures are negative; this result can reflect prior antibiotic administration, the presence of slow-growing or fastidious organisms, or the absence of microbial invasion of the bloodstream. In these cases, Gram's staining and culture of material from the primary site of infection or from infected cutaneous lesions may help establish the microbial etiology. Identification of microbial DNA in peripheral-blood or tissue samples by polymerase chain reaction may also be definitive. The skin and mucosae should be examined carefully and repeatedly for lesions that might yield diagnostic information. With overwhelming bacteremia (e.g., pneumococcal sepsis in splenectomized individuals; fulminant meningococcemia; or infection with *V. vulnificus*, *B. pseudomallei*, or *Y. pestis*), microorganisms are sometimes visible on buffy coat smears of peripheral blood.

TREATMENT **Severe Sepsis and Septic Shock**

Patients in whom sepsis is suspected must be managed expeditiously. This task is best accomplished by personnel who are experienced in the care of the critically ill. Successful management requires urgent measures to treat the infection, to provide hemodynamic and respiratory support, and to eliminate the offending microorganisms. These measures should be initiated within 1 h of the patient's presentation with severe sepsis or septic shock. Rapid assessment and diagnosis are therefore essential.

ANTIMICROBIAL AGENTS Antimicrobial chemotherapy should be started as soon as samples of blood and other relevant sites have been obtained for culture. A large retrospective review of patients who developed septic shock found that the interval between the onset of hypotension and the administration of appropriate antimicrobial chemotherapy was the major determinant of outcome; a delay of as little as 1 h was associated with lower survival rates. Use of inappropriate antibiotics, defined on the basis of local microbial susceptibilities and published guidelines for empirical therapy (see later), was associated with fivefold lower survival rates, even among patients with negative cultures.

It is therefore very important to promptly initiate empirical antimicrobial therapy that is effective against both gram-positive and gram-negative bacteria (Table 28-3). Maximal recommended doses of antimicrobial drugs should be given intravenously, with adjustment for impaired renal function when necessary. Available information about patterns of antimicrobial susceptibility among bacterial isolates from the community, the hospital, and the patient should be taken into account. When culture results become available, the regimen can often be simplified, as a single antimicrobial agent is usually adequate for the treatment of a known pathogen. Meta-analyses have concluded that, with one exception, combination antimicrobial therapy is not superior to monotherapy for treating gram-negative bacteremia; the exception is that aminoglycoside

monotherapy for *P. aeruginosa* bacteremia is less effective than the combination of an aminoglycoside with an antipseudomonal β-lactam agent. Empirical antifungal therapy should be strongly considered if the septic patient is already receiving broad-spectrum antibiotics or parenteral nutrition, has been neutropenic for ≥5 days, has had a long-term central venous catheter, or has been hospitalized in an intensive care unit for a prolonged period. The chosen antimicrobial regimen should be reconsidered daily in order to provide maximal efficacy with minimal resistance, toxicity, and cost.

Most patients require antimicrobial therapy for at least 1 week. The duration of treatment is typically influenced by factors such as the site of tissue infection, the adequacy of surgical drainage, the patient's underlying disease, and the antimicrobial susceptibility of the microbial isolate(s). The absence of an identified microbial pathogen is not necessarily an indication for discontinuing antimicrobial therapy, since "appropriate" antimicrobial regimens seem to be beneficial in both culture-negative and culture-positive cases.

REMOVAL OF THE SOURCE OF INFECTION

Removal or drainage of a focal source of infection is essential. In one series, a focus of ongoing infection

TABLE 28-3

INITIAL ANTIMICROBIAL THERAPY FOR SEVERE SEPSIS WITH NO OBVIOUS SOURCE IN ADULTS WITH NORMAL RENAL FUNCTION

CLINICAL CONDITION	ANTIMICROBIAL REGIMENS (INTRAVENOUS THERAPY)
Immunocompetent adult	The many acceptable regimens include (1) piperacillin-tazobactam (3.375 g q4–6h); (2) imipenem-cilastatin (0.5 g q6h) or meropenem (1 g q8h); or (3) cefepime (2 g q12h). If the patient is allergic to β-lactam agents, use ciprofloxacin (400 mg q12h) or levofloxacin (500–750 mg q12h) plus clindamycin (600 mg q8h). Vancomycin (15 mg/kg q12h) should be added to each of the above regimens.
Neutropenia (<500 neutrophils/μL)	Regimens include (1) imipenem-cilastatin (0.5 g q6h) or meropenem (1 g q8h) or cefepime (2 g q8h); (2) piperacillintazobactam (3.375 g q4h) plus tobramycin (5–7 mg/kg q24h). Vancomycin (15 mg/kg q12h) should be added if the patient has an indwelling vascular catheter, has received quinolone prophylaxis, or has received intensive chemotherapy that produces mucosal damage; if staphylococci are suspected; if the institution has a high incidence of MRSA infections; or if there is a high prevalence of MRSA isolates in the community. Empirical antifungal therapy with an echinocandin (for caspofungin: a 70-mg loading dose, then 50 mg daily) or a lipid formulation of amphotericin B should be added if the patient is hypotensive or has been receiving broad-spectrum antibacterial drugs.
Splenectomy	Cefotaxime (2 g q6–8h) or ceftriaxone (2 g q12h) should be used. If the local prevalence of cephalosporin-resistant pneumococci is high, add vancomycin. If the patient is allergic to β-lactam drugs, vancomycin (15 mg/kg q12h) plus either moxifloxacin (400 mg q24h) or levofloxacin (750 mg q24h) or aztreonam (2 g q8h) should be used.
IV drug user	Vancomycin (15 mg/kg q12h)
AIDS	Cefepime (2 g q8h) or piperacillin-tazobactam (3.375 g q4h) plus tobramycin (5–7 mg/kg q24h) should be used. If the patient is allergic to β-lactam drugs, ciprofloxacin (400 mg q12h) or levofloxacin (750 mg q12h) plus vancomycin (15 mg/kg q12h) plus tobramycin should be used.

Abbreviation: MRSA, methicillin-resistant *Staphylococcus aureus*.
Source: Adapted in part from WT Hughes et al: Clin Infect Dis 25:551, 1997; and DN Gilbert et al: The Sanford Guide to Antimicrobial Therapy, 2009.

was found in ~80% of surgical intensive care patients who died of severe sepsis or septic shock. Sites of occult infection should be sought carefully, particularly in the lungs, abdomen, and urinary tract. Indwelling IV or arterial catheters should be removed and the tip rolled over a blood agar plate for quantitative culture; after antibiotic therapy has been initiated, a new catheter should be inserted at a different site. Foley and drainage catheters should be replaced. The possibility of paranasal sinusitis (often caused by gram-negative bacteria) should be considered if the patient has undergone nasal intubation. Even in patients without abnormalities on chest radiographs, CT of the chest may identify unsuspected parenchymal, mediastinal, or pleural disease. In the neutropenic patient, cutaneous sites of tenderness and erythema, particularly in the perianal region, must be carefully sought. In patients with sacral or ischial decubitus ulcers, it is important to exclude pelvic or other soft tissue pus collections with CT or MRI. In patients with severe sepsis arising from the urinary tract, sonography or CT should be used to rule out ureteral obstruction, perinephric abscess, and renal abscess. Sonographic or CT imaging of the upper abdomen may disclose evidence of cholecystitis, bile duct dilatation, and pus collections in the liver, subphrenic space, or spleen.

HEMODYNAMIC, RESPIRATORY, AND METABOLIC SUPPORT

The primary goals are to restore adequate oxygen and substrate delivery to the tissues as quickly as possible and to improve tissue oxygen utilization and cellular metabolism. Adequate organ perfusion is thus essential. Circulatory adequacy is assessed by measurement of arterial blood pressure and monitoring of parameters such as mentation, urine output, and skin perfusion. Indirect indices of oxygen delivery and consumption, such as central venous oxygen saturation, may also be useful. Initial management of hypotension should include the administration of IV fluids, typically beginning with 1–2 L of normal saline over 1–2 h. To avoid pulmonary edema, the central venous pressure should be maintained at 8–12 cmH$_2$O. The urine output rate should be kept at >0.5 mL/kg per hour by continuing fluid administration; a diuretic such as furosemide may be used if needed. In about one-third of patients, hypotension and organ hypoperfusion respond to fluid resuscitation; a reasonable goal is to maintain a mean arterial blood pressure of >65 mmHg (systolic pressure >90 mmHg). If these guidelines cannot be met by volume infusion, vasopressor therapy is indicated (Chap. 30). Titrated doses of norepinephrine or dopamine should be administered through a central catheter. If myocardial dysfunction produces elevated cardiac filling pressures and low cardiac output, inotropic therapy with dobutamine is recommended.

In patients with septic shock, plasma vasopressin levels increase transiently but then decrease dramatically. Early studies found that vasopressin infusion can reverse septic shock in some patients, reducing or eliminating the need for catecholamine pressors. More recently, a randomized clinical trial that compared vasopressin plus norepinephrine with norepinephrine alone in 776 patients with pressor-dependent septic shock found no difference between treatment groups in the primary study outcome, 28-day mortality. Although vasopressin may have benefited patients who required less norepinephrine, its role in the treatment of septic shock seems to be a minor one overall.

CIRCI should be strongly considered in patients who develop hypotension that does not respond to fluid replacement therapy. Hydrocortisone (50 mg IV every 6 h) should be given; if clinical improvement occurs over 24–48 h, most experts would continue hydrocortisone therapy for 5–7 days before slowly tapering and discontinuing it. Meta-analyses of recent clinical trials have concluded that hydrocortisone therapy hastens recovery from septic shock without increasing long-term survival.

Ventilator therapy is indicated for progressive hypoxemia, hypercapnia, neurologic deterioration, or respiratory muscle failure. Sustained tachypnea (respiratory rate, >30 breaths/min) is frequently a harbinger of impending respiratory collapse; mechanical ventilation is often initiated to ensure adequate oxygenation, to divert blood from the muscles of respiration, to prevent aspiration of oropharyngeal contents, and to reduce the cardiac afterload. The results of recent studies favor the use of low tidal volumes (6 mL/kg of ideal body weight, or as low as 4 mL/kg if the plateau pressure exceeds 30 cmH$_2$O). Patients undergoing mechanical ventilation require careful sedation, with daily interruptions; elevation of the head of the bed helps to prevent nosocomial pneumonia. Stress-ulcer prophylaxis with a histamine H$_2$-receptor antagonist may decrease the risk of gastrointestinal hemorrhage in ventilated patients.

Erythrocyte transfusion is generally recommended when the blood hemoglobin level decreases to ≤7 g/dL, with a target level of 9 g/dL in adults. Erythropoietin is not used to treat sepsis-related anemia. Bicarbonate is sometimes administered for severe metabolic acidosis (arterial pH <7.2), but there is little evidence that it improves either hemodynamics or the response to vasopressor hormones. DIC, if complicated by major bleeding, should be treated with transfusion of fresh-frozen plasma and platelets. Successful treatment of the underlying infection is essential to reverse both acidosis and DIC. Patients who are hypercatabolic and have acute renal failure may benefit greatly from intermittent hemodialysis or continuous veno-venous hemofiltration.

GENERAL SUPPORT

In patients with prolonged severe sepsis (i.e., lasting more than 2 or 3 days), nutritional supplementation may reduce the impact of protein hypercatabolism; the available evidence, which is not strong, favors the enteral delivery route. Prophylactic heparinization to prevent deep venous thrombosis is indicated for patients who do not have active bleeding or coagulopathy; when heparin is contraindicated, compression stockings or an intermittent compression device should be used. Recovery is also assisted by prevention of skin breakdown, nosocomial infections, and stress ulcers.

The role of tight control of the blood glucose concentration in recovery from critical illness has been addressed in numerous controlled trials. Meta-analyses of these trials have concluded that use of insulin to lower blood glucose levels to 100–120 mg/dL is potentially harmful and does not improve survival rates. Most experts now recommend using insulin only if it is needed to maintain the blood glucose concentration below ~150 mg/dL. Patients receiving intravenous insulin must be monitored frequently (every 1–2 h) for hypoglycemia.

OTHER MEASURES Despite aggressive management, many patients with severe sepsis or septic shock die. Numerous interventions have been tested for their ability to improve survival rates among patients with severe sepsis. The list includes endotoxin-neutralizing proteins, inhibitors of cyclooxygenase or nitric oxide synthase, anticoagulants, polyclonal immunoglobulins, glucocorticoids, a phospholipid emulsion, and antagonists to TNF-α, IL-1, platelet-activating factor, and bradykinin. Unfortunately, none of these agents has improved rates of survival among patients with severe sepsis/septic shock in more than one large-scale, randomized, placebo-controlled clinical trial. Many factors have contributed to this lack of reproducibility, including (1) heterogeneity in the patient populations studied, the primary infection sites, the preexisting illnesses, and the inciting microbes; and (2) the nature of the "standard" therapy also used. A dramatic example of this problem was seen in a trial of tissue factor pathway inhibitor (**Fig. 28-1**). Whereas the drug appeared to improve survival rates after 722 patients had been studied ($p = .006$), it did not do so in the next 1032 patients, and the overall result was negative. This inconsistency argues that the results of a clinical trial may not apply to individual patients, even within a carefully selected patient population. It also suggests that, at a minimum, a sepsis intervention should show a significant survival benefit in more than one placebo-controlled, randomized clinical trial before it is accepted as routine clinical practice. In one prominent attempt to reduce patient heterogeneity in clinical trials, experts have called for changes that would restrict these trials to patients who have similar underlying diseases (e.g., major trauma) and inciting infections (e.g., pneumonia). The goal of the predisposition–infection–response–organ

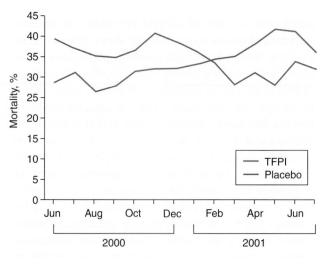

FIGURE 28-1
Mortality rates among patients who received tissue factor pathway inhibitor (TFPI) or placebo, shown as the running average over the course of the clinical trial. The drug seemed highly efficacious at the interim analysis in December 2000, but this trend reversed later in the trial. Demonstrating that therapeutic agents for sepsis have consistent, reproducible efficacy has been extremely difficult, even within well-defined patient populations. (*Reprinted with permission from E Abraham et al: JAMA 290:238, 2003.*)

dysfunction (PIRO) grading system for classification of septic patients (Table 28-1) is similar. Other investigators have used specific biomarkers, such as IL-6 levels in blood or the expression of HLA-DR on peripheral-blood monocytes, to identify the patients most likely to benefit from certain interventions. Multivariate risk stratification based on easily measurable clinical variables should be used with each of these approaches.

Recombinant activated protein C (aPC) was the first drug to be approved by the U.S. Food and Drug Administration for the treatment of patients with severe sepsis or septic shock. Approval was based on the results of a single randomized controlled trial in which the drug was given within 24 h of the patient's first sepsis-related organ dysfunction; the 28-day survival rate was significantly higher among aPC recipients who were very sick (APACHE II score, ≥25) before infusion of the protein than among placebo-treated controls. Subsequent trials failed to show a benefit of aPC treatment in patients who were less sick (APACHE II score, <25) or in children. A second trial of aPC in high-risk patients is now under way in Europe. Given the drug's known toxicity (increased risk of severe bleeding) and uncertain performance in clinical practice, many experts are awaiting the results of the European trial before recommending further use of aPC. Other agents in ongoing or planned clinical trials include intravenous immunoglobulin, a small-molecule endotoxin antagonist (eritoran), and granulocyte-macrophage colony-stimulating factor that was recently reported to restore monocyte immunocompetence in patients with sepsis-associated immunosuppression.

A careful retrospective analysis found that the apparent efficacy of all sepsis therapeutics studied to date has been greatest among the patients at greatest risk of dying before treatment; conversely, use of many of these drugs has been associated with increased mortality rates among patients who are less ill. The authors proposed that neutralizing one of many different mediators may help patients who are very sick, whereas disrupting the mediator balance may be harmful to patients whose adaptive defense mechanisms are working well. This analysis suggests that if more aggressive early resuscitation improves survival rates among sicker patients, it will become more difficult to obtain additional benefit from other therapies; that is, if an intervention improves patients' risk status, moving them into a "less severe illness" category, it will be harder to show that adding another agent to the therapeutic regimen is beneficial.

THE SURVIVING SEPSIS CAMPAIGN An international consortium has advocated "bundling" multiple therapeutic maneuvers into a unified algorithmic approach that will become the standard of care for severe sepsis. In theory, such a strategy could improve care by mandating measures that seem to bring maximal benefit, such as the rapid administration of appropriate antimicrobial therapy; on the other hand, this approach would deemphasize physicians' experience and judgment and minimize the consideration of potentially important differences between patients. Bundling multiple therapies into a single package also obscures the efficacy and toxicity of the individual measures. Caution should be engendered by the fact that two of the key elements of the initial algorithm have now been withdrawn for lack of evidence, while a third remains unproven and controversial.

PROGNOSIS

Approximately 20–35% of patients with severe sepsis and 40–60% of patients with septic shock die within 30 days. Others die within the ensuing 6 months. Late deaths often result from poorly controlled infection, immunosuppression, complications of intensive care, failure of multiple organs, or the patient's underlying disease. Case-fatality rates are similar for culture-positive and culture-negative severe sepsis. Prognostic stratification systems such as APACHE II indicate that factoring in the patient's age, underlying condition, and various physiologic variables can yield estimates of the risk of dying of severe sepsis. Age and prior health status are probably the most important risk factors (Fig. 28-2). In patients with no known preexisting morbidity, the case-fatality rate remains below 10% until the fourth decade of life, after which it gradually increases to exceed 35% in the very elderly. Death is significantly more likely in severely septic patients with preexisting

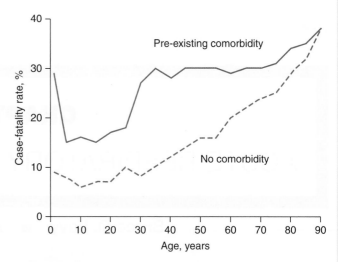

FIGURE 28-2

Influence of age and prior health status on outcome from severe sepsis. With modern therapy, fewer than 10% of previously healthy young individuals (below 35 years of age) die with severe sepsis; the case-fatality rate then increases slowly through middle and old age. The most commonly identified etiologic agents in patients who die are *Staphylococcus aureus*, *Streptococcus pyogenes*, *S. pneumoniae*, and *Neisseria meningitidis*. Individuals with preexisting comorbidities are at greater risk of dying of severe sepsis at any age. The etiologic agents in these cases are likely to be *S. aureus*, *Pseudomonas aeruginosa*, various Enterobacteriaceae, enterococci, or fungi. (*Adapted from DC Angus et al: Crit Care Med 29:1303, 2001.*)

illness, especially during the third to fifth decades. Septic shock is also a strong predictor of short- and long-term mortality.

PREVENTION

Prevention offers the best opportunity to reduce morbidity and mortality from severe sepsis. In developed countries, most episodes of severe sepsis and septic shock are complications of nosocomial infections. These cases might be prevented by reducing the number of invasive procedures undertaken, by limiting the use (and duration of use) of indwelling vascular and bladder catheters, by reducing the incidence and duration of profound neutropenia (<500 neutrophils/μL), and by more aggressively treating localized nosocomial infections. Indiscriminate use of antimicrobial agents and glucocorticoids should be avoided, and optimal infection-control measures should be used. Studies indicate that 50–70% of patients who develop nosocomial severe sepsis or septic shock have experienced a less severe stage of the septic response (e.g., SIRS, sepsis) on at least one previous day in the hospital. Research is needed to identify patients at increased risk and to develop adjunctive agents that can modulate the septic response before organ dysfunction or hypotension occurs.

CHAPTER 29

ACUTE RESPIRATORY DISTRESS SYNDROME

Bruce D. Levy ■ Augustine M. K. Choi

Acute respiratory distress syndrome (ARDS) is a clinical syndrome of severe dyspnea of rapid onset, hypoxemia, and diffuse pulmonary infiltrates leading to respiratory failure. ARDS is caused by diffuse lung injury from many underlying medical and surgical disorders. The lung injury may be direct, as occurs in toxic inhalation, or indirect, as occurs in sepsis (Table 29-1). The clinical features of ARDS are listed in Table 29-2. Acute lung injury (ALI) is a less severe disorder but has the potential to evolve into ARDS (Table 29-2). The arterial (a) PO_2 (in mmHg)/FiO_2 (inspiratory O_2 fraction) <200 mmHg is characteristic of ARDS, while a PaO_2/FiO_2 between 200 and 300 identifies patients with ALI who are likely to benefit from aggressive therapy.

The annual incidences of ALI and ARDS are estimated to be up to 80/100,000 and 60/100,000, respectively. Approximately 10% of all intensive care unit (ICU) admissions suffer from acute respiratory failure, with ~20% of these patients meeting criteria for ALI or ARDS.

TABLE 29-1

CLINICAL DISORDERS COMMONLY ASSOCIATED WITH ARDS	
DIRECT LUNG INJURY	**INDIRECT LUNG INJURY**
Pneumonia	Sepsis
Aspiration of gastric contents	Severe trauma
	Multiple bone fractures
Pulmonary contusion	Flail chest
Near-drowning	Head trauma
Toxic inhalation injury	Burns
	Multiple transfusions
	Drug overdose
	Pancreatitis
	Postcardiopulmonary bypass

TABLE 29-2

DIAGNOSTIC CRITERIA FOR ALI AND ARDS			
OXYGENATION	**ONSET**	**CHEST RADIOGRAPH**	**ABSENCE OF LEFT ATRIAL HYPERTENSION**
ALI: PaO_2/FiO_2 ≤300 mmHg ARDS: PaO_2/FiO_2 ≤200 mmHg	Acute	Bilateral alveolar or interstitial infiltrates	PCWP ≤ 18 mmHg *or* no clinical evidence of increased left atrial pressure

Abbreviations: ALI, acute lung injury; ARDS, acute respiratory distress syndrome; FiO_2, inspired O_2 percentage; PaO_2, arterial partial pressure of O_2; PCWP, pulmonary capillary wedge pressure.

ETIOLOGY

While many medical and surgical illnesses have been associated with the development of ALI and ARDS, most cases (>80%) are caused by a relatively small number of clinical disorders, namely, severe sepsis syndrome and/or bacterial pneumonia (~40–50%), trauma, multiple transfusions, aspiration of gastric contents, and drug overdose. Among patients with trauma, pulmonary contusion, multiple bone fractures, and chest wall trauma/flail chest are the most frequently reported surgical conditions in ARDS, whereas head trauma, near-drowning, toxic inhalation, and burns are rare causes. The risks of developing ARDS are increased in patients suffering from more than one predisposing medical or surgical condition (e.g., the risk for ARDS increases from 25% in patients with severe trauma to 56% in patients with trauma and sepsis).

Several other clinical variables have been associated with the development of ARDS. These include older age, chronic alcohol abuse, metabolic acidosis, and severity of critical illness. Trauma patients with an acute physiology and chronic health evaluation (APACHE) II score ≥16 (Chap. 25) have a 2.5-fold increase in the risk of developing ARDS, and those with a score >20 have an incidence of ARDS that is more than threefold greater than those with APACHE II scores ≤9.

CLINICAL COURSE AND PATHOPHYSIOLOGY

The natural history of ARDS is marked by three phases—exudative, proliferative, and fibrotic—each with characteristic clinical and pathologic features (Fig. 29-1).

Exudative phase

(Figure 29-2) In this phase, alveolar capillary endothelial cells and type I pneumocytes (alveolar epithelial cells) are injured, leading to the loss of the normally tight alveolar barrier to fluid and macromolecules. Edema fluid that is rich in protein accumulates in the interstitial and alveolar spaces. Significant concentrations of cytokines (e.g., interleukin 1, interleukin 8, and tumor necrosis factor α) and lipid mediators (e.g., leukotriene B₄) are present in the lung in this acute phase. In response to proinflammatory mediators, leukocytes (especially neutrophils) traffic into the pulmonary interstitium and alveoli. In addition, condensed plasma proteins aggregate in the air spaces with cellular debris and dysfunctional pulmonary surfactant to form hyaline membrane whorls. Pulmonary vascular injury also occurs early in ARDS, with vascular obliteration by microthrombi and fibrocellular proliferation (Fig. 29-3).

Alveolar edema predominantly involves *dependent* portions of the lung, leading to diminished aeration and atelectasis. Collapse of large sections of dependent lung markedly decreases lung compliance. Consequently, intrapulmonary shunting and hypoxemia develop and the work of breathing rises, leading to dyspnea. The pathophysiologic alterations in alveolar spaces are

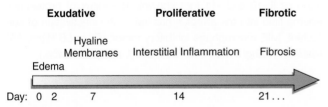

FIGURE 29-1
Diagram illustrating the time course for the development and resolution of ARDS. The exudative phase is notable for early alveolar edema and neutrophil-rich leukocytic infiltration of the lungs with subsequent formation of hyaline membranes from diffuse alveolar damage. Within 7 days, a proliferative phase ensues with prominent interstitial inflammation and early fibrotic changes. Approximately 3 weeks after the initial pulmonary injury, most patients recover. However, some patients enter the fibrotic phase, with substantial fibrosis and bullae formation.

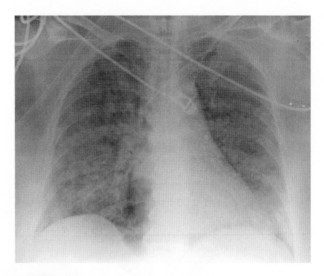

FIGURE 29-2
A representative anteroposterior (AP) chest x-ray in the exudative phase of ARDS that shows diffuse interstitial and alveolar infiltrates, that can be difficult to distinguish from left ventricular failure.

exacerbated by microvascular occlusion that leads to reductions in pulmonary arterial blood flow to ventilated portions of the lung, increasing the dead space, and to pulmonary hypertension. Thus, in addition to severe hypoxemia, hypercapnia secondary to an increase in pulmonary dead space is also prominent in early ARDS.

The exudative phase encompasses the first 7 days of illness after exposure to a precipitating ARDS risk factor, with the patient experiencing the onset of respiratory symptoms. Although usually present within 12–36 h after the initial insult, symptoms can be delayed by 5–7 days. Dyspnea develops with a sensation of rapid shallow breathing and an inability to get enough air. Tachypnea and increased work of breathing frequently result in respiratory fatigue and ultimately in respiratory failure. Laboratory values are generally nonspecific and primarily indicative of underlying clinical disorders. The chest radiograph usually reveals alveolar and interstitial opacities involving at least three-quarters of the lung fields (Fig. 29-2). While characteristic for ARDS or ALI, these radiographic findings are not specific and can be indistinguishable from cardiogenic pulmonary edema (Chap. 30). Unlike the latter, however, the chest x-ray in ARDS rarely shows cardiomegaly, pleural effusions, or pulmonary vascular redistribution. Chest computed tomographic (CT) scanning in ARDS reveals extensive heterogeneity of lung involvement (Fig. 29-4).

Because the early features of ARDS and ALI are nonspecific, alternative diagnoses must be considered. In the differential diagnosis of ARDS, the most common disorders are cardiogenic pulmonary edema, diffuse pneumonia, and alveolar hemorrhage. Less frequent

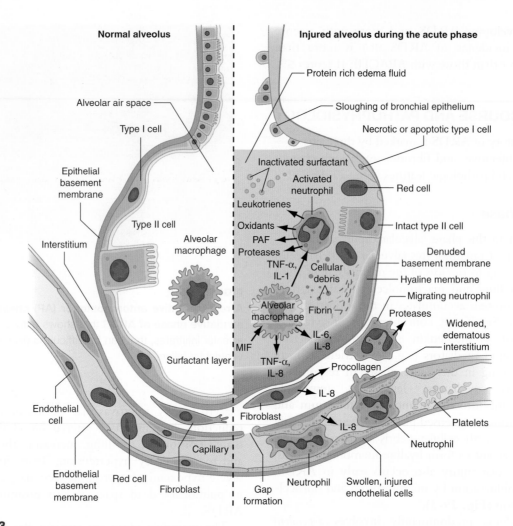

Normal alveolus

Alveolar air space

Type I cell

Epithelial basement membrane

Type II cell

Interstitium

Alveolar macrophage

Endothelial cell

Endothelial basement membrane

Red cell

Fibroblast

Capillary

Surfactant layer

Gap formation

Injured alveolus during the acute phase

Protein rich edema fluid

Sloughing of bronchial epithelium

Necrotic or apoptotic type I cell

Inactivated surfactant

Activated neutrophil

Red cell

Leukotrienes

Oxidants

PAF

Proteases

Intact type II cell

TNF-α, IL-1

Cellular debris

Denuded basement membrane

Hyaline membrane

Alveolar macrophage

Fibrin

Migrating neutrophil

Proteases

MIF

IL-6, IL-8

Widened, edematous interstitium

TNF-α, IL-8

Procollagen

IL-8

Fibroblast

IL-8

Platelets

Neutrophil

Neutrophil

Swollen, injured endothelial cells

FIGURE 29-3

The normal alveolus (left-hand side) and the injured alveolus in the acute phase of acute lung injury and the acute respiratory distress syndrome (right-hand side). In the acute phase of the syndrome (right-hand side), there is sloughing of both the bronchial and alveolar epithelial cells, with the formation of protein-rich hyaline membranes on the denuded basement membrane. Neutrophils are shown adhering to the injured capillary endothelium and marginating through the interstitium into the air space, which is filled with protein-rich edema fluid. In the air space, an alveolar macrophage is secreting cytokines, interleukins 1, 6, 8, and 10 (IL-1, -6, -8, and -10) and tumor necrosis factor α (TNF-α), that act locally to stimulate chemotaxis and activate neutrophils. Macrophages also secrete other cytokines, including IL-1, -6, and -10. IL-1 can also stimulate the production of extracellular matrix by fibroblasts. Neutrophils can release oxidants, proteases, leukotrienes, and other proinflammatory molecules, such as platelet-activating factor (PAF). A number of antiinflammatory mediators are also present in the alveolar milieu, including IL-1–receptor antagonist, soluble TNF-α receptor, autoantibodies against IL-8, and cytokines such as IL-10 and -11 (not shown). The influx of protein-rich edema fluid into the alveolus has led to the inactivation of surfactant. MIF, macrophage inhibitory factor. (*From LB Ware, MA Matthay: N Engl J Med 342:1334, 2000, with permission.*)

diagnoses to consider include acute interstitial lung diseases (e.g., acute interstitial pneumonitis [Chap. 19]), acute immunologic injury (e.g., hypersensitivity pneumonitis [Chap. 9]), toxin injury (e.g., radiation pneumonitis), and neurogenic pulmonary edema.

Proliferative phase

This phase of ARDS usually lasts from day 7 to day 21. Most patients recover rapidly and are liberated from mechanical ventilation during this phase. Despite this improvement, many still experience dyspnea, tachypnea, and hypoxemia. Some patients develop progressive lung injury and early changes of pulmonary fibrosis during the proliferative phase. Histologically, the first signs of resolution are often evident in this phase with the initiation of lung repair, organization of alveolar exudates, and a shift from a neutrophil- to a lymphocyte-predominant pulmonary infiltrate. As part of the reparative process, there is a proliferation of type II pneumocytes along

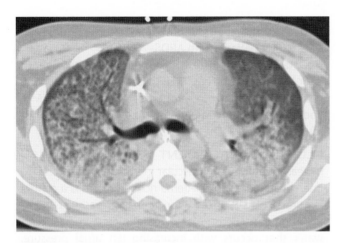

FIGURE 29-4
A representative computed tomographic scan of the chest during the exudative phase of ARDS in which *dependent* alveolar edema and atelectasis predominate.

alveolar basement membranes. These specialized epithelial cells synthesize new pulmonary surfactant and differentiate into type I pneumocytes. The presence of alveolar type III procollagen peptide, a marker of pulmonary fibrosis, is associated with a protracted clinical course and increased mortality from ARDS.

Fibrotic phase

While many patients with ARDS recover lung function 3–4 weeks after the initial pulmonary injury, some will enter a fibrotic phase that may require long-term support on mechanical ventilators and/or supplemental oxygen. Histologically, the alveolar edema and inflammatory exudates of earlier phases are now converted to extensive alveolar duct and interstitial fibrosis. Acinar architecture is markedly disrupted, leading to emphysema-like changes with large bullae. Intimal fibroproliferation in the pulmonary microcirculation leads to progressive vascular occlusion and pulmonary hypertension. The physiologic consequences include an increased risk of pneumothorax, reductions in lung compliance, and increased pulmonary dead space. Patients in this late phase experience a substantial burden of excess morbidity. Lung biopsy evidence for pulmonary fibrosis in any phase of ARDS is associated with increased mortality.

TREATMENT | Acute Respiratory Distress Syndrome

GENERAL PRINCIPLES Recent reductions in ARDS/ALI mortality are largely the result of general advances in the care of critically ill patients (Chap. 25). Thus, caring for these patients requires close attention to (1) the recognition and treatment of the underlying

medical and surgical disorders (e.g., sepsis, aspiration, trauma); (2) minimizing procedures and their complications; (3) prophylaxis against venous thromboembolism, gastrointestinal bleeding, aspiration, excessive sedation, and central venous catheter infections; (4) prompt recognition of nosocomial infections; and (5) provision of adequate nutrition.

MANAGEMENT OF MECHANICAL VENTILATION (See also Chap. 26) Patients meeting clinical criteria for ARDS frequently fatigue from increased work of breathing and progressive hypoxemia, requiring mechanical ventilation for support.

Ventilator-Induced Lung Injury Despite its lifesaving potential, mechanical ventilation can aggravate lung injury. Experimental models have demonstrated that ventilator-induced lung injury appears to require two processes: repeated alveolar overdistention and recurrent alveolar collapse. Clearly evident by chest CT (Fig. 29-4), ARDS is a heterogeneous disorder, principally involving dependent portions of the lung with relative sparing of other regions. Because of their differing compliance, attempts to fully inflate the consolidated lung may lead to overdistention and injury to the more "normal" areas of the lung. Ventilator-induced injury can be demonstrated in experimental models of ALI, with high tidal volume (V_T) ventilation resulting in additional, synergistic alveolar damage. These findings led to the hypothesis that ventilating patients suffering from ALI or ARDS with lower V_Ts would protect against ventilator-induced lung injury and improve clinical outcomes.

A large-scale, randomized controlled trial sponsored by the National Institutes of Health and conducted by the ARDS Network compared low V_T (6 mL/kg predicted body weight) ventilation to conventional V_T (12 mL/kg predicted body weight) ventilation. Mortality was significantly lower in the low V_T patients (31%) compared to the conventional V_T patients (40%). This improvement in survival represents the most substantial benefit in ARDS mortality demonstrated for *any* therapeutic intervention in ARDS to date.

Prevention of Alveolar Collapse In ARDS, the presence of alveolar and interstitial fluid and the loss of surfactant can lead to a marked reduction of lung compliance. Without an increase in end-expiratory pressure, significant alveolar collapse can occur at end-expiration, impairing oxygenation. In most clinical settings, positive end-expiratory pressure (PEEP) is empirically set to minimize Fio_2 and maximize Pao_2. On most modern mechanical ventilators, it is possible to construct a static pressure–volume curve for the respiratory system. The lower inflection point on the curve represents alveolar opening (or "recruitment"). The pressure at this point, usually 12–15 mmHg in ARDS, is a theoretical "optimal PEEP" for alveolar recruitment. Titration of the PEEP to the lower inflection point on the static pressure–volume curve has been hypothesized to keep the lung open, improving oxygenation and protecting against lung injury. Three large randomized trials have investigated the utility of PEEP-based strategies to keep the lung open. In all three trials, improvement in lung function was evident but there were no significant differences in overall mortality. Until more data become available on the clinical utility of high PEEP, it is advisable to set PEEP to minimize Fio_2 and optimize Pao_2 (Chap. 26). Measurement of esophageal pressures to estimate transpulmonary pressure may help identify an optimal PEEP in some patients.

Oxygenation can also be improved by increasing mean airway pressure with "inverse ratio ventilation." In this technique, the inspiratory (*I*) time is lengthened so that it is longer than the expiratory (*E*) time (*I:E* > 1:1). With diminished time to exhale, dynamic hyperinflation leads to increased end-expiratory pressure, similar to ventilator-prescribed PEEP. This mode of ventilation has the advantage of improving oxygenation with lower peak pressures than conventional ventilation. Although inverse ratio ventilation can improve oxygenation and help reduce Fio_2 to ≤0.60 to avoid possible oxygen toxicity, no mortality benefit in ARDS has been demonstrated. Recruitment maneuvers that transiently increase PEEP to "recruit" atelectatic lung can also increase oxygenation, but a mortality benefit has not been established.

In several randomized trials, mechanical ventilation in the prone position improved arterial oxygenation, but its effect on survival and other important clinical outcomes remains uncertain. Moreover, unless the critical-care team is experienced in "proning," repositioning critically ill patients can be hazardous, leading to accidental endotracheal extubation, loss of central venous catheters, and orthopedic injury. Until validation of its efficacy, prone-position ventilation should be reserved for only the most critically ill ARDS patients.

Other Strategies in Mechanical Ventilation

Several additional mechanical ventilation strategies that utilize specialized equipment have been tested in ARDS patients, most with mixed or disappointing results in adults. These include high-frequency ventilation (HFV) (i.e., ventilating at extremely high respiratory rates [5–20 cycles per second] and low V_Ts [1–2 mL/kg]). Partial liquid ventilation (PLV) with perfluorocarbon, an inert, high-density liquid that easily solubilizes oxygen and carbon dioxide, has revealed promising preliminary data on pulmonary function in patients with ARDS but also without survival benefit. Lung-replacement therapy with extracorporeal membrane oxygenation (ECMO), which provides a clear survival benefit in neonatal respiratory distress syndrome, may also have utility in select adult patients with ARDS.

Data in support of the efficacy of "adjunctive" ventilator therapies (e.g., high PEEP, inverse ratio ventilation, recruitment maneuvers, prone positioning, HFV, ECMO, and PLV) remain incomplete, so these modalities are not routinely used.

FLUID MANAGEMENT (See also Chap. 25) Increased pulmonary vascular permeability leading to interstitial and alveolar edema rich in protein is a central feature of ARDS. In addition, impaired vascular integrity augments the normal increase in extravascular lung water that occurs with increasing left atrial pressure. Maintaining a normal or low left atrial filling pressure minimizes pulmonary edema and prevents further decrements in arterial oxygenation and lung compliance, improves pulmonary mechanics, shortens ICU stay and the duration of mechanical ventilation, and is associated with a lower mortality in both medical and surgical ICU patients. Thus, aggressive attempts to reduce left atrial filling pressures with fluid restriction and diuretics should be an important aspect of ARDS management, limited only by hypotension and hypoperfusion of critical organs such as the kidneys.

GLUCOCORTICOIDS Inflammatory mediators and leukocytes are abundant in the lungs of patients with ARDS. Many attempts have been made to treat both early and late ARDS with glucocorticoids to reduce this potentially deleterious pulmonary inflammation. Few studies have shown any benefit. Current evidence does *not* support the use of high-dose glucocorticoids in the care of ARDS patients.

OTHER THERAPIES Clinical trials of surfactant replacement and multiple other medical therapies have proved disappointing. Inhaled nitric oxide (NO) can transiently improve oxygenation but does not improve survival or decrease time on mechanical ventilation. Therefore, the use of NO is *not* currently recommended in ARDS.

RECOMMENDATIONS Many clinical trials have been undertaken to improve the outcome of patients with ARDS; most have been unsuccessful in modifying the natural history. The large number and uncertain clinical efficacy of ARDS therapies can make it difficult for clinicians to select a rational treatment plan, and these patients' critical illnesses can tempt physicians to try unproven and potentially harmful therapies. While results of large clinical trials must be judiciously administered to *individual* patients, evidence-based recommendations are summarized in Table 29-3, and an algorithm for the initial therapeutic goals and limits in ARDS management is provided in Fig. 29-5.

TABLE 29-3

EVIDENCE-BASED RECOMMENDATIONS FOR ARDS THERAPIES

TREATMENT	RECOMMENDATION[a]
Mechanical ventilation:	
Low tidal volume	A
Minimize left atrial filling pressures	B
High-PEEP or "open lung"	C
Prone position	C
Recruitment maneuvers	C
ECMO	C
High-frequency ventilation	D
Glucocorticoids	D
Surfactant replacement, inhaled nitric oxide, and other anti-inflammatory therapy (e.g., ketoconazole, PGE1, NSAIDs)	D

[a]A, recommended therapy based on strong clinical evidence from randomized clinical trials; B, recommended therapy based on supportive but limited clinical data; C, indeterminate evidence: recommended only as alternative therapy; D, not recommended based on clinical evidence against efficacy of therapy.

Abbreviations: ARDS, acute respiratory distress syndrome; ECMO, extracorporeal membrane oxygenation; NSAIDs, nonsteroidal anti-inflammatory drugs; PEEP, positive end-expiratory pressure; PGE_1, prostaglandin E_1.

PROGNOSIS

Mortality

Recent mortality estimates for ARDS range from 26 to 44%. There is substantial variability, but a trend toward improved ARDS outcomes appears evident. Of interest, mortality in ARDS is largely attributable to nonpulmonary causes, with sepsis and nonpulmonary organ failure accounting for >80% of deaths. Thus, improvement in survival is likely secondary to advances in the care of septic/infected patients and those with multiple organ failure (Chap. 25).

Several risk factors for mortality to help estimate prognosis have been identified. Similar to the risk factors for developing ARDS, the major risk factors for ARDS mortality are also nonpulmonary. Advanced age is an important risk factor. Patients >75 years of age have a substantially increased mortality (~60%) compared to those <45 (~20%). Also, patients >60 years of age with ARDS and sepsis have a threefold higher mortality compared to those <60. Preexisting organ dysfunction from chronic medical illness is an important additional risk factor for increased mortality. In particular, chronic liver disease, cirrhosis, chronic alcohol abuse, chronic immunosuppression, sepsis, chronic renal disease, any nonpulmonary organ failure, and increased APACHE III scores (Chap. 25) have also been linked

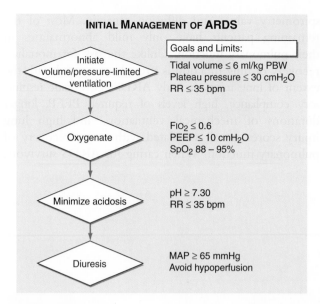

FIGURE 29-5

Algorithm for the initial management of ARDS. Clinical trials have provided evidence-based therapeutic goals for a stepwise approach to the early mechanical ventilation, oxygenation, and correction of acidosis and diuresis of critically ill patients with ARDS.

to increased ARDS mortality. Several factors related to the presenting clinical disorders also increase the risk for ARDS mortality. Patients with ARDS from direct lung injury (including pneumonia, pulmonary contusion, and aspiration; Table 29-1) have nearly twice the mortality of those with indirect causes of lung injury, while surgical and trauma patients with ARDS, especially those without direct lung injury, have a better survival rate than other ARDS patients.

Surprisingly, there is little value in predicting ARDS mortality from the PaO_2/FiO_2 ratio and any of the following measures of the severity of lung injury: the level of PEEP used in mechanical ventilation, the respiratory compliance, the extent of alveolar infiltrates on chest radiography, and the lung injury score (a composite of all these variables). However, recent data indicate that an early (within 24 h of presentation) elevation in dead space and the oxygenation index may predict increased mortality from ARDS.

Functional recovery in ARDS survivors

While it is common for patients with ARDS to experience prolonged respiratory failure and remain dependent on mechanical ventilation for survival, it is a testament to the resolving powers of the lung that the majority of patients recover nearly normal lung function. Patients usually recover their maximum lung function within 6 months. One year after endotracheal extubation, more than one-third of ARDS survivors have normal spirometry values and diffusion capacity. Most of the remaining patients have only mild abnormalities in their pulmonary function. Unlike the risk for mortality, recovery of lung function is strongly associated with the extent of lung injury in early ARDS. Low static respiratory compliance, high levels of required PEEP, longer durations of mechanical ventilation, and high lung injury scores are all associated with worse recovery of pulmonary function. When caring for ARDS survivors, it is important to be aware of the potential for a substantial burden of emotional and respiratory symptoms. There are significant rates of depression and posttraumatic stress disorder in ARDS survivors.

ACKNOWLEDGMENT

The authors acknowledge the contribution to this chapter by the previous author, Dr. Steven D. Shapiro.

CHAPTER 30

CARDIOGENIC SHOCK AND PULMONARY EDEMA

Judith S. Hochman ■ **David H. Ingbar**

Cardiogenic shock and pulmonary edema are life-threatening conditions that should be treated as medical emergencies. The most common etiology for both is severe left ventricular (LV) dysfunction that leads to pulmonary congestion and/or systemic hypoperfusion (**Fig. 30-1**). The pathophysiology of pulmonary edema and shock is discussed in Chaps. 2 and 27, respectively.

CARDIOGENIC SHOCK

Cardiogenic shock (CS) is characterized by systemic hypoperfusion due to severe depression of the cardiac index [<2.2 (L/min)/m^2] and sustained systolic arterial hypotension (<90 mmHg) despite an elevated filling pressure [pulmonary capillary wedge pressure (PCWP) >18 mmHg]. It is associated with in-hospital mortality rates >50%. The major causes of CS are listed in **Table 30-1**. Circulatory failure based on cardiac dysfunction may be caused by primary myocardial failure, most commonly secondary to acute myocardial infarction (MI) (Chap. 33), and less frequently by cardiomyopathy or myocarditis, cardiac tamponade, or critical valvular heart disease.

Incidence

CS is the leading cause of death of patients hospitalized with MI. Early reperfusion therapy for acute MI decreases the incidence of CS. The rate of CS complicating acute MI was 20% in the 1960s, stayed at ~8% for >20 years, but decreased to 5–7% in the first decade of this millennium. Shock typically is associated with ST elevation MI (STEMI) and is less common with non-ST elevation MI (Chap. 33).

LV failure accounts for ~80% of cases of CS complicating acute MI. Acute severe mitral regurgitation (MR), ventricular septal rupture (VSR), predominant right ventricular (RV) failure, and free wall rupture or tamponade account for the remainder.

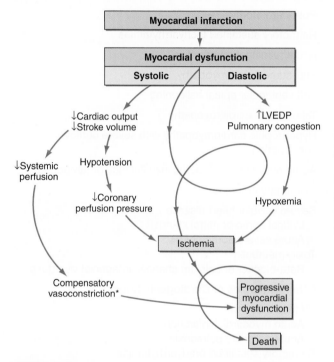

FIGURE 30-1

Pathophysiology of cardiogenic shock. Systolic and diastolic myocardial dysfunction results in a reduction in cardiac output and often pulmonary congestion. Systemic and coronary hypoperfusion occur, resulting in progressive ischemia. Although a number of compensatory mechanisms are activated in an attempt to support the circulation, these compensatory mechanisms may become maladaptive and produce a worsening of hemodynamics. *Release of inflammatory cytokines after myocardial infarction may lead to inducible nitric oxide expression, excess nitric oxide, and inappropriate vasodilation. This causes further reduction in systemic and coronary perfusion. A vicious spiral of progressive myocardial dysfunction occurs that ultimately results in death if it is not interrupted. LVEDP, left ventricular end-diastolic pressure. (*From SM Hollenberg et al: Ann Intern Med 131:47, 1999.*)

TABLE 30-1

ETIOLOGIES OF CARDIOGENIC SHOCK (CS)ᵃ AND CARDIOGENIC PULMONARY EDEMA

Etiologies of Cardiogenic Shock or Pulmonary Edema

Acute myocardial infarction/ischemia
  LV failure
  VSR
  Papillary muscle/chordal rupture—severe MR
  Ventricular free wall rupture with subacute tamponade
  Other conditions complicating large MIs
    Hemorrhage
    Infection
    Excess negative inotropic or vasodilator medications
    Prior valvular heart disease
    Hyperglycemia/ketoacidosis

Post-cardiac arrest

Post-cardiotomy

Refractory sustained tachyarrhythmias

Acute fulminant myocarditis

End-stage cardiomyopathy

Left ventricular apical ballooning

Takotsubo's cardiomyopathy

Hypertrophic cardiomyopathy with severe outflow obstruction

Aortic dissection with aortic insufficiency or tamponade

Pulmonary embolus

Severe valvular heart disease
  Critical aortic or mitral stenosis
  Acute severe aortic or MR
Toxic-metabolic
  Beta-blocker or calcium channel antagonist overdose

Other Etiologies of Cardiogenic Shockᵇ

RV failure due to:
  Acute myocardial infarction
  Acute coronary pulmonale
Refractory sustained bradyarrhythmias
Pericardial tamponade
Toxic/metabolic
  Severe acidosis, severe hypoxemia

ᵃThe etiologies of CS are listed. Most of these can cause pulmonary edema instead of shock or pulmonary edema with CS.
ᵇThese cause CS but not pulmonary edema.
Abbreviations: LV, left ventricular; VSR, ventricular septal rupture; MR, mitral regurgitation; MI, myocardial infarction; RV, right ventricular.

Pathophysiology

CS is characterized by a vicious circle in which depression of myocardial contractility, usually due to ischemia, results in reduced cardiac output and arterial pressure (BP), which result in hypoperfusion of the myocardium and further ischemia and depression of cardiac output (Fig. 30-1). Systolic myocardial dysfunction reduces stroke volume and, together with diastolic dysfunction, leads to elevated LV end-diastolic pressure and PCWP as well as to pulmonary congestion. Reduced coronary perfusion leads to worsening ischemia and progressive myocardial dysfunction and a rapid downward spiral, which, if uninterrupted, is often fatal. A systemic inflammatory response syndrome may accompany large infarctions and shock. Inflammatory cytokines, inducible nitric oxide synthase, and excess nitric oxide and peroxynitrite may contribute to the genesis of CS as they do to that of other forms of shock (Chap. 27). Lactic acidosis from poor tissue perfusion and hypoxemia from pulmonary edema may result from pump failure and then contribute to the vicious circle by worsening myocardial ischemia and hypotension. Severe acidosis (pH <7.25) reduces the efficacy of endogenous and exogenously administered catecholamines. Refractory sustained ventricular or atrial tachyarrhythmias can cause or exacerbate CS.

Patient profile

In patients with acute MI, older age, female sex, prior MI, diabetes, and anterior MI location are all associated with an increased risk of CS. Shock associated with a first inferior MI should prompt a search for a mechanical cause. Reinfarction soon after MI increases the risk of CS. Two-thirds of patients with CS have flow-limiting stenoses in all three major coronary arteries, and 20% have stenosis of the left main coronary artery. CS may rarely occur in the absence of significant stenosis, as seen in LV apical ballooning/Takotsubo's cardiomyopathy.

Timing

Shock is present on admission in only one-quarter of patients who develop CS complicating MI; one-quarter develop it rapidly thereafter, within 6 h of MI onset. Another quarter develop shock later on the first day. Subsequent onset of CS may be due to reinfarction, marked infarct expansion, or a mechanical complication.

Diagnosis

Due to the unstable condition of these patients, supportive therapy must be initiated simultaneously with diagnostic evaluation (Fig. 30-2). A focused history and physical examination should be performed, blood specimens sent to the laboratory, and an electrocardiogram (ECG) and chest x-ray obtained.

Echocardiography is an invaluable diagnostic tool in patients suspected of CS.

Clinical findings

Most patients have continuing chest pain and dyspnea and appear pale, apprehensive, and diaphoretic. Mentation

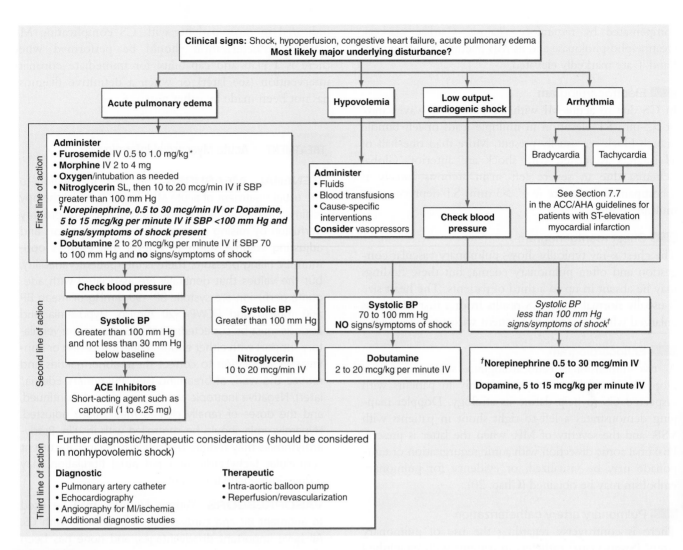

FIGURE 30-2

The emergency management of patients with cardiogenic shock, acute pulmonary edema, or both is outlined. *Furosemide: <0.5 mg/kg for new-onset acute pulmonary edema without hypervolemia; 1 mg/kg for acute on chronic volume overload, renal insufficiency. †Indicates modification from published guidelines. ACE, angiotensin-converting enzyme; BP, blood pressure; MI, myocardial infarction. (*Modified from Guidelines 2000 for Cardiopulmonary Resuscitation and Emergency Cardiovascular Care. Part 7:The era of reperfusion: Section 1: Acute coronary syndromes [acute myocardial infarction]. The American Heart Association in collaboration with the International Liaison Committee on Resuscitation. Circulation 102:I172, 2000.*)

may be altered, with somnolence, confusion, and agitation. The pulse is typically weak and rapid, often in the range of 90–110 beats/min, or severe bradycardia due to high-grade heart block may be present. Systolic blood pressure is reduced (<90 mmHg) with a narrow pulse pressure (<30 mmHg), but occasionally BP may be maintained by very high systemic vascular resistance. Tachypnea, Cheyne-Stokes respirations, and jugular venous distention may be present. The precordium is typically quiet, with a weak apical pulse. S_1 is usually soft, and an S_3 gallop may be audible. Acute, severe MR and VSR usually are associated with characteristic systolic murmurs (Chap. 33). Rales are audible in most

patients with LV failure causing CS. Oliguria (urine output <30 mL/h) is common.

Laboratory findings

The white blood cell count is typically elevated with a left shift. In the absence of prior renal insufficiency, renal function is initially normal, but blood urea nitrogen and creatinine rise progressively. Hepatic transaminases may be markedly elevated due to liver hypoperfusion. Poor tissue perfusion may result in an anion-gap acidosis and elevation of the lactic acid level. Before support with supplemental O_2, arterial blood gases usually demonstrate hypoxemia and metabolic acidosis, which may be compensated by respiratory alkalosis. Cardiac markers, creatine phosphokinase and its MB fraction, and troponins I and T are markedly elevated.

Electrocardiogram

In CS due to acute MI with LV failure, Q waves and/ or >2-mm ST elevation in multiple leads or left bundle branch block are usually present. More than one-half of all infarcts associated with shock are anterior. Global ischemia due to severe left main stenosis usually is accompanied by severe (e.g., >3 mm) ST depressions in multiple leads.

Chest roentgenogram

The chest x-ray typically shows pulmonary vascular congestion and often pulmonary edema, but these findings may be absent in up to a third of patients. The heart size is usually normal when CS results from a first MI but is enlarged when it occurs in a patient with a previous MI.

Echocardiogram

A two-dimensional echocardiogram with color-flow Doppler should be obtained promptly in patients with suspected CS to help define its etiology. Doppler mapping demonstrates a left-to-right shunt in patients with VSR and the severity of MR when the latter is present. Proximal aortic dissection with aortic regurgitation or tamponade may be visualized, or evidence for pulmonary embolism may be obtained (Chap. 20).

Pulmonary artery catheterization

There is controversy regarding the use of pulmonary artery (Swan–Ganz) catheters in patients with established or suspected CS (Chap. 25). Their use is generally recommended for measurement of filling pressures and cardiac output to confirm the diagnosis and optimize the use of IV fluids, inotropic agents, and vasopressors in persistent shock (Table 30-2). Blood samples for O_2 saturation measurement should be obtained from the right atrium, right ventricle, and pulmonary artery to rule out a left-to-right shunt. Mixed venous O_2 saturations are low and arteriovenous (AV) O_2 differences are elevated, reflecting low cardiac index and high fractional O_2 extraction. However, when a systemic inflammatory response syndrome accompanies CS, AV O_2 differences may not be elevated (Chap. 27). The PCWP is elevated. However, use of sympathomimetic amines may return these measurements and the systemic BP to normal. Systemic vascular resistance may be low, normal, or elevated in CS. Equalization of right- and left-sided filling pressures (right atrial and PCWP) suggests cardiac tamponade as the cause of CS.

Left heart catheterization and coronary angiography

Measurement of LV pressure and definition of the coronary anatomy provide useful information and are indicated in most patients with CS complicating MI. Cardiac catheterization should be performed when there is a plan and capability for immediate coronary intervention (see later) or when a definitive diagnosis has not been made by other tests.

TREATMENT   Acute Myocardial Infarction

GENERAL MEASURES (Fig. 30-2) In addition to the usual treatment of acute MI (Chap. 33), initial therapy is aimed at maintaining adequate systemic and coronary perfusion by raising systemic BP with vasopressors and adjusting volume status to a level that ensures optimum LV filling pressure. There is interpatient variability, but the values that generally are associated with adequate perfusion are systolic BP ~90 mmHg or mean BP >60 mmHg and PCWP >20 mmHg. Hypoxemia and acidosis must be corrected; most patients require ventilatory support with either endotracheal intubation or noninvasive ventilation to correct these abnormalities and reduce the work of breathing (see "Pulmonary Edema," later). Negative inotropic agents should be discontinued, and the doses of renally cleared medications adjusted. Hyperglycemia should be controlled with insulin. Bradyarrhythmias may require transvenous pacing. Recurrent ventricular tachycardia or rapid atrial fibrillation may require immediate treatment.

VASOPRESSORS Various IV drugs may be used to augment BP and cardiac output in patients with CS. All have important disadvantages, and none has been shown to change the outcome in patients with established shock. *Norepinephrine* is a potent vasoconstrictor and inotropic stimulant that is useful for patients with CS. As first line of therapy norepinephrine was associated with fewer adverse events, including arrhythmias, compared to a dopamine randomized trial of patients with several eteologies of circulatory shock. Although it did not significantly improve survival compared to dopamine, its relative safety suggests that norepinephrine is reasonable as initial vasopressor therapy. Norepinephrine should be started at a dose of 2 to 4 µg/min and titrated upward as necessary. If systemic perfusion or systolic pressure cannot be maintained at >90 mmHg with a dose of 15 µg/min, it is unlikely that a further increase will be beneficial.

Dopamine has varying hemodynamic effects based on the dose; at low doses (≤ 2 µg/kg per min), it dilates the renal vascular bed, although its outcome benefits at this low dose have not been demonstrated conclusively; at moderate doses (2–10 µg/kg per min), it has positive chronotropic and inotropic effects as a consequence of β-adrenergic receptor stimulation. At higher doses, a vasoconstrictor effect results from α-receptor stimulation. It is started at an infusion rate of 2–5 µg/ kg per min, and the dose is increased every 2–5 min to

TABLE 30-2

HEMODYNAMIC PATTERNS[a]

	RA, mmHg	RVS, mmHg	RVD, mmHg	PAS, mmHg	PAD, mmHg	PCW, mmHg	CI, (L/min)/m²	SVR, (dyn · s)/cm⁵
Normal values	<6	<25	0–12	<25	0–12	<6–12	≥2.5	(800–1600)
MI without pulmonary edema[b]	—	—	—	—	—	~13 (5–18)	~2.7 (2.2–4.3)	—
Pulmonary edema	↔↑	↔↑	↔↑	↑	↑	↑	↔↓	↑
Cardiogenic shock								
LV failure	↔↑	↔↑	↔↑	↔↑	↑	↑	↓	↔↑
RV failure[c]	↑	↓↔↑[d]	↑	↓↔↑[d]	↔↓↑[d]	↓↔↑[d]	↓	↑
Cardiac tamponade	↑	↔↑	↑	↔↑	↔↑	↔↑	↓	↑
Acute mitral regurgitation	↔↑	↑	↔↑	↑	↑	↑	↔↓	↔↑
Ventricular septal rupture	↔↑	↔↑	↑	↔↑	↔↑	↔↑	↑PBF ↓SBF	↔↑
Hypovolemic shock	↓	↔↓	↔↓	↓	↓	↓	↓	↑
Septic shock	↓	↔↓	↔↓	↓	↓	↓	↑	↓

[a]There is significant patient-to-patient variation. Pressure may be normalized if cardiac output is low.

[b]Forrester et al classified nonreperfused MI patients into four hemodynamic subsets. (From Forrester JS et al: N Engl J Med 295:1356, 1976.) PCWP and CI in clinically stable subset 1 patients are shown. Values in parentheses represent range.

[c]"Isolated" or predominant RV failure.

[d]PCW and PA pressures may rise in RV failure after volume loading due to RV dilation, right-to-left shift of the interventricular septum, resulting in impaired LV filling. When biventricular failure is present, the patterns are similar to those shown for LV failure.

Abbreviations: CI, cardiac index; MI, myocardial infarction; P/SBF, pulmonary/systemic blood flow; PAS/D, pulmonary artery systolic/diastolic; PCW, pulmonary capillary wedge; RA, right atrium; RVS/D, right ventricular systolic/diastolic; SVR, systemic vascular resistance.

Source: Table prepared with the assistance of Krishnan Ramanathan, MD.

a maximum of 20–50 μg/kg per min. *Dobutamine* is a synthetic sympathomimetic amine with positive inotropic action and minimal positive chronotropic activity at low doses (2.5 μg/kg per min) but moderate chronotropic activity at higher doses. Although the usual dose is up to 10 μg/kg per min, its vasodilating activity precludes its use when a vasoconstrictor effect is required.

AORTIC COUNTERPULSATION In CS, mechanical assistance with an intraaortic balloon pumping (IABP) system capable of augmenting both arterial diastolic pressure and cardiac output is helpful in rapidly stabilizing patients. A sausage-shaped balloon is introduced percutaneously into the aorta via the femoral artery; the balloon is automatically inflated during early diastole, augmenting coronary blood flow. The balloon collapses in early systole, reducing the afterload against which the LV ejects. IABP improves hemodynamic status temporarily in most patients. In contrast to vasopressors and inotropic agents, myocardial O₂ consumption is reduced, ameliorating ischemia. IABP is useful as a stabilizing measure in patients with CS before and during cardiac catheterization and percutaneous coronary intervention (PCI) or before urgent surgery. IABP is contraindicated if aortic regurgitation is present or aortic dissection is suspected. Ventricular assist devices may be considered for eligible young patients with refractory shock as a bridge to cardiac transplantation.

REPERFUSION-REVASCULARIZATION The rapid establishment of blood flow in the infarct-related artery is essential in the management of CS and forms the centerpiece of management. The randomized SHOCK Trial demonstrated that 132 lives were saved per 1000 patients treated with early revascularization with PCI or coronary artery bypass graft (CABG) compared with initial medical therapy including IABP with fibrinolytics followed by delayed revascularization. The benefit is seen across the risk strata and is sustained up to 11 years after an MI. Early revascularization with PCI or CABG is a class I recommendation for patients age <75 years with ST elevation or left bundle branch block MI who develop CS within 36 h of MI and who can be revascularized within 18 h of the development of CS. When mechanical revascularization is not possible, IABP and fibrinolytic therapy are recommended. Older patients who are suitable candidates for aggressive care also should be offered early revascularization.

Prognosis

Within this high-risk condition, there is a wide range of expected death rates based on age, severity of hemodynamic abnormalities, severity of the clinical manifestations of hypoperfusion, and the performance of early revascularization.

SHOCK SECONDARY TO RIGHT VENTRICULAR INFARCTION

Although transient hypotension is common in patients with RV infarction and inferior MI (Chap. 33), persistent CS due to RV failure accounts for only 3% of CS complicating MI. The salient features of RV shock are absence of pulmonary congestion, high right atrial pressure (which may be seen only after volume loading), RV dilation and dysfunction, only mildly or moderately depressed LV function, and predominance of single-vessel proximal right coronary artery occlusion. Management includes IV fluid administration to optimize right atrial pressure (10–15 mmHg); avoidance of excess fluids, which cause a shift of the interventricular septum into the LV; sympathomimetic amines; IABP; and the early reestablishment of infarct-artery flow.

MITRAL REGURGITATION

(See also Chap. 33) Acute severe MR due to papillary muscle dysfunction and/or rupture may complicate MI and result in CS and/or pulmonary edema. This complication most often occurs on the first day, with a second peak several days later. The diagnosis is confirmed by echo-Doppler. Rapid stabilization with IABP is recommended, with administration of dobutamine as needed to raise cardiac output. Reducing the load against which the LV pumps (afterload) reduces the volume of regurgitant flow of blood into the left atrium. Mitral valve surgery is the definitive therapy and should be performed early in the course in suitable candidates.

VENTRICULAR SEPTAL RUPTURE

(See also Chap. 33) Echo-Doppler demonstrates shunting of blood from the left to the right ventricle and may visualize the opening in the interventricular septum. Timing and management are similar to those for MR with IABP support and surgical correction for suitable candidates.

FREE WALL RUPTURE

Myocardial rupture is a dramatic complication of STEMI that is most likely to occur during the first week after the onset of symptoms; its frequency increases with the age of the patient. The clinical presentation typically is a sudden loss of pulse, blood pressure, and consciousness but sinus rhythm on ECG (pulseless electrical activity) due to cardiac tamponade. Free wall rupture may also result in CS due to subacute tamponade when the pericardium temporarily seals the rupture sites. Definitive surgical repair is required.

ACUTE FULMINANT MYOCARDITIS

Myocarditis can mimic acute MI with ST deviation or bundle branch block on the ECG and marked elevation of cardiac markers. Acute myocarditis causes CS in a small proportion of cases. These patients are typically younger than those with CS due to acute MI and often do not have typical ischemic chest pain. Echocardiography usually shows global LV dysfunction. Initial management is the same as for CS complicating acute MI (Fig. 30-2) but does not involve coronary revascularization.

PULMONARY EDEMA

The etiologies and pathophysiology of pulmonary edema are discussed in Chap. 2.

Diagnosis

Acute pulmonary edema usually presents with the rapid onset of dyspnea at rest, tachypnea, tachycardia, and severe hypoxemia. Rales and wheezing due to airway compression from peribronchial cuffing may be audible. Hypertension is usually present due to release of endogenous catecholamines.

It is often difficult to distinguish between cardiogenic and noncardiogenic causes of acute pulmonary edema. *Echocardiography* may identify systolic and diastolic ventricular dysfunction and valvular lesions. Pulmonary edema associated with electrocardiographic ST elevation and evolving Q waves is usually diagnostic of acute MI and should prompt immediate institution of MI protocols and coronary artery reperfusion therapy (Chap. 33). Brain natriuretic peptide levels, when substantially elevated, support heart failure as the etiology of acute dyspnea with pulmonary edema.

The use of a *Swan-Ganz catheter* permits measurement of PCWP and helps differentiate high-pressure (cardiogenic) from normal-pressure (noncardiogenic) causes of pulmonary edema. Pulmonary artery catheterization is indicated when the etiology of the pulmonary edema is uncertain, when it is refractory to therapy, or when it is accompanied by hypotension. Data derived from use of a catheter often alter the treatment plan, but the impact on mortality rates has not been demonstrated.

TREATMENT Pulmonary Edema

The treatment of pulmonary edema depends on the specific etiology. In light of the acute, life-threatening nature of the condition, a number of measures must be applied immediately to support the circulation, gas exchange, and lung mechanics. In addition, conditions that frequently complicate pulmonary edema, such as infection, acidemia, anemia, and renal failure, must be corrected.

SUPPORT OF OXYGENATION AND VENTILATION Patients with acute cardiogenic pulmonary edema generally have an identifiable cause of acute LV failure—such as arrhythmia, ischemia/infarction, or myocardial decompensation—that can be rapidly treated, with improvement in gas exchange. In contrast, noncardiogenic edema usually resolves much less quickly, and most patients require mechanical ventilation.

Oxygen Therapy Support of oxygenation is essential to ensure adequate O_2 delivery to peripheral tissues, including the heart.

Positive-Pressure Ventilation Pulmonary edema increases the work of breathing and the O_2 requirements of this work, imposing a significant physiologic stress on the heart. When oxygenation or ventilation is not adequate in spite of supplemental O_2, positive-pressure ventilation by face or nasal mask or by endotracheal intubation should be initiated. Noninvasive ventilation (Chap. 26) can rest the respiratory muscles, improve oxygenation and cardiac function, and reduce the need for intubation. In refractory cases, mechanical ventilation can relieve the work of breathing more completely than can noninvasive ventilation. Mechanical ventilation with positive end-expiratory pressure can have multiple beneficial effects on pulmonary edema: (1) decreases both preload and afterload, thereby improving cardiac function, (2) redistributes lung water from the intraalveolar to the extraalveolar space, where the fluid interferes less with gas exchange, and (3) increases lung volume to avoid atelectasis.

REDUCTION OF PRELOAD In most forms of pulmonary edema, the quantity of extravascular lung water is determined by both the PCWP and the intravascular volume status.

Diuretics The "loop diuretics" furosemide, bumetanide, and torsemide are effective in most forms of pulmonary edema, even in the presence of hypoalbuminemia, hyponatremia, or hypochloremia. Furosemide is also a venodilator that reduces preload rapidly, before any diuresis, and is the diuretic of choice. The initial dose of furosemide should be ≤0.5 mg/kg, but a higher dose (1 mg/kg) is required in patients with renal insufficiency, chronic diuretic use, or hypervolemia or after failure of a lower dose.

Nitrates Nitroglycerin and isosorbide dinitrate act predominantly as venodilators but have coronary vasodilating properties as well. They are rapid in onset and effective when administered by a variety of routes. Sublingual nitroglycerin (0.4 mg × 3 every 5 min) is first-line therapy for acute cardiogenic pulmonary edema. If pulmonary edema persists in the absence of hypotension, sublingual may be followed by IV nitroglycerin, commencing at 5–10 μg/min. IV nitroprusside (0.1–5 μg/kg per min) is a potent venous and arterial vasodilator. It is useful for patients with pulmonary edema and hypertension but is not recommended in states of reduced coronary artery perfusion. It requires close monitoring and titration using an arterial catheter for continuous BP measurement.

Morphine Given in 2- to 4-mg IV boluses, morphine is a transient venodilator that reduces preload while relieving dyspnea and anxiety. These effects can diminish stress, catecholamine levels, tachycardia, and ventricular afterload in patients with pulmonary edema and systemic hypertension.

Angiotensin-Converting Enzyme (ACE) Inhibitors ACE inhibitors reduce both afterload and preload and are recommended for hypertensive patients. A low dose of a short-acting agent may be initiated and followed by increasing oral doses. In acute MI with heart failure, ACE inhibitors reduce short- and long-term mortality rates.

Other Preload-Reducing Agents IV recombinant brain natriuretic peptide (nesiritide) is a potent vasodilator with diuretic properties and is effective in the treatment of cardiogenic pulmonary edema. It should be reserved for refractory patients and is not recommended in the setting of ischemia or MI.

Physical Methods Reduction of venous return reduces preload. Patients without hypotension should be maintained in the sitting position with the legs dangling along the side of the bed.

Inotropic and Inodilator Drugs The sympathomimetic amines dopamine and dobutamine (see earlier) are potent inotropic agents. The bipyridine phosphodiesterase-3 inhibitors (inodilators), such as milrinone (50 μg/kg followed by 0.25–0.75 μg/kg per min), stimulate myocardial contractility while promoting peripheral and pulmonary vasodilation. Such agents are indicated in patients with cardiogenic pulmonary edema and severe LV dysfunction.

Digitalis Glycosides Once a mainstay of treatment because of their positive inotropic action, digitalis glycosides are rarely used at present. However, they may be useful for control of ventricular rate in patients with rapid atrial fibrillation or flutter and LV dysfunction, since they do not have the negative inotropic effects of other drugs that inhibit atrioventricular nodal conduction.

Intraaortic Counterpulsation IABP may help relieve cardiogenic pulmonary edema. It is indicated as a stabilizing measure when acute severe mitral regurgitation or ventricular septal rupture causes refractory pulmonary edema, especially in preparation for surgical repair. IABP or LV-assist devices are useful as bridging therapy to cardiac transplantation in patients with refractory pulmonary edema secondary to myocarditis or cardiomyopathy.

Treatment of Tachyarrhythmias and Atrial-Ventricular Resynchronization Sinus tachycardia or atrial fibrillation can result from elevated left atrial pressure and sympathetic stimulation. Tachycardia itself can limit LV filling time and raise left atrial pressure further. Although relief of pulmonary congestion will slow the sinus rate or ventricular response in atrial fibrillation, a primary tachyarrhythmia may require cardioversion. In patients with reduced LV function and without atrial contraction or with lack of synchronized atrioventricular contraction, placement of an atrioventricular sequential pacemaker should be considered.

Stimulation of Alveolar Fluid Clearance Recent mechanistic studies on alveolar epithelial ion transport have defined a variety of ways to upregulate the clearance of solute and water from the alveolar space. In patients with acute lung injury (noncardiogenic pulmonary edema), IV β-adrenergic agonist treatment decreases extravascular lung water, but the outcome benefit is uncertain.

SPECIAL CONSIDERATIONS
The risk of iatrogenic cardiogenic shock
In the treatment of pulmonary edema vasodilators lower BP, and, particularly when used in combination, their use may lead to hypotension, coronary artery hypoperfusion, and shock (Fig. 30-1). In general, patients with a *hypertensive* response to pulmonary edema tolerate and benefit from these medications. In normotensive patients, low doses of single agents should be instituted sequentially, as needed.

Acute Coronary Syndromes (See also Chap. 33) Acute STEMI complicated by pulmonary edema is associated with in-hospital mortality rates of 20–40%. After immediate stabilization, coronary artery blood flow must be reestablished rapidly. When available, primary PCI is preferable; alternatively, a fibrinolytic agent should be administered. Early coronary angiography and revascularization by PCI or CABG also are indicated for patients with non-ST elevation acute coronary syndrome. IABP use may be required to stabilize patients for coronary angiography if hypotension develops or for refractory pulmonary edema in patients with LV failure who are candidates for revascularization.

Unusual Types of Edema Specific etiologies of pulmonary edema may require particular therapy. Reexpansion pulmonary edema can develop after removal of air or fluid that has been in the pleural space for some time. These patients may develop hypotension or oliguria resulting from rapid fluid shifts into the lung. Diuretics and preload reduction are contraindicated, and intravascular volume repletion often is needed while supporting oxygenation and gas exchange.

High-altitude pulmonary edema often can be prevented by use of dexamethasone, calcium channel-blocking drugs, or long-acting inhaled β₂-adrenergic agonists. Treatment includes descent from altitude, bed rest, oxygen, and, if feasible, inhaled nitric oxide; nifedipine may also be effective.

For pulmonary edema resulting from upper airway obstruction, recognition of the obstructing cause is key, since treatment then is to relieve or bypass the obstruction.

CHAPTER 31

CARDIOVASCULAR COLLAPSE, CARDIAC ARREST, AND SUDDEN CARDIAC DEATH

Robert J. Myerburg ■ Agustin Castellanos

OVERVIEW AND DEFINITIONS

Sudden cardiac death (SCD) is defined *as natural death due to cardiac causes* in a person who may or may not have previously recognized heart disease but in whom the time and mode of death are *unexpected*. In the context of time, "sudden" is defined for most clinical and epidemiologic purposes as *1 h or less* between a change in clinical status heralding the onset of the terminal clinical event and the cardiac arrest itself. An exception is unwitnessed deaths, in which pathologists may expand the definition of time to 24 h after the victim was last seen to be alive and stable.

The overwhelming majority of natural deaths are caused by cardiac disorders. However, it is common for underlying heart diseases—often far advanced—to go unrecognized before the fatal event. As a result, up to two-thirds of all SCDs occur as the first clinical expression of previously undiagnosed disease or in patients with known heart disease, the extent of which suggests low risk. The magnitude of sudden *cardiac* death as a public health problem is highlighted by the estimate that ~50% of all cardiac deaths are sudden and unexpected, accounting for a total SCD burden estimated to range from <200,000 to >450,000 deaths each year in the United States. SCD is a direct consequence of cardiac arrest, which may be reversible if addressed promptly. Since resuscitation techniques and emergency rescue systems are available to respond to victims of out-of-hospital cardiac arrest, which was uniformly fatal in the past, understanding the SCD problem has practical clinical importance.

Because of community-based interventions, victims may remain biologically alive for days or even weeks after a cardiac arrest that has resulted in irreversible central nervous system damage. Confusion in terms can be avoided by adhering strictly to definitions of cardiovascular collapse, cardiac arrest, and death (Table 31-1). Although cardiac arrest is often potentially reversible by appropriate and timely interventions, death is biologically, legally, and literally an absolute and irreversible event. Death may be delayed in a survivor of cardiac arrest, but "survival after sudden death" is an irrational term. When biologic death of a cardiac arrest victim is delayed because of interventions, the relevant pathophysiologic event remains the sudden and unexpected cardiac arrest that leads ultimately to death, even though delayed by interventions. The language used should reflect the fact that the index event was a cardiac arrest and that death was due to its delayed consequences. Accordingly, for statistical purposes, deaths that occur during hospitalization or within 30 days after resuscitated cardiac arrest are counted as sudden deaths.

CLINICAL DEFINITION OF FORMS OF CARDIOVASCULAR COLLAPSE

Cardiovascular collapse is a general term connoting loss of sufficient cerebral blood flow to maintain consciousness due to acute dysfunction of the heart and/or peripheral vasculature. It may be caused by vasodepressor syncope (vasovagal syncope, postural hypotension with syncope, neurocardiogenic syncope, a transient severe bradycardia, or cardiac arrest. The latter is distinguished from the transient forms of cardiovascular collapse in that it usually requires an intervention to restore spontaneous blood flow. In contrast, vasodepressor syncope and other primary bradyarrhythmic syncopal events are transient and non-life-threatening, with spontaneous return of consciousness.

The most common electrical mechanism for cardiac arrest is ventricular fibrillation (VF), which is responsible

TABLE 31-1

DISTINCTION BETWEEN CARDIOVASCULAR COLLAPSE, CARDIAC ARREST, AND DEATH

TERM	DEFINITION	QUALIFIERS	MECHANISMS
Cardiovascular collapse	Sudden loss of effective blood flow due to cardiac and/or peripheral vascular factors that may reverse spontaneously (e.g., neurocardiogenic syncope, vasovagal syncope) or require interventions (e.g., cardiac arrest)	Nonspecific term: includes cardiac arrest and its consequences and transient events that characteristically revert spontaneously	Same as "Cardiac Arrest," plus vasodepressor syncope or other causes of transient loss of blood flow
Cardiac arrest	Abrupt cessation of cardiac mechanical function, which may be reversible by a prompt intervention but will lead to death in its absence	Rare spontaneous reversions; likelihood of successful intervention relates to mechanism of arrest, clinical setting, and prompt return of circulation	Ventricular fibrillation, ventricular tachycardia, asystole, bradycardia, pulseless electrical activity, mechanical factors
Sudden cardiac death	Sudden, irreversible cessation of all biological functions	None	

Source: Modified from RJ Myerburg, A Castellanos: Cardiac arrest and sudden cardiac death, in *Braunwald's Heart Disease*, 8th ed, P Libby et al (eds). Philadelphia, Saunders, 2008, with permission of publisher.

for 50–80% of cardiac arrests. Severe persistent bradyarrhythmias, asystole, and pulseless electrical activity (PEA: organized electrical activity, unusually slow, without mechanical response, formerly called electromechanical dissociation [EMD]) cause another 20–30%. Pulseless sustained ventricular tachycardia (a rapid arrhythmia distinct from PEA) is a less common mechanism. Acute low cardiac output states, having a precipitous onset, also may present clinically as a cardiac arrest. These hemodynamic causes include massive acute pulmonary emboli, internal blood loss from a ruptured aortic aneurysm, intense anaphylaxis, and cardiac rupture with tamponade after myocardial infarction (MI). Sudden deaths due to these causes are not included in the SCD category.

ETIOLOGY, INITIATING EVENTS, AND CLINICAL EPIDEMIOLOGY

Clinical, epidemiologic, and pathologic studies have provided information on the underlying *structural abnormalities* in victims of SCD and identified subgroups at high risk for SCD. In addition, studies of clinical physiology have begun to identify *transient functional factors* that may convert a long-standing underlying structural abnormality from a stable to an unstable state, leading to the onset of cardiac arrest (Table 31-2).

Cardiac disorders constitute the most common causes of sudden *natural* death. After an initial peak incidence of sudden death between birth and 6 months of age (the sudden infant death syndrome [SIDS]), the incidence of sudden death declines sharply and remains low through childhood and adolescence. Among adolescents and young adults, the incidence of SCD is approximately 1 per 100,000 population per year. The incidence begins to increase in adults over age 30 years, reaching a second peak in the age range 45–75 years, when it approximates 1–2 per 1000 per year among the unselected adult population. Increasing age within this range is associated with increasing risk for sudden *cardiac* death (Fig. 31-1*A*). From 1 to 13 years of age, only one of five sudden *natural* deaths is due to cardiac causes. Between 14 and 21 years of age, the proportion increases to 30%, and it rises to 88% in the middle-aged and elderly.

Young and middle-aged men and women have different susceptibilities to SCD, but the sex differences decrease with advancing age. The difference in risk for SCD parallels the differences in age-related risks for other manifestations of coronary heart disease (CHD) between men and women. As the gender gap for manifestations of CHD closes in the sixth to eighth decades of life, the excess risk of SCD in males progressively narrows. Despite the lower incidence among younger women, coronary risk factors such as cigarette smoking, diabetes, hyperlipidemia, and hypertension are highly influential, and SCD remains an important clinical and epidemiologic problem. The incidence of SCD among the African-American population appears to be higher than it is among the white population; the reasons remain uncertain.

Genetic factors contribute to the risk of acquiring CHD and its expression as acute coronary syndromes, including SCD. In addition, however, there are data suggesting a familial predisposition to SCD as a specific form of expression of CHD. A parental history of SCD as an initial coronary event increases the probability of a similar expression in the offspring. In a number of less common syndromes, such as hypertrophic

TABLE 31-2

CARDIAC ARREST AND SUDDEN CARDIAC DEATH

Structural Associations and Causes

I. Coronary heart disease
   A. Coronary artery abnormalities
     1. Chronic atherosclerotic lesions
     2. Acute (active) lesions (plaque fissuring, platelet aggregation, acute thrombosis)
     3. Anomalous coronary artery anatomy
   B. Myocardial Infarction
     1. Healed
     2. Acute

II. Myocardial hypertrophy
   A. Secondary
   B. Hypertrophic cardiomyopathy
     1. Obstructive
     2. Nonobstructive

III. Dilated cardiomyopathy—primary muscle disease

IV. Inflammatory and infiltrative disorders.
   A. Myocarditis
   B. Noninfectious inflammatory diseases
   C. Infiltrative diseases

V. Valvular heart disease

VI. Electrophysiologic abnormalities, structural
   A. Anomalous pathways in Wolff-Parkinson-White syndrome
   B. Conducting system disease

VII. Inherited disorders associated with electrophysiological abnormalities (congenital long QT syndromes, right ventricular dysplasia, Brugada syndrome, catecholaminergic polymorphic ventricular tachycardia, etc.)

Functional Contributing Factors

I. Alterations of coronary blood flow
   A. Transient ischemia
   B. Reperfusion after ischemia

II. Low cardiac output states
   A. Heart failure
     1. Chronic
     2. Acute decompensation
   B. Shock

III. Systemic metabolic abnormalities
   A. Electrolyte imbalance (e.g., hypokalemia)
   B. Hypoxemia, acidosis

IV. Neurologic disturbances
   A. Autonomic fluctuations: central, neural, humoral
   B. Receptor function

V. Toxic responses
   A. Proarrhythmic drug effects
   B. Cardiac toxins (e.g., cocaine, digitalis intoxication)
   C. Drug interactions

cardiomyopathy, congenital long QT interval syndromes, right ventricular dysplasia, and the syndrome of right bundle branch block and nonischemic ST-segment elevations (Brugada syndrome), there is a specific inherited risk of ventricular arrhythmias and SCD.

The structural causes of and functional factors contributing to the SCD syndrome are listed in Table 31-2. Worldwide, and especially in Western cultures, coronary atherosclerotic heart disease is the most common structural abnormality associated with SCD in middle-aged and older adults. Up to 80% of all SCDs in the United States are due to the consequences of coronary atherosclerosis. The nonischemic cardiomyopathies (dilated and hypertrophic, collectively) account for another 10–15% of SCDs, and all the remaining diverse etiologies cause only 5–10% of all SCDs. The inherited arrhythmia syndromes (see earlier and Table 31-2) are proportionally more common causes in adolescents and young adults. For some of these syndromes, such as hypertrophic cardiomyopathy, the risk of SCD increases significantly after the onset of puberty.

Transient ischemia in a previously scarred or hypertrophied heart, hemodynamic and fluid and electrolyte disturbances, fluctuations in autonomic nervous system activity, and transient electrophysiologic changes caused by drugs or other chemicals (e.g., proarrhythmia) have all been implicated as mechanisms responsible for the transition from electrophysiologic stability to instability. In addition, reperfusion of ischemic myocardium may cause transient electrophysiologic instability and arrhythmias.

PATHOLOGY

Data from postmortem examinations of SCD victims parallel the clinical observations on the prevalence of CHD as the major structural etiologic factor. More than 80% of SCD victims have pathologic findings of CHD. The pathologic description often includes a combination of long-standing, extensive atherosclerosis of the epicardial coronary arteries and unstable coronary artery lesions, which include various permutations of eroded, fissured, or ruptured plaques; platelet aggregates; hemorrhage; and/or thrombosis. As many as 70–75% of males who die suddenly have preexisting healed MIs, whereas only 20–30% have recent acute MIs, despite the prevalence of unstable plaques and thrombi. The latter suggests transient ischemia as the mechanism of onset. Regional or global left ventricular (LV) hypertrophy often coexists with prior MIs.

PREDICTION AND PREVENTION OF CARDIAC ARREST AND SUDDEN CARDIAC DEATH

SCD accounts for approximately one-half the total number of cardiovascular deaths. As shown in **Fig. 31-1B**, the very high risk subgroups provide more focused populations ("percent per year") for predicting cardiac arrest or SCD, but the representation of such subgroups within

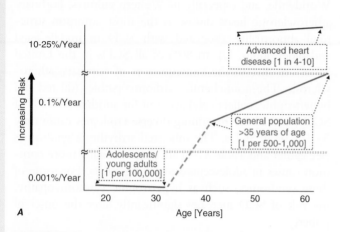

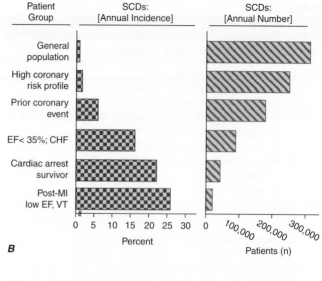

FIGURE 31-1

Panel A demonstrates age-related risk for SCD. For the general population age 35 years and older, SCD risk is 0.1–0.2 percent per year (1 per 500–1000 population). Among the general population of adolescents and adults younger than age 30 years, the overall risk of SCD is 1 per 100,000 population, or 0.001% per year. The risk of SCD increases dramatically beyond age 35 years. The greatest rate of increase is between 40 and 65 years (vertical axis is discontinuous). Among patients older than 30 years of age, with advanced structural heart disease and markers of high risk for cardiac arrest, the event rate may exceed 25% per year, and age-related risk attenuates. (*Modified from Myerburg and Castellanos 2008, with permission of publisher.*) **Panel B demonstrates the incidence of SCD in population subgroups** and the relation of total number of events per year to incidence figures. Approximations of subgroup incidence figures and the related population pool from which they are derived are presented. Approximately 50% of all cardiac deaths are sudden and unexpected. The incidence triangle on the left ("Percent/Year") indicates the approximate percentage of sudden and nonsudden deaths in each of the population subgroups indicated, ranging from the lowest percentage in unselected adult populations (0.1–2% per year) to the highest percentage in patients with VT or VF during convalescence after an MI (approximately 50% per year). The triangle on the right indicates the total number of events per year in each of these groups to reflect incidence in context with the size of the population subgroups. The highest risk categories identify the smallest number of total annual events, and the lowest incidence category accounts for the largest number of events per year. EF, ejection fraction; VT, ventricular tachycardia; VF, ventricular fibrillation; MI, myocardial infarction. (*After RJ Myerburg et al: Circulation 85:2, 1992.*)

the overall population burden of SCD, indicated by the absolute number of events ("events per year"), is relatively small. The requirements for achieving a major population impact are effective prevention of underlying diseases and/or new epidemiologic probes that will allow better resolution of specific high-risk subgroups within the large general populations.

Strategies for predicting and preventing SCD are classified as primary and secondary. *Primary prevention*, as defined in various implantable defibrillator trials, refers to the attempt to identify individual patients at specific risk for SCD and institute preventive strategies. *Secondary prevention* refers to measures taken to prevent recurrent cardiac arrest or death in individuals who have survived a previous cardiac arrest. A third category consists of interventions intended to abort sudden cardiac arrests, thus avoiding their progression to death. This focuses primarily on out-of-hospital response strategies.

The primary prevention strategies currently used depend on the magnitude of risk among the various population subgroups. Because the annual incidence of SCD among the unselected adult population is limited to 1–2 per 1000 population per year (Fig. 31-1) and >30% of all SCDs due to coronary artery disease occur as the first clinical manifestation of the disease **(Fig. 31-2A)**, the only currently practical strategies are profiling for risk of developing CHD and risk factor control **(Fig. 31-2B)**. The most powerful long-term risk factors include age, cigarette smoking, elevated serum cholesterol, diabetes mellitus, elevated blood pressure, LV hypertrophy, and nonspecific electrocardiographic abnormalities. Markers of inflammation (e.g., levels of C-reactive protein) that may predict plaque destabilization have been added to risk classifications. The presence of multiple risk factors progressively increases incidence, but not sufficiently or specifically enough to warrant therapies targeted to potentially fatal arrhythmias (Fig. 31-1A). However, recent studies offer the hope that genetic markers for specific risk may become available. These studies suggest that a family history of SCD associated with acute coronary

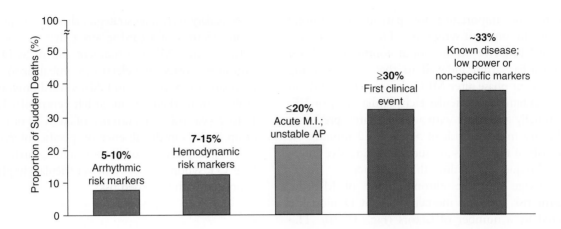

Target	Examples	Goal	Sensitivity
• ASHD risk factors	• Framingham risk index	• Predict evolution of disease	• Very low
• Anatomic screening	• CT imaging	• Identify CAD	• Moderate for anatomy
• Clinical markers	• EF; angiography	• Define extent of disease	• High for extent of disease; variable for specificity of risk
	• AM; EPS	• Identify arrhythmia markers	• Low-to-intermediate for screening
	• History of heart failure	• Define high risk subgroups	• High for specific groups
• Transient risk predictors	• EP and hemodynamic variations	• Clinical markers of instability	• Primary predictive value unknown
	• Autonomic fluctuations	• Quantify autonomic triggers	• Uncertain; some measures useful (?)
	• Predictors of ischemia	• Predict unstable plaques	• Unknown; potentially high
B • Individual risk predictors	• Familial/genetic profiles	• Predict specific SCD risk before disease expression	• High potential for future profiling

FIGURE 31-2

Population subsets, risk predictors, and distribution of sudden cardiac deaths (SCDs) according to clinical circumstances. *A.* The population subset with high-risk arrhythmia markers in conjunction with low ejection fraction is a group at high risk of SCD but accounts for <10% of the total SCD burden attributable to coronary artery disease. In contrast, nearly two-thirds of all SCD victims present with SCD as the first and only manifestation of underlying disease or have known disease but are considered relatively low risk because of the absence of high-risk markers. ***B.*** Risk profile for prediction and prevention of SCD is difficult. The highest absolute numbers of events occur among the general population who may have risk factors for coronary heart disease or expressions of disease that do not predict high risk. This results in a low sensitivity for predicting and preventing SCD. New approaches that include epidemiologic modeling of transient risk factors and methods of predicting individual patient risk offer hope for greater sensitivity in the future. AP, angina pectoris; ASHD, arteriosclerotic heart disease; CAD, coronary artery disease; EPS, electrophysiologic study; HRV, heart rate variability. (*Modified from Myerburg RJ: J Cardiovasc Electrophysiol 2001; 12:369–381, reproduced with permission of the publisher.*)

syndromes predicts a higher likelihood of cardiac arrest as the initial manifestation of coronary artery disease in first-degree family members.

After coronary artery disease has been identified in a patient, additional strategies for risk profiling become available (Fig. 31-2*B*), but the majority of SCDs occur among the large unselected groups rather than in the specific high-risk subgroups that become evident among populations with established disease (compare events per year with percent per year in Fig. 31-1*B*). After a major cardiovascular event, such as acute coronary syndromes, recent onset of heart failure, and survival after out-of-hospital cardiac arrest, the highest risk of death occurs during the initial 6–18 months

after the event and then plateaus toward the baseline risk associated with the extent of underlying disease. However, many of the early deaths are nonsudden, diluting the potential benefit of strategies targeted specifically to SCD. Thus, although post-MI beta-blocker therapy has an identifiable benefit for both early SCD and nonsudden mortality risk, a total mortality benefit for ICD therapy early after MI has not been observed.

Among patients in the acute, convalescent, and chronic phases of myocardial infarction (Chap. 33), subgroups at high absolute risk of SCD can be identified. During the acute phase, the potential risk of cardiac arrest from onset through the first 48 h may be as high as 15%, emphasizing the importance for patients to respond promptly to the onset of symptoms. Those who survive acute-phase VF, however, are not at continuing risk for recurrent cardiac arrest indexed to that event. During the convalescent phase after MI (3 days to ~6 weeks), an episode of sustained ventricular tachycardia (VT) or VF, which is usually associated with a large infarct, predicts a natural history mortality risk of >25% at 12 months. At least one-half of the deaths are sudden. Aggressive intervention techniques may reduce this incidence.

After passage into the chronic phase of MI, the longer-term risk for total mortality and SCD mortality is predicted by a number of factors (Fig. 31-2B). The most important for both SCD and nonsudden death is the extent of myocardial damage sustained as a result of the acute MI. This is measured by the magnitude of reduction of the ejection fraction (EF) and/or the occurrence of heart failure. Various studies have demonstrated that ventricular arrhythmias identified by ambulatory monitoring contribute significantly to this risk, especially in patients with an EF <40%. In addition, inducibility of VT or VF during electrophysiologic testing of patients who have ambient ventricular arrhythmias [premature ventricular contractions (PVCs) and nonsustained VT] and an EF <35 or 40% is a strong predictor of SCD risk. Patients in this subgroup are now considered candidates for implantable cardioverter defibrillators (ICDs) (see later). Risk falls off sharply with EFs >40% after MI and the absence of ambient arrhythmias and conversely is high with EFs <30% even without the ambient arrhythmia markers.

The cardiomyopathies (dilated and hypertrophic) are the second most common category of diseases associated with risk of SCD, after CHD (Table 31-2). Some risk factors have been identified, largely related to extent of disease, documented ventricular arrhythmias, and symptoms of arrhythmias (e.g., syncope). The less common causes of SCD include valvular heart disease (primarily aortic) and inflammatory and infiltrative disorders of the myocardium. The latter include viral myocarditis, sarcoidosis, and amyloidosis.

Among adolescents and young adults, rare inherited disorders such as hypertrophic cardiomyopathy, the long QT interval syndromes, right ventricular dysplasia, and the Brugada syndrome have received attention as important causes of SCD because of advances in genetics and the ability to identify some of those at risk before a fatal event. The subgroup of young competitive athletes has received special attention. The incidence of SCD among athletes appears to be higher than it is for the general adolescent and young adult population, perhaps up to 1 in 75,000. Hypertrophic cardiomyopathy is the most common cause in the United States, compared with Italy, where more comprehensive screening programs remove potential victims from the population of athletes.

Secondary prevention strategies should be applied to surviving victims of a cardiac arrest that was not associated with an acute MI or a transient risk of SCD (e.g., drug exposures, correctable electrolyte imbalances). Multivessel coronary artery disease and dilated cardiomyopathy, especially with markedly reduced left ventricular EF predict a 1- to 2-year risk of recurrence of an SCD or cardiac arrest of up to 30% in the absence of specific interventions (see later). The presence of life-threatening arrhythmias with long QT syndromes or right ventricular dysplasia are also associated with increased risks.

CLINICAL CHARACTERISTICS OF CARDIAC ARREST

PRODROME, ONSET, ARREST, DEATH

SCD may be presaged by days to months of increasing angina, dyspnea, palpitations, easy fatigability, and other nonspecific complaints. However, these *prodromal symptoms* are generally predictive of any major cardiac event; they are not specific for predicting SCD.

The *onset of the clinical transition*, leading to cardiac arrest, is defined as an acute change in cardiovascular status preceding cardiac arrest by up to 1 h. When the onset is instantaneous or abrupt, the probability that the arrest is cardiac in origin is >95%. Continuous electrocardiographic (ECG) recordings fortuitously obtained at the onset of a cardiac arrest commonly demonstrate changes in cardiac electrical activity during the minutes or hours before the event. There is a tendency for the heart rate to increase and for advanced grades of PVCs to evolve. Most cardiac arrests that are caused by VF begin with a run of nonsustained or sustained VT, which then degenerates into VF.

The probability of achieving successful resuscitation from cardiac arrest is related to the interval from onset of loss of circulation to institution of resuscitative efforts, the setting in which the event occurs, the mechanism (VF, VT, PEA, asystole), and the clinical status of the patient before the cardiac arrest. Return of circulation and survival rates as a result of defibrillation decrease almost linearly from the first minute to 10 min. After 5 min, survival rates are no better than 25–30% in out-of-hospital settings. Those settings in which it is possible to institute prompt cardiopulmonary resuscitation (CPR) followed by prompt defibrillation provide a better chance of a successful outcome. However, the outcome in intensive care units and other in-hospital environments is heavily influenced by the patient's preceding clinical status. The immediate outcome is good for cardiac arrest occurring in the intensive care unit in the presence of an acute cardiac event or transient metabolic disturbance, but survival among patients with far-advanced chronic cardiac disease or advanced noncardiac diseases (e.g., renal failure, pneumonia, sepsis, diabetes, cancer) is low and not much better in the in-hospital than in the out-of-hospital setting. Survival from unexpected cardiac arrest in unmonitored areas in a hospital is not much better than that it is for witnessed out-of-hospital arrests. Since implementation of community response systems, survival from out-of-hospital cardiac arrest has improved although it still remains low, under most circumstances. Survival probabilities in public sites exceed those in the home environment.

The success rate for initial resuscitation and survival to hospital discharge after an out-of-hospital cardiac arrest depends heavily on the mechanism of the event. When the mechanism is pulseless VT, the outcome is best; VF is the next most successful; and asystole and PEA generate dismal outcome statistics. Advanced age also adversely influences the chances of successful resuscitation.

Progression to biologic death is a function of the mechanism of cardiac arrest and the length of the delay before interventions. VF or asystole without CPR within the first 4–6 min has a poor outcome even if defibrillation is successful because of superimposed brain damage; there are few survivors among patients who had no life support activities for the first 8 min after onset. Outcome statistics are improved by lay bystander intervention (basic life support—see later) before definitive interventions (advanced life support) especially when followed by early successful defibrillation. In regard to the latter, evaluations of deployment of automatic external defibrillators (AEDs) in communities (e.g., police vehicles, large buildings, airports, and stadiums) are beginning to generate encouraging data. Increased deployment is to be encouraged.

Death during the hospitalization after a successfully resuscitated cardiac arrest relates closely to the severity of central nervous system injury. Anoxic encephalopathy and infections subsequent to prolonged respirator dependence account for 60% of the deaths. Another 30% occur as a consequence of low cardiac output states that fail to respond to interventions. Recurrent arrhythmias are the least common cause of death, accounting for only 10% of in-hospital deaths.

In the setting of acute MI (Chap. 33), it is important to distinguish between primary and secondary cardiac arrests. *Primary cardiac arrests* are those which occur in the absence of hemodynamic instability, and *secondary cardiac arrests* are those which occur in patients in whom abnormal hemodynamics dominate the clinical picture before cardiac arrest. The success rate for immediate resuscitation in primary cardiac arrest during acute MI in a monitored setting should exceed 90%. In contrast, as many as 70% of patients with secondary cardiac arrest succumb immediately or during the same hospitalization.

TREATMENT Cardiac Arrest

An individual who collapses suddenly is managed in five stages: (1) initial evaluation and basic life support if arrest is confirmed, (2) public access defibrillation (when available), (3) advanced life support, (4) postresuscitation care, and (5) long-term management. The initial response, including confirmation of loss of circulation, followed by basic life support and public access defibrillation, can be carried out by physicians, nurses, paramedical personnel, and trained laypersons. There is a requirement for increasingly specialized skills as the patient moves through the stages of advanced life support, postresuscitation care, and long-term management.

INITIAL EVALUATION AND BASIC LIFE SUPPORT Confirmation that a sudden collapse is indeed due to a cardiac arrest includes prompt observations of the state of consciousness, respiratory movements, skin color, and the presence or absence of pulses in the carotid or femoral arteries. For lay responders, the pulse check is no longer recommended. As soon as a cardiac arrest is suspected, confirmed, or even considered to be impending, calling an emergency rescue system (e.g., 911) is the immediate priority. With the development of AEDs that are easily used by nonconventional emergency responders, an additional layer for response has evolved (see later).

Agonal respiratory movements may persist for a short time after the onset of cardiac arrest, but it is important to observe for severe stridor with a persistent pulse as a clue to aspiration of a foreign body or food. If this is suspected, a Heimlich maneuver (see later) may dislodge the obstructing body. A precordial blow, or "thump," delivered firmly with a clenched fist to the junction of the middle and lower thirds of the sternum may occasionally revert VT or VF, but there is concern about converting VT to VF. Therefore, it is recommended to use precordial thumps as a life support technique only when monitoring and defibrillation are available. This conservative application of the technique remains controversial.

The third action during the initial response is to clear the airway. The head is tilted back and the chin lifted so that the oropharynx can be explored to clear the airway. Dentures or foreign bodies are removed, and the Heimlich maneuver is performed if there is reason to suspect that a foreign body is lodged in the oropharynx. If respiratory arrest precipitating cardiac arrest is suspected, a second precordial thump is delivered after the airway is cleared.

Basic life support, more popularly known as CPR, is intended to maintain organ perfusion until definitive interventions can be instituted. The elements of CPR are the maintenance of ventilation of the lungs and compression of the chest. Mouth-to-mouth respiration may be used if no specific rescue equipment is immediately available (e.g., plastic oropharyngeal airways, esophageal obturators, masked Ambu bag). Conventional ventilation techniques during single-responder CPR require that the lungs be inflated twice in succession after every 30 chest compressions. Recent data suggest that interrupting chest compressions to perform mouth-to-mouth respiration may be less effective than a continuous chest compression strategy.

Chest compression is based on the assumption that cardiac compression allows the heart to maintain a pump function by sequential filling and emptying of its chambers, with competent valves maintaining forward direction of flow. The palm of one hand is placed over the lower sternum, with the heel of the other resting on the dorsum of the lower hand. The sternum is depressed, with the arms remaining straight, at a rate of approximately 100 per minute. Sufficient force is applied to depress the sternum 4–5 cm, and relaxation is abrupt.

AUTOMATED EXTERNAL DEFIBRILLATION (AED)
AEDs that are easily used by nonconventional responders, such as nonparamedic firefighters, police officers, ambulance drivers, trained security guards, and minimally trained or untrained laypersons, have been developed. This advance has inserted another level of response into the cardiac arrest paradigm. A number of studies have demonstrated that AED use by nonconventional responders in strategic response systems and public access lay responders can improve cardiac arrest survival rates. This strategy is based on shortening the time to the first defibrillation attempt while awaiting the arrival of advanced life support.

ADVANCED CARDIAC LIFE SUPPORT (ACLS)
ACLS is intended to achieve adequate ventilation, control cardiac arrhythmias, stabilize blood pressure and cardiac output, and restore organ perfusion. The activities carried out to achieve these goals include (1) defibrillation/cardioversion and/or pacing, (2) intubation with an endotracheal tube, and (3) insertion of an intravenous line. The speed with which defibrillation/cardioversion is achieved is an important element in successful resuscitation, both for restoration of spontaneous circulation and for protection of the central nervous system. Immediate defibrillation should precede intubation and insertion of an intravenous line; CPR should be carried out while the defibrillator is being charged. As soon as a diagnosis of VF or VT is established, a shock of at least 300 J should be delivered when one is using a monophasic waveform device or 120–150 J with a biphasic waveform. Additional shocks are escalated to a maximum of 360 J monophasic (200 J biphasic) if the initial shock does not successfully revert VT or VF. However, it is now recommended that five cycles of CPR be carried out before repeated shocks, if the first shock fails to restore an organized rhythm, or 60–90 s of CPR before the first shock if 5 min has elapsed between the onset of cardiac arrest and ability to deliver a shock (see 2005 update of guidelines for cardiopulmonary resuscitation and emergency cardiac care at *http://circ.ahajournals.org/content/112/24_suppl.toc*).

Epinephrine, 1 mg intravenously, is given after failed defibrillation, and attempts to defibrillate are repeated. The dose of epinephrine may be repeated after intervals of 3–5 min (Fig. 31-3A). Vasopressin (a single 40-unit dose given IV) has been suggested as an alternative to epinephrine.

If the patient is less than fully conscious upon reversion or if two or three attempts fail, prompt intubation, ventilation, and arterial blood gas analysis should be carried out. Ventilation with O_2 (room air if O_2 is not immediately available) may promptly reverse hypoxemia and acidosis. A patient who is persistently acidotic after successful defibrillation and intubation should be given 1 meq/kg $NaHCO_3$ initially and an additional 50% of the dose repeated every 10–15 min. However, it should not be used routinely.

After initial unsuccessful defibrillation attempts or with persistent/recurrent electrical instability, antiarrhythmic therapy should be instituted. Intravenous amiodarone has emerged as the initial treatment of choice (150 mg over 10 min, followed by 1 mg/min for up to 6 h and 0.5 mg/min thereafter) (Fig. 31-3A). For cardiac arrest due to VF in the early phase of an acute coronary syndrome, a bolus of 1 mg/kg of lidocaine may be given intravenously as an alternative, and the dose may be repeated in 2 min. It also may be tried in patients in whom amiodarone is unsuccessful. Intravenous procainamide (loading infusion of 100 mg/5 min to a total dose of 500–800 mg, followed by continuous infusion at 2–5 mg/min) is now rarely used in this setting, but may be tried for persisting, hemodynamically stable arrhythmias. Intravenous calcium gluconate is no longer considered safe or necessary for routine administration. It is used only in patients in whom acute hyperkalemia is known to be the triggering event for resistant VF, in the presence of known hypocalcemia, or in patients who have received toxic doses of calcium channel antagonists.

Cardiac arrest due to bradyarrhythmias or asystole (B/A cardiac arrest) is managed differently (Fig. 31-3B). The patient is promptly intubated, CPR is continued, and an attempt is made to control hypoxemia and acidosis. Epinephrine and/or atropine are given intravenously or by an intracardiac route. External pacing devices are used to attempt to establish a regular rhythm. The success rate may be good when B/A arrest is due to acute inferior wall myocardial infarction or to correctable airway obstruction or drug-induced respiratory depression

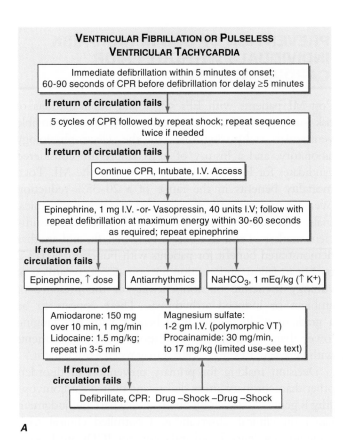

VENTRICULAR FIBRILLATION OR PULSELESS
VENTRICULAR TACHYCARDIA

Immediate defibrillation within 5 minutes of onset;
60-90 seconds of CPR before defibrillation for delay ≥5 minutes

If return of circulation fails

5 cycles of CPR followed by repeat shock; repeat sequence
twice if needed

If return of circulation fails

Continue CPR, Intubate, I.V. Access

Epinephrine, 1 mg I.V. -or- Vasopressin, 40 units I.V; follow with
repeat defibrillation at maximum energy within 30-60 seconds
as required; repeat epinephrine

**If return of
circulation fails**

| Epinephrine, ↑ dose | Antiarrhythmics | NaHCO₃, 1 mEq/kg (↑ K⁺) |

Amiodarone: 150 mg over 10 min, 1 mg/min
Lidocaine: 1.5 mg/kg; repeat in 3-5 min

Magnesium sulfate: 1-2 gm I.V. (polymorphic VT)
Procainamide: 30 mg/min, to 17 mg/kg (limited use-see text)

**If return of
circulation fails**

Defibrillate, CPR: Drug –Shock –Drug –Shock

A

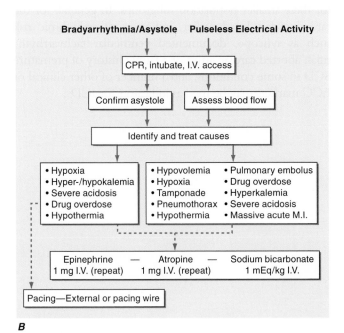

Bradyarrhythmia/Asystole   Pulseless Electrical Activity

CPR, intubate, I.V. access

Confirm asystole   Assess blood flow

Identify and treat causes

• Hypoxia
• Hyper-/hypokalemia
• Severe acidosis
• Drug overdose
• Hypothermia

• Hypovolemia
• Hypoxia
• Tamponade
• Pneumothorax
• Hypothermia

• Pulmonary embolus
• Drug overdose
• Hyperkalemia
• Severe acidosis
• Massive acute M.I.

Epinephrine — Atropine — Sodium bicarbonate
1 mg I.V. (repeat) 1 mg I.V. (repeat) 1 mEq/kg I.V.

Pacing—External or pacing wire

B

FIGURE 31-3

A. **The algorithm of ventricular fibrillation** or pulseless ventricular tachycardia begins with defibrillation attempts. If that fails, it is followed by epinephrine and then antiarrhythmic drugs. See text for details. *B.* **The algorithms for bradyarrhythmia/asystole** (*left*) or pulseless electrical activity (*right*) are dominated first by continued life support and a search for reversible causes. Subsequent therapy is nonspecific and is accompanied by a low success rate. See text for details. CPR, cardiopulmonary resuscitation; MI, myocardial infarction.

or with prompt resuscitation efforts. For acute airway obstruction, prompt removal of foreign bodies by the Heimlich maneuver or, in hospitalized patients, by intubation and suctioning of obstructing secretions in the airway is often successful. The prognosis is generally very poor in other causes of this form of cardiac arrest, such as end-stage cardiac or noncardiac diseases. Treatment of PEA is similar to that for bradyarrhythmias, but its outcome is also dismal.

POSTRESUSCITATION CARE This phase of management is determined by the clinical setting of the cardiac arrest. *Primary VF* in acute MI (not accompanied by low-output states) (Chap. 33) is generally very responsive to life support techniques and easily controlled after the initial event. In the in-hospital setting, respirator support is usually not necessary or is needed for only a short time, and hemodynamics stabilize promptly after defibrillation or cardioversion. In *secondary VF* in acute MI (those events in which hemodynamic abnormalities predispose to the potentially fatal arrhythmia), resuscitative efforts are less often successful, and in patients who are successfully resuscitated, the recurrence rate is high. The clinical picture and outcome are dominated by hemodynamic instability and the ability to control hemodynamic dysfunction. Bradyarrhythmias, asystole, and PEA are commonly secondary events in hemodynamically unstable patients. The in-hospital phase of care of an out-of-hospital cardiac arrest survivor is dictated by specific clinical circumstances. The most difficult is the presence of anoxic encephalopathy, which is a strong predictor of in-hospital death. A recent addition to the management of this condition is induced hypothermia to reduce metabolic demands and cerebral edema.

The outcome after in-hospital cardiac arrest associated with noncardiac diseases is poor, and in the few successfully resuscitated patients, the postresuscitation course is dominated by the nature of the underlying disease. Patients with end-stage cancer, renal failure, acute central nervous system disease, and uncontrolled infections, as a group, have a survival rate of <10% after in-hospital cardiac arrest. Some major exceptions are patients with transient airway obstruction, electrolyte disturbances, proarrhythmic effects of drugs, and severe metabolic abnormalities, most of whom may have a good chance of survival if they can be resuscitated promptly and stabilized while the transient abnormalities are being corrected.

LONG-TERM MANAGEMENT AFTER SURVIVAL OF OUT-OF-HOSPITAL CARDIAC ARREST Patients who survive cardiac arrest without irreversible damage to the central nervous system and who achieve hemodynamic stability should have diagnostic testing to define appropriate therapeutic interventions for their long-term management. This

311

CHAPTER 31 Cardiovascular Collapse, Cardiac Arrest, and Sudden Cardiac Death aggressive approach is driven by the fact that survival after out-of-hospital cardiac arrest is followed by a 10–25% mortality rate during the first 2 years after the event, and there are data suggesting that significant survival benefits can be achieved by prescription of an implantable cardioverter-defibrillator (ICD).

Among patients in whom an acute ST elevation MI, or transient and reversible myocardial ischemia, is identified as the specific mechanism triggering an out-of-hospital cardiac arrest, the management is dictated in part by the transient nature of life-threatening arrhythmia risk during the acute coronary syndrome (ACS) and in part by the extent of permanent myocardial damage that results. Cardiac arrest during the acute ischemic phase is not an ICD indication, but survivors of cardiac arrest not associated with an ACS do benefit. In addition, patients who survive MI with an ejection fraction less than 30–35% appear to benefit from ICDs.

For patients with cardiac arrest determined to be due to a treatable transient ischemic mechanism, particularly with higher EFs, catheter interventional, surgical, and/or pharmacologic anti-ischemic therapy is generally accepted for long-term management.

Survivors of cardiac arrest due to other categories of disease, such as the hypertrophic or dilated cardiomyopathies and the various rare inherited disorders (e.g., right ventricular dysplasia, long QT syndrome, Brugada syndrome, catecholaminergic polymorphic VT, and so-called idiopathic VF), are all considered ICD candidates.

PREVENTION OF SCD IN HIGH-RISK INDIVIDUALS WITHOUT PRIOR CARDIAC ARREST

Post-MI patients with EFs <35% and other markers of risk such as ambient ventricular arrhythmias, inducible ventricular tachyarrhythmias in the electrophysiology laboratory, and a history of heart failure are considered candidates for ICDs 30 days or more after the MI. Total mortality benefits in the range of a 20–35% reduction over 2–5 years have been observed in a series of clinical trials. One study suggested that an EF <30% was a sufficient marker of risk to indicate ICD benefit, and another demonstrated benefit for patients with Functional Class 2 or 3 heart failure and ejection fractions ≤35%, regardless of etiology (ischemic or nonischemic) or the presence of ambient or induced arrhythmias. There appears to be a gradient of increasing ICD benefit with EFs ranging lower than the threshold indications. However, patients with very low EFs (e.g., <20%) may receive less benefit.

Decision making for primary prevention in disorders other than coronary artery disease and dilated cardiomyopathy is generally driven by observational data and judgment based on clinical observations. Controlled clinical trials providing evidence-based indicators for ICDs are lacking for these smaller population subgroups. In general, for the rare disorders listed earlier, indicators of arrhythmic risk such as syncope, documented ventricular tachyarrhythmias, aborted cardiac arrest or a family history of premature SCD in some conditions, and a number of other clinical or ECG markers may be used as indicators for ICDs.

CHAPTER 32

UNSTABLE ANGINA AND NON-ST-SEGMENT ELEVATION MYOCARDIAL INFARCTION

Christopher P. Cannon ■ Eugene Braunwald

Patients with ischemic heart disease fall into two large groups: patients with chronic coronary artery disease (CAD) who most commonly present with stable angina and patients with acute coronary syndromes (ACSs). The latter group, in turn, is composed of patients with acute myocardial infarction (MI) with ST-segment elevation on their presenting electrocardiogram (ECG) (STEMI; Chap. 33) and those with unstable angina (UA) and non-ST-segment elevation MI (UA/NSTEMI; Fig. 33-1). Every year in the United States, approximately 1 million patients are admitted to hospitals with UA/NSTEMI as compared with ~300,000 patients with acute STEMI. The relative incidence of UA/NSTEMI compared to STEMI appears to be increasing. More than one-third of patients with UA/NSTEMI are women, while less than one-fourth of patients with STEMI are women.

DEFINITION

The diagnosis of UA is based largely on the clinical presentation. *Stable* angina pectoris is characterized by chest or arm discomfort that may not be described as pain but is reproducibly associated with physical exertion or stress and is relieved within 5–10 min by rest and/or sublingual nitroglycerin. UA is defined as angina pectoris or equivalent ischemic discomfort with at least one of three features: (1) it occurs at rest (or with minimal exertion), usually lasting >10 min; (2) it is severe and of new onset (i.e., within the prior 4–6 weeks); and/or (3) it occurs with a crescendo pattern (i.e., distinctly more severe, prolonged, or frequent than previously). The diagnosis of NSTEMI is established if a patient with the clinical features of UA develops evidence of myocardial necrosis, as reflected in elevated cardiac biomarkers.

PATHOPHYSIOLOGY

UA/NSTEMI is most commonly caused by a reduction in oxygen supply and/or by an increase in myocardial oxygen demand superimposed on a lesion that causes coronary arterial obstruction, usually an atherothrombotic coronary plaque. Four pathophysiologic processes that may contribute to the development of UA/NSTEMI have been identified: (1) plaque rupture or erosion with a superimposed nonocclusive thrombus, believed to be the most common cause; in such patients, NSTEMI may occur with downstream embolization of platelet aggregates and/or atherosclerotic debris; (2) dynamic obstruction (e.g., coronary spasm, as in Prinzmetal's variant angina [PVA]); (3) progressive mechanical obstruction (e.g., rapidly advancing coronary atherosclerosis or restenosis following percutaneous coronary intervention [PCI]); and (4) UA secondary to increased myocardial oxygen demand and/or decreased supply (e.g., tachycardia, anemia). More than one of these processes may be involved.

Among patients with UA/NSTEMI studied at angiography, approximately 5% have stenosis of the left main coronary artery, 15% have three-vessel CAD, 30% have two-vessel disease, 40% have single-vessel disease, and 10% have no apparent critical epicardial coronary artery stenosis; some of the latter may have obstruction of the coronary microcirculation. The "culprit lesion" may show an eccentric stenosis with scalloped or overhanging edges and a narrow neck on angiography. Angioscopy has been reported to show "white" (platelet-rich) thrombi, as opposed to "red" (fibrin- and cell-rich) thrombi; the latter are more often seen in patients with acute STEMI. Patients with UA/NSTEMI frequently have multiple plaques at risk of disruption (vulnerable plaques).

CLINICAL PRESENTATION

History and physical examination

The clinical hallmark of UA/NSTEMI is chest pain, typically located in the substernal region or sometimes in the epigastrium, that radiates to the neck, left shoulder, and/or the left arm. This discomfort is usually severe enough to be described as frank pain. Anginal "equivalents" such as dyspnea and epigastric discomfort may also occur, and these appear to be more frequent in women. The physical examination resembles that in patients with stable angina and may be unremarkable. If the patient has a large area of myocardial ischemia or a large NSTEMI, the physical findings can include diaphoresis; pale, cool skin; sinus tachycardia; a third and/or fourth heart sound; basilar rales; and, sometimes, hypotension, resembling the findings of large STEMI.

Electrocardiogram

In UA, ST-segment depression, transient ST-segment elevation, and/or T-wave inversion occur in 30 to 50% of patients. In patients with the clinical features of UA, the presence of new ST-segment deviation, even of only 0.05 mV, is an important predictor of adverse outcome. T-wave changes are sensitive for ischemia but less specific unless they are new, deep T-wave inversions (≥0.3 mV).

Cardiac biomarkers

Patients with UA/NSTEMI who have elevated biomarkers of necrosis, such as CK-MB and troponin (a much more specific and sensitive marker of myocardial necrosis), are at increased risk for death or recurrent MI. Elevated levels of these markers distinguish patients with NSTEMI from those with UA. There is a direct relationship between the degree of troponin elevation and mortality. However, in patients *without* a clear clinical history of myocardial ischemia, minor troponin elevations have been reported and can be caused by congestive heart failure (CHF), myocarditis, or pulmonary embolism, or they may be false-positive readings. Thus, in patients with an *unclear* history, small troponin elevations may not be diagnostic of an ACS.

DIAGNOSTIC EVALUATION

Approximately six million persons per year in the United States present to hospital emergency departments (EDs) with a complaint of chest pain or other symptoms suggestive of ACS. A diagnosis of an ACS is established in 20% to 25% of such patients. The first step in evaluating patients with possible UA/NSTEMI is to determine the *likelihood* that CAD is the cause of the presenting symptoms. The American College of Cardiology/American Heart Association (ACC/AHA) Guidelines include, among the factors associated with a high likelihood of ACS, a prior history typical of stable angina, a history of established CAD by angiography, prior MI, CHF, new ECG changes, or elevated cardiac biomarkers.

Diagnostic pathways

Four major diagnostic tools are used in the diagnosis of UA/NSTEMI in the ED: clinical history, the ECG, cardiac markers, and stress testing (coronary imaging is an emerging option). The goals are to: (1) recognize or exclude MI (using cardiac markers), (2) evaluate for rest ischemia (using serial or continuous ECGs), and (3) evaluate for significant CAD (using provocative stress testing). Patients with a low likelihood of ischemia are usually managed with an ED-based critical pathway (which, in some institutions, is carried out in a "chest-pain unit" **Fig. 32-1**). Evaluation of such patients includes clinical monitoring for recurrent ischemic discomfort, serial ECGs, and cardiac markers, typically obtained at baseline and at 4–6 h and 12 h after presentation. If new elevations in cardiac markers or ECG changes are noted, the patient should be admitted to the hospital. If the patient remains pain free and the markers are negative, the patient may proceed to stress testing. CT angiography is used with increasing frequency to exclude obstructive CAD.

RISK STRATIFICATION AND PROGNOSIS

Patients with documented UA/NSTEMI exhibit a wide spectrum of early (30 days) risk of death, ranging from 1 to 10%, and of new or recurrent infarction of 3–5% or recurrent ACS (5-15%). Assessment of risk can be accomplished by clinical risk scoring systems such as that developed from the Thrombolysis in Myocardial Infarction (TIMI) Trials, which includes seven independent risk factors: age ≥ 65 years, three or more risk factors for CAD, documented CAD at catheterization, development of UA/NSTEMI while on aspirin, more than two episodes of angina within the preceding 24 h, ST deviation ≥0.5 mm, and an elevated cardiac marker (**Fig. 32-2**). Other risk factors include diabetes mellitus, left ventricular dysfunction, renal dysfunction and elevated levels of brain natriuretic peptides and C-reactive protein. Multimarker strategies involving several biomarkers are now gaining favor, both to define more fully the pathophysiologic mechanisms underlying a given patient's presentation and to stratify the patient's risk further. Early risk assessment (especially using troponin, ST-segment changes, and/or a global risk-scoring system) is useful both in predicting the risk of recurrent cardiac events and in identifying those

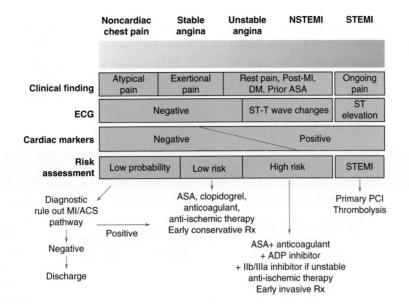

FIGURE 32-1

Algorithm for risk stratification and treatment of patients with suspected coronary artery disease. Using the clinical history of the type of pain and medical history, the ECG, and cardiac markers, one can identify patients who have a low likelihood of UA/NSTEMI, for whom a diagnostic "ruleout myocardial infarction (MI) or acute coronary syndrome (ACS)" is warranted. If this is negative, the patient may be discharged, but if positive, the patient is admitted and treated for UA/NSTEMI. On the other end of the spectrum, patients with acute ongoing pain and ST-segment elevation are treated with percutaneous coronary intervention (PCI) or fibrinolysis (Chap. 33). For those with UA/NSTEMI, risk stratification is used to identify patients at medium to high risk, for whom an early invasive

strategy is warranted. Antithrombotic therapy should include aspirin, an anticoagulant, an ADP antagonist (clopidogrel or prasugrel), with GP IIb/IIIa inhibition considered for use during PCI. For patients at low risk, treatment with aspirin, clopidogrel, an anticoagulant such as unfractionated or low molecular–weight heparin (LMWH) or fondaparinux and anti-ischemic therapy with beta blockers and nitrates, and a conservative strategy are indicated. ASA, aspirin; DM, diabetes mellitus; ECG, electrocardiogram; MI, myocardial infarction; Rx, treatment; STEMI, ST-segment elevation myocardial infarction. (*Adapted from CP Cannon, E Braunwald, in Braunwald's Heart Disease: A Textbook of Cardiovascular Medicine, 9th ed, R Bonow et al [eds]. Philadelphia, Saunders, 2011.*)

patients who would derive the greatest benefit from antithrombotic therapies more potent than unfractionated heparin, such as low molecular–weight heparin (LMWH) and glycoprotein IIb/IIIa inhibitors, and from an early invasive strategy. For example, in the

TACTICS-TIMI 18 Trial, an early invasive strategy conferred a 40% reduction in recurrent cardiac events in patients with a positive troponin level, whereas no benefit was observed in those without detectable troponin.

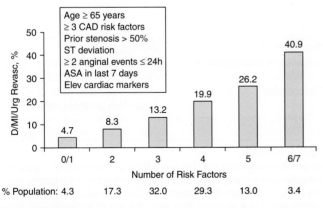

FIGURE 32-2

The TIMI Risk Score for UA/NSTEMI, a simple but comprehensive clinical risk stratification score to identify increasing risk of death, myocardial infarction, or urgent revascularization to day 14. CAD, coronary artery disease; ASA, aspirin. (*Adapted from EM Antman et al: JAMA 284:835, 2000.*)

TREATMENT | **Unstable Angina and Non-ST-Segment Elevation Myocardial Infarction**

MEDICAL TREATMENT Patients with UA/NSTEMI should be placed at bed rest with continuous ECG monitoring for ST-segment deviation and cardiac arrhythmias. Ambulation is permitted if the patient shows no recurrence of ischemia (discomfort or ECG changes) and does not develop a biomarker of necrosis for 12–24 h. Medical therapy involves simultaneous anti-ischemic treatment and antithrombotic treatment.

ANTI-ISCHEMIC TREATMENT (Table 32-1) To provide relief and prevention of recurrence of chest pain, initial treatment should include bed rest, nitrates, and beta blockers.

Nitrates Nitrates should first be given sublingually or by buccal spray (0.3–0.6 mg) if the patient is experiencing ischemic pain. If pain persists after 3 doses given 5 min apart, intravenous nitroglycerin (5–10 µg/min using nonabsorbing tubing) is recommended. The rate of the infusion may be increased by 10 µg/min every 3–5 min until symptoms are relieved or systolic arterial pressure falls to <100 mmHg. Topical or oral nitrates can be used once the pain has resolved or they may replace intravenous nitroglycerin when the patient has been pain-free for 12–24 h. The only absolute contraindications to the use of nitrates are hypotension or the

TABLE 32-1

DRUGS COMMONLY USED IN INTENSIVE MEDICAL MANAGEMENT OF PATIENTS WITH UNSTABLE ANGINA AND NON-ST SEGMENT ELEVATION MI

DRUG CATEGORY	CLINICAL CONDITION	WHEN TO AVOID[a]	DOSAGE
Nitrates	Administer sublingually, and, if symptoms persist, intravenously	Hypotension Patient receiving sildenafil or other PDE-5 inhibitor	Topical, oral, or buccal nitrates are acceptable alternatives for patients without ongoing or refractory symptoms 5–10 µg/min by continuous infusion titrated up to 75–100 µg/min until relief of symptoms or limiting side effects (headache or hypotension with a systolic blood pressure <90 mmHg or more than 30% below starting mean arterial pressure levels if significant hypertension is present)
Beta blockers[b]	Unstable angina	PR interval (ECG) >0.24 s 2° or 3° atrioventricular block Heart rate <60 beats/min Systolic pressure <90 mmHg Shock Left ventricular failure Severe reactive airway disease	Metoprolol 25–50 mg by mouth every 6 h If needed, and no heart failure, 5-mg increments by slow (over 1–2 min) IV administration
Calcium channel blockers	Patients whose symptoms are not relieved by adequate doses of nitrates and beta blockers, or in patients unable to tolerate adequate doses of one or both of these agents, or in patients with variant angina	Pulmonary edema Evidence of left ventricular dysfunction (for diltiazem or verapamil)	Dependent on specific agent
Morphine sulfate	Patients whose symptoms are not relieved after three serial sublingual nitroglycerin tablets or whose symptoms recur with adequate anti-ischemic therapy	Hypotension Respiratory depression Confusion Obtundation	2–5 mg IV dose May be repeated every 5–30 min as needed to relieve symptoms and maintain patient comfort

[a]Allergy or prior intolerance is a contraindication for all categories of drugs listed in this chart.
[b]Choice of the specific agent is not as important as ensuring that appropriate candidates receive this therapy. If there are concerns about patient intolerance owing to existing pulmonary disease, especially asthma, left ventricular dysfunction, risk of hypotension or severe bradycardia, initial selection should favor a short-acting agent, such as propranolol or metoprolol or the ultra-short-acting agent esmolol. Mild wheezing or a history of chronic obstructive pulmonary disease should prompt a trial of a short-acting agent at a reduced dose (e.g., 2.5 mg IV metoprolol, 12.5 mg oral metoprolol, or 25 µg/kg per min esmolol as initial doses) rather than complete avoidance of beta-blocker therapy.
Note: Some of the recommendations in this guide suggest the use of agents for purposes or in doses other than those specified by the U.S. Food and Drug Administration. Such recommendations are made after consideration of concerns regarding nonapproved indications. Where made, such recommendations are based on more recent clinical trials or expert consensus. IV, intravenous; ECG, electrocardiogram; 2°, second-degree; 3°, third-degree.
Source: Modified from E Braunwald et al: Circulation 90:613, 1994.

use of sildenafil or other drugs in that class within the previous 24–48 h.

Beta Adrenergic Blockers and Other Agents

Beta blockers are the other mainstay of anti-ischemic treatment. Oral beta blockade targeted to a heart rate of 50–60 beats/min is recommended as first-line treatment. A caution has been raised in the new ACC/AHA guidelines for use of intravenous beta blockade in patients with any evidence of acute heart failure, where they could increase the risk of cardiogenic shock. Heart rate–slowing calcium channel blockers, e.g., verapamil or diltiazem, are recommended for patients who have persistent or recurrent symptoms after treatment with full-dose nitrates and beta blockers and in patients with contraindications to beta blockade. Additional medical therapy includes angiotensin-converting enzyme (ACE) inhibition and HMG-CoA reductase inhibitors (statins) for long-term secondary prevention. Early administration of intensive statin therapy (e.g., atorvastatin 80 mg) prior to percutaneous coronary intervention (PCI) has been shown to reduce complications, suggesting that high-dose statin therapy should be started at the time of admission.

ANTITHROMBOTIC THERAPY (Table 32-2) This is the other main component of treatment for UA/NSTEMI. Initial treatment should begin with the platelet cyclooxygenase inhibitor aspirin (Fig. 32-3). The typical initial dose is 325 mg/d, with lower doses (75–162 mg/d) recommended for long-term therapy. The OASIS-7 trial randomized 25,087 ACS patients to receive high-dose (300–325 mg/d) vs. low-dose (75-100 mg/d) aspirin for 30 days and reported no differences in the risk of major bleeding or in efficacy over this period of time. "Aspirin resistance" has been noted in 5–10% of patients and more frequently in patients treated with lower doses of aspirin, but frequently has been related to noncompliance.

The thienopyridine, clopidogrel, an inactive prodrug that is converted into an active metabolite, which blocks the platelet $P2Y_{12}$ component or the adenosine diphosphate receptor, in combination with aspirin, was shown in the CURE trial to confer a 20% relative reduction in cardiovascular death, MI, or stroke, compared with aspirin alone in both low- and high-risk patients, but to be associated with a moderate (absolute 1%) increase in major bleeding. Pretreatment with clopidogrel (a 300 or 600 mg loading dose, followed by 75 mg qd) is recommended prior to PCI. The OASIS-7 trial reported that one week of a higher dose of clopidogrel (600 mg loading dose and 150 mg/d for one week) did not result in an overall improvement in outcomes in ACS patients, but did so in patients receiving 325 mg of aspirin, especially those who underwent PCI.

Continued benefit of one year of treatment with the combination of clopidogrel and aspirin has been

TABLE 32-2

CLINICAL USE OF ANTITHROMBOTIC THERAPY

Oral Antiplatelet Therapy

Aspirin	Initial dose of 162–325 mg nonenteric formulation followed by 75–162 mg/d of an enteric or a nonenteric formulation
Clopidogrel	Loading dose of 300-600 mg followed by 75 mg/d
Prasugrel	Pre-PCI: Loading dose 60 mg followed by 10 mg/d

Intravenous Antiplatelet Therapy

Abciximab	0.25 mg/kg bolus followed by infusion of 0.125 µg/kg per min (maximum 10 µg/min) for 12 to 24 h
Eptifibatide	180 µg/kg bolus followed by infusion of 2.0 µg/kg per min for 72 to 96 h
Tirofiban	0.4 µg/kg per min for 30 min followed by infusion of 0.1 µg/kg per min for 48 to 96 h

Heparins[a]

Unfractionated Heparin (UFH)	Bolus 60–70 U/kg (maximum 5000 U) IV followed by infusion of 12–15 U/kg per h (initial maximum 1000 U/h) titrated to a PTT 50–70 s
Enoxaparin	1 mg/kg SC every 12 h; the first dose may be preceded by a 30-mg IV bolus; renal adjustment to 1 mg/kg once daily if creatine Cl < 30 cc/min
Fondaparinux	2.5 mg SC qd
Bivalirudin	Initial bolus intravenous bolus of 0.1 mg/kg and an infusion of 0.25 mg/kg per hour. Before PCI, an additional intravenous bolus of 0.5 mg/kg was administered, and the infusion was increased to 1.75 mg/kg per hour.

[a]Other LMWH exist beyond those listed.
Abbreviations: IV, intravenous; SC, subcutaneously.
Source: Modified from J Anderson et al: JACO 50:e1, 2007.

observed both in patients treated conservatively and in those who underwent PCI and should certainly continue for at least one year in patients with a drug-eluting stent. Up to one-third of patients have low response to clopidogrel, and a substantial proportion of these are related to a genetic variant of the cytochrome P450 system.

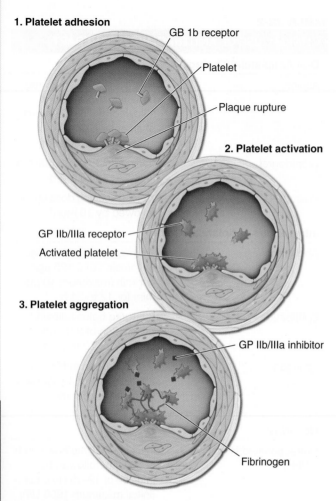

1. Platelet adhesion

GB 1b receptor

Platelet

Plaque rupture

2. Platelet activation

GP IIb/IIIa receptor

Activated platelet

3. Platelet aggregation

GP IIb/IIIa inhibitor

Fibrinogen

FIGURE 32-3

Platelets initiate thrombosis at the site of a ruptured plaque with denuded endothelium: *platelet adhesion* occurs via (1) the GP 1b receptor in conjunction with von Willebrand factor. This is followed by *platelet activation* (2), which leads to a shape change of the platelet, degranulation of the alpha and dense granules, and expression of glycoprotein IIb/IIIa receptors on the platelet surface with activation of the receptor, such that it can bind fibrinogen. The final step is *platelet aggregation* (3), in which fibrinogen (or von Willebrand factor) binds to the activated GP IIb/IIIa receptors. Aspirin (ASA) and clopidogrel act to decrease platelet activation, whereas the GP IIb/IIIa inhibitors inhibit the final step of platelet aggregation. GP, glycoprotein. (*Modified from CP Cannon, E Braunwald, in Braunwald's Heart Disease: A Textbook of Cardiovascular Medicine, 8th ed, R Bonow et al [eds]. Philadelphia, Saunders, 2008.*)

A variant of the 2C19 gene leads to reduced conversion of clopidogrel into its active metabolite, which, in turn, causes lower platelet inhibition and a higher risk of cardiovascular events. Alternate agents, such as prasugrel, should be considered for ACS patients who are hyporesponsive to clopidogrel as identified by platelet and/or genetic testing, although such testing is not yet widespread.

A recently approved thienopyridine, prasugrel, has been shown to achieve a more rapid onset, and higher level of platelet inhibition than clopidogrel. It has been used in ACS patients following angiography in whom PCI is planned at a dose of 60 mg load followed by 10 mg/d for up to 15 months. The TRITON-TIMI 38 trial showed that relative to clopidogrel, prasugrel reduced the risk of cardiovascular death, MI, or stroke significantly by 19%, albeit with an increase in major bleeding. Stent thrombosis was also reduced by 52%. This agent is contraindicated in patients with prior stroke or transient ischemic attack. Ticagrelor is a novel, *reversible* ADP inhibitor that has recently been reported to reduce the risk of cardiovascular death, MI, or stroke by 16% compared with clopidogrel in a broad population of ACS patients. This agent also reduced mortality and did not increase the risk of total bleeding; it is not yet FDA approved at the time of this writing.

Four options are available for anticoagulant therapy to be added to aspirin and clopidogrel. Unfractionated heparin (UFH) is the mainstay of therapy. The low-molecular-weight heparin (LMWH), enoxaparin, has been shown in several studies to be superior to UFH in reducing recurrent cardiac events, especially in conservatively managed patients. The indirect Factor Xa inhibitor, fondaparinux, is equivalent for early efficacy compared with enoxaparin but appears to have a lower risk of major bleeding. Bivalirudin, a direct thrombin inhibitor, is similar in efficacy to either UFH or LMWH among patients treated with a GP IIb/IIIa inhibitor, but use of bivalirudin alone causes less bleeding than the combination of heparin and a GP IIb/IIIa inhibitor in patients with UA/NSTEMI undergoing catheterization and/or PCI.

Prior to the advent of clopidogrel, many trials had shown the benefit of intravenous GP IIb/IIIa inhibitors. The benefit, however, has been small, i.e., only a 9% reduction in death or MI, with a significant increase in major bleeding. Two recent studies also failed to show a benefit for early initiation compared with use only for PCI. The use of these agents may be reserved for unstable patients with recurrent rest pain and ECG changes who undergo PCI.

Excessive bleeding is the most important adverse effect of all antithrombotic agents, including anticoagulants and antiplatelet agents. Therefore, attention must be directed to the doses of antithrombotic agents, accounting for weight, creatinine clearance, and a previous history of excessive bleeding, as a means of reducing the risk of bleeding.

INVASIVE VERSUS CONSERVATIVE STRATEGY Multiple clinical trials have demonstrated the benefit of an early invasive strategy in high-risk patients, i.e., patients with multiple clinical risk factors, ST-segment deviation, and/or positive biomarkers (Table 32-3). In this strategy, following treatment with anti-ischemic and antithrombotic agents, coronary arteriography is carried

TABLE 32-3

CLASS I RECOMMENDATIONS FOR USE OF AN EARLY INVASIVE STRATEGY[a]

Class I (Level of Evidence: A) Indications

Recurrent angina at rest/low-level activity despite Rx
Elevated TnT or TnI
New ST-segment depression
Rec. angina/ischemia with CHF symptoms, rales, MR
Positive stress test
EF < 0.40
Decreased BP
Sustained VT
PCI < 6 months, prior CABG
High-risk score

[a]Any one of the high-risk indicators.
Abbreviations: BP, blood pressure; CABG, coronary artery bypass grafting; CHF, congestive heart failure; EF, ejection fraction; MR, mitral regurgitation; PCI, percutaneous coronary intervention; Rec, recurrent; TnI, troponin I; TnT, troponin T; VT, ventricular tachycardia.
Source: J Anderson et al: JACO 50:e1, 2007.

out within ~48 h of admission, followed by coronary revascularization (PCI or coronary artery bypass grafting), depending on the coronary anatomy.

In low-risk patients, the outcomes from an invasive strategy are similar to those obtained from a conservative strategy, which consists of anti-ischemic and antithrombotic therapy followed by "watchful waiting," and in which coronary arteriography is carried out only if rest pain or ST-segment changes recur or there is evidence of ischemia on a stress test.

LONG-TERM MANAGEMENT

The time of hospital discharge is a "teachable moment" for the patient with UA/NSTEMI, when the physician can review and optimize the medical regimen. Risk-factor modification is key, and the caregiver should discuss with the patient the importance of smoking cessation, achieving optimal weight, daily exercise following an appropriate diet, blood-pressure control, tight control of hyperglycemia (for diabetic patients), and lipid management, as recommended for patients with chronic stable angina.

There is evidence of benefit with long-term therapy with five classes of drugs that are directed at different components of the atherothrombotic process. Beta blockers, statins (at a high dose, e.g., atorvastatin 80 mg/d), and ACE inhibitors or angiotensin receptor blockers are recommended for long-term plaque stabilization. Antiplatelet therapy, now recommended to be the combination of aspirin and clopidogrel (or prasugrel in post PCS patients) for one year, with aspirin continued thereafter, prevents or reduces the severity of any thrombosis that would occur if a plaque were to rupture.

Observational registries have shown that patients with UA/NSTEMI at high risk, including women and the elderly as well as racial minorities, are less likely to receive evidence-based pharmacologic and interventional therapies with resultant poorer clinical outcomes and quality of life.

PRINZMETAL'S VARIANT ANGINA

In 1959 Prinzmetal et al. described a syndrome of severe ischemic pain that occurs at rest but not usually with exertion and is associated with transient ST-segment elevation. This syndrome is due to focal spasm of an epicardial coronary artery, leading to severe myocardial ischemia. The cause of the spasm is not well defined, but it may be related to hypercontractility of vascular smooth muscle due to vasoconstrictor mitogens, leukotrienes, or serotonin.

Clinical and angiographic manifestations

Patients with Prinzmetal's variant angina (PVA) are generally younger and have fewer coronary risk factors (with the exception of cigarette smoking) than patients with UA secondary to coronary atherosclerosis. Cardiac examination is usually unremarkable in the absence of ischemia. The clinical diagnosis of variant angina is made with the detection of transient ST-segment *elevation* with rest pain. Many patients also exhibit multiple episodes of asymptomatic ST-segment elevation (*silent ischemia*). Small elevations of troponin may occur in patients with prolonged attacks of variant angina.

Coronary angiography demonstrates transient coronary spasm as the diagnostic hallmark of PVA. Atherosclerotic plaques, which do not usually cause critical obstruction, in at least one proximal coronary artery occur in the majority of patients, and in them spasm usually occurs within 1 cm of the plaque. Focal spasm is most common in the right coronary artery, and it may occur at one or more sites in one artery or in multiple arteries simultaneously. Ergonovine, acetylcholine, other vasoconstrictor medications, and hyperventilation have been used to provoke focal coronary stenosis on angiography to establish the diagnosis. Hyperventilation has also been used to provoke rest angina, ST-segment elevation, and spasm on coronary arteriography.

TREATMENT   Prinzmetal's Variant Angina

Nitrates and calcium channel blockers are the main agents used to treat acute episodes and to abolish recurrent episodes of PVA. Aspirin may actually increase the severity of ischemic episodes, possibly as a result of the exquisite sensitivity of coronary tone to modest changes in the synthesis of prostacyclin. The response to beta blockers is variable. Coronary revascularization may be helpful in patients who also have discrete, proximal fixed obstructive lesions.

Prognosis

Many patients with PVA pass through an acute, active phase, with frequent episodes of angina and cardiac events during the first 6 months after presentation. Long-term survival at 5 years is excellent (~90–95%). Patients with no or mild fixed coronary obstruction tend to experience a more benign course than do patients with associated severe obstructive lesions. Nonfatal MI occurs in up to 20% of patients by 5 years. Patients with PVA who develop serious arrhythmias during spontaneous episodes of pain are at a higher risk for sudden cardiac death. In most patients who survive an infarction or the initial 3- to 6-month period of frequent episodes, the condition stabilizes, and there is a tendency for symptoms and cardiac events to diminish over time.

CHAPTER 33

ST-SEGMENT ELEVATION MYOCARDIAL INFARCTION

Elliott M. Antman ▪ Joseph Loscalzo

Acute myocardial infarction (AMI) is one of the most common diagnoses in hospitalized patients in industrialized countries. In the United States, approximately 650,000 patients experience a new AMI and 450,000 experience a recurrent AMI each year. The early (30-day) mortality rate from AMI is ~30%, with more than half of these deaths occurring before the stricken individual reaches the hospital. Although the mortality rate after admission for AMI has declined by ~30% over the past two decades, approximately 1 of every 25 patients who survives the initial hospitalization dies in the first year after AMI. Mortality is approximately fourfold higher in elderly patients (over age 75) as compared with younger patients.

When patients with prolonged ischemic discomfort at rest are first seen, the working clinical diagnosis is that they are suffering from an acute coronary syndrome (Fig. 33-1). The 12-lead electrocardiogram (ECG) is a pivotal diagnostic and triage tool because it is at the center of the decision pathway for management; it permits distinction of those patients presenting with ST-segment elevation from those presenting without ST-segment elevation. Serum cardiac biomarkers are obtained to distinguish unstable angina (UA) from non–ST-segment MI (NSTEMI) and to assess the magnitude of an ST-segment elevation MI (STEMI). This chapter focuses on the evaluation and management of patients with STEMI, while Chap. 32 discusses UA/NSTEMI.

PATHOPHYSIOLOGY: ROLE OF ACUTE PLAQUE RUPTURE

STEMI usually occurs when coronary blood flow decreases abruptly after a thrombotic occlusion of a coronary artery previously affected by atherosclerosis. Slowly developing, high-grade coronary artery stenoses do not typically precipitate STEMI because of the

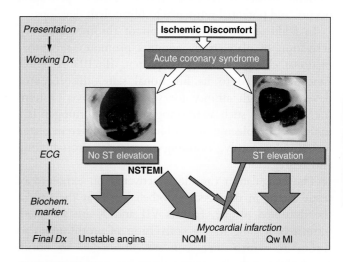

FIGURE 33-1

Acute coronary syndromes. Following disruption of a vulnerable plaque, patients experience ischemic discomfort resulting from a reduction of flow through the affected epicardial coronary artery. The flow reduction may be caused by a completely occlusive thrombus (***right***) or subtotally occlusive thrombus (***left***). Patients with ischemic discomfort may present with or without ST-segment elevation. Of patients with ST-segment elevation, the majority (*wide red arrow*) ultimately develop a Q wave on the ECG (QwMI), while a minority (*thin red arrow*) do not develop Q wave and, in older literature, were said to have sustained a non-Q-wave MI (NQMI). Patients who present without ST-segment elevation are suffering from either unstable angina or a non-ST-segment elevation MI (NSTEMI) (*wide green arrows*), a distinction that is ultimately made on the presence or absence of a serum cardiac marker such as CKMB or a cardiac troponin detected in the blood. The majority of patients presenting with NSTEMI do not develop a Q wave on the ECG; a minority develop a QwMI (*thin green arrow*). (*Adapted from CW Hamm et al: Lancet 358:1533, 2001, and MJ Davies: Heart 83:361, 2000; with permission from the BMJ Publishing Group.*)

development of a rich collateral network over time. Instead, STEMI occurs when a coronary artery thrombus develops rapidly at a site of vascular injury. This injury is produced or facilitated by factors such as cigarette smoking, hypertension, and lipid accumulation. In most cases, STEMI occurs when the surface of an atherosclerotic plaque becomes disrupted (exposing its contents to the blood) and conditions (local or systemic) favor thrombogenesis. A mural thrombus forms at the site of plaque disruption, and the involved coronary artery becomes occluded. Histologic studies indicate that the coronary plaques prone to disruption are those with a rich lipid core and a thin fibrous cap. After an initial platelet monolayer forms at the site of the disrupted plaque, various agonists (collagen, ADP, epinephrine, serotonin) promote platelet activation. After agonist stimulation of platelets, thromboxane A_2 (a potent local vasoconstrictor) is released, further platelet activation occurs, and potential resistance to fibrinolysis develops.

In addition to the generation of thromboxane A_2, activation of platelets by agonists promotes a conformational change in the glycoprotein IIb/IIIa receptor. Once converted to its functional state, this receptor develops a high affinity for soluble adhesive proteins (i.e., integrins) such as fibrinogen. Since fibrinogen is a multivalent molecule, it can bind to two different platelets simultaneously, resulting in platelet cross-linking and aggregation.

The coagulation cascade is activated on exposure of tissue factor in damaged endothelial cells at the site of the disrupted plaque. Factors VII and X are activated, ultimately leading to the conversion of prothrombin to thrombin, which then converts fibrinogen to fibrin. Fluid-phase and clot-bound thrombin participate in an autoamplification reaction leading to further activation of the coagulation cascade. The culprit coronary artery eventually becomes occluded by a thrombus containing platelet aggregates and fibrin strands.

In rare cases, STEMI may be due to coronary artery occlusion caused by coronary emboli, congenital abnormalities, coronary spasm, and a wide variety of systemic—particularly inflammatory—diseases. The amount of myocardial damage caused by coronary occlusion depends on (1) the territory supplied by the affected vessel, (2) whether or not the vessel becomes totally occluded, (3) the duration of coronary occlusion, (4) the quantity of blood supplied by collateral vessels to the affected tissue, (5) the demand for oxygen of the myocardium whose blood supply has been suddenly limited, (6) endogenous factors that can produce early spontaneous lysis of the occlusive thrombus, and (7) the adequacy of myocardial perfusion in the infarct zone when flow is restored in the occluded epicardial coronary artery.

Patients at increased risk for developing STEMI include those with multiple coronary risk factors and those with unstable angina (Chap. 32). Less common underlying medical conditions predisposing patients to STEMI include hypercoagulability, collagen vascular disease, cocaine abuse, and intracardiac thrombi or masses that can produce coronary emboli.

There have been major advances in the management of STEMI with recognition that the "chain of survival" involves a highly integrated system starting with prehospital care and extending to early hospital management so as to provide expeditious implementation of a reperfusion strategy.

CLINICAL PRESENTATION

In up to one-half of cases, a precipitating factor appears to be present before STEMI, such as vigorous physical exercise, emotional stress, or a medical or surgical illness. Although STEMI may commence at any time of the day or night, circadian variations have been reported such that clusters are seen in the morning within a few hours of awakening.

Pain is the most common presenting complaint in patients with STEMI. The pain is deep and visceral; adjectives commonly used to describe it are *heavy*, *squeezing*, and *crushing*, although, occasionally, it is described as stabbing or burning. It is similar in character to the discomfort of angina pectoris but commonly occurs at rest, is usually more severe, and lasts longer. Typically, the pain involves the central portion of the chest and/or the epigastrium, and, on occasion, it radiates to the arms. Less common sites of radiation include the abdomen, back, lower jaw, and neck. The frequent location of the pain beneath the xiphoid and epigastrium and the patients' denial that they may be suffering a heart attack are chiefly responsible for the common mistaken impression of indigestion. The pain of STEMI may radiate as high as the occipital area but not below the umbilicus. It is often accompanied by weakness, sweating, nausea, vomiting, anxiety, and a sense of impending doom. The pain may commence when the patient is at rest, but when it begins during a period of exertion, it does not usually subside with cessation of activity, in contrast to angina pectoris.

The pain of STEMI can simulate pain from acute pericarditis, pulmonary embolism (Chap. 20), acute aortic dissection, costochondritis, and gastrointestinal disorders. These conditions should therefore be considered in the differential diagnosis. Radiation of discomfort to the trapezius is not seen in patients with STEMI and may be a useful distinguishing feature that suggests pericarditis is the correct diagnosis. However, *pain is not uniformly present in patients with STEMI*. The proportion of painless STEMIs is greater in patients with diabetes mellitus, and it increases with age. In the elderly, STEMI may present as sudden-onset breathlessness, which may progress to pulmonary edema. Other less common presentations, with or without pain, include sudden loss of consciousness, a confusional state, a sensation of profound weakness, the appearance of an arrhythmia, evidence of peripheral embolism, or merely an unexplained drop in arterial pressure.

PHYSICAL FINDINGS

Most patients are anxious and restless, attempting unsuccessfully to relieve the pain by moving about in bed, altering their position, and stretching. Pallor associated with perspiration and coolness of the extremities occurs commonly. The combination of substernal chest pain persisting for >30 min and diaphoresis strongly suggests STEMI. Although many patients have a normal pulse rate and blood pressure within the first hour of STEMI, about one-fourth of patients with anterior infarction have manifestations of sympathetic nervous system hyperactivity (tachycardia and/or hypertension), and up to one-half with inferior infarction show evidence of parasympathetic hyperactivity (bradycardia and/or hypotension).

The precordium is usually quiet, and the apical impulse may be difficult to palpate. In patients with anterior wall infarction, an abnormal systolic pulsation caused by dyskinetic bulging of infarcted myocardium may develop in the periapical area within the first days of the illness and then may resolve. Other physical signs of ventricular dysfunction include fourth and third heart sounds, decreased intensity of the first heart sound, and paradoxical splitting of the second heart sound. A transient midsystolic or late systolic apical systolic murmur due to dysfunction of the mitral valve apparatus may be present. A pericardial friction rub is heard in many patients with transmural STEMI at some time in the course of the disease, if the patients are examined frequently. The carotid pulse is often decreased in volume, reflecting reduced stroke volume. Temperature elevations up to 38°C may be observed during the first week after STEMI. The arterial pressure is variable; in most patients with transmural infarction, systolic pressure declines by approximately 10–15 mmHg from the preinfarction state.

LABORATORY FINDINGS

Myocardial infarction (MI) progresses through the following temporal stages: (1) acute (first few hours–7 days), (2) healing (7–28 days), and (3) healed (≥29 days). When evaluating the results of diagnostic tests for STEMI, the temporal phase of the infarction must be considered. The laboratory tests of value in confirming the diagnosis may be divided into four groups: (1) ECG, (2) serum cardiac biomarkers, (3) cardiac imaging, and (4) nonspecific indices of tissue necrosis and inflammation.

ELECTROCARDIOGRAM

During the initial stage, total occlusion of an epicardial coronary artery produces ST-segment elevation. Most patients initially presenting with ST-segment elevation ultimately evolve Q waves on the ECG. However, Q waves in the leads overlying the infarct zone may vary in magnitude and even appear only transiently, depending on the reperfusion status of the ischemic myocardium and restoration of transmembrane potentials over time. A small proportion of patients initially presenting with ST-segment elevation will not develop Q waves when the obstructing thrombus is not totally occlusive, obstruction is transient, or if a rich collateral network is present. Among patients presenting with ischemic discomfort but *without* ST-segment elevation, if a serum cardiac biomarker of necrosis (see later) is detected, the diagnosis of NSTEMI is ultimately made (Fig. 33-1). A minority of patients who present initially without ST-segment elevation may develop a Q-wave MI. Previously, it was believed that transmural MI is present if the ECG demonstrates Q waves or loss of R waves, and nontransmural MI may be present if the ECG shows only transient ST-segment and T-wave changes. However, electrocardiographic-pathologic correlations are far from perfect and terms such as *Q-wave MI*, *non-Q-wave MI*, *transmural MI*, and *nontransmural MI*, have been replaced by STEMI and NSTEMI (Fig. 33-1). Contemporary studies using MRI suggest that the development of a Q wave on the ECG is more dependent on the volume of infarcted tissue rather than the transmurality of infarction.

SERUM CARDIAC BIOMARKERS

Certain proteins, called serum cardiac biomarkers, are released from necrotic heart muscle after STEMI. The rate of liberation of specific proteins differs depending on their intracellular location, their molecular weight, and the local blood and lymphatic flow. Cardiac biomarkers become detectable in the peripheral blood once the capacity of the cardiac lymphatics to clear the interstitium of the infarct zone is exceeded and spillover into the venous circulation occurs. The temporal pattern of protein release is of diagnostic importance, but contemporary urgent reperfusion strategies necessitate making a decision (based largely on a combination of clinical and ECG findings) before the results of blood tests have returned from the laboratory. Rapid whole-blood bedside assays for serum cardiac markers are now available

324

and may facilitate management decisions, particularly in patients with nondiagnostic ECGs.

Cardiac-specific troponin T (cTnT) and *cardiac-specific troponin I* (cTnI) have amino-acid sequences different from those of the skeletal muscle forms of these proteins. These differences permitted the development of quantitative assays for cTnT and cTnI with highly specific monoclonal antibodies. Since cTnT and cTnI are not normally detectable in the blood of healthy individuals but may increase after STEMI to levels >20 times higher than the upper reference limit (the highest value seen in 99% of a reference population not suffering from MI), the measurement of cTnT or cTnI is of considerable diagnostic usefulness, and they are now the preferred biochemical markers for MI (Fig. 33-2).

The cardiac troponins are particularly valuable when there is clinical suspicion of either skeletal muscle injury or a small MI that may be below the detection limit for creatine phosphokinase (CK) and its MB isoenzyme (CKMB) measurements, and they are, therefore, of particular value in distinguishing UA from NSTEMI. Levels of cTnI and cTnT may remain elevated for 7–10 days after STEMI.

CK rises within 4–8 h and generally returns to normal by 48–72 h (Fig. 33-2). An important drawback of total CK measurement is its lack of specificity for STEMI, as CK may be elevated with skeletal muscle disease or trauma, including intramuscular injection. The MB isoenzyme of CK has the advantage over total CK that it is not present in significant concentrations in

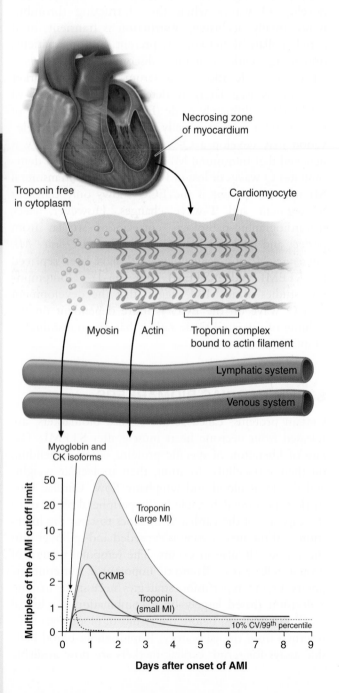

FIGURE 33-2

The zone of necrosing myocardium is shown at the top of the figure, followed in the middle portion of the figure by a diagram of a cardiomyocyte that is in the process of releasing biomarkers. The biomarkers that are released into the interstitium are first cleared by lymphatics followed subsequently by spillover into the venous system. After disruption of the sarcolemmal membrane of the cardiomyocyte, the cytoplasmic pool of biomarkers is released first (left-most arrow in bottom portion of figure). Markers such as myoglobin and CK isoforms are rapidly released, and blood levels rise quickly above the cutoff limit; this is then followed by a more protracted release of biomarkers from the disintegrating myofilaments that may continue for several days. Cardiac troponin levels rise to about 20 to 50 times the upper reference limit (the 99th percentile of values in a reference control group) in patients who have a "classic" acute myocardial infarction (MI) and sustain sufficient myocardial necrosis to result in abnormally elevated levels of the MB fraction of creatine kinase (CKMB). Clinicians can now diagnose episodes of microinfarction by sensitive assays that detect cardiac troponin elevations above the upper reference limit, even though CKMB levels may still be in the normal reference range (not shown). CV = coefficient of variation. (*Modified from Antman EM: Decision making with cardiac troponin tests. N Engl J Med 346:2079, 2002 and Jaffe AS, Babiun L, Apple FS: Biomarkers in acute cardiac disease: The present and the future. J Am Coll Cardiol 48:1, 2006.*)

extracardiac tissue and, therefore, is considerably more specific. However, cardiac surgery, myocarditis, and electrical cardioversion often result in elevated serum levels of the MB isoenzyme. A ratio (relative index) of CKMB mass: CK activity ≥2.5 suggests but is not diagnostic of a myocardial rather than a skeletal muscle source for the CKMB elevation.

Many hospitals are using cTnT or cTnI rather than CKMB as the routine serum cardiac marker for diagnosis of STEMI, although any of these analytes remain clinically acceptable. It is *not* cost-effective to measure both a cardiac-specific troponin and CKMB at all time points in every patient.

While it has long been recognized that the total quantity of protein released correlates with the size of the infarct, the peak protein concentration correlates only weakly with infarct size. Recanalization of a coronary artery occlusion (either spontaneously or by mechanical or pharmacologic means) in the early hours of STEMI causes earlier peaking of biomarker measurements (Fig. 33-2) because of a rapid washout from the interstitium of the infarct zone, quickly overwhelming lymphatic clearance of the proteins.

The *nonspecific reaction* to myocardial injury is associated with polymorphonuclear leukocytosis, which appears within a few hours after the onset of pain and persists for 3–7 days; the white blood cell count often reaches levels of 12,000–15,000/μL. The erythrocyte sedimentation rate rises more slowly than the white blood cell count, peaking during the first week and sometimes remaining elevated for one or two weeks.

CARDIAC IMAGING

Abnormalities of wall motion on *two-dimensional echocardiography* are almost universally present. Although acute STEMI cannot be distinguished from an old myocardial scar or from acute severe ischemia by echocardiography, the ease and safety of the procedure make its use appealing as a screening tool in the Emergency Department setting. When the ECG is not diagnostic of STEMI, early detection of the presence or absence of wall motion abnormalities by echocardiography can aid in management decisions, such as whether the patient should receive reperfusion therapy (e.g., fibrinolysis or a percutaneous coronary intervention [PCI]). Echocardiographic estimation of left ventricular (LV) function is useful prognostically; detection of reduced function serves as an indication for therapy with an inhibitor of the renin-angiotensin–aldosterone system. Echocardiography may also identify the presence of right ventricular (RV) infarction, ventricular aneurysm, pericardial effusion, and LV thrombus. In addition, Doppler echocardiography is useful in the detection and quantitation of a ventricular septal defect and mitral regurgitation, two serious complications of STEMI.

Several *radionuclide imaging techniques* are available for evaluating patients with suspected STEMI. However, these imaging modalities are used less often than echocardiography because they are more cumbersome and lack sensitivity and specificity in many clinical circumstances. Myocardial perfusion imaging with [^{201}Tl] or [^{99m}Tc]-sestamibi, which are distributed in proportion to myocardial blood flow and concentrated by viable myocardium, reveal a defect ("cold spot") in most patients during the first few hours after development of a transmural infarct. Although perfusion scanning is extremely sensitive, it cannot distinguish acute infarcts from chronic scars and, thus, is not specific for the diagnosis of *acute* MI. Radionuclide ventriculography, carried out with [^{99m}Tc]-labeled red blood cells, frequently demonstrates wall motion disorders and reduction in the ventricular ejection fraction in patients with STEMI. While of value in assessing the hemodynamic consequences of infarction and in aiding in the diagnosis of RV infarction when the RV ejection fraction is depressed, this technique is nonspecific, as many cardiac abnormalities other than MI alter the radionuclide ventriculogram.

Myocardial infarction can be detected accurately with high-resolution cardiac MRI using a technique referred to as late enhancement. A standard imaging agent (gadolinium) is administered and images are obtained after a 10-min delay. Since little gadolinium enters normal myocardium, where there are tightly packed myocytes, but does percolate into the expanded intercellular region of the infarct zone, there is a bright signal in areas of infarction that appears in stark contrast to the dark areas of normal myocardium.

INITIAL MANAGEMENT

PREHOSPITAL CARE

The prognosis in STEMI is largely related to the occurrence of two general classes of complications: (1) electrical complications (arrhythmias) and (2) mechanical complications ("pump failure"). Most out-of-hospital deaths from STEMI are due to the sudden development of ventricular fibrillation. The vast majority of deaths due to ventricular fibrillation occur within the first 24 h of the onset of symptoms, and of these, over half occur in the first hour. Therefore, the major elements of prehospital care of patients with suspected STEMI include (1) recognition of symptoms by the patient and prompt seeking of medical attention; (2) rapid deployment of an emergency medical team capable of performing resuscitative maneuvers, including defibrillation;

(3) expeditious transportation of the patient to a hospital facility that is continuously staffed by physicians and nurses skilled in managing arrhythmias and providing advanced cardiac life support; and (4) expeditious implementation of reperfusion therapy (Fig. 33-3). The greatest delay usually occurs not during transportation to the hospital but, rather, between the onset of pain and the patient's decision to call for help. This delay can best be reduced by health care professionals educating the public concerning the significance of chest discomfort and the importance of seeking early medical attention. Regular office visits with patients having a history of or who are at risk for ischemic heart disease are important "teachable moments" for clinicians to review the symptoms of STEMI and the appropriate action plan.

Increasingly, monitoring and treatment are carried out by trained personnel in the ambulance, further shortening the time between the onset of the infarction and appropriate treatment. General guidelines for initiation of fibrinolysis in the prehospital setting include the ability to transmit 12-lead ECGs to confirm the diagnosis, the presence of paramedics in the ambulance, training of paramedics in the interpretation of ECGs and management of STEMI, and online medical command and control that can authorize the initiation of treatment in the field.

MANAGEMENT IN THE EMERGENCY DEPARTMENT

In the Emergency Department, the goals for the management of patients with suspected STEMI include control of cardiac discomfort, rapid identification of patients who are candidates for urgent reperfusion therapy, triage of lower-risk patients to the appropriate location in the hospital, and avoidance of inappropriate discharge of patients with STEMI. Many aspects of the treatment of STEMI are initiated in the Emergency Department and then continued during the in-hospital phase of management.

Aspirin is essential in the management of patients with suspected STEMI and is effective across the entire spectrum of acute coronary syndromes (Fig. 33-1). Rapid inhibition of cyclooxygenase-1 in platelets followed by a reduction of thromboxane A_2 levels is achieved by buccal absorption of a chewed 160–325-mg tablet in the Emergency Department. This measure should be followed by daily oral administration of aspirin in a dose of 75–162 mg.

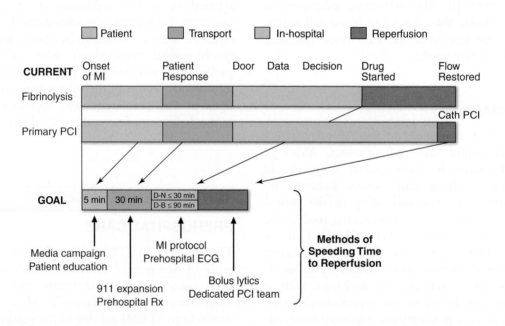

FIGURE 33-3

Major components of time delay between onset of symptoms from STEMI and restoration of flow in the infarct-related artery. Plotted sequentially from left to right are the times for patients to recognize symptoms and seek medical attention, transportation to the hospital, in-hospital decision making, implementation of reperfusion strategy, and restoration of flow once the reperfusion strategy has been initiated. The time to initiate fibrinolytic therapy is the "door-to-needle" (D-N) time; this is followed by the period of time required for pharmacologic restoration of flow. More time is required to move the patient to the catheterization laboratory for a percutaneous coronary interventional (PCI) procedure, referred to as the "door-to-balloon" (D-B) time, but restoration of flow in the epicardial infarct–related artery occurs promptly after PCI. At the bottom is a variety of methods for speeding the time to reperfusion along with the goals for the time intervals for the various components of the time delay. (*Adapted from CP Cannon et al: J Thromb Thrombol 1:27, 1994.*)

In patients whose arterial O_2 saturation is normal, supplemental O_2 is of limited if any clinical benefit and therefore is not cost-effective. However, when hypoxemia is present, O_2 should be administered by nasal prongs or face mask (2–4 L/min) for the first 6–12 h after infarction; the patient should then be reassessed to determine if there is a continued need for such treatment.

CONTROL OF DISCOMFORT

Sublingual *nitroglycerin* can be given safely to most patients with STEMI. Up to three doses of 0.4 mg should be administered at about 5-min intervals. In addition to diminishing or abolishing chest discomfort, nitroglycerin may be capable of both decreasing myocardial oxygen demand (by lowering preload) and increasing myocardial oxygen supply (by dilating infarct-related coronary vessels or collateral vessels). In patients whose initially favorable response to sublingual nitroglycerin is followed by the return of chest discomfort, particularly if accompanied by other evidence of ongoing ischemia such as further ST-segment or T-wave shifts, the use of intravenous nitroglycerin should be considered. Therapy with nitrates should be avoided in patients who present with low systolic arterial pressure (<90 mmHg) or in whom there is clinical suspicion of right ventricular infarction (inferior infarction on ECG, elevated jugular venous pressure, clear lungs, and hypotension). Nitrates should not be administered to patients who have taken the phosphodiesterase-5 inhibitor sildenafil for erectile dysfunction within the preceding 24 h, because it may potentiate the hypotensive effects of nitrates. An idiosyncratic reaction to nitrates, consisting of sudden marked hypotension, sometimes occurs but can usually be reversed promptly by the rapid administration of intravenous atropine.

Morphine is a very effective analgesic for the pain associated with STEMI. However, it may reduce sympathetically mediated arteriolar and venous constriction, and the resulting venous pooling may reduce cardiac output and arterial pressure. These hemodynamic disturbances usually respond promptly to elevation of the legs, but in some patients volume expansion with intravenous saline is required. The patient may experience diaphoresis and nausea, but these events usually pass and are replaced by a feeling of well-being associated with the relief of pain. Morphine also has a vagotonic effect and may cause bradycardia or advanced degrees of heart block, particularly in patients with inferior infarction. These side effects usually respond to atropine (0.5 mg intravenously). Morphine is routinely administered by repetitive (every 5 min) intravenous injection of small doses (2–4 mg), rather than by the subcutaneous administration of a larger quantity, because absorption may be unpredictable by the latter route.

Intravenous *beta blockers* are also useful in the control of the pain of STEMI. These drugs control pain effectively in some patients, presumably by diminishing myocardial O_2 demand and hence ischemia. More important, there is evidence that intravenous beta blockers reduce the risks of reinfarction and ventricular fibrillation (see "Beta-Adrenoceptor Blockers," later). However, patient selection is important when considering beta blockers for STEMI. Oral beta-blocker therapy should be initiated in the first 24 h for patients who do not have any of the following: (1) signs of heart failure, (2) evidence of a low-output state, (3) increased risk for cardiogenic shock, or (4) other relative contraindications to beta blockade (PR interval greater than 0.24 s, second- or third-degree heart block, active asthma, or reactive airway disease). A commonly employed regimen is metoprolol, 5 mg every 2–5 min for a total of 3 doses, provided the patient has a heart rate >60 beats per minute (bpm), systolic pressure >100 mmHg, a PR interval <0.24 s, and rales that are no higher than 10 cm up from the diaphragm. Fifteen minutes after the last intravenous dose, an oral regimen is initiated of 50 mg every 6 h for 48 h, followed by 100 mg every 12 h.

Unlike beta blockers, calcium antagonists are of little value in the acute setting, and there is evidence that short-acting dihydropyridines may be associated with an increased mortality risk.

MANAGEMENT STRATEGIES

The primary tool for screening patients and making triage decisions is the initial 12-lead ECG. When ST-segment elevation of at least 2 mm in 2 contiguous precordial leads and 1 mm in 2 adjacent limb leads is present, a patient should be considered a candidate for *reperfusion therapy* (Fig. 33-4). The process of selecting patients for fibrinolysis versus primary PCI (angioplasty, or stenting) is discussed later. In the absence of ST-segment elevation, fibrinolysis is not helpful, and evidence exists suggesting that it may be harmful.

LIMITATION OF INFARCT SIZE

The quantity of myocardium that becomes necrotic as a consequence of a coronary artery occlusion is determined by factors other than just the site of occlusion. While the central zone of the infarct contains necrotic tissue that is irretrievably lost, the fate of the surrounding ischemic myocardium (ischemic penumbra) may be improved by timely restoration of coronary perfusion, reduction of myocardial O_2 demands, prevention of the accumulation of noxious metabolites, and blunting

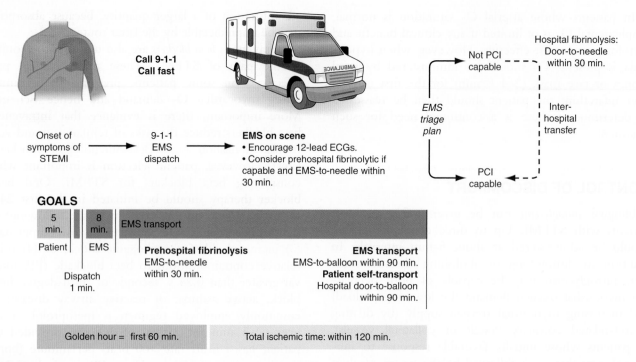

Call 9-1-1
Call fast

FIGURE 33-4

Options for transportation of patients with STEMI and initial reperfusion treatment. Patient transported by EMS after calling 911: Reperfusion in patients with STEMI can be accomplished by the pharmacologic (fibrinolysis) or catheter-based (primary PCI) approaches. Implementation of these strategies varies based on the mode of transportation of the patient and capabilities at the receiving hospital. Transport time to the hospital is variable from case to case, but the goal is to keep total ischemic time within 120 min. There are three possible scenarios: (1) If EMS has fibrinolytic capability and the patient qualifies for therapy, prehospital fibrinolysis should be started within 30 min of EMS arrival on scene. (2) If EMS is not capable of administering prehospital fibrinolysis and the patient is transported to a non-PCI-capable hospital, the hospital door-to-needle time should be within 30 min for patients in whom fibrinolysis is indicated. (3) If EMS is not capable of administering prehospital fibrinolysis and the patient is transported to a PCI-capable hospital, the hospital door-to-balloon time should be within 90 min. *Interhospital transfer*: It is also appropriate to consider emergency interhospital transfer of the patient to a PCI-capable hospital for mechanical revascularization if: (1) there is a contraindication to fibrinolysis, (2) PCI can be initiated promptly (within 90 min after the patient presented to the initial receiving hospital or within 60 min compared to when fibrinolysis with a fibrin-specific agent could be initiated at the initial receiving hospital), (3) fibrinolysis is administered and is unsuccessful (i.e., "rescue PCI"). Secondary nonemergency interhospital transfer can be considered for recurrent ischemia. *Patient self-transport*: Patient self-transportation is discouraged. If the patient arrives at a non-PCI-capable hospital, the door-to-needle time should be within 30 min. If the patient arrives at a PCI-capable hospital, the door-to-balloon time should be within 90 min. The treatment options and time recommended after first hospital arrival are the same. (*Adapted with permission from Antman et al: ACC/AHA guidelines for the management of patients with ST-elevation myocardial infarction: A report of the American College of Cardiology/American Heart Association Task Force on Practice Guidelines [Committee to Revise the 1999 Guidelines for the Management of Patients with Acute Myocardial Infarction]. Circulation 110:e82, 2004.*)

of the impact of mediators of reperfusion injury (e.g., calcium overload and oxygen-derived free radicals). Up to one-third of patients with STEMI may achieve *spontaneous* reperfusion of the infarct-related coronary artery within 24 h and experience improved healing of infarcted tissue. Reperfusion, either pharmacologically (by fibrinolysis) or by PCI, accelerates the opening of infarct-related arteries in those patients in whom spontaneous fibrinolysis ultimately would have occurred and also greatly increases the number of patients in whom restoration of flow in the infarct-related artery is accomplished. Timely restoration of flow in the epicardial infarct–related artery combined with improved perfusion of the downstream zone of infarcted myocardium results in a limitation of infarct size. Protection of the ischemic myocardium by the maintenance of an optimal balance between myocardial O_2 supply and demand through pain control, treatment of congestive heart failure (CHF), and minimization of tachycardia and hypertension extends the "window" of time for the salvage of myocardium by reperfusion strategies.

Glucocorticoids and nonsteroidal anti-inflammatory agents, with the exception of aspirin, should be avoided in patients with STEMI. They can impair infarct healing and increase the risk of myocardial rupture, and their use may result in a larger infarct scar. In addition, they can increase coronary vascular resistance, thereby potentially reducing flow to ischemic myocardium.

Primary percutaneous coronary intervention

PCI, usually angioplasty and/or stenting without preceding fibrinolysis, referred to as *primary PCI*, is effective in restoring perfusion in STEMI when carried out on an emergency basis in the first few hours of MI. It has the advantage of being applicable to patients who have contraindications to fibrinolytic therapy (see later) but otherwise are considered appropriate candidates for reperfusion. It appears to be more effective than fibrinolysis in opening occluded coronary arteries and, *when performed by experienced operators (≥75 PCI cases [not necessarily primary] per year) in dedicated medical centers (≥36 primary PCI cases per year)*, is associated with better short-term and long-term clinical outcomes. Compared with fibrinolysis, primary PCI is generally preferred when the diagnosis is in doubt, cardiogenic shock is present, bleeding risk is increased, or symptoms have been present for at least 2–3 h when the clot is more mature and less easily lysed by fibrinolytic drugs. However, PCI is expensive in terms of personnel and facilities, and its applicability is limited by its availability, around the clock, in only a minority of hospitals.

Fibrinolysis

If no contraindications are present (see later), fibrinolytic therapy should ideally be initiated within 30 min of presentation (i.e., door-to-needle time ≤30 min). The principal goal of fibrinolysis is prompt restoration of full coronary arterial patency. The fibrinolytic agents tissue plasminogen activator (tPA), streptokinase, tenecteplase (TNK), and reteplase (rPA) have been approved by the U.S. Food and Drug Administration for intravenous use in patients with STEMI. These drugs all act by promoting the conversion of plasminogen to plasmin, which subsequently lyses fibrin thrombi. Although considerable emphasis was first placed on a distinction between more fibrin-specific agents, such as tPA, and non-fibrin-specific agents, such as streptokinase, it is now recognized that these differences are only relative, as some degree of systemic fibrinolysis occurs with the former agents. TNK and rPA

are referred to as *bolus fibrinolytics* since their administration does not require a prolonged intravenous infusion.

When assessed angiographically, flow in the culprit coronary artery is described by a simple qualitative scale called the *thrombolysis in myocardial infarction (TIMI) grading system*: grade 0 indicates complete occlusion of the infarct-related artery; grade 1 indicates some penetration of the contrast material beyond the point of obstruction but without perfusion of the distal coronary bed; grade 2 indicates perfusion of the entire infarct vessel into the distal bed, but with flow that is delayed compared with that of a normal artery; and grade 3 indicates full perfusion of the infarct vessel with normal flow. The latter is the goal of reperfusion therapy, because full perfusion of the infarct-related coronary artery yields far better results in terms of limiting infarct size, maintenance of LV function, and reduction of both short- and long-term mortality rates. Additional methods of angiographic assessment of the efficacy of fibrinolysis include counting the number of frames on the cine film required for dye to flow from the origin of the infarct-related artery to a landmark in the distal vascular bed (*TIMI frame count*) and determining the rate of entry and exit of contrast dye from the microvasculature in the myocardial infarct zone (*TIMI myocardial perfusion grade*). These methods have an even tighter correlation with outcomes after STEMI than the more commonly employed TIMI flow grade.

Fibrinolytic therapy can reduce the relative risk of in-hospital death by up to 50% when administered within the first hour of the onset of symptoms of STEMI, and much of this benefit is maintained for at least 10 years. When appropriately used, fibrinolytic therapy appears to reduce infarct size, limit LV dysfunction, and reduce the incidence of serious complications such as septal rupture, cardiogenic shock, and malignant ventricular arrhythmias. Since myocardium can be salvaged only before it has been irreversibly injured, the timing of reperfusion therapy, by fibrinolysis or a catheter-based approach, is of extreme importance in achieving maximum benefit. While the upper time limit depends on specific factors in individual patients, it is clear that every minute counts and that patients treated within 1–3 h of the onset of symptoms generally benefit most. Although reduction of the mortality rate is more modest, the therapy remains of benefit for many patients seen 3–6 h after the onset of infarction, and some benefit appears to be possible up to 12 h, especially if chest discomfort is still present and ST segments remain elevated. Compared with PCI for STEMI (primary PCI), fibrinolysis is generally the preferred reperfusion strategy for patients presenting in the first hour of symptoms, if there are logistical concerns about transportation of the patient to a suitable PCI center (experienced operator and team with a track record for a "door-to-balloon" time of <2 h), or there is an anticipated delay of at least 1 h between the time that fibrinolysis could be started versus implementation of PCI. Although patients <75 years achieve a greater relative reduction in the mortality rate with fibrinolytic therapy than do older patients, the higher *absolute* mortality rate (15–25%) in the latter results in similar absolute reductions in the mortality rates for both age groups.

tPA and the other relatively fibrin-specific plasminogen activators, rPA and TNK, are more effective than streptokinase at restoring full perfusion—i.e., TIMI grade 3 coronary flow—and have a small edge in improving survival as well. The current recommended regimen of tPA consists of a 15-mg bolus followed by 50 mg intravenously over the first 30 min, followed by 35 mg over the next 60 min. Streptokinase is administered as 1.5 million units (MU) intravenously over 1 h. rPA is administered in a double-bolus regimen consisting of a 10-MU bolus given over 2–3 min, followed by a second 10-MU bolus 30 min later. TNK is given as a single weight-based intravenous bolus of 0.53 mg/kg over 10 s. In addition to the fibrinolytic agents discussed above, pharmacologic reperfusion typically involves adjunctive antiplatelet and antithrombotic drugs, as discussed subsequently.

Alternative pharmacologic regimens for reperfusion combine an intravenous glycoprotein IIb/IIIa inhibitor with a reduced dose of a fibrinolytic agent. Compared with fibrinolytic agents that involve a prolonged infusion (e.g., tPA), such combination reperfusion regimens facilitate the rate and extent of fibrinolysis by inhibiting platelet aggregation, weakening the clot structure, and allowing penetration of the fibrinolytic agent deeper into the clot. However, combination reperfusion regimens have similar efficacy as compared with bolus fibrinolytics and are associated with an increased risk of bleeding, especially in patients >75 years. Therefore, combination reperfusion regimens are not recommended for routine use. Glycoprotein IIb/IIIa inhibitors, given alone or in combination with a reduced dose of a fibrinolytic agent as part of a preparatory regimen before planned immediate PCI (facilitated PCI), have not been shown to reduce infarct size or improve outcomes and, furthermore, are associated with increased bleeding. Facilitated PCI is, therefore, also not a strategy that is recommended for routine use.

Integrated reperfusion strategy

Evidence has emerged that suggests PCI plays an increasingly important role in the management of STEMI. Prior approaches that segregated the pharmacologic and catheter-based approaches to reperfusion have now been replaced with an integrated approach to triage and transfer of STEMI patients to receive PCI (Fig. 33-5).

Contraindications and complications

Clear contraindications to the use of fibrinolytic agents include a history of cerebrovascular hemorrhage at any time, a nonhemorrhagic stroke or other cerebrovascular event within the past year, marked hypertension (a reliably determined systolic arterial pressure >180 mmHg and/or a diastolic pressure >110 mmHg) at any time during the acute presentation, suspicion of aortic dissection, and active internal bleeding (excluding menses). While advanced age is associated with an increase in hemorrhagic complications, the benefit of fibrinolytic therapy in the elderly appears to justify its use if no other contraindications are present and the amount of myocardium in jeopardy appears to be substantial.

Relative contraindications to fibrinolytic therapy, which require assessment of the risk:benefit ratio, include current use of anticoagulants (international normalized ratio ≥2), a recent (<2 weeks) invasive or surgical procedure or prolonged (>10 min) cardiopulmonary resuscitation, known bleeding diathesis, pregnancy, a hemorrhagic ophthalmic condition (e.g., hemorrhagic diabetic retinopathy), active peptic ulcer disease, and a history of severe hypertension that is currently adequately controlled. Because of the risk of an allergic reaction, patients should not receive streptokinase if that agent had been received within the preceding five days to two years.

Allergic reactions to streptokinase occur in ~2% of patients who receive it. While a minor degree of hypotension occurs in 4–10% of patients given this agent, marked hypotension occurs, although rarely, in association with severe allergic reactions.

Hemorrhage is the most frequent and potentially the most serious complication. Because bleeding episodes that require transfusion are more common when patients require invasive procedures, unnecessary venous or arterial interventions should be avoided in patients receiving fibrinolytic agents. Hemorrhagic stroke is the most serious complication and occurs in ~0.5–0.9% of patients being treated with these agents. This rate increases with advancing age, with patients >70 years experiencing roughly twice the rate of intracranial hemorrhage as those <65 years. Large-scale trials have suggested that the rate of intracranial hemorrhage with tPA or rPA is slightly higher than with streptokinase.

Cardiac catheterization and coronary angiography should be carried out after fibrinolytic therapy if there is evidence of either (1) failure of reperfusion (persistent chest pain and ST-segment elevation >90 min), in which case a *rescue PCI* should be considered; or (2) coronary artery reocclusion (re-elevation of ST segments and/or recurrent chest pain) or the development of recurrent ischemia (such as recurrent angina in the early hospital course or a positive exercise stress test before discharge), in which case an *urgent PCI*

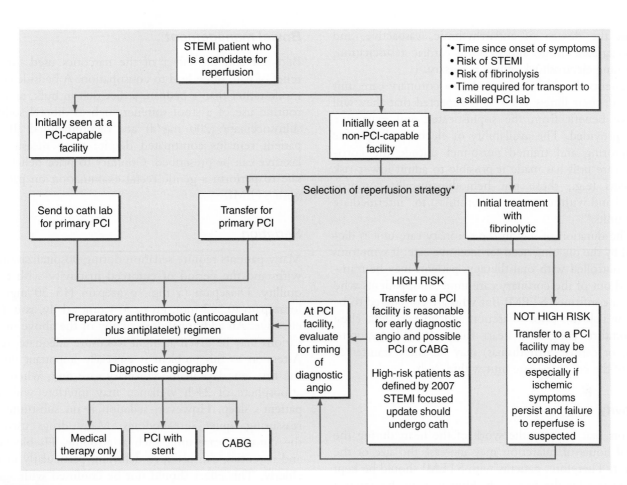

FIGURE 33-5
Each community and each facility in that community should have an agreed-upon plan for how STEMI patients are to be treated that includes which hospitals should receive STEMI patients from EMS units capable of obtaining diagnostic ECGs, management at the initial receiving hospital, and written criteria and agreements for expeditious transfer of patients from non-PCI-capable facilities. Patients initially seen at a PCI-capable facility (left side of diagram) should be sent promptly to the cardiac catheterization laboratory with the intent to perform primary PCI. Patients initially seen at a non-PCI-capable facility (right side of diagram) should rapidly be assessed for the optimum reperfusion therapy (see box in top right corner for assessment criteria). This may include transfer for primary PCI or initial treatment with a fibrinolytic. Following administration of a fibrinolytic, management is dictated by the patient's overall risk for death/serious complications of STEMI, and whether or not they experience recurrent ischemic symptoms or left-ventricular failure (see the two boxes at the bottom right of diagram). (*Adapted from Kushner FG et al: 2009 focused update of the ACC/AHA Guidelines for the Management of Patients with ST-Elevation Myocardial Infarction [updating the 2004 guideline and 2007 focused update]: a report of the American College of Cardiology Foundation/American Heart Association Task Force on Practice Guidelines. Circulation 120:2271, 2009.*)

should be considered. The potential benefits of routine angiography and *elective* PCI even in asymptomatic patients following administration of fibrinolytic therapy are controversial, but such an approach may have merit given the numerous technological advances that have occurred in the catheterization laboratory and the increasing number of skilled interventionalists. Coronary artery bypass surgery should be reserved for patients whose coronary anatomy is unsuited to PCI but in whom revascularization appears to be advisable because of extensive jeopardized myocardium or recurrent ischemia.

HOSPITAL PHASE MANAGEMENT

CORONARY CARE UNITS

These units are routinely equipped with a system that permits continuous monitoring of the cardiac rhythm of each patient and hemodynamic monitoring in selected patients. Defibrillators, respirators, noninvasive transthoracic pacemakers, and facilities for introducing pacing catheters and flow-directed, balloon-tipped catheters are also usually available. Equally important is the organization of a highly trained team of nurses who can recognize arrhythmias;

adjust the dosage of antiarrhythmic, vasoactive, and anticoagulant drugs; and perform cardiac resuscitation, including electroshock, when necessary.

Patients should be admitted to a coronary care unit early in their illness when it is expected that they will derive benefit from the sophisticated and expensive care provided. The availability of electrocardiographic monitoring and trained personnel outside the coronary care unit has made it possible to admit lower-risk patients (e.g., those not hemodynamically compromised and without active arrhythmias) to "intermediate care units."

The duration of stay in the coronary care unit is dictated by the ongoing need for intensive care. If symptoms are controlled with oral therapy, patients may be transferred out of the coronary care unit. Also, patients who have a confirmed STEMI but who are considered to be at low risk (no prior infarction and no persistent chest discomfort, congestive heart failure [CHF], hypotension, or cardiac arrhythmias) may be safely transferred out of the coronary care unit within 24 h.

Activity

Factors that increase the work of the heart during the initial hours of infarction may increase the size of the infarct. Therefore, patients with STEMI should be kept at bed rest for the first 12 h. However, in the absence of complications, patients should be encouraged, under supervision, to resume an upright posture by dangling their feet over the side of the bed and sitting in a chair within the first 24 h. This practice is psychologically beneficial and usually results in a reduction in the pulmonary capillary wedge pressure. In the absence of hypotension and other complications, by the second or third day, patients typically are ambulating in their room with increasing duration and frequency, and they may shower or stand at the sink to bathe. By day 3 after infarction, patients should be increasing their ambulation progressively to a goal of 185 m (600 ft) at least 3 times a day.

Diet

Because of the risk of emesis and aspiration soon after STEMI, patients should receive either nothing or only clear liquids by mouth for the first 4–12 h. The typical coronary care unit diet should provide ≤30% of total calories as fat and have a cholesterol content of ≤300 mg/d. Complex carbohydrates should make up 50–55% of total calories. Portions should not be unusually large, and the menu should be enriched with foods that are high in potassium, magnesium, and fiber, but low in sodium. Diabetes mellitus and hypertriglyceridemia are managed by restriction of concentrated sweets in the diet.

Bowel management

Bed rest and the effect of the narcotics used for the relief of pain often lead to constipation. A bedside commode rather than a bedpan, a diet rich in bulk, and the routine use of a stool softener such as dioctyl sodium sulfosuccinate (200 mg/d) are recommended. If the patient remains constipated despite these measures, a laxative can be prescribed. Contrary to prior belief, it is safe to perform a gentle rectal examination on patients with STEMI.

Sedation

Many patients require sedation during hospitalization to withstand the period of enforced inactivity with tranquillity. Diazepam (5 mg), oxazepam (15–30 mg), or lorazepam (0.5–2 mg), given 3–4 times daily, is usually effective. An additional dose of any of the above medications may be given at night to ensure adequate sleep. Attention to this problem is especially important during the first few days in the coronary care unit, where the atmosphere of 24-h vigilance may interfere with the patient's sleep. However, sedation is no substitute for reassuring, quiet surroundings. Many drugs used in the coronary care unit, such as atropine, H_2 blockers, and narcotics, can produce delirium, particularly in the elderly. This effect should not be confused with agitation, and it is wise to conduct a thorough review of the patient's medications before arbitrarily prescribing additional doses of anxiolytics.

PHARMACOTHERAPY

ANTITHROMBOTIC AGENTS

The use of antiplatelet and anticoagulant therapy during the initial phase of STEMI is based on extensive laboratory and clinical evidence that thrombosis plays an important role in the pathogenesis of this condition. The primary goal of treatment with antiplatelet and anticoagulant agents is to maintain patency of the infarct-related artery, in conjunction with reperfusion strategies. A secondary goal is to reduce the patient's tendency to thrombosis and, thus, the likelihood of mural thrombus formation or deep venous thrombosis, either of which could result in pulmonary embolization. The degree to which antiplatelet and anticoagulant therapy achieves these goals partly determines how effectively it reduces the risk of mortality from STEMI.

As noted previously (see "Management in the Emergency Department," earlier), aspirin is the standard antiplatelet agent for patients with STEMI. The most compelling evidence for the benefits of antiplatelet therapy (mainly with aspirin) in STEMI is found in the comprehensive overview by the Antiplatelet Trialists' Collaboration. Data from nearly 20,000 patients with MI enrolled in 15 randomized trials were pooled and revealed a relative reduction of 27% in the mortality rate, from 14.2% in control patients to 10.4% in patients receiving antiplatelet agents.

Inhibitors of the P2Y12 ADP receptor prevent activation and aggregation of platelets. The addition of the P2Y12 inhibitor clopidogrel to background treatment with aspirin to STEMI patients reduces the risk of clinical events (death, reinfarction, stroke) and, in patients receiving fibrinolytic therapy, has been shown to prevent reocclusion of a successfully reperfused infarct artery. New P2Y12 ADP receptor antagonists, such as prasugrel and ticagrelor, are more effective than clopidogrel in preventing ischemic complications in STEMI patients undergoing PCI, but are associated with an increased risk of bleeding. Glycoprotein IIb/IIIa receptor inhibitors appear useful for preventing thrombotic complications in patients with STEMI undergoing PCI.

The standard anticoagulant agent used in clinical practice is unfractionated heparin (UFH). The available data suggest that when UFH is added to a regimen of aspirin and a non-fibrin-specific thrombolytic agent such as streptokinase, additional mortality benefit occurs (about 5 lives saved per 1000 patients treated). It appears that the immediate administration of intravenous UFH, in addition to a regimen of aspirin and relatively fibrin-specific fibrinolytic agents (tPA, rPA, or TNK), helps to maintain patency of the infarct-related artery. This effect is achieved at the cost of a small increased risk of bleeding. The recommended dose of UFH is an initial bolus of 60 U/kg (maximum 4000 U) followed by an initial infusion of 12 U/kg per hour (maximum 1000 U/h). The activated partial thromboplastin time during maintenance therapy should be 1.5–2 times the control value.

Alternatives to UFH for anticoagulation of patients with STEMI are the low-molecular-weight heparin (LMWH) preparations, a synthetic version of the critical pentasaccharide sequence (fondaparinux), and the direct antithrombin bivalirudin. Advantages of LMWHs include high bioavailability permitting administration subcutaneously, reliable anticoagulation without monitoring, and greater antiXa:IIa activity. Enoxaparin has been shown to reduce significantly the composite endpoints of death/nonfatal reinfarction and death/nonfatal reinfarction/urgent revascularization compared with UFH in STEMI patients who receive fibrinolysis. Treatment with enoxaparin is associated with higher rates of serious bleeding, but net clinical benefit—a composite endpoint that combines efficacy and safety—still favors enoxaparin over UFH. Interpretation of the data on fondaparinux is difficult because of the complex nature of the pivotal clinical trial evaluating it in STEMI (OASIS-6). Fondaparinux appears superior to placebo in STEMI patients not receiving reperfusion therapy, but its relative efficacy and safety compared with UFH is less certain. Owing to the risk of catheter thrombosis, fondaparinux should not be used alone at the time of coronary angiography and PCI but should be combined with another anticoagulant with antithrombin activity such as UFH or bivalirudin. Contemporary trials of bivalirudin used an open-label design to evaluate its efficacy and safety compared with UFH plus a glycoprotein IIb/IIIa inhibitor. Bivalirudin was associated with a lower rate of bleeding, largely driven by reductions in vascular access site hematomas ≥5 cm or the administration of blood transfusions.

Patients with an anterior location of the infarction, severe LV dysfunction, heart failure, a history of embolism, two-dimensional echocardiographic evidence of mural thrombus, or atrial fibrillation are at increased risk of systemic or pulmonary thromboembolism. Such individuals should receive full therapeutic levels of anticoagulant therapy (LMWH or UFH) while hospitalized, followed by at least three months of warfarin therapy.

BETA-ADRENOCEPTOR BLOCKERS

The benefits of beta blockers in patients with STEMI can be divided into those that occur immediately when the drug is given acutely and those that accrue over the long term when the drug is given for secondary prevention after an infarction. Acute intravenous beta blockade improves the myocardial O_2 supply-demand relationship, decreases pain, reduces infarct size, and decreases the incidence of serious ventricular arrhythmias. In patients who undergo fibrinolysis soon after the onset of chest pain, no incremental reduction in mortality rate is seen with beta blockers, but recurrent ischemia and reinfarction are reduced.

Thus, beta-blocker therapy after STEMI is useful for most patients (including those treated with an angiotensin-converting enzyme [ACE] inhibitor) except those in whom it is specifically contraindicated (patients with heart failure or severely compromised LV function, heart block, orthostatic hypotension, or a history of asthma) and perhaps those whose excellent long-term prognosis (defined as an expected mortality rate of <1% per year, patients <55 years, no previous MI, with normal ventricular function, no complex ventricular ectopy, and no angina) markedly diminishes any potential benefit.

INHIBITION OF THE RENIN-ANGIOTENSIN-ALDOSTERONE SYSTEM

ACE inhibitors reduce the mortality rate after STEMI, and the mortality benefits are additive to those achieved with aspirin and beta blockers. The maximum benefit is seen in high-risk patients (those who are elderly or who have an anterior infarction, a prior infarction, and/or globally depressed LV function), but evidence suggests that a short-term benefit occurs when ACE inhibitors are prescribed unselectively to all hemodynamically stable patients with STEMI (i.e., those with a systolic pressure >100 mmHg). The mechanism involves a reduction in ventricular remodeling after infarction (see "Ventricular Dysfunction," later) with a subsequent reduction in the risk of CHF. The rate of recurrent infarction may also be lower in patients treated chronically with ACE inhibitors after infarction.

Before hospital discharge, LV function should be assessed with an imaging study. ACE inhibitors should be continued indefinitely in patients who have clinically evident CHF, in patients in whom an imaging study shows a reduction in global LV function or a large regional wall motion abnormality, or in those who are hypertensive.

Angiotensin receptor blockers (ARBs) should be administered to STEMI patients who are intolerant of ACE inhibitors and who have either clinical or radiological signs of heart failure. Long-term aldosterone blockade should be prescribed for STEMI patients without significant renal dysfunction (creatinine ≥2.5 mg/dL in men and ≥2.0 mg/dL in women) or hyperkalemia (potassium ≥5.0 mEq/L) who are already receiving therapeutic doses of an ACE inhibitor, an LV ejection fraction ≤40 percent, and either symptomatic heart failure or diabetes mellitus. A multidrug regimen for inhibiting the renin-angiotensin-aldosterone system has been shown to reduce both heart failure–related and sudden cardiac death–related cardiovascular mortality after STEMI, but has not been as thoroughly explored as ACE inhibitors in STEMI patients.

OTHER AGENTS

Favorable effects on the ischemic process and ventricular remodeling (see later) previously led many physicians to routinely use *intravenous nitroglycerin* (5–10 μg/min initial dose and up to 200 μg/min as long as hemodynamic stability is maintained) for the first 24–48 h after the onset of infarction. However, the benefits of routine use of intravenous nitroglycerin are less in the contemporary era where beta-adrenoceptor blockers and ACE inhibitors are routinely prescribed for patients with STEMI.

Results of multiple trials of different calcium antagonists have failed to establish a role for these agents in the treatment of most patients with STEMI. Therefore, the routine use of calcium antagonists cannot be recommended. Strict control of blood glucose in diabetic patients with STEMI has been shown to reduce the

mortality rate. Serum magnesium should be measured in all patients on admission, and any demonstrated deficits should be corrected to minimize the risk of arrhythmias.

COMPLICATIONS AND THEIR MANAGEMENT

VENTRICULAR DYSFUNCTION

After STEMI, the left ventricle undergoes a series of changes in shape, size, and thickness in both the infarcted and noninfarcted segments. This process is referred to as *ventricular remodeling* and generally precedes the development of clinically evident CHF in the months to years after infarction. Soon after STEMI, the left ventricle begins to dilate. Acutely, this results from expansion of the infarct, i.e., slippage of muscle bundles, disruption of normal myocardial cells, and tissue loss within the necrotic zone, resulting in disproportionate thinning and elongation of the infarct zone. Later, lengthening of the noninfarcted segments occurs as well. The overall chamber enlargement that occurs is related to the size and location of the infarct, with greater dilation following infarction of the anterior wall and apex of the left ventricle and causing more marked hemodynamic impairment, more frequent heart failure, and a poorer prognosis. Progressive dilation and its clinical consequences may be ameliorated by therapy with ACE inhibitors and other vasodilators (e.g., nitrates). In patients with an ejection fraction <40%, regardless of whether or not heart failure is present, ACE inhibitors or ARBs should be prescribed (see "Inhibition of the Renin-Angiotensin-Aldosterone System").

HEMODYNAMIC ASSESSMENT

Pump failure is now the primary cause of in-hospital death from STEMI. The extent of infarction correlates well with the degree of pump failure and with mortality, both early (within 10 days of infarction) and later. The most common clinical signs are pulmonary rales and S_3 and S_4 gallop sounds. Pulmonary congestion is also frequently seen on the chest roentgenogram. Elevated LV filling pressure and elevated pulmonary artery pressure are the characteristic hemodynamic findings, but these findings may result from a reduction of ventricular compliance (diastolic failure) and/or a reduction of stroke volume with secondary cardiac dilation (systolic failure).

A classification originally proposed by Killip divides patients into four groups: class I, no signs of pulmonary or venous congestion; class II, moderate heart failure as evidenced by rales at the lung bases, S_3 gallop, tachypnea, or signs of failure of the right side of the heart, including venous and hepatic congestion; class III, severe heart failure, pulmonary edema; and class IV, shock with systolic pressure <90 mmHg and evidence of peripheral vasoconstriction, peripheral cyanosis, mental confusion, and oliguria. When this classification was established in 1967, the expected hospital mortality rate of patients in these classes was as follows: class I, 0–5%; class II, 10–20%; class III, 35–45%; and class IV, 85–95%. With advances in management, the mortality rate in each class has fallen, perhaps by as much as one-third to one-half.

Hemodynamic evidence of abnormal global LV function appears when contraction is seriously impaired in 20–25% of the left ventricle. Infarction of ≥40% of the left ventricle usually results in cardiogenic shock (Chap. 30). Positioning of a balloon flotation (Swan-Ganz) catheter in the pulmonary artery permits monitoring of LV filling pressure; this technique is useful in patients who exhibit hypotension and/or clinical evidence of CHF. Cardiac output can also be determined with a pulmonary artery catheter. With the addition of intra-arterial pressure monitoring, systemic vascular resistance can be calculated as a guide to adjusting vasopressor and vasodilator therapy. Some patients with STEMI have markedly elevated LV filling pressures (>22 mmHg) and normal cardiac indices (2.6–3.6 L/[min/m^2]), while others have relatively low LV filling pressures (<15 mmHg) and reduced cardiac indices. The former patients usually benefit from diuresis, while the latter may respond to volume expansion.

HYPOVOLEMIA

This is an easily corrected condition that may contribute to the hypotension and vascular collapse associated with STEMI in some patients. It may be secondary to previous diuretic use, to reduced fluid intake during the early stages of the illness, and/or to vomiting associated with pain or medications. Consequently, hypovolemia should be identified and corrected in patients with STEMI and hypotension before more vigorous forms of therapy are begun. Central venous pressure reflects RV rather than LV filling pressure and is an inadequate guide for adjustment of blood volume, because LV function is almost always affected much more adversely than RV function in patients with STEMI. The optimal LV filling or pulmonary artery wedge pressure may vary considerably among patients. Each patient's ideal level (generally ~20 mmHg) is reached by cautious fluid administration during careful monitoring of oxygenation and cardiac output. Eventually, the cardiac output level plateaus, and further increases in LV filling pressure only increase congestive symptoms and decrease systemic oxygenation without raising arterial pressure.

TREATMENT   Congestive Heart Failure

The management of CHF in association with STEMI is similar to that of acute heart failure secondary to other forms of heart disease (avoidance of hypoxemia, diuresis, afterload reduction, inotropic support), except that the benefits of digitalis administration to patients with STEMI are unimpressive. By contrast, diuretic agents are extremely effective, as they diminish pulmonary congestion in the presence of systolic and/or diastolic heart failure. LV filling pressure falls and orthopnea and dyspnea improve after the intravenous administration of furosemide or other loop diuretics. These drugs should be used with caution, however, as they can result in a massive diuresis with associated decreases in plasma volume, cardiac output, systemic blood pressure, and, hence, coronary perfusion. Nitrates in various forms may be used to decrease preload and congestive symptoms. Oral isosorbide dinitrate, topical nitroglycerin ointment, or intravenous nitroglycerin all have the advantage over a diuretic of lowering preload through venodilation without decreasing the total plasma volume. In addition, nitrates may improve ventricular compliance if ischemia is present, as ischemia causes an elevation of LV filling pressure. Vasodilators must be used with caution to prevent serious hypotension. As noted earlier, ACE inhibitors are an ideal class of drugs for management of ventricular dysfunction after STEMI, especially for the long term. (See "Inhibition of the Renin-Angiotensin-Aldosterone System," earlier.)

CARDIOGENIC SHOCK

Prompt reperfusion, efforts to reduce infarct size and treatment of ongoing ischemia and other complications of MI appear to have reduced the incidence of cardiogenic shock from 20% to about 7%. Only 10% of patients with this condition present with it on admission, while 90% develop it during hospitalization. Typically, patients who develop cardiogenic shock have severe multivessel coronary artery disease with evidence of "piecemeal" necrosis extending outward from the original infarct zone. The evaluation and management of cardiogenic shock and severe power failure after STEMI are discussed in detail in Chap. 30.

RIGHT VENTRICULAR INFARCTION

Approximately one-third of patients with inferior infarction demonstrate at least a minor degree of RV necrosis. An occasional patient with inferoposterior LV infarction also has extensive RV infarction, and rare patients present with infarction limited primarily to the

RV. Clinically significant RV infarction causes signs of severe RV failure (jugular venous distention, Kussmaul's sign, hepatomegaly) with or without hypotension. ST-segment elevations of right-sided precordial ECG leads, particularly lead V_4R, are frequently present in the first 24 h in patients with RV infarction. Two-dimensional echocardiography is helpful in determining the degree of RV dysfunction. Catheterization of the right side of the heart often reveals a distinctive hemodynamic pattern resembling constrictive pericarditis (steep right atrial "y" descent and an early diastolic dip and plateau in RV waveforms). Therapy consists of volume expansion to maintain adequate RV preload and efforts to improve LV performance with attendant reduction in pulmonary capillary wedge and pulmonary arterial pressures.

ARRHYTHMIAS

The incidence of arrhythmias after STEMI is higher in patients seen early after the onset of symptoms. The mechanisms responsible for infarction-related arrhythmias include autonomic nervous system imbalance, electrolyte disturbances, ischemia, and slowed conduction in zones of ischemic myocardium. An arrhythmia can usually be managed successfully if trained personnel and appropriate equipment are available when it develops. Since most deaths from arrhythmia occur during the first few hours after infarction, the effectiveness of treatment relates directly to the speed with which patients come under medical observation. The prompt management of arrhythmias constitutes a significant advance in the treatment of STEMI.

Ventricular premature beats

Infrequent, sporadic ventricular premature depolarizations occur in almost all patients with STEMI and do not require therapy. Whereas in the past, frequent, multifocal, or early diastolic ventricular extrasystoles (so-called warning arrhythmias) were routinely treated with antiarrhythmic drugs to reduce the risk of development of ventricular tachycardia and ventricular fibrillation, pharmacologic therapy is now reserved for patients with sustained ventricular arrhythmias. Prophylactic antiarrhythmic therapy (either intravenous lidocaine early or oral agents later) is contraindicated for ventricular premature beats in the absence of clinically important ventricular tachyarrhythmias, as such therapy may actually increase the mortality rate. Beta-adrenoceptor blocking agents are effective in abolishing ventricular ectopic activity in patients with STEMI and in the prevention of ventricular fibrillation. As described earlier (see "Beta-Adrenoceptor Blockers"), they should be used routinely in patients without contraindications. In addition, hypokalemia and hypomagnesemia are risk factors for ventricular fibrillation in patients with STEMI; to reduce the risk, the serum potassium concentration should be adjusted to approximately 4.5 mmol/L and magnesium to about 2.0 mmol/L.

Ventricular tachycardia and fibrillation

Within the first 24 h of STEMI, ventricular tachycardia and fibrillation can occur without prior warning arrhythmias. The occurrence of ventricular fibrillation can be reduced by prophylactic administration of intravenous lidocaine. However, prophylactic use of lidocaine has not been shown to reduce overall mortality from STEMI. In fact, in addition to causing possible noncardiac complications, lidocaine may predispose to an excess risk of bradycardia and asystole. For these reasons, and with earlier treatment of active ischemia, more frequent use of beta-blocking agents, and the nearly universal success of electrical cardioversion or defibrillation, routine prophylactic antiarrhythmic drug therapy *is no longer recommended*.

Sustained ventricular tachycardia that is well tolerated hemodynamically should be treated with an intravenous regimen of amiodarone (bolus of 150 mg over 10 min, followed by infusion of 1.0 mg/min for 6 h and then 0.5 mg/min) or procainamide (bolus of 15 mg/kg over 20–30 min; infusion of 1–4 mg/min); if it does not stop promptly, electroversion should be used. An unsynchronized discharge of 200–300 J (monophasic wave form; approximately 50% of these energies with biphasic wave forms) is used immediately in patients with ventricular fibrillation or when ventricular tachycardia causes hemodynamic deterioration. Ventricular tachycardia or fibrillation that is refractory to electroshock may be more responsive after the patient is treated with epinephrine (1 mg intravenously or 10 mL of a 1:10,000 solution via the intracardiac route) or amiodarone (a 75–150-mg bolus).

Ventricular arrhythmias, including the unusual form of ventricular tachycardia known as torsades des pointes, may occur in patients with STEMI as a consequence of other concurrent problems (such as hypoxia, hypokalemia, or other electrolyte disturbances) or of the toxic effects of an agent being administered to the patient (such as digoxin or quinidine). A search for such secondary causes should always be undertaken.

Although the in-hospital mortality rate is increased, the long-term survival is excellent in patients who survive to hospital discharge after *primary* ventricular fibrillation; i.e., ventricular fibrillation that is a primary response to acute ischemia that occurs during the first 48 h and is not associated with predisposing factors such as CHF, shock, bundle branch block, or ventricular aneurysm. This result is in sharp contrast to the poor prognosis for patients who develop ventricular fibrillation *secondary* to severe pump failure. For patients who develop ventricular tachycardia or ventricular fibrillation late in their hospital course (i.e., after the first 48 h), the mortality rate is increased both in-hospital and during long-term follow-up. Such patients should be considered for electrophysiologic study and implantation of a cardioverter/defibrillator (ICD). A more challenging issue is the prevention of sudden cardiac death from ventricular fibrillation late after STEMI in patients who have not exhibited sustained ventricular tachyarrhythmias during their index hospitalization. An algorithm for selection of patients who warrant prophylactic implantation of an ICD is shown in **Fig. 33-6**.

Accelerated idioventricular rhythm

Accelerated idioventricular rhythm (AIVR, "slow ventricular tachycardia"), a ventricular rhythm with a rate of 60–100 bpm, often occurs transiently during

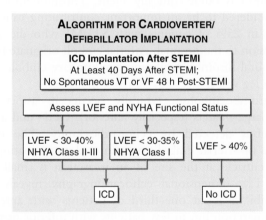

ALGORITHM FOR CARDIOVERTER/ DEFIBRILLATOR IMPLANTATION

ICD Implantation After STEMI
At Least 40 Days After STEMI;
No Spontaneous VT or VF 48 h Post-STEMI

Assess LVEF and NYHA Functional Status

LVEF < 30-40% NHYA Class II-III | LVEF < 30-35% NHYA Class I | LVEF > 40%

ICD | No ICD

FIGURE 33-6

Algorithm for assessment of need for implantation of a cardioverter/defibrillator. The appropriate management is selected based upon measurement of left ventricular ejection fraction and assessment of the NYHA functional class. Patients with depressed left ventricular function at least 40 days post-STEMI are referred for insertion of an implantable cardioverter/defibrillator (ICD) if the LVEF is <30–40% and they are in NYHA class II–III or if the LVEF is <30–35% and they are in NYHA class I functional status. Patients with preserved left ventricular function (LVEF >40%) do not receive an ICD regardless of NYHA functional class. All patients are treated with medical therapy post-STEMI. (*Adapted from data contained in Zipes DP, et al: ACC/AHA/ESC 2006 guidelines for management of patients with ventricular arrhythmias and the prevention of sudden cardiac death; a report of the American College of Cardiology/American Heart Association Task Force and the European Society of Cardiology Committee for Practice Guidelines [Writing Committee to Develop Guidelines for Management of Patients with Ventricular Arrhythmias and the Prevention of Sudden Cardiac Death]. J Am Coll Cardiol 48:1064, 2006.*)

fibrinolytic therapy at the time of reperfusion. For the most part, AIVR, whether it occurs in association with fibrinolytic therapy or spontaneously, is benign and does not presage the development of classic ventricular tachycardia. Most episodes of AIVR do not require treatment if the patient is monitored carefully, as degeneration into a more serious arrhythmia is rare.

Supraventricular arrhythmias

Sinus tachycardia is the most common supraventricular arrhythmia. If it occurs secondary to another cause (such as anemia, fever, heart failure, or a metabolic derangement), the primary problem should be treated first. However, if it appears to be due to sympathetic overstimulation (e.g., as part of a hyperdynamic state), then treatment with a beta blocker is indicated. Other common arrhythmias in this group are atrial flutter and atrial fibrillation, which are often secondary to LV failure. Digoxin is usually the treatment of choice for supraventricular arrhythmias if heart failure is present. If heart failure is absent, beta blockers, verapamil, or diltiazem are suitable alternatives for controlling the ventricular rate, as they may also help to control ischemia. If the abnormal rhythm persists for >2 h with a ventricular rate >120 bpm, or if tachycardia induces heart failure, shock, or ischemia (as manifested by recurrent pain or ECG changes), a synchronized electroshock (100–200 J monophasic wave form) should be used.

Accelerated junctional rhythms have diverse causes but may occur in patients with inferoposterior infarction. Digitalis excess must be ruled out. In some patients with severely compromised LV function, the loss of appropriately timed atrial systole results in a marked reduction of cardiac output. Right atrial or coronary sinus pacing is indicated in such instances.

Sinus bradycardia

Treatment of sinus bradycardia is indicated if hemodynamic compromise results from the slow heart rate. Atropine is the most useful drug for increasing heart rate and should be given intravenously in doses of 0.5 mg initially. If the rate remains <50–60 bpm, additional doses of 0.2 mg, up to a total of 2.0 mg, may be given. Persistent bradycardia (<40 bpm) despite atropine may be treated with electrical pacing. Isoproterenol should be avoided.

Atrioventricular and intraventricular conduction disturbances

Both the in-hospital mortality rate and the post-discharge mortality rate of patients who have complete atrioventricular (AV) block in association with anterior infarction are markedly higher than those of patients who develop AV block with inferior infarction. This difference is related to the fact that heart block in inferior infarction is commonly a result of increased vagal tone and/or the release of adenosine and therefore is transient. In anterior wall infarction, however, heart block is usually related to ischemic malfunction of the conduction system, which is commonly associated with extensive myocardial necrosis.

Temporary electrical pacing provides an effective means of increasing the heart rate of patients with bradycardia due to AV block. However, acceleration of the heart rate may have only a limited impact on prognosis in patients with anterior wall infarction and complete heart block in whom the large size of the infarct is the major factor determining outcome. It should be carried out if it improves hemodynamics. Pacing does appear to be beneficial in patients with inferoposterior infarction who have complete heart block associated with heart failure, hypotension, marked bradycardia, or significant ventricular ectopic activity. A subgroup of these patients, those with RV infarction, often respond poorly to ventricular pacing because of the loss of the atrial contribution to ventricular filling. In such patients, dual-chamber AV sequential pacing may be required.

External noninvasive pacing electrodes should be positioned in a "demand" mode for patients with sinus bradycardia (rate <50 bpm) that is unresponsive to drug therapy, Mobitz II second-degree AV block, third-degree heart block, or bilateral bundle branch block (e.g., right bundle branch block plus left anterior fascicular block). Retrospective studies suggest that permanent pacing may reduce the long-term risk of sudden death due to bradyarrhythmias in the rare patient who develops combined persistent bifascicular and transient third-degree heart block during the acute phase of MI.

OTHER COMPLICATIONS
Recurrent chest discomfort

Recurrent angina develops in ~25% of patients hospitalized for STEMI. This percentage is even higher in patients who undergo successful fibrinolysis. Because recurrent or persistent ischemia often heralds extension of the original infarct or reinfarction in a new myocardial zone and is associated with a near tripling of mortality after STEMI, patients with these symptoms should be referred for prompt coronary arteriography and mechanical revascularization. Repeat administration of a fibrinolytic agent is an alternative to early mechanical revascularization.

Pericarditis

Pericardial friction rubs and/or pericardial pain are frequently encountered in patients with STEMI involving the epicardium. This complication can usually be managed with aspirin (650 mg 4 times daily). It is important to diagnose the chest pain of pericarditis accurately, because failure to recognize it may lead to the erroneous diagnosis of recurrent ischemic pain and/or infarct extension, with resulting inappropriate use of anticoagulants, nitrates, beta blockers, or coronary arteriography. When it occurs, complaints of pain radiating to either trapezius muscle is helpful, because such a pattern of discomfort is typical of pericarditis but rarely occurs with ischemic discomfort. Anticoagulants potentially could cause tamponade in the presence of acute pericarditis (as manifested by either pain or persistent rub) and therefore should not be used unless there is a compelling indication.

Thromboembolism

Clinically apparent thromboembolism complicates STEMI in ~10% of cases, but embolic lesions are found in 20% of patients in necropsy series, suggesting that thromboembolism is often clinically silent. Thromboembolism is considered to be an important contributing cause of death in 25% of patients with STEMI who die after admission to the hospital. Arterial emboli originate from LV mural thrombi, while most pulmonary emboli arise in the leg veins.

Thromboembolism typically occurs in association with large infarcts (especially anterior), CHF, and a LV thrombus detected by echocardiography. The incidence of arterial embolism from a clot originating in the ventricle at the site of an infarction is small but real. Two-dimensional echocardiography reveals LV thrombi in about one-third of patients with anterior wall infarction but in few patients with inferior or posterior infarction. Arterial embolism often presents as a major complication, such as hemiparesis when the cerebral circulation is involved or hypertension if the renal circulation is compromised. When a thrombus has been clearly demonstrated by echocardiographic or other techniques or when a large area of regional wall motion abnormality is seen even in the absence of a detectable mural thrombus, systemic anticoagulation should be undertaken (in the absence of contraindications), as the incidence of embolic complications appears to be markedly lowered by such therapy. The appropriate duration of therapy is unknown, but 3–6 months is probably prudent.

Left ventricular aneurysm

The term *ventricular aneurysm* is usually used to describe *dyskinesis* or local expansile paradoxical wall motion. Normally functioning myocardial fibers must shorten more if stroke volume and cardiac output are to be maintained in patients with ventricular aneurysm; if they cannot, overall ventricular function is impaired. True aneurysms are composed of scar tissue and neither predispose to nor are associated with cardiac rupture.

The complications of LV aneurysm do not usually occur for weeks to months after STEMI; they include CHF, arterial embolism, and ventricular arrhythmias. Apical aneurysms are the most common and the most easily detected by clinical examination. The physical finding of greatest value is a double, diffuse, or displaced apical impulse. Ventricular aneurysms are readily detected by two-dimensional echocardiography, which may also reveal a mural thrombus in an aneurysm.

Rarely, myocardial rupture may be contained by a local area of pericardium, along with organizing thrombus and hematoma. Over time, this *pseudoaneurysm* enlarges, maintaining communication with the LV cavity through a narrow neck. Because a pseudoaneurysm often ruptures spontaneously, it should be surgically repaired if recognized.

POSTINFARCTION RISK STRATIFICATION AND MANAGEMENT

Many clinical and laboratory factors have been identified that are associated with an increase in cardiovascular risk after initial recovery from STEMI. Some of the most important factors include persistent ischemia (spontaneous or provoked), depressed LV ejection fraction (<40%), rales above the lung bases on physical examination or congestion on chest radiograph, and symptomatic ventricular arrhythmias. Other features associated with increased risk include a history of previous MI, age >75, diabetes mellitus, prolonged sinus tachycardia, hypotension, ST-segment changes at rest without angina ("silent ischemia"), an abnormal signal-averaged ECG, nonpatency of the infarct-related coronary artery (if angiography is undertaken), and persistent advanced heart block or a new intraventricular conduction abnormality on the ECG. Therapy must be individualized on the basis of the relative importance of the risk(s) present.

The goal of preventing reinfarction and death after recovery from STEMI has led to strategies to evaluate risk after infarction. In stable patients, submaximal exercise stress testing may be carried out before hospital discharge to detect residual ischemia and ventricular ectopy and to provide the patient with a guideline for exercise in the early recovery period. Alternatively, or in addition, a maximal (symptom-limited) exercise stress test may be carried out 4–6 weeks after infarction. Evaluation of LV function is usually warranted as well. Recognition of a depressed LV ejection fraction by echocardiography or radionuclide ventriculography identifies patients who should receive medications to inhibit the renin-angiotensin-aldosterone system. Patients in whom angina is induced at relatively low workloads, those who have a large reversible defect on perfusion imaging or a depressed ejection fraction, those with demonstrable ischemia, and those in whom exercise provokes symptomatic ventricular arrhythmias should be considered at high risk for recurrent MI or death from arrhythmia (Fig. 33-6). Cardiac catheterization with coronary angiography and/or invasive electrophysiologic evaluation is advised.

Exercise tests also aid in formulating an individualized exercise prescription, which can be much more vigorous in patients who tolerate exercise without any of the earlier-mentioned adverse signs. In addition, predischarge stress testing may provide an important psychological benefit, building the patient's confidence by demonstrating a reasonable exercise tolerance.

In many hospitals, a cardiac rehabilitation program with progressive exercise is initiated in the hospital and continued after discharge. Ideally, such programs should include an educational component that informs patients about their disease and its risk factors.

The usual duration of hospitalization for an uncomplicated STEMI is about 5 days. The remainder of the convalescent phase may be accomplished at home. During the first 1–2 weeks, the patient should be encouraged to increase activity by walking about the house and outdoors in good weather. Normal sexual activity may be resumed during this period. After 2 weeks, the physician must regulate the patient's activity on the basis of exercise tolerance. Most patients will be able to return to work within 2–4 weeks.

SECONDARY PREVENTION

Various secondary preventive measures are at least partly responsible for the improvement in the long-term mortality and morbidity rates after STEMI. Long-term treatment with an antiplatelet agent (usually aspirin) after STEMI is associated with a 25% reduction in the risk of recurrent infarction, stroke, or cardiovascular mortality (36 fewer events for every 1000 patients treated). An alternative antiplatelet agent that may be used for secondary prevention in patients intolerant of aspirin is clopidogrel (75 mg orally daily). ACE inhibitors or ARBs and, in appropriate patients, aldosterone antagonists should be used indefinitely by patients with clinically evident heart failure, a moderate decrease in global ejection fraction, or a large regional wall motion abnormality to prevent late ventricular remodeling and recurrent ischemic events.

The chronic routine use of oral beta-adrenoceptor blockers for at least two years after STEMI is supported by well-conducted, placebo-controlled trials.

Evidence suggests that warfarin lowers the risk of late mortality and the incidence of reinfarction after STEMI. Most physicians prescribe aspirin routinely for all patients without contraindications and add warfarin for patients at increased risk of embolism (see "Thromboembolism," earlier). Several studies suggest that in patients <75 years a low dose of aspirin (75–81 mg/d) in combination with warfarin administered to achieve an INR >2.0 is more effective than aspirin alone for preventing recurrent MI and embolic cerebrovascular accident. However, there is an increased risk of bleeding and a high rate of discontinuation of warfarin that has limited clinical acceptance of combination

antithrombotic therapy. There is increased risk of bleeding when warfarin is added to dual antiplatelet therapy (aspirin and clopidogrel). However, patients who have had a stent implanted and have an indication for anticoagulation should receive dual antiplatelet therapies in combination with warfarin. Such patients should also receive a proton pump inhibitor to minimize the risk of gastrointestinal bleeding and should have regular monitoring of their hemoglobin levels and stool hematest while on combination antithrombotic therapy.

Finally, risk factors for *atherosclerosis* should be discussed with the patient, and, when possible, favorably modified.

CHAPTER 34

COMA

Allan H. Ropper

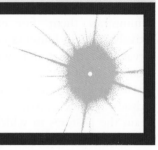

Coma is among the most common and striking problems in general medicine. It accounts for a substantial portion of admissions to emergency wards and occurs on all hospital services. Coma demands immediate attention and requires an organized approach.

There is a continuum of states of reduced alertness, the most severe form being *coma*, defined as a deep sleeplike state from which the patient cannot be aroused. *Stupor* refers to a higher degree of arousability in which the patient can be transiently awakened only by vigorous stimuli, accompanied by motor behavior that leads to avoidance of uncomfortable or aggravating stimuli. *Drowsiness*, which is familiar to all persons, simulates light sleep and is characterized by easy arousal and the persistence of alertness for brief periods. Drowsiness and stupor are usually accompanied by some degree of confusion. A precise narrative description of the level of arousal and of the type of responses evoked by various stimuli as observed at the bedside is preferable to ambiguous terms such as *lethargy*, *semicoma*, or *obtundation*.

Several other conditions that render patients unresponsive and thereby simulate coma are considered separately because of their special significance. The *vegetative state* signifies an awake but nonresponsive state in a patient who has emerged from coma. In the vegetative state, the eyelids may open, giving the appearance of wakefulness. Respiratory and autonomic functions are retained. Yawning, coughing, swallowing, as well as limb and head movements persist and the patient may follow visually presented objects, but there are few, if any, meaningful responses to the external and internal environment—in essence, an "awake coma." The term *vegetative* is unfortunate as it is subject to misinterpretation. There are always accompanying signs that indicate extensive damage in both cerebral hemispheres, e.g., decerebrate or decorticate limb posturing and absent responses to visual stimuli (see later). In the closely related but less severe *minimally conscious state*,

the patient has rudimentary vocal or motor behaviors, often spontaneous, but some in response to touch, visual stimuli, or command. Cardiac arrest with cerebral hypoperfusion and head injuries are the most common causes of the vegetative and minimally conscious states (Chaps. 31 and 35). The prognosis for regaining mental faculties once the vegetative state has supervened for several months is very poor, and after a year, almost nil, hence the term *persistent vegetative state*. Most reports of dramatic recovery, when investigated carefully, are found to yield to the usual rules for prognosis but there have been rare instances in which recovery has occurred to a severely disabled condition and, in rare childhood cases, to an even better state. The possibility of incorrectly attributing meaningful behavior to patients in the vegetative and minimally conscious states has created inordinate problems and anguish for families. On the other hand, the question of whether these patients lack any capability for cognition has been reopened by functional imaging studies demonstrating, in a small proportion of posttraumatic cases, cerebral activation in response to external stimuli.

Apart from the earlier mentioned conditions, several syndromes that affect alertness are prone to be misinterpreted as stupor or coma. *Akinetic mutism* refers to a partially or fully awake state in which the patient is able to form impressions and think, as demonstrated by later recounting of events, but remains virtually immobile and mute. The condition results from damage in the regions of the medial thalamic nuclei or the frontal lobes (particularly lesions situated deeply or on the orbitofrontal surfaces) or from extreme hydrocephalus. The term *abulia* describes a milder form of akinetic mutism characterized by mental and physical slowness and diminished ability to initiate activity. It is also usually the result of damage to the frontal lobes and its connections. *Catatonia* is a curious hypomobile and mute syndrome that occurs as part of a major psychosis, usually schizophrenia or major depression. Catatonic patients make few voluntary or responsive movements, although they blink, swallow, and may not appear distressed. There are nonetheless signs that the patient is responsive, although it may take ingenuity on the part of the examiner to demonstrate them. For example, eyelid elevation is actively resisted, blinking occurs in response to a visual threat, and the eyes move concomitantly with head rotation, all of which are inconsistent with the presence of a brain lesion causing unresponsiveness. It is characteristic but not invariable in catatonia for the limbs to retain the postures in which they have been placed by the examiner ("waxy flexibility," or catalepsy). With recovery, patients often have some memory of events that occurred during their catatonic stupor. Catatonia is superficially similar to akinetic mutism, but clinical evidence of cerebral damage such as Babinski signs and hypertonicity of the limbs is lacking. The special problem of coma in brain death is discussed later.

The *locked-in state* describes yet another type of pseudocoma in which an awake patient has no means of producing speech or volitional movement but retains voluntary vertical eye movements and lid elevation, thus allowing the patient to signal with a clear mind. The pupils are normally reactive. Such individuals have written entire treatises using Morse code. The usual cause is an infarction or hemorrhage of the ventral pons that transects all descending motor (corticospinal and corticobulbar) pathways. A similar awake but de-efferented state occurs as a result of total paralysis of the musculature in severe cases of Guillain-Barré syndrome, critical illness neuropathy (Chap. 35), and pharmacologic neuromuscular blockade.

THE ANATOMY AND PHYSIOLOGY OF COMA

Almost all instances of diminished alertness can be traced to widespread abnormalities of the cerebral hemispheres or to reduced activity of a special thalamocortical alerting system termed the *reticular activating system* (RAS). The proper functioning of this system, its ascending projections to the cortex, and the cortex itself are required to maintain alertness and coherence of thought. It follows that the principal causes of coma are (1) lesions that damage the RAS in the upper midbrain or its projections; (2) destruction of large portions of both cerebral hemispheres; and (3) suppression of reticulocerebral function by drugs, toxins, or metabolic derangements such as hypoglycemia, anoxia, uremia, and hepatic failure.

The proximity of the RAS to midbrain structures that control pupillary function and eye movements permits clinical localization of the cause of coma in many cases. Pupillary enlargement with loss of light reaction and loss of vertical and adduction movements of the eyes suggests that the lesion is in the upper brainstem.

Conversely, preservation of pupillary light reactivity and of eye movements absolves the upper brainstem and indicates that widespread structural lesions or metabolic suppression of the cerebral hemispheres is responsible for coma.

Coma due to cerebral mass lesions and herniations

The cranial cavity is separated into compartments by infoldings of the dura. The two cerebral hemispheres are separated by the falx, and the anterior and posterior fossae by the tentorium. Herniation refers to displacement of brain tissue into a compartment that it normally does not occupy. Coma and many of its associated signs can be attributed to these tissue shifts, and certain clinical features are characteristic of specific herniations (Fig. 34-1). They are in essence "false localizing" signs since they derive from compression of brain structures at a distance from the mass.

The most common herniations are those in which a part of the brain is displaced from the supratentorial to the infratentorial compartment through the tentorial opening; this is referred to as *transtentorial* herniation. *Uncal transtentorial* herniation refers to impaction of the anterior medial temporal gyrus (the uncus) into the tentorial opening just anterior to and adjacent to the midbrain (Fig. 34-1A). The uncus compresses the third nerve as it traverses the subarachnoid space, causing enlargement of the ipsilateral pupil (putatively because the fibers subserving parasympathetic pupillary function

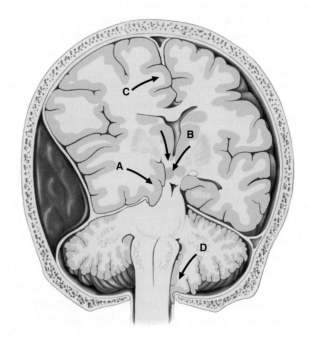

FIGURE 34-1

Types of cerebral herniation. (*A*) uncal; (*B*) central; (*C*) transfalcial; (*D*) foraminal.

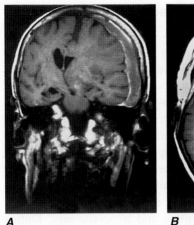 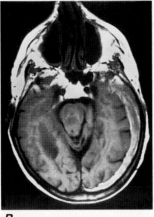

A B

FIGURE 34-2
Coronal (**A**) and axial (**B**) magnetic resonance images from a stuporous patient with a left third nerve palsy as a result of a large left-sided subdural hematoma (seen as a gray-white rim). The upper midbrain and lower thalamic regions are compressed and displaced horizontally away from the mass, and there is transtentorial herniation of the medial temporal lobe structures, including the uncus anteriorly. The lateral ventricle opposite to the hematoma has become enlarged as a result of compression of the third ventricle.

are located peripherally in the nerve). The coma that follows is due to compression of the midbrain against the opposite tentorial edge by the displaced parahippocampal gyrus (**Fig. 34-2**). Lateral displacement of the midbrain may compress the opposite cerebral peduncle, producing a Babinski's sign and hemiparesis contralateral to the original hemiparesis (the Kernohan-Woltman sign). Herniation may also compress the anterior and posterior cerebral arteries as they pass over the tentorial reflections, with resultant brain infarction. The distortions may also entrap portions of the ventricular system, resulting in hydrocephalus.

Central transtentorial herniation denotes a symmetric downward movement of the thalamic medial structures through the tentorial opening with compression of the upper midbrain (**Fig. 34-1B**). Miotic pupils and drowsiness are the heralding signs. Both temporal and central transtentorial herniations have been considered causes of progressive compression of the brainstem, with initial damage to the midbrain, then the pons, and finally the medulla. The result is a sequence of neurologic signs that corresponds to each affected level. Other forms of herniation are *transfalcial herniation* (displacement of the cingulate gyrus under the falx and across the midline, **Fig. 34-1C**), and *foraminal herniation* (downward forcing of the cerebellar tonsils into the foramen magnum, **Fig. 34-1D**), which causes compression of the medulla, respiratory arrest, and death.

A direct relationship between the various configurations of transtentorial herniation and coma is not always

found. Drowsiness and stupor can occur with moderate horizontal displacement of the diencephalon (thalamus), before transtentorial herniation is evident. This lateral shift may be quantified on axial images of CT and MRI scans (**Fig. 34-2**). In cases of *acutely appearing masses*, horizontal displacement of the pineal calcification of 3–5 mm is generally associated with drowsiness, 6–8 mm with stupor, and >9 mm with coma. Intrusion of the medial temporal lobe into the tentorial opening is also apparent on MRI and CT scans as obliteration of the cisterna that surround the upper brainstem.

Coma due to metabolic disorders

Many systemic metabolic abnormalities cause coma by interrupting the delivery of energy substrates (e.g., hypoxia, ischemia, hypoglycemia) or by altering neuronal excitability (drug and alcohol intoxication, anesthesia, and epilepsy). The same metabolic abnormalities that produce coma may, in milder forms, induce an acute confusional state. Thus, in metabolic encephalopathies, clouded consciousness and coma are in a continuum.

Cerebral neurons are fully dependent on cerebral blood flow (CBF) and the delivery of oxygen and glucose. CBF is ~75 mL per 100g/min in gray matter and 30 mL per 100 g/min in white matter (mean ~55 mL per 100 g/min); oxygen consumption is 3.5 mL per 100 g/min, and glucose utilization is 5 mg per 100 g/min. Brain stores of glucose provide energy for ~2 min after blood flow is interrupted, and oxygen stores last 8–10 s after the cessation of blood flow. Simultaneous hypoxia and ischemia exhaust glucose more rapidly. The electroencephalogram (EEG) rhythm in these circumstances becomes diffusely slowed, typical of metabolic encephalopathies, and as conditions of substrate delivery worsen, eventually brain electrical activity ceases.

Unlike hypoxia-ischemia, which causes neuronal destruction, most metabolic disorders such as hypoglycemia, hyponatremia, hyperosmolarity, hypercapnia, hypercalcemia, and hepatic and renal failure cause only minor neuropathologic changes. The causes of the reversible effects of these conditions on the brain are not understood but may result from impaired energy supplies, changes in ion fluxes across neuronal membranes, and neurotransmitter abnormalities. For example, the high ammonia concentration of hepatic coma interferes with cerebral energy metabolism and with the Na^+, K^+-ATPase pump, increases the number and size of astrocytes, and causes increased concentrations of potentially toxic products of ammonia metabolism; it may also affect neurotransmitters, including the production of putative "false" neurotransmitters that are active at receptor sites. Apart from hyperammonemia, which of these mechanisms is of critical importance is not clear. The mechanism of the encephalopathy of renal failure is also not known. Unlike ammonia, urea does not produce central nervous system (CNS) toxicity and a multifactorial causation has been proposed for the encephalopathy, including increased permeability of the blood-brain barrier to toxic substances such as organic acids and an increase in brain calcium and cerebrospinal fluid (CSF) phosphate content.

Coma and seizures are common accompaniments of large shifts in sodium and water balance in the brain. These changes in osmolarity arise from systemic medical disorders, including diabetic ketoacidosis, the nonketotic hyperosmolar state, and hyponatremia from any cause (e.g., water intoxication, excessive secretion of antidiuretic hormone, or atrial natriuretic peptides). Sodium levels <125 mmol/L induce confusion, and <115 mmol/L are associated with coma and convulsions. In hyperosmolar coma, the serum osmolarity is generally >350 mosmol/L. Hypercapnia depresses the level of consciousness in proportion to the rise in carbon dioxide (co_2) tension in the blood. *In all of these metabolic encephalopathies, the degree of neurologic change depends to a large extent on the rapidity with which the serum changes occur.* The pathophysiology of other metabolic encephalopathies such as hypercalcemia, hypothyroidism, vitamin B_{12} deficiency, and hypothermia are incompletely understood but must also reflect derangements of CNS biochemistry, membrane function, and neurotransmitters.

Epileptic coma

Generalized electrical discharges of the cortex (*seizures*) are associated with coma, even in the absence of epileptic motor activity (*convulsions*). The self-limited coma that follows a seizure, the *postictal state*, may be due to exhaustion of energy reserves or effects of locally toxic molecules that are the by-product of seizures. The postictal state produces a pattern of continuous, generalized slowing of the background EEG activity similar to that of other metabolic encephalopathies.

Toxic (including drug–induced) coma

This common class of encephalopathy is in large measure reversible and leaves no residual damage provided there has not been cardiorespiratory failure. Many drugs and toxins are capable of depressing nervous system function. Some produce coma by affecting both the brainstem nuclei, including the RAS, and the cerebral cortex. The combination of cortical and brainstem signs, which occurs in certain drug overdoses, may lead to an incorrect diagnosis of structural brainstem disease. Overdose of medications that have atropinic actions produces signs such as dilated pupils, tachycardia, and dry skin; opiate overdose produces pinpoint pupils <1 mm in diameter.

Coma due to widespread damage to the cerebral hemispheres

This category, comprising a number of unrelated disorders, results from widespread structural cerebral damage, thereby simulating a metabolic disorder of the cortex. Hypoxia-ischemia is perhaps the best known and one in which it is not possible initially to distinguish the acute reversible effects of hypoperfusion and oxygen deprivation of the brain from the subsequent effects of neuronal damage. Similar bihemispheral damage is produced by disorders that occlude small blood vessels throughout the brain; examples include cerebral malaria, thrombotic thrombocytopenic purpura, and hyperviscosity. Diffuse white matter damage from cranial trauma or inflammatory demyelinating diseases causes a similar syndrome of coma.

APPROACH TO THE PATIENT | **Coma**

Acute respiratory and cardiovascular problems should be attended to prior to neurologic assessment. In most instances, a complete medical evaluation, except for vital signs, funduscopy, and examination for nuchal rigidity, may be deferred until the neurologic evaluation has established the severity and nature of coma.

HISTORY In many cases, the cause of coma is immediately evident (e.g., trauma, cardiac arrest, or reported drug ingestion). In the remainder, certain points are especially useful: (1) the circumstances and rapidity with which neurologic symptoms developed; (2) the antecedent symptoms (confusion, weakness, headache, fever, seizures, dizziness, double vision, or vomiting); (3) the use of medications, illicit drugs, or alcohol; and (4) chronic liver, kidney, lung, heart, or other medical disease. Direct interrogation of family, observers, and ambulance technicians on the scene, in person or by telephone, is an important part of the evaluation.

GENERAL PHYSICAL EXAMINATION Fever suggests a systemic infection, bacterial meningitis, encephalitis, heat stroke, neuroleptic malignant syndrome, malignant hyperthermia due to anesthetics or anticholinergic drug intoxication; only rarely is it attributable to a lesion that has disturbed hypothalamic temperature-regulating centers ("*central fever*"). A slight elevation in temperature may follow vigorous convulsions. Hypothermia is observed with exposure; alcoholic, barbiturate, sedative, or phenothiazine intoxication; hypoglycemia; peripheral circulatory failure; or extreme hypothyroidism. Hypothermia itself causes coma only when the temperature is <31°C (87.8°F). Tachypnea may indicate systemic acidosis or pneumonia or rarely infiltration of the brain with lymphoma. Aberrant respiratory patterns that reflect brainstem disorders are discussed later. Marked hypertension suggests hypertensive encephalopathy, but it may also be secondary to a rapid rise in intracranial pressure (ICP) (the Cushing response) most often after cerebral hemorrhage or head injury. Hypotension is characteristic of coma from alcohol or barbiturate intoxication, internal hemorrhage, myocardial infarction, sepsis, profound hypothyroidism, or Addisonian crisis.

The funduscopic examination can detect subarachnoid hemorrhage (subhyaloid hemorrhages), hypertensive encephalopathy (exudates, hemorrhages, vessel-crossing changes, papilledema), and increased ICP (papilledema). Cutaneous petechiae suggest thrombotic thrombocytopenic purpura, meningococcemia, or a bleeding diathesis associated with an intracerebral hemorrhage. Cyanosis, reddish or anemic skin coloration are other indications of an underlying systemic disease responsible for the coma.

NEUROLOGIC EXAMINATION The patient should first be observed without intervention by the examiner. Tossing about in the bed, reaching up toward the face, crossing legs, yawning, swallowing, coughing, or moaning reflect a drowsy state that is close to normal awakeness. Lack of restless movements on one side or an outturned leg suggests a hemiplegia. Intermittent twitching movements of a foot, finger, or facial muscle may be the only sign of seizures. Multifocal myoclonus almost always indicates a metabolic disorder, particularly uremia, anoxia, drug intoxication (especially with lithium or haloperidol), or a prion disease. In a drowsy and confused patient, bilateral *asterixis* is a certain sign of metabolic encephalopathy or drug intoxication.

Decorticate rigidity and *decerebrate rigidity*, or "posturing," describe stereotyped arm and leg movements occurring spontaneously or elicited by sensory stimulation. Flexion of the elbows and wrists and supination of the arm (decortication) suggests bilateral damage rostral to the midbrain, whereas extension of the elbows and wrists with pronation (decerebration) indicates damage to motor tracts in the midbrain or caudal diencephalon. The less frequent combination of arm extension with leg flexion or flaccid legs is associated with lesions in the pons. These concepts have been adapted from animal work and cannot be applied with precision to coma in humans. In fact, acute and widespread disorders of any type, regardless of location, frequently cause limb extension, and almost all extensor posturing becomes predominantly flexor as time passes.

LEVEL OF AROUSAL A sequence of increasingly intense stimuli is used to determine the threshold for arousal and the motor response of each side of the body. The results of testing may vary from minute to minute, and serial examinations are most useful. Tickling the nostrils with a cotton wisp is a moderate stimulus to arousal—all but deeply stuporous and comatose patients will move the head away and arouse to some degree. An even greater degree of responsiveness is present if the patient uses his hand to remove an offending stimulus. Pressure on the knuckles or bony prominences and pinprick stimulation are humane forms of noxious stimuli; pinching the skin causes unsightly ecchymoses and is generally not necessary but may be useful in eliciting abduction withdrawal movements of the limbs. Posturing in response to noxious stimuli indicates severe damage to the corticospinal system, whereas abduction-avoidance movement of a limb is usually purposeful and denotes an intact corticospinal system. Posturing may also be unilateral and coexists with purposeful limb movements, reflecting incomplete damage to the motor system.

BRAINSTEM REFLEXES Assessment of brainstem function is essential to localization of the lesion in coma (Fig. 34-3). The brainstem reflexes that are conveniently examined are pupillary size and reaction to light, spontaneous and elicited eye movements, corneal responses, and the respiratory pattern. As a rule, coma is due to bilateral hemispheral disease when these brainstem activities are preserved, particularly the pupillary reactions and eye movements. However, the presence of abnormal brainstem signs does not always indicate that the primary lesion is in the brainstem because hemispheral masses can cause secondary brainstem pathology by transtentorial herniation.

Pupillary Signs Pupillary reactions are examined with a bright, diffuse light (not an ophthalmoscope). Reactive and round pupils of midsize (2.5–5 mm) essentially exclude midbrain damage, either primary or secondary to compression. A response to light may be difficult to appreciate in pupils <2 mm in diameter, and bright room lighting mutes pupillary reactivity. One enlarged and poorly reactive pupil (>6 mm) signifies compression or stretching of the third nerve from the effects of a cerebral mass above. Enlargement of the pupil contralateral to a hemispheral mass may occur but is infrequent. An oval and slightly eccentric pupil is a transitional sign that accompanies early midbrain–third nerve compression. The most extreme pupillary sign, bilaterally dilated and unreactive pupils, indicates severe midbrain damage, usually from compression by a supratentorial mass. Ingestion of drugs with anticholinergic activity, the use of mydriatic eye drops, and direct ocular trauma are among the causes of misleading pupillary enlargement.

Unilateral miosis in coma has been attributed to dysfunction of sympathetic efferents originating in the posterior hypothalamus and descending in the tegmentum of the brainstem to the cervical cord. It is therefore of

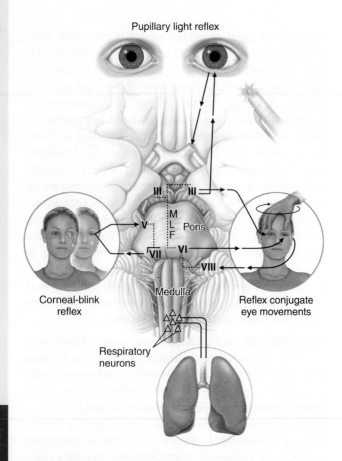

Pupillary light reflex

III III
M
L Pons
F
V
VII VI
VIII

Corneal-blink
reflex

Medulla

Reflex conjugate
eye movements

Respiratory
neurons

FIGURE 34-3

Examination of brainstem reflexes in coma. Midbrain and third nerve function are tested by pupillary reaction to light, pontine function by spontaneous and reflex eye movements and corneal responses, and medullary function by respiratory and pharyngeal responses. Reflex conjugate, horizontal eye movements are dependent on the medial longitudinal fasciculus (MLF) interconnecting the sixth and contralateral third nerve nuclei. Head rotation (oculocephalic reflex) or caloric stimulation of the labyrinths (oculovestibular reflex) elicits contraversive eye movements (for details see text).

limited localizing value but is an occasional finding in patients with a large cerebral hemorrhage that affects the thalamus. Reactive and bilaterally small (1–2.5 mm) but not pinpoint pupils are seen in metabolic encephalopathies or in deep bilateral hemispheral lesions such as hydrocephalus or thalamic hemorrhage. Even smaller reactive pupils (<1 mm) characterize narcotic or barbiturate overdoses but also occur with extensive pontine hemorrhage. The response to naloxone and the presence of reflex eye movements (see later) assist in distinguishing these.

Ocular Movements The eyes are first observed by elevating the lids and noting the resting position and spontaneous movements of the globes. Lid tone, tested by lifting the eyelids and noting their resistance

to opening and the speed of closure, is progressively reduced as unresponsiveness progresses. Horizontal divergence of the eyes at rest is normal in drowsiness. As coma deepens, the ocular axes may become parallel again.

Spontaneous eye movements in coma often take the form of conjugate horizontal roving. This finding alone exonerates damage in the midbrain and pons and has the same significance as normal reflex eye movements (see later). Conjugate horizontal ocular deviation to one side indicates damage to the pons on the opposite side or alternatively, to the frontal lobe on the same side. This phenomenon is summarized by the following maxim: *The eyes look toward a hemispheral lesion and away from a brainstem lesion.* Seizures also drive the eyes to one side but usually with superimposed clonic movements of the globes. The eyes may occasionally turn paradoxically away from the side of a deep hemispheral lesion ("wrong-way eyes"). The eyes turn down and inward with thalamic and upper midbrain lesions, typically thalamic hemorrhage. "Ocular bobbing" describes brisk downward and slow upward movements of the eyes associated with loss of horizontal eye movements and is diagnostic of bilateral pontine damage, usually from thrombosis of the basilar artery. "Ocular dipping" is a slower, arrhythmic downward movement followed by a faster upward movement in patients with normal reflex horizontal gaze; it indicates diffuse cortical anoxic damage.

The oculocephalic reflexes, elicited by moving the head from side to side or vertically and observing eye movements in the direction opposite to the head movement, depend on the integrity of the ocular motor nuclei and their interconnecting tracts that extend from the midbrain to the pons and medulla (Fig. 34-3). The movements, called somewhat inappropriately "doll's eyes" (which refers more accurately to the reflex elevation of the eyelids with flexion of the neck), are normally suppressed in the awake patient. The ability to elicit them therefore indicates both reduced cortical influence on the brainstem and intact brainstem pathways, indicating that coma is caused by a lesion or dysfunction in the cerebral hemispheres. The opposite, an absence of reflex eye movements, usually signifies damage within the brainstem but can result infrequently from overdoses of certain drugs. Normal pupillary size and light reaction distinguishes most drug-induced comas from structural brainstem damage.

Thermal, or "caloric," stimulation of the vestibular apparatus (oculovestibular response) provides a more intense stimulus for the oculocephalic reflex but provides essentially the same information. The test is performed by irrigating the external auditory canal with cool water in order to induce convection currents in the labyrinths. After a brief latency, the result is tonic deviation of both eyes to the side of cool-water irrigation and nystagmus in the opposite direction. (The acronym "COWS" has been used to remind generations of medical students of the direction of nystagmus—"cold water opposite, warm water same.") The loss of induced conjugate ocular movements indicates brainstem damage. The presence of corrective nystagmus indicates that the frontal lobes are functioning and connected to the brainstem; thus functional or hysterical coma is likely.

By touching the cornea with a wisp of cotton, a response consisting of brief bilateral lid closure is normally observed. The corneal reflex depends on the integrity of pontine pathways between the fifth (afferent) and both seventh (efferent) cranial nerves; in conjunction with reflex eye movements, it is a useful test of pontine function. CNS-depressant drugs diminish or eliminate the corneal responses soon after reflex eye movements are paralyzed but before the pupils become unreactive to light. The corneal (and pharyngeal) response may be lost for a time on the side of an acute hemiplegia.

Respiratory Patterns These are of less localizing value in comparison to other brainstem signs. Shallow, slow, but regular breathing suggests metabolic or drug depression. Cheyne-Stokes respiration in its classic cyclic form, ending with a brief apneic period, signifies bihemispheral damage or metabolic suppression and commonly accompanies light coma. Rapid, deep (Kussmaul) breathing usually implies metabolic acidosis but may also occur with pontomesencephalic lesions. Tachypnea occurs with lymphoma of the CNS. Agonal gasps are the result of lower brainstem (medullary) damage and are recognized as the terminal respiratory pattern of severe brain damage. A number of other cyclic breathing variations have been described but are of lesser significance.

LABORATORY STUDIES AND IMAGING

The studies that are most useful in the diagnosis of coma are: chemical-toxicologic analysis of blood and urine, cranial CT or MRI, EEG, and CSF examination. Arterial blood gas analysis is helpful in patients with lung disease and acid-base disorders. The metabolic aberrations commonly encountered in clinical practice require measurement of electrolytes, glucose, calcium, osmolarity, and renal (blood urea nitrogen) and hepatic (NH_3) function. Toxicologic analysis is necessary in any case of acute coma where the diagnosis is not immediately clear. However, the presence of exogenous drugs or toxins, especially alcohol, does not exclude the possibility that other factors, particularly head trauma, are also contributing to the clinical state. An ethanol level of 43 mmol/L (0.2 g/dL) in nonhabituated patients generally causes impaired mental activity; a level of >65 mmol/L

(0.3 g/dL) is associated with stupor. The development of tolerance may allow the chronic alcoholic to remain awake at levels >87 mmol/L (0.4 g/dL).

The availability of CT and MRI has focused attention on causes of coma that are detectable by imaging (e.g., hemorrhage, tumor, or hydrocephalus). Resorting primarily to this approach, although at times expedient, is imprudent because most cases of coma (and confusion) are metabolic or toxic in origin. Furthermore, the notion that a normal CT scan excludes anatomic lesion as the cause of coma is erroneous. Bilateral hemisphere infarction, acute brainstem infarction, encephalitis, meningitis, mechanical shearing of axons as a result of closed head trauma, sagittal sinus thrombosis, and subdural hematoma isodense to adjacent brain are some of the disorders that may not be detected. Nevertheless, if the source of coma remains unknown, a scan should be obtained.

The EEG is useful in metabolic or drug-induced states but is rarely diagnostic, except when coma is due to clinically unrecognized seizure, to herpesvirus encephalitis, or to prion (Creutzfeldt-Jakob) disease. The amount of background slowing of the EEG is a reflection of the severity of an encephalopathy. Predominant high-voltage slowing (δ or triphasic waves) in the frontal regions is typical of metabolic coma, as from hepatic failure, and widespread fast (β) activity implicates sedative drugs (e.g., diazepines, barbiturates). A special pattern of "alpha coma," defined by widespread, variable 8- to 12-Hz activity, superficially resembles the normal α rhythm of waking but, unlike normal α activity, is not altered by environmental stimuli. Alpha coma results from pontine or diffuse cortical damage and is associated with a poor prognosis. Normal α activity on the EEG, which is suppressed by stimulating the patient, also alerts the clinician to the locked-in syndrome or to hysteria or catatonia. The most important use of EEG recordings in coma is to reveal clinically inapparent epileptic discharges.

Lumbar puncture is performed less frequently than in the past for coma diagnosis because neuroimaging effectively excludes intracerebral and extensive subarachnoid hemorrhage. However, examination of the CSF remains indispensable in the diagnosis of meningitis and encephalitis. For patients with an altered level of consciousness, it is generally recommended that an imaging study be performed prior to lumbar puncture to exclude a large intracranial mass lesion. Blood culture and antibiotic administration usually precede the imaging study if meningitis is suspected.

DIFFERENTIAL DIAGNOSIS OF COMA

(Table 34-1) The causes of coma can be divided into three broad categories: those without focal neurologic signs (e.g., metabolic and toxic encephalopathies);

TABLE 34-1

DIFFERENTIAL DIAGNOSIS OF COMA

1. Diseases that cause no focal or lateralizing neurologic signs, usually with normal brainstem functions; CT scan and cellular content of the CSF are normal
   a. Intoxications: alcohol, sedative drugs, opiates, etc.
   b. Metabolic disturbances: anoxia, hyponatremia, hypernatremia, hypercalcemia, diabetic acidosis, non-ketotic hyperosmolar hyperglycemia, hypoglycemia, uremia, hepatic coma, hypercarbia, addisonian crisis, hypo- and hyperthyroid states, profound nutritional deficiency
   c. Severe systemic infections: pneumonia, septicemia, typhoid fever, malaria, Waterhouse-Friderichsen syndrome
   d. Shock from any cause
   e. Postseizure states, status epilepticus, subclinical epilepsy
   f. Hypertensive encephalopathy, eclampsia
   g. Severe hyperthermia, hypothermia
   h. Concussion
   i. Acute hydrocephalus
2. Diseases that cause meningeal irritation with or without fever, and with an excess of WBCs or RBCs in the CSF, usually without focal or lateralizing cerebral or brainstem signs; CT or MRI shows no mass lesion
   a. Subarachnoid hemorrhage from ruptured aneurysm, arteriovenous malformation, trauma
   b. Acute bacterial meningitis
   c. Viral encephalitis
   d. Miscellaneous: fat embolism, cholesterol embolism, carcinomatous and lymphomatous meningitis, etc.
3. Diseases that cause focal brainstem or lateralizing cerebral signs, with or without changes in the CSF; CT and MRI are abnormal
   a. Hemispheral hemorrhage (basal ganglionic, thalamic) or infarction (large middle cerebral artery territory) with secondary brainstem compression
   b. Brainstem infarction due to basilar artery thrombosis or embolism
   c. Brain abscess, subdural empyema
   d. Epidural and subdural hemorrhage, brain contusion
   e. Brain tumor with surrounding edema
   f. Cerebellar and pontine hemorrhage and infarction
   g. Widespread traumatic brain injury
   h. Metabolic coma (see above) with preexisting focal damage
   i. Miscellaneous: Cortical vein thrombosis, herpes simplex encephalitis, multiple cerebral emboli due to bacterial endocarditis, acute hemorrhagic leuko-encephalitis, acute disseminated (postinfectious) encephalomyelitis, thrombotic thrombocytopenic purpura, cerebral vasculitis, gliomatosis cerebri, pituitary apoplexy, intravascular lymphoma, etc.

Abbreviations: CSF, cerebrospinal fluid; RBCs, red blood cells; WBCs, white blood cells.

meningitis syndromes, characterized by fever or stiff neck and an excess of cells in the spinal fluid (e.g., bacterial meningitis, subarachnoid hemorrhage); and conditions associated with prominent focal signs (e.g., stroke, cerebral hemorrhage). In most instances, coma is part of an obvious medical problem, such as drug ingestion, hypoxia, stroke, trauma, or liver or kidney failure. Conditions that cause sudden coma include drug ingestion, cerebral hemorrhage, trauma, cardiac arrest, epilepsy, or basilar artery embolism. Coma that appears subacutely is usually related to a preexisting medical or neurologic problem or, less often, to secondary brain swelling of a mass such as tumor or cerebral infarction.

When cerebrovascular disease is the cause of coma, diagnosis can be difficult. The most common diseases are (1) basal ganglia and thalamic hemorrhage (acute but not instantaneous onset, vomiting, headache, hemiplegia, and characteristic eye signs); (2) pontine hemorrhage (sudden onset, pinpoint pupils, loss of reflex eye movements and corneal responses, ocular bobbing, posturing, hyperventilation, and excessive sweating); (3) cerebellar hemorrhage (occipital headache, vomiting, gaze paresis, and inability to stand); (4) basilar artery thrombosis (neurologic prodrome or warning spells, diplopia, dysarthria, vomiting, eye movement and corneal response abnormalities, and asymmetric limb paresis); and (5) subarachnoid hemorrhage (precipitous coma after headache and vomiting). The most common stroke, infarction in the territory of the middle cerebral artery, does not generally cause coma, but edema surrounding large infarctions may expand during the first few days and act as a mass.

The syndrome of acute hydrocephalus accompanies many intracranial diseases, particularly subarachnoid hemorrhage. It is characterized by headache and sometimes vomiting that may progress quickly to coma with extensor posturing of the limbs, bilateral Babinski signs, small unreactive pupils, and impaired oculocephalic movements in the vertical direction.

If the history and examination do not indicate the cause of coma, then information obtained from CT or MRI is needed. The majority of medical causes of coma can be established without a neuroimaging study. Sometimes imaging results can be misleading such as when small subdural hematomas or old strokes are found, but the patient's coma is due to intoxication.

BRAIN DEATH

This is a state of cessation of cerebral function with preservation of cardiac activity and maintenance of somatic function by artificial means. It is the only type of brain damage recognized as equivalent to death. Several sets of criteria have been advanced for the diagnosis of brain death and it is essential to adhere to those standards endorsed by the local medical community. Ideal criteria are simple, can be assessed at the bedside, and allow no chance of diagnostic error. They contain three essential elements: (1) widespread cortical destruction that is reflected by deep coma and unresponsiveness to all forms of stimulation; (2) global brainstem damage demonstrated by absent pupillary light reaction and by the loss of oculovestibular and corneal reflexes; and (3) destruction of the medulla, manifested by complete apnea. The heart rate is invariant and unresponsive to atropine. Diabetes insipidus is often present but may only develop hours or days after the other clinical signs of brain death. The pupils are usually midsized but may be enlarged; they should not, however, be small. Loss of deep tendon reflexes is not required because the spinal cord remains functional. Babinski signs are generally absent and the toe response is often flexor.

Demonstration that apnea is due to irreversible medullary damage requires that the P_{CO_2} be high enough to stimulate respiration during a test of spontaneous breathing. *Apnea testing* can be done safely by the use of diffusion oxygenation prior to removing the ventilator. This is accomplished by preoxygenation with 100% oxygen, which is then sustained during the test by oxygen administered through a tracheal cannula. CO_2 tension increases ~0.3–0.4 kPa/min (2–3 mmHg/min) during apnea. At the end of a period of observation, typically several minutes, arterial P_{CO_2} should be at least >6.6–8.0 kPa (50–60 mmHg) for the test to be valid. Apnea is confirmed if no respiratory effort has been observed in the presence of a sufficiently elevated P_{CO_2}. Other techniques, including the administration of CO_2 to accelerate the test, are used in special circumstances. The test is usually stopped if there is serious cardiovascular instability.

An isoelectric EEG may be used as a confirmatory test for total cerebral damage. Radionuclide brain scanning, cerebral angiography, or transcranial Doppler measurements may also be included to demonstrate the absence of CBF but they have not been extensively correlated with pathologic changes.

The possibility of profound drug-induced or hypothermic depression of the nervous system should be excluded, and some period of observation, usually 6–24 h, is desirable, during which the clinical signs of brain death are sustained. It is advisable to delay clinical testing for at least 24 h if a cardiac arrest has caused brain death or if the inciting disease is not known.

Although it is largely accepted in Western society that the respirator can be disconnected from a brain-dead patient, problems frequently arise because of poor communication and inadequate preparation of the family by the physician. Reasonable medical practice, ideally with the agreement of the family, allows the removal of support or transfer out of an intensive care unit of patients who are not brain dead but whose neurologic conditions are nonetheless hopeless.

TREATMENT   Coma

The immediate goal in a comatose patient is prevention of further nervous system damage. Hypotension, hypoglycemia, hypercalcemia, hypoxia, hypercapnia, and hyperthermia should be corrected rapidly. An oropharyngeal airway is adequate to keep the pharynx open in a drowsy patient who is breathing normally. Tracheal intubation is indicated if there is apnea, upper airway obstruction, hypoventilation, or emesis, or if the patient is liable to aspirate because of coma. Mechanical ventilation is required if there is hypoventilation or a need to induce hypocapnia in order to lower ICP. IV access is established, and naloxone and dextrose are administered if narcotic overdose or hypoglycemia are possibilities; thiamine is given along with glucose to avoid provoking Wernicke's disease in malnourished patients. In cases of suspected basilar thrombosis with brainstem ischemia, IV heparin or a thrombolytic agent is often utilized, after cerebral hemorrhage has been excluded by a neuroimaging study. Physostigmine may awaken patients with anticholinergic-type drug overdose but should be used only with careful monitoring; many physicians believe that it should only be used to treat anticholinergic overdose–associated cardiac arrhythmias. The use of benzodiazepine antagonists offers some prospect of improvement after overdose of soporific drugs and has transient benefit in hepatic encephalopathy.

Administration of hypotonic solutions should be monitored carefully in any serious acute brain illness because of the potential for exacerbating brain swelling. Cervical spine injuries must not be overlooked, particularly before attempting intubation or evaluation of oculocephalic responses. Fever and meningismus indicate an urgent need for examination of the CSF to diagnose meningitis. If the lumbar puncture in a case of suspected meningitis is delayed, an antibiotic such as a third-generation cephalosporin may be administered, preferably after obtaining blood cultures. The management of raised ICP is discussed in Chap. 35.

PROGNOSIS

One hopes to avoid the anguishing outcome of a patient who is left severely disabled or vegetative. The uniformly poor outcome of the persistent vegetative state has already been mentioned. Children and young adults may have ominous early clinical findings such as abnormal brainstem reflexes and yet recover; temporization in offering a prognosis in this group of patients is wise. Metabolic comas have a far better prognosis than traumatic ones. All systems for estimating prognosis in adults should be taken as approximations, and medical judgments must be tempered by factors such as age, underlying systemic disease, and general medical condition. In an attempt to collect prognostic information from large numbers of patients with head injury, the Glasgow Coma Scale was devised; empirically, it has predictive value in cases of brain trauma. For anoxic and metabolic coma, clinical signs such as the pupillary and motor responses after 1 day, 3 days, and 1 week have been shown to have predictive value (Fig. 35-4). Other studies suggest that the absence of corneal responses may have the most discriminative value. The absence of the cortical waves of the somatosensory evoked potentials has also proved a strong indicator of poor outcome in coma from any cause.

There have been recent advances using functional imaging that demonstrate some preserved cognitive abilities of vegetative and minimally conscious patients. In one series, about 10% of such patients could be trained to activate the frontal or temporal lobes in response to requests by an examiner to imagine certain visuospatial tasks. In one case, a rudimentary form of one-way communication could be established. There are also reports in a limited number of patients of improvement in cognitive function with the implantation of thalamic-stimulating electrodes. It is prudent to avoid generalizations from these experiments.

CHAPTER 35

NEUROLOGIC CRITICAL CARE, INCLUDING HYPOXIC-ISCHEMIC ENCEPHALOPATHY, AND SUBARACHNOID HEMORRHAGE

J. Claude Hemphill, III ■ Wade S. Smith ■ Daryl R. Gress

Life-threatening neurologic illness may be caused by a primary disorder affecting any region of the neuraxis or may occur as a consequence of a systemic disorder such as hepatic failure, multisystem organ failure, or cardiac arrest (Table 35-1). Neurologic critical care focuses on preservation of neurologic tissue and prevention of secondary brain injury caused by ischemia, edema, and elevated intracranial pressure (ICP). Management of other organ systems proceeds concurrently and may need to be modified in order to maintain the overall focus on neurologic issues.

PATHOPHSIOLOGY

Brain edema

Swelling, or edema, of brain tissue occurs with many types of brain injury. The two principal types of edema are vasogenic and cytotoxic. *Vasogenic edema* refers to the influx of fluid and solutes into the brain through an incompetent blood-brain barrier (BBB). In the normal cerebral vasculature, endothelial tight junctions associated with astrocytes create an impermeable barrier (the BBB), through which access into the brain interstitium is dependent upon specific transport mechanisms. The BBB may be compromised in ischemia, trauma, infection, and metabolic derangements. Typically, vasogenic edema develops rapidly following injury. *Cytotoxic edema* refers to cellular swelling and occurs in a variety of settings, including brain ischemia and trauma. Early astrocytic swelling is a hallmark of ischemia. Brain edema that is clinically significant usually represents a combination of vasogenic and cellular components. Edema can lead to increased ICP as well as tissue shifts and brain displacement from focal processes (Chap. 34). These tissue shifts can cause injury by mechanical distention and compression in addition to the ischemia of impaired perfusion consequent to the elevated ICP.

Ischemic cascade and cellular injury

When delivery of substrates, principally oxygen and glucose, is inadequate to sustain cellular function, a series of interrelated biochemical reactions known as the *ischemic cascade* is initiated. The release of excitatory amino acids, especially glutamate, leads to influx of calcium and sodium ions, which disrupt cellular homeostasis. An increased intracellular calcium concentration may activate proteases and lipases, which then lead to lipid peroxidation and free radical–mediated cell membrane injury. Cytotoxic edema ensues, and ultimately necrotic cell death and tissue infarction occur. This pathway to irreversible cell death is common to ischemic stroke, global cerebral ischemia, and traumatic brain injury. *Penumbra* refers to areas of ischemic brain tissue that have not yet undergone irreversible infarction, implying that these regions are potentially salvageable if ischemia can be reversed. Factors that may exacerbate ischemic brain injury include systemic hypotension and hypoxia, which further reduce substrate delivery to vulnerable brain tissue, and fever, seizures, and hyperglycemia, which can increase cellular metabolism, outstripping compensatory processes. Clinically, these events are known as *secondary brain insults* because they lead to exacerbation of the primary brain injury. Prevention, identification, and treatment of secondary brain insults are fundamental goals of management.

An alternative pathway of cellular injury is *apoptosis*. This process implies programmed cell death, which may

TABLE 35-1

NEUROLOGIC DISORDERS IN CRITICAL ILLNESS

LOCALIZATION ALONG NEUROAXIS	SYNDROME
Central Nervous System	
Brain: Cerebral hemispheres	Global encephalopathy
	Delirium
	Sepsis
	Organ failure—hepatic, renal
	Medication related—sedatives, hypnotics, analgesics, H_2 blockers, antihypertensives
	Drug overdose
	Electrolyte disturbance—hyponatremia, hypoglycemia
	Hypotension/hypoperfusion
	Hypoxia
	Meningitis
	Subarachnoid hemorrhage
	Wernicke's disease
	Seizure—postictal or nonconvulsive status
	Hypertensive encephalopathy
	Hypothyroidism—myxedema
	Focal deficits
	Ischemic stroke
	Tumor
	Abscess, subdural empyema
	Subdural/epidural hematoma
Brainstem	Mass effect and compression
	Ischemic stroke, intraparenchymal hemorrhage
	Hypoxia
Spinal cord	Mass effect and compression
	Disk herniation
	Epidural hematoma
	Ischemia—hypotension/embolic
	Epidural abscess
	Trauma, central cord syndrome
Peripheral Nervous System	
Peripheral nerve	
Axonal	Critical illness polyneuropathy
	Possible neuromuscular blocking agent complication
	Metabolic disturbances, uremia, hyperglycemia
	Medication effects—chemotherapeutic, antiretroviral
Demyelinating	Guillain-Barré syndrome
	Chronic inflammatory demyelinating polyneuropathy
Neuromuscular junction	Prolonged effect of neuromuscular blockade
	Medication effects—aminoglycosides
	Myasthenia gravis, Lambert-Eaton sydrome
Muscle	Critical illness myopathy
	Septic myopathy
	Cachectic myopathy—with or without disuse atrophy
	Electrolyte disturbances—hypokalemia/hyperkalemia, hypophosphatemia
	Acute quadriplegic myopathy

occur in the setting of ischemic stroke, global cerebral ischemia, traumatic brain injury, and possibly intracerebral hemorrhage. Apoptotic cell death can be distinguished histologically from the necrotic cell death of ischemia and is mediated through a different set of biochemical pathways. At present, interventions for prevention and treatment of apoptotic cell death remain less well defined than those for ischemia.

Cerebral perfusion and autoregulation

Brain tissue requires constant perfusion in order to ensure adequate delivery of substrate. The hemodynamic response of the brain has the capacity to preserve perfusion across a wide range of systemic blood pressures. Cerebral perfusion pressure (CPP), defined as the mean systemic arterial pressure (MAP) minus the ICP, provides the driving force for circulation across the capillary beds of the brain. *Autoregulation* refers to the physiologic response whereby cerebral blood flow (CBF) is regulated via alterations in cerebrovascular resistance in order to maintain perfusion over wide physiologic changes such as neuronal activation or changes in hemodynamic function. If systemic blood pressure drops, cerebral perfusion is preserved through vasodilation of arterioles in the brain; likewise, arteriolar vasoconstriction occurs at high systemic pressures to prevent hyperperfusion, resulting in fairly constant perfusion across a wide range of systemic blood pressures **(Fig. 35-1)**. At the extreme limits of MAP or CPP (high or low), flow becomes directly related to perfusion pressure. These autoregulatory changes occur in the microcirculation and are mediated by vessels below the resolution of those seen on angiography. CBF is also strongly influenced by pH and Pa_{CO_2}. CBF increases with hypercapnia and acidosis and decreases with hypocapnia and alkalosis. This forms the basis for the use of hyperventilation to lower ICP, and this effect on ICP is mediated through a decrease in intracranial blood volume. Cerebral autoregulation is a complex process critical to the normal homeostatic functioning of the brain, and this process may be disordered focally and unpredictably in disease states such as traumatic brain injury and severe focal cerebral ischemia.

Cerebrospinal fluid and intracranial pressure

The cranial contents consist essentially of brain, cerebrospinal fluid (CSF), and blood. CSF is produced principally in the choroid plexus of each lateral ventricle, exits the brain via the foramens of Luschka and Magendi, and flows over the cortex to be absorbed into the venous system along the superior sagittal sinus. Approximately 150 mL of CSF are contained within the ventricles and surrounding the brain and spinal cord; the cerebral blood volume is also ~150 mL. The bony skull offers excellent protection for the brain but allows little tolerance for additional volume. Significant increases in volume eventually result in increased ICP. Obstruction of CSF outflow, edema of cerebral tissue, or increases in volume from tumor or hematoma may increase ICP. Elevated ICP diminishes cerebral perfusion and can lead to tissue ischemia. Ischemia in turn may lead to vasodilation via autoregulatory mechanisms designed to restore cerebral perfusion. However, vasodilation also increases cerebral blood volume, which in turn then increases ICP, lowers CPP, and provokes further ischemia **(Fig. 35-2)**. This vicious cycle is commonly seen in traumatic brain injury, massive intracerebral hemorrhage, and large hemispheric infarcts with significant tissue shifts.

APPROACH TO THE PATIENT	Severe CNS Dysfunction

Critically ill patients with severe central nervous system dysfunction require rapid evaluation and intervention in order to limit primary and secondary brain injury. Initial neurologic evaluation should be performed concurrent with stabilization of basic respiratory, cardiac,

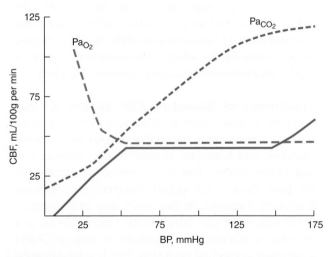

FIGURE 35-1

Autoregulation of cerebral blood flow (*solid line*). Cerebral perfusion is constant over a wide range of systemic blood pressure. Perfusion is increased in the setting of hypoxia or hypercarbia. BP, blood pressure; CBF, cerebral blood flow. (*Reprinted with permission from HM Shapiro: Anesthesiology 43:447, 1975. Copyright 1975, Lippincott Company.*)

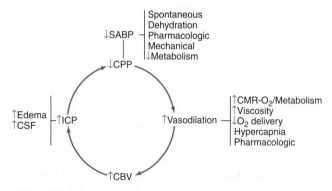

FIGURE 35-2

Ischemia and vasodilatation. Reduced cerebral perfusion pressure (CPP) leads to increased ischemia, vasodilation, increased intracranial pressure (ICP), and further reductions in CPP, a cycle leading to further neurologic injury. CBV, cerebral blood volume; CMR, cerebral metabolic rate; CSF, cerebrospinal fluid; SABP, systolic arterial blood pressure. (*Adapted from MJ Rosner et al: J Neurosurg 83:949, 1995; with permission.*)

and hemodynamic parameters. Significant barriers may exist to neurologic assessment in the critical care unit, including endotracheal intubation and the use of sedative or paralytic agents to facilitate procedures.

An impaired level of consciousness is common in critically ill patients. The essential first task in assessment is to determine whether the cause of dysfunction is related to a diffuse, usually metabolic, process or whether a focal, usually structural, process is implicated. Examples of diffuse processes include metabolic encephalopathies related to organ failure, drug overdose, or hypoxia-ischemia. Focal processes include ischemic and hemorrhagic stroke and traumatic brain injury, especially with intracranial hematomas. Since these two categories of disorders have fundamentally different causes, treatments, and prognoses, the initial focus is on making this distinction rapidly and accurately. The approach to the comatose patient is discussed in Chap. 34; etiologies are listed in Table 34-1.

Minor focal deficits may be present on the neurologic examination in patients with metabolic encephalopathies. However, the finding of prominent focal signs such as pupillary asymmetry, hemiparesis, gaze palsy, or paraplegia should suggest the possibility of a structural lesion. All patients with a decreased level of consciousness associated with focal findings should undergo an urgent neuroimaging procedure, as should all patients with coma of unknown etiology. CT scanning is usually the most appropriate initial study because it can be performed quickly in critically ill patients and demonstrates hemorrhage, hydrocephalus, and intracranial tissue shifts well. MRI may provide more specific information in some situations, such as acute ischemic stroke (diffusion-weighted imaging, DWI) and cerebral venous sinus thrombosis (magnetic resonance venography, MRV). Any suggestion of trauma from the history or examination should alert the examiner to the possibility of cervical spine injury and prompt an imaging evaluation using plain x-rays, CT, or MRI.

Other diagnostic studies are best utilized in specific circumstances, usually when neuroimaging studies fail to reveal a structural lesion and the etiology of the altered mental state remains uncertain. Electroencephalography (EEG) can be important in the evaluation of critically ill patients with severe brain dysfunction. The EEG of metabolic encephalopathy typically reveals generalized slowing. One of the most important uses of EEG is to help exclude inapparent seizures, especially nonconvulsive status epilepticus. Untreated continuous or frequently recurrent seizures may cause neuronal injury, making the diagnosis and treatment of seizures crucial in this patient group. Lumbar puncture (LP) may be necessary to exclude infectious processes, and an elevated opening pressure may be an important clue to cerebral venous sinus thrombosis. In patients with coma or profound encephalopathy,

it is preferable to perform a neuroimaging study prior to LP. If bacterial meningitis is suspected, an LP may be performed first or antibiotics may be empirically administered before the diagnostic studies are completed. Standard laboratory evaluation of critically ill patients should include assessment of serum electrolytes (especially sodium and calcium), glucose, renal and hepatic function, complete blood count, and coagulation. Serum or urine toxicology screens should be performed in patients with encephalopathy of unknown cause. EEG, LP, and other specific laboratory tests are most useful when the mechanism of the altered level of consciousness is uncertain; they are not routinely performed in clear-cut cases of stroke or traumatic brain injury.

Monitoring of ICP can be an important tool in selected patients. In general, patients who should be considered for ICP monitoring are those with primary neurologic disorders, such as stroke or traumatic brain injury, who are at significant risk for secondary brain injury due to elevated ICP and decreased CPP. Included are patients with the following: severe traumatic brain injury (Glasgow Coma Scale [GCS] score $\leq$ 8); large tissue shifts from supratentorial ischemic or hemorrhagic stroke; or hydrocephalus from subarachnoid hemorrhage (SAH), intraventricular hemorrhage, or posterior fossa stroke. An additional disorder in which ICP monitoring can add important information is fulminant hepatic failure, in which elevated ICP may be treated with barbiturates or, eventually, liver transplantation. In general, ventriculostomy is preferable to ICP monitoring devices that are placed in the brain parenchyma, because ventriculostomy allows CSF drainage as a method of treating elevated ICP. However, parenchymal ICP monitoring is most appropriate for patients with diffuse edema and small ventricles (which may make ventriculostomy placement more difficult) or any degree of coagulopathy (in which ventriculostomy carries a higher risk of hemorrhagic complications) (Fig 35-3).

Treatment of Elevated ICP Elevated ICP may occur in a wide range of disorders, including head trauma, intracerebral hemorrhage, SAH with hydrocephalus, and fulminant hepatic failure. Because CSF and blood volume can be redistributed initially, by the time elevated ICP occurs, intracranial compliance is severely impaired. At this point, any small increase in the volume of CSF, intravascular blood, edema, or a mass lesion may result in a significant increase in ICP and a decrease in cerebral perfusion. This is a fundamental mechanism of secondary ischemic brain injury and constitutes an emergency that requires immediate attention. In general, ICP should be maintained at <20 mmHg and CPP should be maintained at $\geq$60 mmHg.

Interventions to lower ICP are ideally based on the underlying mechanism responsible for the elevated

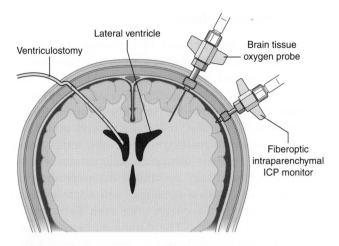

FIGURE 35-3

Intracranial pressure and brain tissue oxygen monitoring.
A ventriculostomy allows for drainage of cerebrospinal fluid to treat elevated intracranial pressure (ICP). Fiberoptic ICP and brain tissue oxygen monitors are usually secured using a screwlike skull bolt. Cerebral blood flow and microdialysis probes (not shown) may be placed in a manner similar to the brain tissue oxygen probe.

ICP (Table 35-2). For example, in hydrocephalus from SAH, the principal cause of elevated ICP is impairment of CSF drainage. In this setting, ventricular drainage of CSF is likely to be sufficient and most appropriate. In head trauma and stroke, cytotoxic edema may be most responsible, and the use of osmotic agents such as mannitol or hypertonic saline becomes an appropriate early step. As described above, elevated ICP may cause tissue ischemia, and, if cerebral autoregulation is intact, the resulting vasodilation can lead to a cycle of worsening ischemia. Paradoxically, administration of vasopressor agents to increase mean arterial pressure may actually lower ICP by improving perfusion, thereby allowing autoregulatory vasoconstriction as ischemia is relieved and ultimately decreasing intracranial blood volume.

Early signs of elevated ICP include drowsiness and a diminished level of consciousness. Neuroimaging studies may reveal evidence of edema and mass effect. Hypotonic IV fluids should be avoided, and elevation of the head of the bed is recommended. Patients must be carefully observed for risk of aspiration and compromise of the airway as the level of alertness declines. Coma and unilateral pupillary changes are late signs and require immediate intervention. Emergent treatment of elevated ICP is most quickly achieved by intubation and hyperventilation, which causes vasoconstriction and reduces cerebral blood volume. In order to avoid provoking or worsening cerebral ischemia, hyperventilation is best used for short periods of time until a more definitive treatment can be instituted. Furthermore, the effects of hyperventilation on

TABLE 35-2

STEPWISE APPROACH TO TREATMENT OF ELEVATED INTRACRANIAL PRESSURE[a]

Insert ICP monitor—ventriculostomy versus parenchymal device
General goals: maintain ICP <20 mmHg and CPP ≥60 mmHg
For ICP >20–25 mmHg for >5 min:

1. Drain CSF via ventriculostomy (if in place)
2. Elevate head of the bed; midline head position
3. Osmotherapy—mannitol 25–100 g q4h as needed (maintain serum osmolality <320 mosmol) or hypertonic saline (30 mL, 23.4% NaCl bolus)
4. Glucocorticoids—dexamethasone 4 mg q6h for vasogenic edema from tumor, abscess (avoid glucocorticoids in head trauma, ischemic and hemorrhagic stroke)
5. Sedation (e.g., morphine, propofol, or midazolam); add neuromuscular paralysis if necessary (patient will require endotracheal intubation and mechanical ventilation at this point, if not before)
6. Hyperventilation—to PaCO$_2$ 30–35 mmHg
7. Pressor therapy—phenylephrine, dopamine, or norepinephrine to maintain adequate MAP to ensure CPP ≥ 60 mmHg (maintain euvolemia to minimize deleterious systemic effects of pressors)
8. Consider second-tier therapies for refractory elevated ICP
   a. High-dose barbiturate therapy ("pentobarb coma")
   b. Aggressive hyperventilation to PaCO$_2$ <30 mmHg
   c. Hypothermia
   d. Hemicraniectomy

[a]Throughout ICP treatment algorithm, consider repeat head CT to identify mass lesions amenable to surgical evacuation.
Abbreviations: CPP, cerebral perfusion pressure; CSF, cerebrospinal fluid; MAP, mean arterial pressure; PaCO$_2$, arterial partial pressure of carbon dioxide.

ICP are short-lived, often lasting only for several hours because of the buffering capacity of the cerebral interstitium, and rebound elevations of ICP may accompany abrupt discontinuation of hyperventilation. As the level of consciousness declines to coma, the ability to follow the neurologic status of the patient by examination deteriorates and measurement of ICP assumes greater importance. If a ventriculostomy device is in place, direct drainage of CSF to reduce ICP is possible. Finally, high-dose barbiturates, decompressive hemicraniectomy, or hypothermia are sometimes used for refractory elevations of ICP, although these have significant side effects and have not been proven to improve outcome.

Secondary Brain Insults Patients with primary brain injuries, whether due to trauma or stroke, are at risk for ongoing secondary ischemic brain injury. Because secondary brain injury can be a major determinant of a poor outcome, strategies for minimizing secondary brain insults are an integral part of the critical care of all patients. While elevated ICP may lead to secondary ischemia, most secondary brain injury is mediated through other clinical events that exacerbate the ischemic cascade already initiated by the primary brain injury. Episodes of secondary brain insults are usually not associated with apparent neurologic worsening. Rather, they lead to cumulative injury limiting eventual recovery, which manifests as higher mortality rate or worsened long-term functional outcome. Thus, close monitoring of vital signs is important, as is early intervention to prevent secondary ischemia. Avoiding hypotension and hypoxia is critical, as significant hypotensive events (systolic blood pressure <90 mmHg) as short as 10 min in duration have been shown to adversely influence outcome after traumatic brain injury. Even in patients with stroke or head trauma who do not require ICP monitoring, close attention to adequate cerebral perfusion is warranted. Hypoxia (pulse oximetry saturation < 90%), particularly in combination with hypotension, also leads to secondary brain injury. Likewise, fever and hyperglycemia both worsen experimental ischemia and have been associated with worsened clinical outcome after stroke and head trauma. Aggressive control of fever with a goal of normothermia is warranted but may be difficult to achieve with antipyretic medications and cooling blankets. The value of newer surface or intravascular temperature control devices for the management of refractory fever is under investigation. The use of IV insulin infusion is encouraged for control of hyperglycemia as this allows better regulation of serum glucose levels than SC insulin. A reasonable goal is to maintain the serum glucose level at <7.8 mmol/L (<140 mg/dL), although episodes of hypoglycemia appear equally detrimental and the optimal targets remain uncertain. New cerebral monitoring tools that allow continuous evaluation of brain tissue oxygen tension, CBF, and metabolism (via microdialysis) may further improve the management of secondary brain injury.

CRITICAL CARE DISORDERS OF THE CENTRAL NERVOUS SYSTEM

HYPOXIC-ISCHEMIC ENCEPHALOPATHY

This occurs from lack of delivery of oxygen to the brain because of hypotension or respiratory failure. Causes include myocardial infarction, cardiac arrest, shock, asphyxiation, paralysis of respiration, and carbon monoxide or cyanide poisoning. In some circumstances, hypoxia may predominate. Carbon monoxide and cyanide poisoning are termed *histotoxic hypoxia* since they cause a direct impairment of the respiratory chain.

Clinical manifestations

Mild degrees of pure hypoxia, such as occur at high altitudes, cause impaired judgment, inattentiveness, motor incoordination, and, at times, euphoria. However, with hypoxia–ischemia, such as occurs with circulatory arrest, consciousness is lost within seconds. If circulation is restored within 3–5 min, full recovery may occur, but if hypoxia–ischemia lasts beyond 3–5 min, some degree of permanent cerebral damage usually results. Except in extreme cases, it may be difficult to judge the precise degree of hypoxia–ischemia, and some patients make a relatively full recovery after even 8–10 min of global cerebral ischemia. The distinction between pure hypoxia and hypoxia–ischemia is important, since a Pa_{O_2} as low as 20 mmHg (2.7 kPa) can be well tolerated if it develops gradually and normal blood pressure is maintained, but short durations of very low or absent cerebral circulation may result in permanent impairment.

Clinical examination at different time points after a hypoxic–ischemic insult (especially cardiac arrest) is useful in assessing prognosis for long-term neurologic outcome. The prognosis is better for patients with intact brainstem function, as indicated by normal pupillary light responses and intact oculocephalic (doll's eyes), oculovestibular (caloric), and corneal reflexes (Fig. 35-4). Absence of these reflexes and the presence of persistently dilated pupils that do not react to light are grave prognostic signs. A uniformly dismal prognosis from hypoxic–ischemic coma is conveyed by an absent pupillary light reflex or extensor or absent motor response to pain on day 3 following the injury. Electrophysiologically, the bilateral absence of the N20 component of the somatosensory evoked potential (SSEP) in the first several days also conveys a poor prognosis. A very elevated serum level (>33 μg/L) of the biochemical marker neuron-specific enolase (NSE) is indicative of brain damage after resuscitation from cardiac arrest and predicts a poor outcome. However, at present, SSEPs and NSE levels may be difficult to obtain in a timely fashion, with SSEP testing requiring substantial expertise in interpretation and NSE measurements not yet standardized. Whether administration of mild hypothermia after cardiac arrest (see "Treatment") will alter the usefulness of these clinical and electrophysiologic predictors is unknown. Long-term consequences of hypoxic–ischemic encephalopathy include persistent coma or a vegetative state (Chap. 34), dementia, visual agnosia, parkinsonism, choreoathetosis, cerebellar ataxia, myoclonus, seizures, and an amnestic state, which may be a consequence of selective damage to the hippocampus.

Pathology

Principal histologic findings are extensive multifocal or diffuse laminar cortical necrosis (Fig. 35-5), with almost

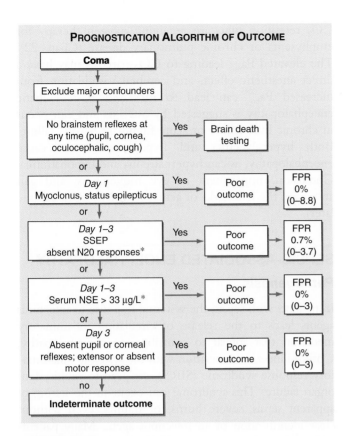

PROGNOSTICATION ALGORITHM OF OUTCOME

FIGURE 35-4
Prognostication of outcome in comatose survivors of cardiopulmonary resuscitation. Numbers in parentheses are 95% confidence intervals. Confounders could include use of sedatives or neuromuscular blocking agents, hypothermia therapy, organ failure, or shock. Tests denoted with an asterisk (*) may not be available in a timely and standardized manner. SSEP, somatosensory evoked potentials; NSE, neuron-specific enolase; FPR, false-positive rate. (*From EFM Wijdicks et al: Neurology 67:203, 2006; with permission.*)

invariable involvement of the hippocampus. The hippocampal CA1 neurons are vulnerable to even brief episodes of hypoxia-ischemia, perhaps explaining why selective persistent memory deficits may occur after brief cardiac arrest. Scattered small areas of infarction or neuronal loss may be present in the basal ganglia, hypothalamus, or brainstem. In some cases, extensive bilateral thalamic scarring may affect pathways that mediate arousal, and this pathology may be responsible for the persistent vegetative state. A specific form of hypoxic-ischemic encephalopathy, so-called watershed infarcts, occurs at the distal territories between the major cerebral arteries and can cause cognitive deficits, including visual agnosia, and weakness that is greater in proximal than in distal muscle groups.

Diagnosis

Diagnosis is based upon the history of a hypoxic-ischemic event such as cardiac arrest. Blood pressure <70 mmHg systolic or Pa_{O_2} <40 mmHg is usually necessary, although

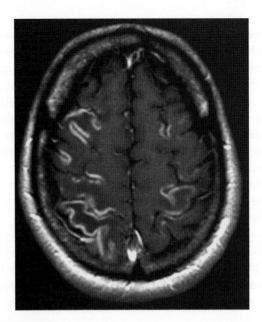

FIGURE 35-5
Cortical laminar necrosis in hypoxic-ischemic encephalopathy. T1-weighted postcontrast MRI shows cortical enhancement in a watershed distribution consistent with laminar necrosis.

both absolute levels as well as duration of exposure are important determinants of cellular injury. Carbon monoxide intoxication can be confirmed by measurement of carboxyhemoglobin and is suggested by a cherry red color of the skin, although the latter is an inconsistent clinical finding.

TREATMENT   **Hypoxic-Ischemic Encephalopathy**

Treatment should be directed at restoration of normal cardiorespiratory function. This includes securing a clear airway, ensuring adequate oxygenation and ventilation, and restoring cerebral perfusion, whether by cardiopulmonary resuscitation, fluid, pressors, or cardiac pacing. Hypothermia may target the neuronal cell injury cascade and has substantial neuroprotective properties in experimental models of brain injury. In two trials, mild hypothermia (33°C) improved functional outcome in patients who remained comatose after resuscitation from a cardiac arrest. Treatment was initiated within minutes of cardiac resuscitation and continued for 12 h in one study and 24 h in the other. Potential complications of hypothermia include coagulopathy and an increased risk of infection. Based upon these studies, the International Liaison Committee on Resuscitation issued the following advisory statement in 2003: "Unconscious adult patients with spontaneous circulation after out-of-hospital cardiac arrest should be cooled to 32°–34°C for 12–24 h when the initial rhythm was ventricular fibrillation."

Severe carbon monoxide intoxication may be treated with hyperbaric oxygen. Anticonvulsants may be needed to control seizures, although these are not usually given prophylactically. Posthypoxic myoclonus may respond to oral administration of clonazepam at doses of 1.5–10 mg daily or valproate at doses of 300–1200 mg daily in divided doses. Myoclonic status epilepticus within 24 h after a primary circulatory arrest generally portends a very poor prognosis, even if seizures are controlled.

Carbon monoxide and cyanide intoxication can also cause a delayed encephalopathy. Little clinical impairment is evident when the patient first regains consciousness, but a parkinsonian syndrome characterized by akinesia and rigidity without tremor may develop. Symptoms can worsen over months, accompanied by increasing evidence of damage in the basal ganglia as seen on both CT and MRI.

METABOLIC ENCEPHALOPATHIES

Altered mental states, variously described as confusion, delirium, disorientation, and encephalopathy, are present in many patients with severe illness in an intensive care unit (ICU). Older patients are particularly vulnerable to delirium, a confusional state characterized by disordered perception, frequent hallucinations, delusions, and sleep disturbance. This is often attributed to medication effects, sleep deprivation, pain, and anxiety. The presence of delirium is associated with worsened outcome in critically ill patients, even in those without an identifiable central nervous system pathology such as stroke or brain trauma. In these patients, the cause of delirium is often multifactorial, resulting from organ dysfunction, sepsis, and especially the use of medications given to treat pain, agitation, or anxiety. Critically ill patients are often treated with a variety of sedative and analgesic medications, including opiates, benzodiazepines, neuroleptics, and sedative-anesthetic medications, such as propofol. Recent studies suggest that in critically ill patients requiring sedation, the use of the centrally acting α_2 agonist dexmedetomidine reduces delirium and shortens the duration of mechanical ventilation compared to the use of benzodiazepines such as lorazepam or midazolam. The presence of family members in the ICU may also help to calm and orient agitated patients, and in severe cases, low doses of neuroleptics (e.g., haloperidol 0.5–1 mg) can be useful. Current strategies focus on limiting the use of sedative medications when this can be done safely.

In the ICU setting, several metabolic causes of an altered level of consciousness predominate. Hypercarbic encephalopathy can present with headache, confusion, stupor, or coma. Hypoventilation syndrome occurs most frequently in patients with a history of chronic CO_2 retention who are receiving oxygen therapy for emphysema or chronic pulmonary disease (Chap. 22). The elevated Pa_{CO_2} leading to CO_2 narcosis may have a direct anesthetic effect, and cerebral vasodilation from increased Pa_{CO_2} can lead to increased ICP. Hepatic encephalopathy is suggested by asterixis and can occur in chronic liver failure or acute fulminant hepatic failure. Both hyperglycemia and hypoglycemia can cause encephalopathy, as can hypernatremia and hyponatremia. Confusion, impairment of eye movements, and gait ataxia are the hallmarks of acute Wernicke's disease (see later).

SEPSIS-ASSOCIATED ENCEPHALOPATHY

Pathogenesis

In patients with sepsis, the systemic response to infectious agents leads to the release of circulating inflammatory mediators that appear to contribute to encephalopathy. Critical illness, in association with the systemic inflammatory response syndrome (SIRS), can lead to multisystem organ failure. This syndrome can occur in the setting of apparent sepsis, severe burns, or trauma, even without clear identification of an infectious agent. Many patients with critical illness, sepsis, or SIRS develop encephalopathy without obvious explanation. This condition is broadly termed *sepsis-associated encephalopathy*. While the specific mediators leading to neurologic dysfunction remain uncertain, it is clear that the encephalopathy is not simply the result of metabolic derangements of multiorgan failure. The cytokines tumor necrosis factor, interleukin (IL)-1, IL-2, and IL-6 are thought to play a role in this syndrome.

Diagnosis

Sepsis-associated encephalopathy presents clinically as a diffuse dysfunction of the brain without prominent focal findings. Confusion, disorientation, agitation, and fluctuations in level of alertness are typical. In more profound cases, especially with hemodynamic compromise, the decrease in level of alertness can be more prominent, at times resulting in coma. Hyperreflexia and frontal release signs such as a grasp or snout reflex can be seen. Abnormal movements such as myoclonus, tremor, or asterixis can occur. Sepsis-associated encephalopathy is quite common, occurring in the majority of patients with sepsis and multisystem organ failure. Diagnosis is often difficult because of the multiple potential causes of neurologic dysfunction in critically ill patients and requires exclusion of structural, metabolic, toxic, and infectious (e.g., meningitis or encephalitis) causes. The mortality rate of patients with sepsis-associated encephalopathy severe enough to produce coma approaches 50%, although this principally reflects the severity of the underlying critical illness and is not a direct result of the encephalopathy. Patients dying from severe sepsis or septic shock may have elevated levels of the serum brain injury biomarker S-100β and neuropathologic findings of neuronal apoptosis and cerebral ischemic injury. However, successful treatment of the underlying critical illness almost always results in complete resolution of the encephalopathy, with profound long-term cognitive disability being uncommon.

CENTRAL PONTINE MYELINOLYSIS

This disorder typically presents in a devastating fashion as quadriplegia and pseudobulbar palsy. Predisposing factors include severe underlying medical illness or nutritional deficiency; most cases are associated with rapid correction of hyponatremia or with hyperosmolar states. The pathology consists of demyelination without inflammation in the base of the pons, with relative sparing of axons and nerve cells. MRI is useful in establishing the diagnosis (Fig. 35-6) and may also identify partial forms that present as confusion, dysarthria, and/or disturbances of conjugate gaze without quadriplegia. Occasional cases present with lesions outside of the brainstem. Therapeutic guidelines for the restoration of severe hyponatremia should aim for gradual correction, i.e., by ≤10 mmol/L (10 meq/L) within 24 h and 20 mmol/L (20 meq/L) within 48 h.

WERNICKE'S DISEASE

Wernicke's disease is a common and preventable disorder due to a deficiency of thiamine. In the United States,

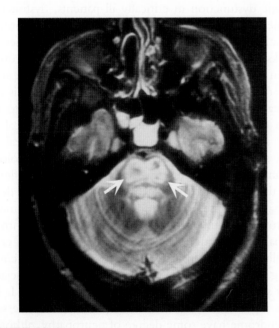

FIGURE 35-6

Central pontine myelinolysis. Axial T2-weighted MR scan through the pons reveals a symmetric area of abnormal high signal intensity within the basis pontis (*arrows*).

alcoholics account for most cases, but patients with malnutrition due to hyperemesis, starvation, renal dialysis, cancer, AIDS, or rarely gastric surgery are also at risk. The characteristic clinical triad is that of ophthalmoplegia, ataxia, and global confusion. However, only one-third of patients with acute Wernicke's disease present with the classic clinical triad. Most patients are profoundly disoriented, indifferent, and inattentive, although rarely they have an agitated delirium related to ethanol withdrawal. If the disease is not treated, stupor, coma, and death may ensue. Ocular motor abnormalities include horizontal nystagmus on lateral gaze, lateral rectus palsy (usually bilateral), conjugate gaze palsies, and rarely ptosis. Gait ataxia probably results from a combination of polyneuropathy, cerebellar involvement, and vestibular paresis. The pupils are usually spared, but they may become miotic with advanced disease.

Wernicke's disease is usually associated with other manifestations of nutritional disease, such as polyneuropathy. Rarely, amblyopia or myelopathy occurs. Tachycardia and postural hypotension may be related to impaired function of the autonomic nervous system or to the coexistence of cardiovascular beriberi. Patients who recover show improvement in ocular palsies within hours after the administration of thiamine, but horizontal nystagmus may persist. Ataxia improves more slowly than the ocular motor abnormalities. Approximately half recover incompletely and are left with a slow, shuffling, wide-based gait and an inability to tandem walk. Apathy, drowsiness, and confusion improve more gradually. As these symptoms recede, an amnestic state with impairment in recent memory and learning may become more apparent (*Korsakoff's psychosis*). Korsakoff's psychosis is frequently persistent; the residual mental state is characterized by gaps in memory, confabulation, and disordered temporal sequencing.

Pathology

Periventricular lesions surround the third ventricle, aqueduct, and fourth ventricle, with petechial hemorrhages in occasional acute cases and atrophy of the mamillary bodies in most chronic cases. There is frequently endothelial proliferation, demyelination, and some neuronal loss. These changes may be detected by MRI scanning (Fig. 35-7). The amnestic defect is related to lesions in the dorsal medial nuclei of the thalamus.

Pathogenesis

Thiamine is a cofactor of several enzymes, including transketolase, pyruvate dehydrogenase, and α-ketoglutarate dehydrogenase. Thiamine deficiency produces a diffuse decrease in cerebral glucose utilization and results in

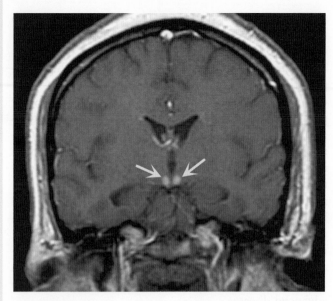

FIGURE 35-7
Wernicke's disease. Coronal T1-weighted postcontrast MRI reveals abnormal enhancement of the mammillary bodies (*arrows*), typical of acute Wernicke's encephalopathy.

mitochondrial damage. Glutamate accumulates owing to impairment of α–ketoglutarate dehydrogenase activity and, in combination with the energy deficiency, may result in excitotoxic cell damage.

TREATMENT   **Wernicke's Disease**

Wernicke's disease is a medical emergency and requires immediate administration of thiamine, in a dose of 100 mg either IV or IM. The dose should be given daily until the patient resumes a normal diet and should be begun prior to treatment with IV glucose solutions. Glucose infusions may precipitate Wernicke's disease in a previously unaffected patient or cause a rapid worsening of an early form of the disease. For this reason, thiamine should be administered to all alcoholic patients requiring parenteral glucose.

CRITICAL CARE DISORDERS OF THE PERIPHERAL NERVOUS SYSTEM

Critical illness with disorders of the peripheral nervous system (PNS) arises in two contexts: (1) primary neurologic diseases that require critical care interventions such as intubation and mechanical ventilation, and (2) secondary PNS manifestations of systemic critical illness, often involving multisystem organ failure. The former include acute polyneuropathies such as Guillain-Barré syndrome, neuromuscular junction disorders

including myasthenia gravis and botulism, and primary muscle disorders such as polymyositis. The latter result either from the systemic disease itself or as a consequence of interventions.

General principles of respiratory evaluation in patients with PNS involvement, regardless of cause, include assessment of pulmonary mechanics, such as maximal inspiratory force (MIF) and vital capacity (VC), and evaluation of strength of bulbar muscles. Regardless of the cause of weakness, endotracheal intubation should be considered when the MIF falls to <-25 cmH$_2$O or the VC is <1 L. Also, patients with severe palatal weakness may require endotracheal intubation in order to prevent acute upper airway obstruction or recurrent aspiration. Arterial blood gases and oxygen saturation from pulse oximetry are used to follow patients with potential respiratory compromise from PNS dysfunction. However, intubation and mechanical ventilation should be undertaken based on clinical assessment rather than waiting until oxygen saturation drops or CO$_2$ retention develops from hypoventilation. Noninvasive mechanical ventilation may be considered initially in lieu of endotracheal intubation but is generally insufficient in patients with severe bulbar weakness or ventilatory failure with hypercarbia. Principles of mechanical ventilation are discussed in Chap. 26.

NEUROPATHY

While encephalopathy may be the most obvious neurologic dysfunction in critically ill patients, dysfunction of the PNS is also quite common. It is typically present in patients with prolonged critical illnesses lasting several weeks and involving sepsis; clinical suspicion is aroused when there is failure to wean from mechanical ventilation despite improvement of the underlying sepsis and critical illness. *Critical illness polyneuropathy* refers to the most common PNS complication related to critical illness; it is seen in the setting of prolonged critical illness, sepsis, and multisystem organ failure. Neurologic findings include diffuse weakness, decreased reflexes, and distal sensory loss. Electrophysiologic studies demonstrate a diffuse, symmetric, distal axonal sensorimotor neuropathy, and pathologic studies have confirmed axonal degeneration. The precise mechanism of critical illness polyneuropathy remains unclear, but circulating factors such as cytokines, which are associated with sepsis and SIRS, are thought to play a role. It has been reported that up to 70% of patients with the sepsis syndrome have some degree of neuropathy, although far fewer have a clinical syndrome profound enough to cause severe respiratory muscle weakness requiring prolonged mechanical ventilation or resulting in failure to wean. Aggressive glycemic control with insulin infusions appears to decrease the risk of critical illness polyneuropathy. Treatment is otherwise supportive, with specific intervention directed at treating the underlying illness. While spontaneous recovery is usually seen, the time course may extend over weeks to months and necessitate long-term ventilatory support and care even after the underlying critical illness has resolved.

DISORDERS OF NEUROMUSCULAR TRANSMISSION

A defect in neuromuscular transmission may be a source of weakness in critically ill patients. Myasthenia gravis may be a consideration; however, persistent weakness secondary to impaired neuromuscular junction transmission is almost always due to administration of drugs. A number of medications impair neuromuscular transmission; these include antibiotics, especially aminoglycosides, and beta-blocking agents. In the ICU, the nondepolarizing neuromuscular blocking agents (nd-NMBAs), also known as muscle relaxants, are most commonly responsible. Included in this group of drugs are such agents as pancuronium, vecuronium, rocuronium, and atracurium. They are often used to facilitate mechanical ventilation or other critical care procedures, but with prolonged use persistent neuromuscular blockade may result in weakness even after discontinuation of these agents hours or days earlier. Risk factors for this prolonged action of neuromuscular blocking agents include female sex, metabolic acidosis, and renal failure.

Prolonged neuromuscular blockade does not appear to produce permanent damage to the PNS. Once the offending medications are discontinued, full strength is restored, although this may take days. In general, the lowest dose of neuromuscular blocking agent should be used to achieve the desired result and, when these agents are used in the ICU, a peripheral nerve stimulator should be used to monitor neuromuscular junction function.

MYOPATHY

Critically ill patients, especially those with sepsis, frequently develop muscle wasting, often in the face of seemingly adequate nutritional support. The assumption has been that this represents a catabolic myopathy brought about as a result of multiple factors, including elevated cortisol and catecholamine release and other circulating factors induced by the SIRS. In this syndrome, known as *cachectic myopathy*, serum creatine kinase levels and electromyography (EMG) are normal. Muscle biopsy shows type II fiber atrophy. Panfascicular muscle fiber necrosis may also occur in the setting of profound sepsis. This so-called *septic myopathy*

is characterized clinically by weakness progressing to a profound level over just a few days. There may be associated elevations in serum creatine kinase and urine myoglobin. Both EMG and muscle biopsy may be normal initially but eventually show abnormal spontaneous activity and panfascicular necrosis with an accompanying inflammatory reaction. Both of these myopathic syndromes may be considered under the broader heading of *critical illness myopathy*.

Acute quadriplegic myopathy describes a clinical syndrome of severe weakness seen in the setting of glucocorticoid and nd-NMBA use. The most frequent scenario in which this is encountered is the asthmatic patient who requires high-dose glucocorticoids and nd-NMBA to facilitate mechanical ventilation. This muscle disorder is not due to prolonged action of nd-NMBAs at the neuromuscular junction but, rather, is an actual myopathy with muscle damage; it has occasionally been described with high-dose glucocorticoid use alone. Clinically this syndrome is most often recognized when a patient fails to wean from mechanical ventilation despite resolution of the primary pulmonary process. Pathologically, there may be vacuolar changes in both type I and type II muscle fibers with evidence of regeneration. Acute quadriplegic myopathy has a good prognosis. If patients survive their underlying critical illness, the myopathy invariably improves and most patients return to normal. However, because this syndrome is a result of true muscle damage, not just prolonged blockade at the neuromuscular junction, this process may take weeks or months, and tracheotomy with prolonged ventilatory support may be necessary. Some patients do have residual long-term weakness, with atrophy and fatigue limiting ambulation. At present, it is unclear how to prevent this myopathic complication, except by avoiding use of nd-NMBAs, a strategy not always possible. Monitoring with a peripheral nerve stimulator can help to avoid the overuse of these agents. However, this is more likely to prevent the complication of prolonged neuromuscular junction blockade than it is to prevent this myopathy.

SUBARACHNOID HEMORRHAGE

Subarachnoid hemorrhage (SAH) renders the brain critically ill from both primary and secondary brain insults. Excluding head trauma, the most common cause of SAH is rupture of a saccular aneurysm. Other causes include bleeding from a vascular malformation (arteriovenous malformation or dural arterial-venous fistula) and extension into the subarachnoid space from a primary intracerebral hemorrhage. Some idiopathic SAHs are localized to the perimesencephalic cisterns and are benign; they probably have a venous or capillary source, and angiography is unrevealing.

Saccular ("berry") aneurysm

Autopsy and angiography studies have found that about 2% of adults harbor intracranial aneurysms, for a prevalence of 4 million persons in the United States; the aneurysm will rupture, producing SAH, in 25,000–30,000 cases per year. For patients who arrive alive at hospital, the mortality rate over the next month is about 45%. Of those who survive, more than half are left with major neurologic deficits as a result of the initial hemorrhage, cerebral vasospasm with infarction, or hydrocephalus. If the patient survives but the aneurysm is not obliterated, the rate of rebleeding is about 20% in the first 2 weeks, 30% in the first month, and about 3% per year afterwards. Given these alarming figures, the major therapeutic emphasis is on preventing the predictable early complications of the SAH.

Unruptured, asymptomatic aneurysms are much less dangerous than a recently ruptured aneurysm. The annual risk of rupture for aneurysms <10 mm in size is ~0.1%, and for aneurysms ≥10 mm in size is ~0.5–1%; the surgical morbidity rate far exceeds these percentages. Because of the longer length of exposure to risk of rupture, younger patients with aneurysms >10 mm in size may benefit from prophylactic treatment. As with the treatment of asymptomatic carotid stenosis, this risk-benefit strongly depends on the complication rate of treatment.

Giant aneurysms, those >2.5 cm in diameter, occur at the same sites (see later) as small aneurysms and account for 5% of cases. The three most common locations are the terminal internal carotid artery, middle cerebral artery (MCA) bifurcation, and top of the basilar artery. Their risk of rupture is ~6% in the first year after identification and may remain high indefinitely. They often cause symptoms by compressing the adjacent brain or cranial nerves.

Mycotic aneurysms are usually located distal to the first bifurcation of major arteries of the circle of Willis. Most result from infected emboli due to bacterial endocarditis causing septic degeneration of arteries and subsequent dilation and rupture. Whether these lesions should be sought and repaired prior to rupture or left to heal spontaneously is controversial.

Pathophysiology

Saccular aneurysms occur at the bifurcations of the large- to medium-sized intracranial arteries; rupture is into the subarachnoid space in the basal cisterns and often into the parenchyma of the adjacent brain. Approximately 85% of aneurysms occur in the anterior circulation, mostly on the circle of Willis. About 20% of patients have multiple aneurysms, many at mirror sites bilaterally. As an aneurysm develops, it typically forms a neck with a dome. The length of the neck and the size of the dome vary greatly and are important factors in planning neurosurgical obliteration or endovascular embolization. The arterial internal elastic lamina disappears at the base of the neck. The media thins, and connective tissue replaces smooth-muscle cells. At the site of rupture (most often the dome) the wall thins, and the tear that allows bleeding is often ≤0.5 mm long. Aneurysm size and site are important in predicting risk of rupture. Those >7 mm in diameter and those at the top of the basilar artery and at the origin of the posterior communicating artery are at greater risk of rupture.

Clinical manifestations

Most unruptured intracranial aneurysms are completely asymptomatic. Symptoms are usually due to rupture and resultant SAH, although some unruptured aneurysms present with mass effect on cranial nerves or brain parenchyma. At the moment of aneurysmal rupture with major SAH, the ICP suddenly rises. This may account for the sudden transient loss of consciousness that occurs in nearly half of patients. Sudden loss of consciousness may be preceded by a brief moment of excruciating headache, but most patients first complain of headache upon regaining consciousness. In 10% of cases, aneurysmal bleeding is severe enough to cause loss of consciousness for several days. In ~45% of cases, severe headache associated with exertion is the presenting complaint. The patient often calls the headache "the worst headache of my life"; however, the most important characteristic is sudden onset. Occasionally, these ruptures may present as headache of only moderate intensity or as a change in the patient's usual headache pattern. The headache is usually generalized, often with neck stiffness, and vomiting is common.

Although sudden headache in the absence of focal neurologic symptoms is the hallmark of aneurysmal rupture, focal neurologic deficits may occur. Anterior communicating artery or MCA bifurcation aneurysms may rupture into the adjacent brain or subdural space and form a hematoma large enough to produce mass effect. The deficits that result can include hemiparesis, aphasia, and abulia.

Occasionally, prodromal symptoms suggest the location of a progressively enlarging unruptured aneurysm. A third cranial nerve palsy, particularly when associated with pupillary dilation, loss of ipsilateral (but retained contralateral) light reflex, and focal pain above or behind the eye, may occur with an expanding aneurysm at the junction of the posterior communicating artery and the internal carotid artery. A sixth nerve palsy may indicate an aneurysm in the cavernous sinus, and visual field defects can occur with an expanding supraclinoid carotid or anterior cerebral artery aneurysm. Occipital and posterior cervical pain may signal a posterior inferior cerebellar artery or anterior inferior cerebellar artery aneurysm. Pain in or behind the eye and in the low temple can occur with an expanding MCA aneurysm. Thunderclap headache is a variant of migraine that simulates an SAH. Before concluding that a patient with sudden, severe headache has thunderclap migraine, a definitive workup for aneurysm or other intracranial pathology is required.

Aneurysms can undergo small ruptures and leaks of blood into the subarachnoid space, so-called *sentinel bleeds*. Sudden unexplained headache at any location should raise suspicion of SAH and be investigated, because a major hemorrhage may be imminent.

The initial clinical manifestations of SAH can be graded using the Hunt-Hess or World Federation of Neurosurgical Societies classification schemes (Table 35-3). For ruptured aneurysms, prognosis for good outcomes falls as the grade increases. For example, it is unusual for a Hunt-Hess grade 1 patient to die if the aneurysm is treated, but the mortality rate for grade 4 and 5 patients may be as high as 80%.

▬▬ Delayed neurologic deficits

There are four major causes of delayed neurologic deficits: reerupture, hydrocephalus, vasospasm, and hyponatremia.

1. *Reerupture.* The incidence of reeruption of an untreated aneurysm in the first month following SAH is ~30%, with the peak in the first 7 days. Reeruption is associated with a 60% mortality rate and poor outcome. Early treatment eliminates this risk.

TABLE 35-3

GRADING SCALES FOR SUBARACHNOID HEMORRHAGE		
GRADE	**HUNT-HESS SCALE**	**WORLD FEDERATION OF NEUROSURGICAL SOCIETIES (WFNS) SCALE**
1	Mild headache, normal mental status, no cranial nerve or motor findings	GCS[a] score 15, no motor deficits
2	Severe headache, normal mental status, may have cranial nerve deficit	GCS score 13–14, no motor deficits
3	Somnolent, confused, may have cranial nerve or mild motor deficit	GCS score 13–14, with motor deficits
4	Stupor, moderate to severe motor deficit, may have intermittent reflex posturing	GCS score 7–12, with or without motor deficits
5	Coma, reflex posturing or flaccid	GCS score 3–6, with or without motor deficits

[a]Glasgow Coma Scale.

2. *Hydrocephalus.* Acute hydrocephalus can cause stupor and coma and can be mitigated by placement of an external ventricular drain. More often, subacute hydrocephalus may develop over a few days or weeks and causes progressive drowsiness or slowed mentation (abulia) with incontinence. Hydrocephalus is differentiated from cerebral vasospasm with a CT scan, CT angiogram, transcranial Doppler (TCD) ultrasound, or conventional x-ray angiography. Hydrocephalus may clear spontaneously or require temporary ventricular drainage. Chronic hydrocephalus may develop weeks to months after SAH and manifest as gait difficulty, incontinence, or impaired mentation. Subtle signs may be a lack of initiative in conversation or a failure to recover independence.

3. *Vasospasm.* Narrowing of the arteries at the base of the brain following SAH causes symptomatic ischemia and infarction in ~30% of patients and is the major cause of delayed morbidity and death. Signs of ischemia appear 4–14 days after the hemorrhage, most often at 7 days. The severity and distribution of vasospasm determine whether infarction will occur.

Delayed vasospasm is believed to result from direct effects of clotted blood and its breakdown products on the arteries within the subarachnoid space. In general, the more blood that surrounds the arteries, the greater the chance of symptomatic vasospasm. Spasm of major arteries produces symptoms referable to the appropriate vascular territory. All of these focal symptoms may present abruptly, fluctuate, or develop over a few days. In most cases, focal spasm is preceded by a decline in mental status.

Vasospasm can be detected reliably with conventional x-ray angiography, but this invasive procedure is expensive and carries the risk of stroke and other complications. TCD ultrasound is based on the principle that the velocity of blood flow within an artery will rise as the lumen diameter is narrowed. By directing the probe along the MCA and proximal anterior cerebral artery (ACA), carotid terminus, and vertebral and basilar arteries on a daily or every-other-day basis, vasospasm can be reliably detected and treatments initiated to prevent cerebral ischemia (see later). CT angiography is another method that can detect vasospasm.

Severe cerebral edema in patients with infarction from vasospasm may increase the ICP enough to reduce cerebral perfusion pressure. Treatment may include mannitol, hyperventilation, and hemicraniectomy; moderate hypothermia may have a role as well.

4. *Hyponatremia.* Hyponatremia may be profound and can develop quickly in the first 2 weeks following SAH. There is both natriuresis and volume depletion with SAH, so that patients become both hyponatremic and hypovolemic. Both atrial natriuretic peptide and

brain natriuretic peptide have a role in producing this "cerebral salt-wasting syndrome." Typically, it clears over the course of 1–2 weeks and, in the setting of SAH, should not be treated with free-water restriction as this may increase the risk of stroke (see later).

Laboratory evaluation and imaging

(**Fig. 35-8**) The hallmark of aneurysmal rupture is blood in the CSF. More than 95% of cases have enough blood to be visualized on a high-quality noncontrast CT scan obtained within 72 h. If the scan fails to establish the diagnosis of SAH and no mass lesion or obstructive hydrocephalus is found, a lumbar puncture should be performed to establish the presence of subarachnoid blood. Lysis of the red blood cells and subsequent conversion of hemoglobin to bilirubin stains the spinal fluid yellow within 6–12 h. This xanthochromic spinal fluid peaks in intensity at 48 h and lasts for 1–4 weeks, depending on the amount of subarachnoid blood.

The extent and location of subarachnoid blood on noncontrast CT scan help locate the underlying aneurysm, identify the cause of any neurologic deficit, and predict delayed vasospasm. A high incidence of symptomatic vasospasm in the MCA and ACA has been found when early CT scans show subarachnoid clots >5 × 3 mm in the basal cisterns or layers of blood >1 mm thick in the cerebral fissures. CT scans less reliably predict vasospasm in the vertebral, basilar, or posterior cerebral arteries.

Lumbar puncture prior to an imaging procedure is indicated only if a CT scan is not available at the time of the suspected SAH. Once the diagnosis of hemorrhage from a ruptured saccular aneurysm is suspected, four-vessel conventional x-ray angiography (both carotids and both vertebrals) is generally performed to localize and define the anatomic details of the aneurysm and to determine if other unruptured aneurysms exist (**Fig. 35-8C**). At some centers, the ruptured aneurysm can be treated using endovascular techniques at the time of the initial angiogram as a way to expedite treatment and minimize the number of invasive procedures. CT angiography is an alternative method for locating the aneurysm and may be sufficient to plan definitive therapy.

Close monitoring (daily or twice daily) of electrolytes is important because hyponatremia can occur precipitously during the first 2 weeks following SAH (see earlier).

The electrocardiogram (ECG) frequently shows ST-segment and T-wave changes similar to those associated with cardiac ischemia. Prolonged QRS complex, increased QT interval, and prominent "peaked" or deeply inverted symmetric T waves are usually secondary to the intracranial hemorrhage. There is evidence that structural myocardial lesions produced by circulating catecholamines and excessive discharge of sympathetic neurons may occur after SAH, causing these ECG changes and a reversible cardiomyopathy sufficient to cause shock or congestive heart failure. Echocardiography reveals a pattern of regional wall motion abnormalities that follow the distribution of sympathetic nerves rather than the major coronary arteries, with relative sparing of the ventricular wall apex. The sympathetic nerves themselves appear to be injured by direct toxicity from the excessive catecholamine release. An asymptomatic troponin elevation is common. Serious ventricular dysrhythmias are unusual.

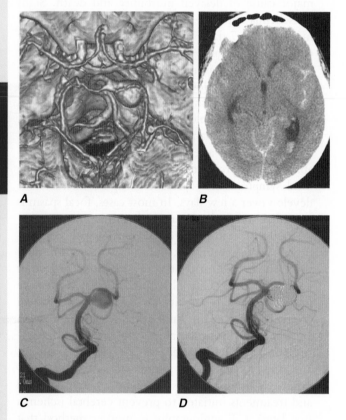

FIGURE 35-8

Subarachnoid hemorrhage. A. CT angiography revealing an aneurysm of the left superior cerebellar artery. **B.** Noncontrast CT scan at the level of the third ventricle revealing subarachnoid blood (*bright*) in the left sylvian fissure and within the left lateral ventricle. **C.** Conventional anteroposterior x-ray angiogram of the right vertebral and basilar artery showing the large aneurysm. **D.** Conventional angiogram following coil embolization of the aneurysm, whereby the aneurysm body is filled with platinum coils delivered through a microcatheter navigated from the femoral artery into the aneurysm neck.

TREATMENT ▶ Subarachnoid Hemorrhage

Early aneurysm repair prevents rerupture and allows the safe application of techniques to improve blood flow (e.g., induced hypertension and hypervolemia) should symptomatic vasospasm develop. An aneurysm can be "clipped" by a neurosurgeon or "coiled" by an endovascular surgeon. Surgical repair involves placing a metal clip across the aneurysm neck, thereby immediately eliminating the risk of rebleeding. This approach requires craniotomy and brain retraction, which is associated with neurologic morbidity. Endovascular techniques involve placing platinum coils, or other embolic material, within the aneurysm via a catheter that is passed from the femoral artery. The aneurysm is packed tightly to enhance thrombosis and over time is walled off from the circulation (Fig. 35-8D). The only prospective randomized trial of surgery versus endovascular treatment for ruptured aneurysm, the International Subarachnoid Aneurysm Trial (ISAT), was terminated early when 24% of patients treated with endovascular therapy were dead or dependent at 1 year compared to 31% treated with surgery, a significant 23% relative reduction. After 5 years, risk of death was lower in the coiling group, although the proportion of survivors who were independent was the same in both groups. Risk of rebleeding was low, but more common in the coiling group. Also, because some aneurysms have a morphology that is not amenable to endovascular treatment, surgery remains an important treatment option. Centers that combine both endovascular and neurosurgical expertise likely offer the best outcomes for patients, and there are reliable data showing that centers that specialize in aneurysm treatment have improved mortality rates.

The medical management of SAH focuses on protecting the airway, managing blood pressure before and after aneurysm treatment, preventing rebleeding prior to treatment, managing vasospasm, treating hydrocephalus, treating hyponatremia, and preventing pulmonary embolus.

Intracranial hypertension following aneurysmal rupture occurs secondary to subarachnoid blood, parenchymal hematoma, acute hydrocephalus, or loss of vascular autoregulation. Patients who are stuporous should undergo emergent ventriculostomy to measure ICP and to treat high ICP in order to prevent cerebral ischemia. Medical therapies designed to combat raised ICP (e.g., mild hyperventilation, mannitol, and sedation) can also be used as needed. High ICP refractory to treatment is a poor prognostic sign.

Prior to definitive treatment of the ruptured aneurysm, care is required to maintain adequate cerebral perfusion pressure while avoiding excessive elevation of arterial pressure. If the patient is alert, it is reasonable to lower the blood pressure to normal using nicardipine, labetolol, or esmolol. If the patient has a depressed level of consciousness, ICP should be measured and the cerebral perfusion pressure targeted to 60–70 mmHg.

If headache or neck pain is severe, mild sedation and analgesia are prescribed. Extreme sedation is avoided because it can obscure changes in neurologic status. Adequate hydration is necessary to avoid a decrease in blood volume predisposing to brain ischemia.

Seizures are uncommon at the onset of aneurysmal rupture. The quivering, jerking, and extensor posturing that often accompany loss of consciousness with SAH are probably related to the sharp rise in ICP rather than seizure. However, anticonvulsants are sometimes given as prophylactic therapy since a seizure could theoretically promote rebleeding.

Glucocorticoids may help reduce the head and neck ache caused by the irritative effect of the subarachnoid blood. There is no good evidence that they reduce cerebral edema, are neuroprotective, or reduce vascular injury, and their routine use therefore is not recommended.

Antifibrinolytic agents are not routinely prescribed but may be considered in patients in whom aneurysm treatment cannot proceed immediately. They are associated with a reduced incidence of aneurysmal rerupture but may also increase the risk of delayed cerebral infarction and deep-vein thrombosis (DVT).

Vasospasm remains the leading cause of morbidity and mortality following aneurysmal SAH. Treatment with the calcium channel antagonist nimodipine (60 mg PO every 4 h) improves outcome, perhaps by preventing ischemic injury rather than reducing the risk of vasospasm. Nimodipine can cause significant hypotension in some patients, which may worsen cerebral ischemia in patients with vasospasm. Symptomatic cerebral vasospasm can also be treated by increasing the cerebral perfusion pressure by raising mean arterial pressure through plasma volume expansion and the judicious use of IV vasopressor agents, usually phenylephrine or norepinephrine. Raised perfusion pressure has been associated with clinical improvement in many patients, but high arterial pressure may promote rebleeding in unprotected aneurysms. Treatment with induced hypertension and hypervolemia generally requires monitoring of arterial and central venous pressures; it is best to infuse pressors through a central venous line as well. Volume expansion helps prevent hypotension, augments cardiac output, and reduces blood viscosity by reducing the hematocrit. This method is called "triple-H" (hypertension, hemodilution, and hypervolemic) therapy.

If symptomatic vasospasm persists despite optimal medical therapy, intraarterial vasodilators and percutaneous transluminal angioplasty are considered. Vasodilatation by direct angioplasty appears to be permanent, allowing triple-H therapy to be tapered sooner. The pharmacologic vasodilators (verapamil and nicardipine) do not last more than about 24 h, and therefore multiple treatments may be required until the subarachnoid blood is reabsorbed. Although intraarterial papaverine is an effective vasodilator, there is evidence that papaverine may be neurotoxic, so its use should generally be avoided.

Acute hydrocephalus can cause stupor or coma. It may clear spontaneously or require temporary ventricular drainage. When chronic hydrocephalus develops, ventricular shunting is the treatment of choice.

Free-water restriction is contraindicated in patients with SAH at risk for vasospasm because hypovolemia and hypotension may occur and precipitate cerebral ischemia. Many patients continue to experience a decline in serum sodium despite receiving parenteral fluids containing normal saline. Frequently, supplemental oral salt coupled with normal saline will mitigate hyponatremia, but often patients also require hypertonic saline. Care must be taken not to correct serum sodium too quickly in patients with marked hyponatremia of several days' duration, as central pontine myelinolysis may occur.

All patients should have pneumatic compression stockings applied to prevent pulmonary embolism. Unfractionated heparin administered subcutaneously for DVT prophylaxis can be initiated immediately following endovascular treatment and within days following craniotomy and surgical clipping and is a useful adjunct to pneumatic compression stockings. Treatment of pulmonary embolus depends on whether the aneurysm has been treated and whether or not the patient has had a craniotomy. Systemic anticoagulation with heparin is contraindicated in patients with ruptured and untreated aneurysms. It is a relative contraindication following craniotomy for several days, and it may delay thrombosis of a coiled aneurysm. Following craniotomy, use of inferior vena cava filters is preferred to prevent further pulmonary emboli, while systemic anticoagulation with heparin is preferred following successful endovascular treatment.

SECTION V

DISORDERS COMPLICATING CRITICAL ILLNESSES AND THEIR MANAGEMENT

CHAPTER 36

DIALYSIS IN THE TREATMENT OF ACUTE RENAL FAILURE

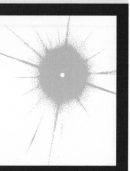

Kathleen D. Liu ■ Glenn M. Chertow

Dialysis may be required for the treatment of either acute or chronic kidney disease. The use of continuous renal replacement therapies (CRRTs) and slow low-efficiency dialysis (SLED) is specific to the management of acute renal failure. These modalities are performed continuously (CRRT) or over 6–12 h per session (SLED), in contrast to the 3–4 h of an intermittent hemodialysis session.

Peritoneal dialysis is rarely used in developed countries for the treatment of acute renal failure because of the increased risk of infection and (as will be discussed in more detail later) less efficient clearance per unit of time. The focus of the majority of this chapter will be on the use of peritoneal and hemodialysis for end-stage renal disease (ESRD).

With the widespread availability of dialysis, the lives of hundreds of thousands of patients with ESRD have been prolonged. In the United States alone, there are now approximately 530,000 patients with ESRD, the vast majority of whom require dialysis. The incidence rate for ESRD is 350 cases per million population per year. The incidence of ESRD is disproportionately higher in African Americans (approximately 1000 per million population per year) as compared with white Americans (275 per million population per year). In the United States, the leading cause of ESRD is diabetes mellitus, currently accounting for nearly 55% of newly diagnosed cases of ESRD. Approximately one-third (33%) of patients have ESRD that has been attributed to hypertension, although it is unclear whether in these cases hypertension is the cause or a consequence of vascular disease or other unknown causes of kidney failure. Other prevalent causes of ESRD include glomerulonephritis, polycystic kidney disease, and obstructive uropathy.

Globally, mortality rates for patients with ESRD are lowest in Europe and Japan but very high in the developing world because of the limited availability of dialysis. In the United States, the mortality rate of patients on dialysis is approximately 18–20% per year, with a 5-year survival rate of approximately 30–35%. Deaths are due mainly to cardiovascular diseases and infections (approximately 50 and 15% of deaths, respectively). Older age, male sex, nonblack race, diabetes mellitus, malnutrition, and underlying heart disease are important predictors of death.

TREATMENT OPTIONS FOR ESRD PATIENTS

Commonly accepted criteria for initiating patients on maintenance dialysis include the presence of uremic symptoms, the presence of hyperkalemia unresponsive to conservative measures, persistent extracellular volume expansion despite diuretic therapy, acidosis refractory to medical therapy, a bleeding diathesis, and a creatinine clearance or estimated glomerular filtration rate (GFR) below 10 mL/min per 1.73 m^2. Timely referral to a nephrologist for advanced planning and creation of a dialysis access, education about ESRD treatment options, and management of the complications of advanced chronic kidney disease (CKD), including hypertension, anemia, acidosis, and secondary hyperparathyroidism, is advisable. Recent data have suggested that a sizable fraction of ESRD cases result following episodes of acute renal failure, particularly among persons with underlying CKD.

In ESRD, treatment options include hemodialysis (in center or at home); peritoneal dialysis, as either continuous ambulatory peritoneal dialysis (CAPD) or continuous cyclic peritoneal dialysis (CCPD); or transplantation. Although there are significant geographic variations and differences in practice patterns, hemodialysis remains the most common therapeutic modality for ESRD (>90% of patients) in the United States. In contrast to hemodialysis, peritoneal dialysis is continuous, but much less efficient, in terms of solute clearance. While no large-scale clinical trials have been completed comparing outcomes among patients randomized to either hemodialysis or peritoneal dialysis, outcomes associated with both therapies are similar in most reports, and the decision of which modality to select is often based on personal preferences and quality-of-life considerations.

HEMODIALYSIS

Hemodialysis relies on the principles of solute diffusion across a semipermeable membrane. Movement of metabolic waste products takes place down a concentration gradient from the circulation into the dialysate. The rate of diffusive transport increases in response to several factors, including the magnitude of the concentration gradient, the membrane surface area, and the mass transfer coefficient of the membrane. The latter is a function of the porosity and thickness of the membrane, the size of the solute molecule, and the conditions of flow on the two sides of the membrane. According to laws of

diffusion, the larger the molecule, the slower its rate of transfer across the membrane. A small molecule, such as urea (60 Da), undergoes substantial clearance, whereas a larger molecule, such as creatinine (113 Da), is cleared less efficiently. In addition to diffusive clearance, movement of waste products from the circulation into the dialysate may occur as a result of ultrafiltration. Convective clearance occurs because of solvent drag, with solutes being swept along with water across the semipermeable dialysis membrane.

THE DIALYZER

There are three essential components to hemodialysis: the dialyzer, the composition and delivery of the dialysate, and the blood delivery system (Fig. 36-1). The dialyzer is a plastic chamber with the ability to perfuse blood and dialysate compartments simultaneously at very high flow rates. The surface area of modern dialysis membranes in adult patients is usually in the range of 1.5–2.0 m². The hollow-fiber dialyzer is the most common in use in the United States. These dialyzers are composed of bundles of capillary tubes through which blood circulates while dialysate travels on the outside of the fiber bundle.

Recent advances have led to the development of many different types of membrane material. Broadly, there are four categories of dialysis membranes: cellulose,

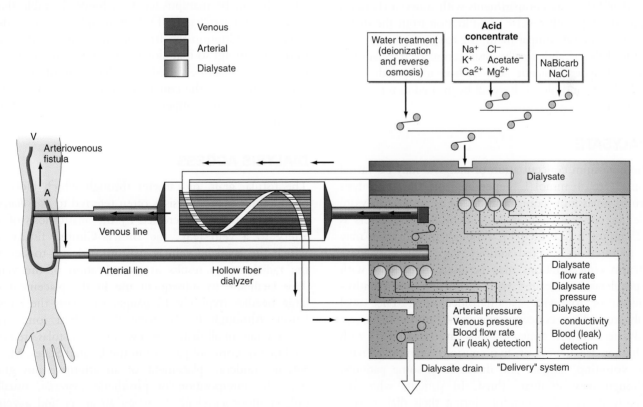

FIGURE 36-1
Schema for hemodialysis.

substituted cellulose, cellulosynthetic, and synthetic. Over the past three decades, there has been a gradual switch from cellulose-derived to synthetic membranes, because the latter are more "biocompatible." *Bioincompatibility* is generally defined as the ability of the membrane to activate the complement cascade. Cellulosic membranes are bioincompatible because of the presence of free hydroxyl groups on the membrane surface. In contrast, with the substituted cellulose membranes (e.g., cellulose acetate) or the cellulosynthetic membranes, the hydroxyl groups are chemically bound to either acetate or tertiary amino groups, resulting in limited complement activation. Synthetic membranes, such as polysulfone, polymethylmethacrylate, and polyacrylonitrile membranes, are even more biocompatible because of the absence of these hydroxyl groups. The majority of dialyzers now manufactured in the United States are derived from polysulfone or newer derivatives (polyarylethersulfone).

Reprocessing and reuse of hemodialyzers are often employed for patients on maintenance hemodialysis in the United States. However, as the manufacturing costs for disposable dialyzers have declined, more and more outpatient dialysis facilities are no longer reprocessing dialyzers. In most centers employing reuse, only the dialyzer unit is reprocessed and reused, whereas in the developing world blood lines are also frequently reused. The reprocessing procedure can be either manual or automated. It consists of the sequential rinsing of the blood and dialysate compartments with water, a chemical cleansing step with reverse ultrafiltration from the dialysate to the blood compartment, the testing of the patency of the dialyzer, and, finally, disinfection of the dialyzer. Formaldehyde, peracetic acid–hydrogen peroxide, glutaraldehyde, and bleach have all been used as reprocessing agents.

DIALYSATE

The potassium concentration of dialysate may be varied from 0 to 4 mmol/L depending on the predialysis serum potassium concentration. The usual dialysate calcium concentration in U.S. hemodialysis centers is 1.25 mmol/L (2.5 meq/L), although modification may be required in selected settings (e.g., higher dialysate calcium concentrations may be used in patients with hypocalcemia associated with secondary hyperparathyroidism or following parathyroidectomy). The usual dialysate sodium concentration is 140 mmol/L. Lower dialysate sodium concentrations are associated with a higher frequency of hypotension, cramping, nausea, vomiting, fatigue, and dizziness in some patients, although may attenuate thirst. In patients who frequently develop hypotension during their dialysis run, "sodium modeling" to counterbalance urea-related osmolar gradients is often employed. With sodium modeling, the dialysate sodium concentration is gradually lowered from the range of 145–155 mmol/L to isotonic concentrations (140 mmol/L) near the end of the dialysis treatment, typically declining either in steps or in a linear or exponential fashion. Higher dialysate sodium concentrations and sodium modeling may predispose patients to positive sodium balance; thus, these strategies to ameliorate intradialytic hypotension may be undesirable in hypertensive patients or in patients with large interdialytic weight gains. Because patients are exposed to approximately 120 L of water during each dialysis treatment, water used for the dialysate is subjected to filtration, softening, deionization, and, ultimately, reverse osmosis. During the reverse osmosis process, water is forced through a semipermeable membrane at very high pressure to remove microbiologic contaminants and >90% of dissolved ions.

BLOOD DELIVERY SYSTEM

The blood delivery system is composed of the extracorporeal circuit in the dialysis machine and the dialysis access. The dialysis machine consists of a blood pump, dialysis solution delivery system, and various safety monitors. The blood pump moves blood from the access site, through the dialyzer, and back to the patient. The blood flow rate may range from 250–500 mL/min, depending largely on the type and integrity of the vascular access. Negative hydrostatic pressure on the dialysate side can be manipulated to achieve desirable fluid removal or *ultrafiltration*. Dialysis membranes have different ultrafiltration coefficients (i.e., mL removed/min per mmHg) so that along with hydrostatic changes, fluid removal can be varied. The dialysis solution delivery system dilutes the concentrated dialysate with water and monitors the temperature, conductivity, and flow of dialysate.

DIALYSIS ACCESS

The fistula, graft, or catheter through which blood is obtained for hemodialysis is often referred to as a *dialysis access*. A native fistula created by the anastomosis of an artery to a vein (e.g., the Brescia-Cimino fistula, in which the cephalic vein is anastomosed end-to-side to the radial artery) results in arterialization of the vein. This facilitates its subsequent use in the placement of large needles (typically 15 gauge) to access the circulation. Although fistulas have the highest long-term patency rate of all dialysis access options, fistulas are created in a minority of patients in the United States. Many patients undergo placement of an arteriovenous graft (i.e., the interposition of prosthetic material, usually polytetrafluoroethylene, between an artery and a vein) or a tunneled dialysis catheter. In recent years, nephrologists, vascular surgeons, and health care policy makers in the United States have encouraged creation of arteriovenous fistulas in a larger fraction of patients (the "fistula first" initiative). Unfortunately, even when created, arteriovenous fistulas may not mature sufficiently to provide reliable access to the circulation, or they may thrombose early in their development. Novel surgical approaches (e.g., brachiobasilic fistula creation with transposition of the basilic vein fistula to the arm surface) have increased options for "native" vascular access.

Grafts and catheters tend to be used among persons with smaller-caliber veins or persons whose veins have been damaged by repeated venipuncture, or after prolonged hospitalization. The most important complication of arteriovenous grafts is thrombosis of the graft and graft failure, due principally to intimal hyperplasia at the anastomosis between the graft and recipient vein. When grafts (or fistulas) fail, catheter-guided angioplasty can be used to dilate stenoses; monitoring of venous pressures on dialysis and of access flow, although not routinely performed, may assist in the early recognition of impending vascular access failure. In addition to an increased rate of access failure, grafts and (in particular) catheters are associated with much higher rates of infection than fistulas.

Intravenous large-bore catheters are often used in patients with acute and chronic kidney disease. For persons on maintenance hemodialysis, tunneled catheters (either two separate catheters or a single catheter with two lumens) are often used when arteriovenous fistulas and grafts have failed or are not feasible due to anatomic considerations. These catheters are tunneled under the skin; the tunnel reduces bacterial translocation from the skin, resulting in a lower infection rate than with nontunneled temporary catheters. Most tunneled catheters are placed in the internal jugular veins; the external jugular, femoral, and subclavian veins may also be used.

Nephrologists, interventional radiologists, and vascular surgeons generally prefer to avoid placement of catheters into the subclavian veins; while flow rates are usually excellent, subclavian stenosis is a frequent complication and, if present, will likely prohibit permanent vascular access (i.e., a fistula or graft) in the ipsilateral extremity. Infection rates may be higher with femoral catheters. For patients with multiple vascular access complications and no other options for permanent vascular access, tunneled catheters may be the last "lifeline" for hemodialysis. Translumbar or transhepatic approaches into the inferior vena cava may be required if the superior vena cava or other central veins draining the upper extremities are stenosed or thrombosed.

GOALS OF DIALYSIS

The hemodialysis procedure is targeted at removing both low- and high-molecular-weight solutes. The procedure consists of pumping heparinized blood through the dialyzer at a flow rate of 300–500 mL/min, while dialysate flows in an opposite *counter-current* direction at 500–800 mL/min. The efficiency of dialysis is determined by blood and dialysate flow through the dialyzer as well as dialyzer characteristics (i.e., its efficiency in removing solute). The *dose* of dialysis, which is currently defined as a derivation of the fractional urea clearance during a single dialysis treatment, is further governed by patient size, residual kidney function, dietary protein intake, the degree of anabolism or catabolism, and the presence of comorbid conditions.

Since the landmark studies of Sargent and Gotch relating the measurement of the dose of dialysis using urea concentrations with morbidity in the National Cooperative Dialysis Study, the *delivered* dose of dialysis has been measured and considered as a quality assurance and improvement tool. While the fractional removal of urea nitrogen and derivations thereof are considered to be the standard methods by which "adequacy of dialysis" is measured, a large multicenter randomized clinical trial (the HEMO Study) failed to show a difference in mortality associated with a large difference in urea clearance. Still, multiple observational studies and widespread expert opinion have suggested that higher dialysis dose is warranted; current targets include a urea reduction ratio (the fractional reduction in blood urea nitrogen per hemodialysis session) of >65–70% and a body water–indexed clearance × time product (KT/V) above 1.2 or 1.05, depending on whether urea concentrations are "equilibrated." For the majority of patients with ESRD, between 9 and 12 h of dialysis are required each week, usually divided into three equal sessions. Several studies have suggested that longer hemodialysis session lengths may be beneficial (independent of urea clearance), although these studies are confounded by a variety of patient characteristics, including body size and nutritional status. Hemodialysis "dose" should be individualized, and factors other than the urea nitrogen should be considered, including the adequacy of ultrafiltration or fluid removal and control of hyperkalemia, hyperphosphatemia, and metabolic acidosis. Several authors have highlighted improved intermediate outcomes associated with more frequent hemodialysis (i.e., more than three times a week), although these studies are also confounded by multiple factors. A randomized clinical trial is currently under way to test whether more frequent dialysis results in differences in a variety of physiologic and functional markers.

COMPLICATIONS DURING HEMODIALYSIS

Hypotension is the most common acute complication of hemodialysis, particularly among patients with diabetes mellitus. Numerous factors appear to increase the risk of hypotension, including excessive ultrafiltration with inadequate compensatory vascular filling, impaired vasoactive or autonomic responses, osmolar shifts, overzealous use of antihypertensive agents, and reduced cardiac reserve. Patients with arteriovenous fistulas and grafts may develop high output cardiac failure due to shunting of blood through the dialysis access; on rare occasions, this may necessitate ligation of the fistula or graft. Because of the vasodilatory and cardiodepressive effects of acetate, its use as the buffer in dialysate was once a common cause of hypotension. Since the introduction of bicarbonate-containing dialysate, dialysis-associated hypotension has become less common. The management of hypotension during dialysis consists of discontinuing ultrafiltration, the administration of 100–250 mL of isotonic saline or 10 mL of 23% saturated hypertonic saline, or administration of salt-poor albumin. Hypotension during dialysis can frequently be prevented by careful evaluation of the dry weight and by ultrafiltration modeling, such that more fluid is removed at the beginning rather than the end of the dialysis procedure. Additional maneuvers include the performance of sequential ultrafiltration followed by dialysis, cooling of the dialysate during dialysis treatment; and avoiding heavy meals during dialysis. Midodrine, a selective α_1 adrenergic pressor agent, has been advocated by some practitioners, although there is insufficient evidence of its safety and efficacy to support its routine use.

Muscle cramps during dialysis are also a common complication of the procedure. The etiology of dialysis-associated cramps remains obscure. Changes in muscle perfusion because of excessively aggressive volume removal, particularly below the estimated dry weight, and the use of low-sodium–containing dialysate, have been proposed as precipitants of dialysis-associated cramps. Strategies that may be used to prevent cramps include reducing volume removal during dialysis, ultrafiltration profiling, and the use of higher concentrations of sodium in the dialysate or sodium modeling (see earlier).

Anaphylactoid reactions to the dialyzer, particularly on its first use, have been reported most frequently with the bioincompatible cellulosic-containing membranes. With the gradual phasing out of cuprophane membranes in the United States, dialyzer reactions have become uncommon. Dialyzer reactions can be divided into two types, A and B. Type A reactions are attributed to an IgE-mediated intermediate hypersensitivity reaction to ethylene oxide used in the sterilization of new dialyzers. This reaction typically occurs soon after the initiation of a treatment (within the first few minutes) and can progress to full-blown anaphylaxis if the therapy is not promptly discontinued. Treatment with steroids or epinephrine may be needed if symptoms are severe. The type B reaction consists of a symptom complex of nonspecific chest and back pain, which appears to result from complement activation and cytokine release. These symptoms typically occur several minutes into the dialysis run and typically resolve over time with continued dialysis.

Cardiovascular disease constitutes the major cause of death in patients with ESRD. Cardiovascular mortality and event rates are higher in dialysis patients than in patients posttransplantation, although rates are extraordinarily high in both populations. The underlying cause of cardiovascular disease is unclear but may be related to shared risk factors (e.g., diabetes mellitus, hypertension, atherosclerotic and arteriosclerotic vascular disease), chronic inflammation, massive changes in extracellular volume (especially with high interdialytic weight gains), inadequate treatment of hypertension, dyslipidemia, anemia, dystrophic vascular calcification, hyperhomocysteinemia, and, perhaps, alterations in cardiovascular dynamics during the dialysis treatment. Few studies have targeted cardiovascular risk reduction in ESRD patients; none have demonstrated consistent benefit. Two clinical trials of statin agents in ESRD demonstrated significant reductions in low-density lipoprotein (LDL) cholesterol concentrations but no significant reductions in death or cardiovascular events (Die Deutsche Diabetes Dialyse Studie [4D] and AURORA studies). Nevertheless, most experts recommend conventional cardioprotective strategies (e.g., lipid-lowering agents, aspirin, β-adrenergic antagonists) in dialysis patients based on the patients' cardiovascular risk profile, which appears to be increased by more than an order of magnitude relative to persons unaffected by kidney disease.

PERITONEAL DIALYSIS

In peritoneal dialysis, 1.5–3 L of a dextrose-containing solution is infused into the peritoneal cavity and allowed to dwell for a set period of time, usually 2–4 h. As with hemodialysis, toxic materials are removed through a combination of convective clearance generated through ultrafiltration and diffusive clearance down a concentration gradient. The clearance of solutes and water during a peritoneal dialysis exchange depends on the balance between the movement of solute and water into the peritoneal cavity versus absorption from the peritoneal cavity. The rate of diffusion diminishes with time and eventually stops when equilibration between plasma and dialysate is reached. Absorption of solutes and water from the peritoneal cavity occurs across the peritoneal membrane into the peritoneal capillary circulation and via peritoneal lymphatics into the lymphatic circulation. The rate of peritoneal solute transport varies from patient to patient and may be altered by the presence of infection (peritonitis), drugs, and physical factors such as position and exercise.

FORMS OF PERITONEAL DIALYSIS

Peritoneal dialysis may be carried out as CAPD, CCPD, or a combination of both. In CAPD, dialysis solution is manually infused into the peritoneal cavity during the day and exchanged three to five times daily. A nighttime dwell is frequently instilled at bedtime and remains in the peritoneal cavity through the night. The drainage of spent dialysate is performed manually with the assistance of gravity to move fluid out of the abdomen. In CCPD, exchanges are performed in an automated fashion, usually at night; the patient is connected to an automated cycler that performs a series of exchange cycles while the patient sleeps. The number of exchange cycles required to optimize peritoneal solute clearance varies by the peritoneal membrane characteristics; as with hemodialysis, experts suggest careful tracking of solute clearances to ensure dialysis "adequacy."

Peritoneal dialysis solutions are available in volumes typically ranging from 1.5 to 3 L. Lactate is the preferred buffer in peritoneal dialysis solutions. The most common additives to peritoneal dialysis solutions are heparin to prevent obstruction of the dialysis catheter lumen with fibrin and antibiotics during an episode of acute peritonitis. Insulin may also be added in patients with diabetes mellitus.

ACCESS TO THE PERITONEAL CAVITY

Access to the peritoneal cavity is obtained through a peritoneal catheter. Catheters used for maintenance peritoneal dialysis are flexible, being made of silicone rubber with numerous side holes at the distal end. These catheters usually have two Dacron cuffs to promote fibroblast proliferation, granulation, and invasion of the cuff. The scarring that occurs around the cuffs anchors the catheter and seals it from bacteria tracking from the skin surface into the peritoneal cavity; it also prevents the external leakage of fluid from the peritoneal cavity. The cuffs are placed in the preperitoneal plane and ~2 cm from the skin surface.

The *peritoneal equilibrium test* is a formal evaluation of peritoneal membrane characteristics that measures the transfer rates of creatinine and glucose across the peritoneal membrane. Patients are classified as low, low–average, high–average, and high transporters. Patients with rapid equilibration (i.e., high transporters) tend to absorb more glucose and lose efficiency of ultrafiltration with long daytime dwells. High transporters also tend to lose larger quantities of albumin and other proteins across the peritoneal membrane. In general, patients with rapid transporting characteristics require more frequent, shorter dwell time exchanges, nearly always obligating use of a cycler for feasibility. Slower (low and low–average) transporters tend to do well with fewer exchanges. The efficiency of solute clearance also depends on the volume of dialysate infused. Larger volumes allow for greater solute clearance, particularly with CAPD in patients with low and low–average transport characteristics. Interestingly, solute clearance also increases with physical activity, presumably related to more efficient flow dynamics within the peritoneal cavity.

As with hemodialysis, the optimal dose of peritoneal dialysis is unknown. Several observational studies have suggested that higher rates of urea and creatinine clearance (the latter generally measured in L/week) are associated with lower mortality rates and fewer uremic complications. However, a randomized clinical trial (Adequacy of Peritoneal Dialysis in Mexico [ADEMEX]) failed to show a significant reduction in mortality or complications with a relatively large increment in urea clearance. In general, patients on peritoneal dialysis do well when they retain residual kidney function. The rates of technique failure increase with years on dialysis and have been correlated with loss of residual function to a greater extent than loss of peritoneal membrane capacity. Recently, a nonabsorbable carbohydrate (icodextrin) has been introduced as an alternative osmotic agent. Studies have demonstrated more efficient ultrafiltration with icodextrin than with dextrose-containing solutions. Icodextrin is typically used as the "last fill" for patients on CCPD or for the longest dwell in patients on CAPD. For some patients in whom CCPD does not provide sufficient solute clearance, a hybrid approach can be adopted where one or more daytime exchanges are added to the CCPD regimen. While this approach can enhance solute clearance and prolong a patient's capacity to remain on peritoneal dialysis, the burden of the hybrid approach can be overwhelming to some.

COMPLICATIONS DURING PERITONEAL DIALYSIS

The major complications of peritoneal dialysis are peritonitis, catheter-associated nonperitonitis infections, weight gain and other metabolic disturbances, and residual uremia (especially among patients with no residual kidney function).

Peritonitis typically develops when there has been a break in sterile technique during one or more of the exchange procedures. Peritonitis is usually defined by an elevated peritoneal fluid leukocyte count ($100/mm^3$, of which at least 50% are polymorphonuclear neutrophils); these cutoffs are lower than in spontaneous bacterial peritonitis because of the presence of dextrose in peritoneal dialysis solutions and rapid bacterial proliferation in this environment without antibiotic therapy. The clinical presentation typically consists of pain and cloudy dialysate, often with fever and other constitutional symptoms. The most common culprit organisms are gram-positive cocci, including *Staphylococcus,* reflecting the origin from the skin. Gram-negative rod infections are less common; fungal and mycobacterial infections can be seen in selected patients, particularly after antibacterial therapy. Most cases of peritonitis can be managed either with intraperitoneal or oral antibiotics, depending on the organism; many patients with peritonitis do not require hospitalization. In cases where peritonitis is due to hydrophilic gram negative rods (e.g., *Pseudomonas* sp.) or yeast, antimicrobial therapy is usually not sufficient, and catheter removal is required to ensure complete eradication of infection. Nonperitonitis catheter-associated infections (often termed *tunnel infections*) vary widely in severity. Some cases can be managed with local antibiotic or silver nitrate administration, while others are severe enough to require parenteral antibiotic therapy and catheter removal.

Peritoneal dialysis is associated with a variety of metabolic complications. As noted earlier, albumin and other proteins can be lost across the peritoneal membrane in concert with the loss of metabolic wastes. The hypoproteinemia induced by peritoneal dialysis obligates a higher dietary protein intake in order to maintain nitrogen balance. Hyperglycemia and weight gain are also common complications of peritoneal dialysis. Several hundred calories in the form of dextrose are absorbed each day, depending on the concentration employed. Peritoneal dialysis patients, particularly those with type II diabetes mellitus, are then prone to other complications of insulin resistance, including hypertriglyceridemia. On the positive side, the continuous nature of peritoneal dialysis usually allows for a more liberal diet, due to continuous removal of potassium and phosphorus—two major dietary components whose accumulation can be hazardous in ESRD.

GLOBAL PERSPECTIVE

The incidence of ESRD is increasing worldwide with longer life expectancies and improved care of infectious and cardiovascular diseases. The management of ESRD varies widely by country and within country by region, and it is influenced by economic and other major factors. In general, peritoneal dialysis is more commonly performed in poorer countries owing to its lower expense and the high cost of establishing in-center hemodialysis units.

ACKNOWLEDGMENTS

We are grateful to Dr. Ajay Singh and Dr. Barry Brenner, authors of "Dialysis in the Treatment of Renal Failure" in the 16th edition of Harrison's Principles of Internal Medicine, for contributions to this chapter.

CHAPTER 37

FLUID AND ELECTROLYTE DISTURBANCES

David B. Mount

SODIUM AND WATER

COMPOSITION OF BODY FLUIDS

Water is the most abundant constituent in the body, accounting for ~50% of body weight in women and 60% in men. Total body water is distributed in two major compartments: 55–75% is intracellular (intracellular fluid [ICF]), and 25–45% is extracellular (extracellular fluid [ECF]). ECF is subdivided into intravascular (plasma water) and extravascular (interstitial) spaces in a ratio of 1:3. Fluid movement between the intravascular and interstitial spaces occurs across the capillary wall and is determined by Starling forces, i.e., capillary hydraulic pressure and colloid osmotic pressure. The transcapillary hydraulic pressure gradient exceeds the corresponding oncotic pressure gradient, thus favoring the movement of plasma ultrafiltrate into the extravascular space. The return of fluid into the intravascular compartment occurs via lymphatic flow.

The solute or particle concentration of a fluid is known as its osmolality and is expressed as milliosmoles per kilogram of water (mosmol/kg). Water easily diffuses across most cell membranes to achieve osmotic equilibrium (ECF osmolality = ICF osmolality). Notably, the extracellular and intracellular solute compositions differ considerably owing to the activity of various transporters, channels, and ATP-driven membrane pumps. The major ECF particles are Na^+ and its accompanying anions Cl^- and HCO_3^-, whereas K^+ and organic phosphate esters (ATP, creatine phosphate, and phospholipids) are the predominant ICF osmoles. Solutes that are restricted to the ECF or the ICF determine the tonicity or effective osmolality of that compartment. Certain solutes, particularly urea, do not contribute to water shifts across most membranes and are thus known as *ineffective osmoles*.

Water balance

Vasopressin secretion, water ingestion, and renal water transport collaborate to maintain human body fluid osmolality between 280 and 295 mosmol/kg. Vasopressin (AVP) is synthesized in magnocellular neurons within the hypothalamus; the distal axons of those neurons project to the posterior pituitary or neurohypophysis, from which AVP is released into the circulation. A network of central osmoreceptor neurons that includes the AVP-expressing magnocellular neurons themselves sense circulating osmolality via nonselective, stretch-activated cation channels. These osmoreceptor neurons are activated or inhibited by modest increases and decreases in circulating osmolality, respectively; activation leads to AVP release and thirst.

AVP secretion is stimulated as systemic osmolality increases above a threshold level of ~285 mosmol/kg, above which there is a linear relationship between osmolality and circulating AVP (Fig. 37-1). Thirst and thus water ingestion also are activated at ~285 mosmol/kg, beyond which there is an equivalent linear increase in the perceived intensity of thirst as a function of circulating osmolality. Changes in blood volume and blood pressure are also direct stimuli for AVP release and thirst, albeit with a less sensitive response profile. Of perhaps greater clinical relevance to the pathophysiology of water homeostasis, ECF volume strongly modulates the relationship between circulating osmolality and AVP release so that *hypovolemia* reduces the osmotic threshold and increases the slope of the response curve to osmolality; *hypervolemia* has the opposite effect, increasing the osmotic threshold and reducing the slope of the response curve (Fig. 37-1). Notably, AVP has a half-life in the circulation of only 10–20 min; thus, changes in extracellular fluid volume and/or circulating osmolality can affect water homeostasis rapidly. In addition to volume status, a number of nonosmotic stimuli have potent activating effects on osmosensitive neurons and AVP release, including nausea, intracerebral angiotensin II, serotonin, and multiple drugs.

The excretion or retention of electrolyte-free water by the kidney is modulated by circulating AVP. AVP

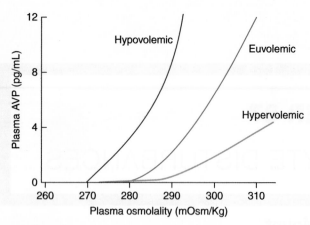

FIGURE 37-1

Circulating levels of vasopressin (AVP) in response to changes in osmolality. Plasma vasopressin becomes detectable in euvolemic, healthy individuals at a threshold of ~285 mOsm/Kg, above which there is a linear relationship between osmolality and circulating AVP. The vasopressin response to osmolality is modulated strongly by volume status. The osmotic threshold is thus slightly lower in hypovolemia, with a steeper response curve; hypervolemia reduces the sensitivity of circulating AVP levels to osmolality.

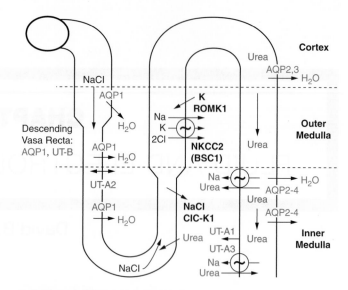

FIGURE 37-2

The renal concentrating mechanism. Water, salt, and solute transport by both proximal and distal nephron segments participates in the renal concentrating mechanism (see text for details). Diagram showing the location of the major transport proteins involved; a loop of Henle is depicted on the left, a collecting duct on the right. UT, urea transporter; AQP, aquaporin; NKCC2, Na-K-2Cl cotransporter; ROMK, renal outer medullary K^+ channel; CLC-K1, chloride channel. (*From JM Sands: J Am Soc Nephrol 13:2795, 2002; with permission.*)

acts on renal V_2-type receptors in the thick ascending limb of Henle and principal cells of the collecting duct (CD), increasing cyclic adenosine monophosphate (AMP) and activating protein kinase A (PKA)–dependent phosphorylation of multiple transport proteins. The AVP- and PKA-dependent activation of Na^+-Cl^- and K^+ transport by the thick ascending limb of the loop of Henle (TALH) is a key participant in the countercurrent mechanism (**Fig. 37-2**). The countercurrent mechanism ultimately increases the interstitial osmolality in the inner medulla of the kidney, driving water absorption across the renal collecting duct. However, water, salt, and solute transport by both proximal and distal nephron segments participates in the renal concentrating mechanism (Fig. 37-2). Water transport across apical and basolateral aquaporin-1 water channels in the descending thin limb of the loop of Henle is thus involved, as is passive absorption of Na^+-Cl^- by the thin ascending limb, via apical and basolateral CLC-K1 chloride channels and paracellular Na^+ transport. Renal urea transport in turn plays important roles in the generation of the medullary osmotic gradient and the ability to excrete solute-free water under conditions of both high and low protein intake (Fig. 37-2).

AVP-induced, PKA-dependent phosphorylation of the aquaporin-2 water channel in principal cells stimulates the insertion of active water channels into the lumen of the collecting duct, resulting in transepithelial water absorption down the medullary osmotic gradient (**Fig. 37-3**). Under antidiuretic conditions, with increased circulating AVP, the kidney reabsorbs water filtered by the

glomerulus, equilibrating the osmolality across the collecting duct epithelium to excrete a hypertonic, concentrated urine (osmolality of up to 1200 mosmol/kg). In the absence of circulating AVP, insertion of aquaporin-2 channels and water absorption across the collecting duct are essentially abolished, resulting in secretion of a hypotonic, dilute urine (osmolality as low as 30–50 mosmol/kg). Abnormalities in this final common pathway are involved in most disorders of water homeostasis, e.g., a reduced or absent insertion of active aquaporin-2 water channels into the membrane of principal cells in diabetes insipidus.

Maintenance of arterial circulatory integrity

Sodium is actively pumped out of cells by the Na^+, K^+-ATPase membrane pump. In consequence, 85–90% of body Na^+ is extracellular, and the extracellular fluid volume (ECFV) is a function of total-body Na^+ content. Arterial perfusion and circulatory integrity are, in turn, determined by renal Na^+ retention or excretion, in addition to the modulation of systemic arterial resistance. Within the kidney, Na^+ is filtered by the glomeruli and then sequentially reabsorbed by the renal tubules. The Na^+ cation typically is reabsorbed with the chloride anion (Cl^-); thus, chloride homeostasis also affects the ECFV. On a quantitative level, at a glomerular filtration rate (GFR) of 180 L/d and serum Na^+ of

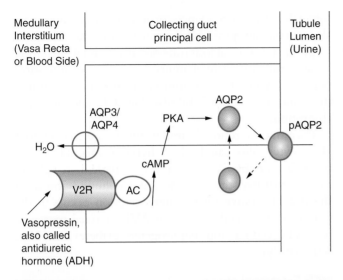

FIGURE 37-3

Vasopressin and the regulation of water permeability in the renal collecting duct. Vasopressin binds to the type 2 vasopressin receptor (V2R) on the basolateral membrane of principal cells, activates adenylyl cyclase (AC), increases intracellular cyclic adenosine monophosphatase (cAMP), and stimulates protein kinase A (PKA) activity. Cytoplasmic vesicles carrying aquaporin-2 (AQP) water channel proteins are inserted into the luminal membrane in response to vasopressin, increasing the water permeability of this membrane. When vasopressin stimulation ends, water channels are retrieved by an endocytic process and water permeability returns to its low basal rate. The AQP3 and AQP4 water channels are expressed on the basolateral membrane and complete the transcellular pathway for water reabsorption. pAQP2 = phosphorylated aquaporin-2. (*From JM Sands, DG Bichet: Ann Intern Med 144:186, 2006; with permission.*)

~140 mM, the kidney filters some 25,200 mmol/d of Na$^+$. This is equivalent to ~1.5 kg of salt, which would occupy roughly 10 times the extracellular space; 99.6% of filtered Na$^+$-Cl$^-$ must be reabsorbed to excrete 100 mM per day. Minute changes in renal Na$^+$-Cl$^-$ excretion will thus have significant effects on the ECFV, leading to edema syndromes or hypovolemia.

Approximately two-thirds of filtered Na$^+$-Cl$^-$ is reabsorbed by the renal proximal tubule via both paracellular and transcellular mechanisms. The TALH subsequently reabsorbs another 25–30% of filtered Na$^+$-Cl$^-$ via the apical, furosemide-sensitive Na$^+$-K$^+$-2Cl$^-$ cotransporter. The adjacent aldosterone-sensitive distal nephron, which encompasses the distal convoluted tubule (DCT), connecting tubule (CNT), and collecting duct, accomplishes the "fine-tuning" of renal Na$^+$-Cl$^-$ excretion. The thiazide-sensitive apical Na$^+$-Cl$^-$ cotransporter (NCC) reabsorbs 5–10% of filtered Na$^+$-Cl$^-$ in the DCT. Principal cells in the CNT and CD reabsorb Na$^+$ via electrogenic, amiloride-sensitive epithelial

Na$^+$ channels (ENaC); Cl$^-$ ions are reabsorbed primarily by adjacent intercalated cells via apical Cl$^-$ exchange (Cl$^-$-OH$^-$ and Cl$^-$-HCO$_3^-$ exchange, mediated by the SLC26A4 anion exchanger) (**Fig. 37-4**).

Renal tubular reabsorption of filtered Na$^+$-Cl$^-$ is regulated by multiple circulating and paracrine hormones in addition to the activity of renal nerves. Angiotensin II activates proximal Na$^+$-Cl$^-$ reabsorption, as do adrenergic receptors under the influence of renal sympathetic innervation; locally generated dopamine, in contrast, has a *natriuretic* effect. Aldosterone primarily activates Na$^+$-Cl$^-$ reabsorption within the aldosterone-sensitive distal nephron. In particular, aldosterone activates the ENaC channel in principal cells, inducing Na$^+$ absorption and promoting K$^+$ excretion (see Fig. 37-4).

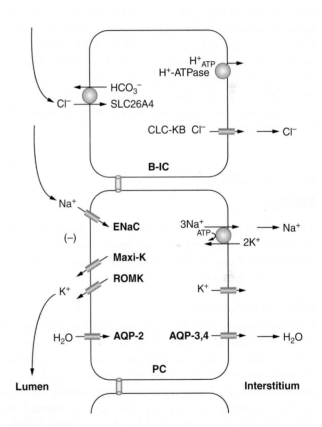

FIGURE 37-4

Sodium, water, and potassium transport in principal cells (PC) and adjacent β-intercalated cells (B-IC). The absorption of Na$^+$ via the amiloride-sensitive epithelial sodium channel (ENaC) generates a lumen-negative potential difference that drives K$^+$ excretion through the apical secretory K$^+$ channel ROMK (renal outer medullary K$^+$ channel) and/or the flow-dependent maxi-K channel. Transepithelial Cl$^-$ transport occurs in adjacent β-intercalated cells via apical Cl$^-$-HCO$_3^-$ and Cl$^-$-OH$^-$ exchange (SLC26A4 anion exchanger, also known as pendrin) basolateral CLC chloride channels. Water is absorbed down the osmotic gradient by principal cells, through the apical aquaporin-2 (AQP-2) and basolateral aquaporin-3 and aquaporin-4 (Fig. 37-3).

Circulatory integrity is critical for the perfusion and function of vital organs. Underfilling of the arterial circulation is sensed by ventricular and vascular pressure receptors, resulting in a neurohumoral activation (increased sympathetic tone, activation of the renin-angiotensin-aldosterone axis, and increased circulating AVP) that synergistically increases renal Na^+-Cl^- reabsorption, vascular resistance, and renal water reabsorption. This occurs in the context of decreased cardiac output, as occurs in hypovolemic states, low-output cardiac failure, decreased oncotic pressure, and/or increased capillary permeability. Alternatively, excessive arterial vasodilation results in *relative* arterial underfilling, leading to neurohumoral activation in the defense of tissue perfusion. These physiologic responses play important roles in many of the disorders discussed in this chapter. In particular, it is important to appreciate that AVP functions in the defense of circulatory integrity, inducing vasoconstriction, increasing sympathetic nervous system tone, increasing renal retention of both water and Na^+-Cl^-, and modulating the arterial baroreceptor reflex. Most of these responses involve activation of systemic V_{1A} AVP receptors, but concomitant activation of V_2 receptors in the kidney can result in renal water retention and hyponatremia.

HYPOVOLEMIA

Etiology

True volume depletion, or hypovolemia, generally refers to a state of combined salt and water loss that leads to contraction of the ECFV. The loss of salt and water may be renal or nonrenal in origin.

Renal causes

Excessive urinary Na^+-Cl^- and water loss is a feature of several conditions. A high filtered load of endogenous solutes, such as glucose and urea, can impair tubular reabsorption of Na^+-Cl^- and water, leading to an osmotic diuresis. Exogenous mannitol, which often is used to decrease intracerebral pressure, is filtered by glomeruli but not reabsorbed by the proximal tubule, thus causing an osmotic diuresis. Pharmacologic diuretics selectively impair Na^+-Cl^- reabsorption at specific sites along the nephron, leading to increased urinary Na^+-Cl^- excretion. Other drugs can induce natriuresis as a side effect. For example, acetazolamide can inhibit proximal tubular Na^+-Cl^- absorption through its inhibition of carbonic anhydrase; other drugs, such as the antibiotics trimethroprim and pentamidine, inhibit distal tubular Na^+ reabsorption through the amiloride-sensitive ENaC channel, leading to urinary Na^+-Cl^- loss. Hereditary defects in renal transport proteins also are associated with reduced reabsorption of filtered Na^+-Cl^- and/or water. Alternatively, mineralocorticoid deficiency,

mineralocorticoid resistance, or inhibition of the mineralocorticoid receptor (MLR) can reduce Na^+-Cl^- reabsorption by the aldosterone-sensitive distal nephron. Finally, tubulointerstitial injury, as occurs in interstitial nephritis, acute tubular injury, or obstructive uropathy, can reduce distal tubular Na^+-Cl^- and/or water absorption.

Excessive excretion of free water, i.e., water without electrolytes, also can lead to hypovolemia. However, the effect on ECFV is usually less marked in light of the fact that two-thirds of the water volume is lost from the ICF. Excessive renal water excretion occurs in the setting of decreased circulating AVP or renal resistance to AVP (central and nephrogenic diabetes insipidus, respectively).

Extrarenal causes

Nonrenal causes of hypovolemia include fluid loss from the gastrointestinal tract, skin, and respiratory system. Accumulations of fluid within specific tissue compartments—typically the interstitium, peritoneum, or gastrointestinal tract—also can cause hypovolemia.

Approximately 9 L of fluid enters the gastrointestinal tract daily, 2 L by ingestion and 7 L by secretion; almost 98% of this volume is absorbed so that daily fecal fluid loss is only 100–200 mL. Impaired gastrointestinal reabsorption or enhanced secretion of fluid can cause hypovolemia. Since gastric secretions have a low pH (high H^+ concentration), whereas biliary, pancreatic, and intestinal secretions are alkaline (high HCO_3^- concentration), vomiting and diarrhea often are accompanied by metabolic alkalosis and acidosis, respectively.

Evaporation of water from the skin and respiratory tract (so-called insensible losses) is the major route for loss of solute-free water, which is typically 500–650 mL/d in healthy adults. This evaporative loss can increase during febrile illness or prolonged heat exposure. Hyperventilation also can increase insensible losses via the respiratory tract, particularly in ventilated patients; the humidity of inspired air is another determining factor. In addition, increased exertion and/or ambient temperature will increase insensible losses via sweat, which is hypotonic to plasma. Profuse sweating without adequate repletion of water and Na^+-Cl^- thus can lead to both hypovolemia and hypertonicity. Alternatively, replacement of these insensible losses with a surfeit of free water without adequate replacement of electrolytes may lead to hypovolemic hyponatremia.

Excessive fluid accumulation in interstitial and/or peritoneal spaces also can cause intravascular hypovolemia. Increases in vascular permeability and/or a reduction in oncotic pressure (hypoalbuminemia) alter Starling forces, resulting in excessive "third spacing" of the ECFV. This occurs in sepsis syndrome, burns, pancreatitis, nutritional hypoalbuminemia, and peritonitis. Alternatively, distributive hypovolemia can result from accumulation of fluid within specific compartments, for example, within the bowel lumen in gastrointestinal obstruction or ileus. Hypovolemia also can occur after extracorporeal hemorrhage or after significant hemorrhage into an expandable space, for example, the retroperitoneum.

Diagnostic evaluation

A careful history usually determines the etiologic cause of hypovolemia. Symptoms of hypovolemia are nonspecific and include fatigue, weakness, thirst, and postural dizziness; more severe symptoms and signs include oliguria, cyanosis, abdominal and chest pain, and confusion or obtundation. Associated electrolyte disorders may cause additional symptoms, for example, muscle weakness in patients with hypokalemia. On examination, diminished skin turgor and dry oral mucous membranes are less than ideal markers of a decreased ECFV in adult patients; reliable signs of hypovolemia include a decreased jugular venous pressure (JVP), orthostatic tachycardia (an increase of >15–20 beats per minute upon standing), and orthostatic hypotension (a >10–20-mmHg drop in blood pressure on standing). More severe fluid loss leads to hypovolemic shock, with hypotension, tachycardia, peripheral vasoconstriction, and peripheral hypoperfusion; these patients may exhibit peripheral cyanosis, cold extremities, oliguria, and altered mental status.

Routine chemistries may reveal an increase in blood urea nitrogen (BUN) and creatinine, reflecting a decrease in GFR. Creatinine is the more dependable measure of GFR, since BUN levels may be influenced by an increase in tubular reabsorption (prerenal azotemia), an increase in urea generation in catabolic states, hyperalimentation, or gastrointestinal bleeding and/or a decreased urea generation in decreased protein intake. In hypovolemic shock, liver function tests and cardiac biomarkers may show evidence of hepatic and cardiac ischemia, respectively. Routine chemistries and/or blood gases may reveal evidence of acid-base disorders. For example, bicarbonate loss due to diarrheal illness is a very common cause of metabolic acidosis; alternatively, patients with severe hypovolemic shock may develop lactic acidosis with an elevated anion gap.

The neurohumoral response to hypovolemia stimulates an increase in renal tubular Na^+ and water reabsorption. Therefore, the urine Na^+ concentration is typically <20 mM in nonrenal causes of hypovolemia, with a urine osmolality of >450 mosmol/kg. The reduction in both GFR and distal tubular Na^+ delivery may cause a defect in renal potassium excretion, with an increase in plasma K^+ concentration. Of note, patients with hypovolemia and a hypochloremic alkalosis due to vomiting, diarrhea, or diuretics typically have a urine Na^+ concentration >20 mM and urine pH >7.0 due to the increase in filtered HCO_3^-; the urine Cl^- concentration in this

setting is a more accurate indicator of volume status, with a level <25 mM suggestive of hypovolemia. The urine Na^+ concentration is often >20 mM in patients with *renal* causes of hypovolemia, such as acute tubular necrosis; similarly, patients with diabetes insipidus will have an inappropriately dilute urine.

> **TREATMENT** Hypovolemia
>
> The therapeutic goals in hypovolemia are to restore normovolemia and replace ongoing fluid losses. Mild hypovolemia usually can be treated with oral hydration and resumption of a normal maintenance diet. More severe hypovolemia requires intravenous hydration, with the choice of solution tailored to the underlying pathophysiology. Isotonic, "normal" saline (0.9% NaCl, 154 mM Na^+) is the most appropriate resuscitation fluid for normonatremic or hyponatremic patients with severe hypovolemia; colloid solutions such as intravenous albumin are not demonstrably superior for this purpose. Hypernatremic patients should receive a hypotonic solution: 5% dextrose if there has been only water loss (as in diabetes insipidus) or hypotonic saline (1/2 or 1/4 normal saline) if there has been water and Na^+-Cl^- loss. Patients with bicarbonate loss and metabolic acidosis, as occurs frequently in diarrhea, should receive intravenous bicarbonate, either an isotonic solution (150 meq of Na^+-HCO_3^- in 5% dextrose) or a more hypotonic bicarbonate solution in dextrose or dilute saline. Patients with severe hemorrhage or anemia should receive red cell transfusions without increasing the hematocrit beyond 35%.

SODIUM DISORDERS

Disorders of serum Na^+ concentration are caused by abnormalities in water homeostasis that lead to changes in the relative ratio of Na^+ to body water. Water intake and circulating AVP constitute the two key effectors in the defense of serum osmolality; defects in one or both of these defense mechanisms cause most cases of hyponatremia and hypernatremia. In contrast, abnormalities in sodium homeostasis per se lead to a deficit or surplus of whole-body Na^+-Cl^- content, a key determinant of the ECFV and circulatory integrity. Notably, volume status also modulates the release of AVP by the posterior pituitary so that hypovolemia is associated with higher circulating levels of the hormone at each level of serum osmolality. Similarly, in hypervolemic causes of arterial underfilling, e.g., heart failure and cirrhosis, the associated neurohumoral activation is associated with an increase in circulating AVP, leading to water retention and hyponatremia. Therefore, a key concept in sodium disorders is that the absolute plasma Na^+ concentration tells one nothing about the volume status of a specific patient; this must be taken into account in the diagnostic and therapeutic approach.

HYPONATREMIA

Hyponatremia, which is defined as a plasma Na^+ concentration <135 mM, is a very common disorder, occurring in up to 22% of hospitalized patients. This disorder is almost always the result of an increase in circulating AVP and/or increased renal sensitivity to AVP, combined with any intake of free water; a notable exception is hyponatremia due to low solute intake (see later). The underlying pathophysiology for the exaggerated or inappropriate AVP response differs in patients with hyponatremia as a function of their ECFV. Hyponatremia thus is subdivided diagnostically into three groups, depending on clinical history and volume status: hypovolemic, euvolemic, and hypervolemic (Fig. 37-5).

Hypovolemic hyponatremia

Hypovolemia causes a marked neurohumoral activation, increasing circulating levels of AVP. The increase in circulating AVP helps preserve blood pressure via vascular and baroreceptor V_{1A} receptors and increases water reabsorption via renal V_2 receptors; activation of V^2 receptors can lead to hyponatremia in the setting of increased free-water intake. Nonrenal causes of hypovolemic hyponatremia include gastrointestinal (GI) loss (vomiting, diarrhea, tube drainage, etc.) and insensible loss (sweating, burns) of Na^+-Cl^- and water in the absence of adequate oral replacement; urine Na^+ concentration is typically <20 mM. Notably, these patients may be clinically classified as euvolemic, with only the reduced urinary Na^+ concentration to indicate the cause of their hyponatremia. Indeed, a urine Na^+ concentration <20 mM in the absence of a cause of hypervolemic hyponatremia predicts a rapid increase in plasma Na^+ concentration in response to intravenous normal saline; saline induces a water diuresis in this setting, as circulating AVP levels plummet.

The *renal* causes of hypovolemic hyponatremia share an inappropriate loss of Na^+-Cl^- in the urine, leading to volume depletion and an increase in circulating AVP; urine Na^+ concentration is typically >20 mM (Fig. 37-5). A deficiency in circulating aldosterone and/or its renal effects can lead to hyponatremia in primary adrenal insufficiency and other causes of hypoaldosteronism; hyperkalemia and hyponatremia in a hypotensive and/or hypovolemic patient with high urine Na^+ concentration (much >20 mM) should strongly suggest this diagnosis. Salt-losing nephropathies may lead to hyponatremia when sodium intake is reduced due to impaired renal tubular function; typical causes include reflux nephropathy, interstitial nephropathies, post-obstructive uropathy, medullary cystic disease, and the recovery phase of acute tubular necrosis. Thiazide diuretics cause hyponatremia via a number of mechanisms, including polydipsia and

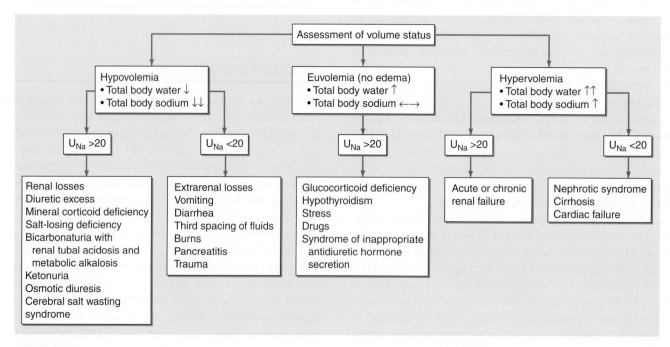

FIGURE 37-5

The diagnostic approach to hyponatremia. (*From S Kumar, T Berl: Diseases of water metabolism, in Atlas of Diseases of the Kidney, RW Schrier [ed]. Philadelphia, Current Medicine, Inc, 1999; with permission.*)

diuretic-induced volume depletion. Notably, thiazides do not inhibit the renal concentrating mechanism so that circulating AVP has a maximal effect on renal water retention. In contrast, loop diuretics, which are associated less frequently with hyponatremia, inhibit Na^+-Cl^- and K^+ absorption by the TALH, blunting the countercurrent mechanism and reducing the ability to concentrate the urine. Increased excretion of an osmotically active nonreabsorbable or poorly reabsorbable solute also can lead to volume depletion and hyponatremia; important causes include glycosuria, ketonuria (e.g., in starvation or in diabetic or alcoholic ketoacidosis), and bicarbonaturia (e.g., in renal tubular acidosis or metabolic alkalosis, in which the associated bicarbonaturia leads to loss of Na^+).

Finally, the syndrome of "cerebral salt wasting" is a rare cause of hypovolemic hyponatremia, encompassing hyponatremia with clinical hypovolemia and inappropriate natriuresis in association with intracranial disease; associated disorders include subarachnoid hemorrhage, traumatic brain injury, craniotomy, encephalitis, and meningitis. Distinction from the more common syndrome of inappropriate antidiuresis (SIAD) is critical, since cerebral salt wasting typically responds to aggressive Na^+-Cl^- repletion.

Hypervolemic hyponatremia

Patients with hypervolemic hyponatremia develop an increase in total body Na^+-Cl^- that is accompanied by a proportionately *greater* increase in total body water, leading to a reduced plasma Na^+ concentration. As in hypovolemic hyponatremia, the causative disorders can be separated by the effect on urine Na^+ concentration, with acute or chronic renal failure uniquely associated with an increase in urine Na^+ concentration (Fig. 37-5). The pathophysiology of hyponatremia in the sodium-avid edematous disorders (congestive heart failure [CHF], cirrhosis, and nephrotic syndrome) is similar to that in hypovolemic hyponatremia except that arterial filling and circulatory integrity are decreased due to the specific etiologic factors, e.g., cardiac dysfunction in CHF and peripheral vasodilation in cirrhosis. Urine Na^+ concentration is typically very low, i.e., <10 mM, even after hydration with normal saline; this Na^+-avid state may be obscured by diuretic therapy. The degree of hyponatremia provides an indirect index of the associated neurohumoral activation and is an important prognostic indicator in hypervolemic hyponatremia.

Euvolemic hyponatremia

Euvolemic hyponatremia can occur in moderate to severe hypothyroidism, with correction after the achievement of a euthyroid state. Severe hyponatremia also can be a consequence of secondary adrenal insufficiency due to pituitary disease; whereas the deficit in circulating aldosterone in primary adrenal insufficiency causes *hypovolemic* hyponatremia, the predominant glucocorticoid deficiency in secondary adrenal failure is associated with *euvolemic* hyponatremia. Glucocorticoids exert a negative feedback on AVP release by the posterior pituitary so that hydrocortisone replacement in these patients will rapidly normalize the AVP response to osmolality, reducing circulating AVP.

The syndrome of inappropriate antidiuresis is the most common cause of euvolemic hyponatremia (Table 37-1). The generation of hyponatremia in SIAD requires an intake of free water, with persistent intake at serum osmolalities that are lower than the usual threshold for thirst; as one would expect, the osmotic threshold and osmotic response curves for the sensation of thirst are shifted downward in patients with SIAD. Four distinct patterns of AVP secretion have been recognized in patients with SIAD, independent for the most part of the underlying cause. Unregulated, erratic AVP secretion is seen in about a third of patients, with no obvious correlation between serum osmolality and circulating AVP levels. Other patients fail to suppress AVP secretion at lower serum osmolalities, with a normal response curve to hyperosmolar conditions; others have a reset osmostat, with a lower threshold osmolality and a left-shifted osmotic response curve. The fourth subset consists of patients who have essentially no detectable circulating AVP, suggesting either a gain in function in renal water reabsorption or a circulating antidiuretic substance that is distinct from AVP. Gain-in-function mutations of a single specific residue in the V_2 vasopressin receptor have been described in some of these patients, leading to constitutive activation of the receptor in the absence of AVP and a nephrogenic subset of SIAD.

Strictly speaking, patients with SIAD are not euvolemic but are subclinically volume expanded due to AVP-induced water and Na^+-Cl^- retention; vasopressin escape mechanisms invoked by sustained increases in AVP serve to limit distal renal tubular transport, preserving a modestly hypervolemic steady state. Serum uric acid is often low (<4 mg/dL) in patients with SIAD, consistent with suppressed proximal tubular transport in the setting of increased distal tubular Na^+-Cl^- and water transport; in contrast, patients with hypovolemic hyponatremia are often hyperuricemic due to a shared activation of proximal tubular Na^+-Cl^- and urate transport.

Common causes of SIAD include pulmonary disease (pneumonia, tuberculosis, pleural effusion, etc.) and central nervous system (CNS) diseases (tumor, subarachnoid hemorrhage, meningitis, etc.). SIAD also occurs with malignancies, most commonly with small cell lung carcinoma (75% of cases of malignancy-associated SIAD); ~10% of patients with this tumor will have a plasma Na^+ concentration <130 mM at presentation.

TABLE 37-1

CAUSES OF THE SYNDROME OF INAPPROPRIATE ANTIDIURESIS

MALIGNANT DISEASES	PULMONARY DISORDERS	DISORDERS OF THE CENTRAL NERVOUS SYSTEM	DRUGS	OTHER CAUSES
Carcinoma	Infections	Infection	Drugs that stimulate release of AVP or enhance its action	Hereditary (gain-of-function mutations in the vasopressin V_2 receptor)
Lung	Bacterial pneumonia	Encephalitis		
Small cell	Viral pneumonia	Meningitis	Chlorpropamide	Idiopathic
Mesothelioma	Pulmonary abscess	Brain abscess	SSRIs	Transient
Oropharynx	Tuberculosis	Rocky Mountain	Tricyclic antidepres-	Endurance exercise
Gastrointestinal tract	Aspergillosis	spotted fever	sants	General anesthesia
Stomach	Asthma	AIDS	Clofibrate	Nausea
Duodenum	Cystic fibrosis	Bleeding and masses	Carbamazepine	Pain
Pancreas	Respiratory failure	Subdural hematoma	Vincristine	Stress
Genitourinary tract	associated with	Subarachnoid	Nicotine	
Ureter	positive-pressure	hemorrhage	Narcotics	
Bladder	breathing	Cerebrovascular	Antipsychotic drugs	
Prostate		accident	Ifosfamide	
Endometrium		Brain tumors	Cyclophosphamide	
Endocrine thymoma		Head trauma	Nonsteroidal anti-	
Lymphomas		Hydrocephalus	inflammatory drugs	
Sarcomas		Cavernous sinus	MDMA (ecstasy)	
Ewing's sarcoma		thrombosis	AVP analogues	
		Other	Desmopressin	
		Multiple sclerosis	Oxytocin	
		Guillain-Barré	Vasopressin	
		syndrome		
		Shy-Drager syndrome		
		Delerium tremens		
		Acute intermittent		
		polyphyria		

Abbreviations: AIDS, acquired immunodeficiency syndrome; AVP, vasopressin; MDMA, 3,4-methylenedioxymethamphetamine (ecstasy); SSRI, selective serotonin reuptake inhibitor.
Source: From DH Ellison, T Berl: N Engl J Med 356:2064, 2007.

SIAD is also a common complication of certain drugs, most commonly the selective serotonin reuptake inhibitors (SSRIs). Other drugs can potentiate the renal effect of AVP without exerting direct effects on circulating AVP levels (Table 37-1).

Low solute intake and hyponatremia

Hyponatremia occasionally can occur in patients with a very low intake of dietary solutes. Classically, this occurs in alcoholics whose sole nutrient is beer, hence the diagnostic label "beer potomania"; beer is very low in protein and salt content, containing only 1–2 millimole per liter of Na$^+$. The syndrome also has been described in nonalcoholic patients with highly restricted solute intake due to nutrient-restricted diets, e.g., extreme vegetarian diets. Patients with hyponatremia due to low solute intake typically present with a very low urine osmolality, <100–200 mosmol/kg, with a urine Na$^+$ concentration that is <10–20 mM. The fundamental abnormality is the inadequate dietary intake of solutes; the reduced urinary solute excretion

limits water excretion so that hyponatremia ensues after relatively modest polydipsia. The ability to excrete a free-water load is thus a function of urinary solute excretion; at a urine osmolality of 80 mosmol/kg, free-water clearance is 2.7 L daily for a solute excretion of 300 mosmol/d, 5.4 L daily at 600 mosmol/d, and 8.1 L at 900 mosmol/d. AVP levels have not been reported in patients with beer potomania but are expected to be suppressed or rapidly suppressible with saline hydration; this fits with the overly rapid correction in plasma Na$^+$ concentration that can be seen with saline hydration. Resumption of a normal diet and/or saline hydration also will correct the causative deficit in urinary solute excretion so that patients with beer potomania typically correct their plasma Na$^+$ concentration promptly after admission to the hospital.

Clinical features of hyponatremia

Hyponatremia induces generalized cellular swelling, a consequence of water movement down the osmotic gradient from the hypotonic ECF to the ICF. The symptoms of hyponatremia are primarily neurologic, reflecting the development of cerebral edema within a rigid skull. The initial CNS response to acute hyponatremia is an increase in interstitial pressure, leading to shunting of ECF and solutes from the interstitial space into the cerebrospinal fluid and then into the systemic circulation. This is accompanied by an efflux of the major intracellular ions, Na^+, K^+, and Cl^-, from brain cells. Acute hyponatremic encephalopathy ensues when these volume regulatory mechanisms are overwhelmed by a rapid decrease in tonicity, resulting in acute cerebral edema. Early symptoms can include nausea, headache, and vomiting. However, severe complications can evolve rapidly, including seizure activity, brainstem herniation, coma, and death. A key complication of acute hyponatremia is normocapnic or hypercapnic respiratory failure; the associated hypoxemia may amplify the neurologic injury. Normocapnic respiratory failure in this setting typically is due to noncardiogenic, neurogenic pulmonary edema, with a normal pulmonary capillary wedge pressure.

Acute symptomatic hyponatremia is a medical emergency that occurs in a number of specific settings (Table 37-2). Women, particularly before menopause, are much more likely to develop encephalopathy and severe neurologic sequelae. Acute hyponatremia often has an iatrogenic component, e.g., when hypotonic intravenous fluids are given to postoperative patients with an increase in circulating AVP. Exercise-associated hyponatremia, an important clinical issue at marathons and other endurance events, similarly has been linked to both a nonosmotic increase in circulating AVP and excessive free-water intake. The recreational drug ecstasy (MDMA, 3,4-methylenedioxymethamphetamine) causes a rapid and potent induction of both thirst and AVP, leading to severe acute hyponatremia.

Persistent, chronic hyponatremia results in an efflux of organic osmolytes (creatine, betaine, glutamate, myoinositol, and taurine) from brain cells; this response reduces intracellular osmolality and the osmotic gradient, favoring water entry. This reduction in intracellular osmolytes is largely complete within 48 h, the time period that clinically defines chronic hyponatremia; this temporal definition has considerable relevance for the treatment of hyponatremia (see later). The cellular response to chronic hyponatremia does not fully protect patients from symptoms, which can include vomiting, nausea, confusion, and seizures, usually at a plasma Na^+ concentration <125 mM. Even patients who are judged asymptomatic can manifest subtle gait and cognitive defects that reverse with correction of hyponatremia; notably, chronic asymptomatic hyponatremia increases the risk of falls. Chronic hyponatremia also increases the risk of bony fractures owing to the associated neurologic dysfunction and to a hyponatremia-associated reduction in bone density. Therefore, every attempt should be made to correct plasma Na^+ concentration safely in patients with chronic hyponatremia, even in the absence of overt symptoms (see the section on treatment of hyponatremia, later).

The management of chronic hyponatremia is complicated significantly by the asymmetry of the cellular response to correction of plasma Na^+ concentration. Specifically, the *reaccumulation* of organic osmolytes by brain cells is attenuated and delayed as osmolality increases after correction of hyponatremia, sometimes resulting in degenerative loss of oligodendrocytes and an osmotic demyelination syndrome (ODS). Overly rapid correction of hyponatremia (>8–10 mM in 24 h or 18 mM in 48 h) also is associated with a disruption in integrity of the blood-brain barrier, allowing the entry of immune mediators that may contribute to demyelination. The lesions of ODS classically affect the pons, a structure in which the delay in the reaccumulation of osmotic osmolytes is particularly pronounced; clinically, patients with central pontine myelinolysis can present one or more days after overcorrection of hyponatremia with para- or quadraparesis, dysphagia, dysarthria, diplopia, a "locked-in syndrome," and/or loss of consciousness. Other regions of the brain also can be involved in ODS, most commonly in association with lesions of the pons but occasionally in isolation; in order of frequency, the lesions of extrapontine myelinolysis can occur in the cerebellum, lateral geniculate body, thalamus, putamen, and cerebral cortex or subcortex. The clinical presentation of ODS therefore can vary as a function of the extent and localization of extrapontine myelinolysis, with the reported development of ataxia, mutism, parkinsonism, dystonia, and catatonia. Relowering of plasma Na^+ concentration after overly rapid correction can prevent or attenuate ODS (see the section on treatment of hyponatremia, later). However, even appropriately slow correction can be associated with ODS, particularly in patients with additional risk factors; these factors include alcoholism, malnutrition, hypokalemia, and liver transplantation.

TABLE 37-2

CAUSES OF ACUTE HYPONATREMIA

Iatrogenic
   Postoperative: premenopausal women
   Hypotonic fluids with cause of ↑ vasopressin
   Glycine irrigation: TURP, uterine surgery
   Colonoscopy preparation
   Recent institution of thiazides
Polydipsia
MDMA ingestion
Exercise-induced
Multifactorial, e.g., thiazide and polydipsia

Abbreviations: MDMA, 3,4-methylenedioxymethamphetamine (ecstasy); TURP, transurethral resection of the prostate.

Diagnostic evaluation of hyponatremia

Clinical assessment of hyponatremic patients should focus on the underlying cause; a detailed drug history is particularly crucial (Table 37-1). A careful clinical assessment of volume status is obligatory for the classical diagnostic approach to hyponatremia (Fig. 37-5). Hyponatremia is frequently multifactorial, particularly when severe; clinical evaluation should consider *all* the possible causes for excessive circulating AVP, including volume status, drugs, and the presence of nausea and/or pain. Radiologic imaging also may be appropriate to assess whether patients have a pulmonary or CNS cause for hyponatremia. A screening chest x-ray may fail to detect a small cell carcinoma of the lung; CT scanning of the thorax should be considered in patients at high risk for this tumor, e.g., patients with a history of smoking.

Laboratory investigation should include a measurement of serum osmolality to exclude pseudohyponatremia, which is defined as the coexistence of hyponatremia with a normal or increased plasma tonicity. Most clinical laboratories measure plasma Na^+ concentration by testing diluted samples with automated ion-sensitive electrodes, correcting for this dilution by assuming that plasma is 93% water; this correction factor can be inaccurate in patients with pseudohyponatremia due to extreme hyperlipidemia and/or hyperproteinemia, in whom serum lipid or protein makes up a greater percentage of plasma volume. The measured osmolality also should be converted to the effective osmolality (tonicity) by subtracting the measured concentration of urea (divided by 2.8 if in mg/dL); patients with hyponatremia have an effective osmolality <275 mosmol/kg.

Elevated BUN and creatinine in routine chemistries also can indicate renal dysfunction as a potential cause of hyponatremia, whereas hyperkalemia may suggest adrenal insufficiency or hypoaldosteronism. Serum glucose also should be measured; plasma Na^+ concentration falls by ~1.6 to 2.4 mM for every 100-mg/dL increase in glucose due to glucose-induced water efflux from cells; this "true" hyponatremia resolves after correction of hyperglycemia. Measurement of serum uric acid also should be performed; whereas patients with SIAD-type physiology typically will be hypouricemic (serum uric acid <4 mg/dL), volume-depleted patients often will be hyperuricemic. In the appropriate clinical setting, thyroid, adrenal, and pituitary function should also be tested; hypothyroidism and secondary adrenal failure due to pituitary insufficiency are important causes of euvolemic hyponatremia, whereas primary adrenal failure causes hypovolemic hyponatremia. A cosyntropin stimulation test is necessary to assess for primary adrenal insufficiency.

Urine electrolytes and osmolality are crucial tests in the initial evaluation of hyponatremia. A urine Na^+ concentration <20–30 mM is consistent with hypovolemic hyponatremia in the clinical absence of a hypervolemic, Na^+-avid syndrome such as CHF (Fig. 37-5). In contrast, patients with SIAD typically excrete urine with a Na^+ concentration that is >30 mM. However, there can be substantial overlap in urine Na^+ concentration values in patients with SIAD and hypovolemic hyponatremia, particularly in the elderly; the ultimate "gold standard" for the diagnosis of hypovolemic hyponatremia is the demonstration that plasma Na^+ concentration corrects after hydration with normal saline. Patients with thiazide-associated hyponatremia also may present with a higher than expected urine Na^+ concentration and other findings suggestive of SIAD; one should defer making a diagnosis of SIAD in these patients until 1–2 weeks after discontinuation of the thiazide. A urine osmolality <100 mosmol/kg is suggestive of polydipsia; urine osmolality >400 mosmol/kg indicates that AVP excess is playing a more dominant role, whereas intermediate values are more consistent with multifactorial pathophysiology (e.g., AVP excess with a significant component of polydipsia). Patients with hyponatremia due to decreased solute intake (beer potomania) typically have urine Na^+ concentration <20 mM and urine osmolality in the range of <100 to the low 200's. Finally, the measurement of urine K^+ concentration is required to calculate the urine:plasma electrolyte ratio, which is useful to predict the response to fluid restriction (see the section on treatment of hyponatremia, later).

TREATMENT   Hyponatremia

Three major considerations guide therapy for hyponatremia. First, the presence and/or severity of symptoms determine the urgency and goals of therapy. Patients with acute hyponatremia (Table 37-2) present with symptoms that can range from headache, nausea, and/or vomiting to seizures, obtundation, and central herniation; patients with chronic hyponatremia that is present for >48 h are less likely to have severe symptoms. Second, patients with chronic hyponatremia are at risk for ODS if plasma Na^+ concentration is corrected by >8–10 mM within the first 24 h and/or by >18 mM within the first 48 h. Third, the response to interventions such as hypertonic saline, isotonic saline, and vasopressin antagonists can be highly unpredictable, and so frequent monitoring of plasma Na^+ concentration during corrective therapy is imperative.

Once the urgency in correcting the plasma Na^+ concentration has been established and appropriate therapy instituted, the focus should be on treatment or withdrawal of the underlying cause. Patients with euvolemic hyponatremia due to SIAD, hypothyroidism, or secondary adrenal failure will respond to successful treatment of the underlying cause, with an increase in plasma Na$^+$ concentration. However, not all causes of SIAD are immediately reversible, necessitating pharmacologic therapy to increase the plasma Na$^+$ concentration (see later). Hypovolemic hyponatremia will respond to intravenous hydration with isotonic normal saline, with a rapid reduction in circulating AVP and a brisk water diuresis; it may be necessary to reduce the rate of correction if the history suggests that hyponatremia has been chronic, i.e., present for more than 48 h (see later). Hypervolemic hyponatremia due to congestive heart failure often responds to improved therapy of the underlying cardiomyopathy, e.g., after the institution or intensification of angiotensin-converting enzyme (ACE) inhibition. Finally, patients with hyponatremia due to beer potomania and low solute intake respond very rapidly to intravenous saline and the resumption of a normal diet. Notably, patients with beer potomania have a very high risk of developing ODS due to the associated hypokalemia, alcoholism, and malnutrition and the high risk of overcorrecting the plasma Na$^+$ concentration.

Water deprivation has long been a cornerstone of therapy for chronic hyponatremia. However, patients who are excreting minimal electrolyte-free water will require aggressive fluid restriction; this can be very difficult for patients with SIAD to tolerate because their thirst is also inappropriately stimulated. The urine:plasma electrolyte ratio (urinary [Na$^+$]+[K$^+$]/plasma [Na$^+$]) can be exploited as a quick indicator of electrolyte-free water excretion (Table 37-3); patients with a ratio >1 should be restricted more aggressively (<500 mL/d), those with a ratio ~1 should be restricted to 500–700 mL/d, and those with a ratio <1 should be restricted to <1 L/d. In hypokalemic patients, potassium replacement will serve to increase plasma Na$^+$ concentration in light of the fact that the plasma Na$^+$ concentration is a function of both exchangeable Na$^+$ and exchangeable K$^+$ divided by total body water; a corollary is that aggressive repletion of K$^+$ has the potential to overcorrect the plasma Na$^+$ concentration even in the absence of hypertonic saline. Plasma Na$^+$ concentration also tends to respond to an increase in dietary solute intake, which increases the ability to excrete free water; however, the use of oral urea and/or salt tablets for this purpose is generally not practical or well tolerated.

Patients in whom therapy with fluid restriction, potassium replacement, and/or increased solute intake fails may require pharmacologic therapy to increase their plasma Na$^+$ concentration. Many patients with SIAD respond to combined therapy with oral furosemide, 20 mg twice a day (higher doses may be necessary in renal insufficiency), and oral salt tablets; furosemide serves to inhibit the renal countercurrent mechanism and blunt urinary concentrating ability,

TABLE 37-3

MANAGEMENT OF HYPERNATREMIA

Water Deficit

1. Estimate total-body water (TBW): 50% of body weight in women and 60% in men
2. Calculate free-water deficit: $\{([Na^+]-140)/140\} \times TBW$
3. Administer deficit over 48–72 h, without decreasing the plasma Na$^+$ concentration by >10 mM/24 h

Ongoing Water Losses

4. Calculate electrolyte-free water clearance, C$_e$H$_2$O:

$$C_eH_2O = \frac{V(1-[U_{Na}+U_K]/P_{Na})}{P_{Na}}$$

where V is urinary volume, U$_{Na}$ is urinary [Na$^+$], U$_K$ is urinary [K$^+$], and P$_{Na}$ is plasma [Na$^+$]

Insensible Losses

5. ~10 mL/kg per day: less if ventilated, more if febrile

Total

6. Add components to determine water deficit and ongoing water loss; correct the water deficit over 48–72 h and replace daily water loss. Avoid correction of plasma [Na$^+$] by >10 mM/d

whereas the salt tablets counteract diuretic-associated natriuresis. Demeclocycline is a potent inhibitor of principal cells and can be utilized in patients whose Na+ levels do not increase in response to furosemide and salt tablets. However, this agent can be associated with a reduction in GFR due to excessive natriuresis and/or direct renal toxicity; it should be avoided in cirrhotic patients in particular, who are at higher risk of nephrotoxicity due to drug accumulation.

Vasopressin antagonists (vaptans) are highly effective in treating SIAD and hypervolemic hyponatremia due to heart failure or cirrhosis, reliably increasing plasma Na$^+$ concentration as a result of their aquaretic effects (augmentation of free-water clearance). Most of these agents specifically antagonize the V$_2$ vasopressin receptor; tolvaptan is currently the only oral V$_2$ antagonist approved by the U.S. Food and Drug Administration. Conivaptan, the only available intravenous vaptan, is a mixed V$_{1A}$/V$_2$ antagonist with a modest risk of hypotension due to V$_{1A}$ receptor inhibition. Therapy with vaptans must be initiated in a hospital setting, with a liberalization of fluid restriction (>2 L/d) and close monitoring of plasma Na$^+$ concentration. Although these agents are approved for the management of all but hypovolemic hyponatremia and acute hyponatremia, the clinical indications for them are not completely clear. Oral tolvaptan is perhaps most appropriate for the management of significant and persistent SIAD (e.g., in small cell lung carcinoma) that has not responded to water restriction and/or oral furosemide and salt tablets.

Treatment of acute symptomatic hyponatremia should include hypertonic 3% saline (513 mM) to acutely increase plasma Na$^+$ concentration by 1–2 mM/h to a total of 4–6 mM; this modest increase is typically sufficient to alleviate severe acute symptoms, after which corrective guidelines for "chronic" hyponatremia are appropriate (see later). A number of equations have been developed to estimate the required rate of hypertonic saline. The traditional approach is to calculate a Na$^+$ deficit, in which the Na$^+$ deficit = 0.6 × body weight × (target plasma Na$^+$ concentration − starting plasma Na$^+$ concentration), followed by a calculation of the required rate. Regardless of the method used to determine the rate of administration, the increase in plasma Na$^+$ concentration can be highly unpredictable during treatment with hypertonic saline due to rapid changes in the underlying physiology; plasma Na$^+$ concentration should be monitored every 2–4 h during treatment, with appropriate changes in therapy based on the observed rate of change. The administration of supplemental oxygen and ventilatory support is also critical in the management of patients with acute hyponatremia who develop acute pulmonary edema or hypercapnic respiratory failure. Intravenous loop diuretics will help treat acute pulmonary edema and also increase free-water excretion by interfering with the renal countercurrent multiplication system. Vasopressin antagonists do *not* have an approved role in the management of acute hyponatremia.

The rate of correction should be comparatively slow in *chronic* hyponatremia (<8–10 mM in the first 24 h and <18 mM in the first 48 h) to avoid ODS. Overcorrection of the plasma Na$^+$ concentration can occur when AVP levels rapidly normalize, for example, after treatment of patients with chronic hypovolemic hyponatremia with intravenous saline or after glucocorticoid replacement in patients with hypopituitarism and secondary adrenal failure. Approximately 10% of patients treated with vaptans will overcorrect; the risk is increased if water intake is not liberalized. If the plasma Na$^+$ concentration overcorrects after therapy—whether with hypertonic saline, isotonic saline, or a vaptan—hyponatremia can be reinduced safely or stabilized by the administration of the vasopressin *agonist* desmopressin acetate (DDAVP) and/or the administration of free water, typically intravenous D5W; the goal is to prevent or reverse the development of ODS.

HYPERNATREMIA

Etiology

Hypernatremia is defined as an increase in the plasma Na$^+$ concentration to >145 mM. Considerably less common than hyponatremia, hypernatremia nonetheless is associated with mortality rates as high as 40–60%, mostly

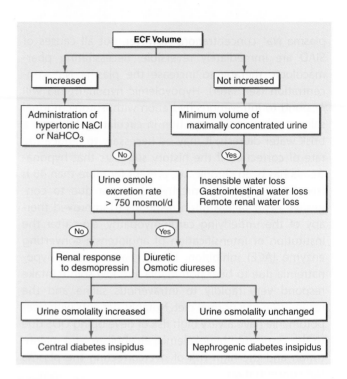

FIGURE 37-6
The diagnostic approach to hypernatremia. ECF, extracellular fluid.

due to the severity of the associated underlying disease processes. Hypernatremia is usually the result of a combined water and electrolyte deficit, with losses of H$_2$O in excess of those of Na$^+$. Less frequently, the ingestion or iatrogenic administration of excess Na$^+$ can be causative, for example, after IV administration of excessive hypertonic Na$^+$-Cl$^-$ or Na$^+$-HCO$_3^-$ (**Fig. 37-6**).

Elderly individuals with reduced thirst and/or diminished access to fluids are at the highest risk of developing hypernatremia. Patients with hypernatremia may rarely have a central defect in hypothalamic osmoreceptor function, with a mixture of both decreased thirst and reduced AVP secretion. Causes of this adipsic diabetes insipidus include primary or metastatic tumor, occlusion or ligation of the anterior communicating artery, trauma, hydrocephalus, and inflammation.

Hypernatremia can develop after the loss of water via both renal and nonrenal routes. Insensible losses of water may increase in the setting of fever, exercise, heat exposure, severe burns, or mechanical ventilation. Diarrhea is the most common gastrointestinal cause of hypernatremia. Notably, osmotic diarrhea and viral gastroenteritis typically generate stools with Na$^+$ and K$^+$ <100 mM, thus leading to water loss and hypernatremia; in contrast, secretory diarrhea typically results in isotonic stool and thus hypovolemia with or without hypovolemic hyponatremia.

Common causes of renal water loss include osmotic diuresis secondary to hyperglycemia, excess urea, post-obstructive diuresis, and mannitol; these disorders share an increase in urinary solute excretion and urinary osmolality (see "Diagnostic Approach," later). Hypernatremia due to a water diuresis occurs in central or nephrogenic diabetes insipidus (DI).

Nephrogenic DI (NDI) is characterized by renal resistance to AVP, which can be partial or complete (see "Diagnostic Approach"). Genetic causes include loss-of-function mutations in the X-linked V_2 receptor; mutations in the AVP-responsive aquaporin-2 water channel can cause autosomal recessive and autosomal dominant nephrogenic DI, whereas recessive deficiency of the aquaporin-1 water channel causes a more modest concentrating defect (Fig. 37-2). Hypercalcemia also can cause polyuria and NDI; calcium signals directly through the calcium-sensing receptor to downregulate Na^+, K^+, and Cl^- transport by the TALH and water transport in principal cells, thus reducing renal concentrating ability in hypercalcemia. Another common acquired cause of NDI is hypokalemia, which inhibits the renal response to AVP and downregulates aquaporin-2 expression. Several drugs can cause acquired NDI, in particular lithium, ifosfamide, and several antiviral agents. Lithium causes NDI by multiple mechanisms, including direct inhibition of renal glycogen synthase kinase-3 (GSK3), a kinase thought to be the pharmacologic target of lithium in bipolar disease; GSK3 is required for the response of principal cells to AVP. The entry of lithium through the amiloride-sensitive Na^+ channel ENaC (Fig. 37-4) is required for the effect of the drug on principal cells; thus, combined therapy with lithium and amiloride can mitigate lithium-associated NDI. However, lithium causes chronic tubulointerstitial scarring and chronic kidney disease after prolonged therapy so that patients may have a persistent NDI long after stopping the drug, with a reduced therapeutic benefit from amiloride.

Finally, gestational diabetes insipidus is a rare complication of late-term pregnancy in which increased activity of a circulating placental protease with vasopressinase activity leads to reduced circulating AVP and polyuria, often accompanied by hypernatremia. DDAVP is an effective therapy for this syndrome because of its resistance to the vasopressinase enzyme.

Clinical features

Hypernatremia increases osmolality of the ECF, generating an osmotic gradient between the ECF and the ICF, an efflux of intracellular water, and cellular shrinkage. As in hyponatremia, the symptoms of hypernatremia are predominantly neurologic. Altered mental status is the most common manifestation, ranging from mild confusion and lethargy to deep coma. The sudden shrinkage of brain cells in acute hypernatremia may lead to parenchymal or subarachnoid hemorrhages and/or subdural hematomas; however, these vascular complications are encountered primarily in pediatric and neonatal patients. Osmotic damage to muscle membranes also can lead to hypernatremic rhabdomyolysis. Brain cells accommodate to a chronic increase in ECF osmolality (>48 h) by activating membrane transporters that mediate influx and intracellular accumulation of organic osmolytes (creatine, betaine, glutamate, *myo*-inositol, and taurine); this results in an increase in ICF water and normalization of brain parenchymal volume. In consequence, patients with *chronic* hypernatremia are less likely to develop severe neurologic compromise. However, the cellular response to chronic hypernatremia predisposes these patients to the development of cerebral edema and seizures during overly rapid hydration (overcorrection of plasma Na^+ concentration by >10 mM/d).

Diagnostic approach

The history should focus on the presence or absence of thirst, polyuria, and/or an extrarenal source for water loss, such as diarrhea. The physical examination should include a detailed neurologic exam and an assessment of the ECFV; patients with a particularly large water deficit and/or a combined deficit in electrolytes and water may be hypovolemic, with reduced JVP and orthostasis. Accurate documentation of daily fluid intake and daily urine output is also critical for the diagnosis and management of hypernatremia.

Laboratory investigation should include a measurement of serum and urine osmolality in addition to urine electrolytes. The appropriate response to hypernatremia and a serum osmolality >295 mosmol/kg is an increase in circulating AVP and the excretion of low volumes (<500 mL/d) of maximally concentrated urine, i.e., urine with osmolality >800 mosmol/kg; if this is the case, an extrarenal source of water loss is primarily responsible for the generation of hypernatremia. Many patients with hypernatremia are polyuric; if an osmotic diuresis is responsible, with excessive excretion of Na^+-Cl^-, glucose, and/or urea, solute excretion will be >750–1000 mosmol/d (>15 mosmol/kg body water per day) (Fig. 37-6). More commonly, patients with hypernatremia and polyuria will have a predominant water diuresis, with excessive excretion of hypotonic, dilute urine.

Adequate differentiation between nephrogenic and central causes of DI requires the measurement of the response in urinary osmolality to DDAVP, combined with measurement of circulating AVP in the setting of hypertonicity. By definition, patients with baseline hypernatremia are hypertonic, with an adequate stimulus for AVP by the posterior pituitary. Therefore, in contrast to polyuric patients with a normal or reduced baseline plasma Na^+ concentration and osmolality, a water deprivation test is unnecessary in hypernatremia; indeed, water deprivation is absolutely contraindicated in this setting because of the risk for worsening the hypernatremia. Patients with NDI will fail to respond to DDAVP, with a urine osmolality that increases by <50% or <150 mosmol/kg from baseline, in combination with a normal or high circulating AVP level; patients with central DI will respond to DDAVP, with a reduced circulating AVP. Patients may exhibit a partial response to DDAVP, with a >50% rise in urine osmolality that nonetheless fails to reach 800 mosmol/kg; the level of circulating AVP will help differentiate the underlying cause, i.e., nephrogenic versus central DI. In pregnant patients, AVP assays should be drawn in tubes containing the protease inhibitor 1,10-phenanthroline to prevent in vitro degradation of AVP by placental vasopressinase.

For patients with hypernatremia due to renal loss of water it is critical to quantify *ongoing* daily losses using the calculated electrolyte-free water clearance in addition to calculation of the baseline water deficit (the relevant formulas are discussed in Table 37-3). This requires daily measurement of urine electrolytes, combined with accurate measurement of daily urine volume.

TREATMENT   Hypernatremia

The underlying cause of hypernatremia should be withdrawn or corrected, whether it is drugs, hyperglycemia, hypercalcemia, hypokalemia, or diarrhea. The approach to the correction of hypernatremia is outlined in Table 37-3. It is imperative tocorrect hypernatremia slowly to avoid cerebral edema, typically replacing the calculated free-water deficit over 48 h. Notably, the plasma Na$^+$ concentration should be corrected by no more than 10 mM/d, which may take longer than 48 h in patients with severe hypernatremia (>160 mM). A rare exception is patients with acute hypernatremia (<48 h) due to sodium loading, who can safely be corrected rapidly at a rate of 1 mM/h.

Water ideally should be administered by mouth or by nasogastric tube as the most direct way to provide free water, i.e., water without electrolytes. Alternatively, patients can receive free water in dextrose-containing IV solutions such as 5% dextrose (D5W); blood glucose should be monitored to avoid hyperglycemia. Depending on the history, blood pressure, or clinical volume status, it may be appropriate to treat initially with hypotonic saline solutions (1/4 or 1/2 normal saline); normal saline is usually inappropriate in the absence of very severe hypernatremia, in which normal saline is proportionally more hypotonic relative to plasma, or frank hypotension. Calculation of urinary electrolyte-free water clearance (see Table 37-3) is required to estimate daily, ongoing loss of free water in patients with nephrogenic or central DI, which should be replenished daily.

Additional therapy may be feasible in specific cases. Patients with central DI should respond to the administration of intravenous, intranasal, or oral DDAVP. Patients with NDI due to lithium may reduce their polyuria with amiloride (2.5–10 mg/d), which decreases entry of lithium into principal cells by inhibiting ENaC (see earlier); in practice, however, most patients with lithium-associated DI are able to compensate for their polyuria simply by increasing their daily water intake. Thiazides may reduce polyuria due to NDI, ostensibly by inducing hypovolemia and increasing proximal tubular water reabsorption. Occasionally, nonsteroidal anti-inflammatory drugs (NSAIDs) have been used to treat polyuria associated with NDI, reducing the negative effect of intrarenal prostaglandins on urinary concentrating mechanisms; however, this creates the risk of NSAID-associated gastric and/or renal toxicity. Furthermore, it must be emphasized that thiazides, amiloride, and NSAIDs are appropriate only for *chronic* management of polyuria from NDI and have *no* role in the acute management of associated hypernatremia, in which the focus is on replacing free-water deficits and ongoing free-water loss.

POTASSIUM DISORDERS

Homeostatic mechanisms maintain plasma K$^+$ concentration between 3.5 and 5.0 mM despite marked variation in dietary K$^+$ intake. In a healthy individual at steady state, the entire daily intake of potassium is excreted, approximately 90% in the urine and 10% in the stool; the kidney thus plays a dominant role in potassium homeostasis. However, more than 98% of total-body potassium is intracellular, chiefly in muscle; buffering of extracellular K$^+$ by this large intracellular pool plays a crucial role in the regulation of plasma K$^+$ concentration. Changes in the exchange and distribution of intra- and extracellular K$^+$ thus can lead to marked hypo- or hyperkalemia. A corollary is that massive necrosis and the attendant release of tissue K$^+$ can cause severe hyperkalemia, particularly in the setting of acute kidney injury and reduced excretion of K$^+$.

Changes in whole-body K$^+$ content are mediated primarily by the kidney, which *reabsorbs* filtered K$^+$ in hypokalemic, K$^+$-deficient states and *secretes* K$^+$ in hyperkalemic, K$^+$-replete states. Although K$^+$ is transported along the entire nephron, it is the principal cells of the connecting tubule (CNT) and cortical collecting duct (CD) that play a dominant role in renal K$^+$ secretion, whereas alpha-intercalated cells of the outer medullary CD function in renal tubular reabsorption of filtered K$^+$ in K$^+$-deficient states. In principal cells, apical Na$^+$ entry via the amiloride-sensitive ENaC generates a lumen-negative potential difference that drives passive K$^+$ exit through apical K$^+$ channels (Fig. 37-4). Two major K$^+$ channels mediate distal tubular K$^+$ secretion: the secretory K$^+$ channel ROMK (the renal outer medullary K$^+$ channel, also known as Kir1.1 or KcnJ1) and the flow-sensitive maxi-K K$^+$ channel (also known as the BK K+ channel). ROMK is thought to mediate the bulk of constitutive K$^+$ secretion, whereas increases in distal flow rate and/or genetic absence of ROMK activate K$^+$ secretion via the maxi-K channel.

An appreciation of the relationship between ENaC-dependent Na$^+$ entry and distal K$^+$ secretion (Fig. 37-4) is required for the bedside interpretation of potassium disorders. For example, decreased distal delivery of Na$^+$, as occurs in hypovolemic, prerenal states, tends to blunt the ability to excrete K$^+$, leading to hyperkalemia; in contrast, an *increase* in distal delivery of Na$^+$ and distal flow rate, as occurs after treatment with thiazide and loop diuretics, can enhance K$^+$ secretion and lead to hypokalemia. Hyperkalemia is also a predictable consequence of drugs that directly inhibit ENaC due to the role of this Na$^+$ channel in generating a lumen-negative potential difference. Aldosterone in turn has a major influence on potassium excretion, increasing the activity of ENaC channels and thus amplifying the driving force for K$^+$ secretion across the luminal membrane of principal cells. Abnormalities in the renin-angiotensin-aldosterone system thus can cause both hypokalemia and hyperkalemia. Notably, however, potassium excess and potassium restriction have opposing, aldosterone-independent effects on the density and activity of apical K$^+$ channels in the distal nephron; i.e., other factors modulate the renal capacity to secrete K$^+$. In addition, potassium restriction and hypokalemia activate aldosterone-independent distal *reabsorption* of filtered K$^+$, activating apical H$^+$/K$^+$-ATPase activity in intercalated cells within the outer medullary CD. Reflective perhaps of this physiology, changes in plasma K$^+$ concentration are not universal in disorders associated with changes in aldosterone activity.

HYPOKALEMIA

Hypokalemia, defined as a plasma K$^+$ concentration <3.6 mM, occurs in up to 20% of hospitalized patients. Hypokalemia is associated with a tenfold increase in in-hospital mortality rates due to adverse effects on cardiac rhythm, blood pressure, and cardiovascular morbidity rate. Mechanistically, hypokalemia can be caused by redistribution of K$^+$ between tissues and the ECF or by renal and nonrenal loss of K$^+$ (**Table 37-4**). Systemic hypomagnesemia also can cause treatment-resistant hypokalemia due to a combination of reduced cellular uptake of K$^+$ and exaggerated renal secretion. Spurious hypokalemia or pseudohypokalemia occasionally can result from in vitro cellular uptake of K$^+$ after venipuncture, for example, due to profound leukocytosis in acute leukemia.

TABLE 37-4

CAUSES OF HYPOKALEMIA

I. Decreased intake
  A. Starvation
  B. Clay ingestion
II. Redistribution into cells
  A. Acid-base
    1. Metabolic alkalosis
  B. Hormonal
    1. Insulin
    2. Increased β$_2$-adrenergic sympathetic activity: post-myocardial infarction, head injury
    3. β$_2$-Adrenergic agonists: bronchodilators, tocolytics
    4. α-Adrenergic antagonists
    5. Thyrotoxic periodic paralysis
    6. Downstream stimulation of Na$^+$/K$^+$-ATPase: theophylline, caffeine
  C. Anabolic state
    1. Vitamin B$_{12}$ or folic acid administration (red blood cell production)
    2. Granulocyte-macrophage colony-stimulating factor (white blood cell production)
    3. Total parenteral nutrition
  D. Other
    1. Pseudohypokalemia
    2. Hypothermia
    3. Familial hypokalemic periodic paralysis
    4. Barium toxicity: systemic inhibition of "leak" K$^+$ channels
III. Increased loss
  A. Nonrenal
    1. Gastrointestinal loss (diarrhea)
    2. Integumentary loss (sweat)
  B. Renal
    1. Increased distal flow and distal Na$^+$ delivery: diuretics, osmotic diuresis, salt-wasting nephropathies
    2. Increased secretion of potassium
      a. Mineralocorticoid excess: primary hyperaldosteronism (aldosterone-producing adenomas [APAs]), primary or unilateral adrenal hyperplasia (PAH), idiopathic hyperaldosteronism (IHA) due to bilateral adrenal hyperplasia, and adrenal carcinoma], familial hyperaldosteronism (FH-I, FH-II, congenital adrenal hyperplasias), secondary hyperaldosteronism (malignant hypertension, renin-secreting tumors, renal artery stenosis, hypovolemia), Cushing's syndrome, Bartter's syndrome, Gitelman's syndrome
      b. Apparent mineralocorticoid excess: genetic deficiency of 11β-dehydrogenase-2 (syndrome of apparent mineralocorticoid excess), inhibition of 11β-dehydrogenase-2 (glycyrrhetinic/glycyrrhizinic acid and/or carbenoxolone; licorice, food products, drugs), Liddle's syndrome (genetic activation of epithelial Na+ channels [ENaC])
      c. Distal delivery of nonreabsorbed anions: vomiting, nasogastric suction, proximal renal tubular acidosis, diabetic ketoacidosis, glue sniffing (toluene abuse), penicillin derivatives (penicillin, nafcillin, dicloxacillin, ticarcillin, oxacillin, and carbenicillin)
    3. Magnesium deficiency

Redistribution and hypokalemia

Insulin, β_2-adrenergic activity, and thyroid hormone promote Na^+,K^+-ATPase-mediated cellular uptake of K^+, leading to hypokalemia. Inhibition of passive *efflux* of K^+ also can cause hypokalemia, albeit rarely; this typically occurs in the setting of systemic inhibition of K^+ channels by toxic barium ions. Exogenous insulin can cause iatrogenic hypokalemia, particularly during the management of K^+-deficient states such as diabetic ketoacidosis. Alternatively, the stimulation of *endogenous* insulin can provoke hypokalemia, hypomagnesemia, and/or hypophosphatemia in malnourished patients who are given a carbohydrate load. Alterations in the activity of the endogenous sympathetic nervous system can cause hypokalemia in several settings, including alcohol withdrawal, hyperthyroidism, acute myocardial infarction, and severe head injury. β_2 agonists, including both bronchodilators and tocolytics (ritodrine), are powerful activators of cellular K^+ uptake; "hidden" sympathomimetics such as pseudoephedrine and ephedrine in cough syrup or dieting agents also may cause unexpected hypokalemia. Finally, xanthine-dependent activation of cyclic AMP–dependent signaling downstream of the β_2 receptor can lead to hypokalemia, usually in the setting of overdose (theophylline) or marked overingestion (dietary caffeine).

Redistributive hypokalemia also can occur in the setting of hyperthyroidism, with periodic attacks of hypokalemic paralysis (thyrotoxic periodic paralysis [TPP]). Similar episodes of hypokalemic weakness in the absence of thyroid abnormalities occur in *familial* hypokalemic periodic paralysis, usually caused by missense mutations of voltage sensor domains within the α^1 subunit of L-type calcium channels or the skeletal Na^+ channel; these mutations generate an abnormal gating pore current activated by hyperpolarization. TPP develops more frequently in patients of Asian or Hispanic origin; this shared predisposition has been linked to genetic variation in Kir2.6, a muscle-specific, thyroid hormone–responsive K^+ channel. Patients typically present with weakness of the extremities and limb girdles, with paralytic episodes that occur most frequently between 1 and 6 A.M. Signs and symptoms of hyperthyroidism are not invariably present. Hypokalemia is usually profound and almost invariably is accompanied by hypophosphatemia and hypomagnesemia. The hypokalemia in TPP is attributed to both direct and indirect activation of Na^+,K^+-ATPase, resulting in increased uptake of K^+ by muscle and other tissues. Increases in β-adrenergic activity play an important role in that high-dose propranolol (3 mg/kg) rapidly reverses the associated hypokalemia, hypophosphatemia, and paralysis.

Nonrenal loss of potassium

The loss of K^+ in sweat is typically low except under extremes of physical exertion. Direct gastric losses of K^+ due to vomiting or nasogastric suctioning are also minimal; however, the ensuing hypochloremic alkalosis results in persistent kaliuresis due to secondary hyperaldosteronism and bicarbonaturia, i.e., a *renal* loss of K^+. Intestinal loss of K^+ due to diarrhea is a globally important cause of hypokalemia in light of the worldwide prevalence of diarrheal disease. Noninfectious gastrointestinal processes such as celiac disease, ileostomy, villous adenomas, VIPomas, and chronic laxative abuse also can cause significant hypokalemia. Colonic pseudo-obstruction (Ogilvie's syndrome) can lead to hypokalemia from secretory diarrhea with an abnormally high potassium content caused by a marked activation of colonic K^+ secretion.

Renal loss of potassium

Drugs can increase renal K^+ excretion by a variety of different mechanisms. Diuretics are a particularly common cause due to associated increases in distal tubular Na^+ delivery and distal tubular flow rate in addition to secondary hyperaldosteronism. Thiazides have an effect on plasma K^+ concentration greater than that of loop diuretics despite their lesser natriuretic effect. The higher propensity of thiazides to cause hypokalemia may be secondary to thiazide-associated hypocalciuria versus the *hypercalciuria* seen with loop diuretics; increases in downstream luminal calcium in response to loop diuretics will inhibit ENaC in principal cells, thus reducing the lumen-negative potential difference and attenuating distal K^+ excretion. High doses of penicillin-related antibiotics (nafcillin, dicloxacillin, ticarcillin, oxacillin, and carbenicillin) can increase obligatory K^+ excretion by acting as nonreabsorbable anions in the distal nephron. Finally, several renal tubular toxins cause renal K^+ and magnesium wasting, leading to hypokalemia and hypomagnesemia; these drugs include aminoglycosides, amphotericin, foscarnet, cisplatin, and ifosfamide (see also "Magnesium Deficiency and Hypokalemia," later).

Aldosterone activates the ENaC channel in principal cells via multiple synergistic mechanisms, thus increasing the driving force for K^+ excretion. In consequence, increases in aldosterone bioactivity and/or gains in function of aldosterone-dependent signaling pathways are associated with hypokalemia. Increases in circulating aldosterone (hyperaldosteronism) may be primary or secondary. Increased levels of circulating renin in secondary forms of hyperaldosteronism lead to increased angiotensin II (AT-II) and thus aldosterone; renal artery stenosis is perhaps the most common cause (Table 37-4). Primary hyperaldosteronism may be genetic or acquired. Hypertension and hypokalemia due to increases in circulating 11-deoxycorticosterone occur in patients with congenital adrenal hyperplasia caused by defects in either steroid 11β-hydroxylase or steroid 17α-hydroxylase;

deficient 11β-hydroxylase results in associated virilization and other signs of androgen excess, whereas reduced sex steroids in 17α-hydroxylase deficiency lead to hypogonadism. The two major forms of *isolated* primary hyperaldosteronism are familial hyperaldosteronism type I (FH-I, also known as glucocorticoid-remediable hyperaldosteronism [GRA]) and familial hyperaldosteronism type II (FH-II), in which aldosterone production is not repressible by exogenous glucocorticoids. FH-I is caused by a chimeric gene duplication between the homologous 11β-hydroxylase (*CYP11B1*) and aldosterone synthase (*CYP11B2*) genes, fusing the adrenocorticotropic hormone (ACTH)-responsive 11β-hydroxylase promoter to the coding region of aldosterone synthase; this chimeric gene is under the control of ACTH and thus is repressible by glucocorticoids.

Acquired causes of primary hyperaldosteronism include aldosterone-producing adenomas (APAs), primary or unilateral adrenal hyperplasia (PAH), idiopathic hyperaldosteronism (IHA) due to bilateral adrenal hyperplasia, and adrenal carcinoma; APA and IHA account for close to 60% and 40%, respectively, of diagnosed cases of hyperaldosteronism. Random testing of plasma renin activity (PRA) and aldosterone is a helpful screening tool in hypokalemic and/or hypertensive patients, with an aldosterone:PRA ratio >50 suggestive of primary hyperaldosteronism.

The glucocorticoid cortisol has affinity for the mineralocorticoid receptor (MLR) equal to that of aldosterone, with resultant mineralocorticoid-like activity. However, cells in the aldosterone-sensitive distal nephron are protected from this illicit activation by the enzyme 11β-hydroxysteroid dehydrogenase-2 (11βHSD-2), which converts cortisol to cortisone; cortisone has minimal affinity for the MLR. Recessive loss-of-function mutations in the *11βHSD-2* gene thus are associated with cortisol-dependent activation of the MLR and the syndrome of apparent mineralocorticoid excess (SAME), encompassing hypertension, hypokalemia, hypercalciuria, and metabolic alkalosis, with suppressed PRA and suppressed aldosterone. A similar syndrome is caused by biochemical inhibition of 11βHSD-2 by glycyrrhetinic/glycyrrhizinic acid and/or carbenoxolone. Glycyrrhizinic acid is a natural sweetener found in licorice root, typically encountered in licorice and its many guises or as a flavoring agent in tobacco and food products.

Finally, hypokalemia may occur with systemic increases in glucocorticoids. In Cushing's syndrome caused by increases in pituitary ACTH the incidence of hypokalemia is only 10%, whereas it is 60–100% in patients with ectopic secretion of ACTH despite a similar incidence of hypertension. Indirect evidence suggests that the activity of renal 11βHSD-2 is reduced in patients with ectopic ACTH compared with Cushing's syndrome, resulting in a syndrome of apparent mineralocorticoid excess.

Finally, defects in multiple renal tubular transport pathways are associated with hypokalemia. For example, loss-of-function mutations in subunits of the acidifying H^+-ATPAse in alpha-intercalated cells cause hypokalemic distal renal tubular acidosis, as do many acquired disorders of the distal nephron. Liddle's syndrome is caused by autosomal dominant gain-in-function mutations of ENaC subunits. Disease-associated mutations either activate the channel directly or abrogate aldosterone-inhibited retrieval of ENaC subunits from the plasma membrane; the end result is increased expression of activated ENaC channels at the plasma membrane of principal cells. Patients classically manifest severe hypertension with hypokalemia that is unresponsive to spironolactone yet sensitive to amiloride. Hypertension and hypokalemia are, however, variable aspects of the Liddle's phenotype; more consistent features include a blunted aldosterone response to ACTH and reduced urinary aldosterone excretion.

Loss of the transport functions of the TALH and DCT nephron segments causes two distinct subtypes of hereditary hypokalemic alkalosis, with TALH dysfunction causing Bartter's syndrome (BS) and DCT dysfunction causing Gitelman's syndrome (GS). Patients with "classic" BS typically have polyuria and polydipsia due to the reduction in renal concentrating ability. They may have an increase in urinary calcium excretion, and 20% are hypomagnesemic. Other features include marked activation of the renin-angiotensin-aldosterone axis. Patients with "antenatal" BS have a severe systemic disorder characterized by marked electrolyte wasting, polyhydramnios, and hypercalciuria with nephrocalcinosis; renal prostaglandin synthesis and excretion are increased significantly, accounting for many of the systemic symptoms. There are five disease genes for BS, all of which function in some aspect of regulated Na^+, K^+, and Cl^- transport by the TALH. Gitelman's syndrome is, in contrast, genetically homogeneous, caused almost exclusively by loss-of-function mutations in the thiazide-sensitive Na^+-Cl^- cotransporter of the DCT. Patients with GS are uniformly hypomagnesemic and exhibit marked hypocalciuria rather than the hypercalciuria typically seen in BS; urinary calcium excretion is thus a critical diagnostic test in GS. GS has a milder phenotype than BS; however, patients with GS may suffer from chondrocalcinosis, an abnormal deposition of calcium pyrophosphate dihydrate (CPPD) in joint cartilage.

Magnesium deficiency and hypokalemia

Magnesium depletion has inhibitory effects on muscle Na^+,K^+-ATPase activity, reducing influx into muscle cells and causing a secondary kaliuresis. In addition, magnesium depletion causes exaggerated K^+ secretion by the distal nephron; this is attributed to a reduction in the magnesium-dependent, intracellular block of K^+ efflux through the secretory K^+ channel of principal cells (ROMK; Fig. 37-4). Regardless of the dominant mechanism(s), hypomagnesemic patients are clinically refractory to K^+ replacement in the absence of Mg^{2+} repletion. Notably, magnesium deficiency is also a common concomitant of hypokalemia, since many disorders of the distal nephron may cause both potassium and magnesium wasting.

Clinical features

Hypokalemia has prominent effects on cardiac, skeletal, and intestinal muscle cells. In particular, it is a major risk factor for both ventricular and atrial arrhythmias. Hypokalemia predisposes to digoxin toxicity by a number of mechanisms, including reduced competition between K^+ and digoxin for shared binding sites on cardiac Na^+,K^+-ATPase subunits. Electrocardiographic changes in hypokalemia include broad flat T waves, ST depression, and QT prolongation; these are most marked when serum K^+ is <2.7 mmol/L. Hypokalemia also results in hyperpolarization of skeletal muscle, thus impairing the capacity to depolarize and contract; weakness and even paralysis may ensue. It also causes a skeletal myopathy and predisposes to rhabdomyolysis. Finally, the paralytic effects of hypokalemia on intestinal smooth muscle may cause intestinal ileus.

The functional effects of hypokalemia on the kidney include Na^+-Cl^- and HCO_3^- retention, polyuria, phosphaturia, hypocitraturia, and an activation of renal ammoniagenesis. Bicarbonate retention and other acid–base effects of hypokalemia can contribute to the generation of metabolic alkalosis. Hypokalemic polyuria is due to a combination of polydipsia and an AVP-resistant renal concentrating defect. Structural changes in the kidney due to hypokalemia include a relatively specific vacuolizing injury to proximal tubular cells, interstitial nephritis, and renal cysts. Hypokalemia also predisposes to acute kidney injury and can lead to end-stage renal disease in patients with long-standing hypokalemia due to eating disorders and/or laxative abuse.

Hypokalemia and/or reduced dietary K^+ are implicated in the pathophysiology and progression of hypertension, heart failure, and stroke. For example, short-term K^+ restriction in healthy humans and patients with essential hypertension induces Na^+-Cl^- retention and hypertension. Correction of hypokalemia is particularly important in hypertensive patients treated with diuretics, in whom blood pressure improves with the establishment of normokalemia.

Diagnostic approach

The cause of hypokalemia is usually evident from history, physical examination, and/or basic laboratory tests. The history should focus on medications (e.g., laxatives, diuretics, antibiotics), diet and dietary habits (e.g., licorice), and/or symptoms that suggest a particular cause (e.g., periodic weakness, diarrhea). The physical examination should pay particular attention to blood pressure, volume status, and signs suggestive of specific hypokalemic disorders, e.g., hyperthyroidism and Cushing's syndrome. Initial laboratory evaluation should include electrolytes, BUN, creatinine, serum osmolality, Mg^{2+}, Ca^{2+}, a complete blood count, and urinary pH (Fig. 37-7). The presence of a non-anion-gap acidosis suggests a distal, hypokalemic renal tubular acidosis or diarrhea; calculation of the urinary anion gap can help differentiate these two diagnoses. Renal K^+ excretion can be assessed with a 24-h urine collection; a 24-h K^+ excretion of <15 mM is indicative of an extrarenal cause of hypokalemia (Fig. 37-7). Alternatively, serum and urine osmolality can be used to calculate the transtubular K^+ gradient (TTKG), which should be <3-4 in the presence of hypokalemia (see the section on hyperkalemia in this chapter). Urine Cl^- is usually decreased in patients with hypokalemia from a nonreabsorbable anion, such as antibiotics or HCO_3^-. Other causes of chronic, hypokalemic alkalosis are surreptitious vomiting, diuretic abuse, and GS. Hypokalemic patients with bulimia thus have a urinary Cl^- <10 mmol/L; urine Na^+, K^+, and Cl^- are persistently elevated in GS due to loss of function in the thiazide-sensitive Na^+-Cl^- cotransporter but less elevated in diuretic abuse and with greater variability. Urine diuretic screens for loop diuretics and thiazides may be necessary to further exclude diuretic abuse.

Other tests, such as urinary Ca^{2+}, thyroid function tests, and/or PRA and aldosterone levels, may be appropriate in specific cases. A plasma aldosterone:PRA ratio >50 is suggestive of hyperaldosteronism. Patients with hyperaldosteronism or apparent mineralocorticoid excess may require further testing, for example, adrenal vein sampling or the clinically available tests for specific genetic causes (FH-I, SAME, Liddle's syndrome, etc.). Patients with primary aldosteronism thus should be tested for the chimeric FH-I/GRA gene (see earlier) if they are younger than 20 years of age or have a family history of primary aldosteronism or stroke at a young age (<40 years). Preliminary differentiation of Liddle's syndrome due to mutant ENaC channels from SAME due to mutant 11βHSD-2 (see earlier)—both of which cause hypokalemia and hypertension with aldosterone suppression—can be made on a clinical basis; patients with Liddle's syndrome should respond to amiloride (ENaC inhibition) but not spironolactone, whereas patients with SAME will respond to spironolactone.

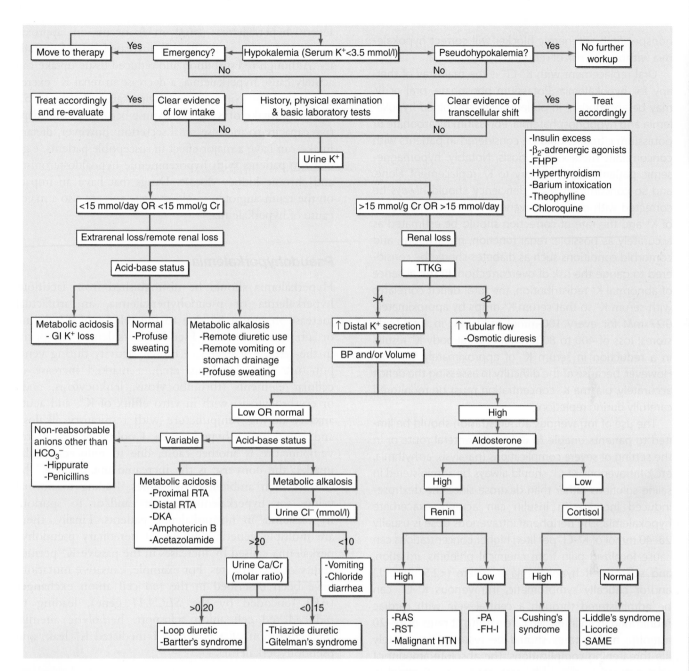

FIGURE 37-7

The diagnostic approach to hypokalemia. See text for details. BP, blood pressure; DKA, diabetic ketoacidosis; FHPP, familial hypokalemic periodic paralysis; FH-I, familial hyperaldosteronism type I; GI, gastrointestinal; HTN, hypertension; PA, primary aldosteronism; RAS, renal artery stenosis; RST, renin-secreting tumor; RTA, renal tubular acidosis; SAME, syndrome of apparent mineralocorticoid excess; TTKG, transtubular potassium gradient. (*From DB Mount, K Zandi-Nejad: Disorders of potassium balance, in Brenner and Rector's The Kidney, 8th ed, BM Brenner [ed]. Philadelphia, W.B. Saunders, 2008, pp 547-587; with permission.*)

TREATMENT Hypokalemia

The goals of therapy for hypokalemia are to prevent life-threatening and/or chronic consequences, replace the associated K⁺ deficit, and correct the underlying cause and/or mitigate future hypokalemia. The urgency of therapy depends on the severity of hypokalemia, associated clinical factors (cardiac disease, digoxin therapy, etc.), and the rate of decline in serum K⁺. Urgent but cautious K⁺ replacement should be considered in patients with severe redistributive hypokalemia (plasma K⁺ concentration <2.5 m*M*) and/or when serious complications ensue; however, this creates a risk of rebound hyperkalemia after resolution of the underlying cause. When excessive activity of the sympathetic nervous system is thought to play a dominant role in redistributive hypokalemia, as in thyrotoxic periodic paralysis, high-dose propranolol (3 mg/kg) should be considered; this nonspecific β-adrenergic blocker will correct hypokalemia without the risk of rebound hyperkalemia.

Oral replacement with K^+-Cl^- is the mainstay of therapy for hypokalemia. Potassium phosphate, oral or IV, may be appropriate in patients with combined hypokalemia and hypophosphatemia. Potassium bicarbonate or potassium citrate should be considered in patients with concomitant metabolic acidosis. Notably, hypomagnesemic patients are refractory to K^+ replacement alone, and so concomitant Mg^{2+} deficiency should *always* be corrected with oral or intravenous repletion. The deficit of K^+ and the rate of correction should be estimated as accurately as possible; renal function, medications, and comorbid conditions such as diabetes should be considered to gauge the risk of overcorrection. In the absence of abnormal K^+ redistribution, the total deficit correlates with serum K^+ so that serum K^+ drops by approximately 0.27 mM for every 100-mmol reduction in total-body stores; loss of 400 to 800 mmol of total-body K^+ results in a reduction in serum K^+ of approximately 2.0 mM. However, because of the difficulty in assessing the deficit accurately, plasma K^+ concentration must be monitored carefully during repletion.

The use of intravenous administration should be limited to patients unable to utilize the enteral route or in the setting of severe complications (paralysis, arrhythmia, etc.). Intravenous K^+-Cl^- should always be administered in saline solutions rather than dextrose since the dextrose-induced increase in insulin can acutely exacerbate hypokalemia. The peripheral intravenous dose is usually 20–40 mmol of K^+-Cl^- per liter; higher concentrations can cause localized pain from chemical phlebitis, irritation, and sclerosis. If hypokalemia is severe (<2.5 mmol/L) and/or critically symptomatic, intravenous K^+-Cl^- can be administered through a central vein with cardiac monitoring in an intensive care setting at rates of 10–20 mmol/h; higher rates should be reserved for acutely life-threatening complications. The absolute amount of administered K^+ should be restricted (e.g., 20 mmol in 100 mL of saline solution) to prevent inadvertent infusion of a large dose. Femoral veins are preferable, since infusion through internal jugular or subclavian central lines can acutely increase the local concentration of K^+ and affect cardiac conduction.

Strategies to minimize K^+ losses also should be considered. These measures may include minimizing the dose of non-K^+-sparing diuretics, restricting Na^+ intake, and using clinically appropriate combinations of non-K^+-sparing and K^+-sparing medications (e.g., loop diuretics with ACE inhibitors).

HYPERKALEMIA

Hyperkalemia is defined as a plasma potassium level of 5.5 mM. It occurs in up to 10% of hospitalized patients;

severe hyperkalemia (>6.0 mM) occurs in approximately 1%, with a significantly increased risk of mortality. Although redistribution and reduced tissue uptake can acutely cause hyperkalemia, a decrease in renal K^+ excretion is the most common underlying cause (Table 37-5). Excessive intake of K^+ is a rare cause because of the adaptive capacity to increase renal secretion; however, dietary intake can have a major effect in susceptible patients, e.g., diabetic patients with hyporeninemic hypoaldosteronism and chronic kidney disease. Drugs that have an impact on the renin–angiotensin–aldosterone axis are also a major cause of hyperkalemia.

Pseudohyperkalemia

Hyperkalemia should be distinguished from factitious hyperkalemia or pseudohyperkalemia, an artifactual increase in serum K^+ due to the release of K^+ during or after venipuncture. Pseudohyperkalemia can occur in the setting of excessive muscle activity during venipuncture (fist clenching, etc.), a marked increase in cellular elements (thrombocytosis, leukocytosis, and/or erythrocytosis) with in vitro efflux of K^+, and acute anxiety during venipuncture with respiratory alkalosis and redistributive hyperkalemia. Cooling of blood after venipuncture is another cause, due to reduced cellular uptake; the converse is the increased uptake of K^+ by cells at high ambient temperatures, leading to normal values for hyperkalemic patients and/or to spurious hypokalemia in normokalemic patients. Finally, there are multiple genetic subtypes of hereditary pseudohyperkalemia caused by increases in the passive K^+ permeability of erythrocytes. For example, causative mutations have been described in the red cell anion exchanger (AE1, encoded by the *SLC4A1* gene), leading to reduced red cell anion transport, hemolytic anemia, the acquisition of a novel AE1-mediated K^+ leak, and pseudohyperkalemia.

Redistribution and hyperkalemia

Several different mechanisms can induce an efflux of intracellular K^+ and hyperkalemia. Hyperkalemia due to hypertonic mannitol, hypertonic saline, and intravenous immunoglobulin generally is attributed to a "solvent drag" effect as water moves out of cells along the osmotic gradient. Diabetic patients are also prone to osmotic hyperkalemia in response to intravenous hypertonic glucose when it is given without adequate insulin. Cationic amino acids—specifically lysine, arginine, and the structurally related drug ε-aminocaproic acid—cause efflux of K^+ and hyperkalemia through an effective cation-K^+ exchange of unknown identity and mechanism. Digoxin inhibits Na^+,K^+-ATPase and impairs the uptake of K^+ by skeletal muscle so that digoxin overdose predictably results in hyperkalemia.

TABLE 37-5

CAUSES OF HYPERKALEMIA

I. "Pseudo" hyperkalemia
   A. Cellular efflux: thrombocytosis, erythrocytosis, leukocytosis, in vitro hemolysis
   B. Hereditary defects in red cell membrane transport
II. Intra- to extracellular shift
   A. Acidosis
   B. Hyperosmolality; radiocontrast, hypertonic dextrose, mannitol
   C. β-adrenergic antagonists (noncardioselective agents)
   D. Digoxin and related glycosides (yellow oleander, foxglove, bufadienolide)
   E. Hyperkalemic periodic paralysis
   F. Lysine, arginine, and ε-aminocaproic acid (structurally similar, positively charged)
   G. Succinylcholine; thermal trauma, neuromuscular injury, disuse atrophy, mucositis, or prolonged immobilization
   H. Rapid tumor lysis
III. Inadequate excretion
   A. Inhibition of the renin-angiotensin-aldosterone axis; ↑ risk of hyperkalemia when used in combination
      1. Angiotensin-converting enzyme (ACE) inhibitors
      2. Renin inhibitors: aliskiren (in combination with ACE-inhibitors or angiotensin receptor blockers [ARBs])
      3. ARBs
      4. Blockade of the mineralocorticoid receptor: spironolactone, eplerenone, drospirenone
      5. Blockade of ENaC: amiloride, triamterene, trimethoprim, pentamidine, nafamostat
   B. Decreased distal delivery
      1. Congestive heart failure
      2. Volume depletion
   C. Hyporeninemic hypoaldosteronism
      1. Tubulointerstitial diseases: systemic lupus erythematosus (SLE), sickle cell anemia, obstructive uropathy
      2. Diabetes, diabetic nephropathy
      3. Drugs: nonsteroidal anti-inflammatory drugs, cyclooxygenase 2 (COX-2) inhibitors, beta blockers, cyclosporine, tacrolimus
      4. Chronic kidney disease, advanced age
      5. Pseudohypoaldosteronism type II: defects in WNK1 or WNK4 kinases
   D. Renal resistance to mineralocorticoid
      1. Tubulointerstitial diseases: SLE, amyloidosis, sickle cell anemia, obstructive uropathy, post-acute tubular necrosis
      2. Hereditary: pseudohypoaldosteronism type I: defects in the mineralocorticoid receptor *or* ENaC
   E. Advanced renal insufficiency
      1. Chronic kidney disease
      2. End-stage renal disease
      3. Acute oliguric kidney injury
   F. Primary adrenal insufficiency
      1. Autoimmune: Addison's disease, polyglandular endocrinopathy
      2. Infectious: HIV, cytomegalovirus, tuberculosis, disseminated fungal infection
      3. Infiltrative: amyloidosis, malignancy, metastatic cancer
      4. Drug-associated: heparin, low-molecular-weight heparin
      5. Hereditary: adrenal hypoplasia congenita, congenital lipoid adrenal hyperplasia, aldosterone synthase deficiency
      6. Adrenal hemorrhage or infarction, including in antiphospholipid syndrome

Structurally related glycosides are found in specific plants (yellow oleander, foxglove, etc.) and in the cane toad, *Bufo marinus* (bufadienolide); ingestion of these substances and extracts from them also can cause hyperkalemia. Finally, fluoride ions also inhibit Na^+,K^+-ATPase, and so fluoride poisoning is typically associated with hyperkalemia.

Succinylcholine depolarizes muscle cells, causing an efflux of K^+ through acetylcholine receptors (AChRs). The use of this agent is contraindicated in patients who have sustained thermal trauma, neuromuscular injury, disuse atrophy, mucositis, or prolonged immobilization. These disorders share a marked increase and redistribution of AChRs at the plasma membrane of muscle cells; depolarization of these upregulated AChRs by succinylcholine leads to an exaggerated efflux of K^+ through the receptor-associated cation channels, resulting in acute hyperkalemia.

Hyperkalemia due to excess intake or tissue necrosis

Increased intake of even small amounts of K^+ may provoke severe hyperkalemia in patients with predisposing factors; hence, an assessment of dietary intake is crucial. Foods rich in potassium include tomatoes, bananas, and citrus fruits; occult sources of K^+, particularly K^+-containing salt substitutes, also may contribute significantly. Iatrogenic causes include simple overreplacement with K^+-Cl^- and the administration of a potassium–containing medication (e.g., K^+-penicillin) to a susceptible patient. Red cell transfusion is a well-described cause of hyperkalemia, typically in the setting of massive transfusions. Finally, tissue necrosis, as in acute tumor lysis syndrome and rhabdomyolysis, predictably causes hyperkalemia from the release of intracellular K^+.

Hypoaldosteronism and hyperkalemia

Aldosterone release from the adrenal gland may be reduced by hyporeninemic hypoaldosteronism, medications, or primary hypoaldosteronism or by isolated deficiency of ACTH (secondary hypoaldosteronism). Primary hypoaldosteronism may be genetic or acquired but is commonly caused by autoimmunity either in Addison's disease or in the context of a polyglandular endocrinopathy. HIV has surpassed tuberculosis as the most important infectious cause of adrenal insufficiency. The adrenal involvement in HIV disease is usually subclinical; however, adrenal insufficiency may be precipitated by stress, drugs such as ketoconazole that inhibit steroidogenesis, or the acute withdrawal of steroid agents such as megestrol.

Hyporeninemic hypoaldosteronism is a very common predisposing factor in several overlapping subsets of hyperkalemic patients: diabetic patients, the elderly, and patients with renal insufficiency. Classically, these patients should have suppressed PRA and aldosterone; approximately 50% have an associated acidosis with a reduced renal excretion of NH_4^+, a positive urinary anion gap, and urine pH <5.5. Most patients are volume expanded, with secondary increases in circulating atrial natriuretic peptide (ANP) that inhibit both renal renin release and adrenal aldosterone release.

Renal disease and hyperkalemia

Chronic kidney disease and end-stage kidney disease are very common causes of hyperkalemia because of the associated deficit or absence of functioning nephrons. Hyperkalemia is more common in oliguric acute kidney injury; distal tubular flow rate and Na^+ delivery is less of a limiting factor in nonoliguric patients. Hyperkalemia out of proportion to GFR can also be seen in the context of tubulointerstitial disease that affects the distal nephron, such as amyloidosis, sickle cell anemia, interstitial nephritis, and obstructive uropathy.

Hereditary renal causes of hyperkalemia have overlapping clinical features with hypoaldosteronism, hence the diagnostic label *pseudohypoaldosteronism* (PHA). PHA-I has both an autosomal recessive and an autosomal dominant form. The autosomal dominant form is due to loss-of-function mutations in MLR; the recessive form is caused by various combinations of mutations in the three subunits of ENaC, resulting in impaired Na^+ channel activity in principal cells and other tissues. Patients with recessive PHA-I experience lifelong salt wasting, hypotension, and hyperkalemia, whereas the phenotype of autosomal dominant PHA-I due to MLR dysfunction improves in adulthood. Pseudohypoaldosteronism type II (PHA-II, also known as hereditary hypertension with hyperkalemia) is in every respect the mirror image of GS caused by loss of function in NCC, the thiazide-sensitive Na^+-Cl^- cotransporter (see earlier); the clinical phenotype includes hypertension, hyperkalemia, hyperchloremic metabolic acidosis, suppressed PRA and aldosterone, hypercalciuria, and reduced bone density. PHA-II thus behaves like a gain of function in NCC, and treatment with thiazides results in resolution of the entire clinical phenotype; however, PHA-II is caused by mutations in the WNK1 and WNK4 serine-threonine kinases, which regulate NCC activity.

Medication-associated hyperkalemia

Most medications associated with hyperkalemia cause inhibition of some component of the renin-angiotensin-aldosterone axis. ACE inhibitors, angiotensin-receptor blockers, renin inhibitors, and mineralocorticoid receptors are predictable and common causes of hyperkalemia, particularly when prescribed in combination. The oral contraceptive agent Yasmin-28 contains the progestin drospirenone, which inhibits the MLR and can cause hyperkalemia in susceptible patients. Cyclosporine, tacrolimus, NSAIDs, and cyclooxygenase 2 (COX-2) inhibitors cause hyperkalemia by multiple mechanisms but share the ability to cause hyporeninemic hypoaldosteronism. Notably, most drugs that affect the renin-angiotensin-aldosterone axis also block the local adrenal response to hyperkalemia, thus attenuating the *direct* stimulation of aldosterone release by increased plasma K^+ concentration.

Inhibition of apical ENaC activity in the distal nephron by amiloride and other K^+-sparing diuretics results in hyperkalemia, often with a voltage-dependent hyperchloremic acidosis and/or hypovolemic hyponatremia. Amiloride is structurally similar to the antibiotics trimethoprim (TMP) and pentamidine, which also block ENaC; risk factors for TMP-associated hyperkalemia include the administered dose, renal insufficiency, and hyporeninemic hypoaldosteronism. Indirect inhibition of ENaC at the plasma membrane is also a cause of hyperkalemia; nafamostat, a protease inhibitor utilized in the management of pancreatitis, inhibits aldosterone-induced proteases that activate ENaC by proteolytic cleavage.

Clinical features

Hyperkalemia is a medical emergency because of its effects on the heart. Cardiac arrhythmias associated with hyperkalemia include sinus bradycardia, sinus arrest, slow idioventricular rhythms, ventricular tachycardia, ventricular fibrillation, and asystole. Mild increases in extracellular K^+ affect the repolarization phase of the cardiac action potential, resulting in changes in T-wave morphology; further increase in plasma K^+ concentration depresses intracardiac conduction, with progressive prolongation of the PR and QRS intervals. Severe hyperkalemia results in loss of the P wave and a progressive widening of the QRS complex; development of a sine-wave sinoventricular rhythm suggests impending ventricular fibrillation or asystole. Classically, the electrocardiographic manifestations in hyperkalemia progress from tall peaked T waves (5.5–6.5 mM), to a loss of P waves (6.5–7.5 mM), to a widened QRS complex (7–8 mM), and ultimately to a sine wave pattern (8 mM). However, these changes are notoriously insensitive, particularly in patients with chronic kidney disease or end-stage renal disease.

Hyperkalemia from a variety of causes can also present with ascending paralysis; this is denoted secondary hyperkalemic paralysis to differentiate it from familial hyperkalemic periodic paralysis (HYPP). The presentation may include diaphragmatic paralysis and respiratory failure. Patients with familial HYPP develop myopathic weakness during hyperkalemia induced by increased K^+ intake or rest after heavy exercise. Depolarization of skeletal muscle by hyperkalemia unmasks an inactivation defect in skeletal Na^+ channels; autosomal dominant mutations in the *SCN4A* gene encoding this channel are the predominant cause.

Within the kidney, hyperkalemia has negative effects on the ability to excrete an acid load, and so hyperkalemia per se can contribute to metabolic acidosis. This defect appears to be due in part to competition between K^+ and NH_4^+ for reabsorption by the TALH and subsequent countercurrent multiplication, ultimately reducing the medullary gradient for NH_3/NH_4 excretion by the distal nephron. Regardless of the underlying mechanism, restoration of normokalemia can in many instances correct hyperkalemic metabolic acidosis.

Diagnostic approach

The first priority in the management of hyperkalemia is to assess the need for emergency treatment, followed by a comprehensive workup to determine the cause (Fig. 37-8). History and physical examination should focus on medications, diet and dietary supplements, risk factors for kidney failure, reduction in urine output, blood pressure, and volume status. Initial laboratory tests should include electrolytes, BUN, creatinine, serum osmolality, Mg^{2+} and Ca^{2+}, a complete blood count, and urinary pH. A urine Na^+ concentration <20 mM indicates that distal Na^+ delivery is a limiting factor in K^+ excretion; volume repletion with 0.9% saline or treatment with furosemide may be effective in reducing plasma K^+ concentration. Serum and urine osmolality is required for calculation of the TTKG (Fig. 37-8). The expected values of the TTKG are largely based on historic data and are <3-4 in the presence of hypokalemia and >6-7 in the presence of hyperkalemia. TTKG is measured as follows:

$$TTKG = \frac{[K^+]_{urine} \times osmol_{serum}}{[K^+]_{serum} \times osmol_{urine}}$$

TREATMENT ▶ **Hyperkalemia**

Electrocardiographic manifestations of hyperkalemia should be considered a medical emergency and treated urgently. However, patients with significant hyperkalemia (plasma K^+ concentration ≤6.5–7 mM) in the absence of ECG changes should be aggressively managed because of the limitations of ECG changes as a predictor of cardiac toxicity. Urgent management of hyperkalemia includes admission to the hospital, continuous cardiac monitoring, and immediate treatment. The treatment of hyperkalemia is divided into three stages:

1. *Immediate antagonism of the cardiac effects of hyperkalemia.* Intravenous calcium serves to protect the heart while measures are taken to correct hyperkalemia. Calcium raises the action potential threshold and reduces excitability without changing the resting membrane potential. By restoring the difference between the resting and threshold potentials, calcium reverses the depolarization blockade caused by hyperkalemia. The recommended dose is 10 mL of 10% calcium gluconate (3–4 mL of calcium chloride), infused intravenously over 2 to 3 min with cardiac monitoring. The effect of the infusion starts in 1–3 min and lasts 30–60 min; the dose should be repeated if there is no change in ECG findings or if they recur after initial improvement. Hypercalcemia potentiates the cardiac toxicity of digoxin; hence, intravenous calcium should be used with extreme caution in patients taking this medication. If judged necessary, 10 mL of 10% calcium gluconate can be added to 100 mL of 5% dextrose in water and infused over 20–30 min to avoid acute hypercalcemia.

2. *Rapid reduction in plasma K^+ concentration by redistribution into cells.* Insulin lowers plasma K^+ concentration by shifting K^+ into cells. The recommended dose is 10 units of IV regular insulin followed immediately by 50 mL of 50% dextrose (D50W, 25 g of glucose total); the effect begins in 10–20 min, peaks at 30–60 min, and lasts 4 to 6 h. Bolus D50W without insulin is *never* appropriate because of the risk of acutely worsening hyperkalemia due to the osmotic effect of hypertonic glucose. Hypoglycemia is common with insulin plus glucose; hence, this should be followed by an infusion of 10% dextrose at 50 to 75 mL/h, with close monitoring of plasma glucose concentration. In hyperkalemic patients with glucose concentrations ≤200–250 mg/dL, insulin should be administered *without* glucose, again with close monitoring of glucose concentrations.

3. β_2-agonists, most commonly albuterol, are effective but underutilized agents for the acute management of hyperkalemia. Albuterol and insulin with glucose have an additive effect on plasma K^+ concentration; however, ~20% of patients with end-stage renal disease are resistant to the effect of β_2-agonists; hence, these drugs should not be used without insulin. The recommended dose for inhaled albuterol is 10–20 mg of nebulized albuterol in 4 mL of normal saline, inhaled over 10 min; the effect starts at about 30 min, reaches its peak at about 90 min, and lasts 2–6 h. Hyperglycemia is a side effect, along with tachycardia; β_2-agonists should be used with caution in hyperkalemic patients with known cardiac disease.

Intravenous bicarbonate has no role in the routine treatment of hyperkalemia. It should be reserved for patients with hyperkalemia and concomitant metabolic acidosis, and only if judged appropriate for management of the acidosis. It should not be given as a hypertonic intravenous bolus in light of the risk of hypernatremia

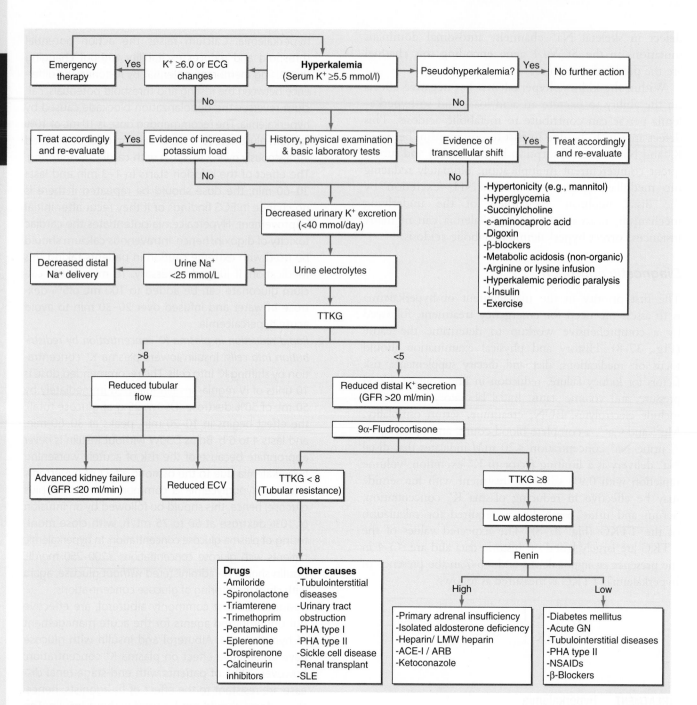

FIGURE 37-8

The diagnostic approach to hyperkalemia. See text for details. ACE-I, angiotensin converting enzyme inhibitor; acute GN, acute glomerulonephritis; ARB, angiotensin II receptor blocker; ECG, electrocardiogram; ECV, effective circulatory volume; GFR, glomerular filtration rate; LMW heparin, low-molecular-weight heparin; NSAIDs, nonsteroidal anti-inflammatory drugs; PHA, pseudohypoaldosteronism; SLE, systemic lupus erythematosus; TTKG, transtubular potassium gradient. (*From DB Mount, K Zandi-Nejad: Disorders of potassium balance, in Brenner and Rector's The Kidney, 8th ed, BM Brenner [ed]. Philadelphia, W.B. Saunders, 2008, pp 547-587; with permission.*)

but should be infused in an isotonic or hypotonic fluid (e.g., 150 meq in 1 L of D5W).

Removal of potassium. This typically is accomplished by using cation exchange resins, diuretics, and/or dialysis. Sodium polystyrene sulfonate (SPS) exchanges Na^+ for K^+ in the gastrointestinal tract and increases the fecal excretion of K^+. The recommended dose of SPS is 15-30 g, typically given in a premade suspension with 33% sorbitol to avoid constipation. The effect of SPS on plasma K^+ concentration is slow; the full effect may take up to 24 h and usually requires repeated doses every 4–6 h. Intestinal necrosis is the most serious complication of SPS.

Studies in experimental animals suggest that sorbitol is required for the intestinal injury; however, SPS crystals can often be detected in the injured human intestine, suggesting a direct role for SPS crystals in this complication. Regardless, in light of the risk of intestinal necrosis, the U.S. Food and Drug Administration has recently stated that the administration of sorbitol with SPS is no longer recommended; however, administering SPS without sorbitol might not eliminate the risk of intestinal necrosis, given the evident role for the SPS resin. Therefore, clinicians must carefully consider whether emergency treatment with SPS is necessary and appropriate for the treatment of hyperkalemia; for example, SPS is unnecessary if acute dialysis is appropriate and immediately available. If SPS is administered, the preparation should ideally not contain sorbitol. Reasonable substitutes for the laxative effect of sorbitol include lactulose and some preparations of polyethylene glycol 3350; however, data demonstrating the efficacy and safety of these laxatives with SPS are not available. SPS should not be administered in patients at higher risk for intestinal necrosis, including postoperative patients, patients with a history of bowel obstruction, patients with slow intestinal transit, patients with ischemic bowel disease, and renal transplant patients. Loop and thiazide diuretics can be utilized to reduce plasma K^+ concentration in volume-replete or hypervolemic patients with sufficient renal function for a diuretic response. Finally, hemodialysis is the most effective and reliable method to reduce plasma K^+ concentration; peritoneal dialysis is considerably less effective. The amount of K^+ removed during hemodialysis depends on the relative distribution of K^+ between ICF and ECF (potentially affected by prior therapy for hyperkalemia), the type and surface area of the dialyzer used, dialysate and blood flow rates, the dialysate flow rate, dialysis duration, and the plasma to dialysate K^+ gradient.

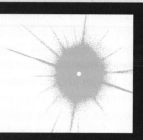

CHAPTER 38

ACIDOSIS AND ALKALOSIS

Thomas D. DuBose, Jr.

NORMAL ACID-BASE HOMEOSTASIS

Systemic arterial pH is maintained between 7.35 and 7.45 by extracellular and intracellular chemical buffering together with respiratory and renal regulatory mechanisms. The control of arterial CO_2 tension (Pa_{CO_2}) by the central nervous system (CNS) and respiratory systems and the control of the plasma bicarbonate by the kidneys stabilize the arterial pH by excretion or retention of acid or alkali. The metabolic and respiratory components that regulate systemic pH are described by the Henderson-Hasselbalch equation:

$$pH = 6.1 + \log \frac{HCO_3^-}{Pa_{CO_2} \times 0.0301}$$

Under most circumstances, CO_2 production and excretion are matched, and the usual steady-state Pa_{CO_2} is maintained at 40 mmHg. Underexcretion of CO_2 produces hypercapnia, and overexcretion causes hypocapnia. Nevertheless, production and excretion are again matched at a new steady-state Pa_{CO_2}. Therefore, the Pa_{CO_2} is regulated primarily by neural respiratory factors and is not subject to regulation by the rate of CO_2 production. Hypercapnia is usually the result of hypoventilation rather than of increased CO_2 production. Increases or decreases in Pa_{CO_2} represent derangements of neural respiratory control or are due to compensatory changes in response to a primary alteration in the plasma $[HCO_3^-]$.

The kidneys regulate plasma $[HCO_3^-]$ through three main processes: (1) "reabsorption" of filtered HCO_3^-, (2) formation of titratable acid, and (3) excretion of NH_4^+ in the urine. The kidney filters ~4000 mmol of HCO_3^- per day. To reabsorb the filtered load of HCO_3^-, the renal tubules must therefore secrete 4000 mmol of hydrogen ions. Between 80 and 90%

of HCO_3^- is reabsorbed in the proximal tubule. The distal nephron reabsorbs the remainder and secretes H^+ to defend systemic pH. While this quantity of protons, 40–60 mmol/d, is small, it must be secreted to prevent chronic positive H^+ balance and metabolic acidosis. This quantity of secreted protons is represented in the urine as titratable acid and NH_4^+. Metabolic acidosis in the face of normal renal function increases NH_4^+ production and excretion. NH_4^+ production and excretion are impaired in chronic renal failure, hyperkalemia, and renal tubular acidosis.

DIAGNOSIS OF GENERAL TYPES OF DISTURBANCES

The most common clinical disturbances are simple acid-base disorders; i.e., metabolic acidosis or alkalosis or respiratory acidosis or alkalosis. Because compensation is not complete, the pH is abnormal in simple disturbances. More complicated clinical situations can give rise to mixed acid-base disturbances.

SIMPLE ACID-BASE DISORDERS

Primary respiratory disturbances (primary changes in Pa_{CO_2}) invoke compensatory metabolic responses (secondary changes in $[HCO_3^-]$), and primary metabolic disturbances elicit predictable compensatory respiratory responses (secondary changes in Pa_{CO_2}). Physiologic compensation can be predicted from the relationships displayed in Table 38-1. Metabolic acidosis due to an increase in endogenous acids (e.g., ketoacidosis) lowers extracellular fluid $[HCO_3^-]$ and decreases extracellular pH. This stimulates the medullary chemoreceptors to increase ventilation and to return the ratio of $[HCO_3^-]$ to Pa_{CO_2}, and thus pH, toward, but not to, normal.

TABLE 38-1

PREDICTION OF COMPENSATORY RESPONSES ON SIMPLE ACID-BASE DISTURBANCES AND PATTERN OF CHANGES

DISORDER	PREDICTION OF COMPENSATION	RANGE OF VALUES		
		pH	HCO$_3^-$	Pa$_{CO_2}$
Metabolic acidosis	Pa$_{CO_2}$ = (1.5 × HCO$_3^-$) + 8 ± 2 *or* Pa$_{CO_2}$ will ↓ 1.25 mmHg per mmol/L ↓ in [HCO$_3^-$] *or* Pa$_{CO_2}$ = [HCO$_3^-$] + 15	Low	Low	Low
Metabolic alkalosis	Pa$_{CO_2}$ will ↑ 0.75 mmHg per mmol/L ↑ in [HCO$_3^-$] *or* Pa$_{CO_2}$ will ↑ 6 mmHg per 10 mmol/L ↑ in [HCO$_3^-$] *or* Pa$_{CO_2}$ = [HCO$_3^-$] + 15	High	High	High
Respiratory alkalosis		High	Low	Low
Acute	[HCO$_3^-$] will ↓ 0.2 mmol/L per mmHg ↓ in Pa$_{CO_2}$			
Chronic	[HCO$_3^-$] will ↓ 0.4 mmol/L per mmHg ↓ in Pa$_{CO_2}$			
Respiratory acidosis		Low	High	High
Acute	[HCO$_3^-$] will ↑ 0.1 mmol/L per mmHg ↑ in Pa$_{CO_2}$			
Chronic	[HCO$_3^-$] will ↑ 0.4 mmol/L per mmHg ↑ in Pa$_{CO_2}$			

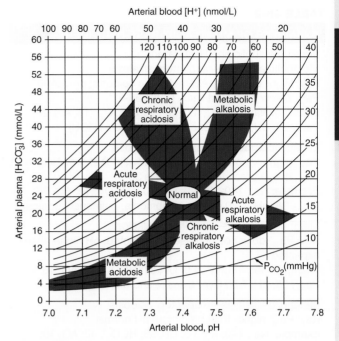

Arterial blood [H⁺] (nmol/L)

FIGURE 38-1

Acid-base nomogram. Shown are the 90% confidence limits (range of values) of the normal respiratory and metabolic compensations for primary acid-base disturbances. (*From TD DuBose: Metabolic alkalosis, in Primer on Kidney Diseases, 5th ed, A Greenberg [ed]. Philadelphia, Saunders Elsevier, 2009, pp 84–90, used with permission.*)

The degree of respiratory compensation expected in a simple form of metabolic acidosis can be predicted from the relationship: Pa$_{CO_2}$ = (1.5 × [HCO$_3^-$]) + 8 ± 2. Thus, a patient with metabolic acidosis and [HCO$_3^-$] of 12 mmol/L would be expected to have a Pa$_{CO_2}$ between 24 and 28 mmHg. Values for Pa$_{CO_2}$ <24 or >28 mmHg define a mixed disturbance (metabolic acidosis and respiratory alkalosis or metabolic alkalosis and respiratory acidosis, respectively). Another way to judge the appropriateness of the response in [HCO$_3^-$] or Pa$_{CO_2}$ is to use

an acid-base nomogram (Fig. 38-1). While the shaded areas of the nomogram show the 95% confidence limits for normal compensation in simple disturbances, finding acid-base values within the shaded area does not necessarily rule out a mixed disturbance. Imposition of one disorder over another may result in values lying within the area of a third. Thus, the nomogram, while convenient, is not a substitute for the equations in Table 38-1.

MIXED ACID-BASE DISORDERS

Mixed acid-base disorders—defined as independently coexisting disorders, not merely compensatory responses—are often seen in patients in critical care units and can lead to dangerous extremes of pH (Table 38-2). A patient with diabetic ketoacidosis (metabolic acidosis) may develop an independent respiratory problem (e.g., pneumonia) leading to respiratory acidosis or alkalosis. Patients with underlying pulmonary disease (e.g., COPD) may not respond to metabolic acidosis with an appropriate ventilatory response because of insufficient respiratory reserve. Such imposition of respiratory acidosis on metabolic acidosis can lead to severe acidemia. When metabolic acidosis and metabolic alkalosis coexist in the same patient, the pH may be normal or near normal. When the pH is normal, an elevated anion gap (AG; see later)

TABLE 38-2

EXAMPLES OF MIXED ACID-BASE DISORDERS

Mixed Metabolic and Respiratory
Metabolic acidosis—respiratory alkalosis
Key: High- or normal-AG metabolic acidosis; prevailing Pa_{CO_2} *below* predicted value (Table 38-1)
Example: Na^+, 140; K^+, 4.0; Cl^-, 106; HCO_3^-, 14; AG, 20; Pa_{CO_2}, 24; pH, 7.39 (lactic acidosis, sepsis in ICU)

Metabolic acidosis—respiratory acidosis
Key: High- or normal-AG metabolic acidosis; prevailing Pa_{CO_2} *above* predicted value (Table 38-1)
Example: Na^+, 140; K^+, 4.0; Cl^-, 102; HCO_3^-, 18; AG, 20; Pa_{CO_2}, 38; pH, 7.30 (severe pneumonia, pulmonary edema)

Metabolic alkalosis—respiratory alkalosis
Key: Pa_{CO_2} does not increase as predicted; pH higher than expected
Example: Na^+, 140; K^+, 4.0; Cl^-, 91; HCO_3^-, 33; AG, 16; Pa_{CO_2}, 38; pH, 7.55 (liver disease and diuretics)

Metabolic alkalosis—respiratory acidosis
Key: Pa_{CO_2} higher than predicted; pH normal
Example: Na^+, 140; K^+, 3.5; Cl^-, 88; HCO_3^-, 42; AG, 10; Pa_{CO_2}, 67; pH, 7.42 (COPD on diuretics)

Mixed Metabolic Disorders
Metabolic acidosis—metabolic alkalosis
Key: Only detectable with high-AG acidosis;
$\Delta AG \gg \Delta HCO_3^-$
Example: Na^+, 140; K^+, 3.0; Cl^-, 95; HCO_3^-, 25; AG, 20; Pa_{CO_2}, 40; pH, 7.42 (uremia with vomiting)

Metabolic acidosis—metabolic acidosis
Key: Mixed high-AG—normal-AG acidosis; ΔHCO_3^- accounted for by combined change in ΔAG and ΔCl^-
Example: Na^+, 135; K^+, 3.0; Cl^-, 110; HCO_3^-, 10; AG, 15; Pa_{CO_2}, 25; pH, 7.20 (diarrhea and lactic acidosis, toluene toxicity, treatment of diabetic ketoacidosis)

Abbreviations: AG, anion gap; COPD, chronic obstructive pulmonary disease; ICU, intensive care unit.

reliably denotes the presence of an AG metabolic acidosis. A discrepancy in the ΔAG (prevailing minus normal AG) and the ΔHCO_3^- (normal minus prevailing HCO_3^-) indicates the presence of a mixed high-gap acidosis—metabolic alkalosis (see example later). A diabetic patient with ketoacidosis may have renal dysfunction resulting in simultaneous metabolic acidosis. Patients who have ingested an overdose of drug combinations such as sedatives and salicylates may have mixed disturbances as a result of the acid-base response to the individual drugs (metabolic acidosis mixed with respiratory acidosis or respiratory alkalosis, respectively). Triple acid-base disturbances are more complex. For example, patients with metabolic acidosis due to alcoholic ketoacidosis may develop metabolic alkalosis due to vomiting and superimposed respiratory alkalosis due to the hyperventilation of hepatic dysfunction or alcohol withdrawal.

Acid-Base Disorders

A stepwise approach to the diagnosis of acid-base disorders follows (Table 38-3). Care should be taken when measuring blood gases to obtain the arterial blood sample without using excessive heparin. Blood for electrolytes and arterial blood gases should be drawn simultaneously prior to therapy, because an increase in $[HCO_3^-]$ occurs with metabolic alkalosis and respiratory acidosis. Conversely, a decrease in $[HCO_3^-]$ occurs in metabolic acidosis and respiratory alkalosis. In the determination of arterial blood gases by the clinical laboratory, both pH and Pa_{CO_2} are measured, and the $[HCO_3^-]$ is calculated from the Henderson-Hasselbalch equation. This calculated value should be compared with the measured $[HCO_3^-]$ (total CO_2) on the electrolyte panel. These two values should agree within 2 mmol/L. If they do not, the values may not have been drawn simultaneously, a laboratory error may be present, or an error could have been made in calculating the $[HCO_3^-]$. After verifying the blood acid-base values, the precise acid-base disorder can then be identified.

CALCULATE THE ANION GAP All evaluations of acid-base disorders should include a simple calculation of the AG; it represents those unmeasured anions in plasma (normally 10 to 12 mmol/L) and is calculated as follows: $AG = Na^+ - (Cl^- + HCO_3^-)$. The unmeasured anions include anionic proteins, (e.g., albumin), phosphate, sulfate, and organic anions. When acid anions, such as acetoacetate and lactate, accumulate in extracellular fluid, the AG increases, causing a high-AG acidosis. An increase in the AG is most often due to an increase in unmeasured anions and, less commonly, is due to a decrease in unmeasured cations (calcium, magnesium, potassium). In addition, the AG may increase with an increase in anionic albumin,

TABLE 38-3

STEPS IN ACID-BASE DIAGNOSIS

1. Obtain arterial blood gas (ABG) and electrolytes simultaneously.
2. Compare $[HCO_3^-]$ on ABG and electrolytes to verify accuracy.
3. Calculate anion gap (AG).
4. Know four causes of high-AG acidosis (ketoacidosis, lactic acid acidosis, renal failure, and toxins).
5. Know two causes of hyperchloremic or nongap acidosis (bicarbonate loss from GI tract, renal tubular acidosis).
6. Estimate compensatory response (Table 38-1).
7. Compare ΔAG and ΔHCO_3^-.
8. Compare change in $[Cl^-]$ with change in $[Na^+]$.

because of either increased albumin concentration or alkalosis, which alters albumin charge. A decrease in the AG can be due to (1) an increase in unmeasured cations; (2) the addition to the blood of abnormal cations, such as lithium (lithium intoxication) or cationic immunoglobulins (plasma cell dyscrasias); (3) a reduction in the major plasma anion albumin concentration (nephrotic syndrome); (4) a decrease in the effective anionic charge on albumin by acidosis; or (5) hyperviscosity and severe hyperlipidemia, which can lead to an underestimation of sodium and chloride concentrations. A fall in serum albumin by 1 g/dL from the normal value (4.5 g/dL) decreases the AG by 2.5 meq/L. Know the common causes of a high-AG acidosis (Table 38-3).

In the face of a normal serum albumin, a high AG is usually due to non-chloride containing acids that contain inorganic (phosphate, sulfate), organic (ketoacids, lactate, uremic organic anions), exogenous (salicylate or ingested toxins with organic acid production), or unidentified anions. The high AG is significant even if an additional acid-base disorder is superimposed to modify the [HCO_3^-] independently. Simultaneous metabolic acidosis of the high-AG variety plus either chronic respiratory acidosis or metabolic alkalosis represents such a situation in which [HCO_3^-] may be normal or even high (Table 38-3). Compare the change in [HCO_3^-] (ΔHCO_3^-) and the change in the AG (ΔAG).

Similarly, normal values for [HCO_3^-], Pa_{CO_2}, and pH do not ensure the absence of an acid-base disturbance. For instance, an alcoholic who has been vomiting may develop a metabolic alkalosis with a pH of 7.55, Pa_{CO_2} of 47 mmHg, [HCO_3^-] of 40 mmol/L, [Na^+] of 135, [Cl^-] of 80, and [K^+] of 2.8. If such a patient were then to develop a superimposed alcoholic ketoacidosis with a β-hydroxybutyrate concentration of 15 mM, arterial pH would fall to 7.40, [HCO_3^-] to 25 mmol/L, and the Pa_{CO_2} to 40 mmHg. Although these blood gases are normal, the AG is elevated at 30 mmol/L, indicating a mixed metabolic alkalosis and metabolic acidosis. A mixture of high-gap acidosis and metabolic alkalosis is recognized easily by comparing the differences (Δ values) in the normal to prevailing patient values. In this example, the ΔHCO_3^- is 0 (25 – 25 mmol/L) but the ΔAG is 20 (30 – 10 mmol/L). Therefore, 20 mmol/L is unaccounted for in the Δ/Δ value (ΔAG to ΔHCO_3^-).

METABOLIC ACIDOSIS

Metabolic acidosis can occur because of an increase in endogenous acid production (such as lactate and ketoacids), loss of bicarbonate (as in diarrhea), or

TABLE 38-4

CAUSES OF HIGH-ANION GAP METABOLIC ACIDOSIS

Lactic acidosis	Toxins
Ketoacidosis	Ethylene glycol
Diabetic	Methanol
Alcoholic	Salicylates
Starvation	Propylene glycol
	Pyroglutamic acid
	Renal failure (acute and chronic)

accumulation of endogenous acids (as in renal failure). Metabolic acidosis has profound effects on the respiratory, cardiac, and nervous systems. The fall in blood pH is accompanied by a characteristic increase in ventilation, especially the tidal volume (Kussmaul respiration). Intrinsic cardiac contractility may be depressed, but inotropic function can be normal because of catecholamine release. Both peripheral arterial vasodilation and central venoconstriction can be present; the decrease in central and pulmonary vascular compliance predisposes to pulmonary edema with even minimal volume overload. CNS function is depressed, with headache, lethargy, stupor, and, in some cases, even coma. Glucose intolerance may also occur.

There are two major categories of clinical metabolic acidosis: high-AG and normal-AG, or hyperchloremic acidosis (Table 38-3 and **Table 38-4**).

TREATMENT	Metabolic Acidosis

Treatment of metabolic acidosis with alkali should be reserved for severe acidemia except when the patient has no "potential HCO_3^-" in plasma. Potential [HCO_3^-] can be estimated from the increment (Δ) in the AG (ΔAG = patient's AG – 10). It must be determined if the acid anion in plasma is metabolizable (i.e., β-hydroxybutyrate, acetoacetate, and lactate) or nonmetabolizable (anions that accumulate in chronic renal failure and after toxin ingestion). The latter requires return of renal function to replenish the [HCO_3^-] deficit, a slow and often unpredictable process. Consequently, patients with a normal AG acidosis (hyperchloremic acidosis), a slightly elevated AG (mixed hyperchloremic and AG acidosis), or an AG attributable to a nonmetabolizable anion in the face of renal failure should receive alkali therapy, either PO ($NaHCO_3$ or Shohl's solution) or IV ($NaHCO_3$), in an amount necessary to slowly increase the plasma [HCO_3^-] into the 20–22 mmol/L range.

Controversy exists, however, in regard to the use of alkali in patients with a pure AG acidosis owing to accumulation of a metabolizable organic acid anion (ketoacidosis or lactic acidosis). In general, severe acidosis (pH < 7.10) warrants the IV administration of 50–100 meq of $NaHCO_3$, over 30–45 min, during the initial 1–2 h of therapy. Provision of such modest quantities of alkali in this situation seems to provide an added measure of safety, but it is essential to monitor plasma electrolytes during the course of therapy, because the $[K^+]$ may decline as pH rises. The goal is to increase the $[HCO_3^-]$ to 10 meq/L and the pH to 7.20, not to increase these values to normal.

HIGH–ANION GAP ACIDOSES

| APPROACH TO THE PATIENT | High–Anion Gap Acidoses |

There are four principal causes of a high-AG acidosis: (1) lactic acidosis, (2) ketoacidosis, (3) ingested toxins, and (4) acute and chronic renal failure (Table 38-4). Initial screening to differentiate the high-AG acidoses should include (1) a probe of the history for evidence of drug and toxin ingestion and measurement of arterial blood gas to detect coexistent respiratory alkalosis (salicylates); (2) determination of whether diabetes mellitus is present (diabetic ketoacidosis); (3) a search for evidence of alcoholism or increased levels of β-hydroxybutyrate (alcoholic ketoacidosis); (4) observation for clinical signs of uremia and determination of the blood urea nitrogen (BUN) and creatinine (uremic acidosis); (5) inspection of the urine for oxalate crystals (ethylene glycol); and (6) recognition of the numerous clinical settings in which lactate levels may be increased (hypotension, shock, cardiac failure, leukemia, cancer, and drug or toxin ingestion).

Lactic acidosis

An increase in plasma L-lactate may be secondary to poor tissue perfusion (type A)—circulatory insufficiency (shock, cardiac failure), severe anemia, mitochondrial enzyme defects, and inhibitors (carbon monoxide, cyanide)—or to aerobic disorders (type B)—malignancies, nucleoside analogue reverse transcriptase inhibitors in HIV, diabetes mellitus, renal or hepatic failure, thiamine deficiency, severe infections (cholera, malaria), seizures, or drugs/toxins (biguanides, ethanol, methanol, propylene glycol, isoniazid, and fructose). Propylene glycol may be used as a vehicle for IV medications including lorazepam, and toxicity has been reported in several settings. Unrecognized bowel ischemia or infarction in a patient with severe atherosclerosis or cardiac decompensation receiving

vasopressors is a common cause of lactic acidosis. Pyroglutamic acidemia has been reported in critically ill patients receiving acetaminophen, which is associated with depletion of glutathione. D-Lactic acid acidosis, which may be associated with jejunoileal bypass, short bowel syndrome, or intestinal obstruction, is due to formation of D-lactate by gut bacteria.

| APPROACH TO THE PATIENT | Lactic Acid Acidosis |

The underlying condition that disrupts lactate metabolism must first be corrected; tissue perfusion must be restored when inadequate. Vasoconstrictors should be avoided, if possible, because they may worsen tissue perfusion. Alkali therapy is generally advocated for acute, severe acidemia (pH < 7.15) to improve cardiac function and lactate use. However, $NaHCO_3$ therapy may paradoxically depress cardiac performance and exacerbate acidosis by enhancing lactate production (HCO_3^- stimulates phosphofructokinase). While the use of alkali in moderate lactic acidosis is controversial, it is generally agreed that attempts to return the pH or $[HCO_3^-]$ to normal by administration of exogenous $NaHCO_3$ are deleterious. A reasonable approach is to infuse sufficient $NaHCO_3$ to raise the arterial pH to no more than 7.2 over 30–40 min.

$NaHCO_3$ therapy can cause fluid overload and hypertension because the amount required can be massive when accumulation of lactic acid is relentless. Fluid administration is poorly tolerated because of central venoconstriction, especially in the oliguric patient. When the underlying cause of the lactic acidosis can be remedied, blood lactate will be converted to HCO_3^- and may result in an overshoot alkalosis.

Ketoacidosis

Diabetic ketoacidosis (DKA)

This condition is caused by increased fatty acid metabolism and the accumulation of ketoacids (acetoacetate and β-hydroxybutyrate). DKA usually occurs in insulin-dependent diabetes mellitus in association with cessation of insulin or an intercurrent illness such as an infection, gastroenteritis, pancreatitis, or myocardial infarction, which increases insulin requirements temporarily and acutely. The accumulation of ketoacids accounts for the increment in the AG and is accompanied most often by hyperglycemia (glucose > 17 mmol/L [300 mg/dL]). The relationship between the ΔAG and ΔHCO₃⁻ is typically ~1:1 in DKA. It should be noted that, because insulin prevents production of ketones, bicarbonate therapy is rarely needed except with extreme acidemia (pH < 7.1), and then in only limited amounts. Patients with DKA are typically volume depleted and require fluid resuscitation with isotonic saline. Volume over-expansion with IV-fluid administration is not uncommon, however, and contributes to the development of a hyperchloremic acidosis during treatment of DKA.

Alcoholic ketoacidosis (AKA)

Chronic alcoholics can develop ketoacidosis when alcohol consumption is abruptly curtailed and nutrition is poor. AKA is usually associated with binge drinking, vomiting, abdominal pain, starvation, and volume depletion. The glucose concentration is variable, and acidosis may be severe because of elevated ketones, predominantly β-hydroxybutyrate. Hypoperfusion may enhance lactic acid production, chronic respiratory alkalosis may accompany liver disease, and metabolic alkalosis can result from vomiting (refer to the relationship between ΔAG and ΔHCO$_3^-$). Thus, mixed acid-base disorders are common in AKA. As the circulation is restored by administration of isotonic saline, the preferential accumulation of β-hydroxybutyrate is then shifted to acetoacetate. This explains the common clinical observation of an increasingly positive nitroprusside reaction as the patient improves. The nitroprusside ketone reaction (Acetest) can detect acetoacetic acid but not β-hydroxybutyrate, so that the degree of ketosis and ketonuria can not only change with therapy, but can be underestimated initially. Patients with AKA usually present with relatively normal renal function, as opposed to DKA, where renal function is often compromised because of volume depletion (osmotic diuresis) or diabetic nephropathy. The AKA patient with normal renal function may excrete relatively large quantities of ketoacids in the urine, therefore, and may have a relatively normal AG and a discrepancy in the ΔAG/ΔHCO$_3^-$ relationship.

TREATMENT   Alcoholic Ketoacidosis

Extracellular fluid deficits almost always accompany AKA and should be repleted by IV administration of saline and glucose (5% dextrose in 0.9% NaCl). Hypophosphatemia, hypokalemia, and hypomagnesemia may coexist and should be corrected. Hypophosphatemia usually emerges 12–24 h after admission, may be exacerbated by glucose infusion, and, if severe, may induce rhabdomyolysis. Upper gastrointestinal hemorrhage, pancreatitis, and pneumonia may accompany this disorder.

Drug- and toxin-induced acidosis

Salicylates

Salicylate intoxication in adults usually causes respiratory alkalosis or a mixture of high-AG metabolic acidosis and respiratory alkalosis. Only a portion of the AG is due to salicylates. Lactic acid production is also often increased.

TREATMENT   Salicylate-Induced Acidosis

Vigorous gastric lavage with isotonic saline (not NaHCO$_3$) should be initiated immediately, followed by administration of activated charcoal per NG tube. In the acidotic patient, to facilitate removal of salicylate, intravenous NaHCO$_3$ is administered in amounts adequate to alkalinize the urine and to maintain urine output (urine pH > 7.5). While this form of therapy is straightforward in acidotic patients, a coexisting respiratory alkalosis may make this approach hazardous. Alkalemic patients should not receive NaHCO$_3$. Acetazolamide may be administered in the face of alkalemia, when an alkaline diuresis cannot be achieved, or to ameliorate volume overload associated with NaHCO$_3$ administration, but this drug can cause systemic metabolic acidosis if HCO$_3^-$ is not replaced. Hypokalemia should be anticipated with an alkaline diuresis and should be treated promptly and aggressively. Glucose-containing fluids should be administered because of the danger of hypoglycemia. Excessive insensible fluid losses may cause severe volume depletion and hypernatremia. If renal failure prevents rapid clearance of salicylate, hemodialysis can be performed against a bicarbonate dialysate.

Alcohols

Under most physiologic conditions, sodium, urea, and glucose generate the osmotic pressure of blood. Plasma osmolality is calculated according to the following expression: $P_{osm} = 2Na^+ + Glu + BUN$ (all in mmol/L), or, using conventional laboratory values in which glucose and BUN are expressed in milligrams per deciliter: $P_{osm} = 2Na^+ + Glu/18 + BUN/2.8$. The calculated and determined osmolality should agree within 10–15 mmol/kg H$_2$O. When the measured osmolality exceeds the calculated osmolality by >15–20 mmol/kg H$_2$O, one of two circumstances prevails. Either the serum sodium is spuriously low, as with hyperlipidemia or hyperproteinemia (pseudohyponatremia), or osmolytes other than sodium salts, glucose, or urea have accumulated in plasma. Examples of such osmolytes include mannitol, radiocontrast media, ethanol, isopropyl alcohol, ethylene glycol, propylene glycol, methanol, and acetone. In this situation, the difference between the calculated osmolality and the measured osmolality (*osmolar gap*) is proportional to the concentration of the unmeasured solute. With an appropriate clinical history and index of suspicion, identification of an osmolar gap is helpful in identifying the presence of poison-associated AG acidosis. Three alcohols may cause fatal intoxications: ethylene glycol, methanol, and isopropyl alcohol. All cause an elevated osmolal gap, but only the first two cause a high-AG acidosis.

Ethylene glycol

Ingestion of ethylene glycol (commonly used in antifreeze) leads to a metabolic acidosis and severe damage to the CNS, heart, lungs, and kidneys. The increased AG and osmolar gap are attributable to ethylene glycol and its metabolites, oxalic acid, glycolic acid, and other organic acids. Lactic acid production increases secondary to inhibition of the tricarboxylic acid cycle and altered intracellular redox state. Diagnosis is facilitated by recognizing oxalate crystals in the urine, the presence of an osmolar gap in serum, and a high-AG acidosis. Treatment should not be delayed while awaiting measurement of ethylene glycol levels in this setting.

TREATMENT   Ethylene Glycol–Induced Acidosis

This includes the prompt institution of a saline or osmotic diuresis, thiamine and pyridoxine supplements, fomepizole or ethanol, and hemodialysis. The IV administration of the alcohol dehydrogenase inhibitor fomepizole (4-methylpyrazole; 15 mg/kg as a loading dose) or ethanol IV to achieve a level of 22 mmol/L (100 mg/dL) serves to lessen toxicity because they compete with ethylene glycol for metabolism by alcohol dehydrogenase. Fomepizole, although expensive, is the agent of choice and offers the advantages of a predictable decline in ethylene glycol levels without excessive obtundation during ethyl alcohol infusion. Hemodialysis is indicated when the arterial pH is <7.3, or the osmolar gap exceeds 20 mOsm/kg.

Methanol

The ingestion of methanol (wood alcohol) causes metabolic acidosis, and its metabolites formaldehyde and formic acid cause severe optic nerve and CNS damage. Lactic acid, ketoacids, and other unidentified organic acids may contribute to the acidosis. Due to its low molecular mass (32 Da), an osmolar gap is usually present.

TREATMENT   Methanol-Induced Acidosis

This is similar to that for ethylene glycol intoxication, including general supportive measures, fomepizole, and hemodialysis (as noted earlier).

Isopropyl alcohol

Ingested isopropanol is absorbed rapidly and may be fatal when as little as 150 mL of rubbing alcohol, solvent, or de-icer is consumed. A plasma level >400 mg/dL is life-threatening. Isopropyl alcohol differs from ethylene glycol and methanol in that the parent compound, not the metabolites, causes toxicity, and an AG acidosis is not present because acetone is rapidly excreted.

TREATMENT   Isopropyl Alcohol Toxicity

Isopropanol alcohol toxicity is treated by watchful waiting and supportive therapy; IV fluids, pressors, ventilatory support if needed, and occasionally hemodialysis for prolonged coma or levels >400 mg/dL.

Renal failure

The hyperchloremic acidosis of moderate renal insufficiency is eventually converted to the high-AG acidosis of advanced renal failure. Poor filtration and reabsorption of organic anions contribute to the pathogenesis. As renal disease progresses, the number of functioning nephrons eventually becomes insufficient to keep pace with net acid production. Uremic acidosis is characterized, therefore, by a reduced rate of NH_4^+ production and excretion. The acid retained in chronic renal disease is buffered by alkaline salts from bone. Despite significant retention of acid (up to 20 mmol/d), the serum $[HCO_3^-]$ does not decrease further, indicating participation of buffers outside the extracellular compartment. Chronic metabolic acidosis results in significant loss of bone mass due to reduction in bone calcium carbonate. Chronic acidosis also increases urinary calcium excretion, proportional to cumulative acid retention.

TREATMENT   Renal Failure

Because of the association of renal failure acidosis with muscle catabolism and bone disease, both uremic acidosis and the hyperchloremic acidosis of renal failure require oral alkali replacement to maintain the $[HCO_3^-]$ between 20 and 24 mmol/L. This can be accomplished with relatively modest amounts of alkali (1.0–1.5 mmol/kg body weight per day). Sodium citrate (Shohl's solution) or $NaHCO_3$ tablets (650-mg tablets contain 7.8 meq) are equally effective alkalinizing salts. Citrate enhances the absorption of aluminum from the gastrointestinal tract and should never be given together with aluminum-containing antacids because of the risk of aluminum intoxication. When hyperkalemia is present, furosemide (60–80 mg/d) should be added.

NON–ANION GAP METABOLIC ACIDOSES

Alkali can be lost from the gastrointestinal tract in diarrhea or from the kidneys (renal tubular acidosis, RTA). In these disorders (Table 38-5), reciprocal changes in $[Cl^-]$ and $[HCO_3^-]$ result in a normal AG. In pure non–AG acidosis, therefore, the increase in $[Cl^-]$ above the normal value approximates the decrease in $[HCO_3^-]$. The absence of such a relationship suggests a mixed disturbance.

TABLE 38-5

CAUSES OF NON–ANION GAP ACIDOSIS

I. Gastrointestinal bicarbonate loss
  A. Diarrhea
  B. External pancreatic or small-bowel drainage
  C. Ureterosigmoidostomy, jejunal loop, ileal loop
  D. Drugs
    1. Calcium chloride (acidifying agent)
    2. Magnesium sulfate (diarrhea)
    3. Cholestyramine (bile acid diarrhea)

II. Renal acidosis
  A. Hypokalemia
    1. Proximal RTA (type 2)
      Drug-induced: acetazolamide, topiramate
    2. Distal (classic) RTA (type 1)
      Drug induced: amphotericin B, ifosfamide
  B. Hyperkalemia
    1. Generalized distal nephron dysfunction (type 4 RTA)
      a. Mineralocorticoid deficiency
      b. Mineralocorticoid resistance (autosomal dominant PHA I)
      c. Voltage defect (autosomal dominant PHA I and PHA II)
      d. Tubulointerstitial disease

III. Drug-induced hyperkalemia (with renal insufficiency)
  A. Potassium-sparing diuretics (amiloride, triamterene, spironolactone)
  B. Trimethoprim
  C. Pentamidine
  D. ACE-Is and ARBs
  E. Nonsteroidal anti-inflammatory drugs
  F. Cyclosporine and tacrolimus

IV. Other
  A. Acid loads (ammonium chloride, hyperalimentation)
  B. Loss of potential bicarbonate: ketosis with ketone excretion
  C. Expansion acidosis (rapid saline administration)
  D. Hippurate
  E. Cation exchange resins

Abbreviations: ACE-I, angiotensin-converting enzyme inhibitor; ARB, angiotensin receptor blocker; PHA, pseudohypoaldosteronism; RTA, renal tubular acidosis.

TREATMENT   Non–Anion Gap Metabolic Acidoses

In diarrhea, stools contain a higher $[HCO_3^-]$ and decomposed HCO_3^- than plasma so that metabolic acidosis develops along with volume depletion. Instead of an acid urine pH (as anticipated with systemic acidosis), urine pH is usually around 6 because metabolic acidosis and hypokalemia increase renal synthesis and excretion of NH_4^+, thus providing a urinary buffer that increases urine pH. Metabolic acidosis due to gastrointestinal losses with a high urine pH can be differentiated from RTA because urinary NH_4^+ excretion is typically low in RTA and high with diarrhea. Urinary NH_4^+ levels can be estimated by calculating the urine anion gap (UAG): $UAG = [Na^+ + K^+]_u - [Cl^-]_u$. When $[Cl^-]_u > [Na^+ + K^+]_u$, the UAG is negative by definition. This indicates that the urine ammonium level is appropriately increased, suggesting an extrarenal cause of the acidosis. Conversely, when the UAG is positive, the urine ammonium level is low, suggesting a renal cause of the acidosis.

Loss of functioning renal parenchyma by progressive renal disease leads to hyperchloremic acidosis when the glomerular filtration rate (GFR) is between 20 and 50 mL/min and to uremic acidosis with a high AG when the GFR falls to <20 mL/min. In advanced renal failure, ammoniagenesis is reduced in proportion to the loss of functional renal mass, and ammonium accumulation and trapping in the outer medullary collecting tubule may also be impaired. Because of adaptive increases in K^+ secretion by the collecting duct and colon, the acidosis of chronic renal insufficiency is typically normokalemic.

Proximal RTA (type 2 RTA) is most often due to generalized proximal tubular dysfunction manifested by glycosuria, generalized aminoaciduria, and phosphaturia (Fanconi syndrome). With a low plasma $[HCO_3^-]$, the urine pH is acid (pH < 5.5). The fractional excretion of $[HCO_3^-]$ may exceed 10–15% when the serum $HCO_3^- > 20$ mmol/L. Because HCO_3^- is not reabsorbed normally in the proximal tubule, therapy with $NaHCO_3$ will enhance renal potassium wasting and hypokalemia.

The typical findings in acquired or inherited forms of classic distal RTA (type 1 RTA) include hypokalemia, non-AG metabolic acidosis, low urinary NH_4^+ excretion (positive UAG, low urine $[NH_4^+]$), and inappropriately high urine pH (pH > 5.5). Most patients have hypocitraturia and hypercalciuria, so nephrolithiasis, nephrocalcinosis, and bone disease are common. In generalized distal nephron dysfunction (type 4 RTA), hyperkalemia is disproportionate to the reduction in GFR because of coexisting dysfunction of potassium and acid secretion. Urinary ammonium excretion is invariably depressed, and renal function may be compromised, for example, due to diabetic nephropathy, obstructive uropathy, or chronic tubulointerstitial disease.

Hyporeninemic hypoaldosteronism typically causes non-AG metabolic acidosis, most commonly in older adults with diabetes mellitus or tubulointerstitial disease and renal insufficiency. Patients usually have mild to moderate CKD (GFR, 20–50 mL/min) and acidosis, with elevation in serum [K+] (5.2–6.0 mmol/L), concurrent hypertension, and congestive heart failure. Both the metabolic acidosis and the hyperkalemia are out of proportion to impairment in GFR. Nonsteroidal anti-inflammatory drugs, trimethoprim, pentamidine, and angiotensin-converting enzyme (ACE) inhibitors can also cause non-AG metabolic acidosis in patients with renal insufficiency (Table 38-5).

METABOLIC ALKALOSIS

Metabolic alkalosis is manifested by an elevated arterial pH, an increase in the serum [HCO_3^-], and an increase in Pa_{CO_2} as a result of compensatory alveolar hypoventilation (Table 38-1). It is often accompanied by hypochloremia and hypokalemia. The arterial pH establishes the diagnosis, because it is increased in metabolic alkalosis and decreased or normal in respiratory acidosis. Metabolic alkalosis frequently occurs in association with other disorders such as respiratory acidosis or alkalosis or metabolic acidosis.

PATHOGENESIS

Metabolic alkalosis occurs as a result of net gain of [HCO_3^-] or loss of nonvolatile acid (usually HCl by vomiting) from the extracellular fluid. For HCO_3^- to be added to the extracellular fluid, it must be administered exogenously or synthesized endogenously, in part or entirely by the kidneys. Because it is unusual for alkali to be added to the body, the disorder involves a generative stage, in which the loss of acid usually causes alkalosis, and a maintenance stage, in which the kidneys fail to compensate by excreting HCO_3^-.

Under normal circumstances, the kidneys have an impressive capacity to excrete HCO_3^-. Continuation of metabolic alkalosis represents a failure of the kidneys to eliminate HCO_3^- in the usual manner. The kidneys will retain, rather than excrete, the excess alkali and maintain the alkalosis if (1) volume deficiency, chloride deficiency, and K^+ deficiency exist in combination with a reduced GFR, which augments distal tubule H^+ secretion; or (2) hypokalemia exists because of autonomous hyperaldosteronism. In the first example, alkalosis is corrected by administration of NaCl and KCl, whereas, in the latter, it is necessary to repair the alkalosis by pharmacologic or surgical intervention, not with saline administration.

DIFFERENTIAL DIAGNOSIS

To establish the cause of metabolic alkalosis (Table 38-6), it is necessary to assess the status of the extracellular fluid volume (ECFV), the recumbent and upright blood pressure, the serum [K^+], and the renin-aldosterone system. For example, the presence of chronic hypertension and chronic hypokalemia in an alkalotic patient suggests either mineralocorticoid excess or that the hypertensive patient is receiving diuretics. Low plasma renin activity and normal urine [Na^+] and [Cl^-] in a patient who is not taking diuretics indicate a primary mineralocorticoid excess syndrome. The combination of hypokalemia and alkalosis in a normotensive, nonedematous patient can be due to Bartter's or Gitelman's syndrome, magnesium deficiency, vomiting, exogenous alkali, or diuretic ingestion. Determination of urine electrolytes (especially the urine [Cl^-]) and screening of the urine for diuretics may be helpful. If the urine is alkaline, with an elevated [Na^+] and [K^+] but low [Cl^-], the diagnosis is usually either vomiting (overt or surreptitious) or alkali ingestion. If the urine is relatively acid and has low concentrations of Na^+, K^+, and Cl^-, the most likely possibilities are prior vomiting, the posthypercapnic state, or prior diuretic ingestion. If, on the other hand, neither the urine sodium, potassium, nor chloride concentrations are depressed, magnesium deficiency, Bartter's or Gitelman's syndrome, or current diuretic ingestion should be considered. Bartter's syndrome is distinguished from Gitelman's syndrome because of hypocalciuria and hypomagnesemia in the latter disorder.

Alkali administration

Chronic administration of alkali to individuals with normal renal function rarely causes alkalosis. However, in patients with coexistent hemodynamic disturbances, alkalosis can develop because the normal capacity to excrete HCO_3^- may be exceeded or there may be enhanced reabsorption of HCO_3^-. Such patients include those who receive HCO_3^- (PO or IV), acetate loads (parenteral hyperalimentation solutions), citrate loads (transfusions), or antacids plus cation-exchange resins (aluminum hydroxide and

TABLE 38-6

CAUSES OF METABOLIC ALKALOSIS

I. Exogenous HCO_3^- loads
  A. Acute alkali administration
  B. Milk-alkali syndrome

II. Effective ECFV contraction, normotension, K^+ deficiency, and secondary hyperreninemic hyperaldosteronism
  A. Gastrointestinal origin
    1. Vomiting
    2. Gastric aspiration
    3. Congenital chloridorrhea
    4. Villous adenoma
  B. Renal origin
    1. Diuretics
    2. Posthypercapnic state
    3. Hypercalcemia/hypoparathyroidism
    4. Recovery from lactic acidosis or ketoacidosis
    5. Nonreabsorbable anions including penicillin, carbenicillin
    6. Mg^{2+} deficiency
    7. K^+ depletion
    8. Bartter's syndrome (loss of function mutations in TALH)
    9. Gitelman's syndrome (loss of function mutation in Na^+-Cl^- cotransporter in DCT)

III. ECFV expansion, hypertension, K^+ deficiency, and mineralocorticoid excess
  A. High renin
    1. Renal artery stenosis
    2. Accelerated hypertension
    3. Renin-secreting tumor
    4. Estrogen therapy
  B. Low renin
    1. Primary aldosteronism
      a. Adenoma
      b. Hyperplasia
      c. Carcinoma
    2. Adrenal enzyme defects
      a. 11 β-Hydroxylase deficiency
      b. 17 α-Hydroxylase deficiency
    3. Cushing's syndrome or disease
    4. Other
      a. Licorice
      b. Carbenoxolone
      c. Chewer's tobacco

IV. Gain-of-function mutation of renal sodium channel with ECFV expansion, hypertension, K^+ deficiency, and hyporeninemic-hypoaldosteronism
  A. Liddle's syndrome

Abbreviations: DCT, distal convoluted tubule; ECFV, extracellular fluid volume; TALH, thick ascending limb of Henle's loop.

sodium polystyrene sulfonate). Nursing-home patients receiving tube feedings have a higher incidence of metabolic alkalosis than nursing-home patients receiving oral feedings.

METABOLIC ALKALOSIS ASSOCIATED WITH ECFV CONTRACTION, K^+ DEPLETION, AND SECONDARY HYPERRENINEMIC HYPERALDOSTERONISM

Gastrointestinal origin

Gastrointestinal loss of H^+ from vomiting or gastric aspiration results in retention of HCO_3^-. The loss of fluid and NaCl in vomitus or nasogastric suction results in contraction of the ECFV and an increase in the secretion of renin and aldosterone. Volume contraction through a reduction in GFR results in an enhanced capacity of the renal tubule to reabsorb HCO_3^-. During active vomiting, however, the filtered load of bicarbonate is acutely increased to the point that the reabsorptive capacity of the proximal tubule for HCO_3^- is exceeded. The excess $NaHCO_3$ issuing out of the proximal tubule reaches the distal tubule, where H^+ secretion is enhanced by an aldosterone and the delivery of the poorly reabsorbed anion, HCO_3^-. Correction of the contracted ECFV with NaCl and repair of K^+ deficits corrects the acid-base disorder, and chloride deficiency.

Renal origin

Diuretics

Drugs that induce chloruresis, such as thiazides and loop diuretics (furosemide, bumetanide, torsemide, and ethacrynic acid), acutely diminish the ECFV without altering the total body bicarbonate content. The serum $[HCO_3^-]$ increases because the reduced ECFV "contracts" the $[HCO_3^-]$ in the plasma (contraction alkalosis). The chronic administration of diuretics tends to generate an alkalosis by increasing distal salt delivery, so that K^+ and H^+ secretion are stimulated. The alkalosis is maintained by persistence of the contraction of the ECFV, secondary hyperaldosteronism, K^+ deficiency, and the direct effect of the diuretic (as long as diuretic administration continues). Repair of the alkalosis is achieved by providing isotonic saline to correct the ECFV deficit.

Nonreabsorbable anions and magnesium deficiency

Administration of large quantities of nonreabsorbable anions, such as penicillin or carbenicillin, can enhance distal acidification and K^+ secretion by increasing the transepithelial potential difference. Mg^{2+} deficiency results in hypokalemic alkalosis by enhancing distal acidification through stimulation of renin and hence aldosterone secretion.

Potassium depletion

Chronic K^+ depletion may cause metabolic alkalosis by increasing urinary acid excretion. Both NH_4^+ production and absorption are enhanced and HCO_3^- reabsorption is stimulated. Chronic K^+ deficiency upregulates the renal H^+, K^+-ATPase to increase K^+ absorption at the expense of enhanced H^+ secretion. Alkalosis associated with severe K^+ depletion is resistant to salt administration, but repair of the K^+ deficiency corrects the alkalosis.

After treatment of lactic acidosis or ketoacidosis

When an underlying stimulus for the generation of lactic acid or ketoacid is removed rapidly, as with repair of circulatory insufficiency or with insulin therapy, the lactate or ketones are metabolized to yield an equivalent amount of HCO_3^-. Other sources of new HCO_3^- are additive with the original amount generated by organic anion metabolism to create a surfeit of HCO_3^-. Such sources include (1) new HCO_3^- added to the blood by the kidneys as a result of enhanced acid excretion during the preexisting period of acidosis, and (2) alkali therapy during the treatment phase of the acidosis. Acidosis-induced contraction of the ECFV and K^+ deficiency act to sustain the alkalosis.

Posthypercapnia

Prolonged CO_2 retention with chronic respiratory acidosis enhances renal HCO_3^- absorption and the generation of new HCO_3^- (increased net acid excretion). If the Pa_{CO_2} is returned to normal, metabolic alkalosis results from the persistently elevated $[HCO_3^-]$. Alkalosis develops if the elevated Pa_{CO_2} is abruptly returned toward normal by a change in mechanically controlled ventilation. Associated ECFV contraction does not allow complete repair of the alkalosis by correction of the Pa_{CO_2} alone, and alkalosis persists until Cl^- supplementation is provided.

METABOLIC ALKALOSIS ASSOCIATED WITH ECFV EXPANSION, HYPERTENSION, AND HYPERALDOSTERONISM

Increased aldosterone levels may be the result of autonomous primary adrenal overproduction or of secondary aldosterone release due to renal overproduction of renin. Mineralocorticoid excess increases net acid excretion and may result in metabolic alkalosis, which may be worsened by associated K^+ deficiency. ECFV expansion from salt retention causes hypertension. The kaliuresis persists because of mineralocorticoid excess and distal Na^+ absorption causing enhanced K^+ excretion, continued K^+ depletion with polydipsia, inability to concentrate the urine, and polyuria.

Liddle's syndrome results from increased activity of the collecting duct Na^+ channel (ENaC) and is a rare monogenic form of hypertension due to volume expansion manifested as hypokalemic alkalosis and normal aldosterone levels.

Symptoms

With metabolic alkalosis, changes in CNS and peripheral nervous system function are similar to those of hypocalcemia; symptoms include mental confusion; obtundation; and a predisposition to seizures, paresthesia, muscular cramping, tetany, aggravation of arrhythmias, and hypoxemia in chronic obstructive pulmonary disease. Related electrolyte abnormalities include hypokalemia and hypophosphatemia.

TREATMENT Metabolic Alkalosis

This is primarily directed at correcting the underlying stimulus for HCO_3^- generation. If primary aldosteronism, renal artery stenosis, or Cushing's syndrome is present, correction of the underlying cause will reverse the alkalosis. $[H^+]$ loss by the stomach or kidneys can be mitigated by the use of proton pump inhibitors or the discontinuation of diuretics. The second aspect of treatment is to remove the factors that sustain the inappropriate increase in HCO_3^- reabsorption, such as ECFV contraction or K^+ deficiency. K^+ deficits should always be repaired. Isotonic saline is usually sufficient to reverse the alkalosis if ECFV contraction is present.

If associated conditions preclude infusion of saline, renal HCO_3^- loss can be accelerated by administration of acetazolamide, a carbonic anhydrase inhibitor, which is usually effective in patients with adequate renal function but can worsen K^+ losses. Dilute hydrochloric acid (0.1 N HCl) is also effective but can cause hemolysis, and must be delivered centrally and slowly. Hemodialysis against a dialysate low in $[HCO_3^-]$ and high in $[Cl^-]$ can be effective when renal function is impaired.

RESPIRATORY ACIDOSIS

Respiratory acidosis can be due to severe pulmonary disease, respiratory muscle fatigue, or abnormalities in ventilatory control and is recognized by an increase in Pa_{CO_2} and decrease in pH (Table 38-7). In acute respiratory acidosis, there is an immediate compensatory elevation (due to cellular buffering mechanisms) in HCO_3^-, which increases 1 mmol/L for every 10-mmHg increase in Pa_{CO_2}. In chronic respiratory acidosis (>24 h), renal adaptation increases the $[HCO_3^-]$ by 4 mmol/L for every 10-mmHg increase in Pa_{CO_2}. The serum HCO_3^- usually does not increase above 38 mmol/L.

TABLE 38-7

RESPIRATORY ACID-BASE DISORDERS

I. Alkalosis
  A. Central nervous system stimulation
    1. Pain
    2. Anxiety, psychosis
    3. Fever
    4. Cerebrovascular accident
    5. Meningitis, encephalitis
    6. Tumor
    7. Trauma
  B. Hypoxemia or tissue hypoxia
    1. High altitude
    2. Pneumonia, pulmonary edema
    3. Aspiration
    4. Severe anemia
  C. Drugs or hormones
    1. Pregnancy, progesterone
    2. Salicylates
    3. Cardiac failure
  D. Stimulation of chest receptors
    1. Hemothorax
    2. Flail chest
    3. Cardiac failure
    4. Pulmonary embolism
  E. Miscellaneous
    1. Septicemia
    2. Hepatic failure
    3. Mechanical hyperventilation
    4. Heat exposure
    5. Recovery from metabolic acidosis

II. Acidosis
  A. Central
    1. Drugs (anesthetics, morphine, sedatives)
    2. Stroke
    3. Infection
  B. Airway
    1. Obstruction
    2. Asthma
  C. Parenchyma
    1. Emphysema
    2. Pneumoconiosis
    3. Bronchitis
    4. Adult respiratory distress syndrome
    5. Barotrauma
  D. Neuromuscular
    1. Poliomyelitis
    2. Kyphoscoliosis
    3. Myasthenia
    4. Muscular dystrophies
  E. Miscellaneous
    1. Obesity
    2. Hypoventilation
    3. Permissive hypercapnia

The clinical features vary according to the severity and duration of the respiratory acidosis, the underlying disease, and whether there is accompanying hypoxemia. A rapid increase in Pa_{CO_2} may cause anxiety, dyspnea, confusion, psychosis, and hallucinations and may progress to coma. Lesser degrees of dysfunction in chronic hypercapnia include sleep disturbances; loss of memory; daytime somnolence; personality changes; impairment of coordination; and motor disturbances such as tremor, myoclonic jerks, and asterixis. Headaches and other signs that mimic raised intracranial pressure, such as papilledema, abnormal reflexes, and focal muscle weakness, are due to vasoconstriction secondary to loss of the vasodilator effects of CO_2.

Depression of the respiratory center by a variety of drugs, injury, or disease can produce respiratory acidosis. This may occur acutely with general anesthetics, sedatives, and head trauma or chronically with sedatives, alcohol, intracranial tumors, and the syndromes of sleep-disordered breathing including the primary alveolar and obesity-hypoventilation syndromes (Chaps. 22 and 23). Abnormalities or disease in the motor neurons, neuromuscular junction, and skeletal muscle can cause hypoventilation via respiratory muscle fatigue. Mechanical ventilation, when not properly adjusted and supervised, may result in respiratory acidosis, particularly if CO_2 production suddenly rises (because of fever, agitation, sepsis, or overfeeding) or alveolar ventilation falls because of worsening pulmonary function. High levels of positive end-expiratory pressure in the presence of reduced cardiac output may cause hypercapnia as a result of large increases in alveolar dead space (Chap. 5). Permissive hypercapnia is being used with increasing frequency because of studies suggesting lower mortality rates than with conventional mechanical ventilation, especially with severe CNS or heart disease. The respiratory acidosis associated with permissive hypercapnia may require administration of $NaHCO_3$ to increase the arterial pH to 7.25 but overcorrection of the acidemia may be deleterious.

Acute hypercapnia follows sudden occlusion of the upper airway or generalized bronchospasm as in severe asthma, anaphylaxis, inhalational burn, or toxin injury. Chronic hypercapnia and respiratory acidosis occur in end-stage obstructive lung disease. Restrictive disorders involving both the chest wall and the lungs can cause respiratory acidosis because the high metabolic cost of respiration causes ventilatory muscle fatigue. Advanced stages of intrapulmonary and extrapulmonary restrictive defects present as chronic respiratory acidosis.

The diagnosis of respiratory acidosis requires the measurement of Pa_{CO_2} and arterial pH. A detailed history and physical examination often indicate the cause. Pulmonary function studies (Chap. 5), including spirometry, diffusion capacity for carbon monoxide, lung volumes, and arterial Pa_{CO_2} and O_2 saturation, usually make it possible to determine if respiratory acidosis is secondary to lung disease. The workup for nonpulmonary causes should include a detailed drug history, measurement of hematocrit, and assessment of upper airway, chest wall, pleura, and neuromuscular function.

TREATMENT   Respiratory Acidosis

The management of respiratory acidosis depends on its severity and rate of onset. Acute respiratory acidosis can be life-threatening, and measures to reverse the underlying cause should be undertaken simultaneously with restoration of adequate alveolar ventilation. This may necessitate tracheal intubation and assisted mechanical ventilation. Oxygen administration should be titrated carefully in patients with severe obstructive pulmonary disease and chronic CO_2 retention who are breathing spontaneously (Chap. 18). When oxygen is used injudiciously, these patients may experience progression of the respiratory acidosis. Aggressive and rapid correction of hypercapnia should be avoided, because the falling Pa_{CO_2} may provoke the same complications noted with acute respiratory alkalosis (i.e., cardiac arrhythmias, reduced cerebral perfusion, and seizures). The Pa_{CO_2} should be lowered gradually in chronic respiratory acidosis, aiming to restore the Pa_{CO_2} to baseline levels and to provide sufficient Cl^- and K^+ to enhance the renal excretion of HCO_3^-.

Chronic respiratory acidosis is frequently difficult to correct, but measures aimed at improving lung function (Chap. 18) can help some patients and forestall further deterioration in most.

RESPIRATORY ALKALOSIS

Alveolar hyperventilation decreases Pa_{CO_2} and increases the HCO_3^-/Pa_{CO_2} ratio, thus increasing pH (Table 38-7). Nonbicarbonate cellular buffers respond by consuming HCO_3^-. Hypocapnia develops when a sufficiently strong ventilatory stimulus causes CO_2 output in the lungs to exceed its metabolic production by tissues. Plasma pH and $[HCO_3^-]$ appear to vary proportionately with Pa_{CO_2} over a range from 40–15 mmHg. The relationship between arterial $[H^+]$ concentration and Pa_{CO_2} is ~0.7 mmol/L per mmHg (or 0.01 pH unit/mmHg), and that for plasma $[HCO_3^-]$ is 0.2 mmol/L per mmHg. Hypocapnia sustained for >2–6 h is further compensated by a decrease in renal ammonium and titratable acid excretion and a reduction in filtered HCO_3^- reabsorption. Full renal adaptation to respiratory alkalosis may take several days and requires normal volume status and renal function. The kidneys appear to respond directly to the lowered Pa_{CO_2} rather than to alkalosis per se. In chronic respiratory alkalosis a 1-mmHg fall in Pa_{CO_2} causes a 0.4- to 0.5-mmol/L drop in $[HCO_3^-]$ and a 0.3-mmol/L fall (or 0.003 rise in pH) in $[H^+]$.

The effects of respiratory alkalosis vary according to duration and severity but are primarily those of the underlying disease. Reduced cerebral blood flow as a consequence of a rapid decline in Pa_{CO_2} may cause dizziness, mental confusion, and seizures, even in the absence of hypoxemia. The cardiovascular effects of acute hypocapnia in the conscious human are generally minimal, but in the anesthetized or mechanically ventilated patient, cardiac output and blood pressure may fall because of the depressant effects of anesthesia and positive-pressure ventilation on heart rate, systemic resistance, and venous return. Cardiac arrhythmias may occur in patients with heart disease as a result of changes in oxygen unloading by blood from a left shift in the hemoglobin-oxygen dissociation curve (Bohr effect). Acute respiratory alkalosis causes intracellular shifts of Na^+, K^+, and PO_4^{2-} and reduces free $[Ca^{2+}]$ by increasing the protein-bound fraction. Hypocapnia-induced hypokalemia is usually minor.

Chronic respiratory alkalosis is the most common acid-base disturbance in critically ill patients and, when severe, portends a poor prognosis. Many cardiopulmonary disorders manifest respiratory alkalosis in their early to intermediate stages, and the finding of normocapnia and hypoxemia in a patient with hyperventilation may herald the onset of rapid respiratory failure and should prompt an assessment to determine if the patient is becoming fatigued. Respiratory alkalosis is common during mechanical ventilation.

The hyperventilation syndrome may be disabling. Paresthesia; circumoral numbness; chest wall tightness or pain; dizziness; inability to take an adequate breath; and, rarely, tetany may be sufficiently stressful to perpetuate the disorder. Arterial blood-gas analysis demonstrates an acute or chronic respiratory alkalosis, often with hypocapnia in the range of 15–30 mmHg and no hypoxemia. CNS diseases or injury can produce several patterns of hyperventilation and sustained Pa_{CO_2} levels of 20–30 mmHg. Hyperthyroidism, high caloric loads, and exercise raise the basal metabolic rate, but ventilation usually rises in proportion so that arterial blood gases are unchanged and respiratory alkalosis does not develop. Salicylates are the most common cause of drug-induced respiratory alkalosis as a result of direct stimulation of the medullary chemoreceptor. The methylxanthines, theophylline, and aminophylline stimulate ventilation and increase the ventilatory response to CO_2. Progesterone increases ventilation and lowers arterial Pa_{CO_2} by as much as 5–10 mmHg. Therefore, chronic respiratory alkalosis is a common feature of pregnancy. Respiratory alkalosis is also prominent in liver failure, and the severity correlates with the degree of hepatic insufficiency. Respiratory alkalosis is often an early finding in gram-negative septicemia, before fever, hypoxemia, or hypotension develops.

The diagnosis of respiratory alkalosis depends on measurement of arterial pH and Pa_{CO_2}. The plasma $[K^+]$ is often reduced and the $[Cl^-]$ increased. In the acute phase, respiratory alkalosis is not associated with increased renal HCO_3^- excretion, but within hours net acid excretion is reduced. In general, the HCO_3^- concentration falls by 2.0 mmol/L for each 10-mmHg decrease in Pa_{CO_2}. Chronic hypocapnia reduces the serum $[HCO_3^-]$ by 4.0 mmol/L for each 10-mmHg decrease in Pa_{CO_2}. It is unusual to observe a plasma HCO_3^- < 12 mmol/L as a result of a pure respiratory alkalosis.

When a diagnosis of respiratory alkalosis is made, its cause should be investigated. The diagnosis of hyperventilation syndrome is made by exclusion. In difficult cases, it may be important to rule out other conditions such as pulmonary embolism, coronary artery disease, and hyperthyroidism.

TREATMENT Respiratory Alkalosis

The management of respiratory alkalosis is directed toward alleviation of the underlying disorder. If respiratory alkalosis complicates ventilator management, changes in dead space, tidal volume, and frequency can minimize the hypocapnia. Patients with the hyperventilation syndrome may benefit from reassurance, rebreathing from a paper bag during symptomatic attacks, and attention to underlying psychological stress. Antidepressants and sedatives are not recommended. β-Adrenergic blockers may ameliorate peripheral manifestations of the hyperadrenergic state.

CHAPTER 39

COAGULATION DISORDERS

Valder R. Arruda ■ Katherine A. High

Deficiencies of coagulation factors have been recognized for centuries. Patients with genetic deficiencies of plasma coagulation factors exhibit life-long recurrent bleeding episodes into joints, muscles, and closed spaces, either spontaneously or following an injury. The most common inherited factor deficiencies are the hemophilias, X-linked diseases caused by deficiency of factor (F) VIII (hemophilia A) or factor IX (FIX, hemophilia B). Rare congenital bleeding disorders due to deficiencies of other factors, including FII (prothrombin), FV, FVII, FX, FXI, FXIII, and fibrinogen are commonly inherited in an autosomal recessive manner (Table 39-1). Advances in characterization of the molecular bases of clotting factor deficiencies have contributed to better understanding of the disease phenotypes and may eventually allow more targeted therapeutic approaches through the development of small molecules, recombinant proteins, or cell and gene-based therapies.

Commonly used tests of hemostasis provide the initial screening for clotting factor activity (Fig. 39-1), and disease phenotype often correlates with the level of clotting activity. An isolated abnormal prothrombin time (PT) suggests FVII deficiency, whereas a prolonged activated partial thromboplastin time (aPTT) indicates most commonly hemophilia or FXI deficiency (Fig. 39-1). The prolongation of both PT and aPTT suggests deficiency of FV, FX, FII, or fibrinogen abnormalities. The addition of the missing factor at a range of doses to the subject's plasma will correct the abnormal clotting times; the result is expressed as a percentage of the activity observed in normal subjects.

Acquired deficiencies of plasma coagulation factors are more frequent than congenital disorders; the most common disorders include hemorrhagic diathesis of liver disease, disseminated intravascular coagulation (DIC), and vitamin K deficiency. In these disorders, blood coagulation is hampered by the deficiency of more than one clotting factor, and the bleeding episodes are the result of perturbation of both primary (coagulation) and secondary (e.g., platelet and vessel wall interactions) hemostasis.

The development of antibodies to coagulation plasma proteins, clinically termed *inhibitors*, is a relatively rare disease that often affects hemophilia A or B and FXI-deficient patients on repetitive exposure to the missing protein to control bleeding episodes. Inhibitors also occur among subjects without genetic deficiency of clotting factors (e.g., in the postpartum setting as a manifestation of underlying autoimmune or neoplastic disease or idiopathically). Rare cases of inhibitors to thrombin or FV have been reported in patients receiving topical bovine thrombin preparation as a local hemostatic agent in complex surgeries. The diagnosis of inhibitors is based on the same tests as those used to diagnose inherited plasma coagulation factor deficiencies. However, the addition of the missing protein to the plasma of a subject with an inhibitor does not correct the abnormal aPTT and/or PT tests. This is the major laboratory difference between deficiencies and inhibitors. Additional tests are required to measure the specificity of the inhibitor and its titer.

The treatment of these bleeding disorders often requires replacement of the deficient protein using recombinant or purified plasma-derived products or fresh-frozen plasma (FFP). Therefore, it is imperative to arrive at a proper diagnosis to optimize patient care without unnecessary exposure to suboptimal treatment and the risks of bloodborne disease.

TABLE 39-1

GENETIC AND LABORATORY CHARACTERISTICS OF INHERITED COAGULATION DISORDERS

CLOTTING FACTOR DEFICIENCY	INHERITANCE	PREVALENCE IN GENERAL POPULATION	LABORATORY ABNORMALITY[a]			MINIMUM HEMOSTATIC LEVELS	TREATMENT	PLASMA HALF-LIFE
			aPTT	PT	TT			
Fibrinogen	AR	1 in 1,000,000	+	+	+	100 mg/dL	Cryoprecipitate	2–4 d
Prothrombin	AR	1 in 2,000,000	+	+	–	20–30%	FFP/PCC	3–4 d
Factor V	AR	1 in 1,000,000	+/–	+/–	–	15–20%	FFP	36 h
Factor VII	AR	1 in 500,000	–	+	–	15–20%	FFP/PCC	4–6 h
Factor VIII	X-linked	1 in 5,000	+	–	–	30%	FVIII concentrates	8–12 h
Factor IX	X-linked	1 in 30,000	+	–	–	30%	FIX concentrates	18–24 h
Factor X	AR	1 in 1,000,000	+/–	+/–	–	15–20%	FFP/PCC	40–60 h
Factor XI	AR	1 in 1,000,000	+	–	–	15–20%	FFP	40–70 h
Factor XII	AR	ND	+	–	–	[b]	[b]	60 h
HK	AR	ND	+	–	–	[b]	[b]	150 h
Prekallikrein	AR	ND	+	–	–	[b]	[b]	35 h
Factor XIII	AR	1 in 2,000,000	–	–	+/–	2–5%	Cryoprecipitate	11–14 d

[a]Values within normal range (–) or prolonged (+).
[b]No risk for bleeding; treatment is not indicated.
Abbreviations: aPTT, activated partial thromboplastin time; AR, autosomal recessive; FFP, fresh-frozen plasma; HK, high-molecular-weight kininogen; ND, not determined; PCC, prothrombin complex concentrates; PT, prothrombin time; TT, thrombin time.

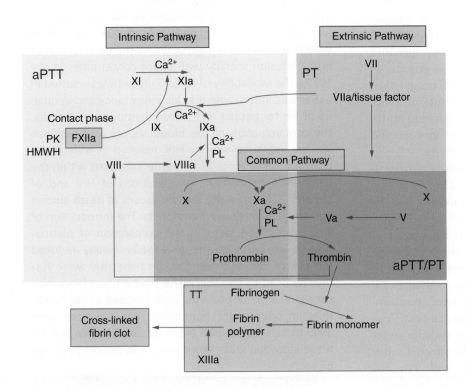

FIGURE 39-1

Coagulation cascade and laboratory assessment of clotting factor deficiency by activated partial prothrombin time (aPTT), prothrombin time (PT), and thrombin time (TT).

HEMOPHILIA

PATHOGENESIS AND CLINICAL MANIFESTATIONS

Hemophilia is an X-linked recessive hemorrhagic disease due to mutations in the *F8* gene (hemophilia A or classic hemophilia) or *F9* gene (hemophilia B). The disease affects 1 in 10,000 males worldwide, in all ethnic groups; hemophilia A represents 80% of all cases. Male subjects are clinically affected; women, who carry a single mutated gene, are generally asymptomatic. Family history of the disease is absent in ~30% of cases and in these cases, 80% of the mothers are carriers of the de novo mutated allele. More than 500 different mutations have been identified in the *F8* or *F9* genes of patients with hemophilia A or B, respectively. One of the most common hemophilia A mutations results from an inversion of the intron 22 sequence, and it is present in 40% of cases of severe hemophilia A. Advances in molecular diagnosis now permit precise identification of mutations, allowing accurate diagnosis of women carriers of the hemophilia gene in affected families.

Clinically, hemophilia A and hemophilia B are indistinguishable. The disease phenotype correlates with the residual activity of FVIII or FIX and can be classified as severe (<1%), moderate (1–5%), or mild (6–30%). In the severe and moderate forms, the disease is characterized by bleeding into the joints (hemarthrosis), soft tissues, and muscles after minor trauma or even spontaneously. Patients with mild disease experience infrequent bleeding that is usually secondary to trauma. Among those with residual FVIII or FIX activity >25% of normal, the disease is discovered only by bleeding after major trauma or during routine presurgery laboratory tests. Typically, the global tests of coagulation show only an isolated prolongation of the aPTT assay. Patients with hemophilia have normal bleeding times and platelet counts. The diagnosis is made after specific determination of FVIII or FIX clotting activity.

Early in life, bleeding may present after circumcision or rarely as intracranial hemorrhages. The disease is more evident when children begin to walk or crawl. In the severe form, the most common bleeding manifestations are the recurrent hemarthroses, which can affect every joint but mainly affect knees, elbows, ankles, shoulders, and hips. Acute hemarthroses are painful, and clinical signs are local swelling and erythema. To avoid pain, the patient may adopt a fixed position, which leads eventually to muscle contractures. Very young children unable to communicate verbally show irritability and a lack of movement of the affected joint. Chronic hemarthroses are debilitating, with synovial thickening and synovitis in response to the intraarticular blood. After a joint has been damaged, recurrent bleeding episodes result in the clinically recognized "target joint," which then establishes a vicious cycle of bleeding, resulting in progressive joint deformity that in critical cases requires surgery as the only therapeutic option. Hematomas into the muscle of distal parts of the limbs may lead to external compression of arteries, veins, or nerves that can evolve to a compartment syndrome.

Bleeding into the oropharyngeal spaces, central nervous system (CNS), or the retroperitoneum is life threatening and requires immediate therapy. Retroperitoneal hemorrhages can accumulate large quantities of blood with formation of masses with calcification and inflammatory tissue reaction (pseudotumor syndrome) and also result in damage to the femoral nerve. Pseudotumors can also form in bones, especially long bones of the lower limbs. Hematuria is frequent among hemophilia patients, even in the absence of genitourinary pathology. It is often self-limited and may not require specific therapy.

TREATMENT   Hemophilia

Without treatment, severe hemophilia has a limited life expectancy. Advances in the blood fractionation industry during World War II resulted in the realization that plasma could be used to treat hemophilia, but the volumes required to achieve even modest elevation of circulating factor levels limit the utility of plasma infusion as an approach to disease management. The discovery in the 1960s that the cryoprecipitate fraction of plasma was enriched for FVIII, and the eventual purification of FVIII and FIX from plasma, led to the introduction of home infusion therapy with factor concentrates in the 1970s. The availability of factor concentrates resulted in a dramatic improvement in life expectancy and in quality of life for people with severe hemophilia. However, the contamination of the blood supply with hepatitis viruses and, subsequently HIV, resulted in widespread transmission of these bloodborne infections within the hemophilia population; complications of HIV and of hepatitis C are now the leading causes of death among U.S. adults with severe hemophilia. The introduction of viral inactivation steps in the preparation of plasma-derived products in the mid-1980s greatly reduced the risk of HIV and hepatitis, and the risks were further reduced by the successful production of recombinant FVIII and FIX proteins, both licensed in the 1990s. It is uncommon for hemophilic patients born after 1985 to have contracted either hepatitis or HIV, and for these individuals, life expectancy is in the range of age 65 years.

Factor replacement therapy for hemophilia can be provided either in response to a bleeding episode or as a prophylactic treatment. Primary prophylaxis is defined as a strategy for maintaining the missing clotting factor at levels ~1% or higher on a regular basis in order to prevent bleeds, especially the onset of hemarthroses. Hemophilic boys receiving regular infusions of FVIII (3 days/week) or FIX (2 days/week) can reach puberty without detectable joint abnormalities.

Prophylaxis has become gradually more common in young patients. The Centers for Disease Control and Prevention reported that 51% of children with severe hemophilia who are younger than age 6 years receive prophylaxis, increasing considerably from 33% in 1995. Although highly recommended, the high cost and difficulties in accessing peripheral veins in young patients and the potential infectious and thrombotic risks of long-term central vein catheters are important limiting factors for many patients.

General considerations regarding the treatment of bleeds in hemophilia include (1) the need to begin the treatment as soon as possible because symptoms often precede objective evidence of bleeding; because of the superior efficacy of early therapeutic intervention, classic symptoms of bleeding into the joint in a reliable patient, headaches, or automobile or other accidents require prompt replacement and further laboratory investigation; and (2) the need to avoid drugs that hamper platelet function, such as aspirin or aspirin-containing drugs; to control pain, drugs such as ibuprofen or propoxyphene are preferred.

Factor VIII and FIX are dosed in units. One unit is defined as amount of FVIII (100 ng/mL) or FIX (5 μg/mL) in 1 mL of normal plasma. One unit of FVIII per kilogram of body weight increases the plasma FVIII level by 2%. One can calculate the dose needed to increase FVIII levels to 100% in a 70-kg severe hemophilia patient (<1%) using the simple formula below. Thus, 3500 units of FVIII will raise the circulating level to 100%.

$$\text{FVIII dose (IU)} = \text{Target FVIII levels} - \text{FVIII baseline levels} \times \text{body weight (kg)} \times 0.5 \text{ unit/kg}$$

The doses for FIX replacement are different from those for FVIII, because FIX recovery postinfusion is usually only 50% of the predicted value. Therefore, the formula for FIX replacement is

$$\text{FIX dose (IU)} = \text{Target FIX levels} - \text{FIX baseline levels} \times \text{body weight (kg)} \times 1 \text{ unit/kg}$$

The FVIII half-life of 8–12 h requires injections twice a day to maintain therapeutic levels, whereas FIX half-life is longer, ~24 h, so that once-a-day injection is sufficient. In specific situations such as postsurgery, continuous infusion of factor may be desirable because of its safety in achieving sustained factor levels at a lower total cost.

Cryoprecipitate is enriched with FVIII protein (each bag contains ~80 IU of FVIII) and was commonly used for the treatment of hemophilia A decades ago; it is still in use in some developing countries, but because of the risk of bloodborne diseases, this product should be avoided in hemophilia patients when factor concentrates are available.

Mild bleeds such as uncomplicated hemarthroses or superficial hematomas require initial therapy with factor levels of 30–50%. Additional doses to maintain levels of 15–25% for 2 or 3 days are indicated for severe hemarthroses, especially when these episodes affect the "target joint." Large hematomas, or bleeds into deep muscles, require factor levels of 50% or even higher if the clinical symptoms do not improve, and factor replacement may be required for a period of 1 week or longer. The control of serious bleeds including those that affect the oropharyngeal spaces, CNS, and the retroperitoneum require sustained protein levels of 50–100% for 7–10 days. Prophylactic replacement for surgery is aimed at achieving normal factor levels (100%) for a period of 7–10 days; replacement can then be tapered depending on the extent of the surgical wounds. Oral surgery is associated with extensive tissue damage that usually requires factor replacement for 1–3 days coupled with oral antifibrinolytic drugs.

NONTRANFUSION THERAPY IN HEMOPHILIA

DDAVP (1-Amino-8-D-Arginine Vasopressin)
DDAVP is a synthetic vasopressin analog that causes a transient rise in FVIII and von Willebrand factor (vWF), but not FIX, through a mechanism involving release from endothelial cells. Patients with moderate or mild hemophilia A should be tested to determine if they respond to DDAVP before a therapeutic application. DDAVP at doses of 0.3 μg/kg body weight, over a 20-min period, is expected to raise FVIII levels by two- to threefold over baseline, peaking between 30 and 60 min postinfusion. DDAVP does not improve FVIII levels in severe hemophilia A patients, since there are no stores to release. Repeated dosing of DDAVP results in tachyphylaxis, since the mechanism is an increase in release rather than de novo synthesis of FVIII and vWF. More than three consecutive doses become ineffective and if further therapy is indicated, FVIII replacement is required to achieve hemostasis.

Antifibrinolytic Drugs. Bleeding in the gums, gastrointestinal tract, and during oral surgery requires the use of oral antifibrinolytic drugs such as ε-amino caproic acid (EACA) or tranexamic acid to control local hemostasis. The duration of the treatment depending on the clinical indication is 1 week or longer. Tranexamic acid is given at doses of 25 mg/kg three to four times a day. EACA treatment requires a loading dose of 200 mg/kg (maximum of 10 g) followed by 100 mg/kg per dose (maximum 30 g/d) every 6 h. These drugs are not indicated to control hematuria because of the risk of formation of an occlusive clot in the lumen of genitourinary tract structures.

COMPLICATIONS

Inhibitor Formation The formation of alloantibodies to FVIII or FIX is currently the major complication of hemophilia treatment. The prevalence of inhibitors to FVIII is estimated to be between 5 and 10% of all cases and ~20% of severe hemophilia A patients. Inhibitors to FIX are detected in only 3–5% of all hemophilia B patients. The high-risk group for inhibitor formation includes severe deficiency (>80% of all cases of inhibitors), familial history of inhibitor, African descent, mutations in the FVIII or FIX gene resulting in deletion of large coding regions, or gross gene rearrangements. Inhibitors usually appear early in life, at a median of 2 years of age, and after 10 cumulative days of exposure. However, intensive replacement therapy such as for major surgery, intracranial bleeding, or trauma increases the risk of inhibitor formation for patients of all ages that requires close laboratory monitoring in the following weeks.

The clinical diagnosis of an inhibitor is suspected when patients do not respond to factor replacement at therapeutic doses. Inhibitors increase both morbidity and mortality in hemophilia. Because early detection of an inhibitor is critical to a successful correction of the bleeding or to eradication of the antibody, most hemophilia centers perform annual screening for inhibitors. The laboratory test required to confirm the presence of an inhibitor is an aPTT with a mix (with normal plasma). In most hemophilia patients, a 1:1 mix with normal plasma completely corrects the aPTT. In inhibitor patients, the aPTT on a 1:1 mix is abnormally prolonged, because the inhibitor neutralizes the FVIII clotting activity of the normal plasma. The Bethesda assay uses a similar principle and defines the specificity of the inhibitor and its titer. The results are expressed in Bethesda units (BU), in which 1 BU is the amount of antibody that neutralizes 50% of the FVIII or FIX present in normal plasma after 2 h of incubation at 37°C. Clinically, inhibitor patients are classified as low responders or high responders, which provides guidelines for optimal therapy. Therapy for inhibitor patients has two goals, the control of acute bleeding episodes and the eradication of the inhibitor. For the control of bleeding episodes, low responders, those with titer <5 BU, respond well to high doses of human or porcine FVIII (50–100 U/kg), with minimal or no increase in the inhibitor titers. However, high-responder patients, those with initial inhibitor titer >10 BU or an anamnestic response

in the antibody titer to >10 BU even if low titer initially, do not respond to FVIII or FIX concentrates. The control of bleeding episodes in high-responder patients can be achieved by using concentrates enriched for prothrombin, FVII, FIX, FX (prothrombin complex concentrates [PCCs] or activated PCCs), and more recently by recombinant activated factor VII (FVIIa) (Fig. 39-1). The rates of therapeutic success have been higher for FVIIa than for PCC or aPCC. For eradication of the inhibitory antibody, immunosuppression alone is not effective. The most effective strategy is the immune tolerance induction (ITI) based on daily infusion of missing protein until the inhibitor disappears, typically requiring periods longer than 1 year, with success rates in the range of 60%. The management of patients with severe hemophilia A and inhibitors resistant to ITI is challenging. The use of anti-CD20 monoclonal antibody (rituximab) combined with FVIII was thought to be effective. Although this therapy may reduce the inhibitor titers, sustained eradication is uncommon and may require two to three infusions weekly of FVIII concentrates.

Infectious Diseases Hepatitis C viral (HCV) infection is the major cause of morbidity and the second leading cause of death in hemophilia patients exposed to older clotting factor concentrates. The vast majority of young patients treated with plasma-derived products from 1970 to 1985 became infected with HCV. It has been estimated that >80% of patients older than 20 years of age are HCV antibody positive as of 2006. The comorbidity of the underlying liver disease in hemophilia patients is clear when these individuals require invasive procedures; correction of both genetic and acquired (secondary to liver disease) deficiencies may be needed. Infection with HIV also swept the population of patients using plasma-derived concentrates 2 decades ago. Co-infection of HCV and HIV, present in almost 50% of hemophilia patients, is an aggravating factor for the evolution of liver disease. The response to HCV antiviral therapy in hemophilia is restricted to <30% of patients and even poorer among those with both HCV and HIV infection. End-stage liver disease requiring organ transplantation may be curative for both the liver disease and for hemophilia.

Emerging Clinical Problems in Aging Hemophilia Patients There has been continuous improvement of the management of hemophilia since the increase in the population of adults living beyond middle age in the developing world. The life expectancy of a patient with severe hemophilia is only ~10 years shorter than the general male population. In patients with mild or moderate hemophilia, life expectancy is approaching that of the male population without coagulopathy. Elderly hemophilia patients have different problems compared to the younger generation; they have more severe arthropathy and chronic pain due to suboptimal treatment, and high rates of HCV and/or HIV infections.

Early data indicate that mortality from coronary artery disease is lower in hemophilia patients than the general male population. The underlying hypocoagulability probably provides a protective effect against thrombus formation, but it does not prevent the development of atherogenesis. Similar to the general population, these patients are exposed to cardiovascular risk factors such as age, obesity, and smoking. Moreover, physical inactivity, hypertension, and chronic renal disease are commonly observed in hemophilia patients. In HIV patients on combined antiretroviral therapy, there may be a further increase in the risk of cardiovascular disease. Therefore, these patients should be carefully considered for preventive and therapeutic approaches to minimize the risk of cardiovascular disease.

Excessive replacement therapy should be avoided, and it is prudent to slowly infuse factor concentrates. Continuous infusion of clotting factor is preferable to bolus dosing in patients with cardiovascular risk factors undergoing invasive procedures. The management of an acute ischemic event and coronary revascularization should include the collaboration of hematologists and internists. The early assumption that hemophilia would protect against occlusive vascular disease may change in this aging population.

Cancer is a common cause of mortality in aging hemophilia patients as they are at risk for HIV- and HCV-related malignancies. Hepatocellular carcinoma (HCC) is the most prevalent primary liver cancer and a common cause of death in HIV-negative patients. The recommendations for cancer screening for the general population should be the same for age-matched hemophilia patients. Among those with high-risk HCV, a semiannual or annual ultrasound and α fetoprotein is recommended for HCC. Screening for urogenital neoplasm in the presence of hematuria or hematochezia may be delayed due to the underlying bleeding disease, thus preventing early intervention. Multidisciplinary interaction should facilitate the attempts to ensure optimal cancer prevention and treatment recommendations for those with hemophilia.

Management of Carriers of Hemophilia

Usually hemophilia carriers, with factor levels of ~50% of normal, have not been considered to be at risk for bleeding. However, a wide range of values (22–116%) have been reported due to random inactivation of the X chromosomes (*lyonization*). Therefore, it is important to measure the factor level of carriers to recognize those at risk of bleeding and to optimize preoperative and postoperative management. During pregnancy, both FVIII and FIX levels increase gradually until delivery. FVIII levels increase approximately two- to threefold compared to nonpregnant women, whereas a FIX increase is less pronounced. After delivery, there is a rapid fall in the pregnancy-induced rise of maternal clotting factor levels. This represents an imminent risk of bleeding that can be prevented by infusion of factor concentrate to levels of 50–70% for 3 days in the setting of vaginal delivery and up to 5 days for cesarean section. In mild cases, the use of DDAVP and/or antifibrinolytic drugs is recommended.

FACTOR XI DEFICIENCY

Factor XI is a zymogen of an active serine protease (FIXa) in the intrinsic pathway of blood coagulation that activates FIX (Fig. 39-1). There are two pathways for the formation of FXIa. In an aPTT-based assay, the protease is the result of activation by FXIIa in conjunction with high-molecular-weight kininogen and kallikrein. In vivo data suggest that thrombin is the physiologic activator of FXI. The generation of thrombin by the tissue-factor/factor VIIa pathway activates FXI on the platelet surface that contributes to additional thrombin generation after the clot has formed and thus augments resistance to fibrinolysis through a thrombin-activated fibrinolytic inhibitor (TAFI).

Factor XI deficiency is a rare bleeding disorder that occurs in the general population at a frequency of one in a million. However, the disease is highly prevalent among Ashkenazi and Iraqi Jewish populations, reaching a frequency of 6% as heterozygotes and 0.1% to 0.3% as homozygotes. More than 65 mutations in the FXI gene have been reported, whereas fewer mutations (two to three) are found among affected Jewish populations.

Normal FXI clotting activity levels range from 70 to 150 U/dL. In heterozygous patients with moderate deficiency, FXI ranges from 20 to 70 U/dL, whereas in homozygous or double heterozygote patients, FXI levels are <1–20 U/dL. Patients with FXI levels <10% of normal have a high risk of bleeding, but the disease phenotype does not always correlate with residual FXI clotting activity. A family history is indicative of the risk of bleeding in the propositus. Clinically, the presence of mucocutaneous hemorrhages such as bruises, gum bleeding, epistaxis, hematuria, and menorrhagia are common, especially following trauma. This hemorrhagic phenotype suggests that tissues rich in fibrinolytic activity are more susceptible to FXI deficiency. Postoperative bleeding is common but not always present, even among patients with very low FXI levels.

FXI replacement is indicated in patients with severe disease required to undergo a surgical procedure. A negative history of bleeding complications following invasive procedures does not exclude the possibility of an increased risk for hemorrhage.

TREATMENT	Factor XI Deficiency

The treatment of FXI deficiency is based on the infusion of FFP at doses of 15 to 20 mL/kg to maintain trough levels ranging from 10% to 20%. Because FXI has a half-life of 40–70 h, the replacement therapy can be given on alternate days. The use of antifibrinolytic drugs is beneficial to control bleeds, with the exception of hematuria or bleeds in the bladder. The development of an FXI inhibitor was observed in 10% of severely FXI-deficient patients who received replacement therapy. Patients with severe FXI deficiency who develop inhibitors usually do not bleed spontaneously. However, bleeding following a surgical procedure or trauma can be severe. In these patients, FFP and FXI concentrates should be avoided. The use of PCC/aPCC or recombinant activated FVII has been effective.

RARE BLEEDING DISORDERS

Collectively, the inherited disorders resulting from deficiencies of clotting factors other than FVIII, FIX, and FXI (Table 39-1) represent a group of rare bleeding diseases. The bleeding symptoms in these patients vary from asymptomatic (dysfibrinogenemia or FVII deficiency) to life-threatening (FX or FXIII deficiency). There is no pathognomonic clinical manifestation that suggests one specific disease, but overall, in contrast to hemophilia, hemarthrosis is a rare event and bleeding in the mucosal tract or after umbilical cord clamping is common. Individuals heterozygous for plasma coagulation deficiencies are often asymptomatic. The laboratory assessment for the specific deficient factor following screening with general coagulation tests (Table 39-1) will define the diagnosis.

Replacement therapy using FFP or prothrombin complex concentrates (containing prothrombin, FVII, FIX, and FX) provides adequate hemostasis in response to bleeds or as prophylactic treatment. The use of PCC should be carefully monitored and avoided in patients with underlying liver disease, or those at high risk for thrombosis because of the risk of disseminated intravascular coagulopathy.

FAMILIAL MULTIPLE COAGULATION DEFICIENCIES

There are several bleeding disorders characterized by the inherited deficiency of more than one plasma coagulation factor. To date, the genetic defects in two of these diseases have been characterized and they provide new insights into the regulation of hemostasis by gene-encoding proteins outside blood coagulation.

Combined deficiency of FV and FVIII

Patients with combined FV and FVIII deficiency exhibit ~5% of residual clotting activity of each factor. Interestingly, the disease phenotype is a mild bleeding tendency, often following trauma. An underlying mutation has been identified in the endoplasmic reticulum/Golgi intermediate compartment (*ERGIC-53*) gene, a mannose-binding protein localized in the Golgi apparatus that functions as a chaperone for both FV and FVIII. In other families, mutations in the multiple coagulation factor deficiency 2 (*MCFD2*) gene have been defined; this gene encodes a protein that forms a Ca^{2+}–dependent complex with *ERGIC-53* and provides cofactor activity in the intracellular mobilization of both FV and FVIII.

Multiple deficiencies of vitamin K–dependent coagulation factors

Two enzymes involved in vitamin K metabolism have been associated with combined deficiency of all vitamin K–dependent proteins, including the procoagulant proteins prothrombin, VII, IX, and X and the anticoagulant proteins C and S. Vitamin K is a fat-soluble vitamin that is a cofactor for carboxylation of the gamma carbon of the glutamic acid residues in the vitamin K–dependent factors, a critical step for calcium and phospholipid binding of these proteins (**Fig. 39-2**). The enzymes γ-glutamylcarboxylase and epoxide reductase are critical for the metabolism and regeneration of vitamin K. Mutations in the genes encoding the gamma-carboxylase (GGCX) or vitamin K epoxide reductase complex 1 (VKORC1)

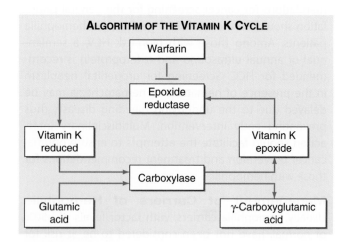

FIGURE 39-2

The vitamin K cycle. Vitamin K is a cofactor for the formation of γ-carboxyglutamic acid residues on coagulation proteins. Vitamin K–dependent γ-glutamylcarboxylase, the enzyme that catalyzes the vitamin K epoxide reductase, regenerates reduced vitamin K. Warfarin blocks the action of the reductase and competitively inhibits the effects of vitamin K.

result in defective enzymes and thus in vitamin K–dependent factors with reduced activity, varying from 1 to 30% of normal. The disease phenotype is characterized by mild to severe bleeding episodes present from birth. Some patients respond to high doses of vitamin K. For severe bleeding, replacement therapy with FFP or PCC may be necessary for achieving full hemostatic control.

DISSEMINATED INTRAVASCULAR COAGULATION

Disseminated intravascular coagulation (DIC) is a clinicopathologic syndrome characterized by widespread intravascular fibrin formation in response to excessive blood protease activity that overcomes the natural anticoagulant mechanisms. There are several underlying pathologies associated with DIC (Table 39-2).

TABLE 39-2

COMMON CLINICAL CAUSES OF DISSEMINATED INTRAVASCULAR COAGULATION

Sepsis	**Immunologic disorders**
• Bacterial: Staphylococci, streptococci, pneumococci, meningococci, gram-negative bacilli	• Acute hemolytic transfusion reaction
• Viral	• Organ or tissue transplant rejection
• Mycotic	• Graft-versus-host disease
• Parasitic	
• Rickettsial	
Trauma and tissue injury	**Drugs**
• Brain injury (gunshot)	• Fibrinolytic agents
• Extensive burns	• Aprotinin
• Fat embolism	• Warfarin (especially in neonates with protein C deficiency)
• Rhabdomyolysis	• Prothrombin complex concentrates
	• Recreational drugs (amphetamines)
Vascular disorders	**Envenomation**
• Giant hemangiomas (Kasabach-Merritt syndrome)	• Snake
• Large vessel aneurysms (e.g., aorta)	• Insects
Obstetrical complications	**Liver disease**
• Abruptio placentae	• Fulminant hepatic failure
• Amniotic-fluid embolism	• Cirrhosis
• Dead fetus syndrome	• Fatty liver of pregnancy
• Septic abortion	
Cancer	**Miscellaneous**
• Adenocarcinoma (prostate, pancreas, etc.)	• Shock
• Hematologic malignancies (acute promyelocytic leukemia)	• Respiratory distress syndrome
	• Massive transfusion

The most common causes are bacterial sepsis, malignant disorders such as solid tumors or acute promyelocytic leukemia, and obstetric causes. DIC is diagnosed in almost one-half of pregnant women with abruptio placentae, or with amniotic fluid embolism. Trauma, particularly to the brain, can also result in DIC. The exposure of blood to phospholipids from damaged tissue, hemolysis, and endothelial damage are all contributing factors to the development of DIC in this setting. Purpura fulminans is a severe form of DIC resulting from thrombosis of extensive areas of the skin; it affects predominantly young children following viral or bacterial infection, particularly those with inherited or acquired hypercoagulability due to deficiencies of the components of the protein C pathway. Neonates homozygous for protein C deficiency also present high risk for purpura fulminans with or without thrombosis of large vessels.

The central mechanism of DIC is the uncontrolled generation of thrombin by exposure of the blood to pathologic levels of tissue factor (Fig. 39-3). Simultaneous suppression of physiologic anticoagulant mechanisms and abnormal fibrinolysis further accelerate the process. Together, these abnormalities contribute to systemic fibrin deposition in small and midsize vessels. The duration and intensity of the fibrin deposition can compromise the blood supply of many organs, especially the lung, kidney, liver, and brain, with consequent organ failure. The sustained activation of coagulation results in consumption of clotting factors and platelets, which in turn leads to systemic bleeding. This is further aggravated by secondary hyperfibrinolysis. Studies in animals demonstrate that the fibrinolytic system is indeed suppressed at the time of maximal activation of coagulation. Interestingly, in patients with acute promyelocytic leukemia, a severe hyperfibrinolytic state often occurs in addition to the coagulation activation. The release of several proinflammatory cytokines such as interleukin-6 and tumor necrosis factor α play central roles in mediating the coagulation defects in DIC and symptoms associated with systemic inflammatory response syndrome (SIRS).

Clinical manifestations of DIC are related to the magnitude of the imbalance of hemostasis, to the underlying disease, or to both. The most common findings are bleeding ranging from oozing from venipuncture sites, petechiae, and ecchymoses to severe hemorrhage from the gastrointestinal tract, lung, or into the CNS. In chronic DIC, the bleeding symptoms are discrete and restricted to skin or mucosal surfaces. The hypercoagulability of DIC manifests as the occlusion of vessels in the microcirculation and resulting organ failure. Thrombosis of large vessels and cerebral embolism can also occur. Hemodynamic complications and shock are common among patients with acute DIC. The mortality ranges from 30% to >80% depending on the

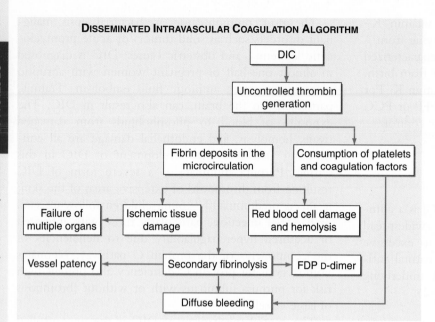

DISSEMINATED INTRAVASCULAR COAGULATION ALGORITHM

FIGURE 39-3

The pathophysiology of disseminated intravascular coagulation (DIC). Interactions between coagulation and fibrinolytic pathways result in bleeding and thrombosis in the microcirculation in patients with DIC.

underlying disease, the severity of the DIC, and the age of the patient.

The diagnosis of clinically significant DIC is based on the presence of clinical and/or laboratory abnormalities of coagulation or thrombocytopenia. The laboratory diagnosis of DIC should prompt a search for the underlying disease if it is not already apparent. There is no single test that establishes the diagnosis of DIC. The laboratory investigation should include coagulation tests (aPTT, PT, thrombin time [TT]) and markers of fibrin degradation products (FDPs), in addition to platelet and red cell count and analysis of the blood smear. These tests should be repeated over a period of 6–8 h because an initially mild abnormality can change dramatically in patients with severe DIC.

Common findings include the prolongation of PT and/or aPTT; platelet counts ≤100,000/μL^3, or a rapid decline in platelet numbers; the presence of schistocytes (fragmented red cells) in the blood smear; and elevated levels of FDP. The most sensitive test for DIC is the FDP level. DIC is an unlikely diagnosis in the presence of normal levels of FDP. The D-dimer test is more specific for detection of fibrin—but not fibrinogen—degradation products and indicates that the cross-linked fibrin has been digested by plasmin. Because fibrinogen has a prolonged half-life, plasma levels diminish acutely only in severe cases of DIC. High-grade DIC is also associated with levels of antithrombin III or plasminogen activity <60% of normal.

Chronic DIC

Low-grade, compensated DIC can occur in clinical situations including giant hemangioma, metastatic carcinoma, or the dead fetus syndrome. Plasma levels of FDP or D-dimers are elevated. aPTT, PT, and fibrinogen values

are within the normal range or high. Mild thrombocytopenia or normal platelet counts are also common findings. Red cell fragmentation is often detected but at a lower degree than in acute DIC.

Differential diagnosis

The differential diagnosis between DIC and severe liver disease is challenging and requires serial measurements of the laboratory parameters of DIC. Patients with severe liver disease are at risk for bleeding and manifest laboratory features including thrombocytopenia (due to platelet sequestration, portal hypertension, or hypersplenism), decreased synthesis of coagulation factors and natural anticoagulants, and elevated levels of FDP due to reduced hepatic clearance. However, in contrast to DIC, these laboratory parameters in liver disease do not change rapidly. Other important differential findings include the presence of portal hypertension or other clinical or laboratory evidence of an underlying liver disease.

Microangiopathic disorders such as thrombotic thrombocytopenic purpura present an acute clinical onset of illness accompanied by thrombocytopenia, red cell fragmentation, and multiorgan failure. However, there is no consumption of clotting factors or hyperfibrinolysis.

| TREATMENT | Disseminated Intravascular Coagulation |

The morbidity and mortality associated with DIC are primarily related to the underlying disease rather than the complications of the DIC. The control or elimination of the underlying cause should therefore be the primary concern. Patients with severe DIC require control of hemodynamic parameters, respiratory support, and sometimes invasive surgical procedures. Attempts to treat DIC without accompanying treatment of the causative disease are likely to fail.

MANAGEMENT OF HEMORRHAGIC SYMPTOMS The control of bleeding in DIC patients with marked thrombocytopenia (platelet counts <10,000–20,000/μL^3) and low levels of coagulation factors will require replacement therapy. The PT (>1.5 times the normal) provides a good indicator of the severity of the clotting factor consumption. Replacement with FFP is indicated (1 unit of FFP increases most coagulation factors by 3% in an adult without DIC). Low levels of fibrinogen (<100 mg/dL) or brisk hyperfibrinolysis will require infusion of cryoprecipitate (plasma fraction enriched for fibrinogen, FVIII, and vWF). The replacement of 10 U of cryoprecipitate for every 2–3 U of FFP is sufficient to correct the hemostasis. The transfusion scheme must be adjusted according to the patient's clinical and laboratory evolution. Platelet concentrates at a dose of 1–2 U/10 kg body weight are sufficient for most DIC patients with severe thrombocytopenia.

Clotting factor concentrates are not recommended for control of bleeding in DIC because of the limited efficacy afforded by replacement of single factors (FVIII or FIX concentrates), and the high risk of products containing traces of aPCCs that further aggravate the disease.

REPLACEMENT OF COAGULATION OR FIBRINOLYSIS INHIBITORS Drugs to control coagulation such as heparin, ATIII concentrates, or antifibrinolytic drugs have all been tried in the treatment of DIC. Low doses of continuous infusion heparin (5–10 U/kg per h) may be effective in patients with low-grade DIC associated with solid tumor, acute promyelocytic leukemia, or in a setting with recognized thrombosis. Heparin is also indicated for the treatment of purpura fulminans during the surgical resection of giant hemangiomas and during removal of a dead fetus. In acute DIC, the use of heparin is likely to aggravate bleeding. To date, the use of heparin in patients with severe DIC has no proven survival benefit.

The use of antifibrinolytic drugs, EACA, or tranexamic acid, to prevent fibrin degradation by plasmin may reduce bleeding episodes in patients with DIC and confirmed hyperfibrinolysis. However, these drugs can increase the risk of thrombosis and concomitant use of heparin is indicated. Patients with acute promyelocytic leukemia or those with chronic DIC associated with giant hemangiomas are among the few patients who may benefit from this therapy.

The use of protein C concentrates to treat purpura fulminans associated with acquired protein C deficiency or meningococcemia has been proven efficacious. The results from the replacement of ATIII in early-phase studies are promising but require further study.

VITAMIN K DEFICIENCY

Vitamin K–dependent proteins are a heterogenous group, including clotting factor proteins and also proteins found in bone, lung, kidney, and placenta. Vitamin K mediates posttranslational modification of glutamate residues to γ-carboxylglutamate, a critical step for the activity of vitamin K–dependent proteins for calcium binding and proper assembly to phospholipid membranes (Fig. 39-2). Inherited deficiency of the functional activity of the enzymes involved in vitamin K metabolism, notably the GGCX or VKORC1 (see earlier), results in bleeding disorders. The amount of vitamin K in the diet is often limiting for the carboxylation reaction; thus recycling of the vitamin K is essential to maintain normal levels of vitamin K–dependent proteins. In adults, low dietary intake alone is seldom reason for severe vitamin K deficiency but may become common in association with the use of broad-spectrum antibiotics. Disease or surgical interventions that affect the ability of the intestinal tract to absorb vitamin K, either through anatomic alterations or by changing the fat content of bile salts and pancreatic juices in the proximal small bowel, can result in significant reduction of vitamin K levels. Chronic liver diseases such as primary biliary cirrhosis also deplete vitamin K stores. Neonatal vitamin K deficiency and the resulting hemorrhagic disease of the newborn have been almost entirely eliminated by routine administration of vitamin K to all neonates. Prolongation of PT values is the most common and earliest finding in vitamin K–deficient patients due to reduction in prothrombin, FVII, FIX, and FX levels. FVII has the shortest half-life among these factors that can prolong the PT before changes in the aPTT. Parenteral administration of vitamin K at a total dose of 10 mg is sufficient to restore normal levels of clotting factor within 8–10 h. In the presence of ongoing bleeding or a need for immediate correction before an invasive procedure, replacement with FFP or PCC is required. The latter should be avoided in patients with severe underlying liver disorders due to high risk of thrombosis. The reversal of excessive anticoagulant therapy with warfarin or warfarin-like drugs can be achieved by minimal doses of vitamin K (1 mg orally or by intravenous injection) for asymptomatic patients. This strategy can diminish the risk of bleeding while maintaining therapeutic anticoagulation for an underlying prothrombotic state.

In patients with life-threatening bleeds, the use of recombinant factor VIIa in nonhemophilia patients on anticoagulant therapy has been shown to be effective at restoring hemostasis rapidly, allowing emergency surgical intervention. However, patients with underlying vascular disease, vascular trauma and other comorbidities are at risk for thromboembolic complications that affect both arterial and venous systems. Thus, the use of factor VIIa in this setting is limited to administration of low doses given for only a limited number of injections. Close monitoring for vascular complications is highly indicated.

COAGULATION DISORDERS ASSOCIATED WITH LIVER FAILURE

The liver is central to hemostasis because it is the site of synthesis and clearance of most procoagulant and natural anticoagulant proteins and of essential components of the fibrinolytic system. Liver failure is associated with a high risk of bleeding due to deficient synthesis of procoagulant factors and enhanced fibrinolysis. Thrombocytopenia is common in patients with liver disease, and may be due to congestive splenomegaly (hypersplenism), or immune-mediated shortened platelet lifespan (primary biliary cirrhosis). In addition, several anatomic abnormalities secondary to underlying liver disease further promote the occurrence of hemorrhage (Table 39-3). Dysfibrinogenemia is a relatively common finding in patients with liver disease due to impaired fibrin polymerization. The development of DIC concomitant to chronic liver disease is not uncommon and may enhance the risk for bleeding. Laboratory evaluation is mandatory for an optimal therapeutic strategy, either to control ongoing bleeding or to prepare patients with liver disease for invasive procedures. Typically, these patients present with prolonged PT, aPTT, and TT depending on the degree of liver damage, thrombocytopenia, and normal or slight increase of FDP. Fibrinogen levels are diminished only in fulminant hepatitis, decompensated cirrhosis or advanced liver disease, or in the presence of DIC. The presence of prolonged TT and normal fibrinogen and FDP levels suggest dysfibrinogenemia. FVIII levels are often normal or elevated in patients with liver failure, and decreased levels suggest superimposing DIC. Because FV is only synthesized in the hepatocyte and is not a vitamin K–dependent protein, reduced levels of FV may be an indicator of hepatocyte failure. Normal levels of FV and low levels of FVII suggest vitamin K deficiency. Vitamin K levels may be reduced in patients with liver failure due to compromised storage in hepatocellular disease, changes in bile acids or cholestasis that can diminish the absorption of vitamin K. Replacement of vitamin K may be desirable (10 mg given by slow intravenous injection) to improve hemostasis.

Treatment with FFP is the most effective to correct hemostasis in patients with liver failure. Infusion of FFP (5–10 mL/kg; each bag contains ~200 mL) is sufficient to ensure 10–20% of normal levels of clotting factors but not correction of PT or aPTT. Even high doses of FFP (20 mL/kg) do not correct the clotting times in all patients. Monitoring for clinical symptoms and clotting times will determine if repeated doses are required 8–12 h after the first infusion. Platelet concentrates are indicated when platelet counts are $<10,000–20,000/\mu L^3$ to control an ongoing bleed or immediately before an invasive procedure if counts are $<50,000/\mu L^3$. Cryoprecipitate is indicated only when fibrinogen levels are less than 100 mg/mL; dosing is six bags for a 70-kg patient daily. Prothrombin complex concentrate infusion in patients with liver failure should be avoided due to the high risk of thrombotic complications. The safety of the use of antifibrinolytic drugs to control bleeding in patients with liver failure is not yet well defined and should be avoided.

Liver disease and thromboembolism

The clinical bleeding phenotype of hemostasis in patients with stable liver disease is often mild or even asymptomatic. However, as the disease progresses, the hemostatic balance is less stable and more easily disturbed than in healthy individuals. Furthermore, the hemostatic balance is compromised by comorbid complications such as infections and renal failure (Fig. 39-4).

Based on the clinical bleeding complications in patients with cirrhosis and laboratory evidence of hypocoagulation such as a prolonged PT/aPTT, it has long been assumed that these patients are protected against thrombotic disease. Cumulative clinical experience,

TABLE 39-3

COAGULATION DISORDERS AND HEMOSTASIS IN LIVER DISEASE

Bleeding

Portal hypertension
    Esophageal varices
Thrombocytopenia
    Splenomegaly
    Chronic or acute DIC
Decreased synthesis of clotting factors
    Hepatocyte failure
    Vitamin K deficiency
Systemic fibrinolysis
DIC
Dysfibrinogenemia

Thrombosis

Decreased synthesis of coagulation inhibitors: protein C, protein S, antithrombin
    Hepatocyte failure
    Vitamin K deficiency (protein C, protein S)
Failure to clear activated coagulation proteins (DIC)
Dysfibrinogenemia
Iatrogenic: Transfusion of prothrombin complex
    concentrates
    Antifibrinolytic agents: EACA, tranexamic acid

Abbreviations: DIC, disseminated intravascular coagulation; EACA, ε-aminocaproic acid.

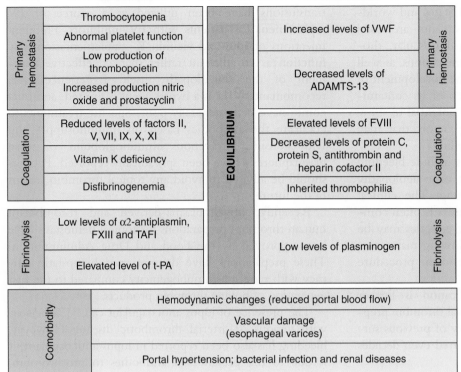

	BLEEDING		**THROMBOSIS**	
Primary hemostasis	Thrombocytopenia	**E**	Increased levels of VWF	**Primary hemostasis**
	Abnormal platelet function	**Q**		
	Low production of thrombopoietin	**U**	Decreased levels of ADAMTS-13	
	Increased production nitric oxide and prostacyclin	**I**		
Coagulation	Reduced levels of factors II, V, VII, IX, X, XI	**L**	Elevated levels of FVIII	**Coagulation**
	Vitamin K deficiency	**I**	Decreased levels of protein C, protein S, antithrombin and heparin cofactor II	
	Disfibrinogenemia	**B**	Inherited thrombophilia	
Fibrinolysis	Low levels of α2-antiplasmin, FXIII and TAFI	**R**	Low levels of plasminogen	**Fibrinolysis**
	Elevated level of t-PA	**I**		
		U		
Comorbidity	Hemodynamic changes (reduced portal blood flow)			
	Vascular damage (esophageal varices)			
	Portal hypertension; bacterial infection and renal diseases			

FIGURE 39-4
Balance of hemostasis in liver disease. TAFI, thrombin-activated fibriolytic inhibitor; t-PA, tissue plasminogen activator; VWF, von Willebrand factor.

however, has demonstrated that these patients are at risk for thrombosis, especially those with advanced liver disease. Although hypercoagulability could explain the occurrence of venous thrombosis, according to Virchow's triad, hemodynamic changes and damaged vasculature may also be a contributing factor, and both processes may potentially also occur in patients with liver disease. Liver-related thrombosis, in particular, thrombosis of the portal and mesenteric veins, is common in patients with advanced cirrhosis. Hemodynamic changes such as decreased portal flow, and evidence that inherited thrombophilia may enhance the risk for portal vein thrombosis in patients with cirrhosis suggest that hypercoagulability may play a role as well. Patients with liver disease develop deep vein thrombosis and pulmonary embolism at appreciable rates (ranging from 0.5% to 1.9%). The implication of these findings is relevant to the erroneous exclusion of thrombosis in patients with advanced liver disease, even in the presence of prolongation of routine clotting times, and caution should be advised on overcorrection of these laboratory abnormalities.

ACQUIRED INHIBITORS OF COAGULATION FACTORS

An acquired inhibitor is an immune-mediated disease characterized by the presence of an autoantibody against a specific clotting factor. FVIII is the most common target of antibody formation, but inhibitors to prothrombin, FV, FIX, FX, and FXI are also reported. The disease occurs predominantly in older adults (median age of 60 years), but occasionally in pregnant or postpartum women with no previous history of bleeding. In 50% of the patients with inhibitors, no underlying disease is identified at the time of diagnosis. In the remaining, the causes are autommimune diseases, malignancies (lymphomas, prostate cancer), dermatologic diseases, and pregnancy. Bleeding episodes occur commonly in soft tissues, in the gastrointestinal or urinary tracts, and skin. In contrast to hemophilia, hemarthrosis is rare in these patients. Retroperitoneal hemorrhages and other life-threatening bleeding may appear suddenly. The overall mortality in untreated patients ranges from 8% to 22%, and most deaths occur within the first few weeks after presentation. The diagnosis is based on the prolonged aPTT with normal PT and TT. The aPTT remains prolonged after mixture of the test plasma with equal amounts of pooled normal plasma for 2 h at 37°C. The Bethesda assay using FVIII-deficient plasma as performed for inhibitor detection in hemophilia will confirm the diagnosis. Major bleeding is treated with high doses of human or porcine FVIII, PCC/PCCa, or recombinant FVIIa. High-dose intravenous gamma globulin, and anti-CD20 monoclonal antibody have been reported to be effective in patients with autoantibodies to FVIII. In contrast to hemophilia, inhibitors in nonhemophilia patients are sometimes responsive to prednisone alone or in association with cytotoxic therapy (e.g., cyclophosphamide).

Topical plasma-derived bovine and human thrombin are commonly used in the United States and worldwide. These effective hemostatic sealants are used during major surgery such as for cardiovascular, thoracic, neurologic, pelvic, and trauma indications, as well as in the setting of extensive burns. The development of antibody formation to the xenoantigen or its contaminant (bovine clotting protein) has the potential to show cross-reactivity with human clotting factors that may hamper their function and induce bleeding.

Clinical features of these antibodies include bleeding from a primary hemostastatic defect or coagulopathy that sometimes can be life threatening. The clinical diagnosis of these acquired coagulopathies is often complicated by the fact that the bleeding episodes may be detectable during or immediately following major surgery that could be assumed to be due to the procedure itself.

Notably, the risk of this complication is further increased by repeated exposure to topical thrombin preparations. Thus, a careful medical history of previous surgical interventions that may have occurred even decades earlier is critical to assessing risk.

The laboratory abnormalities are reflected by combined prolongation of the aPTT and PT that often fail to improve by transfusion of FFP and vitamin K. The abnormal laboratory tests cannot be corrected by mixing a test with equal parts of normal plasma that denotes the presence of inhibitory antibodies. The diagnosis of a specific antibody is obtained by the determination of the residual activity of human FV or other suspected human clotting factor. There are no commercially available assays specific for bovine thrombin coagulopathy.

There are no established treatment guidelines. Platelet transfusions have been utilized as a source of FV replacement for patients with FV inhibitors. Frequent injections of FFP and vitamin K supplementation may function as co-adjuvant rather than an effective treatment of the coagulopathy itself. Experience with recombinant FVIIa as a bypass agent is limited, and outcomes have been generally poor. Specific treatments to eradicate the antibodies based on immunosuppression with steroids, intravenous immunoglobulin, or serial plasmapheresis have been sporadically reported. Patients should be advised to avoid any topical thrombin sealant in the future.

Recently, novel plasma-derived and recombinant human thrombin preparations for topical hemostasis have been approved by the Food and Drug Administration. These preparations have demonstrated hemostatic efficacy with reduced immunogenicity compared to the first generation of bovine thrombin products.

The presence of lupus anticoagulant can be associated with venous or arterial thrombotic disease. However, bleeding has also been reported in lupus anticoagulant; it is due to the presence of antibodies to prothrombin, which results in hypoprothrombinemia. Both disorders show a prolonged PTT that do not correct on mixing. To distinguish acquired inhibitors from lupus anticoagulant, note that the dilute Russell's viper venom test and the hexagonal-phase phospholipids test will be negative in patients with an acquired inhibitor and positive in patients with lupus anticoagulants. Moreover, lupus anticoagulant interferes with the clotting activity of many factors (FVIII, FIX, FXII, FXI), whereas acquired inhibitors are specific to a single factor.

CHAPTER 40

TREATMENT AND PROPHYLAXIS OF BACTERIAL INFECTIONS

Gordon L. Archer ■ Ronald E. Polk

The development of vaccines and drugs that prevent and cure bacterial infections was one of the twentieth century's major contributions to human longevity and quality of life. Antibacterial agents are among the most commonly prescribed drugs of any kind worldwide. Used appropriately, these drugs are lifesaving. However, their indiscriminate use drives up the cost of health care, leads to a plethora of side effects and drug interactions, and fosters the emergence of bacterial resistance, rendering previously valuable drugs useless. The rational use of antibacterial agents depends on an understanding of (1) the drugs' mechanisms of action, spectra of activity, pharmacokinetics, pharmacodynamics, toxicities, and interactions; (2) mechanisms underlying bacterial resistance; and (3) strategies that can be used by clinicians to limit resistance. In addition, patient-associated parameters, such as infection site, other drugs being taken, allergies, and immune and excretory status, are critically important to appropriate therapeutic decisions. This chapter provides specific data required for making an informed choice of antibacterial agent.

MECHANISMS OF ACTION

Antibacterial agents, like all antimicrobial drugs, are directed against unique targets not present in mammalian cells. The goal is to limit toxicity to the host and maximize chemotherapeutic activity affecting invading microbes only. *Bactericidal drugs* kill the bacteria that are within their spectrum of activity; *bacteriostatic drugs* only inhibit bacterial growth. While bacteriostatic activity is adequate for the treatment of most infections, bactericidal activity may be necessary for cure in patients with altered immune systems (e.g., neutropenia), protected infectious foci (e.g., endocarditis or meningitis), or specific infections (e.g., complicated *Staphylococcus aureus*

bacteremia). The mechanisms of action of the antibacterial agents to be discussed in this section are summarized in Table 40-1 and are depicted in Fig. 40-1.

INHIBITION OF CELL-WALL SYNTHESIS

One major difference between bacterial and mammalian cells is the presence in bacteria of a rigid wall external to the cell membrane. The wall protects bacterial cells from osmotic rupture, which would result from the cell's usual marked hyperosmolarity (by up to 20 atm) relative to the host environment. The structure conferring cell-wall rigidity and resistance to osmotic lysis in both gram-positive and gram-negative bacteria is peptidoglycan, a large, covalently linked sacculus that surrounds the bacterium. In gram-positive bacteria, peptidoglycan is the only layered structure external to the cell membrane and is thick (20–80 nm); in gram-negative bacteria, there is an outer membrane external to a very thin (1-nm) peptidoglycan layer.

Chemotherapeutic agents directed at any stage of the synthesis, export, assembly, or cross-linking of peptidoglycan lead to inhibition of bacterial cell growth and, in most cases, to cell death. Peptidoglycan is composed of (1) a backbone of two alternating sugars, *N*-acetylglucosamine and *N*-acetylmuramic acid; (2) a chain of four amino acids that extends down from the backbone (stem peptides); and (3) a peptide bridge that cross-links the peptide chains. Peptidoglycan is formed by the addition of subunits (a sugar with its five attached amino acids) that are assembled in the cytoplasm and transported through the cytoplasmic membrane to the cell surface. Subsequent cross-linking is driven by cleavage of the terminal stem-peptide amino acid.

Virtually all the antibiotics that inhibit bacterial cell-wall synthesis are bactericidal. That is, they eventually result in the cell's death due to osmotic lysis.

TABLE 40-1

MECHANISMS OF ACTION OF AND RESISTANCE TO MAJOR CLASSES OF ANTIBACTERIAL AGENTS

LETTER FOR FIG. 40-1	ANTIBACTERIAL AGENT[a]	MAJOR CELLULAR TARGET	MECHANISM OF ACTION	MAJOR MECHANISMS OF RESISTANCE
A	β-Lactams (penicillins, cephalosporins)	Cell wall	Inhibit cell-wall cross-linking	1. Drug inactivation (β-lactamase) 2. Insensitivity of target (altered penicillin-binding proteins) 3. Decreased permeability (altered gram-negative outer-membrane porins) 4. Active efflux
B	Vancomycin	Cell wall	Interferes with addition of new cell-wall subunits (muramyl pentapeptides)	Alteration of target (substitution of terminal amino acid of peptidoglycan subunit)
	Bacitracin	Cell wall	Prevents addition of cell-wall subunits by inhibiting recycling of membrane lipid carrier	Not defined
C	Macrolides (erythromycin)	Protein synthesis	Bind to 50S ribosomal subunit	1. Alteration of target (ribosomal methylation and mutation of 23S rRNA) 2. Active efflux
	Lincosamides (clindamycin)	Protein synthesis	Bind to 50S ribosomal subunit Block peptide chain elongation	1. Alteration of target (ribosomal methylation) 2. Active efflux
D	Chloramphenicol	Protein synthesis	Binds to 50S ribosomal subunit Blocks aminoacyl tRNA attachment	1. Drug inactivation (chloramphenicol acetyltransferase) 2. Active efflux
E	Tetracycline	Protein synthesis	Binds to 30S ribosomal subunit Blocks binding of aminoacyl tRNA	1. Decreased intracellular drug accumulation (active efflux) 2. Insensitivity of target
F	Aminoglycosides (gentamicin)	Protein synthesis	Bind to 30S ribosomal subunit Inhibit translocation of peptidyl-tRNA	1. Drug inactivation (aminoglycoside-modifying enzyme) 2. Decreased permeability through gram-negative outer membrane 3. Active efflux 4. Ribosomal methylation
G	Mupirocin	Protein synthesis	Inhibits isoleucine tRNA synthetase	Mutation of gene for target protein or acquisition of new gene for drug-insensitive target
H	Streptogramins (quinupristin/dalfopristin [Synercid])	Protein synthesis	Bind to 50S ribosomal subunit Block peptide chain elongation	1. Alteration of target (ribosomal methylation: dalfopristin) 2. Active efflux (quinupristin) 3. Drug inactivation (quinupristin and dalfopristin)
I	Linezolid	Protein synthesis	Binds to 50S ribosomal subunit Inhibits initiation of protein synthesis	Alteration of target (mutation of 23S rRNA)
J	Sulfonamides and trimethoprim	Cell metabolism	Competitively inhibit enzymes involved in two steps of folic acid biosynthesis	Production of insensitive targets (dihydropteroate synthetase [sulfonamides] and dihydrofolate reductase [trimethoprim]) that bypass metabolic block

(continued)

TABLE 40-1

429

CHAPTER 40

MECHANISMS OF ACTION OF AND RESISTANCE TO MAJOR CLASSES OF ANTIBACTERIAL AGENTS *(CONTINUED)*

LETTER FOR FIG. 40-1	ANTIBACTERIAL AGENT*a*	MAJOR CELLULAR TARGET	MECHANISM OF ACTION	MAJOR MECHANISMS OF RESISTANCE
K	Rifampin	Nucleic acid synthesis	Inhibits DNA-dependent RNA polymerase	Insensitivity of target (mutation of polymerase gene)
L	Metronidazole	Nucleic acid synthesis	Intracellularly generates short-lived reactive inter-mediates that damage DNA by electron transfer system	Not defined
M	Quinolones (ciprofloxacin)	DNA synthesis	Inhibit activity of DNA gyrase (A subunit) and topoisomerase IV	1. Insensitivity of target (mutation of gyrase genes) 2. Decreased intracellular drug accumulation (active efflux)
	Novobiocin	DNA synthesis	Inhibits activity of DNA gyrase (B subunit)	Not defined
N	Polymyxins (polymyxin B)	Cell membrane	Disrupt membrane perme-ability by charge alteration	Not defined
	Gramicidin	Cell membrane	Forms pores	Not defined
O	Daptomycin	Cell membrane	Forms channels that disrupt membrane potential	Alteration of membrane charge

*a*Compounds in parentheses are major representatives for the class.

However, much of the loss of cell-wall integrity following treatment with cell wall–active agents is due to the bacteria's own cell-wall remodeling enzymes (autolysins) that cleave peptidoglycan bonds in the normal course of cell growth. In the presence of antibacterial agents that inhibit cell-wall growth, autolysis proceeds without normal cell-wall repair; weakness and eventual cellular lysis occur. Antibacterial agents act to inhibit cell-wall synthesis in several ways, as described below.

Bacitracin

Bacitracin, a cyclic peptide antibiotic, inhibits the conversion to its active form of the lipid carrier that moves the water-soluble cytoplasmic peptidoglycan subunits through the cell membrane to the cell exterior.

Glycopeptides

Glycopeptides (vancomycin, teicoplanin, and telavancin [lipoglycopeptide]) are high-molecular-weight antibiotics that bind to the terminal D-alanine–D-alanine component of the stem peptide while the subunits are external to the cell membrane but still linked to the lipid carrier. This binding sterically inhibits the addition of subunits to the peptidoglycan backbone.

β-Lactam antibiotics

β-Lactam antibiotics (penicillins, cephalosporins, carbapenems, and monobactams; Table 40-2) are characterized by a four-membered β-lactam ring and prevent the cross-linking reaction called *transpeptidation*. The energy for attaching a peptide cross-bridge from the stem peptide of one peptidoglycan subunit to another is derived from the cleavage of a terminal D-alanine residue from the subunit stem peptide. The cross-bridge amino acid is then attached to the penultimate D-alanine by transpeptidase enzymes. The β-lactam ring of the antibiotic forms an irreversible covalent acyl bond with the transpeptidase enzyme (probably because of the antibiotic's steric similarity to the enzyme's D-alanine–D-alanine target), preventing the cross-linking reaction. Transpeptidases and similar enzymes involved in cross-linking are called *penicillin-binding proteins* (PBPs) because they all have active sites that bind β-lactam antibiotics.

INHIBITION OF PROTEIN SYNTHESIS

Most of the antibacterial agents that inhibit protein synthesis interact with the bacterial ribosome. The difference between the composition of bacterial and mammalian ribosomes gives these compounds their selectivity.

Aminoglycosides

Aminoglycosides (gentamicin, kanamycin, tobramycin, streptomycin, neomycin, and amikacin) are a group of structurally related compounds containing three linked hexose sugars. They exert a bactericidal effect by binding irreversibly to the 30S subunit of the bacterial ribosome and inhibiting translocation of peptidyl-tRNA from the A to the P site. Uptake of aminoglycosides and their penetration through the cell membrane

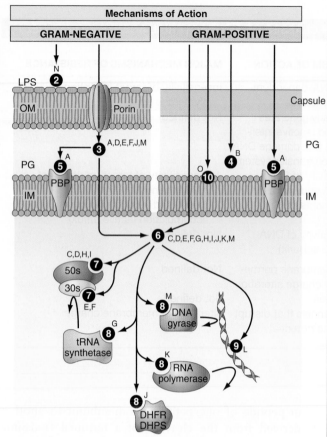

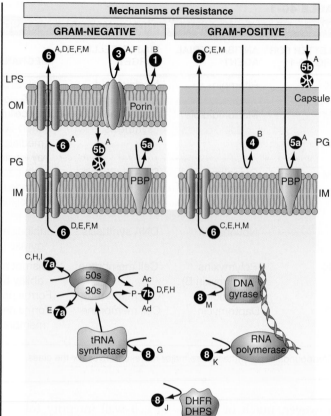

2 Detergent action on lipid gram ⊖ outer membrane.

3 Penetration of hydrophilic drugs through porin channels in gram ⊖ outer membrane.

4 Free diffusion through gram ⊕ cell envelope with binding to cell wall PG **or**

5 Binding to cell membrane PBP. Drug confined to space external to IM.

6 Diffusion or transport of drugs with intracellular target through IM.

7 Binding to ribosomal target for protein synthesis inhibition.

8 Antibiotic interaction with target protein leading to metabolic (DHFR, DHPS), protein synthetic (tRNA synthetase), or nucleic acid (DNA gyrase, RNA polymerase) abnormalities.

9 Direct interaction of reactive intermediates with nucleic acid.

10 Insertion into cell membrane, disrupting membrane potential.

1 **Intrinsic resistance:** Inability of antibiotic to penetrate gram ⊖ envelope (e.g., vancomycin).

3 Mutant porin channels **decrease** antimicrobial **penetration**.

4 **Production of insensitive target** by acquired gene mediating production of altered peptidoglycan.

5a **Production of β-lactam-insensitive PBP target** by mutation of gene or acquisition of new gene.

5b **Inactivation** of β-lactam antibiotic by β-lactamases in periplasm (gram ⊖) or surrounding medium (gram ⊕).

6 **Active efflux** of drugs from cytoplasm or from gram ⊖ periplasm.

7a Decreased ribosomal binding due to **target site alteration**.

7b **Inactivation** of drug by chemical modification leading to decreased ribosomal interaction.

8 Mutation of target gene or acquisition of new gene producing a **drug-insensitive target** protein.

FIGURE 40-1

Mechanisms of action of and resistance to antibacterial agents. Black lines trace the routes of drug interaction with bacterial cells, from entry to target site. The letters in each figure indicate specific antibacterial agents or classes of agents, as shown in Table 40-1. The numbers correspond to mechanisms listed beneath each panel. 50s and 30s, large and small ribosome subunits; Ac, acetylation; Ad, adenylation; DHFR, dihydrofolate reductase; DHPS, dihydropteroate synthetase; IM, inner (cytoplasmic) membrane; LPS, lipopolysaccharide; OM, outer membrane; P, phosphorylation; PBP, penicillin-binding protein; PG, peptidoglycan.

constitute an aerobic, energy-dependent process. Thus, aminoglycoside activity is markedly reduced in an anaerobic environment. *Spectinomycin*, an aminocyclitol antibiotic, also acts on the 30S ribosomal subunit but has a different mechanism of action from the aminoglycosides and is bacteriostatic rather than bactericidal.

Macrolides, ketolides, and lincosamides

Macrolide antibiotics (erythromycin, clarithromycin, and azithromycin) consist of a large lactone ring to which sugars are attached. *Ketolide antibiotics*, including telithromycin, replace the cladinose sugar on the macrolactone ring with a ketone group. These drugs bind specifically

TABLE 40-2

CLASSIFICATION OF β-LACTAM ANTIBIOTICS

	ROUTE OF ADMINISTRATION	
CLASS	PARENTERAL	ORAL
Penicillins		
β-Lactamase-susceptible		
Narrow-spectrum	Penicillin G	Penicillin V
Enteric-active	Ampicillin	Amoxicillin, ampicillin
Enteric-active and antipseudomonal	Ticarcillin, piperacillin	None
β-Lactamase-resistant		
Antistaphylococcal	Oxacillin, nafcillin	Cloxacillin, dicloxacillin
Combined with β-lactamase inhibitors	Ticarcillin plus clavulanic acid, ampicillin plus sulbactam, piperacillin plus tazobactam	Amoxicillin plus clavulanic acid
Cephalosporins		
First-generation	Cefazolin, cephapirin	Cephalexin, cefadroxil
Second-generation		
Haemophilus-active	Cefuroxime, cefonicid, ceforanide	Cefaclor, cefuroxime axetil, ceftibuten, cefdinir, cefprozil, cefditoren, cefpodoxime[a]
Bacteroides-active	Cefoxitin, cefotetan	None
Third-generation		
Extended-spectrum	Ceftriaxone, cefotaxime, ceftizoxime	None
Extended-spectrum and antipseudomonal	Ceftazidime, cefepime	None
Extended-spectrum and anti-MRSA[b]	Ceftobiprole	None
Carbapenems	Imipenem/cilastatin, meropenem, ertapenem, doripenem	None
Monobactams	Aztreonam	None

[a]Some sources classify cefpodoxime as a third-generation oral agent because of a marginally broader spectrum.
[b]Methicillin-resistant *Staphylococcus aureus*.

to the 50S portion of the bacterial ribosome and inhibit protein chain elongation. Although structurally unrelated to the macrolides, *lincosamides* (clindamycin and lincomycin) bind to a site on the 50S ribosome nearly identical to the binding site for macrolides.

Streptogramins

Streptogramins (quinupristin [streptogramin B] and dalfopristin [streptogramin A]), which are supplied as a combination in Synercid, are peptide macrolactones that also bind to the 50S ribosomal subunit and block protein synthesis. Streptogramin B binds to a ribosomal site similar to the binding site for macrolides and lincosamides, whereas streptogramin A binds to a different ribosomal site, blocking the late phase of protein synthesis. The two streptogramins act synergistically to kill bacteria if the strain is susceptible to both components.

Chloramphenicol

Chloramphenicol consists of a single aromatic ring and a short side chain. This antibiotic binds reversibly to the 50S portion of the bacterial ribosome at a site close to but not identical with the binding sites for the macrolides

and lincosamides, inhibiting peptide bond formation by blocking attachment of the amino acid end of aminoacyl-tRNA to the ribosome.

Linezolid

Linezolid is the only commercially available drug in the oxazolidinone class. Linezolid binds to the 50S ribosomal subunit and blocks the initiation of protein synthesis.

Tetracyclines and glycylcyclines

Tetracyclines (tetracycline, doxycycline, and minocycline) and glycylcyclines (tigecycline) consist of four aromatic rings with various substituent groups. They interact reversibly with the bacterial 30S ribosomal subunit, blocking the binding of aminoacyl tRNA to the mRNA-ribosome complex. This mechanism is markedly different from that of the aminoglycosides, which also bind to the 30S subunit.

Mupirocin

Mupirocin (pseudomonic acid) inhibits isoleucine tRNA synthetase by competing with bacterial isoleucine for its binding site on the enzyme and depleting cellular stores of isoleucine-charged tRNA.

INHIBITION OF BACTERIAL METABOLISM

The *antimetabolites* are all synthetic compounds that interfere with bacterial synthesis of folic acid. Products of the folic acid synthesis pathway function as coenzymes for the one-carbon transfer reactions that are essential for the synthesis of thymidine, all purines, and several amino acids. Inhibition of folate synthesis leads to cessation of bacterial cell growth and, in some cases, to bacterial cell death. The principal antibacterial antimetabolites are sulfonamides (sulfisoxazole, sulfadiazine, and sulfamethoxazole) and trimethoprim.

Sulfonamides

Sulfonamides are structural analogues of *p*-aminobenzoic acid (PABA), one of the three structural components of folic acid (the other two being pteridine and glutamate). The first step in the synthesis of folic acid is the addition of PABA to pteridine by the enzyme dihydropteroic acid synthetase. Sulfonamides compete with PABA as substrates for the enzyme. The selective effect of sulfonamides is due to the fact that bacteria synthesize folic acid, while mammalian cells cannot synthesize the cofactor and must use exogenous supplies. However, the activity of sulfonamides can be greatly reduced by the presence of excess PABA or by the exogenous addition of end products of one-carbon transfer reactions (e.g., thymidine and purines). High concentrations of the latter substances may be present in some infections as a result of tissue and white cell breakdown, compromising sulfonamide activity.

Trimethoprim

Trimethoprim is a diaminopyrimidine, a structural analogue of the pteridine moiety of folic acid. Trimethoprim is a competitive inhibitor of dihydrofolate reductase; this enzyme is responsible for reduction of dihydrofolic acid to tetrahydrofolic acid—the essential final component in the folic acid synthesis pathway. Like that of the sulfonamides, the activity of trimethoprim is compromised in the presence of exogenous thymine or thymidine.

INHIBITION OF NUCLEIC ACID SYNTHESIS OR ACTIVITY

Numerous antibacterial compounds have disparate effects on nucleic acids.

Quinolones

The quinolones, including nalidixic acid and its fluorinated derivatives (ciprofloxacin, levofloxacin, and moxifloxacin), are synthetic compounds that inhibit the activity of the A subunit of the bacterial enzyme DNA gyrase as well as topoisomerase IV. DNA gyrase and topoisomerases are responsible for negative supercoiling of DNA—an essential conformation for DNA replication in the intact cell. Inhibition of the activity of DNA gyrase and topoisomerase IV is lethal to bacterial cells. The antibiotic

novobiocin also interferes with the activity of DNA gyrase, but it interferes with the B subunit.

Rifampin

Rifampin, used primarily against *Mycobacterium tuberculosis*, is also active against a variety of other bacteria. Rifampin binds tightly to the B subunit of bacterial DNA-dependent RNA polymerase, thus inhibiting transcription of DNA into RNA. Mammalian-cell RNA polymerase is not sensitive to this compound.

Nitrofurantoin

Nitrofurantoin, a synthetic compound, causes DNA damage. The nitrofurans, compounds containing a single five-membered ring, are reduced by a bacterial enzyme to highly reactive, short-lived intermediates that are thought to cause DNA strand breakage, either directly or indirectly.

Metronidazole

Metronidazole, a synthetic imidazole, is active only against anaerobic bacteria and protozoa. The reduction of metronidazole's nitro group by the bacterial anaerobic electron-transport system produces a transient series of reactive intermediates that are thought to cause DNA damage.

ALTERATION OF CELL-MEMBRANE PERMEABILITY

Polymyxins

The polymyxins (polymyxin B and colistin [polymyxin E]) are cyclic, basic polypeptides. They behave as cationic, surface-active compounds that disrupt the permeability of both the outer and the cytoplasmic membranes of gram-negative bacteria.

Gramicidin A

Gramicidin A is a polypeptide of 15 amino acids that acts as an ionophore, forming pores or channels in lipid bilayers.

Daptomycin

Insertion of daptomycin, a bactericidal lipopeptide antibiotic, into the cell membrane of gram-positive bacteria forms a channel that causes depolarization of the membrane by efflux of intracellular ions, resulting in cell death.

MECHANISMS OF RESISTANCE

Some bacteria exhibit *intrinsic resistance* to certain classes of antibacterial agents (e.g., obligate anaerobic bacteria to aminoglycosides and gram-negative bacteria to vancomycin). In addition, bacteria that are ordinarily susceptible to antibacterial agents can acquire resistance. *Acquired resistance* is a major limitation to effective antibacterial chemotherapy. Resistance can develop by mutation of resident genes or by acquisition of new genes. New genes mediating resistance are usually spread from cell to cell by way of mobile genetic elements such as plasmids, transposons, and bacteriophages. The resistant bacterial populations flourish in areas of high antimicrobial use, where they enjoy a selective advantage over susceptible populations.

The major mechanisms used by bacteria to resist the action of antimicrobial agents are inactivation of the compound, alteration or overproduction of the antibacterial target through mutation of the target protein's gene, acquisition of a new gene that encodes a drug-insensitive target, decreased permeability of the cell envelope to the agent, failure to convert an inactive prodrug to its active derivative, and active efflux of the compound from the periplasm or interior of the cell. Specific mechanisms of bacterial resistance to the major antibacterial agents are outlined below, summarized in Table 40-1, and depicted in Fig. 40-1.

β-LACTAM ANTIBIOTICS

Bacteria develop resistance to β-lactam antibiotics by a variety of mechanisms. Most common is the destruction of the drug by β-lactamases. The β-lactamases of gram-negative bacteria are confined to the periplasm, between the inner and outer membranes, while gram-positive bacteria secrete their β-lactamases into the surrounding medium. These enzymes have a higher affinity for the antibiotic than the antibiotic has for its target. Binding results in hydrolysis of the β-lactam ring. Genes encoding β-lactamases have been found in both chromosomal and extrachromosomal locations and in both gram-positive and gram-negative bacteria; these genes are often on mobile genetic elements. Many "advanced-generation" β-lactam antibiotics, such as ceftriaxone and cefepime, are stable in the presence of plasmid-mediated β-lactamases and are active against bacteria resistant to earlier-generation β-lactam antibiotics. However, extended-spectrum β-lactamases (ESBLs), either acquired on mobile genetic elements by gram-negative bacteria (e.g., *Klebsiella pneumoniae* and *Escherichia coli*) or present as stable chromosomal genes in other gram-negative species (e.g., *Enterobacter* spp.), have broad substrate specificity, hydrolyzing virtually all penicillins and cephalosporins. Carbapenems are generally resistant to ESBL hydrolysis and are the drugs of choice for the treatment of infections caused by ESBL-producing Enterobacteriaceae. However, Enterobacteriaceae (particularly *K. pneumoniae*) that produce carbapenemases and are resistant to virtually all β-lactam antibiotics have now emerged. One strategy that has been devised for circumventing resistance mediated by β-lactamases is to combine the β-lactam agent with an inhibitor that avidly binds the inactivating enzyme, preventing its attack on the antibiotic. Unfortunately, the

inhibitors (e.g., clavulanic acid, sulbactam, and tazobactam) do not bind all chromosomal β-lactamases (e.g., that of *Enterobacter*) or carbapenemases and thus cannot be depended on to prevent the inactivation of β-lactam antibiotics by such enzymes. No β-lactam antibiotic or inhibitor has been produced that can resist all of the many β-lactamases that have been identified.

A second mechanism of bacterial resistance to β-lactam antibiotics is an alteration in PBP targets so that the PBPs have a markedly reduced affinity for the drug. While this alteration may occur by mutation of existing genes, the acquisition of new PBP genes (as in staphylococcal resistance to methicillin) or of new pieces of PBP genes (as in streptococcal, gonococcal, and meningococcal resistance to penicillin) is more important.

A final resistance mechanism is the coupling, in gram-negative bacteria, of a decrease in outer-membrane permeability with rapid efflux of the antibiotic from the periplasm to the cell exterior. Mutations of genes encoding outer-membrane protein channels called *porins* decrease the entry of β-lactam antibiotics into the cell, while additional proteins form channels that actively pump β-lactams out of the cell. Resistance of Enterobacteriaceae to some cephalosporins and resistance of *Pseudomonas* spp. to cephalosporins and piperacillin are the best examples of this mechanism.

VANCOMYCIN

Clinically important resistance to vancomycin was first described among enterococci in France in 1988. Vancomycin-resistant enterococci (VRE) have subsequently become disseminated worldwide. The genes encoding resistance are carried on plasmids that can transfer themselves from cell to cell and on transposons that can jump from plasmids to chromosomes. Resistance is mediated by enzymes that substitute D-lactate for D-alanine on the peptidoglycan stem peptide so that there is no longer an appropriate target for vancomycin binding. This alteration does not appear to affect cell-wall integrity, however. This type of acquired vancomycin resistance was confined for 14 years to enterococci—more specifically, to *Enterococcus faecium* rather than the more common pathogen *E. faecalis*. However, since 2002, *S. aureus* isolates that are highly resistant to vancomycin have been recovered from 11 patients in the United States. All of the isolates contain *vanA*, the gene that mediates vancomycin resistance in enterococci. In addition, since 1996, a few isolates of both *S. aureus* and *Staphylococcus epidermidis* that display a four- to eightfold reduction in susceptibility to vancomycin have been found worldwide; such *S. aureus* strains are termed vancomycin-intermediate-susceptibility *S. aureus*, or VISA. Many more isolates may contain subpopulations with reduced vancomycin susceptibility (heteroVISA, or hVISA). These isolates have not acquired the genes that mediate vancomycin resistance in enterococci but are mutant bacteria with markedly thickened cell walls. These mutants were apparently selected in patients who were undergoing prolonged vancomycin therapy. The failure of vancomycin therapy in some patients infected with *S. aureus* or *S. epidermidis* strains exhibiting only intermediate susceptibility to this drug is thought to have resulted from this resistance.

DAPTOMYCIN

In some *S. aureus* isolates with reduced susceptibility to daptomycin, a mutation in the *mprF* gene leads to an increase in the net positive charge of the bacterial membrane, repelling the antibiotic.

AMINOGLYCOSIDES

The most common aminoglycoside resistance mechanism is inactivation of the antibiotic. Aminoglycoside-modifying enzymes, usually encoded on plasmids, transfer phosphate, adenyl, or acetyl residues from intracellular molecules to hydroxyl or amino side groups on the antibiotic. The modified antibiotic is less active because of diminished binding to its ribosomal target. Modifying enzymes that can inactivate any of the available aminoglycosides have been found in both gram-positive and gram-negative bacteria. A second aminoglycoside resistance mechanism, which has been identified predominantly in clinical isolates of *Pseudomonas aeruginosa*, is decreased antibiotic uptake, presumably due to alterations in the bacterial outer membrane. A third, emerging form of resistance in gram-negative bacteria is methylation of the target 16S ribosomal RNA, which is mediated by plasmid-encoded methylases.

MACROLIDES, KETOLIDES, LINCOSAMIDES, AND STREPTOGRAMINS

Resistance in gram-positive bacteria, which are the usual target organisms for macrolides, ketolides, lincosamides, and streptogramins, can be due to the production of an enzyme—most commonly plasmid-encoded—that methylates ribosomal RNA, interfering with binding of the antibiotics to their target. Methylation mediates resistance to erythromycin, clarithromycin, azithromycin, clindamycin, and streptogramin B. Resistance to streptogramin B converts quinupristin/dalfopristin from a bactericidal to a bacteriostatic antibiotic. Streptococci can also actively cause the efflux of macrolides, and staphylococci can cause the efflux of macrolides, clindamycin, and streptogramin A. Ketolides such as

telithromycin retain activity against most isolates of *Streptococcus pneumoniae* that are resistant to macrolides. In addition, staphylococci can inactivate streptogramin A by acetylation and streptogramin B by either acetylation or hydrolysis. Finally, mutations in 23S ribosomal RNA that alter the binding of macrolides to their targets have been found in both staphylococci and streptococci.

CHLORAMPHENICOL

Most bacteria resistant to chloramphenicol produce a plasmid-encoded enzyme, chloramphenicol acetyltransferase, that inactivates the compound by acetylation.

TETRACYCLINES AND TIGECYCLINE

The most common mechanism of tetracycline resistance in gram-negative bacteria is a plasmid-encoded active-efflux pump that is inserted into the cytoplasmic membrane and extrudes antibiotic from the cell. Resistance in gram-positive bacteria is due either to active efflux or to ribosomal alterations that diminish binding of the antibiotic to its target. Genes involved in ribosomal protection are found on mobile genetic elements. The parenteral tetracycline derivative tigecycline (a glycylcycline) is active against tetracycline-resistant bacteria because it is not removed by efflux and can bind to altered ribosomes.

MUPIROCIN

Although the topical compound mupirocin was introduced into clinical use relatively recently, resistance is already becoming widespread in some areas. The mechanism appears to be either mutation of the target isoleucine tRNA synthetase so that it is no longer inhibited by the antibiotic or plasmid-encoded production of a form of the target enzyme that binds mupirocin poorly.

TRIMETHOPRIM AND SULFONAMIDES

The most prevalent mechanism of resistance to trimethoprim and the sulfonamides in both gram-positive and gram-negative bacteria is the acquisition of plasmid-encoded genes that produce a new, drug-insensitive target—specifically, an insensitive dihydrofolate reductase for trimethoprim and an altered dihydropteroate synthetase for sulfonamides.

QUINOLONES

The most common mechanism of resistance to quinolones is the development of one or more mutations in target DNA gyrases and topoisomerase IV that prevent the antibacterial agent from interfering with the enzymes' activity. Some gram-negative bacteria develop mutations that both decrease outer-membrane porin permeability and cause active drug efflux from the cytoplasm. Mutations that result in active quinolone efflux are also found in gram-positive bacteria.

RIFAMPIN

Bacteria rapidly become resistant to rifampin by developing mutations in the B subunit of RNA polymerase that render the enzyme unable to bind the antibiotic. The rapid selection of resistant mutants is the major limitation to the use of this antibiotic against otherwise-susceptible staphylococci and requires that the drug be used in combination with another antistaphylococcal agent.

LINEZOLID

Enterococci, streptococci, and staphylococci can become resistant to linezolid in vitro by mutation of the 23S rRNA binding site. Clinical isolates of *E. faecium* and *E. faecalis* acquire resistance to linezolid readily by this mechanism, often during therapy. A new plasmid-encoded resistance gene has been found in staphylococci that methylates the linezolid ribosomal binding site. At least one outbreak of linezolid-resistant S. aureus infections caused by isolates carrying this gene has been described.

MULTIPLE ANTIBIOTIC RESISTANCE

The acquisition by one bacterium of resistance to multiple antibacterial agents is becoming increasingly common. The two major mechanisms are the acquisition of multiple unrelated resistance genes and the development of mutations in a single gene or gene complex that mediate resistance to a series of unrelated compounds. The construction of multiresistant strains by acquisition of multiple genes occurs by sequential steps of gene transfer and environmental selection in areas of high-level antimicrobial use. In contrast, mutations in a single gene can conceivably be selected in a single step. Bacteria that are multiresistant by virtue of the acquisition of new genes include hospital-associated strains of gram-negative bacteria, enterococci, and staphylococci and community-acquired strains of salmonellae, gonococci, and pneumococci. Mutations that confer resistance to multiple unrelated antimicrobial agents occur in the genes encoding outer-membrane porins and efflux proteins of gram-negative bacteria. These mutations decrease bacterial intracellular and periplasmic accumulation of β-lactams, quinolones, tetracyclines, chloramphenicol, and aminoglycosides. Multiresistant bacterial isolates pose increasing problems in U.S. hospitals; strains resistant to all available antibacterial chemotherapy have already been identified.

PHARMACOKINETICS OF ANTIBIOTICS

The *pharmacokinetic profile* of an antibacterial agent refers to its concentrations in serum and tissue versus time and reflects the processes of absorption, distribution, metabolism, and excretion. Important characteristics include peak and trough serum concentrations and mathematically derived parameters such as half-life, clearance, and distribution volume. Pharmacokinetic information is useful for estimating the appropriate antibacterial dose and frequency of administration, for adjusting dosages in patients with impaired excretory capacity, and for comparing one drug with another. In contrast, the *pharmacodynamic profile* of an antibiotic refers to the relationship between the pharmacokinetics of the antibiotic and its minimal inhibitory concentrations (MICs) for bacteria (see "Principles of Antibacterial Chemotherapy," later).

ABSORPTION

Antibiotic *absorption* refers to the rate and extent of a drug's systemic bioavailability after oral, IM, or IV administration.

Oral administration

Most patients with infection are treated with oral antibacterial agents in the outpatient setting. Advantages of oral therapy over parenteral therapy include lower cost, generally fewer adverse effects (including complications of indwelling lines), and greater acceptance by patients. The percentage of an orally administered antibacterial agent that is absorbed (i.e., its *bioavailability*) ranges from as little as 10–20% (erythromycin and penicillin G) to nearly 100% (amoxicillin, clindamycin, metronidazole, doxycycline, trimethoprim-sulfamethoxazole [TMP-SMX], linezolid, and most fluoroquinolones). These differences in bioavailability are not clinically important as long as drug concentrations at the site of infection are sufficient to inhibit or kill the pathogen. However, therapeutic efficacy may be compromised when absorption is reduced as a result of physiologic or pathologic conditions (such as the presence of food for some drugs or the shunting of blood away from the gastrointestinal tract in patients with hypotension), drug interactions (e.g., of quinolones and metal cations), or noncompliance. The oral route is usually used for patients with relatively mild infections in whom absorption is not thought to be compromised by the preceding conditions. In addition, the oral route can often be used in more severely ill patients after they have responded to parenteral therapy and can take oral medications.

Intramuscular administration

Although the IM route of administration usually results in 100% bioavailability, it is not as widely used in the United States as the oral and IV routes, in part because of the pain often associated with IM injections and the relative ease of IV access in the hospitalized patient. IM injection may be suitable for specific indications requiring an "immediate" and reliable effect (e.g., with long-acting forms of penicillin, including benzathine and procaine, and with single doses of ceftriaxone for acute otitis media or uncomplicated gonococcal infection).

Intravenous administration

The IV route is appropriate when oral antibacterial agents are not effective against a particular pathogen, when bioavailability is uncertain, or when larger doses are required than are feasible with the oral route. After IV administration, bioavailability is 100%; serum concentrations are maximal at the end of the infusion. For many patients in whom long-term antimicrobial therapy is required and oral therapy is not feasible, outpatient parenteral antibiotic therapy (OPAT), including the use of convenient portable pumps, may be cost-effective and safe. Alternatively, some oral antibacterial drugs (e.g., fluoroquinolones) are sufficiently active against many Enterobacteriaceae to provide potency equal to that of parenteral therapy; oral use of such drugs may allow the patient to return home from the hospital earlier or to avoid hospitalization entirely.

DISTRIBUTION

To be effective, concentrations of an antibacterial agent must exceed the pathogen's MIC. Serum antibiotic concentrations usually exceed the MIC for susceptible bacteria, but since most infections are extravascular, the antibiotic must also distribute to the site of the infection. Concentrations of most antibacterial agents in interstitial fluid are similar to free-drug concentrations in serum. However, when the infection is located in a "protected" site where penetration is poor, such as cerebrospinal fluid (CSF), the eye, the prostate, or infected cardiac vegetations, high parenteral doses or local administration for prolonged periods may be required for cure. In addition, even though an antibacterial agent may penetrate to the site of infection, its activity may be antagonized by factors in the local environment, such as an unfavorable pH or inactivation by cellular degradation products.

For example, daptomycin's binding to pulmonary surfactant is believed to account for its poor efficacy in the treatment of pneumonia. In addition, the abscess milieu reduces the penetration and local activity of many antibacterial compounds, so that surgical drainage may be required for cure.

Most bacteria that cause human infections are located extracellularly. Intracellular pathogens such as *Legionella*, *Chlamydia*, *Brucella*, and *Salmonella* may persist or cause relapse if the antibacterial agent does not enter the cell. In general, β-lactams, vancomycin, and aminoglycosides penetrate cells poorly, whereas macrolides, ketolides, tetracyclines, metronidazole, chloramphenicol, rifampin, TMP-SMX, and quinolones penetrate cells well.

METABOLISM AND ELIMINATION

Like other drugs, antibacterial agents are disposed of by hepatic elimination (metabolism or biliary elimination), by renal excretion of the unchanged or metabolized form, or by a combination of the two processes. For most of the antibacterial drugs, metabolism leads to loss of in vitro activity, although some agents, such as cefotaxime, rifampin, and clarithromycin, have bioactive metabolites that may contribute to their overall efficacy.

The most practical application of information on the mode of excretion of an antibacterial agent is in adjusting dosage when elimination capability is impaired (Table 40-3). Direct, nonidiosyncratic toxicity from antibacterial drugs may result from failure to reduce the dosage given to patients with impaired elimination. For agents that are primarily cleared intact by glomerular filtration, drug clearance is correlated with creatinine clearance, and estimates of the latter can be used to guide dosage. For drugs, the elimination of which is primarily hepatic, no simple marker is useful for dosage adjustment in patients with liver disease. However, in patients with severe hepatic disease, residual metabolic capability is usually sufficient to preclude accumulation and toxic effects.

PRINCIPLES OF ANTIBACTERIAL CHEMOTHERAPY

The choice of an antibacterial compound for a particular patient and a specific infection involves more than just a knowledge of the agent's pharmacokinetic profile and in vitro activity. The basic tenets of chemotherapy, to be elaborated below, include the following: When appropriate, material containing the infecting organism(s) should be obtained before the start of treatment so that presumptive identification can be made by microscopic examination of stained specimens and the organism can be grown for definitive identification and susceptibility

TABLE 40-3

ANTIBACTERIAL DRUG DOSE ADJUSTMENTS IN PATIENTS WITH RENAL IMPAIRMENT

ANTIBIOTIC	MAJOR ROUTE OF EXCRETION	DOSAGE ADJUSTMENT WITH RENAL IMPAIRMENT
Aminoglycosides	Renal	Yes
Azithromycin	Biliary	No
Cefazolin	Renal	Yes
Cefepime	Renal	Yes
Ceftazidime	Renal	Yes
Ceftriaxone	Renal/biliary	Modest reduction in severe renal impairment
Ciprofloxacin	Renal/biliary	Only in severe renal insufficiency
Clarithromycin	Renal/biliary	Only in severe renal insufficiency
Daptomycin	Renal	Yes
Erythromycin	Biliary	Only when given in high IV doses
Levofloxacin	Renal	Yes
Linezolid	Metabolism	No
Metronidazole	Biliary	No
Nafcillin	Biliary	No
Penicillin G	Renal	Yes (when given in high IV doses)
Piperacillin	Renal	Only with Cl_{cr} of <40 mL/min
Quinupristin/dalfopristin	Metabolism	No
Tigecycline	Biliary	No
TMP-SMX	Renal/biliary	Only in severe renal insufficiency
Vancomycin	Renal	Yes

Note: Cl_{cr}, creatinine clearance rate; TMP-SMX, trimethoprim-sulfamethoxazole.

testing. Awareness of local susceptibility patterns is useful when the patient is treated empirically. Once the organism is identified and its susceptibility to antibacterial agents is determined, the regimen with the narrowest effective spectrum should be chosen. The choice of antibacterial agent is guided by the pharmacokinetic and adverse-reaction profile of active compounds, the site of infection, the immune status of the host, and evidence of efficacy from well-performed clinical trials. If all other factors are equal, the least expensive antibacterial regimen should be chosen.

SUSCEPTIBILITY OF BACTERIA TO ANTIBACTERIAL DRUGS IN VITRO

Determination of the susceptibility of the patient's infecting organism to a panel of appropriate antibacterial agents is an essential first step in devising a chemotherapeutic regimen. Susceptibility testing is designed to estimate the susceptibility of a bacterial isolate to an antibacterial drug under standardized conditions. These conditions favor rapidly growing aerobic or facultative organisms and assess bacteriostasis only. Specialized testing is required for the assessment of bactericidal antimicrobial activity; for the detection of resistance among such fastidious organisms as obligate anaerobes, *Haemophilus* spp., and pneumococci; and for the determination of resistance phenotypes with variable expression, such as resistance to methicillin or oxacillin

among staphylococci. Antimicrobial susceptibility testing is important when susceptibility is unpredictable, most often as a result of increasing acquired resistance among bacteria infecting hospitalized patients.

PHARMACODYNAMICS: RELATIONSHIP OF PHARMACOKINETICS AND IN VITRO SUSCEPTIBILITY TO CLINICAL RESPONSE

Bacteria have historically been considered *susceptible* to an antibacterial drug if the achievable peak serum concentration exceeds the MIC by approximately fourfold. Each antibiotic has a *breakpoint* concentration that separates susceptible from resistant bacteria (Fig. 40-2). When a majority of isolates of a given bacterial species are inhibited at concentrations below the breakpoint, the species is considered to be within the spectrum of the antibiotic.

The *pharmacokinetic-pharmacodynamic (PK-PD) profile* of an antibiotic refers to the quantitative relationships between the time course of antibiotic concentrations in serum and tissue, in vitro susceptibility (MIC), and microbial response (inhibition of growth or rate of killing). Three PK-PD parameters quantify these relationships: the ratio of the area under the plasma concentration vs. time curve to the MIC (AUC/MIC), the ratio of the maximal serum concentration to the MIC (C_{max}/MIC), and the time during a dosing interval that plasma concentrations exceed the MIC ($T > $ MIC). The PK-PD profile of an antibiotic class

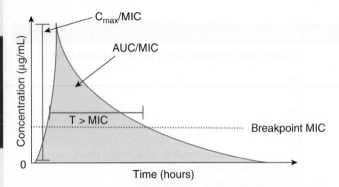

FIGURE 40-2

Relationship between the pharmacokinetic-pharmacodynamic (PK-PD) properties of an antibiotic and susceptibility. An organism is considered "susceptible" to an antibiotic if the drug's minimal inhibitory concentration (MIC) is below its "breakpoint" concentration (see text). PK-PD investigations explore various pharmacodynamic indices and clinical responses, including the ratio of the maximal serum concentration to the MIC (C_{max}/MIC), the ratio of the area under the serum concentration vs. time curve to the MIC (AUC/MIC), and the time during which serum concentrations exceed the MIC (T > MIC). See Table 40-4.

is characterized as either *concentration dependent* (fluoroquinolones, aminoglycosides), such that an increase in antibiotic concentration leads to a more rapid rate of bacterial death, or *time dependent* (β-lactams), such that the reduction in bacterial density is proportional to the time that concentrations exceed the MIC. For concentration-dependent antibiotics, the C_{max}/MIC or AUC/MIC ratio correlates best with the reduction in microbial density in vitro and in animal investigations. Dosing strategies attempt to maximize these ratios by the administration of a large dose relative to the MIC for anticipated pathogens, often at long intervals (relative to the serum half-life). Once-daily dosing of aminoglycoside antibiotics is one practical consequence of these relationships. Another is the administration of larger doses of vancomycin than have been used in the past (e.g., >2 g/d for an adult with normal renal function) to increase the AUC/MIC ratio in an effort to improve the response rates of patients infected with methicillin-resistant *S. aureus* (MRSA). In contrast, dosage strategies for time-dependent antibiotics emphasize the maintenance of serum concentrations above the MIC for 30–50% of the dose interval. For example, some clinicians advocate prolonged—or even constant—infusions of some β-lactam antibiotics, such as the carbapenems and the β-lactam/β-lactamase inhibitors, to increase the T > MIC between doses. The clinical implications of these pharmacodynamic relationships continue to be elucidated; their consideration has led to more rational antibacterial dosage

TABLE 40-4

PHARMACODYNAMIC INDICES OF MAJOR ANTIMICROBIAL CLASSES

PARAMETER PREDICTING RESPONSE	DRUG OR DRUG CLASS
Time above the MIC	Penicillins, cephalosporins, carbapenems, aztreonam
24-h AUC/MIC	Aminoglycosides, fluoroquinolones, tetracyclines, vancomycin, macrolides, clindamycin, quinupristin/dalfopristin, tigecycline, daptomycin
Peak to MIC	Aminoglycosides, fluoroquinolones

Note: MIC, minimal inhibitory concentration; AUC, area under the concentration curve.

regimens. Table 40-4 summarizes the pharmacodynamic properties of the major antibiotic classes.

STATUS OF THE HOST

Various host factors must be considered in the devising of antibacterial chemotherapy. The host's antibacterial *immune function* is of importance, particularly as it relates to opsonophagocytic function. Since the major host defense against acute, overwhelming bacterial infection is the polymorphonuclear leukocyte, patients with neutropenia must be treated aggressively and empirically with bactericidal drugs for suspected infection. Likewise, patients who have deficient humoral immunity (e.g., those with chronic lymphocytic leukemia and multiple myeloma) and individuals with surgical or functional asplenia (e.g., those with sickle cell disease) should be treated empirically for infections with encapsulated organisms, especially the pneumococcus.

Pregnancy increases the risk of toxicity of certain antibacterial drugs for the mother (e.g., hepatic toxicity of tetracycline), affects drug disposition and pharmacokinetics, and—because of the risk of fetal toxicity—severely limits the choice of agents for treating infections. Certain antibacterial agents are contraindicated in pregnancy either because their safety has not been established (categories B and C) or because they are known to be toxic (categories D and X). Table 40-5 summarizes antibacterial drug safety in pregnancy.

In patients with *concomitant viral infections*, the incidence of adverse reactions to antibacterial drugs may be unusually high. For example, persons with infectious mononucleosis and those infected with HIV experience skin reactions more often to penicillins and folic acid synthesis inhibitors such as TMP-SMX, respectively.

TABLE 40-5

ANTIBACTERIAL DRUGS IN PREGNANCY

ANTIBACTERIAL DRUG (PREGNANCY CLASS[a])	TOXICITY IN PREGNANCY	RECOMMENDATION
Aminoglycosides (C/D)	Possible 8th-nerve toxicity	Caution[b]
Chloramphenicol (C)	Gray syndrome in newborn	Caution at term
Fluoroquinolones (C)	Arthropathy in immature animals	Caution
Clarithromycin (C)	Teratogenicity in animals	Contraindicated
Ertapenem (B)	Decreased weight in animals	Caution
Erythromycin estolate (B)	Cholestatic hepatitis	Contraindicated
Imipenem/cilastatin (C)	Toxicity in some pregnant animals	Caution
Linezolid (C)	Embryonic and fetal toxicity in rats	Caution
Meropenem (B)	Unknown	Caution
Metronidazole (B)	None known, but carcinogenic in rats	Caution
Nitrofurantoin (B)	Hemolytic anemia in newborns	Caution; contraindicated at term[c]
Quinupristin/dalfopristin (B)	Unknown	Caution
Sulfonamides (C/D)	Hemolysis in newborn with G6PD[d] deficiency; kernicterus in newborn	Caution; contraindicated at term[c]
Telavancin (C)	Unknown (adverse development in animals)	Pregnancy test before use
Tetracyclines/tigecycline (D)	Tooth discoloration, inhibition of bone growth in fetus; hepatotoxicity	Contraindicated
Vancomycin (C)	Unknown	Caution

[a]**Category A:** Controlled studies in women fail to demonstrate a risk to the fetus; the possibility of fetal harm appears remote.
Category B: Either (1) animal reproduction studies have not demonstrated a fetal risk but there are no controlled studies in pregnant women or (2) animal reproduction studies have shown an adverse effect (other than a decrease in fertility) that was not confirmed in controlled studies of women in the first trimester (and there is no evidence of risk in later trimesters).
Category C: Studies in animals have revealed adverse effects on the fetus (teratogenic, embryocidal, or other), but no controlled studies of women have been conducted. Drug should be given only if the potential benefit justifies the potential risk to the fetus.
Category D: There is positive evidence of human fetal risk, but the benefits from use in pregnant women may nevertheless be acceptable (e.g., if the drug is needed in a life-threatening situation or for a serious disease against which safer drugs cannot be used or are ineffective).
[b]Use only for strong clinical indication in the absence of a suitable alternative.
[c]See KS Crider et al: Arch Pediatr Adolesc Med 163:978, 2009.
[d]G6PD, glucose-6-phosphate dehydrogenase.

In addition, the patient's age, sex, racial heritage, genetic background, concomitant drugs, and excretory status all determine the incidence and type of side effects that can be expected with certain antibacterial agents.

SITE OF INFECTION

The location of the infected site may play a major role in the choice and dose of antimicrobial drug. Patients with suspected *meningitis* should receive drugs that can cross the blood-CSF barrier; in addition, because of the relative paucity of phagocytes and opsonins at the site of infection, the agents should be bactericidal. β-Lactam drugs are the mainstay of therapy for most of these infections, even though they do not normally reach high concentrations in CSF. Their efficacy is based on the increased permeability of the blood-brain and blood-CSF barriers to hydrophilic molecules during inflammation and the low minimal bactericidal concentrations (MBCs) for most infectious organisms.

The vegetation, which is the major site of infection in *bacterial endocarditis*, is also a focus that is protected from normal host-defense mechanisms. Antibacterial therapy needs to be bactericidal, with the selected agent administered parenterally over a long period and at a dose that can eradicate the infecting organism. Likewise, *osteomyelitis* involves a site that is resistant to opsonophagocytic removal of infecting bacteria; furthermore, avascular bone (sequestrum) represents a foreign body that thwarts normal host-defense mechanisms. *Chronic prostatitis* is exceedingly difficult to cure because most antibiotics do not penetrate through the capillaries serving the prostate, especially when acute inflammation is absent. *Intraocular infections*, especially endophthalmitis, are difficult to treat because retinal capillaries lacking fenestration hinder drug penetration into the vitreous from blood. Inflammation does little to disrupt this barrier. Thus, direct injection into the vitreous is necessary in many cases. Antibiotic penetration into *abscesses* is usually poor, and local conditions (e.g., low pH or the presence of enzymes that hydrolyze the drug) may further antagonize antibacterial activity.

In contrast, *urinary tract infections* (UTIs), when confined to the bladder, are relatively easy to cure, in part because of the higher concentration of most antibiotics in urine than in blood. Since blood is the usual reference fluid in defining susceptibility (Fig. 40-2), even organisms found to be resistant to achievable serum concentrations may be susceptible to achievable urine concentrations. For drugs that are used only for the treatment of UTIs, such as the urinary tract antiseptics nitrofurantoin and methenamine salts, achievable urine concentrations are used to determine susceptibility.

COMBINATION CHEMOTHERAPY

One of the tenets of antibacterial chemotherapy is that if the infecting bacterium has been identified, the most specific chemotherapy possible should be used. The use of a single agent with a narrow spectrum of activity against the pathogen diminishes the alteration of normal flora and thus limits the overgrowth of resistant nosocomial organisms (e.g., *Candida albicans*, enterococci, *Clostridium difficile*, or MRSA), avoids the potential toxicity of multiple-drug regimens, and reduces cost. However, certain circumstances call for the use of more than one antibacterial agent. These are summarized below.

1. *Prevention of the emergence of resistant mutants.* Spontaneous mutations occur at a detectable frequency in certain genes encoding the target proteins for some antibacterial agents. The use of these agents can eliminate the susceptible population, select out resistant mutants at the site of infection, and result in the failure of chemotherapy. Resistant mutants are usually selected when the MIC of the antibacterial agent for the infecting bacterium is close to achievable levels in serum or tissues and/or when the site of infection limits the access or activity of the agent. Among the most common examples are rifampin for staphylococci, imipenem for *Pseudomonas*, and fluoroquinolones for staphylococci and *Pseudomonas*. Small-colony variants of staphylococci resistant to aminoglycosides also emerge during monotherapy with these antibiotics. A second antibacterial agent with a mechanism of action different from that of the first is added in an attempt to prevent the emergence of resistant mutants (e.g., imipenem plus an aminoglycoside or a fluoroquinolone for systemic *Pseudomonas* infections). However, since resistant mutants have emerged following combination chemotherapy, this approach clearly is not uniformly successful.

2. *Synergistic or additive activity.* Synergistic or additive activity involves a lowering of the MIC or MBC of each or all of the drugs tested in combination against a specific bacterium. In *synergy*, each agent is more active when combined with a second drug than it would be alone, and the drugs' combined activity is therefore greater than the sum of the individual activities of each drug. In an *additive relationship*, the combined activity of the drugs is equal to the sum of their individual activities. Among the best examples of a synergistic or additive effect, confirmed both in vitro and by animal studies, are the enhanced bactericidal activities of certain β-lactam/aminoglycoside combinations against enterococci, viridans streptococci, and *P. aeruginosa*. The synergistic or additive activity of these combinations has also been demonstrated against selected isolates of enteric gram-negative bacteria and staphylococci. The combination of trimethoprim and sulfamethoxazole has synergistic or additive activity against many enteric gram-negative bacteria. Most other antimicrobial combinations display indifferent activity (i.e., the combination is *no better* than the more active of the two agents alone), and some combinations (e.g., penicillin plus tetracycline against pneumococci) may be antagonistic (i.e., the combination is *worse* than either drug alone).

3. *Therapy directed against multiple potential pathogens.* For certain infections, either a mixture of pathogens is suspected or the patient is desperately ill with an as-yet-unidentified infection (see "Empirical Therapy," next). In these situations, the most important of the likely infecting bacteria must be covered by therapy until culture and susceptibility results become available. Examples of the former infections are intraabdominal or brain abscesses and infections of limbs in diabetic patients with microvascular disease. The latter situations include fevers in neutropenic patients, acute pneumonia from aspiration of oral flora by hospitalized patients, and septic shock or sepsis syndrome.

EMPIRICAL THERAPY

In most situations, antibacterial therapy is begun before a specific bacterial pathogen has been identified. The choice of agent is guided by the results of studies identifying the usual pathogens at that site or in that clinical setting, by pharmacodynamic considerations, and by the resistance profile of the expected pathogens in a particular hospital or geographic area. Situations in which empirical therapy is appropriate include the following:

1. *Life-threatening infection.* Any suspected bacterial infection in a patient with a life-threatening illness should be treated presumptively. Therapy is usually begun with more than one agent and is later tailored to a specific pathogen if one is eventually identified. Early therapy with an effective antimicrobial regimen has consistently been demonstrated to improve survival rates.

2. *Treatment of community-acquired infections.* In most situations, it is appropriate to treat non-life-threatening infections without obtaining cultures. These situations include outpatient infections such as community-acquired upper and lower respiratory tract infections, cystitis, cellulitis or local wound infection, urethritis, and prostatitis. However, if any of these infections recurs or fails to respond to initial therapy, every effort should be made to obtain cultures to guide re-treatment.

CHOICE OF ANTIBACTERIAL THERAPY

Infections for which specific antibacterial agents are among the drugs of choice are detailed in Table 40-6. No attempt has been made to include all of the potential situations in which antibacterial agents may be used. A more detailed discussion of specific bacteria and infections that they cause can be found elsewhere in this volume.

The choice of antibacterial therapy increasingly involves an assessment of the acquired resistance of major microbial pathogens to the antimicrobial agents available to treat them. Resistance rates are dynamic (Table 40-6), both increasing and decreasing in response to the environmental pressure applied by antimicrobial use. For example, increased fluoroquinolone use in the community is associated with increasing rates of quinolone resistance in community-acquired strains of *S. pneumoniae*, *E. coli*, *Neisseria gonorrhoeae*, and *K. pneumoniae*. Fluoroquinolone resistance has also emerged rapidly among nosocomial isolates of *S. aureus* and *Pseudomonas* spp. as hospital use of this drug class has increased. It is important to note that, in many cases, wide variations in worldwide antimicrobial-resistance trends may not be reflected in the values recorded at U.S. hospitals. Therefore, the most important factor in choosing initial therapy for an infection in which the susceptibility of the specific pathogen(s) is not known is information on local resistance rates. This information can be obtained from local clinical microbiology laboratories in the annual hospital "antibiogram," from state health departments, or from publications of the Centers for Disease Control and Prevention (e.g., *Antimicrobial Resistance in Healthcare Settings; www.cdc.gov/ncidod/dhqp/ar.html*).

ADVERSE REACTIONS

Adverse drug reactions are frequently classified by mechanism as either *dose-related* ("toxic") or *unpredictable*. Unpredictable reactions are either idiosyncratic or allergic. Dose-related reactions include aminoglycoside-induced nephrotoxicity, linezolid-induced thrombocytopenia, penicillin-induced seizures, and vancomycin-induced anaphylactoid reactions. Many of these reactions can be avoided by reducing dosage in patients with impaired renal function, limiting the duration of therapy, or reducing the rate of administration. Adverse reactions to antibacterial agents are a common cause of morbidity, requiring alteration in therapy and additional expense, and they occasionally result in death. The elderly, often those with the more severe infections, may be especially prone to certain adverse reactions. The most clinically relevant adverse reactions to common antibacterial drugs are listed in Table 40-7.

DRUG INTERACTIONS

Antimicrobial drugs are a common cause of drug-drug interactions. Table 40-8 lists the most common and best-documented interactions of antibacterial agents with other drugs and characterizes the clinical relevance of these interactions. Coadministration of drugs paired in the table does not necessarily result in clinically important adverse consequences in all cases. The information in Table 40-8 is intended only to heighten awareness of the potential for an interaction. Additional sources should be consulted to identify appropriate options.

MACROLIDES AND KETOLIDES

Erythromycin, clarithromycin, and telithromycin inhibit CYP3A4, the hepatic P450 enzyme that metabolizes many drugs. In ~10% of patients receiving digoxin, concentrations increase significantly when erythromycin or telithromycin is coadministered, and this increase may lead to digoxin toxicity. Azithromycin has little effect on the metabolism of other drugs.

Many drugs, such as the azole antifungals, can also increase erythromycin serum concentrations, leading to prolongation of the QT interval and a fivefold increase in mortality rate. This example serves as a reminder that the true significance of drug-drug interactions may be subtle yet profound and that close attention to the evolving safety literature is important.

TABLE 40-6

INFECTIONS FOR WHICH SPECIFIC ANTIBACTERIAL AGENTS ARE AMONG THE DRUGS OF CHOICE

AGENT	INFECTIONS	COMMON PATHOGEN(S) (RESISTANCE RATE,%)[a]
Penicillin G	Syphilis, yaws, leptospirosis, groups A and B streptococcal infections, pneumococcal infections, actinomycosis, oral and periodontal infections, meningococcal meningitis and meningococcemia, viridans streptococcal endocarditis, clostridial myonecrosis, tetanus, anthrax, rat-bite fever, *Pasteurella multocida* infections, and erysipeloid (*Erysipelothrix rhusiopathiae*)	*Neisseria meningitidis*[b] (intermediate,[c] 15–30; resistant, 0; geographic variation) Viridans streptococci (intermediate, 15–30; resistant, 5–10) *Streptococcus pneumoniae* (intermediate, 23; resistant, 17)
Ampicillin, amoxicillin	Salmonellosis, acute otitis media, *Haemophilus influenzae* meningitis and epiglottitis, *Listeria monocytogenes* meningitis, *Enterococcus faecalis* UTI	*Escherichia coli* (37) *H. influenzae* (35) *Salmonella* spp.[b] (30–50; geographic variation) *Enterococcus* spp. (24)
Nafcillin, oxacillin	*Staphylococcus aureus* (non-MRSA) bacteremia and endocarditis	*S. aureus* (46; MRSA) *Staphylococcus epidermidis* (78; MRSE)
Piperacillin plus tazobactam	Intraabdominal infections (facultative enteric gram-negative bacilli plus obligate anaerobes); infections caused by mixed flora (aspiration pneumonia, diabetic foot ulcers); infections caused by *Pseudomonas aeruginosa*	*P. aeruginosa* (6)
Cefazolin	*E. coli* UTI, surgical prophylaxis, *S. aureus* (non-MRSA) bacteremia and endocarditis	*E. coli* (7) *S. aureus* (46; MRSA)
Cefoxitin, cefotetan	Intraabdominal infections and pelvic inflammatory disease	*Bacteroides fragilis* (12)
Ceftriaxone	Gonococcal infections, pneumococcal meningitis, viridans streptococcal endocarditis, salmonellosis and typhoid fever, hospital-acquired infections caused by nonpseudomonal facultative gram-negative enteric bacilli	*S. pneumoniae* (intermediate, 16; resistant, 0) *E. coli* and *Klebsiella pneumoniae* (1; ESBL producers)
Ceftazidime, cefepime	Hospital-acquired infections caused by facultative gram-negative enteric bacilli and *Pseudomonas*	*P. aeruginosa* (16) (See ceftriaxone for ESBL producers)
Imipenem, meropenem	Intraabdominal infections, hospital-acquired infections (non-MRSA), infections caused by *Enterobacter* spp. and ESBL-producing gram-negative bacilli	*P. aeruginosa* (6) *Acinetobacter* spp. (35)
Aztreonam	Hospital-acquired infections caused by facultative gram-negative bacilli and *Pseudomonas* in penicillin-allergic patients	*P. aeruginosa* (16)
Vancomycin	Bacteremia, endocarditis, and other serious infections due to MRSA; pneumococcal meningitis; antibiotic-associated pseudomembranous colitis[d]	*Enterococcus* spp. (24)
Daptomycin	VRE infections; MRSA bacteremia	Rare
Gentamicin, amikacin, tobramycin	Combined with a penicillin for staphylococcal, enterococcal, or viridans streptococcal endocarditis; combined with a β-lactam antibiotic for gram-negative bacteremia; pyelonephritis	Gentamicin: *E. coli* (6) *P. aeruginosa* (17) *Acinetobacter* spp. (32)
Erythromycin, clarithromycin, azithromycin	*Legionella, Campylobacter,* and *Mycoplasma* infections; CAP; group A streptococcal pharyngitis in penicillin-allergic patients; bacillary angiomatosis (*Bartonella henselae*); gastric infections due to *Helicobacter pylori*; *Mycobacterium avium-intracellulare* infections	*S. pneumoniae* (28) *Streptococcus pyogenes*[b] (0–10; geographic variation) *H. pylori*[b] (2–20; geographic variation)

(continued)

INFECTIONS FOR WHICH SPECIFIC ANTIBACTERIAL AGENTS ARE AMONG THE DRUGS OF CHOICE *(CONTINUED)*

AGENT	INFECTIONS	COMMON PATHOGEN(S) (RESISTANCE RATE,%)[a]
Clindamycin	Severe, invasive group A streptococcal infections; infections caused by obligate anaerobes; infections caused by susceptible staphylococci	*S. aureus* (nosocomial = 58; CA-MRSA = 10b)
Doxycycline, minocycline	Acute bacterial exacerbations of chronic bronchitis, granuloma inguinale, brucellosis (with streptomycin), tularemia, glanders, melioidosis, spirochetal infections caused by *Borrelia* (Lyme disease and relapsing fever; doxycycline), infections caused by *Vibrio vulnificus*, some *Aeromonas* infections, infections due to *Stenotrophomonas* (minocycline), plague, ehrlichiosis, chlamydial infections (doxycycline), granulomatous skin infections due to *Mycobacterium marinum* (minocycline), rickettsial infections, mild CAP, skin and soft tissue infections caused by gram-positive cocci (CA-MRSA infections, leptospirosis, syphilis, actinomycosis in the penicillin-allergic patient)	*S. pneumoniae* (17) MRSA (5)
Trimethoprim-sulfamethoxazole	Community-acquired UTI; *S. aureus* skin and soft tissue infections (CA-MRSA)	*E. coli* (19) MRSA (3)
Sulfonamides	Nocardial infections, leprosy (dapsone, a sulfone), and toxoplasmosis (sulfadiazine)	UNK
Ciprofloxacin, levofloxacin, moxifloxacin	CAP (levofloxacin and moxifloxacin); UTI; bacterial gastroenteritis; hospital-acquired gram-negative enteric infections; Pseudomonas infections (ciprofloxacin and levofloxacin)	*S. pneumoniae* (1) *E. coli* (13) *P. aeruginosa* (23) *Salmonella* spp. (10–50; geographic variation) *Neisseria gonorrhoeae*[b] (0–5, non–West Coast U.S.; 10–15, California and Hawaii; 20–70, Asia, England, Wales)
Rifampin	Staphylococcal foreign body infections, in combination with other antistaphylococcal agents; *Legionella* pneumonia	Staphylococci rapidly develop resistance during rifampin monotherapy.
Metronidazole	Obligate anaerobic gram-negative bacteria (Bacteroides spp.): abscess in lung, brain, or abdomen; bacterial vaginosis; antibiotic-associated *Clostridium difficile* disease	UNK
Linezolid	VRE; staphylococcal skin and soft tissue infection (CA-MRSA)	Rare
Polymyxin E (colistin)	Hospital-acquired infection due to gram-negative bacilli resistant to all other chemotherapy: *P. aeruginosa*, *Acinetobacter* spp., *Stenotrophomonas maltophilia*	UNK
Quinupristin/dalfopristin	VRE	Vancomycin-resistant *E. faecalis*[b] (100) Vancomycin-resistant *E. faecium* (10)
Mupirocin	Topical application to nares to eradicate *S. aureus* carriage	UNK

[a]Unless otherwise noted, resistance rates are based on all isolates tested in 2008 in the clinical microbiology laboratory at Virginia Commonwealth University Medical Center. The rates are consistent with those reported by the National Nosocomial Infections Surveillance System (Am J Infect Control 32:470, 2004).
[b]Data from recent literature sources.
[c]Intermediate resistance.
[d]Drug is given orally for this indication.
Abbreviations: CA-MRSA, community-acquired methicillin-resistant *S. aureus*; CAP, community-acquired pneumonia; ESBL, extended-spectrum β-lactamase; MRSA, methicillin-resistant *S. aureus*; MRSE, methicillin-resistant *S. epidermidis*; UNK, resistance rates unknown: UTI, urinary tract infection; VRE, vancomycin-resistant enterococci.

TABLE 40-7

MOST CLINICALLY RELEVANT ADVERSE REACTIONS TO COMMON ANTIBACTERIAL DRUGS

DRUG	ADVERSE EVENT	COMMENTS
β-Lactams	Allergies in ~1–4% of treatment courses	Cephalosporins cause allergy in 2–4% of penicillin-allergic patients. Aztreonam is safe in β-lactam-allergic patients.
	Nonallergic skin reactions	Ampicillin "rash" is common among patients with Epstein-Barr virus infection.
	Diarrhea, including Clostridium *difficile* colitis	—
Vancomycin	Anaphylactoid reaction ("red man syndrome")	Give as a 1- to 2-h infusion.
	Nephrotoxicity, ototoxicity, allergy, neutropenia	Thought to be rare, but appear to be increasing as larger dosages are used
Telavancin	Taste disturbance, foamy urine, gastrointestinal distress	New drug; full spectrum of adverse reactions unclear
Aminoglycosides	Nephrotoxicity (generally reversible)	Greatest with prolonged therapy in the elderly or with preexisting renal insufficiency. Monitor serum creatinine every 2–3 days.
	Ototoxicity (often irreversible)	Risk factors similar to those for nephrotoxicity; both vestibular and hearing toxicities
Macrolides/ ketolides	Gastrointestinal distress	Most common with erythromycin
	Ototoxicity	High-dose IV erythromycin
	Cardiac toxicity	QTc prolongation and torsades de pointes, especially when inhibitors of erythromycin metabolism are given simultaneously
	Hepatic toxicity (telithromycin)	Warning added to prescribing information (July 2006)
	Respiratory failure in patients with myasthenia gravis (telithromycin)	Warning added to prescribing information (July 2006)
Clindamycin	Diarrhea, including *C. difficile colitis*	—
Sulfonamides	Allergic reactions	Rashes (more common in HIV-infected patients); serious dermal reactions, including erythema multiforme, Stevens-Johnson syndrome, toxic epidermal necrolysis
	Hematologic reactions	Uncommon; include agranulocytosis and granulocytopenia (more common in HIV-infected patients), hemolytic and megaloblastic anemia, thrombocytopenia
	Renal insufficiency	Crystalluria with sulfadiazine therapy
Fluoroquinolones	Diarrhea, including *C. difficile colitis*	—
	Contraindicated for general use in patients <18 years old and pregnant women	Appear safe in treatment of pulmonary infections in children with cystic fibrosis
	Central nervous system adverse effects (e.g., insomnia)	—
	Miscellaneous: allergies, tendon rupture, dysglycemias, QTc prolongation	Rare, although warnings for tendon rupture have been added to prescribing information
Rifampin	Hepatotoxicity	Rare
	Orange discoloration of urine and body fluids	Common
	Miscellaneous: flu-like symptoms, hemolysis, renal insufficiency	Uncommon; usually related to intermittent administration
Metronidazole	Metallic taste	Common
Tetracyclines/ glycylcyclines	Gastrointestinal distress	Up to 20% with tigecycline
	Esophageal ulceration	Doxycycline (take in A.M. with fluids)
Linezolid	Myelosuppression	Follows long-term treatment
	Ocular and peripheral neuritis	Follows long-term treatment
Daptomycin	Distal muscle pain or weakness	Weekly creatine phosphokinase measurements, especially in patients also receiving statins

TABLE 40-8

INTERACTIONS OF ANTIBACTERIAL AGENTS WITH OTHER DRUGS

ANTIBIOTIC	INTERACTS WITH	POTENTIAL CONSEQUENCE (CLINICAL SIGNIFICANCE[a])
Erythromycin/clarithromycin/telithromycin	Theophylline	Theophylline toxicity (1)
	Carbamazepine	CNS depression (1)
	Digoxin	Digoxin toxicity (2)
	Triazolam/midazolam	CNS depression (2)
	Ergotamine	Ergotism (1)
	Warfarin	Bleeding (2)
	Cyclosporine/tacrolimus	Nephrotoxicity (1)
	Cisapride	Cardiac arrhythmias (1)
	Statins[b]	Rhabdomyolysis (2)
	Valproate	Valproate toxicity (2)
	Vincristine/vinblastine	Excess neurotoxicity (2)
Quinupristin/dalfopristin	Similar to erythromycin[c]	
Fluoroquinolones	Theophylline	Theophylline toxicity (2)[d]
	Antacids/sucralfate/iron	Subtherapeutic antibiotic levels (1)
Tetracycline	Antacids/sucralfate/iron	Subtherapeutic antibiotic levels (1)
Trimethoprim-sulfamethoxazole	Phenytoin	Phenytoin toxicity (2)
	Oral hypoglycemics	Hypoglycemia (2)
	Warfarin	Bleeding (1)
	Digoxin	Digoxin toxicity (2)
Metronidazole	Ethanol	Disulfiram-like reactions (2)
	Fluorouracil	Bone marrow suppression (1)
	Warfarin	Bleeding (2)
Rifampin	Warfarin	Clot formation (1)
	Oral contraceptives	Pregnancy (1)
	Cyclosporine/tacrolimus	Rejection (1)
	HIV-1 protease inhibitors	Increased viral load, resistance (1)
	Nonnucleoside reverse-transcriptase inhibitors	Increased viral load, resistance (1)
	Glucocorticoids	Loss of steroid effect (1)
	Methadone	Narcotic withdrawal symptoms (1)
	Digoxin	Subtherapeutic digoxin levels (1)
	Itraconazole	Subtherapeutic itraconazole levels (1)
	Phenytoin	Loss of seizure control (1)
	Statins	Hypercholesterolemia (1)
	Diltiazem	Subtherapeutic diltiazem levels (1)
	Verapamil	Subtherapeutic verapamil levels (1)

[a]1 = a well-documented interaction with clinically important consequences; 2 = an interaction of uncertain frequency but of potential clinical importance.

[b]Lovastatin and simvastatin are most affected; pravastatin and atorvastatin are less prone to clinically important effects.

[c]The macrolide antibiotics and quinupristin/dalfopristin inhibit the same human metabolic enzyme, CYP3A4, and similar interactions are anticipated.

[d]Ciprofloxacin only. Levofloxacin and moxifloxacin do not inhibit theophylline metabolism.

Note: New interactions are commonly reported after marketing. Consult the most recent prescribing information for updates. CNS, central nervous system.

QUINUPRISTIN/DALFOPRISTIN

Quinupristin/dalfopristin is an inhibitor of CYP3A4. Its interactions with other drugs are similar to those of erythromycin.

LINEZOLIDS

Linezolid is a monoamine oxidase inhibitor. Its concomitant administration with sympathomimetics (e.g.,

phenylpropanolamine) and with foods with high concentrations of tyramine should be avoided. Many case reports describe serotonin syndrome following coadministration of linezolid with selective serotonin reuptake inhibitors.

TETRACYCLINES

The most important interaction involving tetracyclines is reduced absorption when these drugs are coadministered with divalent and trivalent cations, such as antacids, iron compounds, or dairy products.

SULFONAMIDES

Sulfonamides, including TMP-SMX, increase the hypoprothrombinemic effect of warfarin by inhibition of its metabolism or by protein-binding displacement. This interaction is a relatively common cause of bleeding in patients also taking warfarin, and the incidence may be increasing as more TMP-SMX is used to treat community-acquired infections caused by MRSA.

FLUOROQUINOLONES

Chelation of all fluoroquinolones with divalent and trivalent cations leads to a significant reduction in absorption. Scattered case reports suggest that quinolones can also potentiate the effects of warfarin, but this effect has not been observed in most controlled trials. Patients receiving glucocorticoids are at increased risk of tendon rupture.

RIFAMPIN

Rifampin is an excellent inducer of many cytochrome P450 enzymes and increases the hepatic clearance of a large number of drugs. Before rifampin is prescribed for any patient, a review of concomitant drug therapy is essential.

METRONIDAZOLE

Metronidazole has been reported to cause a disulfiram-like syndrome when alcohol is ingested. The true frequency and significance of this reaction are unknown, and it is not well documented; however, patients for whom metronidazole is prescribed are usually instructed to avoid alcohol. Inhibition of the metabolism of warfarin by metronidazole leads to significant rises in prothrombin times.

PROPHYLAXIS OF BACTERIAL INFECTIONS

Antibacterial agents are occasionally indicated for use in patients who have no evidence of infection but who have been or are expected to be exposed to bacterial pathogens under circumstances that constitute a major risk of infection. The basic tenets of antimicrobial prophylaxis are as follows: (1) The risk or potential severity of infection should outweigh the risk of side effects from the antibacterial agent. (2) The antibacterial agent should be given for the shortest period necessary to prevent target infections. (3) The antibacterial agent should

be given before the expected period of risk (e.g., within 1 h of incision before elective surgery) or as soon as possible after contact with an infected individual (e.g., prophylaxis for meningococcal meningitis).

Table 40-9 lists the major indications for antibacterial prophylaxis in adults. The table includes only those indications that are widely accepted, supported by well-designed studies, or recommended by expert panels. Prophylaxis is also used but is less widely accepted for recurrent cellulitis in conjunction with lymphedema, recurrent pneumococcal meningitis in conjunction with deficiencies in humoral immunity or CSF leaks, traveler's diarrhea, gram-negative sepsis in conjunction with neutropenia, and spontaneous bacterial peritonitis in conjunction with ascites. The use of antibacterial agents in children to prevent rheumatic fever is also common practice.

The major use of antibacterial prophylaxis is to prevent infections following surgical procedures. Antibacterial agents are administered just before the surgical procedure—and, for long operations, during the procedure as well—to ensure high drug concentrations in serum and tissues during surgery. The objective is to eradicate bacteria originating from the air of the operating suite, the skin of the surgical team, or the patient's own flora that may contaminate the wound. In all but colorectal surgical procedures, prophylaxis is predominantly directed against staphylococci and cefazolin is the drug most commonly recommended. Prophylaxis is intended to prevent wound infection or infection of implanted devices, not all infections that may occur during the postoperative period (e.g., UTIs or pneumonia). Prolonged prophylaxis (beyond 24 h) merely alters the normal flora and favors infections with organisms resistant to the antibacterial agents used. National efforts to reduce surgical-site infections were begun in 2002 by the Surgical Infection Prevention Project (SIPP) sponsored by the Centers for Medicare and Medicaid Services. Additional initiatives by the American College of Surgeons–National Surgical Quality Improvement Program have been undertaken to further characterize best practices and to reduce surgical-site infections.

DURATION OF THERAPY AND TREATMENT FAILURE

Until recently, there was little incentive to establish the most appropriate duration of treatment; patients were instructed to take a 7- or 10-day course of treatment for most common infections. A number of recent investigations have evaluated shorter durations of therapy than have been used in the past, including treatment of patients with community-acquired pneumonia (5 days) and those with ventilator-associated pneumonia (7 or 8 days).

TABLE 40-9

PROPHYLAXIS OF BACTERIAL INFECTIONS IN ADULTS

CONDITION	ANTIBACTERIAL AGENT	TIMING OR DURATION OF PROPHYLAXIS
Nonsurgical		
Cardiac lesions highly susceptible to bacterial endocarditis (prosthetic valves, previous endocarditis, congenital heart defects)	Amoxicillin	Before and after dental procedures that manipulate gingival tissue
Recurrent *S. aureus* infections	Mupirocin	5 days (intranasal)
Contact with patient with meningococcal meningitis	Rifampin	2 days
	Fluoroquinolone	Single dose
Bite wounds[a]	Amoxicillin/clavulanic acid (alternatives: amoxicillin, doxycycline, or moxifloxacin)	3–5 days
Recurrent cystitis	Trimethoprim-sulfamethoxazole or a fluoroquinolone or nitrofurantoin	3 times per week for up to 1 year or after sexual intercourse
Surgical		
Clean (cardiac, vascular, neurologic, or orthopedic surgery)	Cefazolin (vancomycin)[b]	Before and during procedure
Ocular	Topical combinations and subconjunctival cefazolin	During and at end of procedure
Clean-contaminated (head and neck, high-risk gastroduodenal or biliary tract surgery; high-risk cesarean section; hysterectomy)	Cefazolin (or clindamycin for head and neck)	Before and during procedure
Clean-contaminated (vaginal or abdominal hysterectomy)	Cefazolin or cefoxitin or cefotetan or ampicillin-sulbactam	Before and during procedure
Clean-contaminated (high-risk genitourinary surgery)	Fluoroquinolone	Before and during procedure
Clean-contaminated (colorectal surgery or appendectomy)	Oral: neomycin plus erythromycin or metronidazole Parenteral: cefoxitin *or* cefotetan *or* cefazolin plus metronidazole *or* ampicillin-sulbactam	Before and during procedure
Dirty[a] (ruptured viscus)	Cefoxitin or cefotetan ± gentamicin, clindamycin + gentamicin, or another appropriate regimen directed at anaerobes and gram-negative aerobes	Before and for 3–5 days after procedure
Dirty[a] (traumatic wound)	Cefazolin	Before and for 3–5 days after trauma

[a]In these cases, use of antibacterial agents actually constitutes treatment of infection rather than prophylaxis.
[b]Vancomycin is recommended only in institutions that have a high incidence of infection with methicillin-resistant staphylococci.

Table 40-10 lists common bacterial infections for which treatment duration guidelines have been established or for which there is sufficient clinical experience to establish treatment durations. The ultimate test of cure for a bacterial infection is the absence of relapse when therapy is discontinued. *Relapse* is defined as a recurrence of infection with the identical organism that caused the first infection. In general, therefore, the duration of therapy should be long enough to prevent relapse yet not excessive. Extension of therapy beyond the limit of effectiveness will increase the medication's side effects and encourage the selection of resistant bacteria. The art of treating bacterial infections lies in the ability to determine the appropriate duration of therapy for infections that are not covered by established guidelines. Re-treatment of serious infections for which therapy has failed usually requires a prolonged course (>4 weeks) with combinations of antibacterial agents.

STRATEGIES TO OPTIMIZE ANTIMICROBIAL USE

Antibiotic use is often not "rational," and it is easy to understand why. The diagnosis of bacterial infection is often uncertain, patients may expect or demand antimicrobial agents in this tenuous situation, and clinicians wish to provide effective therapy even when the cause remains uncertain. Furthermore, the rates

TABLE 40-10

DURATION OF THERAPY FOR BACTERIAL INFECTIONS

DURATION OF THERAPY	INFECTIONS
Single dose	Gonococcal urethritis, streptococcal pharyngitis (penicillin G benzathine), primary and secondary syphilis (penicillin G benzathine)
3 days	Cystitis in young women, community- or travel-acquired diarrhea
3–10 days	Community-acquired pneumonia (3–5 days), community-acquired meningitis (pneumococcal or meningococcal), antibiotic-associated diarrhea (10 days), *Giardia* enteritis, cellulitis, epididymitis
2 weeks	*Helicobacter pylori*–associated peptic ulcer, neurosyphilis (penicillin IV), penicillin-susceptible viridans streptococcal endocarditis (penicillin plus aminoglycoside), disseminated gonococcal infection with arthritis, acute pyelonephritis, uncomplicated *S. aureus* catheter-associated bacteremia
3 weeks	Lyme disease, septic arthritis (nongonococcal)
4 weeks	Acute and chronic prostatitis, infective endocarditis (penicillin-resistant streptococcal)
>4 weeks	Acute and chronic osteomyelitis, *S. aureus* endocarditis, foreign-body infections (prosthetic-valve and joint infections), relapsing pseudomembranous colitis

of resistance for many bacterial pathogens are ever-changing, and even experts may not agree on the appropriate therapy or the clinical significance of resistance in some pathogens. Consequently, investigators report that ~50% of antibiotic use is in some way "inappropriate." Aside from the monetary cost of using unnecessary or expensive antibiotics, there are the more serious costs associated with excess morbidity from superinfections such as *C. difficile* disease, adverse drug reactions, drug interactions, and selection of resistant organisms. It is increasingly recognized that these costs add substantially to the overall costs of medical care.

At a time when fewer new antimicrobial drugs are entering the worldwide market than in the past, much has been written about the continued rise in rates of resistant microorganisms, its causes, and the solutions. The message seems clear: the use of existing and new antimicrobial agents must be more judicious and infection control efforts more effective if we are to slow or reverse trends in resistance. The phrase *antimicrobial stewardship* is used to describe the new attitude toward antibacterial agents that must be adopted to preserve their usefulness, and hospitals have been encouraged by professional organizations to implement multidisciplinary antimicrobial stewardship programs. These programs are designed to improve the quality of patient care by adopting best practices at the local level to ensure that antimicrobial drugs are used only when necessary, at the most appropriate dosage, and for the most appropriate duration. While some newer antibacterial drugs undeniably represent important advances in therapy, many offer no advantage over older, less expensive agents. With rare exceptions, newer drugs are usually found to be no more effective than the comparison antibiotic in controlled trials, despite the "high

prevalence of resistance" often touted to market the advantage of the new antibiotic over older therapies.

The following suggestions are intended to provide guidance through the antibiotic maze. First, objective evaluation of the merits of newer and older drugs is available. Online references such as the Johns Hopkins website (*www.hopkins-abxguide.org*) offer current and practical information regarding antimicrobial drugs and treatment regimens. Evidence-based practice guidelines for the treatment of most infections are available from the Infectious Diseases Society of America (*www.idsociety.org*). Furthermore, specialty texts such as *Principles and Practice of Infectious Diseases* are available online. Second, clinicians should become comfortable using a few drugs recommended by independent experts and professional organizations and should resist the temptation to use a new drug unless the merits are clear. A new antibacterial agent with a "broader spectrum and greater potency" or a "higher serum concentration-to-MIC ratio" will not necessarily be more clinically efficacious. Third, clinicians should become familiar with local bacterial susceptibility profiles available via annual "antibiograms" published by hospital clinical microbiology laboratories. It may not be necessary to use a new drug with "improved activity against *P. aeruginosa*" if that pathogen is rarely encountered or if it retains full susceptibility to older drugs. Fourth, a skeptical attitude toward manufacturers' claims is still appropriate. For example, rising rates of penicillin resistance in *S. pneumoniae* have been used to promote the use of broader-spectrum drugs, notably the fluoroquinolones. However, except in patients with meningitis, amoxicillin is still effective for infections caused by these "penicillin-resistant" strains. Finally, with regard to inpatient treatment with antibacterial drugs, a number of efforts to improve use are under study. The strategy of antibiotic "cycling" or rotation has not proved effective, but other strategies, such as reductions in the duration of therapy, hold promise. Adoption of other evidence-based strategies to improve antimicrobial use may be the best way to retain the utility of existing compounds. For example, appropriate empirical treatment of the seriously ill patient with one or more broad-spectrum agents is important for improving survival rates, but therapy may often be simplified by switching to a narrower-spectrum agent or even an oral drug once the results of cultures and susceptibility tests become available. While there is an understandable temptation not to alter effective empirical broad-spectrum therapy, switching to a more specific agent once the patient's clinical condition has improved does not compromise outcome. A promising and active area of research includes the use of shorter courses of antimicrobial therapy, perhaps guided by markers of infection such as serum concentrations of procalcitonin. Many antibiotics that once were given for 7–14 days can be given for 3–5 days with no apparent loss of efficacy and no increase in relapse rates (Table 40-10). Shorter durations of therapy, once proven as effective as longer durations, offer an opportunity to decrease overall drug use and may result in decreased resistance. Adoption of new guidelines for shorter-course therapy will not undermine the care of patients, many unnecessary complications and expenses will be avoided, and the useful life of these valuable drugs will perhaps be extended.

CHAPTER 41

ANTIVIRAL CHEMOTHERAPY, EXCLUDING ANTIRETROVIRAL DRUGS

Lindsey R. Baden ■ Raphael Dolin

The field of antiviral therapy—both the number of antiviral drugs and our understanding of their optimal use—historically has lagged behind that of antibacterial drug treatment, but significant progress has been made in recent years on new drugs for several viral infections. The development of antiviral drugs poses several challenges. Viruses replicate intracellularly and often employ host cell enzymes, macromolecules, and organelles for synthesis of viral particles. Therefore, useful antiviral compounds must discriminate between host and viral functions with a high degree of specificity; agents without such selectivity are likely to be too toxic for clinical use.

Significant progress has also been made in the development of laboratory assays to assist clinicians in the appropriate use of antiviral drugs. Phenotypic and genotypic assays for resistance to antiviral drugs are becoming more widely available, and correlations of laboratory results with clinical outcomes are being better defined. Of particular note has been the development of highly sensitive and specific methods that measure the concentration of virus in blood (*virus load*) and permit direct assessment of the antiviral effect of a given drug regimen in that host site. Virus load measurements have been useful in recognizing the risk of disease progression in patients with certain viral infections and in identifying patients for whom antiviral chemotherapy might be of greatest benefit. As with any in vitro laboratory test, results are highly dependent on (and likely to vary with) the laboratory techniques employed.

Information regarding the pharmacokinetics of some antiviral drugs, particularly in diverse clinical settings, is limited. Assays to measure the concentrations of these drugs, especially of their active moieties within cells, are primarily research procedures and are not widely available to clinicians. Thus, there are relatively few guidelines for adjusting dosages of antiviral agents to maximize antiviral activity and minimize toxicity.

Consequently, clinical use of antiviral drugs must be accompanied by particular vigilance with regard to unanticipated adverse effects.

Like that of other infections, the course of viral infections is profoundly affected by an interplay of the pathogen with a complex set of host defenses. The presence or absence of preexisting immunity, the ability to mount humoral and/or cell-mediated immune responses, and the stimulation of innate immunity are important determinants of the outcome of viral infections. The state of the host's defenses needs to be considered when antiviral agents are used or evaluated.

As with any therapy, the optimal use of antiviral compounds requires a specific and timely diagnosis. For some viral infections, such as herpes zoster, the clinical manifestations are so characteristic that a diagnosis can be made on clinical grounds alone. For other viral infections, such as influenza A, epidemiologic information (e.g., the documentation of a community-wide outbreak) can be used to make a presumptive diagnosis with a high degree of accuracy. However, for most of the remaining viral infections, including herpes simplex encephalitis, cytomegaloviral infections other than retinitis, and enteroviral infections, diagnosis on clinical grounds alone cannot be accomplished with certainty. For such infections, rapid viral diagnostic techniques are of great importance. Considerable progress has also been made in recent years in the development of such tests, which are now widely available for a number of viral infections.

Despite these complexities, the efficacy of a number of antiviral compounds has been clearly established in rigorously conducted and controlled studies. As summarized in Table 41-1, this chapter reviews the antiviral drugs that are currently approved or are likely to be considered for approval in the near future for use against viral infections other than those caused by HIV.

TABLE 41-1

ANTIVIRAL CHEMOTHERAPY AND CHEMOPROPHYLAXIS

INFECTION	DRUG	ROUTE	DOSAGE	COMMENT
Influenza A and B: Treatment	Oseltamivir	Oral	Adults: 75 mg bid × 5 d Children 1–12 years: 30–75 mg bid, depending on weight,[a] × 5 d	When started within 2 days of onset in uncomplicated disease, zanamivir and oseltamivir reduce symptom duration by 1.0–1.5 and 1.3 d, respectively. Their effectiveness in prevention or treatment of complications is unclear, although some analyses suggest that oseltamivir may reduce the frequency of respiratory tract complications and hospitalizations. Oseltamivir's side effects of nausea and vomiting can be reduced in frequency by drug administration with food. Zanamivir may exacerbate bronchospasm in patients with asthma. Amantadine and rimantadine are not recommended for routine use unless antiviral susceptibilities are known because of widespread resistance in A/H3N2 viruses since 2005–2006 and in pandemic A/H1N1 viruses in 2009–2010. Their efficacy in treatment of uncomplicated disease caused by sensitive viruses has been similar to that of neuraminidase inhibitors.
	Zanamivir	Inhaled orally	Adults and children ≥7 years: 10 mg bid × 5 d	
	Amantadine[b]	Oral	Adults: 100 mg qd or bid × 5–7 d Children 1–9 years: 5 mg/kg per day (maximum, 150 mg/d) × 5–7 d	
	Rimantadine[b]	Oral	100 mg qd or bid × 5–7 d in adults	
Influenza A and B: Prophylaxis	Oseltamivir	Oral	Adults: 75 mg/d Children ≥1 year: 30–75 mg/d, depending on weight[a]	Prophylaxis must be continued for the duration of exposure and can be administered simultaneously with inactivated vaccine. Unless the sensitivity of isolates is known, neither amantadine nor rimantadine is currently recommended for prophylaxis or therapy.
	Zanamivir	Inhaled orally	Adults and children ≥5 years: 10 mg/d	
	Amantadine[b] or rimantadine[b]	Oral	Adults: 200 mg/d Children 1–9 years: 5 mg/kg per day (maximum, 150 mg/d)	
RSV infection	Ribavirin	Small-particle aerosol	Administered 12–18 h/d from reservoir containing 20 mg/mL × 3–6 d	Use of ribavirin is to be "considered" for treatment of infants and young children hospitalized with RSV pneumonia and bronchiolitis, according to the American Academy of Pediatrics.
CMV disease	Ganciclovir	IV	5 mg/kg bid × 14–21 d; then 5 mg/kg per day as maintenance dose	Ganciclovir, valganciclovir, foscarnet, and cidofovir are approved for treatment of CMV retinitis in patients with AIDS. They are also used for colitis, pneumonia, or "wasting" syndrome associated with CMV and for prevention of CMV disease in transplant recipients. Valganciclovir has largely supplanted oral ganciclovir and is frequently used in place of IV ganciclovir. Foscarnet is not myelosuppressive and is active against acyclovir- and ganciclovir-resistant herpesviruses.
	Valganciclovir	Oral	900 mg bid × 21 d; then 900 mg/d as maintenance dose	
	Foscarnet	IV	60 mg/kg q8h × 14–21 d; then 90–120 mg/kg per day as maintenance dose	
	Cidofovir	IV	5 mg/kg once weekly × 2 weeks, then once every other week; given with probenecid and hydration	

(continued)

TABLE 41-1

ANTIVIRAL CHEMOTHERAPY AND CHEMOPROPHYLAXIS *(CONTINUED)*

INFECTION	DRUG	ROUTE	DOSAGE	COMMENT
	Fomivirsen	Intravitreal	330 mg on days 1 and 15 followed by 330 mg monthly as maintenance	Fomivirsen has reduced the rate of progression of CMV retinitis in patients in whom other regimens have failed or have not been well tolerated. The major form of toxicity is ocular inflammation.
Varicella: Immuno-competent host	Acyclovir	Oral	20 mg/kg (maximum, 800 mg) 4 or 5 times daily × 5 d	Treatment confers modest clinical benefit when administered within 24 h of rash onset.
	Valacyclovir	Oral	Children 2–18 years: 20 mg/kg tid, not to exceed 1 g tid, × 5 d	
Varicella: Immu-nocompromised host	Acyclovir	IV	10 mg/kg q8h × 7 d	A change to oral valacyclovir can be considered once fever has subsided if there is no evidence of visceral involvement.
Herpes simplex encephalitis	Acyclovir	IV	10 mg/kg q8h × 14–21 d	Results are optimal when therapy is initiated early. Some authorities recommend treatment for 21 d to prevent relapses.
Neonatal herpes simplex	Acyclovir	IV	20 mg/kg q8h × 14–21 d	Serious morbidity is common despite therapy. Prolonged oral administration after initial IV therapy has been suggested because of long-term sequelae associated with cutaneous recurrences of HSV infection.
Genital herpes simplex: Primary (treatment)	Acyclovir	IV	5 mg/kg q8h × 5–10 d	The IV route is preferred for infections severe enough to warrant hospitalization or with neurologic complications.
		Oral	400 mg tid or 200 mg 5 times daily × 7–10 d or 800 mg tid × 2 d	The oral route is preferred for patients whose condition does not warrant hospitalization. Adequate hydration must be maintained.
		Topical	5% ointment; 4–6 applications daily × 7–10 d	Topical use—largely supplemented by oral therapy—may obviate systemic administration to pregnant women. Systemic symptoms and untreated areas are not affected.
	Valacyclovir	Oral	1 g bid × 7–10 d	Valacyclovir appears to be as effective as acyclovir but can be administered less frequently.
	Famciclovir	Oral	250 mg tid × 7–10 d[c]	Famciclovir appears to be similar in effectiveness to acyclovir.
Genital herpes simplex: Recurrent (treatment)	Acyclovir	Oral	400 mg tid or 800 mg bid × 5 d	The clinical effect is modest and is enhanced if therapy is initiated early. Treatment does not affect recurrence rates.
	Famciclovir	Oral	125 mg bid × 5 d or 1000 mg bid × 1 d	
	Valacyclovir	Oral	500 mg bid × 3 d or 1 g once a day × 5 d	
Genital herpes simplex: Recurrent (suppression)	Acyclovir	Oral	400 mg bid	Suppressive therapy is recommended only for patients with at least 6–10 recurrences per year. "Breakthrough" occasionally takes place, and asymptomatic shedding of virus occurs. The need for suppressive therapy should be reevaluated after 1 year. Suppression with valacyclovir reduces transmission of genital HSV among discordant couples.
	Valacyclovir	Oral	500–1000 mg/d	
	Famciclovir	Oral	250 mg bid	

(continued)

TABLE 41-1

ANTIVIRAL CHEMOTHERAPY AND CHEMOPROPHYLAXIS (CONTINUED)

INFECTION	DRUG	ROUTE	DOSAGE	COMMENT
Mucocutaneous herpes simplex in immunocom- promised host: Treatment	Acyclovir	IV	5 mg/kg q8h × 7–14 d	The choice of the IV or oral route and the duration of therapy depend on the severity of infection and the patient's ability to take oral medication. Oral or IV treatment has supplanted topical therapy except for small, easily accessible lesions. Foscarnet is used for acyclovir-resistant viruses.
		Oral	400 mg 5 times daily × 10–14 d	
		Topical	5% ointment; 4–6 applications daily × 7 d or until healed	
	Valacyclovir	Oral	1 g tid × 7–10 d[c]	
	Famciclovir	Oral	500 mg bid × 7–10 d[d]	
Mucocutaneous herpes simplex in immunocompro- mised host: Prevention of recurrence during intense immuno- suppression	Acyclovir	Oral	400 mg 2–5 times daily or 800 mg bid	Treatment is administered during periods when intense immunosuppression is expected— e.g., during antitumor chemotherapy or after transplantation—and is usually continued for 2–3 months.
		IV	5 mg/kg q12h	
	Valacyclovir	Oral	500 mg to 1 g bid or tid	
	Famciclovir	Oral	500 mg bid[c]	
Herpes simplex orolabialis (recurrent)[e]	Penciclovir	Topical	1.0% cream applied q2h during waking hours × 4 d	Treatment shortens healing time and symptom duration by 0.5–1.0 d (compared with placebo).
	Valacyclovir	Oral	2 g q12h × 1 d	Therapy begun at the earliest symptom reduces disease duration by 1 d.
	Famciclovir[c]	Oral	1500 mg once or 750 bid × 1 d	Therapy begun within 1 h of prodrome decreased time to healing by 1.8–2.2 d.
	Docosanol[f]	Topical	10% cream 5 times daily until healed	Application at initial symptoms reduces healing time by 1 d.
Herpes simplex keratitis	Trifluridine	Topical	1 drop of 1% ophthal- mic solution q2h while awake (maximum, 9 drops daily)	Therapy should be undertaken in consultation with an ophthalmologist.
	Vidarabine	Topical	0.5-in. ribbon of 3% ophthalmic ointment 5 times daily	
Herpes zoster: Immunocompe- tent host	Valacyclovir	Oral	1 g tid × 7 d	Valacyclovir may be more effective than acy- clovir for pain relief; otherwise, it has a similar effect on cutaneous lesions and should be given within 72 h of rash onset.
	Famciclovir	Oral	500 mg q8h × 7 d	The duration of postherpetic neuralgia is shorter than with placebo. Famciclovir showed overall efficacy similar to that of acy- clovir in a comparative trial. It should be given ≤72 h after rash onset.
	Acyclovir	Oral	800 mg 5 times daily × 7–10 d	Acyclovir causes faster resolution of skin lesions than placebo and provides some relief of acute symptoms if given within 72 h of rash onset. Combined with tapering doses of prednisone, acyclovir improves quality-of-life outcomes.
Herpes zoster: Immunocompro- mised host	Acyclovir	IV	10 mg/kg q8h × 7 d	Effectiveness in localized zoster is most marked when treatment is given early. Fos- carnet may be used for acyclovir-resistant VZV infections.
		Oral	800 mg 5 times daily × 7 d	
	Famciclovir	Oral	500 mg tid × 10 d[c]	

(continued)

TABLE 41-1

ANTIVIRAL CHEMOTHERAPY AND CHEMOPROPHYLAXIS (CONTINUED)

INFECTION	DRUG	ROUTE	DOSAGE	COMMENT
Herpes zoster ophthalmicus	Acyclovir	Oral	600–800 mg 5 times daily × 10 d	Treatment reduces ocular complications, including ocular keratitis and uveitis.
	Valacyclovir	Oral	1 g tid × 7 d	
	Famciclovir	Oral	500 mg tid × 7 d	
Condyloma acuminatum	IFN-α2b	Intralesional	1 million units per wart (maximum of 5) thrice weekly × 3 weeks	Intralesional treatment frequently results in regression of warts, but lesions often recur. Parenteral administration may be useful if lesions are numerous.
	IFN-αn3	Intralesional	250,000 units per wart (maximum of 10) twice weekly × up to 8 weeks	
Chronic hepatitis B	IFN-α2b	SC	5 million units daily or 10 million units thrice weekly × 16–24 weeks	HBeAg and DNA are eliminated in 33–37% of cases. Histopathologic improvement is also seen.
	Pegylated IFN-α2a	SC	180 μg weekly × 48 weeks	ALT levels return to normal in 39% of patients, and histologic improvement occurs in 38%.
	Lamivudine	Oral	100 mg/d × 12–18 months; 150 mg bid as part of therapy for HIV infection	Lamivudine monotherapy is well tolerated and effective in reduction of HBV DNA levels, normalization of ALT levels, and improvement in histopathology. However, resistance develops in 24% of recipients when lamivudine is used as monotherapy for 1 year.
	Adefovir dipivoxil	Oral	10 mg/d × 48 weeks	A return of ALT levels to normal is documented in 48–72% of recipients and improved liver histopathology in 53–64%. Adefovir is effective in lamivudine-resistant hepatitis B. Renal function should be monitored.
	Entecavir	Oral	0.5 mg/d × 48 weeks (1 mg/d if HBV is resistant to lamivudine)	Normalization of ALT is seen in 68–78% of recipients and loss of HBeAg in 21%. Entecavir is active against lamivudine-resistant HBV.
	Telbivudine	Oral	600 mg/d × 52 weeks	HBV DNA is reduced by >5 log10 copies/mL along with normalization of ALT levels in 74–77% of patients and improved histopathology in 65–67%. Resistance develops in 9–22% of patients after 2 years of therapy. Elevated CPK levels and myopathy may occur.
	Tenofovir	Oral	300 mg/d × 48 weeks	ALT levels return to normal in 68–76% of patients, and liver histopathology improves in 72–74%. Resistance is uncommon with up to 2 years of therapy.
Chronic hepatitis C	IFN-α2a or IFN-α2b	SC	3 million units thrice weekly × 12–24 months	SVRs are noted in 20–30% of patients. Normalization of ALT levels and improvements in liver histopathology are also seen.
	IFN-α2b/ ribavirin	SC (IFN)/oral (ribavirin)	3 million units thrice weekly (IFN)/1000–1200 mg daily (ribavirin) × 6–12 months	Combination therapy results in SVR in up to 40–50% of recipients.

(continued)

ANTIVIRAL CHEMOTHERAPY AND CHEMOPROPHYLAXIS *(CONTINUED)*

INFECTION	DRUG	ROUTE	DOSAGE	COMMENT
	Pegylated IFN-α2b	SC	1.5 µg weekly × 48 weeks	The slower clearance of pegylated IFNs than of standard IFNs permits once-weekly administration. Pegylated formulations appear to be superior to standard IFNs in efficacy, both as monotherapy and in combination with ribavirin, and have largely supplanted standard IFNs in treatment of hepatitis C. SVRs were seen in 42–51% of patients infected with genotype 1 and in 76–82% of those infected with genotype 2 or 3.
	Pegylated IFN-α2a	SC	180 µg weekly × 48 weeks	
	Pegylated IFN-α2b/ ribavirin	SC (IFN)/oral (ribavirin)	1.5 µg/kg weekly (IFN)/800–1400 mg daily (ribavirin) × 24–48 weeks	
	Pegylated IFN-α2a/ ribavirin	SC (IFN)/oral (ribavirin)	180 µg weekly (IFN)/800–1200 mg daily (ribavirin) × 24–48 weeks	
	IFN-alfacon	SC	9–15 µg thrice weekly × 6–12 months	Doses of 9 and 15 µg are equivalent to IFN-α2a and IFN-α2b doses of 3 million and 5 million units, respectively.
Chronic hepatitis D	IFN-α2a or IFN-α2b	SC	9 million units thrice weekly × 12 months	The overall efficacy and the optimal regimen and duration of therapy have not been established. Response rates have varied among studies.
	Pegylated IFN-α2b	SC	1.5 µg weekly × 48 weeks	
	Pegylated IFN-α2a	SC	180 µg weekly × 48 weeks	

[a]For detailed weight recommendations and for children ≥1 year of age, see *www.cdc.gov/flu/professionals/antivirals/summary-clinicians.htm*.
[b]Amantadine and rimantadine are not recommended for routine use because of widespread resistance in A/H3N2 and pandemic A/H1N1 viruses in 2009–2010. Their use may be considered if sensitivities become reestablished.
[c]Not approved for this indication by the U.S. Food and Drug Administration (FDA).
[d]Approved by the FDA for treatment of HIV-infected individuals.
[e]Acyclovir suspension (15 mg/kg PO to a maximum of 200 mg per dose) given for 7 d has been reported to be effective in treatment of primary herpetic gingivostomatitis in children.
[f]Active ingredient: benzyl alcohol. Available without prescription.
Abbreviations: ALT, alanine aminotransferase; CMV, cytomegalovirus; CPK, creatine phosphokinase; HBeAg, hepatitis B e antigen; HBV, hepatitis B virus; HSV, herpes simplex virus; IFN, interferon; RSV, respiratory syncytial virus; SVR, sustained virologic response; UV, ultraviolet; VZV, varicella-zoster virus.

ANTIVIRAL DRUGS ACTIVE AGAINST RESPIRATORY INFECTIONS (ALSO SEE CHAP. 13)

ZANAMIVIR, OSELTAMIVIR, AND PERAMIVIR

Zanamivir and oseltamivir are inhibitors of the influenza viral neuraminidase enzyme, which is essential for release of the virus from infected cells and for its subsequent spread throughout the respiratory tract of the infected host. The enzyme cleaves terminal sialic acid residues and thus destroys the cellular receptors to which the viral hemagglutinin attaches. Zanamivir and oseltamivir are sialic acid transition-state analogues and are highly active and specific inhibitors of the neuraminidases of both influenza A and B viruses. The antineuraminidase activity of the two drugs is similar, although zanamivir has somewhat greater in vitro activity against influenza B. Both zanamivir and oseltamivir act through competitive and reversible inhibition of the active site of influenza A and B viral neuraminidases and have relatively little effect on mammalian cell enzymes.

Oseltamivir phosphate is an ethyl ester prodrug that is converted to oseltamivir carboxylate by esterases in the liver. Orally administered oseltamivir has a bioavailability of >60% and a plasma half-life of 7–9 h. The drug is excreted unmetabolized, primarily by the kidneys. Zanamivir has low oral bioavailability and is administered orally via a hand-held inhaler. By this route, ~15% of the dose is deposited in the lower respiratory tract, and low plasma levels of the drug are detected.

Orally inhaled zanamivir is generally well tolerated, although exacerbations of asthma may occur. The toxicities most frequently encountered with orally administered oseltamivir are nausea, gastrointestinal discomfort, and (less commonly) vomiting. Gastrointestinal discomfort is usually transient and is less likely if the drug is administered with food. Neuropsychiatric events (delirium, self-injury) have been reported in children who have been taking oseltamivir, primarily in Japan. An IV formulation of zanamivir is under development and is available from GlaxoSmith Kline as part of clinical trials.

Inhaled zanamivir and orally administered oseltamivir have been effective in the treatment of naturally occurring, uncomplicated influenza A or B in otherwise healthy adults. In placebo-controlled studies, illness has been shortened by 1.0–1.5 days of therapy with either of these drugs when treatment is administered within 2 days of onset. Pooled analyses of clinical studies of oseltamivir suggest that treatment may reduce the likelihood of hospitalizations and of certain respiratory tract complications associated with influenza (Chap. 13). Once-daily inhaled zanamivir or once-daily orally administered oseltamivir can provide prophylaxis against laboratory-documented influenza A– and influenza B–associated illness.

Resistance to the neuraminidase inhibitors may develop by changes in the viral neuraminidase enzyme, by changes in the hemagglutinin that make it more resistant to the actions of the neuraminidase, or by both mechanisms. Isolates that are resistant to oseltamivir—most commonly through the H275Y mutation, which leads to a change from histidine to tyrosine at that residue in the neuraminidase—remain sensitive to zanamivir. Certain mutations impart resistance to both oseltamivir and zanamivir (e.g., I223R, which leads to a change from isoleucine to arginine). Since the mechanisms of action of the neuraminidase inhibitors differ from those of the adamantanes (see later), zanamivir and oseltamivir are active against strains of influenza A virus that are resistant to amantadine and rimantadine.

Appropriate use of antiviral agents against influenza viruses depends on a knowledge of the resistance patterns of circulating viruses. For example, in the 2008–2009 influenza season, the circulating influenza A/H3N2 viruses were sensitive to both oseltamivir and zanamivir, whereas the seasonal A/H1N1 viruses, although also sensitive to zanamivir, were resistant to oseltamivir. Moreover, the pandemic A/H1N1 viruses that circulated in 2009–2010 remained sensitive to zanamivir and oseltamivir, with a few exceptions in the latter case. Up-to-date information on resistance patterns to antiviral drugs is available from the Centers for Disease Control and Prevention (CDC) at *www.cdc.gov/flu*.

Zanamivir and oseltamivir have been approved by the U.S. Food and Drug Administration (FDA) for treatment of influenza in adults and in children (those ≥7 years old for zanamivir and those ≥1 year old for oseltamivir) who have been symptomatic for ≤2 days. Oseltamivir is approved for prophylaxis of influenza in individuals ≥1 year of age and zanamivir for those ≥5 years of age (Table 41-1). Guidelines for use of oseltamivir in children <1 year of age can be accessed through the CDC website, as noted in the footnote to Table 41-1.

Peramivir, an investigational neuraminidase inhibitor that can be administered intravenously to patients for whom such an intervention is considered necessary, is available as part of clinical trials through BioCryst Pharmaceuticals. Oseltamivir-resistant viruses generally exhibit reduced sensitivity to peramivir.

AMANTADINE AND RIMANTADINE

Amantadine and the closely related compound rimantadine are primary symmetric amines that have antiviral activity limited to influenza A viruses. Amantadine and rimantadine have been shown to be efficacious in the prophylaxis and treatment of influenza A infections in humans for >45 years. High frequencies of resistance to these drugs were noted among influenza A/H3N2 viruses in the 2005–2006 influenza season and continued to be seen in 2008–2009. The pandemic A/H1N1 viruses that circulated in 2009–2010 were also resistant to amantadine and rimantadine. Therefore, these agents are no longer recommended for use unless the sensitivity of the individual influenza A isolate is known, in which case their use may be considered. Amantadine and rimantadine act through inhibition of the ion channel function of the influenza A M2 matrix protein, on which uncoating of the virus depends. A substitution of a single amino acid at critical sites in the M2 protein can result in a virus that is resistant to amantadine and rimantadine.

Amantadine and rimantadine have been shown to be effective in the prophylaxis of influenza A in large-scale studies of young adults and in less extensive studies of children and elderly persons. In such studies, efficacy rates of 55–80% in the prevention of influenza-like illness were noted, and even higher rates were reported when virus-specific attack rates were calculated. Amantadine and rimantadine have also been found to be effective in the treatment of influenza A infection in studies involving predominantly young adults and, to a lesser extent, children. Administration of these compounds within 24–72 h after the onset of illness has resulted in a reduction of the duration of signs and symptoms by ~50% compared to that in placebo recipients. The effect on signs and symptoms of illness is superior to that of commonly used antipyretic-analgesic agents. Only anecdotal reports are available concerning the efficacy of amantadine or rimantadine in the prevention or treatment of complications of influenza (e.g., pneumonia).

Amantadine and rimantadine are available only in oral formulations and are ordinarily administered to adults once or twice daily, with a dosage of 100–200 mg/d. Despite their structural similarities, the two compounds have different pharmacokinetics. Amantadine is not metabolized and is excreted almost entirely by the kidneys, with a half-life of 12–17 h and peak plasma concentrations of 0.4 μg/mL. In contrast, rimantadine is extensively metabolized to hydroxylated derivatives and has a half-life of 30 h. Only 30–40% of an orally administered dose of rimantadine is recovered in the urine. The peak plasma levels of rimantadine are approximately half those of amantadine, but rimantadine is concentrated in respiratory secretions to a greater extent than amantadine. For prophylaxis, the compounds must be administered daily for the period at risk (i.e., duration of the exposure). For therapy, amantadine or rimantadine is generally administered for 5–7 days.

Although these compounds are generally well tolerated, 5–10% of amantadine recipients experience mild central nervous system side effects consisting primarily of dizziness, anxiety, insomnia, and difficulty in concentrating. These effects are rapidly reversible upon cessation of the drug's administration. At a dose of 200 mg/d, rimantadine is better tolerated than amantadine; in a large-scale study of young adults, adverse effects were no more frequent among rimantadine recipients than among placebo recipients. Seizures and worsening of congestive heart failure have also been reported in patients treated with amantadine, although a causal relationship has not been established. The dosage of amantadine should be reduced to 100 mg/d in patients with renal insufficiency (i.e., a creatinine clearance rate [Cr_{Cl}] of <50 mL/min) and in the elderly. A rimantadine dose of 100 mg/d should be used for patients with a Cr_{Cl} of <10 mL/min and for the elderly.

RIBAVIRIN

Ribavirin is a synthetic nucleoside analogue that inhibits a wide range of RNA and DNA viruses. The mechanism of action of ribavirin is not completely defined and may be different for different groups of viruses. Ribavirin-5′-monophosphate blocks the conversion of inosine-5′-monophosphate to xanthosine–5′-monophosphate and interferes with the synthesis of guanine nucleotides as well as that of both RNA and DNA. Ribavirin-5′-monophosphate also inhibits capping of virus-specific messenger RNA in certain viral systems.

Ribavirin administered as a small-particle aerosol to young children hospitalized with RSV infection has been clinically beneficial and has improved oxygenation in some studies (7 of 11). Although ribavirin has been approved for treatment of infants hospitalized with respiratory syncytial virus (RSV) infection, the American Academy of Pediatrics has recommended that its use be considered on an individual basis rather than routinely in that setting. Aerosolized ribavirin has also been administered to older children and adults (including immunosuppressed patients) with severe RSV and parainfluenza virus infections and to older children and

adults with influenza A or B infection, but the benefit of this treatment, if any, is unclear. In RSV infections in immunosuppressed patients, ribavirin is often given in combination with anti-RSV immunoglobulins.

Orally administered ribavirin has not been effective in the treatment of influenza A virus infections. IV or oral ribavirin has reduced mortality rates among patients with Lassa fever; it has been particularly effective in this regard when given within the first 6 days of illness. IV ribavirin has been reported to be of clinical benefit in the treatment of hemorrhagic fever with renal syndrome caused by Hantaan virus and as therapy for Argentinean hemorrhagic fever. Oral ribavirin has also been recommended for the treatment and prophylaxis of Congo-Crimean hemorrhagic fever. An open-label trial suggested that oral ribavirin may be beneficial in the treatment of Nipah virus encephalitis. Use of IV ribavirin in patients with hantavirus pulmonary syndrome in the United States has not been associated with clear-cut benefits. Oral administration of ribavirin reduces serum aminotransferase levels in patients with chronic hepatitis C virus (HCV) infection; since it appears not to reduce serum HCV RNA levels, the mechanism of this effect is unclear. The drug provides added benefit when given by mouth in doses of 800–1200 mg/d in combination with interferon (IFN) α2b or α2a (see next), and the ribavirin/IFN combination has been approved for the treatment of patients with chronic HCV infection. Large oral doses of ribavirin (800–1000 mg/d) have been associated with reversible hematopoietic toxicity. This effect has not been observed with aerosolized ribavirin, apparently because little drug is absorbed systemically. Aerosolized administration of ribavirin is generally well tolerated but occasionally is associated with bronchospasm, rash, or conjunctival irritation. It should be administered under close supervision—particularly in the setting of mechanical ventilation, where precipitation of the drug is possible. Health care workers exposed to the drug have experienced minor toxicity, including eye and respiratory tract irritation. Because ribavirin is mutagenic, teratogenic, and embryotoxic, its use is generally contraindicated in pregnancy. Its administration as an aerosol poses a risk to pregnant health care workers. Because clearance of ribavirin is primarily renal, dose reduction is required in the setting of significant renal dysfunction.

ANTIVIRAL DRUGS ACTIVE AGAINST HERPESVIRUS INFECTIONS

ACYCLOVIR AND VALACYCLOVIR

Acyclovir is a highly potent and selective inhibitor of the replication of certain herpesviruses, including herpes simplex virus (HSV) types 1 and 2, varicella-zoster virus (VZV), and Epstein-Barr virus (EBV). It is relatively ineffective in the treatment of human cytomegalovirus (CMV) infections; however, some studies have indicated effectiveness in the prevention of CMV-associated disease in immunosuppressed patients. Valacyclovir, the L-valyl ester of acyclovir, is converted almost entirely to acyclovir by intestinal and hepatic hydrolysis after oral administration. Valacyclovir has pharmacokinetic advantages over orally administered acyclovir: it exhibits significantly greater oral bioavailability, results in higher blood levels, and can be given less frequently than acyclovir (two or three rather than five times daily).

The high degree of selectivity of acyclovir is related to its mechanism of action, which requires that the compound first be phosphorylated to acyclovir monophosphate. This phosphorylation occurs efficiently in herpesvirus-infected cells by means of a virus-coded thymidine kinase. In uninfected mammalian cells, little phosphorylation of acyclovir occurs, and the drug is therefore concentrated in herpesvirus-infected cells. Acyclovir monophosphate is subsequently converted by host cell kinases to a triphosphate that is a potent inhibitor of virus-induced DNA polymerase but has relatively little effect on host cell DNA polymerase. Acyclovir triphosphate can also be incorporated into viral DNA, with early chain termination.

Acyclovir is available in IV, oral, and topical forms, while valacyclovir is available in an oral formulation. IV acyclovir is effective in the treatment of mucocutaneous HSV infections in immunocompromised hosts, in whom it reduces time to healing, duration of pain, and virus shedding. When administered prophylactically during periods of intense immunosuppression (e.g., related to chemotherapy for leukemia or transplantation) and before the development of lesions, IV acyclovir reduces the frequency of HSV-associated disease. After prophylaxis is discontinued, HSV lesions recur. IV acyclovir is also effective in the treatment of HSV encephalitis.

Because VZV is generally less sensitive to acyclovir than is HSV, higher doses of acyclovir must be used to treat VZV infections. In immunocompromised patients with herpes zoster, IV acyclovir reduces the frequency of cutaneous dissemination and visceral complications and—in one comparative trial—was more effective than vidarabine. Acyclovir, administered at oral doses of 800 mg five times a day, had a modest beneficial effect on localized herpes zoster lesions in both immunocompromised and immunocompetent patients. Combination of acyclovir with a tapering regimen of prednisone appeared to be more effective than acyclovir alone in terms of quality-of-life outcomes in immunocompetent patients over age 50 with herpes zoster. A comparative study of acyclovir (800 mg PO five times daily) and valacyclovir (1 g PO three times daily) in immunocompetent patients with herpes zoster indicated that the latter drug may be more effective in eliciting the resolution of zoster-associated pain. Orally administered acyclovir (600 mg five times a day) reduced complications of herpes zoster ophthalmicus in a placebo-controlled trial.

In chickenpox, a modest overall clinical benefit is attained when oral acyclovir therapy is begun within 24 h of the onset of rash in otherwise healthy children (20 mg/kg, up to a maximum of 800 mg, four times a day) or adults (800 mg five times a day). IV acyclovir has also been reported to be effective in the treatment of immunocompromised children with chickenpox.

The most widespread use of acyclovir is in the treatment of genital HSV infections. IV or oral acyclovir or oral valacyclovir has shortened the duration of symptoms, reduced virus shedding, and accelerated healing when employed for the treatment of primary genital HSV infections. Oral acyclovir and valacyclovir have also had a modest effect in treatment of recurrent genital HSV infections. However, the failure of treatment of either primary or recurrent disease to reduce the frequency of subsequent recurrences has indicated that acyclovir is ineffective in eliminating latent infection. Chronic oral administration of acyclovir for ≥1–6 years or of valacyclovir for ≥1 year has reduced the frequency of recurrences markedly during therapy; once the drug is discontinued, lesions recur. In one study, suppressive therapy with valacyclovir (500 mg once daily for 8 months) reduced transmission of HSV-2 genital infections among discordant couples by 50%. A modest effect on herpes labialis (i.e., a reduction of disease duration by 1 day) was seen when valacyclovir was administered upon detection of the first symptom of a lesion at a dose of 2 g every 12 h for 1 day. In AIDS patients, chronic or intermittent administration of acyclovir has been associated with the development of HSV and VZV strains resistant to the action of the drug and with clinical failures. The most common mechanism of resistance is a deficiency of the virus-induced thymidine kinase. Patients with HSV or VZV infections resistant to acyclovir have frequently responded to foscarnet.

With the availability of the oral and IV forms, there are few indications for topical acyclovir, although treatment with this formulation has been modestly beneficial in primary genital HSV infections and in mucocutaneous HSV infections in immunocompromised hosts.

Overall, acyclovir is remarkably well tolerated and is generally free of toxicity. The most frequently encountered form of toxicity is renal dysfunction because of drug crystallization, particularly after rapid IV administration or with inadequate hydration. Central nervous system changes, including lethargy and tremors, are occasionally reported, primarily in immunosuppressed patients. However, whether these changes are related to acyclovir, to concurrent administration of other therapy, or to underlying infection remains unclear. Acyclovir is excreted primarily unmetabolized by the kidneys via both glomerular filtration and tubular secretion. Approximately 15% of a dose of acyclovir is metabolized to 9-([carboxymethoxy]methyl)guanine or other minor metabolites. Reduction in dosage is indicated in patients with a Cr_{Cl} of <50 mL/min. The half-life of acyclovir is ~3 h in normal adults, and the peak plasma concentration after a 1-h infusion of a dose of 5 mg/kg is 9.8 μg/mL. Approximately 22% of an orally administered acyclovir dose is absorbed, and peak plasma concentrations of 0.3–0.9 μg/mL are attained after administration of a 200-mg dose. Acyclovir penetrates relatively well into the cerebrospinal fluid (CSF), with concentrations approaching half of those found in plasma.

Acyclovir causes chromosomal breakage at high doses, but its administration to pregnant women has not been associated with fetal abnormalities. Nonetheless, the potential risks and benefits of acyclovir should be carefully assessed before the drug is used in pregnancy.

Valacyclovir exhibits three to five times greater bioavailability than acyclovir. The concentration-time curve for valacyclovir, given as 1 g PO three times daily, is similar to that for acyclovir, given as 5 mg/kg IV every 8 h. The safety profiles of valacyclovir and acyclovir are similar, although thrombotic thrombocytopenic purpura/hemolytic-uremic syndrome has been reported in immunocompromised patients who have received high doses of valacyclovir (8 g/d). Valacyclovir is approved for the treatment of herpes zoster, of initial and recurrent episodes of genital HSV infection, and of herpes labialis in immunocompetent adults as well as for suppressive treatment of genital herpes. Although it has not been extensively studied in other clinical settings involving HSV or VZV infections, many consultants use valacyclovir rather than oral acyclovir in settings where only the latter has been approved because of valacyclovir's superior pharmacokinetics and more convenient dosing schedule.

CIDOFOVIR

Cidofovir is a phosphonate nucleotide analogue of cytosine. Its major use is in CMV infections, particularly retinitis, but it is active against a broad range of herpesviruses, including HSV, human herpesvirus (HHV) type 6, HHV-8, and certain other DNA viruses such as polyomaviruses, papillomaviruses, adenoviruses, and poxviruses, including variola (smallpox) and vaccinia. Cidofovir does not require initial phosphorylation by virus-induced kinases; the drug is phosphorylated by host cell enzymes to cidofovir diphosphate, which is a competitive inhibitor of viral DNA polymerases and, to a lesser extent, of host cell DNA polymerases.

Incorporation of cidofovir diphosphate slows or terminates nascent DNA chain elongation. Cidofovir is active against HSV isolates that are resistant to acyclovir because of absent or altered thymidine kinase and against CMV isolates that are resistant to ganciclovir because of UL97 phosphotransferase mutations. CMV isolates resistant to ganciclovir on the basis of UL54 mutations are usually resistant to cidofovir as well. Cidofovir is usually active against foscarnet-resistant CMV, although cross-resistance to foscarnet has also been described.

Cidofovir has poor oral availability and is administered intravenously. It is excreted primarily by the kidney and has a plasma half-life of 2.6 h. Cidofovir diphosphate's intracellular half-life of >48 h is the basis for the recommended dosing regimen of 5 mg/kg once a week for the initial 2 weeks and then 5 mg/kg every other week. The major toxic effect of cidofovir is proximal renal tubular injury, as manifested by elevated serum creatinine levels and proteinuria. The risk of nephrotoxicity can be reduced by vigorous saline hydration and by concomitant oral administration of probenecid. Neutropenia, rashes, and gastrointestinal tolerance may also occur.

IV cidofovir has been approved for the treatment of CMV retinitis in AIDS patients who are intolerant of ganciclovir or foscarnet or in whom those drugs have failed. In a controlled study, a maintenance dosage of 5 mg/kg per week administered to AIDS patients reduced the progression of CMV retinitis from that seen at 3 mg/kg. Intravitreal cidofovir has been used to treat CMV retinitis but has been associated with significant toxicity. IV cidofovir has been reported anecdotally to be effective for treatment of acyclovir-resistant mucocutaneous HSV infections. Likewise, topically administered cidofovir is reportedly beneficial against mucocutaneous HSV infections in HIV-infected patients. Anecdotal use of IV cidofovir has been described in disseminated adenoviral infections in immunosuppressed patients and in genitourinary infections with BK virus in renal transplant recipients; however, its efficacy, if any, in these circumstances is not established.

FOMIVIRSEN

Fomivirsen is the first antisense oligonucleotide approved by the FDA for therapy in humans. This phosphorothioate oligonucleotide, 21 nucleotides in length, inhibits CMV replication through interaction with CMV messenger RNA. Fomivirsen is complementary to messenger transcripts of the major immediate early region 2 (IE2) of CMV, which codes for proteins regulating viral gene expression. In addition to its antisense mechanism of action, fomivirsen may exert activity against CMV through inhibition of viral adsorption to cells as well as direct inhibition of viral replication. Because of its different mechanism of action, fomivirsen is active against

CMV isolates that are resistant to nucleoside or nucleotide analogues, such as ganciclovir, foscarnet, or cidofovir.

Fomivirsen has been approved for intravitreal administration in the treatment of CMV retinitis in AIDS patients who have failed to respond to other treatments or cannot tolerate them. Injections of 330 mg for two doses 2 weeks apart, followed by maintenance doses of 330 mg monthly, significantly reduce the rate of progression of CMV retinitis. The major toxicity is ocular inflammation, including vitritis and iritis, which usually responds to topically administered glucocorticoids.

GANCICLOVIR AND VALGANCICLOVIR

An analogue of acyclovir, ganciclovir is active against HSV and VZV and is markedly more active than acyclovir against CMV. Ganciclovir triphosphate inhibits CMV DNA polymerase and can be incorporated into CMV DNA, whose elongation it eventually terminates. In HSV- and VZV-infected cells, ganciclovir is phosphorylated by virus-encoded thymidine kinases; in CMV-infected cells, it is phosphorylated by a viral kinase encoded by the UL97 gene. Ganciclovir triphosphate is present in tenfold higher concentrations in CMV-infected cells than in uninfected cells. Ganciclovir is approved for the treatment of CMV retinitis in immunosuppressed patients and for the prevention of CMV disease in transplant recipients. It is widely used for the treatment of other CMV-associated syndromes, including pneumonia, esophagogastrointestinal infections, hepatitis, and "wasting" illness.

Ganciclovir is available for IV or oral administration. Because its oral bioavailability is low (5–9%), relatively large doses (1 g three times daily) must be administered by this route. Oral ganciclovir has largely been supplanted by valganciclovir, which is the L-valyl ester of ganciclovir. Valganciclovir is well absorbed orally, with a bioavailability of 60%, and is rapidly hydrolyzed to ganciclovir in the intestine and liver. The area under the curve for a 900-mg dose of valganciclovir is equivalent to that for 5 mg/kg of IV ganciclovir, although peak serum concentrations are ~40% lower for valganciclovir. The serum half-life is 3.5 h after IV administration of ganciclovir and 4.0 h after PO administration of valganciclovir. Ganciclovir is excreted primarily by the kidneys in an unmetabolized form, and its dosage should be reduced in cases of renal failure. Ganciclovir therapy at the most commonly employed initial IV dosage—i.e., 5 mg/kg every 12 h for 14–21 days—can be changed to valganciclovir (900 mg PO twice daily) when the patient can tolerate oral therapy. The maintenance dose is 5 mg/kg IV daily or five times per week for ganciclovir and 900 mg by mouth once a day for valganciclovir. Dose adjustment in patients with renal dysfunction is required. Intraocular ganciclovir, given by either intravitreal injection or intraocular implantation, has also been used to treat CMV retinitis.

Ganciclovir is effective as prophylaxis against CMV-associated disease in organ and bone marrow transplant recipients. Oral ganciclovir administered prophylactically to AIDS patients with CD4+ T cell counts of <100/μL has provided protection against the development of CMV retinitis. However, the long-term benefits of this approach to prophylaxis in AIDS patients have not been established, and most experts do not recommend the use of oral ganciclovir for this purpose. As already mentioned, valganciclovir has supplanted oral ganciclovir in settings where oral prophylaxis or therapy is considered.

The administration of ganciclovir has been associated with profound bone marrow suppression, particularly neutropenia, which significantly limits the drug's use in many patients. Bone marrow toxicity is potentiated in the setting of renal dysfunction and when other bone marrow suppressants, such as zidovudine or mycophenolate mofetil, are used concomitantly.

Resistance has been noted in CMV isolates obtained after therapy with ganciclovir, especially in patients with AIDS. Such resistance may develop through a mutation in either the viral UL97 gene or the viral DNA polymerase. Ganciclovir-resistant isolates are usually sensitive to foscarnet (see later) or cidofovir (see earlier).

FAMCICLOVIR AND PENCICLOVIR

Famciclovir is the diacetyl 6-deoxyester of the guanosine analogue penciclovir. Famciclovir is well absorbed orally, has a bioavailability of 77%, and is rapidly converted to penciclovir by deacetylation and oxidation in the intestine and liver. Penciclovir's spectrum of activity and mechanism of action are similar to those of acyclovir. Thus, penciclovir usually is not active against acyclovir-resistant viruses. However, some acyclovir-resistant viruses with altered thymidine kinase or DNA polymerase substrate specificity may be sensitive to penciclovir. This drug is phosphorylated initially by a virus-encoded thymidine kinase and subsequently by cellular kinases to penciclovir triphosphate, which inhibits HSV-1, HSV-2, VZV, and EBV as well as hepatitis B virus (HBV). The serum half-life of penciclovir is 2 h, but the intracellular half-life of penciclovir triphosphate is 7–20 h—markedly longer than that of acyclovir triphosphate. The latter is the basis for the less frequent (twice-daily) dosing schedule for famciclovir than for acyclovir. Penciclovir is eliminated primarily in the urine by both glomerular filtration and tubular secretion. The usually recommended dosage interval should be adjusted for renal insufficiency.

Clinical trials involving immunocompetent adults with herpes zoster showed that famciclovir was superior to placebo in eliciting the resolution of skin lesions and virus shedding and in shortening the duration of postherpetic neuralgia; moreover, administered at 500 mg every 8 h, famciclovir was at least as effective as acyclovir administered at an oral dose of 800 mg five times daily. Famciclovir was also effective in the treatment of herpes zoster in immunosuppressed patients. Clinical trials have demonstrated its effectiveness in the suppression of genital HSV infections for up to 1 year and in the treatment of initial and recurrent episodes of genital herpes. Famciclovir is effective as therapy for mucocutaneous HSV infections in HIV-infected patients. Application of a 1% penciclovir cream reduces the duration of signs and symptoms of herpes labialis in immunocompetent patients (by 0.5–1 day) and has been approved for that purpose by the FDA. Famciclovir is generally well tolerated, with occasional headache, nausea, and diarrhea reported in frequencies similar to those among placebo recipients. The administration of high doses of famciclovir for 2 years was associated with an increased incidence of mammary adenocarcinomas in female rats, but the clinical significance of this effect is unknown.

FOSCARNET

Foscarnet (phosphonoformic acid) is a pyrophosphate-containing compound that potently inhibits herpesviruses, including CMV. This drug inhibits DNA polymerases at the pyrophosphate binding site at concentrations that have relatively little effect on cellular polymerases. Foscarnet does not require phosphorylation to exert its antiviral activity and is therefore active against HSV and VZV isolates that are resistant to acyclovir because of deficiencies in thymidine kinase as well as against most ganciclovir-resistant strains of CMV. Foscarnet also inhibits the reverse transcriptase of HIV and is active against HIV in vivo.

Foscarnet is poorly soluble and must be administered intravenously via an infusion pump in a dilute solution over 1–2 h. The plasma half-life of foscarnet is 3–5 h and increases with decreasing renal function, since the drug is eliminated primarily by the kidneys. It has been estimated that 10–28% of a dose may be deposited in bone, where it can persist for months. The most common initial dosage of foscarnet–60 mg/kg every 8 h for 14–21 days—is followed by a maintenance dose of 90–120 mg/kg once a day.

Foscarnet is approved for the treatment of CMV retinitis in patients with AIDS and of acyclovir-resistant mucocutaneous HSV infections. In a comparative clinical trial, the drug appeared to be about as efficacious as ganciclovir against CMV retinitis but was associated with a longer survival period, possibly because of its activity against HIV. Intraocular foscarnet has been used to treat CMV retinitis. Foscarnet has also been employed to treat acyclovir-resistant HSV and VZV infections as well as ganciclovir-resistant CMV infections, although resistance to foscarnet has been reported in CMV isolates obtained during therapy. Foscarnet has also been used to treat HHV-6 infections in immunosuppressed patients.

The major form of toxicity associated with foscarnet is renal impairment. Thus renal function should be monitored closely, particularly during the initial phase of therapy. Since foscarnet binds divalent metal ions, hypocalcemia, hypomagnesemia, hypokalemia, and hypo- or hyperphosphatemia can develop. Saline hydration and slow infusion appear to protect the patient against nephrotoxicity and electrolyte disturbances. Although hematologic abnormalities have been documented (most commonly anemia), foscarnet is not generally myelosuppressive and can be administered concomitantly with myelosuppressive medications such as zidovudine.

TRIFLURIDINE

Trifluridine is a pyrimidine nucleoside active against HSV-1, HSV-2, and CMV. Trifluridine monophosphate irreversibly inhibits thymidylate synthetase, and trifluridine triphosphate inhibits viral and, to a lesser extent, cellular DNA polymerases. Because of systemic toxicity, its use is limited to topical therapy. Trifluridine is approved for treatment of HSV keratitis, against which trials have shown that it is more effective than topical idoxuridine but similar in efficacy to topical vidarabine. The drug has benefited some patients with HSV keratitis who have failed to respond to idoxuridine or vidarabine. Topical application of trifluridine to sites of acyclovir-resistant HSV mucocutaneous infections has also been beneficial in some cases.

VIDARABINE

Vidarabine is a purine nucleoside analogue with activity against HSV-1, HSV-2, VZV, and EBV. Vidarabine inhibits viral DNA synthesis through its 5′-triphosphorylated metabolite, although its precise molecular mechanisms of action are not completely understood. IV-administered vidarabine has been shown to be effective in the treatment of herpes simplex encephalitis, mucocutaneous HSV infections, herpes zoster in immunocompromised patients, and neonatal HSV infections. Its use has been supplanted by that of IV acyclovir, which is more effective and easier to administer. Production of the IV preparation has been discontinued by the manufacturer, but vidarabine is available as an ophthalmic ointment, which is effective in the treatment of HSV keratitis.

ANTIVIRAL DRUGS ACTIVE AGAINST HEPATITIS VIRUSES

LAMIVUDINE

Lamivudine is a pyrimidine nucleoside analogue that is used primarily in combination therapy against HIV infection. Its activity against hepatitis B virus (HBV) is attributable to inhibition of the viral DNA polymerase. This drug has also been approved for the treatment of chronic HBV infection. At doses of 100 mg/d given for 1 year to patients positive for hepatitis B e antigen (HBeAg), lamivudine is well tolerated and results in suppression of HBV DNA levels, normalization of serum aminotransferase levels in 40–75% of patients, and reduction of hepatic inflammation and fibrosis in 50–60% of patients. Loss of HBeAg occurs in 30% of patients. Lamivudine also appears to be useful in the prevention or suppression of HBV infection associated with liver transplantation. Resistance to lamivudine develops in 24% of patients treated for 1 year and is associated with changes in the YMDD motif of HBV DNA polymerase. Because of the frequency of development of resistance, lamivudine has been largely supplanted by less-resistance-prone drugs for the treatment of HBV infection.

ADEFOVIR DIPIVOXIL

Adefovir dipivoxil is the oral prodrug of adefovir, an acyclic nucleotide analogue of adenosine monophosphate that has activity against HBV, HIV, HSV, CMV, and poxviruses. It is phosphorylated by cellular kinases to the active triphosphate moiety, which is a competitive inhibitor of HBV DNA polymerase and results in chain termination after incorporation into nascent viral DNA. Adefovir is administered orally and is eliminated primarily by the kidneys, with a plasma half-life of 5–7.5 h. In clinical studies, therapy with adefovir at a dose of 10 mg/d for 48 weeks resulted in normalization of serum alanine aminotransferase (ALT) levels in 48–72% of patients and improved liver histology in 53–64%; it also resulted in a 3.5- to 3.9-$\log_{10}$ reduction in the number of HBV DNA copies per milliliter of plasma. Adefovir was effective in treatment-naïve patients as well as in those infected with lamivudine-resistant HBV. Resistance to adefovir appears to develop less readily than that to lamivudine, but adefovir resistance rates of 15–18% have been reported after 192 weeks of treatment and may reach 30% after 5 years. This agent is generally well tolerated. Significant nephrotoxicity attributable to adefovir is uncommon at the dose employed in the treatment of HBV infections (10 mg/d) but is a treatment-limiting adverse effect at the higher doses used in therapy for HIV infections (30–120 mg/d).

In any case, renal function should be monitored in patients taking adefovir, even at the lower dose. Adefovir is approved only for treatment of chronic HBV infection.

TENOFOVIR

Tenofovir disoproxil fumarate is a prodrug of tenofovir, a nucleotide analogue of adenosine monophosphate with activity against both retroviruses and hepadnaviruses. In both immunocompetent and immunocompromised patients (including those co-infected with HIV and HBV), tenofovir given at a dose of 300 mg/d for 48 weeks reduced HBV replication by 4.6–6 $\log_{10}$, normalized ALT levels in 68–76% of patients, and improved liver histopathology in 72–74% of patients. Resistance develops uncommonly during ≥2 years of therapy, and tenofovir is active against lamivudine-resistant HBV. The safety profile of tenofovir is similar to that of adefovir, but nephrotoxicity has not been encountered at the dose used for HBV therapy. Tenofovir is approved for the treatment of HIV and chronic HBV infections.

ENTECAVIR

Entecavir is a cyclopentyl 2′-deoxyguanosine analogue that inhibits HBV through interaction of entecavir triphosphate with several HBV DNA polymerase functions. At a dose of 0.5 mg/d given for 48 weeks, entecavir reduced HBV DNA copies by 5.0–6.9 $\log_{10}$, normalized serum aminotransferase levels in 68–78% of patients, and improved histopathology in 70–72% of patients. Entecavir inhibits lamivudine-resistant viruses that have M550I or M550V/L526M mutations but only at serum concentrations 20- or 30-fold higher than those obtained with the 0.5-mg/d dose. Thus, higher doses of entecavir (1 mg/d) are recommended for the treatment of patients infected with lamivudine-resistant HBV. Development of resistance to entecavir is uncommon in treatment-naïve patients but does occur at unacceptably high rates (43% after 4 years) in patients previously infected with lamivudine-resistant virus. Entecavir-resistant strains appear to be sensitive to adefovir and tenofovir.

Entecavir is highly bioavailable but should be taken on an empty stomach since food interferes with its absorption. The drug is eliminated primarily in unchanged form by the kidneys, and its dosage should be adjusted for patients with Cr_{Cl} values of <50 mL/min. Overall, entecavir is well tolerated, with a safety profile similar to that of lamivudine. As with other anti-HBV treatments, exacerbation of hepatitis may occur when entecavir therapy is stopped. Entecavir is approved for treatment of chronic hepatitis B, including infection with lamivudine-resistant viruses, in adults.

Entecavir has some activity against HIV-1 (median effective concentration, 0.026 to >10 μM) but should not be used as monotherapy in HIV-positive patients because of the potential for development of HIV resistance due to the M184V mutation.

TELBIVUDINE

Telbivudine is a β-L enantiomer of thymidine and is a potent, selective inhibitor of HBV. Its active form is telbivudine triphosphate, which inhibits HBV DNA polymerase and causes chain termination but has little or no activity against human DNA polymerase. Administration of telbivudine at an oral dose of 600 mg/d for 52 weeks to patients with chronic hepatitis B resulted in reduction of HBV DNA by 5.2–6.4 $\log_{10}$ copies/mL along with normalization of ALT levels in 74–77% of recipients and improved histopathology in 65–67% of patients. Telbivudine-resistant HBV is generally cross-resistant with lamivudine-resistant virus but is usually susceptible to adefovir. After 2 years of therapy, resistance to telbivudine was noted in isolates from 22% of HBeAg-positive patients and in those from 9% of HBeAg-negative patients.

Orally administered telbivudine is rapidly absorbed; because it is eliminated primarily by the kidneys, its dosage should be reduced in patients with a Cr_{Cl} value of <50 mL/min. Telbivudine is generally well tolerated, but increases in serum levels of creatinine kinases as well as fatigue and myalgias have been observed. As with other anti-HBV drugs, hepatitis may be exacerbated in patients who discontinue telbivudine therapy. Telbivudine has been approved for the treatment of adults with chronic hepatitis B who have evidence of viral replication and either persistently elevated serum aminotransferase levels or histopathologically active disease, but it has not been widely used because of the frequency of development of resistance noted earlier.

INTERFERONS

IFNs are cytokines that exhibit a broad spectrum of antiviral activities as well as immunomodulating and antiproliferative properties. IFNs are not available for oral administration but must be given IM, SC, or IV. Early studies with human leukocyte IFN demonstrated an effect in the prophylaxis of experimentally induced rhinovirus infections in humans and in the treatment of VZV infections in immunosuppressed patients. DNA recombinant technology has made available highly purified α, β, and γ IFNs that have been evaluated in a variety of viral infections. Results of such trials have confirmed the effectiveness of intranasally administered IFN in the prophylaxis of rhinovirus infections, although its use has been associated with nasal mucosal irritation. Studies have also demonstrated a beneficial effect of intralesionally or systemically administered IFNs on genital warts. The effect of systemic administration consists primarily of a reduction in the size of the warts, and this mode of therapy may be useful in persons who have numerous warts that cannot easily be treated by individual intralesional injections. However, lesions frequently recur after either intralesional or systemic IFN therapy is discontinued.

IFNs have undergone extensive study in the treatment of chronic HBV infection. The administration of standard IFN-α2b (5 million units daily or 10 million units three times a week for 16–24 weeks) to patients with stable chronic HBV infection resulted in loss of markers of HBV replication, such as HBeAg and HBV DNA, in 33–37% of cases; 8% of patients also became negative for hepatitis B surface antigen. In most patients who lose HBeAg and HBV DNA markers, serum aminotransferases return to normal levels, and both short- and long-term improvements in liver histopathology have been described. Predictors of a favorable response to standard IFN therapy include low pretherapy levels of HBV DNA, high pretherapy serum levels of ALT, a short duration of chronic HBV infection, and active inflammation in liver histopathology. Poor responses are seen in immunosuppressed patients, including those with HIV infection.

In pegylated IFNs, IFN alphas are linked to polyethylene glycol. This linkage results in slower absorption, decreased clearance, and more sustained serum concentrations, thereby permitting a more convenient, once-weekly dosing schedule; in many instances, pegylated IFN has supplanted standard IFN. After 48 weeks of treatment with 180 μg of pegylated IFN-α2a, HBV DNA was reduced by 4.1–4.5 $\log_{10}$ copies/mL, with normalization of serum ALT levels in 39% of patients and improved histology in 38%. Response rates were somewhat higher when lamivudine was administered with pegylated IFN-α2a. Adverse effects of IFN are common and include fever, chills, myalgia, fatigue, neurotoxicity (manifested primarily as somnolence, depression, anxiety, and confusion), and leukopenia. Autoantibodies (e.g., antithyroid antibodies) can also develop. IFN-α2b and pegylated IFN-α2a are approved for the treatment of patients with chronic hepatitis B. Data supporting the therapeutic efficacy of pegylated interferon-α2b in HBV infection have been published; the drug has not been approved for this indication in the United States but has been approved for treatment of chronic HBV infection in other countries.

Several IFN preparations, including IFN-α2a, IFN-α2b, IFN-alfacon-1, and IFN-αm1 (lymphoblastoid), have been studied as therapy for chronic HCV infections. A variety of monotherapy regimens have been studied, of which the most common for standard IFN is IFN-α2b or -α2a at 3 million units three times per week for 12–18 months. The addition of oral ribavirin to IFN-α2b—either as initial therapy or after failure of IFN therapy alone—results in significantly higher rates of sustained virologic and/or serum ALT responses (40–50%) than are obtained with monotherapy. Comparative studies indicate that pegylated IFN-α2b or -α2a therapy is more effective than standard IFN treatment against chronic HCV infection. The combination of SC pegylated IFN and oral ribavirin is more convenient and appears to be the most effective regimen for treatment of chronic hepatitis C. With this combination regimen, sustained virologic responses (SVRs) were seen in 42–51% of patients with genotype 1 infection and in 76–82% of patients with genotype 2 or 3 infection. Ribavirin appears to have a small antiviral effect in HCV infection but may also be working through an immunomodulatory effect in combination with IFN. Optimal results with ribavirin appear to be associated with weight-based dosing. Prognostic factors for a favorable response include an age of <40 years, a short duration of infection, low levels of HCV RNA, a lesser degree of liver histopathology, and infection with HCV genotypes other than 1. IFN-alfacon, a synthetic "consensus" α interferon, appears to produce response rates similar to those elicited by standard IFN-α2a or -α2b alone and is also approved in the United States for the treatment of chronic hepatitis C.

The efficacy of IFN-α treatment for chronic hepatitis D remains unestablished. Anecdotal reports suggested that doses ranging from 5 million units daily to 9 million units three times per week for 12 months elicit biochemical and virologic responses. Results from small controlled trials have been inconsistent, and observed responses have not generally been sustained. Limited experience has been published with the use of pegylated IFN-α2a or -α2b for treatment of hepatitis D, but some consultants prefer these agents for this indication because of their pharmacologic advantages over standard IFN.

PROTEASE INHIBITORS

This drug class is specifically designed to inhibit the 3/4A (NS3/4A) HCV protease. These agents resemble the HCV polypeptide and, when processed by the viral protease, form a covalent bond with the catalytic serine residues and block further activity. The most clinically advanced compound in this class is telaprevir. In initial phase 1 and 2 clinical studies, telaprevir monotherapy decreased the HCV load by 2–5 $\log_{10}$. Telaprevir in combination with IFN and ribavirin increased the SVR rate from ~40% to 60% when used as primary therapy for genotype 1 infections. For re-treatment of HCV-infected patients in whom prior IFN/ribavirin therapy had failed, the addition of telaprevir plus pegylated IFN/ribavirin increased the SVR rate to 51–53%. The combination of telaprevir/pegylated IFN and ribavirin is superior to this combination without ribavirin. Typically, an oral loading dose of 1125 mg is followed by 750 mg every 8 h orally for 12–24 weeks. Monotherapy is associated with the rapid emergence of antiviral resistance; substitutions are found in the NS3 protease, especially double variants at positions V35M and R155K. Telaprevir therapy is associated with rashes in ~50% of patients; these eruptions are severe in ~5% of cases and often develop weeks after therapy has begun. Data suggest that telaprevir has the potential to increase the SVR rate and may shorten the overall duration of HCV therapy from 48 to 24 weeks when used in conjunction with pegylated IFN and ribavirin. As of this writing (February 2011), protease inhibitors have not been approved for treatment of HCV.

CHAPTER 42

DIAGNOSIS AND TREATMENT OF FUNGAL INFECTIONS

John E. Edwards, Jr.

TERMINOLOGY AND MICROBIOLOGY

Traditionally, fungal infections have been classified into specific categories based on both anatomic location and epidemiology. The most common general anatomic categories are mucocutaneous and deep organ infection; the most common general epidemiologic categories are endemic and opportunistic. Although *mucocutaneous infections* can cause serious morbidity, they are rarely fatal. *Deep organ infections* also cause severe illness in many cases and, in contrast to mucocutaneous infections, are often fatal. The *endemic mycoses* (e.g., coccidioidomycosis) are infections caused by fungal organisms that are not part of the normal human microbial flora and are acquired from environmental sources. In contrast, *opportunistic mycoses* are caused by organisms (e.g., *Candida* and *Aspergillus*) that commonly are components of the normal human flora and whose ubiquity in nature renders them easily acquired by the immunocompromised host. Opportunistic fungi cause serious infections when the immunologic response of the host becomes ineffective, allowing the organisms to transition from harmless commensals to invasive pathogens. Frequently, the diminished effectiveness of the immune system is a result of advanced modern therapies that coincidentally either unbalance the host's microflora or directly interfere with immunologic responses. Endemic mycoses cause more severe illness in immunocompromised patients than in immunocompetent individuals.

Patients acquire deep organ infection with endemic fungi almost exclusively by inhalation. Cutaneous infections result either from hematogenous dissemination or, more often, from direct contact with soil—the natural reservoir for the vast majority of endemic mycoses. The dermatophytic fungi may be acquired by human-to-human transmission, but the majority of infections result from environmental contact. In contrast, the opportunistic fungus *Candida* invades the host from normal sites of colonization, usually the mucous membranes of the gastrointestinal tract. In general, innate immunity is the primary defense mechanism against fungi. Although antibodies are formed during many fungal infections (and even during commensalism), they generally do not constitute the primary mode of defense. Nevertheless, in selected infections, as discussed later, measurement of antibody titers may be a useful diagnostic test.

Three other terms frequently used in clinical discussions of fungal infections are *yeast*, *mold*, and *dimorphic fungus*. *Yeasts* are seen as rounded single cells or as budding organisms. *Candida* and *Cryptococcus* are traditionally classified as yeasts. *Molds* grow as filamentous forms called *hyphae* both at room temperature and in invaded tissue. *Aspergillus*, *Rhizopus* (the species that causes mucormycosis [zygomycosis]), and fungi commonly infecting the skin to cause ringworm and related cutaneous conditions are classified as molds. Variations occur within this classification of yeasts and molds. For instance, when *Candida* infects tissue, both yeasts and filamentous forms may occur (except with *C. glabrata*, which forms only yeasts in tissue); in contrast, *Cryptococcus* exists only in yeast form. *Dimorphic* is the term used to describe fungi that grow as yeasts or large spherical structures in tissue but as filamentous forms at room temperature in the environment. Classified in this group are the organisms causing blastomycosis, paracoccidioidomycosis, coccidioidomycosis, histoplasmosis, and sporotrichosis.

The incidence of nearly all fungal infections has risen substantially. Opportunistic infections have increased in frequency as a consequence of intentional immunosuppression in organ and stem cell transplantation and other diseases, the administration of cytotoxic chemotherapy for cancers, and the liberal use of antibacterial agents. The incidence of endemic mycoses has increased in geographic locations where there has been substantial population growth.

DIAGNOSIS

The definitive diagnosis of any fungal infection requires histopathologic identification of the fungus invading tissue, accompanied by evidence of an inflammatory response. The identification of an inflammatory response has been especially important with regard to *Aspergillus* infection. *Aspergillus* is ubiquitous and can float from the air onto biopsy material. Therefore, in rare but important instances, this fungus is an ex vivo contaminant during processing of a specimen for microscopy, with a consequent incorrect diagnosis. The stains most commonly used to identify fungi are periodic acid–Schiff and Gomori methenamine silver. *Candida*, unlike other fungi, is visible on gram-stained tissue smears. Hematoxylin and eosin stain is not sufficient to identify *Candida* in tissue specimens. When positive, an India ink preparation of cerebrospinal fluid (CSF) is diagnostic for cryptococcosis. Most laboratories now use calcofluor white staining coupled with fluorescent microscopy to identify fungi in fluid specimens.

Extensive investigations of the diagnosis of deep organ fungal infections have yielded a variety of tests with different degrees of specificity and sensitivity. The most reliable tests are the detection of antibody to *Coccidioides immitis* in serum and CSF; of *Histoplasma capsulatum* antigen in urine, serum, and CSF; and of cryptococcal polysaccharide antigen in serum and CSF. These tests have a general sensitivity and specificity of 90%; however, because there is variability among laboratories, testing on multiple occasions is advisable. The test for galactomannan has been used extensively in Europe and is now approved in the United States for diagnosis of aspergillosis. Sources of concern regarding galactomannan are the incidence of false-negative results and the need for multiple serial tests to reduce this incidence. The β-glucan test for *Candida* is also under evaluation but, like the galactomannan test, requires additional validation; this test has a negative predictive value of ~90%. Numerous polymerase chain reaction assays to detect antigens are in the developmental stages, as are nucleic acid hybridization techniques.

Of the fungal organisms, *Candida* is by far the most frequently recovered from blood. Although *Candida* species can be detected with any of the automated blood culture systems widely used at present, the lysis-centrifugation technique increases the sensitivity of blood cultures for *Candida* and for less common organisms (e.g., *H. capsulatum*). Lysis-centrifugation should be used when disseminated fungal infection is suspected.

Except in the cases of coccidioidomycosis, cryptococcosis, and histoplasmosis, there are no fully validated

and widely used tests for serodiagnosis of disseminated fungal infection. Skin tests for the endemic mycoses are no longer available.

TREATMENT	Fungal Infections

This discussion is intended as a brief overview of general strategies for the use of antifungal agents in the treatment of fungal infections. Regimens, schedules, and strategies are detailed in the chapters on specific mycoses that follow in this section.

Since fungal organisms are eukaryotic cells that contain most of the same organelles (with many of the same physiologic functions) as human cells, the identification of drugs that selectively kill or inhibit fungi but are not toxic to human cells has been highly problematic. Far fewer antifungal than antibacterial agents have been introduced into clinical medicine.

AMPHOTERICIN B The introduction of amphotericin B (AmB) in the late 1950s revolutionized the treatment of fungal infections in deep organs. Before AmB became available, cryptococcal meningitis and other disseminated fungal infections were nearly always fatal. For nearly a decade after AmB was introduced, it was the only effective agent for the treatment of life-threatening fungal infections. AmB remains the broadest-spectrum antifungal agent but carries several disadvantages, including significant nephrotoxicity, lack of an oral preparation, and unpleasant side effects (fever, chills, and nausea) during treatment. To circumvent nephrotoxicity and infusion side effects, lipid formulations of AmB were developed and have virtually replaced the original colloidal deoxycholate formulation in clinical use (although the older formulation is still available). The lipid formulations include liposomal AmB (L-AmB; 3–5 mg/kg per day) and AmB lipid complex (ABLC; 5 mg/kg per day). A third preparation, AmB colloidal dispersion (ABCD; 3–4 mg/kg per day), is rarely used because of the high incidence of side effects associated with infusion. (The doses listed are standard doses for adults with invasive infection.)

The lipid formulations of AmB have the disadvantage of being considerably more expensive than the deoxycholate formulation. Experience is still accumulating on the comparative efficacy, toxicity, and advantages of the different formulations for specific clinical fungal infections (e.g., central nervous system [CNS] infection). Whether there is a clinically significant difference in these drugs with respect to CNS penetration or nephrotoxicity remains controversial. Despite these issues and despite the expense, the lipid formulations are now much more commonly used than AmB deoxycholate in developed countries. In developing countries, AmB deoxycholate is still preferred because of the expense of the lipid formulations.

AZOLES This class of antifungal drugs offers important advantages over AmB: The azoles cause little or no nephrotoxicity and are available in oral preparations. Early azoles included ketoconazole and miconazole, which have been replaced by newer agents for the treatment of deep organ fungal infections. The azoles' mechanism of action is inhibition of ergosterol synthesis in the fungal cell wall. Unlike AmB, these drugs are considered fungistatic, not fungicidal.

Fluconazole Since its introduction, fluconazole has played an extremely important role in the treatment of a wide variety of serious fungal infections. Its major advantages are the availability of both oral and IV formulations, a long half-life, satisfactory penetration of most body fluids (including ocular fluid and CSF), and minimal toxicity (especially relative to that of AmB). Its disadvantages include (usually reversible) hepatotoxicity and—at high doses—alopecia, muscle weakness, and dry mouth with a metallic taste. Fluconazole is not effective for the treatment of aspergillosis, mucormycosis, or *Scedosporium apiospermum* infections. It is less effective than the newer azoles against *C. glabrata* and *C. krusei*.

Fluconazole has become the agent of choice for the treatment of coccidioidal meningitis, although relapses have followed therapy with this drug. In addition, fluconazole is useful for both consolidation and maintenance therapy for cryptococcal meningitis. This agent has been shown to be as efficacious as AmB in the treatment of candidemia. The effectiveness of fluconazole in candidemia and the drug's relatively minimal toxicity, in conjunction with the inadequacy of diagnostic tests for widespread hematogenously disseminated candidiasis, have led to a change in the paradigm for candidemia management. The standard of care is now to treat all candidemic patients with an antifungal agent and to change all their intravascular lines, if feasible, rather than merely to remove a singular suspect intravascular line and then observe the patient. The usual fluconazole regimen for treatment of candidemia is 400 mg/d given until 2 weeks after the last positive blood culture.

Fluconazole is considered effective as fungal prophylaxis in bone marrow transplant recipients and high-risk liver transplant patients. Its general use for prophylaxis in patients with leukemia, in AIDS patients with low CD4+ T cell counts, and in patients on surgical intensive care units remains controversial.

Voriconazole Voriconazole, which is available in both oral and IV formulations, has a broader spectrum than fluconazole against *Candida* species (including *C. glabrata* and *C. krusei*) and is active against *Aspergillus*, *Scedosporium*, and *Fusarium*. It is generally considered the first-line drug of choice for treatment of aspergillosis. A few case reports have shown voriconazole to be effective in individual patients with coccidioidomycosis, blastomycosis, and histoplasmosis, but because of limited data this agent is not recommended for treatment of the endemic mycoses. Among the disadvantages of voriconazole (compared with fluconazole) are its more numerous interactions with many of the drugs used in patients predisposed to fungal infections. Hepatotoxicity, skin rashes (including photosensitivity), and visual disturbances are relatively common. Skin cancer surveillance is now recommended for patients taking voriconazole. Voriconazole is also considerably more expensive than fluconazole. Moreover, it is advisable to monitor voriconazole levels in certain patients since (1) this drug is completely metabolized in the liver by CYP2C9, CYP3A4, and CYP2C19; and (2) human genetic variability in CYP2C19 activity exists. Dosages should be reduced accordingly in those patients with liver failure. Dose adjustments for renal insufficiency are not necessary; however, because the IV formulation is prepared in cyclodextrin, it should not be given to patients with severe renal insufficiency.

Itraconazole Itraconazole is available in IV and oral (capsule and suspension) formulations. Varying blood levels among patients taking oral itraconazole reflect a disadvantage compared with the other azoles. Itraconazole is the drug of choice for mild to moderate histoplasmosis and blastomycosis and has often been used for chronic mucocutaneous candidiasis. It has been approved by the U.S. Food and Drug Administration (FDA) for use in febrile neutropenic patients. Itraconazole has also proved useful for the treatment of chronic coccidioidomycosis, sporotrichosis, and *S. apiospermum* infection. The mucocutaneous and cutaneous fungal infections that have been treated successfully with itraconazole include oropharyngeal candidiasis (especially in AIDS patients), tinea versicolor, tinea capitis, and onychomycosis. Disadvantages of itraconazole include its poor penetration into CSF, the use of cyclodextrin in both the oral suspension and the IV preparation, the variable absorption of the drug in capsule form, and the need for monitoring of blood levels in patients taking capsules for disseminated mycoses. Reported cases of severe congestive heart failure in patients taking itraconazole have been a source of concern. Like the other azoles, itraconazole can cause hepatic toxicity.

Posaconazole Posaconazole is approved by the FDA for prophylaxis of aspergillosis and candidiasis in patients at high risk for developing these infections because of severe immunocompromise. It has also been approved for the treatment of oropharyngeal candidiasis and has been evaluated for the treatment of zygomycosis, fusariosis, aspergillosis, cryptococcosis, and various other forms of candidal infection. The relevant studies of posaconazole in zygomycosis, fusariosis, and aspergillosis have examined salvage therapy. A study of >90 patients whose zygomycosis was refractory to other therapy yielded encouraging results. No trials of posaconazole for the treatment of candidemia have yet been reported. Case reports have described the drug's efficacy in coccidioidomycosis and histoplasmosis. Controlled trials have shown its effectiveness as a prophylactic agent in patients with acute leukemia and in bone marrow transplant recipients. In addition, posaconazole has been found to be effective against fluconazole-resistant *Candida* species. The results of a large-scale study of the use of posaconazole as salvage therapy for aspergillosis indicated that it is an alternative to other agents for salvage therapy; however, that study predated the use of voriconazole and the echinocandins.

ECHINOCANDINS The echinocandins, including the FDA-approved drugs caspofungin, anidulafungin, and micafungin, have added considerably to the antifungal armamentarium. All three of these agents inhibit β-1,3-glucan synthase, which is necessary for cell wall synthesis in fungi and is not a component of human cells. None of these agents is currently available in an oral formulation. The echinocandins are considered fungicidal for *Candida* and fungistatic for *Aspergillus*. Their greatest use to date is against candidal infections. They offer two advantages: broad-spectrum activity against all *Candida* species and relatively low toxicity. The minimal inhibitory concentrations (MICs) of all the echinocandins are highest against *C. parapsilosis*; it is not clear whether these higher MIC values represent less clinical effectiveness against this species. The echinocandins are among the safest antifungal agents.

In controlled trials, *caspofungin* has been at least as efficacious as AmB for the treatment of candidemia and invasive candidiasis and as efficacious as fluconazole for the treatment of candidal esophagitis. In addition, caspofungin has been efficacious as salvage therapy for aspergillosis. *Anidulafungin* has been approved by the FDA as therapy for candidemia in nonneutropenic patients and for *Candida* esophagitis, intraabdominal infection, and peritonitis. In controlled trials, anidulafungin has been shown to be noninferior and possibly superior to fluconazole against candidemia and invasive candidiasis. It is as efficacious as fluconazole against candidal esophagitis. When anidulafungin is used with cyclosporine, tacrolimus, or voriconazole, no dosage adjustment is required for either drug in the combination. *Micafungin* has been approved for the treatment of esophageal candidiasis and candidemia and for prophylaxis in patients receiving stem cell transplants. In a head-to-head trial, micafungin was noninferior to caspofungin for the treatment of candidemia. Studies thus far have shown that coadministration of micafungin and cyclosporine does not require dose adjustments for either drug. When micafungin is given with sirolimus, the AUC rises for sirolimus, usually necessitating a reduction in its dose. In open-label trials, favorable results have been obtained with micafungin for the treatment of deep-seated *Aspergillus* and *Candida* infections.

FLUCYTOSINE (5-FLUOROCYTOSINE) The use of flucytosine has diminished as newer antifungal drugs have been developed. Flucytosine has a unique mechanism of action based on intrafungal conversion to 5-fluorouracil, which is toxic to the fungal cell. Development of resistance to the compound has limited its use as a single agent. Flucytosine is nearly always used in combination with AmB. Its good penetration into the CSF makes it attractive for use with AmB for treatment of cryptococcal meningitis. Flucytosine has also been recommended for the treatment of candidal meningitis in combination with AmB; comparative trials with AmB alone have not been done. Significant and frequent bone marrow depression is seen with flucytosine when this drug is used with AmB.

GRISEOFULVIN AND TERBINAFINE Historically, griseofulvin has been useful primarily for ringworm infection. This agent is usually given for relatively long periods. Terbinafine has been used primarily for onychomycosis but also for ringworm. In comparative studies, terbinafine has been as effective as itraconazole and more effective than griseofulvin for both conditions.

TOPICAL ANTIFUNGAL AGENTS A detailed discussion of the agents used for the treatment of cutaneous fungal infections and onychomycosis is beyond the scope of this chapter; the reader is referred to the dermatology literature. Many classes of compounds have been used to treat the common fungal infections of the skin. Among the azoles used are clotrimazole, econazole, miconazole, oxiconazole, sulconazole, ketoconazole, tioconazole, butoconazole, and terconazole. In general, topical treatment of vaginal candidiasis has been successful. Since there is considered to be little difference in the efficacy of the various vaginal preparations, the choice of agent is made by the physician and/or the patient on the basis of preference and availability. Fluconazole given orally at 150 mg has the advantage of not requiring repeated intravaginal application. Nystatin is a polyene that has been used for both oropharyngeal thrush and vaginal candidiasis. Useful agents in other classes include ciclopirox olamine, haloprogin, terbinafine, naftifine, tolnaftate, and undecylenic acid.

CHAPTER 43
ONCOLOGIC EMERGENCIES

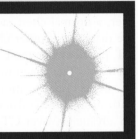

Rasim Gucalp ■ Janice Dutcher

Emergencies in patients with cancer may be classified into three groups: pressure or obstruction caused by a space-occupying lesion, metabolic or hormonal problems (paraneoplastic syndromes), and treatment-related complications.

STRUCTURAL-OBSTRUCTIVE ONCOLOGIC EMERGENCIES

SUPERIOR VENA CAVA SYNDROME

Superior vena cava syndrome (SVCS) is the clinical manifestation of superior vena cava (SVC) obstruction, with severe reduction in venous return from the head, neck, and upper extremities. Malignant tumors, such as lung cancer, lymphoma, and metastatic tumors, are responsible for the majority of SVCS cases. With the expanding use of intravascular devices (e.g., permanent central venous access catheters, pacemaker/defibrillator leads), the prevalence of benign causes of SVCS is increasing now, accounting for at least 40% of cases. Lung cancer, particularly of small cell and squamous cell histologies, accounts for approximately 85% of all cases of malignant origin. In young adults, malignant lymphoma is a leading cause of SVCS. Hodgkin's lymphoma involves the mediastinum more commonly than other lymphomas but rarely causes SVCS. When SVCS is noted in a young man with a mediastinal mass, the differential diagnosis is lymphoma vs primary mediastinal germ cell tumor. Metastatic cancers to the mediastinum, such as testicular and breast carcinomas, account for a small proportion of cases. Other causes include benign tumors, aortic aneurysm, thyromegaly, thrombosis, and fibrosing mediastinitis from prior irradiation, histoplasmosis, or Behçet's syndrome. SVCS as the initial manifestation of Behçet's syndrome may be due to inflammation of the SVC associated with thrombosis.

Patients with SVCS usually present with neck and facial swelling (especially around the eyes), dyspnea, and cough. Other symptoms include hoarseness, tongue swelling, headaches, nasal congestion, epistaxis, hemoptysis, dysphagia, pain, dizziness, syncope, and lethargy. Bending forward or lying down may aggravate the symptoms. The characteristic physical findings are dilated neck veins; an increased number of collateral veins covering the anterior chest wall; cyanosis; and edema of the face, arms, and chest. More severe cases include proptosis, glossal and laryngeal edema, and obtundation. The clinical picture is milder if the obstruction is located above the azygos vein. Symptoms are usually progressive, but in some cases they may improve as collateral circulation develops.

Signs and symptoms of cerebral and/or laryngeal edema, though rare, are associated with a poorer prognosis and require urgent evaluation. Seizures are more likely related to brain metastases than to cerebral edema from venous occlusion. Patients with small cell lung cancer and SVCS have a higher incidence of brain metastases than those without SVCS.

Cardiorespiratory symptoms at rest, particularly with positional changes, suggest significant airway and vascular obstruction and limited physiologic reserve. Cardiac arrest or respiratory failure can occur, particularly in patients receiving sedatives or undergoing general anesthesia.

Rarely, esophageal varices may develop. These are "downhill" varices based on the direction of blood flow from cephalad to caudad (in contrast to "uphill" varices associated with caudad to cephalad flow from portal hypertension). If the obstruction to the SVC is proximal to the azygous vein, varices develop in the upper one-third of the esophagus. If the obstruction involves or is distal to the azygous vein, varices occur in the entire length of the esophagus. Variceal bleeding may be a late complication of chronic SVCS.

The diagnosis of SVCS is a clinical one. The most significant chest radiographic finding is widening of the superior mediastinum, most commonly on the right side. Pleural effusion occurs in only 25% of patients, often on the right side. The majority of these effusions are exudative and occasionally chylous. However, a normal chest radiograph is still compatible with the diagnosis if other characteristic findings are present. CT provides the most reliable view of the mediastinal anatomy. The diagnosis of SVCS requires diminished or absent opacification of central venous structures with prominent collateral venous circulation. MRI has no advantages over CT. Invasive procedures, including bronchoscopy, percutaneous needle biopsy, mediastinoscopy, and even thoracotomy, can be performed by a skilled clinician without any major risk of bleeding. For patients with a known cancer, a detailed workup usually is not necessary, and appropriate treatment may be started after obtaining a CT scan of the thorax. For those with no history of malignancy, a detailed evaluation is essential to rule out benign causes and determine a specific diagnosis to direct the appropriate therapy.

TREATMENT Superior Vena Cava Syndrome

The one potentially life-threatening complication of a superior mediastinal mass is tracheal obstruction. Upper airway obstruction demands emergent therapy. Diuretics with a low-salt diet, head elevation, and oxygen may produce temporary symptomatic relief. Glucocorticoids may be useful at shrinking lymphoma masses; they are of no benefit in patients with lung cancer.

Radiation therapy is the primary treatment for SVCS caused by non-small cell lung cancer and other metastatic solid tumors. Chemotherapy is effective when the underlying cancer is small cell carcinoma of the lung, lymphoma, or germ cell tumor. SVCS recurs in 10–30% of patients; it may be palliated with the use of intravascular self-expanding stents (Fig. 43-1). Early stenting may be necessary in patients with severe symptoms; however, the prompt increase in venous return after stenting may precipitate heart failure and pulmonary edema. Surgery may provide immediate relief for patients in whom a benign process is the cause.

Clinical improvement occurs in most patients, although this improvement may be due to the development of adequate collateral circulation. The mortality associated with SVCS does not relate to caval obstruction but rather to the underlying cause.

SVCS AND CENTRAL VENOUS CATHETERS IN ADULTS The use of long-term central venous catheters has become common practice in patients with cancer. Major vessel thrombosis may occur. In these cases, catheter removal should be combined with anticoagulation to prevent embolization. SVCS in this setting, if detected early, can be treated by fibrinolytic therapy without sacrificing the catheter. The routine use of low-dose warfarin or low-molecular-weight heparin to prevent thrombosis related to permanent central venous access catheters in cancer patients is not recommended.

PERICARDIAL EFFUSION/TAMPONADE

Malignant pericardial disease is found at autopsy in 5–10% of patients with cancer, most frequently with lung cancer, breast cancer, leukemias, and lymphomas. Cardiac tamponade as the initial presentation of extrathoracic malignancy is rare. The origin is not malignancy in about 50% of cancer patients with symptomatic pericardial disease, but it can be related to irradiation, drug-induced pericarditis, hypothyroidism, idiopathic pericarditis, infection, or autoimmune diseases. Two types of radiation pericarditis occur: an acute inflammatory, effusive pericarditis occurring within months of irradiation, which usually resolves spontaneously, and a chronic effusive pericarditis that may appear up to 20 years after radiation therapy and is accompanied by a thickened pericardium.

Most patients with pericardial metastasis are asymptomatic. However, the common symptoms are dyspnea, cough, chest pain, orthopnea, and weakness. Pleural effusion, sinus tachycardia, jugular venous distention, hepatomegaly, peripheral edema, and cyanosis are the most frequent physical findings. Relatively specific diagnostic findings, such as paradoxical pulse, diminished heart sounds, pulsus alternans (pulse waves alternating between those of greater and lesser amplitude with successive beats), and friction rub are less common than with nonmalignant pericardial disease. Chest radiographs and ECG reveal abnormalities in 90% of patients, but half of these abnormalities are nonspecific. Echocardiography is the most helpful diagnostic test. Pericardial fluid may be serous, serosanguineous, or hemorrhagic, and cytologic examination of pericardial fluid is diagnostic in most patients. Cancer patients with pericardial effusion containing malignant cells on cytology have a very poor survival, about 7 weeks.

TREATMENT Pericardial Effusion/Tamponade

Pericardiocentesis with or without the introduction of sclerosing agents, the creation of a pericardial window, complete pericardial stripping, cardiac irradiation, or systemic chemotherapy are effective treatments. Acute pericardial tamponade with life-threatening hemodynamic instability requires immediate drainage of fluid.

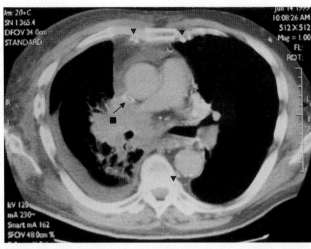

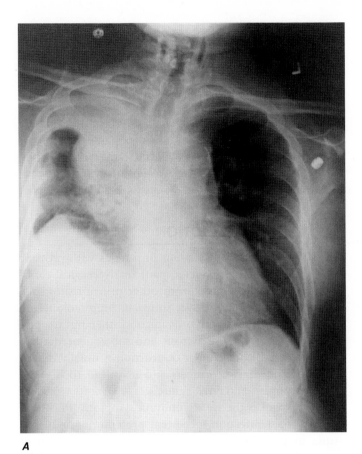

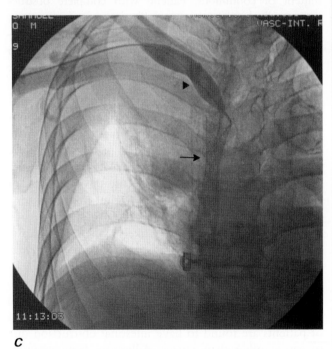

FIGURE 43-1
Superior vena cava syndrome. *A.* Chest radiographs of a 59-year-old man with recurrent SVCS caused by non-small cell lung cancer showing right paratracheal mass with right pleural effusion. ***B.*** CT of same patient demonstrating obstruction of SVC with thrombosis (*arrow*) by the lung cancer (*square*) and collaterals (*arrowheads*). ***C.*** Balloon angioplasty (*arrowhead*) with Wallstent (*arrow*) in same patient.

This can be quickly achieved by pericardiocentesis. The recurrence rate after percutaneous catheter drainage is about 20%. Sclerotherapy (pericardial instillation of bleomycin, mitomycin C, or tetracycline) may decrease recurrences. Alternatively, subxiphoid pericardiotomy can be performed in 45 min under local anesthesia. Thoracoscopic pericardial fenestration can be employed for benign causes; however, 60% of malignant pericardial effusions recur after this procedure.

INTESTINAL OBSTRUCTION

Intestinal obstruction and reobstruction are common problems in patients with advanced cancer, particularly colorectal or ovarian carcinoma. However, other cancers, such as lung or breast cancer and melanoma, can metastasize within the abdomen, leading to intestinal obstruction. Typically, obstruction occurs at multiple sites in peritoneal carcinomatosis. Melanoma has a predilection to involve the small bowel; this involvement may be isolated and resection may result in prolonged survival. Intestinal pseudoobstruction is caused by infiltration of the mesentery or bowel muscle by tumor, involvement of the celiac plexus, or paraneoplastic neuropathy in patients with small cell lung cancer. Paraneoplastic neuropathy is associated with IgG antibodies reactive to neurons of the myenteric and submucosal plexuses of the jejunum and stomach. Ovarian cancer can lead to authentic luminal obstruction or to pseudoobstruction that results when circumferential invasion of a bowel segment arrests the forward progression of peristaltic contractions.

The onset of obstruction is usually insidious. Pain is the most common symptom and is usually colicky in nature. Pain can also be due to abdominal distention, tumor masses, or hepatomegaly. Vomiting can be intermittent or continuous. Patients with complete obstruction usually have constipation. Physical examination may reveal abdominal distention with tympany, ascites, visible peristalsis, high-pitched bowel sounds, and tumor masses. Erect plain abdominal films may reveal multiple air-fluid levels and dilation of the small or large bowel. Acute cecal dilation to >12–14 cm is considered a surgical emergency because of the high likelihood of rupture. CT scan is useful in differentiating benign from malignant causes of obstruction in patients who have undergone surgery for malignancy. Malignant obstruction is suggested by a mass at the site of obstruction or prior surgery, adenopathy, or an abrupt transition zone and irregular bowel thickening at the obstruction site. Benign obstruction is more likely when CT shows mesenteric vascular changes, a large volume of ascites, or a smooth transition zone and smooth bowel thickening at the obstruction site. The prognosis for the patient with cancer who develops intestinal obstruction is poor; median survival is 3–4 months. About 25–30% of patients are found to have intestinal obstruction due to causes other than cancer. Adhesions from previous operations are a common benign cause. Ileus induced by vinca alkaloids, narcotics, or other drugs is another reversible cause.

TREATMENT   Intestinal Obstruction

The management of intestinal obstruction in patients with advanced malignancy depends on the extent of the underlying malignancy and the functional status of the major organs. The initial management should include surgical evaluation. Operation is not always successful and may lead to further complications with a substantial mortality rate (10–20%). Laparoscopy can diagnose and treat malignant bowel obstruction in some cases. Self-expanding metal stents placed in the gastric outlet, duodenum, proximal jejunum, colon, or rectum may palliate obstructive symptoms at those sites without major surgery. Patients known to have advanced intraabdominal malignancy should receive a prolonged course of conservative management, including nasogastric decompression. Percutaneous endoscopic or surgical gastrostomy tube placement is an option for palliation of nausea and vomiting, the so-called "venting gastrostomy." Treatment with antiemetics, antispasmodics, and analgesics may allow patients to remain outside the hospital. Octreotide may relieve obstructive symptoms through its inhibitory effect on gastrointestinal secretion.

URINARY OBSTRUCTION

Urinary obstruction may occur in patients with prostatic or gynecologic malignancies, particularly cervical carcinoma; metastatic disease from other primary sites such as carcinomas of the breast, stomach, lung, colon, and pancreas; or lymphomas. Radiation therapy to pelvic tumors may cause fibrosis and subsequent ureteral obstruction. Bladder outlet obstruction is usually due to prostate and cervical cancers and may lead to bilateral hydronephrosis and renal failure.

Flank pain is the most common symptom. Persistent urinary tract infection, persistent proteinuria, or hematuria in patients with cancer should raise suspicion of ureteral obstruction. Total anuria and/or anuria alternating with polyuria may occur. A slow, continuous rise in the serum creatinine level necessitates immediate evaluation. Renal ultrasound is the safest and cheapest way to identify hydronephrosis. The function of an obstructed kidney can be evaluated by a nuclear scan. CT scan can reveal the point of obstruction and identify a retroperitoneal mass or adenopathy.

TREATMENT   Urinary Obstruction

Obstruction associated with flank pain, sepsis, or fistula formation is an indication for immediate palliative urinary diversion. Internal ureteral stents can be placed under local anesthesia. Percutaneous nephrostomy offers an alternative approach for drainage. In the case of bladder outlet obstruction due to malignancy, a suprapubic cystostomy can be used for urinary drainage.

MALIGNANT BILIARY OBSTRUCTION

This common clinical problem can be caused by a primary carcinoma arising in the pancreas, ampulla of Vater, bile duct, or liver or by metastatic disease to the periductal lymph nodes or liver parenchyma. The most common metastatic tumors causing biliary obstruction are gastric, colon, breast, and lung cancers. Jaundice, light-colored stools, dark urine, pruritus, and weight loss due to malabsorption are usual symptoms. Pain and secondary infection are uncommon in malignant biliary obstruction. Ultrasound, CT scan, or percutaneous transhepatic or endoscopic retrograde cholangiography will identify the site and nature of the biliary obstruction.

TREATMENT	Malignant Biliary Obstruction

Palliative intervention is indicated only in patients with disabling pruritus resistant to medical treatment, severe malabsorption, or infection. Stenting under radiographic control, surgical bypass, or radiation therapy with or without chemotherapy may alleviate the obstruction. The choice of therapy should be based on the site of obstruction (proximal vs distal), the type of tumor (sensitive to radiotherapy, chemotherapy, or neither), and the general condition of the patient. In the absence of pruritus, biliary obstruction may be a largely asymptomatic cause of death.

SPINAL CORD COMPRESSION

Malignant spinal cord compression (MSCC) is defined as compression of the spinal cord and/or cauda equina by an extradural tumor mass. The minimum radiologic evidence for cord compression is indentation of the theca at the level of clinical features. Spinal cord compression occurs in 5–10% of patients with cancer. Epidural tumor is the first manifestation of malignancy in about 10% of patients. The underlying cancer is usually identified during the initial evaluation; lung cancer is the most common cause of MSCC.

Metastatic tumor involves the vertebral column more often than any other part of the bony skeleton. Lung, breast, and prostate cancer are the most frequent offenders. Multiple myeloma also has a high incidence of spine involvement. Lymphomas, melanoma, renal cell cancer, and genitourinary cancers also cause cord compression. The thoracic spine is the most common site (70%), followed by the lumbosacral spine (20%) and the cervical spine (10%). Involvement of multiple sites is most frequent in patients with breast and prostate carcinoma. Cord injury develops when metastases to the vertebral body or pedicle enlarge and compress the underlying dura. Another cause of cord compression is direct extension of a paravertebral lesion through the intervertebral foramen. These cases usually involve a lymphoma, myeloma, or pediatric neoplasm. Parenchymal spinal cord metastasis due to hematogenous spread is rare. Intramedullary metastases can be seen in lung cancer, multiple myeloma, renal cell cancer, and breast cancer and are frequently associated with brain metastases and leptomeningeal disease.

Expanding extradural tumors induce injury through several mechanisms. Obstruction of the epidural venous plexus leads to edema. Local production of inflammatory cytokines enhances blood flow and edema formation. Compression compromises blood flow leading to ischemia. Production of vascular endothelial growth factor is associated with spinal cord hypoxia and has been implicated as a potential cause of damage after spinal cord injury.

The most common initial symptom in patients with spinal cord compression is localized back pain and tenderness due to involvement of vertebrae by tumor. Pain is usually present for days or months before other neurologic findings appear. It is exacerbated by movement and by coughing or sneezing. It can be differentiated from the pain of disk disease by the fact that it worsens when the patient is supine. Radicular pain is less common than localized back pain and usually develops later. Radicular pain in the cervical or lumbosacral areas may be unilateral or bilateral. Radicular pain from the thoracic roots is often bilateral and is described by patients as a feeling of tight, band-like constriction around the thorax and abdomen. Typical cervical radicular pain radiates down the arm; in the lumbar region, the radiation is down the legs. *Lhermitte's sign*, a tingling or electric sensation down the back and upper and lower limbs upon flexing or extending the neck, may be an early sign of cord compression. Loss of bowel or bladder control may be the presenting symptom but usually occurs late in the course. Occasionally patients present with ataxia of gait without motor and sensory involvement due to involvement of the spinocerebellar tract.

On physical examination, pain induced by straight leg raising, neck flexion, or vertebral percussion may help to determine the level of cord compression. Patients develop numbness and paresthesias in the extremities or trunk. Loss of sensibility to pinprick is as common as loss of sensibility to vibration or position. The upper limit of the zone of sensory loss is often one or two vertebrae below the site of compression. Motor findings include weakness, spasticity, and abnormal muscle stretching. An extensor plantar reflex reflects significant compression. Deep tendon reflexes may be brisk. Motor and sensory loss usually precedes sphincter disturbance. Patients with autonomic dysfunction may present with decreased anal tonus, decreased perineal sensibility, and a distended bladder. The absence of the anal wink reflex or the bulbocavernosus reflex confirms cord involvement. In doubtful cases, evaluation of postvoiding urinary residual volume can be helpful. A residual volume of >150 mL suggests bladder dysfunction. Autonomic dysfunction is an unfavorable prognostic factor. Patients with progressive neurologic symptoms should have frequent neurologic examinations and rapid therapeutic intervention. Other illnesses that may mimic cord compression include osteoporotic vertebral collapse, disk disease, pyogenic abscess or vertebral tuberculosis, radiation myelopathy, neoplastic leptomeningitis, benign tumors, epidural hematoma, and spinal lipomatosis.

Cauda equina syndrome is characterized by low back pain; diminished sensation over the buttocks, posterior-superior thighs, and perineal area in a saddle distribution; rectal and bladder dysfunction; sexual impotence; absent bulbocavernous, patellar, and Achilles' reflexes; and variable amount of lower-extremity weakness. This reflects compression of nerve roots as they form the cauda equina after leaving the spinal cord.

Patients with cancer who develop back pain should be evaluated for spinal cord compression as quickly as possible (Fig. 43-2). Treatment is more often successful in patients who are ambulatory and still have sphincter control at the time treatment is initiated. Patients should have a neurologic examination and plain films of the spine. Those whose physical examination suggests cord compression should receive dexamethasone (6 mg intravenously every 6 h), starting immediately.

Erosion of the pedicles (the "winking owl" sign) is the earliest radiologic finding of vertebral tumor. Other radiographic changes include increased intrapedicular distance, vertebral destruction, lytic or sclerotic lesions, scalloped vertebral bodies, and vertebral body collapse. Vertebral collapse is not a reliable indicator of the presence of tumor; about 20% of cases of vertebral collapse, particularly those in older patients and postmenopausal women, are due not to cancer but to osteoporosis. Also, a normal appearance on plain films of the spine does not exclude the diagnosis of cancer. The role of bone scans in the detection of cord compression is not clear; this method is sensitive but less specific than spinal radiography.

The full-length image of the cord provided by MRI is the imaging procedure of choice. Multiple epidural metastases are noted in 25% of patients with cord compression, and their presence influences treatment plans. On T1-weighted images, good contrast is noted between the cord, cerebrospinal fluid, and extradural lesions. Owing to its sensitivity in demonstrating the replacement of bone marrow by tumor, MRI can

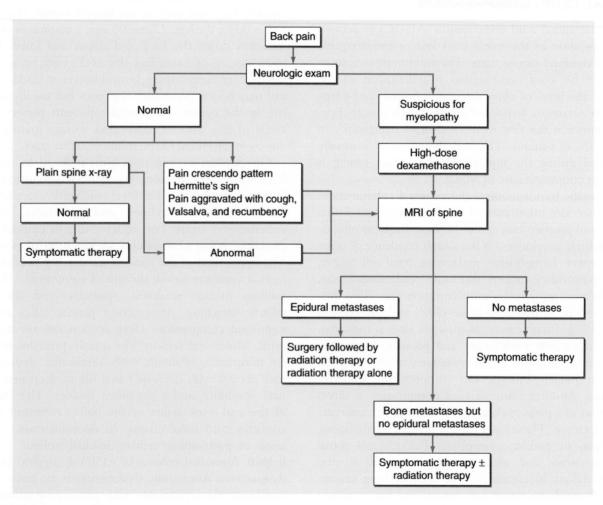

FIGURE 43-2
Management of cancer patients with back pain.

show which parts of a vertebra are involved by tumor. MRI also visualizes intraspinal extradural masses compressing the cord. T2-weighted images are most useful for the demonstration of intramedullary pathology. Gadolinium-enhanced MRI can help to delineate intramedullary disease. MRI is as good as or better than myelography plus postmyelogram CT scan in detecting metastatic epidural disease with cord compression. Myelography should be reserved for patients who have poor MR images or who cannot undergo MRI promptly. CT scan in conjunction with myelography enhances the detection of small areas of spinal destruction.

In patients with cord compression and an unknown primary tumor, a simple workup including chest radiography, mammography, measurement of prostate-specific antigen, and abdominal CT usually reveals the underlying malignancy.

TREATMENT   Spinal Cord Compression

The treatment of patients with spinal cord compression is aimed at relief of pain and restoration/preservation of neurologic function (Fig. 43-2).

Radiation therapy plus glucocorticoids is generally the initial treatment of choice for most patients with spinal cord compression. Up to 75% of patients treated when still ambulatory remain ambulatory, but only 10% of patients with paraplegia recover walking capacity. Indications for surgical intervention include unknown etiology, failure of radiation therapy, a radioresistant tumor type (e.g., melanoma or renal cell cancer), pathologic fracture dislocation, and rapidly evolving neurologic symptoms. Laminectomy is done for tissue diagnosis and for the removal of posteriorly localized epidural deposits in the absence of vertebral body disease. Because most cases of epidural spinal cord compression are due to anterior or anterolateral extradural disease, resection of the anterior vertebral body along with the tumor, followed by spinal stabilization, has achieved good results. A randomized trial showed that patients who underwent an operation followed by radiotherapy (within 14 days) retained the ability to walk significantly longer than those treated with radiotherapy alone. Surgically treated patients also maintained continence and neurologic function significantly longer than patients in the radiation group. The length of survival was not significantly different in the two groups, although there was a trend toward longer survival in the surgery group. The study drew some criticism for the poorer than expected results in the patients who did not go to surgery. However, patients should be evaluated for surgery if they are expected to survive longer than 3 months. Conventional radiotherapy has a role after surgery. Chemotherapy may have a role in patients with chemosensitive tumors who have had prior radiotherapy to the same region and who are not candidates for surgery. Most patients with prostate cancer who develop cord compression have already had hormonal therapy; however, for those who have not, androgen deprivation is combined with surgery and radiotherapy.

Patients with metastatic vertebral tumors may benefit from percutaneous vertebroplasty or kyphoplasty, the injection of acrylic cement into a collapsed vertebra to stabilize the fracture. Pain palliation is common, and local antitumor effects have been noted. Cement leakage may cause symptoms in about 10% of patients. Bisphosphonates may be helpful in prevention of SCC in patients with bony involvement.

The histology of the tumor is an important determinant of both recovery and survival. Rapid onset and progression of signs and symptoms are poor prognostic features.

INCREASED INTRACRANIAL PRESSURE

About 25% of patients with cancer die with intracranial metastases. The cancers that most often metastasize to the brain are lung and breast cancers and melanoma. Brain metastases often occur in the presence of systemic disease, and they frequently cause major symptoms, disability, and early death. The initial presentation of brain metastases from a previously unknown primary cancer is common. Lung cancer is most commonly the primary malignancy. Chest CT scans and brain MRI as the initial diagnostic studies can identify a biopsy site in most patients.

The signs and symptoms of a metastatic brain tumor are similar to those of other intracranial expanding lesions: headache, nausea, vomiting, behavioral changes, seizures, and focal, progressive neurologic changes. Occasionally the onset is abrupt, resembling a stroke, with the sudden appearance of headache, nausea, vomiting, and neurologic deficits. This picture is usually due to hemorrhage into the metastasis. Melanoma, germ cell tumors, and renal cell cancers have a particularly high incidence of intracranial bleeding. The tumor mass and surrounding edema may cause obstruction of the circulation of cerebrospinal fluid, with resulting hydrocephalus. Patients with increased intracranial pressure may have papilledema with visual disturbances and neck stiffness. As the mass enlarges, brain tissue may be displaced through the fixed cranial openings, producing various herniation syndromes.

CT scan and MRI are equally effective in the diagnosis of brain metastases. CT scan with contrast should be used as a screening procedure. The CT scan shows brain metastases as multiple enhancing lesions of various sizes with surrounding areas of low-density edema. If a single lesion or no metastases are visualized by contrast-enhanced CT, MRI of the brain should be performed. Gadolinium-enhanced MRI is more sensitive than CT at revealing meningeal involvement and small lesions, particularly in the brainstem or cerebellum.

Intracranial hypertension secondary to tretinoin therapy has been reported.

TREATMENT — Increased Intracranial Pressure

Dexamethasone is the best initial treatment for all symptomatic patients with brain metastases. If signs and symptoms of brain herniation (particularly headache, drowsiness, and papilledema) are present, the patient should be intubated and hyperventilated to maintain P_{CO_2} between 25 and 30 mmHg and should receive infusions of mannitol (1–1.5 g/kg) every 6 h. Other measures include head elevation, fluid restriction, and hypertonic saline with diuretics. Patients with multiple lesions should receive whole-brain radiation. Patients with a single brain metastasis and with controlled extracranial disease may be treated with surgical excision followed by whole-brain radiation therapy, especially if they are younger than 60 years. Radioresistant tumors should be resected if possible. Stereotactic radiosurgery is an effective treatment for inaccessible or recurrent lesions. With a gamma knife or linear accelerator, multiple small, well-collimated beams of ionizing radiation destroy lesions seen on MRI. Some patients with increased intracranial pressure associated with hydrocephalus may benefit from shunt placement. If neurologic deterioration is not reversed with medical therapy, ventriculotomy to remove cerebrospinal fluid (CSF) or craniotomy to remove tumors or hematomas may be necessary.

NEOPLASTIC MENINGITIS

Tumor involving the leptomeninges is a complication of both primary central nervous system (CNS) tumors and tumors that metastasize to the CNS. The incidence is estimated at 3–8% of patients with cancer. Melanoma, breast and lung cancer, lymphoma (including AIDS-associated), and acute leukemia are the most common causes. Synchronous intraparenchymal brain metastases are evident in 11–31% of patients with neoplastic meningitis.

Patients typically present with multifocal neurologic signs and symptoms, including headache, gait abnormality, mental changes, nausea, vomiting, seizures, back or radicular pain, and limb weakness. Signs include cranial nerve palsies, extremity weakness, paresthesia, and decreased deep tendon reflexes.

Diagnosis is made by demonstrating malignant cells in the CSF; however, up to 40% of patients may have false-negative CSF cytology. An elevated CSF protein level is nearly always present (except in HTLV-1–associated adult T cell leukemia). Patients with neurologic signs and symptoms consistent with neoplastic meningitis who have a negative CSF cytology but an elevated CSF protein level should have the spinal tap repeated at least three times for cytologic examination before the diagnosis is rejected. MRI findings suggestive of neoplastic meningitis include leptomeningeal, subependymal, dural, or cranial nerve enhancement; superficial cerebral lesions; and communicating hydrocephalus. Spinal cord imaging by MRI is a necessary component of the evaluation of nonleukemia neoplastic meningitis as ~20% of patients have cord abnormalities, including intradural enhancing nodules that are diagnostic for leptomeningeal involvement. Cauda equina lesions are common, but lesions may be seen anywhere in the spinal canal. Radiolabeled CSF flow studies are abnormal in up to 70% of patients with neoplastic meningitis; ventricular outlet obstruction, abnormal flow in the spinal canal, or impaired flow over the cerebral convexities may affect distribution of intrathecal chemotherapy resulting in decreased efficacy or increased toxicity. Radiation therapy may correct CSF flow abnormalities before use of intrathecal chemotherapy. Neoplastic meningitis can also lead to intracranial hypertension and hydrocephalus. Placement of a ventriculoperitoneal shunt may effectively palliate symptoms in these patients.

The development of neoplastic meningitis usually occurs in the setting of uncontrolled cancer outside the CNS; thus, prognosis is poor (median survival 10–12 weeks). However, treatment of the neoplastic meningitis may successfully alleviate symptoms and control the CNS spread.

TREATMENT — Neoplastic Meningitis

Intrathecal chemotherapy, usually methotrexate, cytarabine, or thiotepa, is delivered by lumbar puncture or by an intraventricular reservoir (Ommaya) three times a week until the CSF is free of malignant cells. Injections are given twice a week for a month and then weekly for a month. An extended-release preparation of cytarabine (Depocyte) has a longer half-life and is more effective than other formulations. Among solid tumors, breast cancer responds best to therapy. Patients with neoplastic meningitis from either acute leukemia or lymphoma may be cured of their CNS disease if the systemic disease can be eliminated.

SEIZURES

Seizures occurring in a patient with cancer can be caused by the tumor itself, by metabolic disturbances, by radiation injury, by cerebral infarctions, by chemotherapy-related encephalopathies, or by CNS infections. Metastatic disease to the CNS is the most common cause of seizures in patients with cancer. However, seizures occur more frequently in primary brain tumors than in metastatic brain lesions. Seizures are a presenting symptom of CNS metastasis in 6–29% of cases. Approximately 10% of patients with CNS metastasis eventually develop seizures. Tumors that affect the frontal, temporal, and parietal lobes are more commonly associated with seizures than are occipital lesions. The presence of frontal lesions correlates with early seizures, and the presence of hemispheric symptoms increases the risk for late seizures. Both early and late seizures are uncommon in patients with posterior fossa and sellar lesions. Seizures are common in patients with CNS metastases from melanoma and low-grade primary brain tumors. Very rarely, cytotoxic drugs such as etoposide, busulfan, and chlorambucil cause seizures. Another cause of seizures related to drug therapy is reversible posterior leukoencephalopathy syndrome (RPLS). RPLS is associated with administration of cisplatin, 5-fluorouracil, bleomycin, vinblastine, vincristine, etoposide, paclitaxel, ifosfamide, cyclophosphamide, doxorubicin, cytarabine, methotrexate, oxaliplatin, cyclosporine, tacrolimus, and bevacizumab. RPLS is characterized by headache, altered consciousness, generalized seizures, visual disturbances, hypertension, and posterior cerebral white matter vasogenic edema on CT/MRI. Seizures may begin focally but are typically generalized.

TREATMENT   Seizures

Patients in whom seizures due to CNS metastases have been demonstrated should receive anticonvulsive treatment with phenytoin. Prophylactic anticonvulsant therapy is not recommended unless the patient is at high risk for late seizures (melanoma primary, hemorrhagic metastases, treatment with radiosurgery). Serum phenytoin levels should be monitored closely and the dosage adjusted according to serum levels. Phenytoin induces the hepatic metabolism of dexamethasone, reducing its half-life, while dexamethasone may decrease phenytoin levels. Most antiseizure medications induce CYP450, which alters the metabolism of antitumor agents, including irinotecan, taxanes, and etoposide as well as molecular targeted agents, including imatinib, gefitinib, erlotinib, and tipifarnib. Levetiracetam and topiramate are anticonvulsant agents not metabolized by the hepatic cytochrome P450 system and do not alter the metabolism of antitumor agents.

PULMONARY AND INTRACEREBRAL LEUKOSTASIS

Hyperleukocytosis and the leukostasis syndrome associated with it is a potentially fatal complication of acute leukemia (particularly myeloid leukemia) that can occur when the peripheral blast cell count is >100,000/mL. The frequency of hyperleukocytosis is 5–13% in acute myelid leukemia (AML) and 10–30% in acute lymphoid leukemia; however, leukostasis is rare in lymphoid leukemia. At such high blast cell counts, blood viscosity is increased, blood flow is slowed by aggregates of tumor cells, and the primitive myeloid leukemic cells are capable of invading through the endothelium and causing hemorrhage. Brain and lung are most commonly affected. Patients with brain leukostasis may experience stupor, headache, dizziness, tinnitus, visual disturbances, ataxia, confusion, coma, or sudden death. Administration of 600 cGy of whole-brain irradiation can protect against this complication and can be followed by rapid institution of antileukemic therapy. Hydroxyurea, 3-5 grams, can rapidly reduce a high blast cell count while the accurate diagnostic workup is in progress. Pulmonary leukostasis may present as respiratory distress, hypoxemia, and progress to respiratory failure. Chest radiographs may be normal but usually show interstitial or alveolar infiltrates. Arterial blood gas results should be interpreted cautiously. Rapid consumption of plasma oxygen by the markedly increased number of white blood cells can cause spuriously low arterial oxygen tension. Pulse oximetry is the most accurate way of assessing oxygenation in patients with hyperleukocytosis. Leukapheresis may be helpful in decreasing circulating blast counts. Treatment of the leukemia can result in pulmonary hemorrhage from lysis of blasts in the lung, called *leukemic cell lysis pneumopathy*. Intravascular volume depletion and unnecessary blood transfusions may increase blood viscosity and worsen the leukostasis syndrome. Leukostasis is very rarely a feature of the high white cell counts associated with chronic lymphoid or chronic myeloid leukemia.

When acute promyelocytic leukemia is treated with differentiating agents like tretinoin and arsenic trioxide, cerebral or pulmonary leukostasis may occur as tumor cells differentiate into mature neutrophils. This complication can be largely avoided by using cytotoxic chemotherapy together with the differentiating agents.

HEMOPTYSIS

Hemoptysis may be caused by nonmalignant conditions, but lung cancer accounts for a large proportion of cases. Up to 20% of patients with lung cancer have hemoptysis some time in their course. Endobronchial metastases from carcinoid tumors, breast cancer, colon cancer, kidney cancer, and melanoma may also cause hemoptysis. The volume of bleeding is often difficult to gauge. Massive hemoptysis is defined as >200–600 mL of blood produced in 24 h. However, any hemoptysis should be considered massive if it threatens life. When respiratory difficulty occurs, hemoptysis should be treated emergently. The first priorities are to maintain the airway, optimize oxygenation, and stabilize the hemodynamic status. *Often patients can tell where the bleeding is occurring.* They should be placed bleeding side down and given supplemental oxygen. If large-volume bleeding continues or the airway is compromised, the patient should be intubated and undergo emergency bronchoscopy. If the site of bleeding is detected, either the patient undergoes a definitive surgical procedure or the lesion is treated with a neodymium:yttrium–aluminum–garnet (Nd:YAG) laser. The surgical option is preferred. Bronchial artery embolization may control brisk bleeding in 75–90% of patients, permitting the definitive surgical procedure to be done more safely. Embolization without definitive surgery is associated with rebleeding in 20–50% of patients. Recurrent hemoptysis usually responds to a second embolization procedure. A postembolization syndrome characterized by pleuritic pain, fever, dysphagia, and leukocytosis may occur; it lasts 5–7 days and resolves with symptomatic treatment. Bronchial or esophageal wall necrosis, myocardial infarction, and spinal cord infarction are rare complications.

Pulmonary hemorrhage with or without hemoptysis in hematologic malignancies is often associated with fungal infections, particularly *Aspergillus* sp. After granulocytopenia resolves, the lung infiltrates in aspergillosis may cavitate and cause massive hemoptysis. Thrombocytopenia and coagulation defects should be corrected, if possible. Surgical evaluation is recommended in patients with aspergillosis-related cavitary lesions.

Bevacizumab, an antibody to vascular endothelial growth factor (VEGF) that inhibits angiogenesis, has been associated with life-threatening hemoptysis in patients with non-small cell lung cancer, particularly squamous cell histology. Non-small cell lung cancer patients with cavitary lesions have higher risk for pulmonary hemorrhage.

AIRWAY OBSTRUCTION

Airway obstruction refers to a blockage at the level of the mainstem bronchi or above. It may result either from intraluminal tumor growth or from extrinsic compression of the airway. The most common cause of malignant upper airway obstruction is invasion from an adjacent primary tumor, most commonly lung cancer, followed by esophageal, thyroid, and mediastinal malignancies. Extrathoracic primary tumors such as renal, colon, or breast cancer can cause airway obstruction through endobronchial and/or mediastinal lymph node metastases.

Patients may present with dyspnea, hemoptysis, stridor, wheezing, intractable cough, postobstructive pneumonia, or hoarseness. Chest radiographs usually demonstrate obstructing lesions. CT scans reveal the extent of tumor. Cool, humidified oxygen, glucocorticoids, and ventilation with a mixture of helium and oxygen (Heliox) may provide temporary relief. If the obstruction is proximal to the larynx, a tracheostomy may be lifesaving. For more distal obstructions, particularly intrinsic lesions incompletely obstructing the airway, bronchoscopy with laser treatment, photodynamic therapy, or stenting can produce immediate relief in most patients (**Fig. 43-3**). However, radiation therapy (either external-beam irradiation or brachytherapy) given together with glucocorticoids may also open the airway. Symptomatic extrinsic compression may be palliated by stenting. Patients with primary airway tumors such as squamous cell carcinoma, carcinoid tumor, adenocystic carcinoma, or non-small cell lung cancer should have surgery.

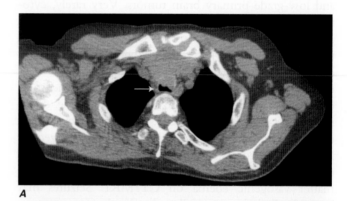

A

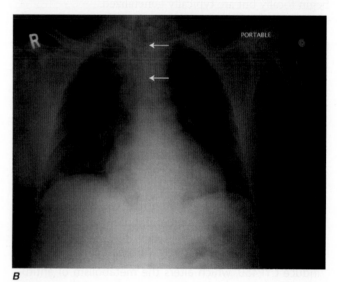

B

FIGURE 43-3

Airway obstruction. A. CT scan of a 62-year-old man with tracheal obstruction caused by renal carcinoma showing paratracheal mass (**A**) with tracheal invasion/obstruction (*arrow*). **B.** Chest x-ray of same patient after stent (*arrows*) placement.

METABOLIC EMERGENCIES

HYPERCALCEMIA

Hypercalcemia is the most common paraneoplastic syndrome.

SYNDROME OF INAPPROPRIATE SECRETION OF ANTIDIURETIC HORMONE (SIADH)

Hyponatremia is a common electrolyte abnormality in cancer patients, and SIADH is the most common cause among patients with cancer.

LACTIC ACIDOSIS

Lactic acidosis is a rare and potentially fatal metabolic complication of cancer. The body produces about 1500 mmols of lactic acid per day, most of which is metabolized by the liver. Normally, this lactate is generated by the skin (25%), muscle (25%), red cells (20%), brain (20%), and gut (10%). Lactic acidosis may occur as a consequence of increased production or decreased hepatic metabolism. Normal venous levels of lactate are 0.5–2.2 mmol/L (4.5–19.8 mg/dL). Lactic acidosis associated with sepsis and circulatory failure is a common preterminal event in many malignancies. Lactic acidosis in the absence of hypoxemia may occur in patients with leukemia, lymphoma, or solid tumors. Extensive involvement of the liver by tumor is often present. In most cases, decreased metabolism and increased production by the tumor both contribute to lactate accumulation. Tumor cell overexpression of certain glycolytic enzymes and mitochondrial dysfunction can contribute to its increased lactate production. HIV-infected patients have an increased risk of aggressive lymphoma; lactic acidosis that occurs in such patients may be related either to the rapid growth of the tumor or from toxicity of nucleoside reverse transcriptase inhibitors. Symptoms of lactic acidosis include tachypnea, tachycardia, change of mental status, and hepatomegaly. The serum level of lactic acid may reach 10–20 mmol/L (90–180 mg/dL). Treatment is aimed at the underlying disease. *The danger from lactic acidosis is from the acidosis, not the lactate.* Sodium bicarbonate should be added if acidosis is very severe or if hydrogen ion production is very rapid and uncontrolled. The prognosis is poor.

HYPOGLYCEMIA

Persistent hypoglycemia is occasionally associated with tumors other than pancreatic islet cell tumors. Usually these tumors are large; tumors of mesenchymal origin, hepatomas, or adrenocortical tumors may cause hypoglycemia. Mesenchymal tumors are usually located in the retroperitoneum or thorax. Obtundation, confusion, and behavioral aberrations occur in the postabsorptive period and may precede the diagnosis of the tumor. These tumors often secrete incompletely processed insulin-like growth factor II (IGF-II), a hormone capable of activating insulin receptors and causing hypoglycemia. Tumors secreting incompletely processed big IGF-II are characterized by an increased IGF-II to IGF-I ratio, suppressed insulin and C-peptide level, and inappropriately low growth hormone and β-hydroxybutyrate concentrations. Rarely, hypoglycemia is due to insulin secretion by a non-islet cell carcinoma. The development of hepatic dysfunction from liver metastases and increased glucose consumption by the tumor can contribute to hypoglycemia. If the tumor cannot be resected, hypoglycemia symptoms may be relieved by the administration of glucose, glucocorticoids, or glucagon.

Hypoglycemia can be artifactual; hyperleukocytosis from leukemia, myeloproliferative diseases, leukemoid reactions, or colony-stimulating factor treatment can increase glucose consumption in the test tube after blood is drawn, leading to pseudohypoglycemia.

ADRENAL INSUFFICIENCY

In patients with cancer, adrenal insufficiency may go unrecognized because the symptoms, such as nausea, vomiting, anorexia, and orthostatic hypotension, are nonspecific and may be mistakenly attributed to progressive cancer or to therapy. Primary adrenal insufficiency may develop owing to replacement of both glands by metastases (lung, breast, colon, or kidney cancer; lymphoma), to removal of both glands, or to hemorrhagic necrosis in association with sepsis or anticoagulation. Impaired adrenal steroid synthesis occurs in patients being treated for cancer with mitotane, ketoconazole, or aminoglutethimide or undergoing rapid reduction in glucocorticoid therapy. Rarely, metastatic replacement causes primary adrenal insufficiency as the first manifestation of an occult malignancy. Metastasis to the pituitary or hypothalamus is found at autopsy in up to 5% of patients with cancer, but associated secondary adrenal insufficiency is rare. Megestrol acetate, used to manage cancer and HIV-related cachexia, may suppress plasma levels of cortisol and adrenocorticotropic hormone (ACTH). Patients taking megestrol may develop adrenal insufficiency, and even those whose adrenal dysfunction is not symptomatic may have inadequate adrenal reserve if they become seriously ill. Paradoxically, some patients may develop Cushing's syndrome and/or hyperglycemia because of the glucocorticoid-like activity of megestrol acetate. Cranial irradiation for childhood brain tumors may affect the hypothalamus-pituitary-adrenal axis, resulting in secondary adrenal insufficiency.

Acute adrenal insufficiency is potentially lethal. Treatment of suspected adrenal crisis is initiated after the sampling of serum cortisol and ACTH levels.

TREATMENT-RELATED EMERGENCIES

TUMOR LYSIS SYNDROME

Tumor lysis syndrome (TLS) is characterized by hyperuricemia, hyperkalemia, hyperphosphatemia, and hypocalcemia and is caused by the destruction of a large number of rapidly proliferating neoplastic cells. Acidosis may also develop. Acute renal failure occurs frequently.

TLS is most often associated with the treatment of Burkitt's lymphoma, acute lymphoblastic leukemia, and other rapidly proliferating lymphomas, but it also may be seen with chronic leukemias and, rarely, with solid tumors. This syndrome has been seen in patients with chronic lymphocytic leukemia after treatment with nucleosides like fludarabine. TLS has been observed with administration of glucocorticoids, hormonal agents such as letrozole and tamoxifen, and monoclonal antibodies such as rituximab and gemtuzumab. TLS usually occurs during or shortly (1–5 days) after chemotherapy. Rarely, spontaneous necrosis of malignancies causes TLS.

Hyperuricemia may be present at the time of chemotherapy. Effective treatment kills malignant cells and leads to increased serum uric acid levels from the turnover of nucleic acids. Owing to the acidic local environment, uric acid can precipitate in the tubules, medulla, and collecting ducts of the kidney, leading to renal failure. Lactic acidosis and dehydration may contribute to the precipitation of uric acid in the renal tubules. The finding of uric acid crystals in the urine is strong evidence for uric acid nephropathy. The ratio of urinary uric acid to urinary creatinine is >1 in patients with acute hyperuricemic nephropathy and <1 in patients with renal failure due to other causes.

Hyperphosphatemia, which can be caused by the release of intracellular phosphate pools by tumor lysis, produces a reciprocal depression in serum calcium, which causes severe neuromuscular irritability and tetany. Deposition of calcium phosphate in the kidney and hyperphosphatemia may cause renal failure. Potassium is the principal intracellular cation, and massive destruction of malignant cells may lead to hyperkalemia. Hyperkalemia in patients with renal failure may rapidly become life-threatening by causing ventricular arrhythmias and sudden death.

The likelihood that TLS will occur in patients with Burkitt's lymphoma is related to the tumor burden and renal function. Hyperuricemia and high serum levels of lactate dehydrogenase (LDH >1500 U/L), both of which correlate with total tumor burden, also correlate with the risk of TLS. In patients at risk for TLS, pretreatment evaluations should include a complete blood count, serum chemistry evaluation, and urine analysis. High leukocyte and platelet counts may artificially elevate potassium levels ("pseudohyperkalemia") due to lysis of these cells after the blood is drawn. In these cases, plasma potassium instead of serum potassium should be followed. In pseudohyperkalemia, no electrocardiographic abnormalities are present. In patients with abnormal baseline renal function, the kidneys and retroperitoneal area should be evaluated by sonography and/or CT to rule out obstructive uropathy. Urine output should be watched closely.

> **TREATMENT** Tumor Lysis Syndrome
>
> Recognition of risk and prevention are the most important steps in the management of this syndrome (Fig. 43-4). The standard preventive approach consists of allopurinol, urinary alkalinization, and aggressive hydration. Intravenous allopurinol may be given in patients who cannot tolerate oral therapy. In some cases, uric acid levels cannot be lowered sufficiently with the standard preventive approach. Rasburicase (recombinant urate oxidase) can be effective in these instances. Urate oxidase is missing from primates and catalyzes the conversion of poorly soluble uric acid to readily soluble allantoin. Rasburicase acts rapidly, decreasing uric acid levels within hours; however, it may cause hypersensitivity reactions such as bronchospasm, hypoxemia, and hypotension. Rasburicase should also be administered to high-risk patients for TLS prophylaxis. Rasburicase is contraindicated in patients with glucose-6-phosphate dehydrogenase deficiency who are unable to break down hydrogen peroxide, an end product of the urate oxidase reaction. Despite aggressive prophylaxis, TLS and/or oliguric or anuric renal failure may occur. Care should be taken to prevent worsening of symptomatic hypocalcemia by induction of alkalosis during bicarbonate infusion. Administration of sodium bicarbonate may also lead to urinary precipitation of calcium phosphate, which is less soluble at alkaline pH. Dialysis is often necessary and should be considered early in the course. Hemodialysis is preferred. Hemofiltration offers a gradual, continuous method of removing cellular byproducts and fluid. The prognosis is excellent, and renal function recovers after the uric acid level is lowered to ≤10 mg/dL.

HUMAN ANTIBODY INFUSION REACTIONS

The initial infusion of human or humanized antibodies (e.g., rituximab, gemtuzumab, trastuzumab) is associated

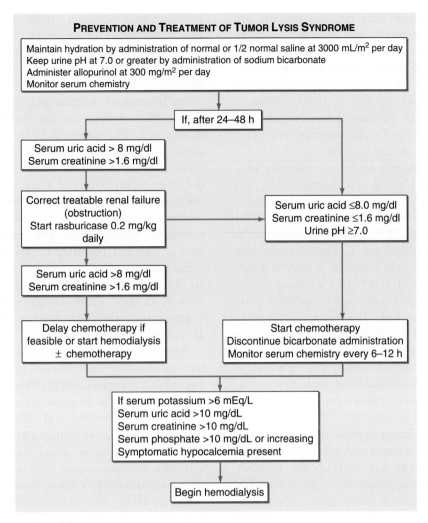

FIGURE 43-4
Management of patients at high risk for the tumor lysis syndrome.

with fever, chills, nausea, asthenia, and headache in up to half of treated patients. Bronchospasm and hypotension occur in 1% of patients. Severe manifestations including pulmonary infiltrates, acute respiratory distress syndrome, and cardiogenic shock occur rarely. Laboratory manifestations include elevated hepatic aminotransferase levels, thrombocytopenia, and prolongation of prothrombin time. The pathogenesis is thought to be activation of immune effector processes (cells and complement) and release of inflammatory cytokines, such as tumor necrosis factor α and interleukin 6 (cytokine release syndrome). Severe reactions from rituximab have occurred with high numbers (more than 50×10^9 lymphocytes) of circulating cells bearing the target antigen (CD 20) and have been associated with a rapid fall in circulating tumor cells, mild electrolyte evidence of TLS, and very rarely, with death. In addition, increased liver enzymes, D-dimer, LDH, and prolongation of the prothrombin time may occur. Diphenhydramine, hydrocortisone, and acetaminophen can often prevent or suppress the infusion-related symptoms. If they occur, the infusion is stopped and restarted at

half the initial infusion rate after the symptoms have abated. Severe "cytokine release syndrome" may require intensive support for acute respiratory distress syndrome (ARDS) and resistant hypotension.

HEMOLYTIC-UREMIC SYNDROME

Hemolytic-uremic syndrome (HUS) and, less commonly, thrombotic thrombocytopenic purpura (TTP) may rarely occur after treatment with antineoplastic drugs including mitomycin, cisplatin, bleomycin, and gemcitabine. It occurs most often in patients with gastric, lung, colorectal, pancreatic, and breast carcinoma. In one series, 35% of patients were without evident cancer at the time this syndrome appeared. Secondary HUS/TTP has also been reported as a rare but sometimes fatal complication of bone marrow transplantation.

HUS usually has its onset 4–8 weeks after the last dose of chemotherapy, but it is not rare to detect it several months later. HUS is characterized by microangiopathic hemolytic anemia, thrombocytopenia, and renal failure.

Dyspnea, weakness, fatigue, oliguria, and purpura are also common initial symptoms and findings. Systemic hypertension and pulmonary edema frequently occur. Severe hypertension, pulmonary edema, and rapid worsening of hemolysis and renal function may occur after a blood or blood product transfusion. Cardiac findings include atrial arrhythmias, pericardial friction rub, and pericardial effusion. Raynaud's phenomenon is part of the syndrome in patients treated with bleomycin.

Laboratory findings include severe to moderate anemia associated with red blood cell fragmentation and numerous schistocytes on peripheral smear. Reticulocytosis, decreased plasma haptoglobin, and an LDH level document hemolysis. The serum bilirubin level is usually normal or slightly elevated. The Coombs' test is negative. The white cell count is usually normal, and thrombocytopenia ($<100,000/\mu L$) is almost always present. Most patients have a normal coagulation profile, although some have mild elevations in thrombin time and in levels of fibrin degradation products. The serum creatinine level is elevated at presentation and shows a pattern of subacute worsening within weeks of the initial azotemia. The urinalysis reveals hematuria, proteinuria, and granular or hyaline casts; and circulating immune complexes may be present.

The basic pathologic lesion appears to be deposition of fibrin in the walls of capillaries and arterioles, and these deposits are similar to those seen in HUS due to other causes. These microvascular abnormalities involve mainly the kidneys and rarely occur in other organs. The pathogenesis of chemotherapy-related HUS is unknown. Other forms of HUS/TTP are related to a decrease in processing of von Willebrand factor by a protease called ADAMTS13.

The case fatality rate is high; most patients die within a few months. There is no consensus on the optimal treatment for chemotherapy-induced HUS. Treatment modalities for HUS/TTP including immunocomplex removal (plasmapheresis, immunoadsorption, or exchange transfusion), antiplatelet/anticoagulant therapies, immunosuppressive therapies, and plasma exchange employed varying degrees of success. Rituximab is successfully used in patients with chemotherapy-induced HUS as well as in ADAMTS13-deficient TTP.

NEUTROPENIA AND INFECTION

These remain the most common serious complications of cancer therapy.

PULMONARY INFILTRATES

Patients with cancer may present with dyspnea associated with diffuse interstitial infiltrates on chest radiographs. Such infiltrates may be due to progression of the underlying malignancy, treatment-related toxicities, infection, and/or unrelated diseases. The cause may be multifactorial; however, most commonly they occur as a consequence of treatment. Infiltration of the lung by malignancy has been described in patients with leukemia, lymphoma, and breast and other solid cancers. Pulmonary lymphatics may be involved diffusely by neoplasm (pulmonary lymphangitic carcinomatosis), resulting in a diffuse increase in interstitial markings on chest radiographs. The patient is often mildly dyspneic at the onset, but pulmonary failure develops over a period of weeks. In some patients, dyspnea precedes changes on the chest radiographs and is accompanied by a nonproductive cough. This syndrome is characteristic of solid tumors. In patients with leukemia, diffuse microscopic neoplastic peribronchial and peribronchiolar infiltration is frequent but may be asymptomatic. However, some patients present with diffuse interstitial infiltrates, an alveolar capillary block syndrome, and respiratory distress. In these situations, glucocorticoids can provide symptomatic relief, but specific chemotherapy should always be started promptly.

Several cytotoxic agents, such as bleomycin, methotrexate, busulfan, nitrosoureas, gemcitabine, mitomycin, vinorelbine, docetaxel, and ifosfamide may cause pulmonary damage. The most frequent presentations are interstitial pneumonitis, alveolitis, and pulmonary fibrosis. Some cytotoxic agents, including methotrexate and procarbazine, may cause an acute hypersensitivity reaction. Cytosine arabinoside has been associated with noncardiogenic pulmonary edema. Administration of multiple cytotoxic drugs, as well as radiotherapy and preexisting lung disease, may potentiate the pulmonary toxicity. Supplemental oxygen may potentiate the effects of drugs and radiation injury. Patients should always be managed with the lowest FiO_2 that is sufficient to maintain hemoglobin saturation.

The onset of symptoms may be insidious, with symptoms including dyspnea, nonproductive cough, and tachycardia. Patients may have bibasilar crepitant rales, end-inspiratory crackles, fever, and cyanosis. The chest radiograph generally shows an interstitial and sometimes an intraalveolar pattern that is strongest at the lung bases and may be symmetric. A small effusion may occur. Hypoxemia with decreased carbon monoxide diffusing capacity is always present. Glucocorticoids may be helpful in patients in whom pulmonary toxicity is related to radiation therapy or to chemotherapy. Treatment is otherwise supportive.

Molecular targeted agents, imatinib, erlotinib, and gefitinib are potent inhibitors of tyrosine kinases. These drugs may cause interstitial lung disease. In the case of gefitinib, preexisting fibrosis, poor performance status, and prior thoracic irradiation are independent risk factors; this complication has a high fatality rate. In Japan, incidence of interstitial lung disease associated with gefitinib was about 4.5% compared to 0.5% in the United States. Temsirolimus, a derivative of rapamycin, is an agent that blocks the effects of mTOR, an enzyme that has an important role in regulating the synthesis of proteins that control cell division. It may cause ground-glass opacities in the lung with or without diffuse interstitial disease and lung parenchymal consolidation.

Radiation pneumonitis and/or fibrosis is a relatively frequent side effect of thoracic radiation therapy. It may be acute or chronic. Radiation-induced lung toxicity is a function of the irradiated lung volume, dose per fraction, and radiation dose. The larger the irradiated lung field, the higher the risk for radiation pneumonitis. The use of concurrent chemoradiation increases pulmonary toxicity. Radiation pneumonitis usually develops from 2 to 6 months after completion of radiotherapy. The clinical syndrome, which varies in severity, consists of dyspnea, cough with scanty sputum, low-grade fever, and an initial hazy infiltrate on chest radiographs. The infiltrate and tissue damage usually are confined to the radiation field. The patients subsequently may develop a patchy alveolar infiltrate and air bronchograms, which may progress to acute respiratory failure that is sometimes fatal. A lung biopsy may be necessary to make the diagnosis. Asymptomatic infiltrates found incidentally after radiation therapy need not be treated. However, prednisone should be administered to patients with fever or other symptoms. The dosage should be tapered slowly after the resolution of radiation pneumonitis, as abrupt withdrawal of glucocorticoids may cause an exacerbation of pneumonia. Delayed radiation fibrosis may occur years after radiation therapy and is signaled by dyspnea on exertion. Often it is mild, but it can progress to chronic respiratory failure. Therapy is supportive.

Classical radiation pneumonitis that leads to pulmonary fibrosis is due to radiation-induced production of local cytokines such as platelet-derived growth factor β, tumor necrosis factor, interleukins, and transforming growth factor β in the radiation field. An immunologically mediated sporadic radiation pneumonitis occurs in about 10% of patients; bilateral alveolitis mediated by T cells results in infiltrates outside the radiation field. This form of radiation pneumonitis usually resolves without sequelae.

Pneumonia is a common problem in patients undergoing treatment for cancer. Bacterial pneumonia typically causes a localized infiltrate on chest radiographs. Therapy is tailored to the causative organism. When diffuse interstitial infiltrates appear in a febrile patient, the differential diagnosis is extensive and includes pneumonia due to infection with *Pneumocystis carinii*; viral infections including cytomegalovirus, adenovirus, herpes simplex virus, herpes zoster, respiratory syncytial virus, or intracellular pathogens such as *Mycoplasma* and *Legionella*; effects of drugs or radiation; tumor progression; nonspecific pneumonitis; and fungal disease. Detection of opportunistic pathogens in pulmonary

infections is still a challenge. Diagnostic tools include chest radiographs, CT scans, bronchoscopy with bronchoalveolar lavage, brush cytology, transbronchial biopsy, fine-needle aspiration, and open lung biopsy. In addition to the culture, evaluation of bronchoalveolar lavage fluid for *P. carinii* by polymerase chain reaction (PCR) and serum galactomannan test improve the diagnostic yield. Patients with cancer who are neutropenic and have fever and local infiltrates on chest radiograph should be treated initially with broad-spectrum antibiotics. A new or persistent focal infiltrate not responding to broad-spectrum antibiotics argues for initiation of empiric antifungal therapy. When diffuse bilateral infiltrates develop in patients with febrile neutropenia, broad-spectrum antibiotics plus trimethoprim-sulfamethoxazole, with or without erythromycin, should be initiated. Addition of an antiviral agent is necessary in some settings, such as patients undergoing allogeneic hematopoietic stem cell transplantation. If the patient does not improve in 4 days, open lung biopsy is the procedure of choice. Bronchoscopy with bronchoalveolar lavage may be used in patients who are poor candidates for surgery.

In patients with pulmonary infiltrates who are afebrile, heart failure and multiple pulmonary emboli are in the differential diagnosis.

NEUTROPENIC ENTEROCOLITIS

Neutropenic enterocolitis (typhlitis) is the inflammation and necrosis of the cecum and surrounding tissues that may complicate the treatment of acute leukemia. Nevertheless, it may involve any segment of the gastrointestinal tract including small intestine, appendix, and colon. This complication has also been seen in patients with other forms of cancer treated with taxanes and in patients receiving high-dose chemotherapy (Fig. 43-5). The patient develops right lower quadrant abdominal pain, often with rebound tenderness and a tense, distended abdomen, in a setting of fever and neutropenia. Watery diarrhea (often containing sloughed mucosa) and bacteremia are common, and bleeding may occur. Plain abdominal films are generally of little value in the diagnosis; CT scan may show marked bowel wall thickening, particularly in the cecum, with bowel wall edema, mesenteric stranding, and ascites. Patients with bowel wall thickness >10 mm on ultrasonogram have higher mortality rates. However, bowel wall thickening is significantly more prominent in patients with *Clostridium difficile* colitis. Pneumatosis intestinalis is a more specific finding, seen only in those with neutropenic enterocolitis and ischemia. The combined involvement of the small and large bowel suggests a diagnosis of neutropenic enterocolitis. Rapid institution of broad-spectrum antibiotics and nasogastric suction may reverse the process. Surgical intervention is reserved for severe cases of neutropenic enterocolitis with evidence of perforation,

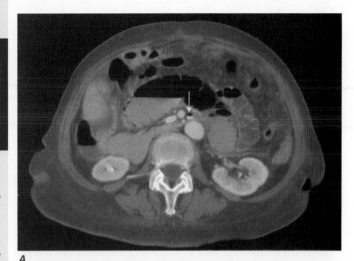

A

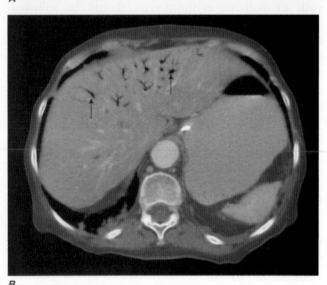

B

FIGURE 43-5

Abdominal CT scans of a 72-year-old woman with neutropenic enterocolitis secondary to chemotherapy. *A.* Air in inferior mesenteric vein (*arrow*) and bowel wall with pneumatosis intestinalis. ***B.*** CT scans of upper abdomen demonstrating air in portal vein (*arrows*).

peritonitis, gangrenous bowel, or gastrointestinal hemorrhage despite correction of any coagulopathy.

C. difficile colitis is increasing in incidence. Newer strains of *C. difficile* produce about 20 times more of toxins A and B compared to previously studied strains. *C. difficile* risk is also increased with chemotherapy. Antibiotic coverage for *C. difficile* should be added if pseudomembranous colitis cannot be excluded.

HEMORRHAGIC CYSTITIS

Hemorrhagic cystitis can develop in patients receiving cyclophosphamide or ifosfamide. Both drugs are metabolized to acrolein, which is a strong chemical irritant that is excreted in the urine. Prolonged contact or high concentrations may lead to bladder irritation and hemorrhage. Symptoms include gross hematuria, frequency, dysuria, burning, urgency, incontinence, and nocturia. The best management is prevention. Maintaining a high rate of urine flow minimizes exposure. In addition, 2-mercaptoethanesulfonate (mesna) detoxifies the metabolites and can be coadministered with the instigating drugs. Mesna usually is given three times on the day of ifosfamide administration in doses that are each 20% of the total ifosfamide dose. If hemorrhagic cystitis develops, the maintenance of a high urine flow may be sufficient supportive care. If conservative management is not effective, irrigation of the bladder with a 0.37–0.74% formalin solution for 10 min stops the bleeding in most cases. *N*-acetylcysteine may also be an effective irrigant. Prostaglandin (carboprost) can inhibit the process. In extreme cases, ligation of the hypogastric arteries, urinary diversion, or cystectomy may be necessary.

Hemorrhagic cystitis also occurs in patients who undergo bone marrow transplantation (BMT). In the BMT setting, early-onset hemorrhagic cystitis is related to drugs in the treatment regimen (e.g., cyclophosphamide), and late-onset hemorrhagic cystitis is usually due to the polyoma virus BKV or adenovirus type 11. BKV load in urine alone or in combination with acute graft-versus-host disease correlate with development of hemorrhagic cystitis. Viral causes are usually detected by PCR-based diagnostic tests. Treatment of viral hemorrhagic cystitis is largely supportive, with reduction in doses of immunosuppressive agents, if possible. No antiviral therapy is approved, though cidofovir is reported to be effective in small series.

HYPERSENSITIVITY REACTIONS TO ANTINEOPLASTIC DRUGS

Many antineoplastic drugs may cause hypersensitivity reaction (HSR). These reactions are unpredictable and potentially life-threatening. Most reactions occur during or within hours of parenteral drug administration. Taxanes, platinum compounds, asparaginase, etoposide, and biologic agents, including rituximab, bevacizumab, trastuzumab, gemtuzumab, cetuximab, and alemtuzumab, are more commonly associated with acute HSR than are other agents. Acute hypersensitivity reactions to some drugs, such as taxanes, occur during the first or second dose administered. HSR from platinum compounds occurs after prolonged exposure. Skin testing may identify patients with high risk for HSR after carboplatin exposure. Premedication with histamine H_1 and H_2 receptor antagonists and glucocorticoids reduce the incidence of hypersensitivity reaction to taxanes, particularly paclitaxel. Despite premedication, HSR may still occur. In these cases, re-treatment may be attempted with care, but use of alternative agents may be required.

APPENDIX

LABORATORY VALUES OF CLINICAL IMPORTANCE

Alexander Kratz ■ Michael A. Pesce ■ Robert C. Basner
■ Andrew J. Einstein

This Appendix contains tables of reference values for laboratory tests, special analytes, and special function tests. A variety of factors can influence reference values. Such variables include the population studied, the duration and means of specimen transport, laboratory methods and instrumentation, and even the type of container used for the collection of the specimen. The reference or "normal" ranges given in this appendix may therefore not be appropriate for all laboratories, and these values should only be used as general guidelines. Whenever possible, reference values provided by the laboratory performing the testing should be utilized in the interpretation of laboratory data. Values supplied in this Appendix reflect typical reference ranges in adults. Pediatric reference ranges may vary significantly from adult values.

In preparing the Appendix, the authors have taken into account the fact that the system of international units (SI, système international d'unités) is used in most countries and in some medical journals. However, clinical laboratories may continue to report values in "traditional" or conventional units. Therefore, both systems are provided in the Appendix. The dual system is also used in the text except for (1) those instances in which the numbers remain the same but only the terminology is changed (mmol/L for meq/L or IU/L for mIU/mL), when only the SI units are given; and (2) most pressure measurements (e.g., blood and cerebrospinal fluid pressures), when the traditional units (mmHg, mmH_2O) are used. In all other instances in the text the SI unit is followed by the traditional unit in parentheses.

REFERENCE VALUES FOR LABORATORY TESTS

TABLE 1

HEMATOLOGY AND COAGULATION

ANALYTE	SPECIMEN	SI UNITS	CONVENTIONAL UNITS
Activated clotting time	WB	70–180 s	70–180 s
Activated protein C resistance (factor V Leiden)	P	Not applicable	Ratio >2.1
ADAMTS13 activity	P	≥0.67	≥67%
ADAMTS13 inhibitor activity	P	Not applicable	≤0.4 U
ADAMTS13 antibody	P	Not applicable	≤18 U
Alpha$_2$ antiplasmin	P	0.87–1.55	87–155%
Antiphospholipid antibody panel			
PTT-LA (lupus anticoagulant screen)	P	Negative	Negative
Platelet neutralization procedure	P	Negative	Negative
Dilute viper venom screen	P	Negative	Negative
Anticardiolipin antibody	S		
IgG		0–15 arbitrary units	0–15 GPL
IgM		0–15 arbitrary units	0–15 MPL

(continued)

TABLE 1

HEMATOLOGY AND COAGULATION (*CONTINUED*)

ANALYTE	SPECIMEN	SI UNITS	CONVENTIONAL UNITS
Antithrombin III	P		
Antigenic		220–390 mg/L	22–39 mg/dL
Functional		0.7–1.30 U/L	70–130%
Anti-Xa assay (heparin assay)	P		
Unfractionated heparin		0.3–0.7 kIU/L	0.3–0.7 IU/mL
Low-molecular-weight heparin		0.5–1.0 kIU/L	0.5–1.0 IU/mL
Danaparoid (Orgaran)		0.5–0.8 kIU/L	0.5–0.8 IU/mL
Autohemolysis test	WB	0.004–0.045	0.4–4.50%
Autohemolysis test with glucose	WB	0.003–0.007	0.3–0.7%
Bleeding time (adult)		<7.1 min	<7.1 min
Bone marrow: See Table 7			
Clot retraction	WB	0.50–1.00/2 h	50–100%/2 h
Cryofibrinogen	P	Negative	Negative
D-dimer	P	220–740 ng/mL FEU	220–740 ng/mL FEU
Differential blood count	WB		
Relative counts:			
Neutrophils		0.40–0.70	40–70%
Bands		0.0–0.05	0–5%
Lymphocytes		0.20–0.50	20–50%
Monocytes		0.04–0.08	4–8%
Eosinophils		0.0–0.6	0–6%
Basophils		0.0–0.02	0–2%
Absolute counts:			
Neutrophils		1.42–6.34 × 10^9/L	1420–6340/mm^3
Bands		0–0.45 × 10^9/L	0–450/mm^3
Lymphocytes		0.71–4.53 × 10^9/L	710–4530/mm^3
Monocytes		0.14–0.72 × 10^9/L	140–720/mm^3
Eosinophils		0–0.54 × 10^9/L	0–540/mm^3
Basophils		0–0.18 × 10^9/L	0–180/mm^3
Erythrocyte count	WB		
Adult males		4.30–5.60 × 10^12/L	4.30–5.60 × 10^6/mm^3
Adult females		4.00–5.20 × 10^12/L	4.00–5.20 × 10^6/mm^3
Erythrocyte life span	WB		
Normal survival		120 days	120 days
Chromium labeled, half-life ($t_{1/2}$)		25–35 days	25–35 days
Erythrocyte sedimentation rate	WB		
Females		0–20 mm/h	0–20 mm/h
Males		0–15 mm/h	0–15 mm/h
Euglobulin lysis time	P	7200–14,400 s	120–240 min
Factor II, prothrombin	P	0.50–1.50	50–150%
Factor V	P	0.50–1.50	50–150%
Factor VII	P	0.50–1.50	50–150%
Factor VIII	P	0.50–1.50	50–150%
Factor IX	P	0.50–1.50	50–150%
Factor X	P	0.50–1.50	50–150%
Factor XI	P	0.50–1.50	50–150%
Factor XII	P	0.50–1.50	50–150 %
Factor XIII screen	P	Not applicable	Present
Factor inhibitor assay	P	<0.5 Bethesda Units	<0.5 Bethesda Units
Fibrin(ogen) degradation products	P	0–1 mg/L	0–1 µg/mL
Fibrinogen	P	2.33–4.96 g/L	233–496 mg/dL
Glucose-6-phosphate dehydrogenase (erythrocyte)	WB	<2400 s	<40 min
Ham's test (acid serum)	WB	Negative	Negative

(continued)

TABLE 1

487

HEMATOLOGY AND COAGULATION (*CONTINUED*)

ANALYTE	SPECIMEN	SI UNITS	CONVENTIONAL UNITS
Hematocrit	WB		
Adult males		0.388–0.464	38.8–46.4
Adult females		0.354–0.444	35.4–44.4
Hemoglobin			
Plasma	P	6–50 mg/L	0.6–5.0 mg/dL
Whole blood:	WB		
Adult males		133–162 g/L	13.3–16.2 g/dL
Adult females		120–158 g/L	12.0–15.8 g/dL
Hemoglobin electrophoresis	WB		
Hemoglobin A		0.95–0.98	95–98%
Hemoglobin A_2		0.015–0.031	1.5–3.1%
Hemoglobin F		0–0.02	0–2.0%
Hemoglobins other than A, A_2, or F		Absent	Absent
Heparin-induced thrombocytopenia antibody	P	Negative	Negative
Immature platelet fraction (IPF)	WB	0.011–0.061	1.1–6.1%
Joint fluid crystal	JF	Not applicable	No crystals seen
Joint fluid mucin	JF	Not applicable	Only type I mucin present
Leukocytes			
Alkaline phosphatase (LAP)	WB	0.2–1.6 μkat/L	13–100 μ/L
Count (WBC)	WB	$3.54–9.06 \times 10^9$/L	$3.54–9.06 \times 10^3$/mm^3
Mean corpuscular hemoglobin (MCH)	WB	26.7–31.9 pg/cell	26.7–31.9 pg/cell
Mean corpuscular hemoglobin concentration (MCHC)	WB	323–359 g/L	32.3–35.9 g/dL
Mean corpuscular hemoglobin of reticulocytes (CH)	WB	24–36 pg	24–36 pg
Mean corpuscular volume (MCV)	WB	79–93.3 fL	79–93.3 μm^3
Mean platelet volume (MPV)	WB	9.00–12.95 fL	9.00–12.95
Osmotic fragility of erythrocytes	WB		
Direct		0.0035–0.0045	0.35–0.45%
Indirect		0.0030–0.0065	0.30–0.65%
Partial thromboplastin time, activated	P	26.3–39.4 s	26.3–39.4 s
Plasminogen	P		
Antigen		84–140 mg/L	8.4–14.0 mg/dL
Functional		0.70–1.30	70–130%
Plasminogen activator inhibitor 1	P	4–43 μg/L	4–43 ng/mL
Platelet aggregation	PRP	Not applicable	>65% aggregation in response to adenosine diphosphate, epinephrine, collagen, ristocetin, and arachidonic acid
Platelet count	WB	$165–415 \times 10^9$/L	$165–415 \times 10^3$/mm^3
Platelet, mean volume	WB	6.4–11 fL	6.4–11.0 μm^3
Prekallikrein assay	P	0.50–1.5	50–150%
Prekallikrein screen	P		No deficiency detected
Protein C	P		
Total antigen		0.70–1.40	70–140%
Functional		0.70–1.30	70–130%
Protein S	P		
Total antigen		0.70–1.40	70–140%
Functional		0.65–1.40	65–140%
Free antigen		0.70–1.40	70–140%
Prothrombin gene mutation G20210A	WB	Not applicable	Not present
Prothrombin time	P	12.7–15.4 s	12.7–15.4 s

(continued)

TABLE 1

HEMATOLOGY AND COAGULATION (*CONTINUED*)

ANALYTE	SPECIMEN	SI UNITS	CONVENTIONAL UNITS
Protoporphyrin, free erythrocyte	WB	0.28–0.64 μmol/L of red blood cells	16–36 μg/dL of red blood cells
Red cell distribution width	WB	<0.145	<14.5%
Reptilase time	P	16–23.6 s	16–23.6 s
Reticulocyte count	WB		
Adult males		0.008–0.023 red cells	0.8–2.3% red cells
Adult females		0.008–0.020 red cells	0.8–2.0% red cells
Reticulocyte hemoglobin content	WB	>26 pg/cell	>26 pg/cell
Ristocetin cofactor (functional von Willebrand factor)	P		
Blood group O		0.75 mean of normal	75% mean of normal
Blood group A		1.05 mean of normal	105% mean of normal
Blood group B		1.15 mean of normal	115% mean of normal
Blood group AB		1.25 mean of normal	125% mean of normal
Serotonin release assay	S	<0.2 release	<20% release
Sickle cell test	WB	Negative	Negative
Sucrose hemolysis	WB	<0.1	<10% hemolysis
Thrombin time	P	15.3–18.5 s	15.3–18.5 s
Total eosinophils	WB	150–300 × 10^6/L	150–300/mm^3
Transferrin receptor	S, P	9.6–29.6 nmol/L	9.6–29.6 nmol/L
Viscosity			
Plasma	P	1.7–2.1	1.7–2.1
Serum	S	1.4–1.8	1.4–1.8
von Willebrand factor (vWF) antigen (factor VIII:R antigen)			
Blood group O		0.75 mean of normal	75% mean of normal
Blood group A		1.05 mean of normal	105% mean of normal
Blood group B		1.15 mean of normal	115% mean of normal
Blood group AB		1.25 mean of normal	125% mean of normal
von Willebrand factor multimers	P	Normal distribution	Normal distribution
White blood cells: see "Leukocytes"			

Abbreviations: JF, joint fluid; P, plasma; PRP, platelet-rich plasma; S, serum; WB, whole blood.

TABLE 2

CLINICAL CHEMISTRY AND IMMUNOLOGY

ANALYTE	SPECIMEN	SI UNITS	CONVENTIONAL UNITS
Acetoacetate	P	49–294 μmol/L	0.5–3.0 mg/dL
Adrenocorticotropin (ACTH)	P	1.3–16.7 pmol/L	6.0–76.0 pg/mL
Alanine aminotransferase (ALT, SGPT)	S	0.12–0.70 μkat/L	7–41 U/L
Albumin	S	40–50 g/L	4.0–5.0 mg/dL
Aldolase	S	26–138 nkat/L	1.5–8.1 U/L
Aldosterone (adult)			
Supine, normal sodium diet	S, P	<443 pmol/L	<16 ng/dL
Upright, normal	S, P	111–858 pmol/L	4–31 ng/dL
Alpha fetoprotein (adult)	S	0–8.5 μg/L	0–8.5 ng/mL
Alpha_1 antitrypsin	S	1.0–2.0 g/L	100–200 mg/dL
Ammonia, as NH_3	P	11–35 μmol/L	19–60 μg/dL
Amylase (method dependent)	S	0.34–1.6 μkat/L	20–96 U/L

(continued)

TABLE 2 489

ANALYTE	SPECIMEN	SI UNITS	CONVENTIONAL UNITS
Androstendione (adult)	S		
Males		0.81–3.1 nmol/L	23–89 ng/dL
Females			
Premenopausal		0.91–7.5 nmol/L	26–214 ng/dL
Postmenopausal		0.46–2.9 nmol/L	13–82 ng/dL
Angiotensin-converting enzyme (ACE)	S	0.15–1.1 μkat/L	9–67 U/L
Anion gap	S	7–16 mmol/L	7–16 mmol/L
Apolipoprotein A-1	S		
Male		0.94–1.78 g/L	94–178 mg/dL
Female		1.01–1.99 g/L	101–199 mg/dL
Apolipoprotein B	S		
Male		0.55–1.40 g/L	55–140 mg/dL
Female		0.55–1.25 g/L	55–125 mg/dL
Arterial blood gases	WB		
$[HCO_3^-]$		22–30 mmol/L	22–30 meq/L
Pco_2		4.3–6.0 kPa	32–45 mmHg
pH		7.35–7.45	7.35–7.45
Po_2		9.6–13.8 kPa	72–104 mmHg
Aspartate aminotransferase (AST, SGOT)	S	0.20–0.65 μkat/L	12–38 U/L
Autoantibodies	S		
Anti-centromere antibody IgG		≤29 AU/mL	≤29 AU/mL
Anti-double-strand (native) DNA		<25 IU/L	<25 IU/L
Anti-glomerular basement membrane antibodies			
Qualitative IgG, IgA		Negative	Negative
Quantitative IgG antibody		≤19 AU/mL	≤19 AU/mL
Anti-histone antibodies		<1.0 U	<1.0 U
Anti-Jo-1 antibody		≤29 AU/mL	≤29 AU/mL
Anti-mitochondrial antibody		Not applicable	<20 Units
Anti-neutrophil cytoplasmic autoantibodies		Not applicable	<1:20
Serine proteinase 3 antibodies		≤19 AU/mL	≤19 AU/mL
Myeloperoxidase antibodies		≤19 AU/mL	≤19 AU/mL
Antinuclear antibody		Not applicable	Negative at 1:40
Anti-parietal cell antibody		Not applicable	None detected
Anti-RNP antibody		Not applicable	<1.0 U
Anti-Scl 70 antibody		Not applicable	<1.0 U
Anti-Smith antibody		Not applicable	<1.0 U
Anti-smooth muscle antibody		Not applicable	<1.0 U
Anti-SSA antibody		Not applicable	<1.0 U
Anti-SSB antibody		Not applicable	Negative
Anti-thyroglobulin antibody		<40 kIU/L	<40 IU/mL
Anti-thyroid peroxidase antibody		<35 kIU/L	<35 IU/mL
B-type natriuretic peptide (BNP)	P	Age and gender specific: <100 ng/L	Age and gender specific: <100 pg/mL
Bence Jones protein, serum qualitative	S	Not applicable	None detected
Bence Jones protein, serum quantitative	S		
Free kappa		3.3–19.4 mg/L	0.33–1.94 mg/dL
Free lambda		5.7–26.3 mg/L	0.57–2.63 mg/dL
K/L ratio		0.26–1.65	0.26–1.65
Beta-2-microglobulin	S	1.1–2.4 mg/L	1.1–2.4 mg/L
Bilirubin	S		
Total		5.1–22 μmol/L	0.3–1.3 mg/dL
Direct		1.7–6.8 μmol/L	0.1–0.4 mg/dL
Indirect		3.4–15.2 μmol/L	0.2–0.9 mg/dL

(continued)

TABLE 2

CLINICAL CHEMISTRY AND IMMUNOLOGY (*CONTINUED*)

ANALYTE	SPECIMEN	SI UNITS	CONVENTIONAL UNITS
C peptide	S	0.27–1.19 nmol/L	0.8–3.5 ng/mL
C1-esterase-inhibitor protein	S	210–390 mg/L	21–39 mg/dL
CA 125	S	<35 kU/L	<35 U/mL
CA 19-9	S	<37 kU/L	<37 U/mL
CA 15-3	S	<33 kU/L	<33 U/mL
CA 27-29	S	0–40 kU/L	0–40 U/mL
Calcitonin 　Male 　Female	S 	 0–7.5 ng/L 0–5.1 ng/L	 0–7.5 pg/mL 0–5.1 pg/mL
Calcium	S	2.2–2.6 mmol/L	8.7–10.2 mg/dL
Calcium, ionized	WB	1.12–1.32 mmol/L	4.5–5.3 mg/dL
Carbon dioxide content (TCO$_2$)	P (sea level)	22–30 mmol/L	22–30 meq/L
Carboxyhemoglobin (carbon monoxide content) 　Nonsmokers 　Smokers 　Loss of consciousness and death	WB 	 0.0–0.015 0.04–0.09 >0.50	 0–1.5% 4–9% >50%
Carcinoembryonic antigen (CEA) 　Nonsmokers 　Smokers	S 	 0.0–3.0 μg/L 0.0–5.0 μg/L	 0.0–3.0 ng/mL 0.0–5.0 ng/mL
Ceruloplasmin	S	250–630 mg/L	25–63 mg/dL
Chloride	S	102–109 mmol/L	102–109 meq/L
Cholesterol: see Table 5			
Cholinesterase	S	5–12 kU/L	5–12 U/mL
Chromogranin A	S	0–50 μg/L	0–50 ng/mL
Complement 　C3 　C4 　Complement total	S 	 0.83–1.77 g/L 0.16–0.47 g/L 60–144 CAE units	 83–177 mg/dL 16–47 mg/dL 60–144 CAE units
Cortisol 　Fasting, 8 A.M.–12 noon 　12 noon–8 P.M. 　8 P.M.–8 A.M.	 S 	 138–690 nmol/L 138–414 nmol/L 0–276 nmol/L	 5–25 μg/dL 5–15 μg/dL 0–10 μg/dL
C-reactive protein	S	<10 mg/L	<10 mg/L
C-reactive protein, high sensitivity	S	Cardiac risk 　Low: <1.0 mg/L 　Average: 1.0–3.0 mg/L 　High: >3.0 mg/L	Cardiac risk 　Low: <1.0 mg/L 　Average: 1.0–3.0 mg/L 　High: >3.0 mg/L
Creatine kinase (total) 　Females 　Males	S 	 0.66–4.0 μkat/L 0.875.0 μkat/L	 39–238 U/L 51–294 U/L
Creatine kinase-MB 　Mass 　Fraction of total activity (by electrophoresis)	S 	 0.0–5.5 μg/L 0–0.04	 0.0–5.5 ng/mL 0–4.0%
Creatinine 　Female 　Male	S 	 44–80 μmol/L 53–106 μmol/L	 0.5–0.9 mg/dL 0.6–1.2 mg/dL
Cryoglobulins	S	Not applicable	None detected
Cystatin C	S	0.5–1.0 mg/L	0.5–1.0 mg/L

(continued)

TABLE 2

CLINICAL CHEMISTRY AND IMMUNOLOGY (*CONTINUED*)

ANALYTE	SPECIMEN	SI UNITS	CONVENTIONAL UNITS
Dehydroepiandrosterone (DHEA) (adult)			
Male	S	6.2–43.4 nmol/L	180–1250 ng/dL
Female		4.5–34.0 nmol/L	130–980 ng/dL
Dehydroepiandrosterone (DHEA) sulfate	S		
Male (adult)		100–6190 µg/L	10–619 µg/dL
Female (adult, premenopausal)		120–5350 µg/L	12–535 µg/dL
Female (adult, postmenopausal)		300–2600 µg/L	30–260 µg/dL
11-Deoxycortisol (adult) (compound S)	S	0.34–4.56 nmol/L	12–158 ng/dL
Dihydrotestosterone			
Male	S, P	1.03–2.92 nmol/L	30–85 ng/dL
Female		0.14–0.76 nmol/L	4–22 ng/dL
Dopamine	P	0–130 pmol/L	0–20 pg/mL
Epinephrine	P		
Supine (30 min)		<273 pmol/L	<50 pg/mL
Sitting		<328 pmol/L	<60 pg/mL
Standing (30 min)		<491 pmol/L	<90 pg/mL
Erythropoietin	S	4–27 U/L	4–27 U/L
Estradiol	S, P		
Female			
Menstruating:			
Follicular phase		74–532 pmol/L	<20–145 pg/mL
Midcycle peak		411–1626 pmol/L	112–443 pg/mL
Luteal phase		74–885 pmol/L	<20–241 pg/mL
Postmenopausal		217 pmol/L	<59 pg/mL
Male		74 pmol/L	<20 pg/mL
Estrone	S, P		
Female			
Menstruating:			
Follicular phase		<555 pmol/L	<150 pg/mL
Luteal phase		<740 pmol/L	<200 pg/mL
Postmenopausal		11–118 pmol/L	3–32 pg/mL
Male		33–133 pmol/L	9–36 pg/mL
Fatty acids, free (nonesterified)	P	0.1–0.6 mmol/L	2.8–16.8 mg/dL
Ferritin	S		
Female		10–150 µg/L	10–150 ng/mL
Male		29–248 µg/L	29–248 ng/mL
Follicle-stimulating hormone (FSH)	S, P		
Female			
Menstruating:			
Follicular phase		3.0–20.0 IU/L	3.0–20.0 mIU/mL
Ovulatory phase		9.0–26.0 IU/L	9.0–26.0 mIU/mL
Luteal phase		1.0–12.0 IU/L	1.0–12.0 mIU/mL
Postmenopausal		18.0–153.0 IU/L	18.0–153.0 mIU/mL
Male		1.0–12.0 IU/L	1.0–12.0 mIU/mL
Fructosamine	S	<285 umol/L	<285 umol/L
Gamma glutamyltransferase	S	0.15–0.99 µkat/L	9–58 U/L
Gastrin	S	<100 ng/L	<100 pg/mL
Glucagon	P	40–130 ng/L	40–130 pg/mL

(*continued*)

TABLE 2

CLINICAL CHEMISTRY AND IMMUNOLOGY (*CONTINUED*)

ANALYTE	SPECIMEN	SI UNITS	CONVENTIONAL UNITS
Glucose	WB	3.6–5.3 mmol/L	65–95 mg/dL
Glucose (fasting)	P		
Normal		4.2–5.6 mmol/L	75–100 mg/dL
Increased risk for diabetes		5.6–6.9 mmol/L	100–125 mg/dL
Diabetes mellitus		Fasting >7.0 mmol/L	Fasting >126 mg/dL
		A 2-hour level of >11.1 mmol/L during an oral glucose tolerance test	A 2-hour level of ≥200 mg/dL during an oral glucose tolerance test
		A random glucose level of ≥11.1 mmol/L in patients with symptoms of hyperglycemia	A random glucose level of ≥200 mg/dL in patients with symptoms of hyperglycemia
Growth hormone	S	0–5 μg/L	0–5 ng/mL
Hemoglobin A_{1c}	WB	0.04–0.06 HgB fraction	4.0–5.6%
Pre-diabetes		0.057–0.064 HgB fraction	5.7–6.4%
Diabetes mellitus		A hemoglobin A_{1c} level of ≥0.065 Hgb fraction as suggested by the American Diabetes Association	A hemoglobin A_{1c} level of ≥6.5% as suggested by the American Diabetes Association
Hemoglobin A_{1c} with estimated average glucose (eAg)	WB	eAg mmoL/L = 1.59 × HbA_{1c} − 2.59	eAg (mg/dL) = 28.7 × HbA_{1c} − 46.7
High-density lipoprotein (HDL) (see Table 5)			
Homocysteine	P	4.4–10.8 μmol/L	4.4–10.8 μmol/L
Human chorionic gonadotropin (HCG)	S		
Nonpregnant female		<5 IU/L	<5 mIU/mL
1–2 weeks postconception		9–130 IU/L	9–130 mIU/mL
2–3 weeks postconception		75–2600 IU/L	75–2600 mIU/mL
3–4 weeks postconception		850–20,800 IU/L	850–20,800 mIU/mL
4–5 weeks postconception		4000–100,200 IU/L	4000–100,200 mIU/mL
5–10 weeks postconception		11,500–289,000 IU/L	11,500–289,000 mIU/mL
10–14 weeks post conception		18,300–137,000 IU/L	18,300–137,000 mIU/mL
Second trimester		1400–53,000 IU/L	1400–53,000 mIU/mL
Third trimester		940–60,000 IU/L	940–60,000 mIU/mL
β-Hydroxybutyrate	P	60–170 μmol/L	0.6–1.8 mg/dL
17-Hydroxyprogesterone (adult)	S		
Male		<4.17 nmol/L	<139 ng/dL
Female			
Follicular phase		0.45–2.1 nmol/L	15–70 ng/dL
Luteal phase		1.05–8.7 nmol/L	35–290 ng/dL
Immunofixation	S	Not applicable	No bands detected
Immunoglobulin, quantitation (adult)			
IgA	S	0.70–3.50 g/L	70–350 mg/dL
IgD	S	0–140 mg/L	0–14 mg/dL
IgE	S	1–87 kIU/L	1–87 IU/mL
IgG	S	7.0–17.0 g/L	700–1700 mg/dL
IgG_1	S	2.7–17.4 g/L	270–1740 mg/dL
IgG_2	S	0.3–6.3 g/L	30–630 mg/dL
IgG_3	S	0.13–3.2 g/L	13–320 mg/dL
IgG_4	S	0.11–6.2 g/L	11–620 mg/dL
IgM	S	0.50–3.0 g/L	50–300 mg/dL
Insulin	S, P	14.35–143.5 pmol/L	2–20 μU/mL
Iron	S	7–25 μmol/L	41–141 μg/dL

(continued)

TABLE 2

CLINICAL CHEMISTRY AND IMMUNOLOGY (*CONTINUED*)

ANALYTE	SPECIMEN	SI UNITS	CONVENTIONAL UNITS
Iron-binding capacity	S	45–73 µmol/L	251–406 µg/dL
Iron-binding capacity saturation	S	0.16–0.35	16–35%
Ischemia modified albumin	S	<85 kU/L	<85 U/mL
Joint fluid crystal	JF	Not applicable	No crystals seen
Joint fluid mucin	JF	Not applicable	Only type I mucin present
Ketone (acetone)	S	Negative	Negative
Lactate	P, arterial	0.5–1.6 mmol/L	4.5–14.4 mg/dL
	P, venous	0.5–2.2 mmol/L	4.5–19.8 mg/dL
Lactate dehydrogenase	S	2.0–3.8 µkat/L	115–221 U/L
Lipase	S	0.51–0.73 µkat/L	3–43 U/L
Lipids: see Table 5			
Lipoprotein (a)	S	0–300 mg/L	0–30 mg/dL
Low-density lipoprotein (LDL) (see Table 5)			
Luteinizing hormone (LH)	S, P		
Female			
Menstruating:			
Follicular phase		2.0–15.0 U/L	2.0–15.0 mIU/mL
Ovulatory phase		22.0–105.0 U/L	22.0–105.0 mIU/mL
Luteal phase		0.6–19.0 U/L	0.6–19.0 mIU/mL
Postmenopausal		16.0–64.0 U/L	16.0–64.0 mIU/mL
Male		2.0–12.0 U/L	2.0–12.0 mIU/mL
Magnesium	S	0.62–0.95 mmol/L	1.5–2.3 mg/dL
Metanephrine	P	<0.5 nmol/L	<100 pg/mL
Methemoglobin	WB	0.0–0.01	0–1%
Myoglobin	S		
Male		20–71 µg/L	20–71 µg/L
Female		25–58 µg/L	25–58 µg/L
Norepinephrine	P		
Supine (30 min)		650–2423 pmol/L	110–410 pg/mL
Sitting		709–4019 pmol/L	120–680 pg/mL
Standing (30 min)		739–4137 pmol/L	125–700 pg/mL
N-telopeptide (cross-linked), NTx	S		
Female, premenopausal		6.2–19.0 nmol BCE	6.2–19.0 nmol BCE
Male		5.4–24.2 nmol BCE	5.4–24.2 nmol BCE
BCE = bone collagen equivalent			
NT-Pro BNP	S, P	<125 ng/L up to 75 years	<125 pg/mL up to 75 years
		<450 ng/L >75 years	<450 pg/mL >75 years
5′ Nucleotidase	S	0.00–0.19 µkat/L	0–11 U/L
Osmolality	P	275–295 mOsmol/kg serum water	275–295 mOsmol/kg serum water
Osteocalcin	S	11–50 µg/L	11–50 ng/mL
Oxygen content	WB		
Arterial (sea level)		17–21	17–21 vol%
Venous (sea level)		10–16	10–16 vol%
Oxygen saturation (sea level)	WB	Fraction:	Percent:
Arterial		0.94–1.0	94–100%
Venous, arm		0.60–0.85	60–85%
Parathyroid hormone (intact)	S	8–51 ng/L	8–51 pg/mL

(continued)

TABLE 2

CLINICAL CHEMISTRY AND IMMUNOLOGY (*CONTINUED*)

ANALYTE	SPECIMEN	SI UNITS	CONVENTIONAL UNITS
Phosphatase, alkaline	S	0.56–1.63 μkat/L	33–96 U/L
Phosphorus, inorganic	S	0.81–1.4 mmol/L	2.5–4.3 mg/dL
Potassium	S	3.5–5.0 mmol/L	3.5–5.0 meq/L
Prealbumin	S	170–340 mg/L	17–34 mg/dL
Procalcitonin	S	<0.1 μg/L	<0.1 ng/mL
Progesterone	S, P		
Female: Follicular		<3.18 nmol/L	<1.0 ng/mL
Midluteal		9.54–63.6 nmol/L	3–20 ng/mL
Male		<3.18 nmol/L	<1.0 ng/mL
Prolactin	S		
Male		53–360 mg/L	2.5–17 ng/mL
Female		40–530 mg/L	1.9–25 ng/mL
Prostate-specific antigen (PSA)	S	0.0–4.0 μg/L	0.0–4.0 ng/mL
Prostate-specific antigen, free	S	With total PSA between 4 and 10 μg/L and when the free PSA is: >0.25 decreased risk of prostate cancer <0.10 increased risk of prostate cancer	With total PSA between 4 and 10 ng/mL and when the free PSA is: >25% decreased risk of prostate cancer <10% increased risk of prostate cancer
Protein fractions:	S		
Albumin		35–55 g/L	3.5–5.5 g/dL (50–60%)
Globulin		20–35 g/L	2.0–3.5 g/dL (40–50%)
Alpha$_1$		2–4 g/L	0.2–0.4 g/dL (4.2–7.2%)
Alpha$_2$		5–9 g/L	0.5–0.9 g/dL (6.8–12%)
Beta		6–11 g/L	0.6–1.1 g/dL (9.3–15%)
Gamma		7–17 g/L	0.7–1.7 g/dL (13–23%)
Protein, total	S	67–86 g/L	6.7–8.6 g/dL
Pyruvate	P	40–130 μmol/L	0.35–1.14 mg/dL
Rheumatoid factor	S	<15 kIU/L	<15 IU/mL
Serotonin	WB	0.28–1.14 umol/L	50–200 ng/mL
Serum protein electrophoresis	S	Not applicable	Normal pattern
Sex hormone–binding globulin (adult)	S		
Male		11–80 nmol/L	11–80 nmol/L
Female		30–135 nmol/L	30–135 nmol/L
Sodium	S	136–146 mmol/L	136–146 meq/L
Somatomedin-C (IGF-1) (adult)	S		
16 years		226–903 μg/L	226–903 ng/mL
17 years		193–731 μg/L	193–731 ng/mL
18 years		163–584 μg/L	163–584 ng/mL
19 years		141–483 μg/L	141–483 ng/mL
20 years		127–424 μg/L	127–424 ng/mL
21–25 years		116–358 μg/L	116–358 ng/mL
26–30 years		117–329 μg/L	117–329 ng/mL
31–35 years		115–307 μg/L	115–307 ng/mL
36–40 years		119–204 μg/L	119–204 ng/mL
41–45 years		101–267 μg/L	101–267 ng/mL
46–50 years		94–252 μg/L	94–252 ng/mL
51–55 years		87–238 μg/L	87–238 ng/mL
56–60 years		81–225 μg/L	81–225 ng/mL
61–65 years		75–212 μg/L	75–212 ng/mL

(*continued*)

TABLE 2

495

CLINICAL CHEMISTRY AND IMMUNOLOGY (*CONTINUED*)

ANALYTE	SPECIMEN	SI UNITS	CONVENTIONAL UNITS
66–70 years		69–200 µg/L	69–200 ng/mL
71–75 years		64–188 µg/L	64–188 ng/mL
76–80 years		59–177 µg/L	59–177 ng/mL
81–85 years		55–166 µg/L	55–166 ng/mL
Somatostatin	P	<25 ng/L	<25 pg/mL
Testosterone, free			
Female, adult	S	10.4–65.9 pmol/L	3–19 pg/mL
Male, adult		312–1041 pmol/L	90–300 pg/mL
Testosterone, total,	S		
Female		0.21–2.98 nmol/L	6–86 ng/dL
Male		9.36–37.10 nmol/L	270–1070 ng/dL
Thyroglobulin	S	1.3–31.8 µg/L	1.3–31.8 ng/mL
Thyroid-binding globulin	S	13–30 mg/L	1.3–3.0 mg/dL
Thyroid-stimulating hormone	S	0.34–4.25 mIU/L	0.34–4.25 µIU/mL
Thyroxine, free (fT4)	S	9.0–16 pmol/L	0.7–1.24 ng/dL
Thyroxine, total (T4)	S	70–151 nmol/L	5.4–11.7 µg/dL
Thyroxine index (free)	S	6.7–10.9	6.7–10.9
Transferrin	S	2.0–4.0 g/L	200–400 mg/dL
Triglycerides (see Table 5)	S	0.34–2.26 mmol/L	30–200 mg/dL
Triiodothyronine, free (fT3)	S	3.7–6.5 pmol/L	2.4–4.2 pg/mL
Triiodothyronine, total (T3)	S	1.2–2.1 nmol/L	77–135 ng/dL
Troponin I (method dependent)	S, P		
99th percentile of a healthy population		0–0.04 µg/L	0–0.04 ng/mL
Troponin T	S, P		
99th percentile of a healthy population		0–0.01 µg/L	0–0.01 ng/mL
Urea nitrogen	S	2.5–7.1 mmol/L	7–20 mg/dL
Uric acid	S		
Females		0.15–0.33 mmol/L	2.5–5.6 mg/dL
Males		0.18–0.41 mmol/L	3.1–7.0 mg/dL
Vasoactive intestinal polypeptide	P	0–60 ng/L	0–60 pg/mL
Zinc protoporphyrin	WB	0–400 µg/L	0–40 µg/dL
Zinc protoporphyrin (ZPP)-to-heme ratio	WB	0–69 µmol ZPP/mol heme	0–69 µmol ZPP/mol heme

Abbreviations: P, plasma; S, serum; WB, whole blood.

TABLE 3

TOXICOLOGY AND THERAPEUTIC DRUG MONITORING

DRUG	THERAPEUTIC RANGE		TOXIC LEVEL	
	SI UNITS	CONVENTIONAL UNITS	SI UNITS	CONVENTIONAL UNITS
Acetaminophen	66–199 µmol/L	10–30 µg/mL	>1320 µmol/L	>200 µg/mL
Amikacin				
Peak	34–51 µmol/L	20–30 µg/mL	>60 µmol/L	>35 µg/mL
Trough	0–17 µmol/L	0–10 µg/mL	>17 µmol/L	>10 µg/mL
Amitriptyline/nortriptyline (total drug)	430–900 nmol/L	120–250 ng/mL	>1800 nmol/L	>500 ng/mL
Amphetamine	150–220 nmol/L	20–30 ng/mL	>1500 nmol/L	>200 ng/mL
Bromide	9.4–18.7 mmol/L	75–150 mg/dL	>18.8 mmol/L	>150 mg/dL
Mild toxicity			6.4–18.8 mmol/L	51–150 mg/dL
Severe toxicity			>18.8 mmol/L	>150 mg/dL
Lethal			>37.5 mmol/L	>300 mg/dL
Caffeine	25.8–103 µmol/L	5–20 µg/mL	>206 µmol/L	>40 µg/mL
Carbamazepine	17–42 µmol/L	4–10 µg/mL	>85 µmol/L	>20 µg/mL
Chloramphenicol				
Peak	31–62 µmol/L	10–20 µg/mL	>77 µmol/L	>25 µg/mL
Trough	15–31 µmol/L	5–10 µg/mL	>46 µmol/L	>15 µg/mL
Chlordiazepoxide	1.7–10 µmol/L	0.5–3.0 µg/mL	>17 µmol/L	>5.0 µg/mL
Clonazepam	32–240 nmol/L	10–75 ng/mL	>320 nmol/L	>100 ng/mL
Clozapine	0.6–2.1 µmol/L	200–700 ng/mL	>3.7 µmol/L	>1200 ng/mL
Cocaine			>3.3 µmol/L	>1.0 µg/mL
Codeine	43–110 nmol/mL	13–33 ng/mL	>3700 nmol/mL	>1100 ng/mL (lethal)
Cyclosporine				
Renal transplant				
0–6 months	208–312 nmol/L	250–375 ng/mL	>312 nmol/L	>375 ng/mL
6–12 months after transplant	166–250 nmol/L	200–300 ng/mL	>250 nmol/L	>300 ng/mL
>12 months	83–125 nmol/L	100–150 ng/mL	>125 nmol/L	>150 ng/mL
Cardiac transplant				
0–6 months	208–291 nmol/L	250–350 ng/mL	>291 nmol/L	>350 ng/mL
6–12 months after transplant	125–208 nmol/L	150–250 ng/mL	>208 nmol/L	>250 ng/mL
>12 months	83–125 nmol/L	100–150 ng/mL	>125 nmol/L	150 ng/mL
Lung transplant				
0–6 months	250–374 nmol/L	300–450 ng/mL	>374 nmol/L	>450 ng/mL
Liver transplant				
Initiation	208–291 nmol/L	250–350 ng/mL	>291 nmol/L	>350 ng/mL
Maintenance	83–166 nmol/L	100–200 ng/mL	>166 nmol/L	>200 ng/mL
Desipramine	375–1130 nmol/L	100–300 ng/mL	>1880 nmol/L	>500 ng/mL
Diazepam (and metabolite)				
Diazepam	0.7–3.5 µmol/L	0.2–1.0 µg/mL	>7.0 µmol/L	>2.0 µg/mL
Nordiazepam	0.4–6.6 µmol/L	0.1–1.8 µg/mL	>9.2 µmol/L	>2.5 µg/mL
Digoxin	0.64–2.6 nmol/L	0.5–2.0 ng/mL	>5.0 nmol/L	>3.9 ng/mL
Disopyramide	5.3–14.7 µmol/L	2–5 µg/mL	>20.6 µmol/L	>7 µg/mL
Doxepin and nordoxepin				
Doxepin	0.36–0.98 µmol/L	101–274 ng/mL	>1.8 µmol/L	>503 ng/mL
Nordoxepin	0.38–1.04 µmol/L	106–291 ng/mL	>1.9 µmol/L	>531 ng/mL
Ethanol				
Behavioral changes			>4.3 mmol/L	>20 mg/dL
Legal limit			≥17 mmol/L	≥80 mg/dL
Critical with acute exposure			>54 mmol/L	>250 mg/dL
Ethylene glycol				
Toxic			>2 mmol/L	>12 mg/dL
Lethal			>20 mmol/L	>120 mg/dL

(continued)

TABLE 3

497

TOXICOLOGY AND THERAPEUTIC DRUG MONITORING (*CONTINUED*)

DRUG	THERAPEUTIC RANGE		TOXIC LEVEL	
	SI UNITS	CONVENTIONAL UNITS	SI UNITS	CONVENTIONAL UNITS
Ethosuximide	280–700 µmol/L	40–100 µg/mL	>700 µmol/L	>100 µg/mL
Everolimus	3.13–8.35 nmol/L	3–8 ng/mL	>12.5 nmol/L	>12 ng/mL
Flecainide	0.5–2.4 µmol/L	0.2–1.0 µg/mL	>3.6 µmol/L	>1.5 µg/mL
Gentamicin				
Peak	10–21 µmol/mL	5–10 µg/mL	>25 µmol/mL	>12 µg/mL
Trough	0–4.2 µmol/mL	0–2 µg/mL	>4.2 µmol/mL	>2 µg/mL
Heroin (diacetyl morphine)			>700 µmol/L	>200 ng/mL (as morphine)
Ibuprofen	49–243 µmol/L	10–50 µg/mL	>970 µmol/L	>200 µg/mL
Imipramine (and metabolite)				
Desimipramine	375–1130 nmol/L	100–300 ng/mL	>1880 nmol/L	>500 ng/mL
Total imipramine + desimipramine	563–1130 nmol/L	150–300 ng/mL	>1880 nmol/L	>500 ng/mL
Lamotrigine	11.7–54.7 µmol/L	3–14 µg/mL	>58.7 µmol/L	>15 µg/mL
Lidocaine	5.1–21.3 µmol/L	1.2–5.0 µg/mL	>38.4 µmol/L	>9.0 µg/mL
Lithium	0.5–1.3 mmol/L	0.5–1.3 meq/L	>2 mmol/L	>2 meq/L
Methadone	1.0–3.2 µmol/L	0.3–1.0 µg/mL	>6.5 µmol/L	>2 µg/mL
Methamphetamine	0.07–0.34 µmol/L	0.01–0.05 µg/mL	>3.35 µmol/L	>0.5 µg/mL
Methanol			>6 mmol/L	>20 mg/dL
Methotrexate				
Low-dose	0.01–0.1 µmol/L	0.01–0.1 µmol/L	>0.1 mmol/L	>0.1 mmol/L
High-dose (24 h)	<5.0 µmol/L	<5.0 µmol/L	>5.0 µmol/L	>5.0 µmol/L
High-dose (48 h)	<0.50 µmol/L	<0.50 µmol/L	>0.5 µmol/L	>0.5 µmol/L
High-dose (72 h)	<0.10 µmol/L	<0.10 µmol/L	>0.1 µmol/L	>0.1 µmol/L
Morphine	232–286 µmol/L	65–80 ng/mL	>720 µmol/L	>200 ng/mL
Mycophenolic acid	3.1–10.9 µmol/L	1.0–3.5 ng/mL	>37 µmol/L	>12 ng/mL
Nitroprusside (as thiocyanate)	103–499 µmol/L	6–29 µg/mL	860 µmol/L	>50 µg/mL
Nortriptyline	190–569 nmol/L	50–150 ng/mL	>1900 nmol/L	>500 ng/mL
Phenobarbital	65–172 µmol/L	15–40 µg/mL	>258 µmol/L	>60 µg/mL
Phenytoin	40–79 µmol/L	10–20 µg/mL	>158 µmol/L	>40 µg/mL
Phenytoin, free	4.0–7.9 µg/mL	1–2 µg/mL	>13.9 µg/mL	>3.5 µg/mL
% Free	0.08–0.14	8–14%		
Primidone and metabolite				
Primidone	23–55 µmol/L	5–12 µg/mL	>69 µmol/L	>15 µg/mL
Phenobarbital	65–172 µmol/L	15–40 µg/mL	>215 µmol/L	>50 µg/mL
Procainamide				
Procainamide	17–42 µmol/L	4–10 µg/mL	>43 µmol/L	>10 µg/mL
NAPA (*N*-acetylprocainamide)	22–72 µmol/L	6–20 µg/mL	>126 µmol/L	>35 µg/mL
Quinidine	6.2–15.4 µmol/L	2.0–5.0 µg/mL	>19 µmol/L	>6 µg/mL
Salicylates	145–2100 µmol/L	2–29 mg/dL	>2900 µmol/L	>40 mg/dL
Sirolimus (trough level)				
Kidney transplant	4.4–15.4 nmol/L	4–14 ng/mL	>16 nmol/L	>15 ng/mL
Tacrolimus (FK506) (trough)				
Kidney and liver				
Initiation	12–19 nmol/L	10–15 ng/mL	>25 nmol/L	>20 ng/mL
Maintenance	6–12 nmol/L	5–10 ng/mL	>25 nmol/L	>20 ng/mL
Heart				
Initiation	19–25 nmol/L	15–20 ng/mL		
Maintenance	6–12 nmol/L	5–10 ng/mL		

(*continued*)

TABLE 3

TOXICOLOGY AND THERAPEUTIC DRUG MONITORING (*CONTINUED*)

DRUG	THERAPEUTIC RANGE		TOXIC LEVEL	
	SI UNITS	CONVENTIONAL UNITS	SI UNITS	CONVENTIONAL UNITS
Theophylline	56–111 µg/mL	10–20 µg/mL	>168 µg/mL	>30 µg/mL
Thiocyanate				
After nitroprusside infusion	103–499 µmol/L	6–29 µg/mL	860 µmol/L	>50 µg/mL
Nonsmoker	17–69 µmol/L	1–4 µg/mL		
Smoker	52–206 µmol/L	3–12 µg/mL		
Tobramycin				
Peak	11–22 µg/L	5–10 µg/mL	>26 µg/L	>12 µg/mL
Trough	0–4.3 µg/L	0–2 µg/mL	>4.3 µg/L	>2 µg/mL
Valproic acid	346–693 µmol/L	50–100 µg/mL	>693 µmol/L	>100 µg/mL
Vancomycin				
Peak	14–28 µmol/L	20–40 µg/mL	>55 µmol/L	>80 µg/mL
Trough	3.5–10.4 µmol/L	5–15 µg/mL	>14 µmol/L	>20 µg/mL

TABLE 4

VITAMINS AND SELECTED TRACE MINERALS

SPECIMEN	ANALYTE	REFERENCE RANGE	
		SI UNITS	CONVENTIONAL UNITS
Aluminum	S	<0.2 µmol/L	<5.41 µg/L
Arsenic	WB	0.03–0.31 µmol/L	2–23 µg/L
Cadmium	WB	<44.5 nmol/L	<5.0 µg/L
Coenzyme Q10 (ubiquinone)	P	433–1532 µg/L	433–1532 µg/L
β-Carotene	S	0.07–1.43 µmol/L	4–77 µg/dL
Copper	S	11–22 µmol/L	70–140 µg/dL
Folic acid	RC	340–1020 nmol/L cells	150–450 ng/mL cells
Folic acid	S	12.2–40.8 nmol/L	5.4–18.0 ng/mL
Lead (adult)	S	<0.5 µmol/L	<10 µg/dL
Mercury	WB	3.0–294 nmol/L	0.6–59 µg/L
Selenium	S	0.8–2.0 umol/L	63–160 µg/L
Vitamin A	S	0.7–3.5 µmol/L	20–100 µg/dL
Vitamin B_1 (thiamine)	S	0–75 nmol/L	0–2 µg/dL
Vitamin B_2 (riboflavin)	S	106–638 nmol/L	4–24 µg/dL
Vitamin B_6	P	20–121 nmol/L	5–30 ng/mL
Vitamin B_{12}	S	206–735 pmol/L	279–996 pg/mL
Vitamin C (ascorbic acid)	S	23–57 µmol/L	0.4–1.0 mg/dL
Vitamin D_3,1,25-dihydroxy, total	S, P	36–180 pmol/L	15–75 pg/mL
Vitamin D_3,25-hydroxy, total	P	75–250 nmol/L	30–100 ng/mL
Vitamin E	S	12–42 µmol/L	5–18 µg/mL
Vitamin K	S	0.29–2.64 nmol/L	0.13–1.19 ng/mL
Zinc	S	11.5–18.4 µmol/L	75–120 µg/dL

Abbreviations: P, plasma; RC, red cells; S, serum; WB, whole blood.

TABLE 5

CLASSIFICATION OF LDL, TOTAL, AND HDL CHOLESTEROL

LDL Cholesterol

<70 mg/dL	Therapeutic option for very high risk patients
<100 mg/dL	Optimal
100–129 mg/dL	Near optimal/above optimal
130–159 mg/dL	Borderline high
160–189 mg/dL	High
≥190 mg/dL	Very high

Total Cholesterol

<200 mg/dL	Desirable
200–239 mg/dL	Borderline high
≥240 mg/dL	High

HDL Cholesterol

<40 mg/dL	Low
≥60 mg/dL	High

Abbreviations: LDL, low-density lipoprotein; HDL, high-density lipoprotein.

Source: Executive summary of the third report of the National Cholesterol Education Program (NCEP) expert panel on detection, evaluation, and treatment of high blood cholesterol in adults (adult treatment panel III). JAMA 2001; 285:2486–97. Implications of Recent Clinical Trials for the National Cholesterol Education Program Adult Treatment Panel III Guidelines. SM Grundy et al for the Coordinating Committee of the National Cholesterol Education Program: Circulation 110:227, 2004.

REFERENCE VALUES FOR SPECIFIC ANALYTES

TABLE 6

CEREBROSPINAL FLUID[a]

	REFERENCE RANGE	
CONSTITUENT	**SI UNITS**	**CONVENTIONAL UNITS**
Osmolarity	292–297 mmol/kg water	292–297 mOsm/L
Electrolytes		
Sodium	137–145 mmol/L	137–145 meq/L
Potassium	2.7–3.9 mmol/L	2.7–3.9 meq/L
Calcium	1.0–1.5 mmol/L	2.1–3.0 meq/L
Magnesium	1.0–1.2 mmol/L	2.0–2.5 meq/L
Chloride	116–122 mmol/L	116–122 meq/L
CO_2 content	20–24 mmol/L	20–24 meq/L
P_{CO_2}	6–7 kPa	45–49 mmHg
pH	7.31–7.34	
Glucose	2.22–3.89 mmol/L	40–70 mg/dL
Lactate	1–2 mmol/L	10–20 mg/dL
Total protein:		
Lumbar	0.15–0.5 g/L	15–50 mg/dL
Cisternal	0.15–0.25 g/L	15–25 mg/dL
Ventricular	0.06–0.15 g/L	6–15 mg/dL
Albumin	0.066–0.442 g/L	6.6–44.2 mg/dL
IgG	0.009–0.057 g/L	0.9–5.7 mg/dL
IgG index[b]	0.29–0.59	
Oligoclonal bands (OGB)	<2 bands not present in matched serum sample	
Ammonia	15–47 μmol/L	25–80 μg/dL
Creatinine	44–168 μmol/L	0.5–1.9 mg/dL
Myelin basic protein	<4 μg/L	
CSF pressure		50–180 mmH₂O
CSF volume (adult)	~150 mL	
Red blood cells	0	0
Leukocytes		
Total	0–5 mononuclear cells per μL	
Differential		
Lymphocytes	60–70%	
Monocytes	30–50%	
Neutrophils	None	

[a]Since cerebrospinal fluid concentrations are equilibrium values, measurements of the same parameters in blood plasma obtained at the same time are recommended. However, there is a time lag in attainment of equilibrium, and cerebrospinal levels of plasma constituents that can fluctuate rapidly (such as plasma glucose) may not achieve stable values until after a significant lag phase.

[b]IgG index = CSF IgG (mg/dL) × serum albumin (g/dL)/serum IgG (g/dL) × CSF albumin (mg/dL).

TABLE 7A

DIFFERENTIAL NUCLEATED CELL COUNTS OF BONE MARROW ASPIRATES[a]

	OBSERVED RANGE (%)	95% RANGE (%)	MEAN (%)
Blast cells	0–3.2	0–3.0	1.4
Promyelocytes	3.6–13.2	3.2–12.4	7.8
Neutrophil myelocytes	4–21.4	3.7–10.0	7.6
Eosinophil myelocytes	0–5.0	0–2.8	1.3
Metamyelocytes	1–7.0	2.3–5.9	4.1
Neutrophils			
Males	21.0–45.6	21.9–42.3	32.1
Females	29.6–46.6	28.8–45.9	37.4
Eosinophils	0.4–4.2	0.3–4.2	2.2
Eosinophils plus eosinophil myelocytes	0.9–7.4	0.7–6.3	3.5
Basophils	0–0.8	0–0.4	0.1
Erythroblasts			
Male	18.0–39.4	16.2–40.1	28.1
Females	14.0–31.8	13.0–32.0	22.5
Lymphocytes	4.6–22.6	6.0–20.0	13.1
Plasma cells	0–1.4	0–1.2	0.6
Monocytes	0–3.2	0–2.6	1.3
Macrophages	0–1.8	0–1.3	0.4
M:E ratio			
Males	1.1–4.0	1.1–4.1	2.1
Females	1.6–5.4	1.6–5.2	2.8

[a]Based on bone marrow aspirate from 50 healthy volunteers (30 men, 20 women).

Abbreviation: M:E, myeloid to erythroid ratio.

Source: BJ Bain: Br J Haematol 94:206, 1996.

TABLE 7B

BONE MARROW CELLULARITY

AGE	OBSERVED RANGE	95% RANGE	MEAN
Under 10 years	59.0–95.1%	72.9–84.7%	78.8%
10–19 years	41.5–86.6%	59.2–69.4%	64.3%
20–29 years	32.0–83.7%	54.1–61.9%	58.0%
30–39 years	30.3–81.3%	41.1–54.1%	47.6%
40–49 years	16.3–75.1%	43.5–52.9%	48.2%
50–59 years	19.7–73.6%	41.2–51.4%	46.3%
60–69 years	16.3–65.7%	40.8–50.6%	45.7%
70–79 years	11.3–47.1%	22.6–35.2%	28.9%

Source: From RJ Hartsock et al: Am J Clin Pathol 1965; 43:326, 1965.

TABLE 8

STOOL ANALYSIS

	REFERENCE RANGE	
	SI UNITS	CONVENTIONAL UNITS
Alpha-1-antitrypsin	≤540 mg/L	≤54 mg/dL
Amount	0.1–0.2 kg/d	100–200 g/24 h
Coproporphyrin	611–1832 nmol/d	400–1200 µg/24 h
Fat		
Adult		<7 g/d
Adult on fat-free diet		<4 g/d
Fatty acids	0–21 mmol/d	0–6 g/24 h
Leukocytes	None	None
Nitrogen	<178 mmol/d	<2.5 g/24 h
pH	7.0–7.5	
Potassium	14–102 mmol/L	14–102 mmol/L
Occult blood	Negative	Negative
Osmolality	280–325 mOsmol/kg	280–325 mOsmol/kg
Sodium	7–72 mmol/L	7–72 mmol/L
Trypsin		20–95 U/g
Urobilinogen	85–510 µmol/d	50–300 mg/24 h
Uroporphyrins	12–48 nmol/d	10–40 µg/24 h
Water	<0.75	<75%

Source: Modified from: FT Fishbach, MB Dunning III: *A Manual of Laboratory and Diagnostic Tests*, 7th ed. Philadelphia, Lippincott Williams & Wilkins, 2004.

TABLE 9

URINE ANALYSIS AND RENAL FUNCTION TESTS

	REFERENCE RANGE	
	SI UNITS	CONVENTIONAL UNITS
Acidity, titratable	20–40 mmol/d	20–40 meq/d
Aldosterone	Normal diet: 6–25 µg/d	Normal diet: 6–25 µg/d
	Low-salt diet: 17–44 µg/d	Low-salt diet: 17–44 µg/d
	High-salt diet: 0–6 µg/d	High-salt diet: 0–6 µg/d
Aluminum	0.19–1.11 µmol/L	5–30 µg/L
Ammonia	30–50 mmol/d	30–50 meq/d
Amylase		4–400 U/L
Amylase/creatinine clearance ratio $[(Cl_{am}/Cl_{cr}) \times 100]$	1–5	1–5
Arsenic	0.07–0.67 µmol/d	5–50 µg/d
Bence Jones protein, urine, qualitative	Not applicable	None detected
Bence Jones protein, urine, quantitative		
Free Kappa	1.4–24.2 mg/L	0.14–2.42 mg/dL
Free Lambda	0.2–6.7 mg/L	0.02–0.67 mg/dL
K/L ratio	2.04–10.37	2.04–10.37
Calcium (10 meq/d or 200 mg/d dietary calcium)	<7.5 mmol/d	<300 mg/d
Chloride	140–250 mmol/d	140–250 mmol/d
Citrate	320–1240 mg/d	320–1240 mg/d
Copper	<0.95 µmol/d	<60 µg/d
Coproporphyrins (types I and III)	0–20 µmol/mol creatinine	0–20 µmol/mol creatinine
Cortisol, free	55–193 nmol/d	20–70 µg/d
Creatine, as creatinine		
Female	<760 µmol/d	<100 mg/d
Male	<380 µmol/d	<50 mg/d
Creatinine	8.8–14 mmol/d	1.0–1.6 g/d
Dopamine	392–2876 nmol/d	60–440 µg/d
Eosinophils	<100 eosinophils/mL	<100 eosinophils/mL
Epinephrine	0–109 nmol/d	0–20 µg/d
Glomerular filtration rate	>60 mL/min/1.73 m²	>60 mL/min/1.73 m²
	For African Americans multiply the result by 1.21	For African Americans multiply the result by 1.21
Glucose (glucose oxidase method)	0.3–1.7 mmol/d	50–300 mg/d
5-Hydroindoleacetic acid [5-HIAA]	0–78.8 µmol/d	0–15 mg/d
Hydroxyproline	53–328 µmol/d	53–328 µmol/d
Iodine, spot urine		
WHO classification of iodine deficiency:		
Not iodine deficient	>100 µg/L	>100 µg/L
Mild iodine deficiency	50–100 µg/L	50–100 µg/L
Moderate iodine deficiency	20–49 µg/L	20–49 µg/L
Severe iodine deficiency	<20 µg/L	<20 µg/L
Ketone (acetone)	Negative	Negative
17 Ketosteroids	3–12 mg/d	3–12 mg/d
Metanephrines		
Metanephrine	30–350 µg/d	30–350 µg/d
Normetanephrine	50–650 µg/d	50–650 µg/d

(continued)

TABLE 9

URINE ANALYSIS AND RENAL FUNCTION TESTS (*CONTINUED*)

	REFERENCE RANGE	
	SI UNITS	CONVENTIONAL UNITS
Microalbumin		
Normal	0.0–0.03 g/d	0–30 mg/d
Microalbuminuria	0.03–0.30 g/d	30–300 mg/d
Clinical albuminuria	>0.3 g/d	>300 mg/d
Microalbumin/creatinine ratio		
Normal	0–3.4 g/mol creatinine	0–30 µg/mg creatinine
Microalbuminuria	3.4–34 g/mol creatinine	30–300 µg/mg creatinine
Clinical albuminuria	>34 g/mol creatinine	>300 µg/mg creatinine
β_2-Microglobulin	0–160 µg/L	0–160 µg/L
Norepinephrine	89–473 nmol/d	15–80 µg/d
N-telopeptide (cross-linked), NTx		
Female, premenopausal	17–94 nmol BCE/mmol creatinine	17–94 nmol BCE/mmol creatinine
Female, postmenopausal	26–124 nmol BCE/mmol creatinine	26–124 nmol BCE/mmol creatinine
Male	21–83 nmol BCE/mmol creatinine	21–83 nmol BCE/mmol creatinine
BCE = bone collagen equivalent		
Osmolality	100–800 mOsm/kg	100–800 mOsm/kg
Oxalate		
Male	80–500 µmol/d	7–44 mg/d
Female	45–350 µmol/d	4–31 mg/d
pH	5.0–9.0	5.0–9.0
Phosphate (phosphorus) (varies with intake)	12.9–42.0 mmol/d	400–1300 mg/d
Porphobilinogen	None	None
Potassium (varies with intake)	25–100 mmol/d	25–100 meq/d
Protein	<0.15 g/d	<150 mg/d
Protein/creatinine ratio	Male: 15–68 mg/g Female: 10–107 mg/g	Male: 15–68 mg/g Female: 10–107 mg/g
Sediment		
Red blood cells	0–2/high-power field	
White blood cells	0–2/high-power field	
Bacteria	None	
Crystals	None	
Bladder cells	None	
Squamous cells	None	
Tubular cells	None	
Broad casts	None	
Epithelial cell casts	None	
Granular casts	None	
Hyaline casts	0–5/low-power field	
Red blood cell casts	None	
Waxy casts	None	
White cell casts	None	
Sodium (varies with intake)	100–260 mmol/d	100–260 meq/d
Specific gravity:		
After 12-h fluid restriction	>1.025	>1.025
After 12-h deliberate water intake	≤1.003	≤1.003
Tubular reabsorption, phosphorus	0.79–0.94 of filtered load	79–94% of filtered load
Urea nitrogen	214–607 mmol/d	6–17 g/d
Uric acid (normal diet)	1.49–4.76 mmol/d	250–800 mg/d
Vanillylmandelic acid (VMA)	<30 µmol/d	<6 mg/d

TABLE 10

NORMAL PRESSURES IN HEART AND GREAT VESSELS

PRESSURE (mmHg)	AVERAGE	RANGE
Right Atrium		
Mean	2.8	1–5
a wave	5.6	2.5–7
c wave	3.8	1.5–6
x wave	1.7	0–5
v wave	4.6	2–7.5
y wave	2.4	0–6
Right Ventricle		
Peak systolic	25	17–32
End-diastolic	4	1–7
Pulmonary Artery		
Mean	15	9–19
Peak systolic	25	17–32
End-diastolic	9	4–13
Pulmonary Artery Wedge		
Mean	9	4.5–13
Left Atrium		
Mean	7.9	2–12
a wave	10.4	4–16
v wave	12.8	6–21
Left Ventricle		
Peak systolic	130	90–140
End-diastolic	8.7	5–12
Brachial Artery		
Mean	85	70–105
Peak systolic	130	90–140
End-diastolic	70	60–90

Source: Reproduced from: MJ Kern *The Cardiac Catheterization Handbook*, 4th ed. Philadelphia, Mosby, 2003.

TABLE 11

CIRCULATORY FUNCTION TESTS

TEST	RESULTS: REFERENCE RANGE	
	SI UNITS (RANGE)	CONVENTIONAL UNITS (RANGE)
Arteriovenous oxygen difference	30–50 mL/L	30–50 mL/L
Cardiac output (Fick)	2.5–3.6 L/m^2 of body surface area per min	2.5–3.6 L/m^2 of body surface area per min
Contractility indexes		
Max. left ventricular dp/dt (dp/dt)	220 kPa/s (176–250 kPa/s)	1650 mmHg/s (1320–1880 mmHg/s)
DP when DP = 5.3 kPa	(37.6 ± 12.2)/s	(37.6 ± 12.2)/s
(40 mmHg) (DP, developed LV pressure)	3.32 ± 0.84 end-diastolic volumes per second	3.32 ± 0.84 end-diastolic volumes per second
Mean normalized systolic ejection rate (angiography)	1.83 ± 0.56 circumferences per second	1.83 ± 0.56 circumferences per second
Mean velocity of circumferential fiber shortening (angiography)		
Ejection fraction: stroke volume/ end-diastolic volume (SV/EDV)	0.67 ± 0.08 (0.55–0.78)	0.67 ± 0.08 (0.55–0.78)
End-diastolic volume	70 ± 20.0 mL/m^2 (60–88 mL/m^2)	70 ± 20.0 mL/m^2 (60–88 mL/m^2)
End-systolic volume	25 ± 5.0 mL/m^2 (20–33 mL/m^2)	25 ± 5.0 mL/m^2 (20–33 mL/m^2)
Left ventricular work		
Stroke work index	50 ± 20.0 (g·m)/m^2 (30–110)	50 ± 20.0 (g·m)/m^2 (30–110)
Left ventricular minute work index	1.8–6.6 [(kg·m)/m^2]/min	1.8–6.6 [(kg·m)/m^2]/min
Oxygen consumption index	110–150 mL	110–150 mL
Maximum oxygen uptake	35 mL/min (20–60 mL/min)	35 mL/min (20–60 mL/min)
Pulmonary vascular resistance	2–12 (kPa·s)/L	20–130 (dyn·s)/cm^5
Systemic vascular resistance	77–150 (kPa·s)/L	770–1600 (dyn·s)/cm^5

Source: E Braunwald et al: *Heart Disease*, 6th ed. Philadelphia, W.B. Saunders Co., 2001.

TABLE 12

NORMAL ECHOCARDIOGRAPHIC REFERENCE LIMITS AND PARTITION VALUES IN ADULTS

	WOMEN REFERENCE RANGE	MILDLY ABNORMAL	MODERATELY ABNORMAL	SEVERELY ABNORMAL	MEN REFERENCE RANGE	MILDLY ABNORMAL	MODERATELY ABNORMAL	SEVERELY ABNORMAL
Left ventricular dimensions								
Septal thickness, cm	0.6–0.9	1.0–1.2	1.3–1.5	≥1.6	0.6–1.0	1.1–1.3	1.4–1.6	≥1.7
Posterior wall thickness, cm	0.6–0.9	1.0–1.2	1.3–1.5	≥1.6	0.6–1.0	1.1–1.3	1.4–1.6	≥1.7
Diastolic diameter, cm	3.9–5.3	5.4–5.7	5.8–6.1	≥6.2	4.2–5.9	6.0–6.3	6.4–6.8	≥6.9
Diastolic diameter/BSA, cm/m²	2.4–3.2	3.3–3.4	3.5–3.7	≥3.8	2.2–3.1	3.2–3.4	3.5–3.6	≥3.7
Diastolic diameter/height, cm/m	2.5–3.2	3.3–3.4	3.5–3.6	≥3.7	2.4–3.3	3.4–3.5	3.6–3.7	≥3.8
Left ventricular volumes								
Diastolic, mL	56–104	105–117	118–130	≥131	67–155	156–178	179–201	≥202
Diastolic/BSA, mL/m²	35–75	76–86	87–96	≥97	35–75	76–86	87–96	≥97
Systolic, mL	19–49	50–59	60–69	≥70	22–58	59–70	71–82	≥83
Systolic/BSA, mL/m²	12–30	31–36	37–42	≥43	12–30	31–36	37–42	≥43
Left ventricular mass, 2D method								
Mass, g	66–150	151–171	172–182	≥183	96–200	201–227	228–254	≥255
Mass/BSA, g/m²	44–88	89–100	101–112	≥113	50–102	103–116	117–130	≥131
Left ventricular function								
Endocardial fractional shortening (%)	27–45	22–26	17–21	≤16	25–43	20–24	15–19	≤14
Midwall fractional shortening (%)	15–23	13–14	11–12	≤10	14–22	12–13	10–11	≤9
Ejection fraction, 2D method (%)	≥55	45–54	30–44	≤29	≥55	45–54	30–44	≤29
Right heart dimensions (cm)								
Basal RV diameter	2.0–2.8	2.9–3.3	3.4–3.8	≥3.9	2.0–2.8	2.9–3.3	3.4–3.8	≥3.9
Mid-RV diameter	2.7–3.3	3.4–3.7	3.8–4.1	≥4.2	2.7–3.3	3.4–3.7	3.8–4.1	≥4.2
Base-to-apex length	7.1–7.9	8.0–8.5	8.6–9.1	≥9.2	7.1–7.9	8.0–8.5	8.6–9.1	≥9.2
RVOT diameter above aortic valve	2.5–2.9	3.0–3.2	3.3–3.5	≥3.6	2.5–2.9	3.0–3.2	3.3–3.5	≥3.6
RVOT diameter above pulmonic valve	1.7–2.3	2.4–2.7	2.8–3.1	≥3.2	1.7–2.3	2.4–2.7	2.8–3.1	≥3.2
Pulmonary artery diameter below pulmonic valve	1.5–2.1	2.2–2.5	2.6–2.9	≥3.0	1.5–2.1	2.2–2.5	2.6–2.9	≥3.0
Right ventricular size and function in 4-chamber view								
Diastolic area, cm²	11–28	29–32	33–37	≥38	11–28	29–32	33–37	≥38
Systolic area, cm²	7.5–16	17–19	20–22	≥23	7.5–16	17–19	20–22	≥23
Fractional area change, %	32–60	25–31	18–24	≤17	32–60	25–31	18–24	≤17
Atrial sizes								
LA diameter, cm	2.7–3.8	3.9–4.2	4.3–4.6	≥4.7	3.0–4.0	4.1–4.6	4.7–5.2	≥5.3
LA diameter/BSA, cm/m²	1.5–2.3	2.4–2.6	2.7–2.9	≥3.0	1.5–2.3	2.4–2.6	2.7–2.9	≥3.0
RA minor axis, cm	2.9–4.5	4.6–4.9	5.0–5.4	≥5.5	2.9–4.5	4.6–4.9	5.0–5.4	≥5.5
RA minor axis/BSA, cm/m²	1.7–2.5	2.6–2.8	2.9–3.1	≥3.2	1.7–2.5	2.6–2.8	2.9–3.1	≥3.2

(continued)

TABLE 12

NORMAL ECHOCARDIOGRAPHIC REFERENCE LIMITS AND PARTITION VALUES IN ADULTS (CONTINUED)

	WOMEN REFERENCE RANGE	MILDLY ABNORMAL	MODERATELY ABNORMAL	SEVERELY ABNORMAL	MEN REFERENCE RANGE	MILDLY ABNORMAL	MODERATELY ABNORMAL	SEVERELY ABNORMAL
LA area, cm²	<20	20–30	30–40	≥41	<20	20–30	30–40	≥41
LA volume, mL	22–52	53–62	63–72	≥73	18–58	59–68	69–78	≥79
LA volume/BSA, mL/m²	16–28	29–33	34–39	≥40	16–28	29–33	34–39	≥40
Aortic stenosis, classification of severity								
Aortic jet velocity, m/s		2.6–2.9	3.0–4.0	>4.0		2.6–2.9	3.0–4.0	>4.0
Mean gradient, mmHg		<20	20–40	>40		<20	20–40	>40
Valve area, cm²		>1.5	1.0–1.5	<1.0		>1.5	1.0–1.5	<1.0
Indexed valve area, cm²/m²		>0.85	0.60–0.85	<0.6		>0.85	0.60–0.85	<0.6
Velocity ratio		>0.50	0.25–0.50	<0.25		>0.50	0.25–0.50	<0.25
Mitral stenosis, classification of severity								
Valve area, cm²		>1.5	1.0–1.5	<1.0		>1.5	1.0–1.5	<1.0
Mean gradient, mmHg		<5	5–10	>10		<5	5–10	>10
Pulmonary artery pressure, mmHg		<30	30–50	>50		<30	30–50	>50
Aortic regurgitation, indices of severity								
Vena contracta width, cm		<0.30	0.30–0.60	≥0.60		<0.30	0.30–0.60	≥0.60
Jet width/LVOT width, %		<25	25–64	≥65		<25	25–64	≥65
Jet CSA/LVOT CSA, %		<5	5–59	≥60		<5	5–59	≥60
Regurgitant volume, mL/beat		<30	30–59	≥60		<30	30–59	≥60
Regurgitant fraction, %		<30	30–49	≥50		<30	30–49	≥50
Effective regurgitant orifice area, cm²		<0.10	0.10–0.29	≥0.30		<0.10	0.10–0.29	≥0.30
Mitral regurgitation, indices of severity								
Vena contracta width, cm		<0.30	0.30–0.69	≥0.70		<0.30	0.30–0.69	≥0.70
Regurgitant volume, mL/beat		<30	30–59	≥60		<30	30–59	≥60
Regurgitant fraction, %		<30	30–49	≥50		<30	30–49	≥50
Effective regurgitant orifice area, cm²		<0.20	0.20–0.39	≥0.40		<0.20	0.20–0.39	≥0.40

Abbreviations: BSA, body surface area; CSA, cross-sectional area; LA, left atrium; LVOT, left ventricular outflow tract; RA, right atrium; RV, right ventricle; RVOT, right ventricular outflow tract; 2D, 2-dimensional.

Source: Values adapted from: American Society of Echocardiography, Guidelines and Standards. *http://www.asecho.org/i4a/pages/index.cfm?pageid=3317.* Accessed Feb 23, 2010.

TABLE 13

507

SUMMARY OF VALUES USEFUL IN PULMONARY PHYSIOLOGY

		TYPICAL VALUES	
	SYMBOL	MAN AGED 40, 75 kg, 175 cm TALL	WOMAN AGED 40, 60 kg, 160 cm TALL
Pulmonary Mechanics			
Spirometry—volume-time curves			
Forced vital capacity	FVC	5.0 L	3.4 L
Forced expiratory volume in 1 s	FEV_1	4.0 L	2.8 L
FEV_1/FVC	FEV_1%	80%	78%
Maximal midexpiratory flow rate	MMEF (FEF 25–75)	4.1 L/s	3.2 L/s
Maximal expiratory flow rate	MEFR (FEF 200–1200)	9.0 L/s	6.1 L/s
Spirometry—flow-volume curves			
Maximal expiratory flow at 50% of expired vital capacity	V_{max} 50 (FEF 50%)	5.0 L/s	4.0 L/s
Maximal expiratory flow at 75% of expired vital capacity	V_{max} 75 (FEF 75%)	2.1 L/s	2.0 L/s
Resistance to airflow:			
Pulmonary resistance	RL (R_L)	<3.0 $(cmH_2O/s)/L$	
Airway resistance	Raw	<2.5 $(cmH_2O/s)/L$	
Specific conductance	SGaw	>0.13 cmH_2O/s	
Pulmonary compliance			
Static recoil pressure at total lung capacity	Pst TLC	25 ± 5 cmH_2O	
Compliance of lungs (static)	CL	0.2 L cmH_2O	
Compliance of lungs and thorax	C(L + T)	0.1 L cmH_2O	
Dynamic compliance of 20 breaths per minute	C dyn 20	0.25 ± 0.05 L/cmH_2O	
Maximal static respiratory pressures:			
Maximal inspiratory pressure	MIP	>110 cmH_2O	>70 cmH_2O
Maximal expiratory pressure	MEP	>200 cmH_2O	>140 cmH_2O
Lung Volumes			
Total lung capacity	TLC	6.9 L	4.9 L
Functional residual capacity	FRC	3.3 L	2.6 L
Residual volume	RV	1.9 L	1.5 L
Inspiratory capacity	IC	3.7 L	2.3 L
Expiratory reserve volume	ERV	1.4 L	1.1 L
Vital capacity	VC	5.0 L	3.4 L
Gas Exchange (Sea Level)			
Arterial O_2 tension	Pa_{O_2}	12.7 ± 0.7 kPa (95 ± 5 mmHg)	
Arterial CO_2 tension	Pa_{CO_2}	5.3 ± 0.3 kPa (40 ± 2 mmHg)	
Arterial O_2 saturation	Sa_{O_2}	0.97 ± 0.02 (97 ± 2%)	
Arterial blood pH	pH	7.40 ± 0.02	
Arterial bicarbonate	HCO_3^-	24 + 2 meq/L	
Base excess	BE	0 ± 2 meq/L	
Diffusing capacity for carbon monoxide (single breath)	DL_{CO}	37 mL CO/min/mmHg	27 mL CO/min/mmHg
Dead space volume	V_D	2 mL/kg body wt	
Physiologic dead space; dead space-tidal volume ratio	V_D/V_T		
Rest		≤35% V_T	
Exercise		≤20% V_T	
Alveolar-arterial difference for O_2	$P(A - a)_{O_2}$	≤2.7 kPa ≤20 kPa (≤24 mmHg)	

Source: Based on: AH Morris et al: *Clinical Pulmonary Function Testing. A Manual of Uniform Laboratory Procedures*, 2nd ed. Salt Lake City, Utah, Intermountain Thoracic Society, 1984.

TABLE 14

GASTROINTESTINAL TESTS

| | RESULTS | |
TEST	SI UNITS	CONVENTIONAL UNITS
Absorption tests		
D-Xylose: after overnight fast, 25 g xylose given in oral aqueous solution		
Urine, collected for following 5 h	25% of ingested dose	25% of ingested dose
Serum, 2 h after dose	2.0–3.5 mmol/L	30–52 mg/dL
Vitamin A: a fasting blood specimen is obtained and 200,000 units of vitamin A in oil is given orally	Serum level should rise to twice fasting level in 3–5 h	Serum level should rise to twice fasting level in 3–5 h
Bentiromide test (pancreatic function): 500 mg bentiromide (chymex) orally; *p*-aminobenzoic acid (PABA) measured		
Plasma		>3.6 (±1.1) μg/mL at 90 min
Urine	>50% recovered in 6 h	>50% recovered in 6 h
Gastric juice		
Volume		
24 h	2–3 L	2–3 L
Nocturnal	600–700 mL	600–700 mL
Basal, fasting	30–70 mL/h	30–70 mL/h
Reaction		
pH	1.6–1.8	1.6–1.8
Titratable acidity of fasting juice	4–9 μmol/s	15–35 meq/h
Acid output		
Basal		
Females (mean ± 1 SD)	0.6 ± 0.5 μmol/s	2.0 ± 1.8 meq/h
Males (mean ± 1 SD)	0.8 ± 0.6 μmol/s	3.0 ± 2.0 meq/h
Maximal (after SC histamine acid phosphate, 0.004 mg/kg body weight, and preceded by 50 mg promethazine, or after betazole, 1.7 mg/kg body weight, or pentagastrin, 6 μg/kg body weight)		
Females (mean ± 1 SD)	4.4 ± 1.4 μmol/s	16 ± 5 meq/h
Males (mean ± 1 SD)	6.4 ± 1.4 μmol/s	23 ± 5 meq/h
Basal acid output/maximal acid output ratio	≤0.6	≤0.6
Gastrin, serum	0–200 μg/L	0–200 pg/mL
Secretin test (pancreatic exocrine function): 1 unit/kg body weight, IV		
Volume (pancreatic juice) in 80 min	>2.0 mL/kg	>2.0 mL/kg
Bicarbonate concentration	>80 mmol/L	>80 meq/L
Bicarbonate output in 30 min	>10 mmol	>10 meq

MISCELLANEOUS

TABLE 15

BODY FLUIDS AND OTHER MASS DATA

	REFERENCE RANGE	
	SI UNITS	CONVENTIONAL UNITS
Ascitic fluid		
Body fluid		
Total volume (lean) of body weight	50% (in obese) to 70%	
Intracellular	30–40% of body weight	
Extracellular	20–30% of body weight	
Blood		
Total volume		
Males	69 mL/kg body weight	
Females	65 mL/kg body weight	
Plasma volume		
Males	39 mL/kg body weight	
Females	40 mL/kg body weight	
Red blood cell volume		
Males	30 mL/kg body weight	1.15–1.21 L/m² of body surface area
Females	25 mL/kg body weight	0.95–1.00 L/m² of body surface area
Body mass index	$18.5–24.9 \ kg/m^2$	$18.5–24.9 \ kg/m^2$

TABLE 16

RADIATION-DERIVED UNITS

QUANTITY	MEASURES	OLD UNIT	SI UNIT	SPECIAL NAME FOR SI UNIT (ABBREVIATION)	CONVERSION
Activity	Rate of radioactive decay	curie (Ci)	Disintegrations per second (dps)	becquerel (Bq)	$1 \ Ci = 3.7 \times 10^{10} \ Bq$ $1 \ mCi = 37 \ MBq$ $1 \ Bq = 2.703 \times 10^{-11} \ Ci$
Exposure	Amount of ionizations produced in dry air by x-rays or gamma rays, per unit of mass	roentgen (R)	Coulomb per kilogram (C/kg)	none	$1 \ C/kg = 3876 \ R$ $1 \ R = 2.58 \times 10^{-4} \ C/kg$ $1 \ mR = 258 \ pC/kg$
Air kerma	Sum of initial energies of charged particles liberated by ionizing radiation in air, per unit of mass	rad	Joule per kilogram (J/kg)	gray (Gy)	$1 \ Gy = 100 \ rad$ $1 \ rad = 0.01 \ Gy$ $1 \ mrad = 10 \ \mu Gy$
Absorbed dose	Energy deposited per unit of mass in a medium, e.g., an organ/tissue	rad	Joule per kilogram (J/kg)	gray (Gy)	$1 \ Gy = 100 \ rad$ $1 \ rad = 0.01 \ Gy$ $1 \ mrad = 10 \ \mu Gy$
Equivalent dose	Energy deposited per unit of mass in a medium, e.g., an organ/tissue, weighted to reflect type(s) of radiation	rem	Joule per kilogram (J/kg)	sievert (Sv)	$1 \ Sv = 100 \ rem$ $1 \ rem = 0.01 \ Sv$ $1 \ mrem = 10 \ \mu Sv$
Effective dose	Energy deposited per unit of mass in a reference individual, doubly weighted to reflect type(s) of radiation and organ(s) irradiated	rem	Joule per kilogram (J/kg)	sievert (Sv)	$1 \ Sv = 100 \ rem$ $1 \ rem = 0.01 \ Sv$ $1 \ mrem = 10 \ \mu Sv$

The contributions of Drs. Daniel J. Fink, Patrick M. Sluss, James L. Januzzi, and Kent B. Lewandrowski to this chapter in previous editions of Harrison's Principles of Internal Medicine are gratefully acknowledged. We also express our gratitude to Drs. Amudha Palanisamy and Scott Fink for careful review of tables and helpful suggestions.

REVIEW AND SELF-ASSESSMENT[a]

Charles Wiener ■ Cynthia D. Brown ■ Anna R. Hemnes

QUESTIONS

DIRECTIONS: Choose the **one best** response to each question.

1. Which of the following statements regarding auscultation of the chest is TRUE?

   A. Absence of breath sounds in a hemithorax is almost always associated with a pneumothorax.
   B. An astute clinician should be able to differentiate "wet" from "dry" crackles.
   C. "Cardiac asthma" refers to wheezing associated with alveolar edema in congestive heart failure.
   D. Rhonchi are a manifestation of obstruction of medium-sized airways.
   E. The presence of egophony can be used to distinguish pulmonary fibrosis from alveolar filling.

2. A 72-year-old male with a long history of tobacco use is seen in the clinic for 3 weeks of progressive dyspnea on exertion. He has had a mild non-productive cough and anorexia but denies fevers, chills, or sweats. On physical examination, he has normal vital signs and normal oxygen saturation on room air. Jugular venous pressure is normal, and cardiac examination shows decreased heart sounds but no other abnormality. The trachea is midline, and there is no associated lymphadenopathy. On pulmonary examination, the patient has dullness over the left lower lung field, decreased tactile fremitus, decreased breath sounds, and no voice transmission. The right lung examination is normal. After obtaining chest plain film, appropriate initial management at this point would include which of the following?

   A. Intravenous antibiotics
   B. Thoracentesis
   C. Bronchoscopy
   D. Deep suctioning
   E. Bronchodilator therapy

3. A 62-year-old man presents to his physician complaining of shortness of breath. All of the following

3. (*Continued*)
   findings are consistent with left ventricular dysfunction as a cause of the patient's dyspnea EXCEPT:

   A. Feeling of chest tightness
   B. Nocturnal dyspnea
   C. Orthopnea
   D. Pulsus paradoxus greater than 10 mmHg
   E. Sensation of air hunger

4. A 32-year-old woman seeks evaluation for cough that has been present for 4 months. She reports that the cough is present day and night. It does awaken her from sleep and is worse in the early morning hours. She also notes the cough to be worse in cold weather and after exercise. She describes the cough as dry and has no associated shortness of breath or wheezing. She gives no antecedent history of an upper respiratory tract infection that preceded the onset of cough. She has a medical history of pulmonary embolus occurring in the postpartum period 6 years previously. Her only medication is norgestimate/ethinyl estradiol. She works as an elementary school teacher. On review of systems, she reports intermittent itchy eyes and runny nose that is worse in the spring and fall. She denies postnasal drip and heartburn. Her physical examination findings are normal with the exception of coughing when breathing through an open mouth. A chest radiograph is also normal. Spirometry demonstrates a forced expiratory volume in 1 second (FEV_1) of 3.0 L (85% predicted), forced vital capacity (FVC) of 3.75 L (88% predicted), and FEV_1/FVC ratio of 80%. After administration of a bronchodilator, the FEV_1 increases to 3.3 L (10% change). What would you recommend next in the evaluation and treatment of this patient?

   A. Initiate a nasal corticosteroid.
   B. Initiate a proton pump inhibitor.
   C. Perform a methacholine challenge test.
   D. Perform a nasopharyngeal culture for *Bordetella pertussis*.
   E. Reassure the patient that there are no pulmonary abnormalities and continue supportive care.

[a]Questions and answers were taken from Wiener C et al (eds): *Harrison's Principles of Internal Medicine Self-Assessment and Board Review*, 18th ed. New York: McGraw-Hill, 2012.

5. A 56-year-old man presents to his primary care physician complaining of coughing up blood. He has felt ill for the past 4 days with a low-grade fever and cough. The cough was initially productive of yellow-green sputum, but it now is sputum mixed with red blood. He estimates that he has produced about 1–2 tsp (5–10 mL) of blood in the past day. He smokes 1 pack of cigarettes daily and has done so since the 15 years of age. He is known to have moderate chronic obstructive pulmonary disease and coronary artery disease. He takes aspirin, metoprolol, lisinopril, tiotropium, and albuterol as needed. His physical examination is notable for a temperature of 37.8°C (100.0°F). Bilateral expiratory wheezing and coarse rhonchi are heard on examination. Chest radiograph is normal. What is the most likely cause of hemoptysis in this individual?

A. Acute bronchitis
B. Infection with tuberculosis
C. Lung abscess
D. Lung cancer
E. Medications

6. A 65-year-old man with a known squamous cell carcinoma near the right upper lobe bronchus is admitted to intensive care after coughing up more than 100 mL of bright red blood. He appears in significant respiratory distress with an oxygen saturation of 78% on room air. He continues to have violent coughing with ongoing hemoptysis. He had a prior pulmonary embolus and is being treated with warfarin. His last INR was therapeutic at 2.5 three days previously. All of the following would be useful in the immediate management of this patient EXCEPT:

A. Consultation with anesthesia for placement of a dual-lumen endotracheal tube.
B. Consultation with interventional radiology for embolization.
C. Consultation with thoracic surgery for urgent surgical intervention if conservative management fails.
D. Correction of the patient's coagulopathy.
E. Positioning of the patient in the left lateral decubitus position.

7. A 48-year-old man is evaluated for hypoxia of unknown etiology. He recently has noticed shortness of breath that is worse with exertion and in the upright position. It is relieved with lying down. On physical examination, he is visibly dyspneic with minimal exertion. He is noted to have a resting oxygen saturation of 89% on room air. When lying down, his oxygen saturation increases to 93%. His pulmonary examination shows no wheezes or crackles. His cardiac examination findings are normal without murmur.

7. (Continued)
His chest radiograph reports a possible 1-cm lung nodule in the right lower lobe. On 100% oxygen and in the upright position, the patient has an oxygen saturation of 90%. What is the most likely cause of the patient's hypoxia?

A. Circulatory hypoxia
B. Hypoventilation
C. Intracardiac right-to-left shunting
D. Intrapulmonary right-to-left shunting
E. Ventilation–perfusion mismatch

8. A patient is evaluated in the emergency department for peripheral cyanosis. All of the following are potential etiologies EXCEPT:

A. Cold exposure
B. Deep venous thrombosis
C. Methemoglobinemia
D. Peripheral vascular disease
E. Raynaud's phenomenon

9. At what lung volume does the outward recoil of the chest wall equal the inward elastic recoil of the lung?

A. Expiratory reserve volume
B. Functional residual capacity
C. Residual volume
D. Tidal volume
E. Total lung capacity

10. A 65-year-old man is evaluated for progressive dyspnea on exertion that has occurred over the course of the past 3 months. His medical history is significant for an episode of necrotizing pancreatitis that resulted in multiorgan failure and acute respiratory distress syndrome. He required mechanical ventilation for 6 weeks prior to his recovery. He also has a history of 30 pack-years of tobacco, quitting 15 years previously. He is not known to have chronic obstructive pulmonary disease. On physical examination, a low-pitched inspiratory and expiratory wheeze is heard that is loudest over the mid-chest area. On pulmonary function testing, the forced expiratory volume in 1 second is 2.5 L (78% predicted), forced vital capacity is 4.00 L (94% predicted), and the FEV_1/FVC ratio is 62.5%. The flow volume curve is shown in **Figure 10**. What is the most likely cause of the patient's symptoms?

A. Aspirated foreign body
B. Chronic obstructive pulmonary disease
C. Idiopathic pulmonary fibrosis
D. Subglottic stenosis
E. Unilateral vocal cord paralysis

10. (*Continued*)

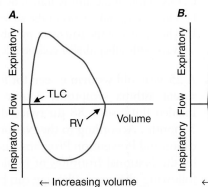

A.

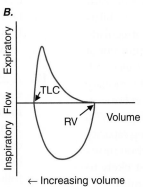

B.

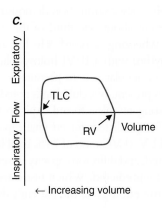

C.

FIGURE 10

11. A 32-year-old woman presents to the emergency department in her 36th week of pregnancy complaining of acute dyspnea. She has had an uncomplicated pregnancy and has no other medical problems. She is taking no medications other than prenatal vitamins. On examination, she appears dyspneic. Her vital signs are as follows: blood pressure 128/78 mmHg, heart rate 126 beats/min, respiratory rate 28 breaths/min, and oxygen saturation is 96% on room air. She is afebrile. Her lung and cardiac examinations are normal. There is trace bilateral pitting pedal edema. A chest x-ray performed with abdominal shielding is normal, and the ECG demonstrates sinus tachycardia. An arterial blood gas is performed. The pH is 7.52, $PaCO_2$ is 26 mmHg, and PaO_2 is 85 mmHg. What is the next best step in the diagnosis and management of this patient?

A. Initiate therapy with amoxicillin for acute bronchitis.
B. Perform a CT pulmonary angiogram.
C. Perform an echocardiogram.
D. Reassure the patient that dyspnea is normal during this stage of pregnancy and no abnormalities are seen on testing.
E. Treat with clonazepam for a panic attack.

12. Match each of the following pulmonary function test results with the respiratory disorder for which they are the most likely findings.

A. Increased total lung capacity (TLC), decreased vital capacity (VC), decreased FEV_1/FVC ratio
B. Decreased TLC, decreased VC, decreased residual volume (RV), increased FEV_1/FVC ratio, normal maximum inspiratory pressure (MIP)
C. Decreased TLC, increased RV, normal FEV_1/FVC ratio, decreased MIP
D. Normal TLC, normal RV, normal FEV_1/FVC ratio, normal MIP

12. (*Continued*)
   1. Myasthenia gravis
   2. Idiopathic pulmonary fibrosis
   3. Familial pulmonary hypertension
   4. Chronic obstructive pulmonary disease

13. A 78-year-old woman is admitted to the medical intensive care unit with multilobar pneumonia. On initial presentation to the emergency room, her initial oxygen saturation was 60% on room air and only increased to 82% on a non-rebreather face mask. She was in marked respiratory distress and intubated in the emergency room. Upon admission to the intensive care unit, she was sedated and paralyzed. The ventilator is set in the assist-control mode with a respiratory rate of 24, tidal volume of 6 mL/kg, FiO_2 of 1.0, and positive end-expiratory pressure of 12 cmH$_2$O. An arterial blood gas measurement is performed on these settings; the results are pH 7.20, PCO_2 of 32 mmHg, and PO_2 of 54 mmHg. What is the cause of the hypoxemia?

A. Hypoventilation alone
B. Hypoventilation and ventilation-perfusion mismatch
C. Shunt
D. Ventilation-perfusion mismatch

14. A 65-year-old man is evaluated for progressive dyspnea on exertion and dry cough that have worsened over the course of 6 months. He has not had dyspnea at rest and denies wheezing. He has not experienced chest pain. He has a history of coronary artery disease and atrial fibrillation, and underwent coronary artery bypass surgery 12 years ago. His medications include metoprolol, aspirin, warfarin, and enalapril. He previously smoked one pack of cigarettes daily for 40 years, quitting 5 years previously. His vital signs are blood pressure 122/68 mmHg, heart rate 68 beats/min, respiratory rate 18 breaths/min, and oxygen saturation 92% on

14. (*Continued*)

room air. His chest examination demonstrates bibasilar crackles present about one-third of the way up bilaterally. No wheezing is heard. He has an irregularly irregular rhythm with a II/VI holosystolic murmur at the apex. The jugular venous pressure is not elevated. No edema is present, but clubbing is noted. Pulmonary function testing reveals a forced expiratory volume in 1 second 65% predicted, forced vital capacity of 67% predicted, FEV_1/FVC ratio of 74%, total lung capacity 68% predicted, and diffusion capacity for carbon monoxide of 62% predicted. Which test is most likely to determine the etiology of the patient's dyspnea?

A. Bronchoscopy with transbronchial lung biopsy
B. CT pulmonary angiography
C. Echocardiography
D. High-resolution CT scan of the chest
E. Nuclear medicine stress test

15. A 24-year-old woman is seen for a complaint of shortness of breath and wheezing. She reports the symptoms to be worse when she has exercised outdoors and is around cats. She has had allergic rhinitis in the spring and summer for many years and suffered from eczema as a child. On physical examination, she is noted to have expiratory wheezing. Her pulmonary function tests demonstrate a forced expiratory volume in 1 second (FEV_1) of 2.67 (79% predicted), forced vital capacity of 3.81 L (97% predicted), and an FEV_1/FVC ratio of 70% (predicted value 86%). Following administration of albuterol, the FEV_1 increases to 3.0 L (12.4%). Which of the following statements regarding the patient's disease process is TRUE?

A. Confirmation of the diagnosis will require methacholine challenge testing.
B. Mortality due to the disease has been increasing over the past decade.
C. The most common risk factor in individuals with the disorder is genetic predisposition.
D. The prevalence of the disorder has not changed in the last several decades.
E. The severity of the disease does not vary significantly within a given patient with the disease.

16. A 38-year-old woman is brought to the emergency room for status asthmaticus. She rapidly deteriorates and dies of her disease. All of the following pathologic findings would likely be seen in this individual EXCEPT:

A. Infiltration of the airway mucosa with eosinophils and activated T-lymphocytes
B. Infiltration of the alveolar spaces with eosinophils and neutrophils

16. (*Continued*)

C. Occlusion of the airway lumen by mucous plugs
D. Thickening and edema of the airway wall
E. Thickening of the basement membrane of the airways with subepithelial collagen deposition

17. A 25-year-old woman is seen for follow-up of persistent asthma symptoms despite treatment with inhaled fluticasone 88 μg twice daily for the past 3 months. According to the National Asthma Education and Prevention Program guidelines endorsed by the National Institutes of Health, which of the following changes in therapy can be considered?

A. Addition of a leukotriene antagonist.
B. Addition of a long-acting beta-agonist.
C. Addition of low-dose theophylline.
D. Increase the dosage of inhaled corticosteroid.
E. Any of the above can be considered.

18. Which of the following patients is appropriately diagnosed with asthma?

A. A 24-year-old woman treated with inhaled corticosteroids for cough and wheezing that has persisted for 6 weeks following a viral upper respiratory infection.
B. A 26-year-old man who coughs and occasionally wheezes following exercise in cold weather.
C. A 34-year-old woman evaluated for chronic cough with an FEV_1/FVC ratio of 68% with an FEV_1 that increases from 1.68 L (52% predicted) to 1.98 L (61% predicted) after albuterol (18% change in FEV_1).
D. A 44-year-old man who works as a technician caring for the mice in a medical research laboratory complains of wheezing, shortness of breath, and cough that are most severe at the end of the week.
E. A 60-year-old man who has smoked two packs of cigarettes per day for 40 years who has dyspnea and cough, and airway hyperreactivity in response to methacholine.

19. A 40-year-old woman with moderate persistent asthma has been under good control for 3 months and is currently using her albuterol MDI for symptomatic control once weekly. She awakens at night twice monthly with asthma symptoms, but continues to exercise regularly without difficulties. Her other medications include fluticasone inhaled 88 μg/puff twice daily and salmeterol 50 μg twice daily. Her FEV_1 is currently at 83% of her personal best. Which action is most appropriate at the present time?

A. Add montelukast 10 mg once daily, as the current albuterol usage suggests poor asthma control.
B. Decrease the fluticasone to 44 μg/puff twice daily.
C. Discontinue the fluticasone.

19. *(Continued)*

    D. Discontinue the salmeterol.

    E. Do nothing, as the current albuterol usage suggests poor asthma control.

20. You are considering omalizumab therapy for a patient with severe persistent asthma who is requiring oral prednisone at 5–10 mg daily in addition to high-dose inhaled corticosteroids, long-acting bronchodilators, and montelukast to control her symptoms. Which of the following is necessary prior to initiating omalizumab?

    A. Discontinuation of oral prednisone

    B. Demonstrated elevation in immunoglobulin E levels to greater than 1000 IU/L

    C. Normalization of FEV_1 or peak expiratory flow rates

    D. Presence of sensitivity to a perennial aeroallergen

    E. Switch oral prednisone to intravenous prednisolone

21. A 76-year-old woman is evaluated for acute onset of shortness of breath and dry cough for the past 2 days. She also has had a fever to as high as 102.5°F (39.2°C). Her past medical history includes hypothyroidism and diabetes mellitus. She currently is taking metformin 1000 mg twice daily. Her levothyroxine dose was increased to 100 μg daily 1 month ago, and she was prescribed nitrofurantoin 100 mg twice daily 3 days ago for a urinary tract infection. Her vital signs show a blood pressure of 115/82 mmHg, heart rate of 96 beats per minute, respiratory rate of 24 breaths per minute, temperature of 101.3°F (38.5°C), and oxygen saturation of 94% on room air. There is dullness to percussion and decreased breath sounds at the right lung base. Crackles are heard bilaterally as well. A chest radiograph shows a moderate right-sided pleural effusion, and patchy bilateral lung infiltrates are seen. The patient is admitted to the hospital. A thoracentesis is performed demonstrating an exudative effusion. The fluid has a white cell count of 3500/mm³ with a differential of 60% polymorphonuclear cells, 30% eosinophils, and 10% lymphocytes. A bronchoscopy is performed that shows a differential of 50% polymorphonuclear cells, 15% eosinophils, and 35% alveolar macrophages. Which of the following would be the most important next step in the treatment of this patient?

    A. Await pleural fluid cultures before making a treatment recommendation.

    B. Decrease levothyroxine dose.

    C. Discontinue nitrofurantoin.

    D. Increase levothyroxine dose.

    E. Initiate treatment with high-dose steroid therapy (methylprednisolone 1 g daily).

22. A 75-year-old man is evaluated for a new left-sided pleural effusion and shortness of breath. He worked as an insulation worker at a shipyard for more than 30 years and did not wear protective respiratory equipment. He has a 50 pack-year history of tobacco with known moderate COPD (FEV_1 55% predicted) and prior history of myocardial infarction 10 years previously. His current medications include aspirin, atenolol, benazepril, tiotropium, and albuterol. His physical examination is consistent with a left-sided effusion with dullness to percussion and decreased breath sounds occurring over one-half of the hemithorax. On chest x-ray, there is a moderate left-sided pleural effusion with bilateral pleural calcifications and left apical pleural thickening. No lung mass is seen. A chest CT confirms the findings on chest x-ray and also fails to show a mass. There is compressive atelectasis of the left lower lobe. A thoracentesis is performed that demonstrates an exudative effusion with 65% lymphocytes, 25% mesothelial cells, and 10% neutrophils. Cytology does not demonstrate any malignancy. Which of the following statements regarding the most likely cause of the patient's effusion is TRUE?

    A. Cigarette smoking increases the likelihood of developing the condition.

    B. Death in this disease is usually related to diffuse metastatic disease.

    C. Exposure to the causative agent can be as little as 1–2 years, and latency to expression of disease may be as great as 40 years.

    D. Repeated pleural fluid cytology will most likely lead to a definitive diagnosis.

    E. Therapy with a combination of surgical resection and adjuvant chemotherapy significantly improves long-term survival.

23. Chronic silicosis is related to an increased risk of which of the following conditions?

    A. Infection with invasive *Aspergillus*

    B. Infection with *Mycobacterium tuberculosis*

    C. Lung cancer

    D. Rheumatoid arthritis

    E. All of the above

24. All of the following occupational lung diseases are correctly matched with their exposure EXCEPT:

    A. Berylliosis—High-technology electronics

    B. Byssinosis—Cotton milling

    C. Farmer's lung—Moldy hay

    D. Progressive massive fibrosis—Shipyard workers

    E. Metal fume fever—Welding

25. A 45-year-old male is evaluated in the clinic for asthma. His symptoms began 2 years ago and are characterized by an episodic cough and wheezing that responded initially to inhaled bronchodilators and inhaled corticosteroids but now require nearly constant prednisone tapers. He notes that the symptoms are worst on weekdays but cannot pinpoint specific triggers. His medications are an albuterol MDI, a fluticasone MDI, and prednisone 10 mg po daily. The patient has no habits and works as a textile worker. Physical examination is notable for mild diffuse polyphonic expiratory wheezing but no other abnormality. Which of the following is the most appropriate next step?

A. Exercise physiology testing
B. Measurement of FEV_1 before and after work
C. Methacholine challenge testing
D. Skin testing for allergies
E. Sputum culture for *Aspergillus fumigatus*

26. A 53-year-old male is seen in the emergency department with sudden-onset fever, chills, malaise, and shortness of breath, but no wheezing. He has no significant past medical history and is a farmer. Of note, he worked earlier in the day stacking hay. PA and lateral chest radiography show bilateral upper lobe infiltrates. Which organism is most likely to be responsible for this presentation?

A. *Nocardia asteroides*
B. *Histoplasma capsulatum*
C. *Cryptococcus neoformans*
D. *Actinomyces*
E. *Aspergillus fumigatus*

27. All of the following conditions are associated with an increased risk of methicillin-resistant *Staphylococcus aureus* as a cause of health care–associated pneumonia EXCEPT:

A. Antibiotic therapy in the preceding 3 months
B. Chronic dialysis
C. Home wound care
D. Hospitalization for more than 2 days in the preceding 3 months
E. Nursing home residence

28. Which of the following statements regarding the diagnosis of community-acquired pneumonia is TRUE?

A. Directed therapy specific to the causative organism is more effective than empirical therapy in hospitalized patients who are not in intensive care.

28. *(Continued)*

B. Five percent to 15% of patients hospitalized with community-acquired pneumonia will have positive blood cultures.
C. In patients who have bacteremia caused by *Streptococcus pneumoniae*, sputum cultures are positive in more than 80% of cases.
D. Polymerase chain reaction tests for identification of *Legionella pneumophila* and *Mycoplasma pneumoniae* are widely available and should be utilized for diagnosis in patients hospitalized with community-acquired pneumonia.
E. The etiology of community-acquired pneumonia is typically identified in about 70% of cases.

29. A 55-year-old man presents to his primary care physician with a 2-day history of cough and fever. His cough is productive of thick, dark green sputum. His past medical history is significant for hypercholesterolemia treated with rosuvastatin. He does not smoke cigarettes and is generally quite healthy, exercising several times weekly. He has no ill contacts and cannot recall the last time he was treated with any antibiotics. On presentation, his vital signs are as follows: temperature 102.1°F (38.9°C), blood pressure 132/78 mmHg, heart rate 87 beats/min, respiratory rate 20 breaths/min, and oxygen saturation 95% on room air. Crackles are present in the right lung base with egophony. A chest radiograph demonstrates segmental consolidation of the right lower lobe with air bronchograms. What is the most appropriate approach to the ongoing care of this patient?

A. Obtain a sputum culture and await results prior to initiating treatment.
B. Perform a chest CT to rule out postobstructive pneumonia.
C. Refer to the emergency department for admission and treatment with intravenous antibiotics.
D. Treat with doxycycline 100 mg twice daily.
E. Treat with moxifloxacin 400 mg daily.

30. A 65-year-old woman is admitted to the intensive care unit for management of septic shock associated with an infected hemodialysis catheter. She was initially intubated on hospital day 1 for acute respiratory distress syndrome. She has slowly been improving such that her FiO_2 was weaned to 0.40, and she was no longer febrile or requiring vasopressors. On hospital day 7, she develops a new fever to 39.4°C (102.9°F) with increased thick, yellow-green sputum from her endotracheal tube. You suspect the patient has ventilator-associated pneumonia. What is the best way to make a definitive diagnosis in this patient?

30. (*Continued*)

A. Endotracheal aspirate yielding a new organism typical of a ventilator-associated pneumonia.

B. Presence of a new infiltrate on chest radiograph.

C. Quantitative cultures from an endotracheal aspirate yielding more than 106 organisms typical of ventilator-associated pneumonia.

D. Quantitative culture from a protected brush specimen yielding more than 103 organisms typical of ventilator-associated pneumonia.

E. There is no single set of criteria that is reliably diagnostic of pneumonia in a ventilated patient.

31. Which of the following associations correctly pairs clinical scenarios and community-acquired pneumonia (CAP) pathogens?

A. Aspiration pneumonia: *Streptococcus pyogenes*

B. Heavy alcohol use: Atypical pathogens and *Staphylococcus aureus*

C. Poor dental hygiene: *Chlamydia pneumoniae, Klebsiella pneumoniae*

D. Structural lung disease: *Pseudomonas aeruginosa, S. aureus*

E. Travel to southwestern United States: *Aspergillus* spp.

32. All of the following factors influence the likelihood of transmitting active tuberculosis EXCEPT:

A. Duration of contact with an infected person

B. Environment in which contact occurs

C. Presence of extrapulmonary tuberculosis

D. Presence of laryngeal tuberculosis

E. Probability of contact with an infectious person

33. Which of the following individuals with a known history of prior latent tuberculosis infection (without therapy) has the *lowest* likelihood of developing reactivation tuberculosis?

A. A 28-year-old woman with anorexia nervosa, a body mass index of 16 kg/m², and a serum albumin of 2.3 g/dL

B. A 36-year-old intravenous drug user who does not have HIV but is homeless

C. A 42-year-old man who is HIV-positive with a CD4 count of 350/µL on highly active antiretroviral therapy

D. A 52-year-old man who works as a coal miner

E. An 83-year-old man who was infected while stationed in Korea in 1958

34. A 42-year-old Nigerian man comes to the emergency department because of fevers, fatigue, weight loss, and cough for 3 weeks. He complains of fevers and a 4.5-kg weight loss. He describes his sputum as yellow in color. It has rarely been blood streaked.

34. (*Continued*)

He emigrated to the United States 1 year ago and is an undocumented alien. He has never been treated for tuberculosis, has never had a purified protein derivative (PPD) skin test placed, and does not recall receiving BCG vaccination. He denies HIV risk factors. He is married and reports no ill contacts. He smokes 1 pack of cigarettes daily and drinks 1 pint of vodka on a daily basis. On physical examination, he appears chronically ill with temporal wasting. His body mass index is 21 kg/m². Vital signs are blood pressure of 122/68 mmHg, heart rate of 89 beats/min, respiratory rate of 22 breaths/min, SaO₂ of 95% on room air, and temperature of 37.9°C. There are amphoric breath sounds posteriorly in the right upper lung field with a few scattered crackles in this area. No clubbing is present. The examination is otherwise unremarkable. His chest radiograph is shown in **Figure 34**. A stain for acid-fast bacilli is negative. What is the most appropriate approach to the ongoing care of this patient?

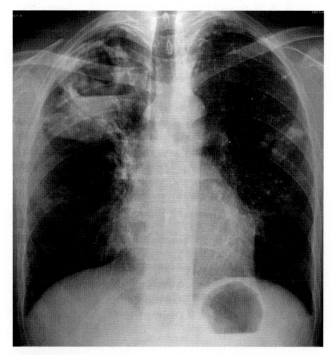

FIGURE 34

A. Admit the patient on airborne isolation until three expectorated sputums show no evidence of acid-fast bacilli.

B. Admit the patient without isolation as he is unlikely to be infectious with a negative acid-fast smear.

C. Perform a biopsy of the lesion and consult oncology.

D. Place a PPD test on his forearm and have him return for evaluation in 3 days.

E. Start a 6-week course of antibiotic treatment for anaerobic bacterial abscess.

35. A 50-year-old man is admitted to the hospital for active pulmonary tuberculosis with a positive sputum acid-fast bacilli smear. He is HIV positive with a CD4 count of 85/μL and is not on highly active antiretroviral therapy. In addition to pulmonary disease, he is found to have disease in the L4 vertebral body. What is the most appropriate initial therapy?

A. Isoniazid, rifampin, ethambutol, and pyrazinamide
B. Isoniazid, rifampin, ethambutol, and pyrazinamide; initiate antiretroviral therapy
C. Isoniazid, rifampin, ethambutol, pyrazinamide, and streptomycin
D. Isoniazid, rifampin, and ethambutol
E. Withhold therapy until sensitivities are available.

36. All of the following individuals receiving tuberculin skin purified protein derivative (PPD) reactions should be treated for latent tuberculosis EXCEPT:

A. A 23-year-old injection drug user who is HIV negative has a 12-mm PPD reaction.
B. A 38-year-old fourth grade teacher has a 7-mm PPD reaction and no known exposures to active tuberculosis. She has never been tested with a PPD previously.
C. A 43-year-old individual in the Peace Corps working in sub-Saharan Africa has a 10-mm PPD reaction. Eighteen months ago, the PPD reaction was 3 mm.
D. A 55-year-old man who is HIV positive has a negative PPD result. His partner was recently diagnosed with cavitary tuberculosis.
E. A 72-year-old man who is receiving chemotherapy for non-Hodgkin's lymphoma has a 16-mm PPD reaction.

37. All of the following statements regarding interferon-gamma release assays for the diagnosis of latent tuberculosis are true EXCEPT:

A. There is no booster phenomenon.
B. They are more specific than tuberculin skin testing.
C. They have a higher sensitivity than tuberculin skin testing in high HIV-burden areas.
D. They have less cross reactivity with BCG and non-tuberculous mycobacteria than tuberculin skin testing.
E. They may be used to screen for latent tuberculosis in adults working in low prevalence U.S. settings.

38. All of the following statements regarding BCG vaccination are true EXCEPT:

A. BCG dissemination may occur in severely immune-suppressed patients.
B. BCG vaccination is recommended at birth in countries with high TB prevalence.
C. BCG vaccination may cause a false-positive tuberculin skin test result.

38. (*Continued*)
D. BCG vaccine provides protection for infants and children from TB meningitis and miliary disease.
E. BCG vaccine provides protection from TB in HIV-infected patients.

39. A 32-year-old woman experiences an upper respiratory illness that began with rhinorrhea and nasal congestion. She also is complaining of a sore throat but has no fever. Her illness lasts for about 5 days and resolves. Just before her illness, her 4-year-old child who attends daycare also experienced a similar illness. All of the following statements regarding the most common etiologic agent causing this illness are true EXCEPT:

A. After the primary illness in a household, a secondary case of illness will occur in 25% to 70% of cases.
B. The seasonal peak of the infection is in early fall and spring in temperate climates.
C. The virus can be isolated from plastic surfaces up to 3 hours after exposure.
D. The virus grows best at a temperature of 37°C, the temperature within the nasal passages.
E. The virus is a single-stranded RNA virus of the Picornaviridae family.

40. All of the following respiratory viruses is a cause of the common cold syndrome in children or adults EXCEPT:

A. Adenoviruses
B. Coronaviruses
C. Enteroviruses
D. Human respiratory syncytial viruses
E. Rhinoviruses

41. All of the following viruses are correctly matched with their primary clinical manifestations EXCEPT:

A. Adenovirus—Gingivostomatitis
B. Coronavirus—Severe acute respiratory syndrome
C. Human respiratory syncytial virus—Bronchiolitis in infants and young children
D. Parainfluenza—Croup
E. Rhinovirus—Common cold

42. A 9-month-old infant is admitted to the hospital with a febrile respiratory illness with wheezing and cough. Upon admission to the hospital, the baby is tachypneic and tachycardic with an oxygen saturation of 75% on room air. Rapid viral diagnostic testing confirms the presence of human respiratory syncytial virus. All of the following treatments should be used as part of the treatment plan for this child EXCEPT:

42. (*Continued*)
  A. Aerosolized ribavirin
  B. Hydration
  C. Immunoglobulin with high titers of antibody directed against human respiratory syncytial virus
  D. Nebulized albuterol
  E. Oxygen therapy to maintain oxygen saturation greater than 90%

43. In March 2009, the H1N1 strain of the influenza A virus emerged in Mexico and quickly spread worldwide over the next several months. Ultimately, more than 18,000 people died from the pandemic. This virus had genetic components of swine influenza viruses, an avian virus, and a human influenza virus. The genetic process by which this pandemic strain of influenza A emerged is an example of:

  A. Antigenic drift
  B. Antigenic shift
  C. Genetic reassortment
  D. Point mutation
  E. B and C

44. A 65-year-old woman is admitted to the hospital in January with a 2-day history of fevers, myalgias, headache, and cough. She has a history of end-stage kidney disease, diabetes mellitus, and hypertension. Her medications include darbepoetin, selamaver, calcitriol, lisinopril, aspirin, amlodipine, and insulin. She receives hemodialysis three times weekly. Upon admission, her blood pressure is 138/65 mmHg, heart rate is 122 beats/min, temperature is 39.4°C, respiratory rate is 24 breaths/min, and oxygen saturation is 85% on room air. On physical examination, diffuse crackles are heard, and a chest radiograph confirms the presence of bilateral lung infiltrates concerning for pneumonia. It is known that the most common cause of seasonal influenza in this area is an H3N2 strain of influenza A. All of the following should be included in the initial management of this patient EXCEPT:

  A. Amantadine
  B. Assessment of the need for close household contacts to receive chemoprophylaxis if influenza swab result is positive
  C. Droplet precautions
  D. Nasal swab for influenza
  E. Oxygen therapy

45. In which of the following individuals has the intranasal influenza vaccine been determined to be safe and effective?

  A. A 3-year-old child who was hospitalized on one occasion for wheezing in association with human respiratory syncytial virus infection at 9 months of age

45. (*Continued*)
  B. A 32-year-old woman who is currently 32 weeks pregnant
  C. A 42-year-old registered nurse who had a known exposure to an individual with pandemic H1N1 who is currently receiving chemoprophylaxis with oseltamivir. He does not have contact with transplant, oncology, or HIV-positive patients.
  D. A 48-year-old hematologist whose primary specialty is bone marrow transplant
  E. A 69-year-old man with hypertension

46. A 17-year-old woman with a medical history of mild intermittent asthma presents to your clinic in February with several days of cough, fever, malaise, and myalgias. She notes that her symptoms started 3 days earlier with a headache and fatigue and that several students and teachers at her high school have been diagnosed recently with "the flu." She did not receive a flu shot this year. Which of the following medication treatment plans is the best option for this patient?

  A. Aspirin and a cough suppressant with codeine
  B. Oseltamivir, 75 mg PO bid for 5 days
  C. Rimantadine, 100 mg PO bid for 1 week
  D. Symptom-based therapy with over-the-counter agents
  E. Zanamivir, 10 mg inhaled bid for 5 days

47. A 35-year-old woman with long-standing rheumatoid arthritis has been treated with infliximab for the past 6 months with improvement of her joint disease. She has a history of positive PPD and takes INH prophylaxis. For the past week, she reports worsening dyspnea on exertion with low-grade fevers and a nonproductive cough. On examination, her vital signs are notable for normal blood pressure, temperature of 38.0°C, heart rate of 105 beats/min, respiratory rate of 22 breaths/min, and SaO$_2$ of 91% on room air. Her lungs are clear. Within one flight of steps, she becomes dyspneic, and her SaO$_2$ falls to 80%. A chest CT scan is shown in **Figure 47**. Which of the following is the most likely diagnosis?

  A. *Aspergillus fumigatus* pneumonia
  B. *Nocardia asteroides* pneumonia
  C. *Pneumocystis jiroveci* pneumonia
  D. Rheumatoid nodules
  E. Staphylococcal bacteremia and septic pulmonary emboli

48. Which of the following patients should receive prophylaxis against *Pneumocystis jiroveci* pneumonia?

  A. A 19-year-old woman with acute myelogenous leukemia initiating induction chemotherapy

47. (*Continued*)

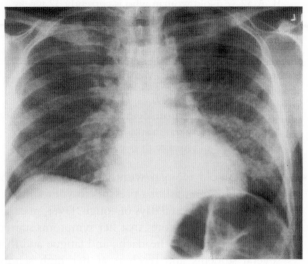
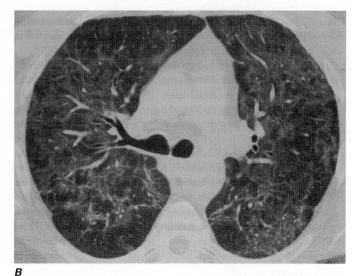

A

B

FIGURE 47

48. (*Continued*)

    B. A 24-year-old man with HIV initiated on HAART therapy 9 months ago when his CD4 count was 100/μL and now has a CD4 count of 500/μL for the past 4 months

    C. A 36-year-old man with newly diagnosed HIV and a CD4 count of 300/μL

    D. A 42-year-old woman with rheumatoid arthritis who recovered from an episode of *Pneumocystis* pneumonia while taking infliximab who is now initiating therapy with abatacept

    E. A 56-year-old man with COPD receiving prednisone for an acute exacerbation

49. A 45-year-old woman with known HIV infection and medical nonadherence to therapy is admitted to the hospital with 2 to 3 weeks of increasing dyspnea on exertion and malaise. A chest radiograph shows bilateral alveolar infiltrates, and induced sputum is positive for *Pneumocystis jiroveci*. Which of the following clinical conditions is an indication for administration of adjunct glucocorticoids?

    A. Acute respiratory distress syndrome

    B. CD4+ lymphocyte count <100/μL

    C. No clinical improvement 5 days into therapy

    D. Pneumothorax

    E. Room air PaO_2 <70 mmHg

50. Which of the following is the most common cause of diffuse bronchiectasis worldwide?

    A. Cystic fibrosis

    B. Immunoglobulin deficiency

    C. *Mycobacterium avium-intracellulare* infection

50. (*Continued*)

    D. *Mycobacterium tuberculosis* infection

    E. Rheumatoid arthritis

51. A 54-year-old woman presents complaining of chronic cough that has worsened over a period of 6–12 months. She reports the cough to be present day and night, and productive of a thick green sputum. Over the course of the day, she estimates that she produces as much as 100 mL of sputum daily. Bilateral coarse crackles are heard in the lower lung zones. Pulmonary function tests demonstrate an FEV_1 of 1.68 L (53.3% predicted), FVC of 3.00 L (75% predicted), and FEV_1/FVC ratio of 56%. A chest radiograph is unremarkable. What would you recommend as the next step in the evaluation of this patient?

    A. Bronchoscopy with bronchoalveolar lavage

    B. Chest CT with intravenous contrast

    C. High-resolution chest CT

    D. Serum immunoglobulin levels

    E. Treatment with a long-acting bronchodilator and inhaled corticosteroid

52. A 48-year-old man is admitted to the hospital with fever and cough. He suffers from alcoholism and is homeless. He does not routinely obtain any health care. He reports that he has felt poorly for about 8 weeks. He has fatigue and generalized malaise. He states that he lost weight over this period as his clothing is very loose, but he cannot quantify the weight loss. He has felt feverish at times. During this period, he has been having increasing cough with

52. (*Continued*)

malodorous sputum production. He coughs at least 3 tablespoons of dark sputum daily that has been blood streaked at times. He takes no medications, but drinks about 1 L of vodka daily. He also smokes one pack of cigarettes daily. On physical examination, the patient is disheveled and appears chronically ill. His vital signs are heart rate 98 beats/min, blood pressure 110/73 mmHg, respiratory rate 20 breaths/min, temperature 38.2°C (100.8°F), and oxygen saturation of 94% on room air. He has evidence of temporal wasting with very poor dentition. A foul odor is present on his breath. Amphoric breath sounds are heard posteriorly in the right lower lung field. A chest x-ray shows a 4-cm cavitary lung lesion in the right lower lobe. The patient is admitted and placed on respiratory isolation. Sputum cultures for bacteria, mycobacteria, and fungus are ordered. What is the best initial choice for therapy in this patient?

A. Ampicillin–sulbactam 3 g intravenously every 6 hours
B. Isoniazid, rifampin, pyrazinamide, and ethambutol orally
C. Metronidazole 500 mg orally four times daily
D. Percutaneous drainage of the cavity
E. Piperacillin–tazobactam 2.25 g intravenously every 4 hours in combination with tobramycin 5 mg/kg intravenously daily

53. A 35-year-old male is seen in the clinic for evaluation of infertility. He has never fathered any children, and after 2 years of unprotected intercourse his wife has not achieved pregnancy. Sperm analysis shows a normal number of sperm, but they are immotile. Past medical history is notable for recurrent sinopulmonary infections, and the patient recently was told that he has bronchiectasis. Chest radiography is likely to show which of the following?

A. Bihilar lymphadenopathy
B. Bilateral upper lobe infiltrates
C. Normal findings
D. Situs inversus
E. Water balloon–shaped heart

54. A 28-year-old woman is evaluated for recurrent lung and sinus infections. She recalls having at least yearly episodes of bronchitis beginning in her early teens. She states that for the past 5 years she has been on antibiotics at least three times yearly for respiratory or sinus infections. She also reports that she has had difficulty gaining weight and has always felt short compared to her peers. On physical examination, the patient has a body mass index of 18.5 kg/m². Her oxygen saturation is 94% on room air at rest. Nasal polyps are present. Coarse rhonchi

54. (*Continued*)

and crackles are heard in the bilateral upper lung zones. Mild clubbing is seen. A chest radiograph shows bilateral upper lobe bronchiectasis with areas of mucous plugging. You are concerned about the possibility of undiagnosed cystic fibrosis (CF). Which of the following tests would provide the strongest support for the diagnosis of CF in this individual?

A. DNA analysis demonstrating one copy of the delta F508 allele
B. Decreased baseline nasal potential difference
C. Presence of *Pseudomonas aeruginosa* on repeated sputum cultures
D. Sweat chloride values greater than 35 meq/L
E. Sweat chloride values greater than 70 meq/L

55. A 22-year-old man with cystic fibrosis is seen for a routine follow-up exam. He is currently treated with recombinant human DNAse and albuterol by nebulization twice daily. His primary sputum clearance technique is aerobic exercise five times weekly and autogenic drainage. He is feeling well overall, and his examination is normal. Pulmonary function testing demonstrates an FEV_1 of 4.48 L (97% predicted), an FVC of 5.70 L (103% predicted), and an FEV_1/FVC ratio of 79%. A routine sputum culture grows *Pseudomonas aeruginosa*. The only organism isolated on prior cultures has been *Staphylococcus aureus*. What do you recommend for this patient?

A. High-frequency chest wall oscillation
B. Hypertonic saline (7%) nebulized twice daily
C. Inhaled tobramycin 300 mg twice daily every other month
D. Intravenous cefepime and tobramycin for 14 days
E. Return visit in 3 months with repeat sputum cultures and treatment only if there is persistent *P. aeruginosa*

56. Which of the following organisms is unlikely to be found in the sputum of a patient with cystic fibrosis?

A. *Haemophilus influenzae*
B. *Acinetobacter baumannii*
C. *Burkholderia cepacia*
D. *Aspergillus fumigatus*
E. *Staphylococcus aureus*

57. All of the following are risk factors for chronic obstructive pulmonary disease EXCEPT:

A. Airway hyperresponsiveness
B. Coal dust exposure
C. Passive cigarette smoke exposure
D. Recurrent respiratory infections
E. Use of biomass fuels in poorly ventilated areas

58. A 65-year-old woman is evaluated for dyspnea on exertion and chronic cough. She has a long history of tobacco use, smoking 1.5 packs of cigarettes daily since the age of 20. She is a thin woman in no obvious distress. Her oxygen saturation on room air is 93% with a respiratory rate of 22/min. The lungs are hyperexpanded on percussion with decreased breath sounds in the upper lung fields. You suspect chronic obstructive pulmonary disease. What are the expected findings on pulmonary function testing? (See **Table 58**.)

TABLE 58

	FEV$_1$	FVC	FEV$_1$/FVC RATIO	TLC	DLCO
A.	Decreased	Normal or decreased	Decreased	Decreased	Decreased
B.	Decreased	Normal or decreased	Decreased	Increased	Decreased
C.	Decreased	Decreased	Normal	Decreased	Decreased
D.	Decreased	Normal or decreased	Decreased	Increased	Normal or increased

59. A 70-year-old man with known chronic obstructive pulmonary disease is seen for follow-up. He has been clinically stable without an exacerbation for the past 6 months. However, he generally feels in poor health and is limited in what he can do. He reports dyspnea with usual activities. He is currently being managed with an albuterol metered-dose inhaler twice daily and as needed. He has a 50 pack-year history of smoking and quit 5 years previously. His other medical problems include peripheral vascular disease, hypertension, and benign prostatic hyperplasia. He is managed with aspirin, lisinopril, hydrochlorothiazide, and tamsulosin. On examination, the patient has a resting oxygen saturation of 93% on room air. He is hyperinflated to percussion with decreased breath sounds at the apices and faint expiratory wheezing. His pulmonary function tests demonstrate an FEV$_1$ of 55% predicted, an FVC of 80% predicted, and an FEV$_1$/FVC ratio of 50%. What is the next best step in the management of this patient?

A. Initiate a trial of oral glucocorticoids for a period of 4 weeks and initiate inhaled fluticasone if there is a significant improvement in pulmonary function.

B. Initiate treatment with inhaled fluticasone 110 μg/puff twice daily.

C. Initiate treatment with inhaled fluticasone 250 μg/puff in combination with inhaled salmeterol 50 mg/puff twice daily.

D. Initiate treatment with inhaled tiotropium 18 μg/daily.

E. Perform exercise and nocturnal oximetry, and initiate oxygen therapy if these demonstrate significant hypoxemia.

60. A 56-year-old woman is admitted to the intensive care unit with a 4-day history of increasing shortness of breath and cough with copious sputum production. She has known severe COPD with an FEV$_1$

60. (*Continued*)
of 42% predicted. On presentation, she has a room air blood gas with a pH 7.26, PaCO$_2$ 78 mmHg, and PaO$_2$ 50 mmHg. She is in obvious respiratory distress with the use of accessory muscles and retractions. Breath sounds are quiet with diffuse expiratory wheezing and rhonchi. No infiltrates are present on chest radiograph. Which of the following therapies has been demonstrated to have the greatest reduction in mortality for patients with these findings?

A. Administration of inhaled bronchodilators

B. Administration of intravenous glucocorticoids

C. Early administration of broad-spectrum antibiotics with coverage of *Pseudomonas aeruginosa*

D. Early intubation with mechanical ventilation

E. Use of noninvasive positive pressure ventilation

61. A 63-year-old male with a long history of cigarette smoking comes to see you for a 4-month history of progressive shortness of breath and dyspnea on exertion. The symptoms have been indolent, with no recent worsening. He denies fever, chest pain, or hemoptysis. He has a daily cough of 3–6 tablespoons of yellow phlegm. The patient says he has not seen a physician for over 10 years. Physical examination is notable for normal vital signs, a prolonged expiratory phase, scattered rhonchi, elevated jugular venous pulsation, and moderate pedal edema. Hematocrit is 49%. Which of the following therapies is most likely to prolong his survival?

A. Atenolol

B. Enalapril

C. Oxygen

D. Prednisone

E. Theophylline

62. A 62-year-old man is evaluated for dyspnea on exertion that has progressively worsened over a period of

62. (*Continued*)

10 months. He has a 50 pack-year history of tobacco, quitting 10 years ago. His physiologic and radiologic evaluation demonstrates a restrictive ventilatory defect with diffuse fibrosis that is worse in the subpleural region and at the bases. A surgical lung biopsy is performed, which is consistent with usual interstitial pneumonia. No autoimmune or drug-related cause is found. What is the recommended treatment for this patient?

A. Azathioprine 125 mg daily plus prednisone 60 mg daily
B. Cyclophosphamide 100 mg daily
C. N-acetylcysteine 600 mg twice daily plus prednisone 60 mg daily
D. Prednisone 60 mg daily
E. Referral for lung transplantation

63. What would be the expected finding on bronchoalveolar lavage in a patient with diffuse alveolar hemorrhage?

A. Atypical hyperplastic type II pneumocytes
B. Ferruginous bodies
C. Hemosiderin laden macrophages
D. Lymphocytosis with an elevated CD4:CD8 ratio
E. Milky appearance with foamy macrophages

64. A 42-year-old male presents with progressive dyspnea on exertion, low-grade fevers, and weight loss over 6 months. He also is complaining of a primarily dry cough, although occasionally he coughs up thick mucoid sputum. There is no past medical history. He does not smoke cigarettes. On physical examination, the patient appears dyspneic with minimal exertion. The patient's temperature is 37.9°C (100.3°F). Oxygen saturation is 91% on room air at rest. Faint basilar crackles are heard. On laboratory studies, the patient has polyclonal hypergammaglobulinemia and a hematocrit of 52%. A CT scan reveals bilateral alveolar infiltrates that are primarily perihilar in nature with a mosaic pattern. The patient undergoes bronchoscopy with bronchoalveolar lavage. The effluent appears milky. The cytopathology shows amorphous debris with periodic acid–Schiff (PAS)-positive macrophages. What is the diagnosis?

A. Bronchiolitis obliterans organizing pneumonia
B. Desquamative interstitial pneumonitis
C. Nocardiosis
D. *Pneumocystis carinii* pneumonia
E. Pulmonary alveolar proteinosis

65. What treatment is most appropriate at this time for the patient in question 64?

65. (*Continued*)

A. Doxycycline
B. Prednisone
C. Prednisone and cyclophosphamide
D. Trimethoprim-sulfamethoxazole
E. Whole-lung saline lavage

66. A 68-year-old man presents for evaluation of dyspnea on exertion. He states that he first noticed the symptoms about 2 years ago. At that time, he had to stop walking the golf course and began to use a cart, but he was still able to complete a full 18 holes. Over the past year, he has stopped golfing altogether because of breathlessness and states that he has difficulty walking to and from his mailbox, which is about 50 yards from his house. He also has a dry cough that occurs on most days. It is not worse at night, and he can identify no triggers. He denies wheezing. He has had no fevers, chills, or weight loss. He denies any joint symptoms. He is a former smoker of about 50 pack-years, but quit 8 years previously after being diagnosed with coronary artery disease. On physical examination, he appears breathless after walking down the hallway to the examination room, but quickly recovers upon resting. Vital signs are as follows: blood pressure 118/67 mmHg, heart rate 88 beats/min, respiratory rate 20 breaths/min. His SaO$_2$ is 94% at rest and decreases to 86% after ambulating 300 ft. His lung examination shows normal percussion and expansion. There are Velcro-like crackles at both bases, and they are distributed halfway through both lung fields. No wheezing is noted. Cardiovascular examination is normal. Digital clubbing is present. A chest CT is performed and is shown in **Figure 66**. He is referred for surgical lung biopsy. Which pathologic description is most likely to be seen in this patient's disease?

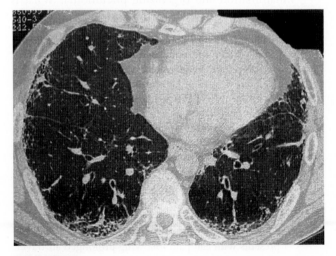

FIGURE 66

66. (*Continued*)

   A. Dense amorphous fluid within the alveoli diffusely that stains positive with periodic acid–Schiff stain

   B. Destruction of alveoli with resultant emphysematous areas, predominantly in the upper lobes

   C. Diffuse alveolar damage

   D. Formation of noncaseating granulomas

   E. Heterogeneous collagen deposition with fibroblast foci and honeycombing

67. All the following are pulmonary manifestations of systemic lupus erythematosus EXCEPT:

   A. Cavitary lung nodules

   B. Diaphragmatic dysfunction with loss of lung volumes

   C. Pleuritis

   D. Pulmonary hemorrhage

   E. Pulmonary vascular disease

68. A 56-year-old woman presents for evaluation of dyspnea and cough for 2 months. During this time, she has also had intermittent fevers, malaise, and a 5.5-kg (12-lb) weight loss. She denies having any ill contacts and has not recently traveled. She works as a nurse, and a yearly PPD test performed 3 months ago was negative. She denies any exposure to organic dusts and does not have any birds as pets. She has a history of rheumatoid arthritis and is currently taking hydroxychloroquine, 200 mg twice daily. There has been no worsening in her joint symptoms. On physical examination, diffuse inspiratory crackles and squeaks are heard. A CT scan of the chest reveals patchy alveolar infiltrates and bronchial wall thickening. Pulmonary function testing reveals mild restriction. She undergoes a surgical lung biopsy. The pathology shows granulation tissue filling the small airways, alveolar ducts, and alveoli. The alveolar interstitium has chronic inflammation and organizing pneumonia. What is the most appropriate therapy for this patient?

   A. Azathioprine 100 mg daily

   B. Discontinuation of hydroxychloroquine and observation

   C. Infliximab IV once monthly

   D. Methotrexate 15 mg weekly

   E. Prednisone 1 mg/kg daily

69. In which of the following patients presenting with acute dyspnea would a positive D-dimer prompt additional testing for a pulmonary embolus?

   A. A 24-year-old woman who is 32 weeks pregnant.

   B. A 48-year-old man with no medical history who presents with calf pain following prolonged air travel. The alveolar-arterial oxygen gradient is normal.

69. (*Continued*)

   C. A 56-year-old woman undergoing chemotherapy for breast cancer.

   D. A 62-year-old man who underwent hip replacement surgery 4 weeks previously.

   E. A 72-year-old man who had an acute myocardial infarction 2 weeks ago.

70. A 62-year-old woman is hospitalized following an acute pulmonary embolism. All of the following would typically indicate a massive pulmonary embolism EXCEPT:

   A. Elevated serum troponin levels

   B. Initial presentation with hemoptysis

   C. Initial presentation with syncope

   D. Presence of right ventricular enlargement on CT scan of the chest

   E. Presence of right ventricular hypokinesis on echocardiogram

71. Which of the following statements regarding diagnostic imaging in pulmonary embolism is TRUE?

   A. A high probability ventilation-perfusion scan is one that has at least one segmental perfusion defect in the setting of normal ventilation.

   B. If a patient has a high probability ventilation-perfusion scan, there is a 90% likelihood that the patient does indeed have a pulmonary embolism.

   C. Magnetic resonance angiography provides excellent resolution for both large proximal and smaller segmental pulmonary emboli.

   D. Multidetector-row spiral CT imaging is suboptimal for detecting small peripheral emboli, necessitating the use of invasive pulmonary angiography.

   E. None of the routinely used imaging techniques provide adequate evaluation of the right ventricle to assist in risk stratification of the patient.

72. A 53-year-old woman presents to the hospital following an episode of syncope, with ongoing lightheadedness and shortness of breath. She had a history of antiphospholipid syndrome with prior pulmonary embolism and has been nonadherent to her anticoagulation medication recently. She has been prescribed warfarin, 7.5 mg daily, but reports taking it only intermittently. She does not know her most recent INR. On presentation to the emergency room, she appears diaphoretic and tachypneic. Her vital signs are as follows: blood pressure 86/44 mmHg, heart rate 130 beats/min, respiratory rate 30 breaths/min, and oxygen saturation of 85% on room air. Cardiovascular examination shows a regular tachycardia without murmurs, rubs, or gallops. The lungs are clear to auscultation.

72. (*Continued*)

On extremity examination, there is swelling of her left thigh with a positive Homan's sign. Chest CT angiography confirms a saddle pulmonary embolus with ongoing clot seen in the pelvic veins on the left. Anticoagulation with unfractionated heparin is administered. After a fluid bolus of 1 L, the patient's blood pressure remains low at 88/50 mmHg. Echocardiogram demonstrates hypokinesis of the right ventricle. On 100% non-rebreather mask, the oxygen saturation is 92%. What is the next best step in the management of this patient?

A. Continue current management.
B. Continue IV fluids at 500 mL/h for a total of 4 L of fluid resuscitation.
C. Refer for inferior vena cava filter placement and continue current management.
D. Refer for surgical embolectomy.
E. Treat with dopamine and recombinant tissue plasminogen activator, 100 mg IV.

73. A 42-year-old woman presents to the emergency room with acute onset of shortness of breath. She recently had been to visit her parents out of state and rode in a car for about 9 hours each way. Two days ago, she developed mild calf pain and swelling, but she thought that this was not unusual after having been sitting with her legs dependent for the recent trip. On arrival to the emergency room, she is noted to be tachypneic. The vital signs are as follows: blood pressure 98/60 mmHg, heart rate 114 beats/min, respiratory rate 28 breaths/min, oxygen saturation of 92% on room air, weight 89 kg. The lungs are clear bilaterally. There is pain in the right calf with dorsiflexion of the foot, and the right leg is more swollen when compared to the left. An arterial blood gas measurement shows a pH of 7.52, PCO_2 25 mmHg, and PO_2 68 mmHg. Kidney and liver function are normal. A helical CT scan confirms a pulmonary embolus. All of the following agents can be used alone as initial therapy in this patient EXCEPT:

A. Enoxaparin 1 mg/kg SC twice daily
B. Fondaparinux 7.5 mg SC once daily
C. Tinzaparin 175 U/kg SC once daily
D. Unfractionated heparin IV adjusted to maintain activated partial thromboplastin time (aPTT) two to three times the upper limit of normal
E. Warfarin 7.5 mg po once daily to maintain INR at 2–3

74. A 62-year-old woman is admitted to the hospital with a community-acquired pneumonia with a

74. (*Continued*)

4-day history of fever, cough, and right-sided pleuritic chest pain. The admission chest x-ray identifies a right lower and middle lobe infiltrate with an associated effusion. All of the following characteristics of the pleural effusion indicate a complicated effusion that may require tube thoracostomy EXCEPT:

A. Loculated fluid
B. Pleural fluid pH less than 7.20
C. Pleural fluid glucose less than 60 mg/dL
D. Positive Gram stain or culture of the pleural fluid
E. Recurrence of fluid following the initial thoracentesis

75. A 58-year-old man is evaluated for dyspnea and is found to have a moderate right-sided pleural effusion. He undergoes thoracentesis with the following characteristics:

APPEARANCE	SEROSANGUINOUS
pH	7.48
Protein	5.8 g/dL (serum protein 7.2 g/dL)
LDH	285 IU/L (serum LDH 320 IU/L)
Glucose	66 mg/dL
WBC	3800/mm³
RBC	24,000/mm³
PMNs	10%
Lymphocytes	80%
Mesothelial cells	10%
Cytology	Lymphocytosis with chronic inflammation and no malignant cells or organisms identified

Which of the following is an unlikely cause of the pleural effusion in this patient?

A. Cirrhosis
B. Lung cancer
C. Mesothelioma
D. Pulmonary embolism
E. Tuberculosis

76. A 66-year-old woman is evaluated for dyspnea. One month previously, she had undergone an esophagectomy for adenocarcinoma of the esophagus. On physical examination, the patient appears tachypneic with difficulty speaking in full sentences. She has a respiratory rate of 28/min and an oxygen saturation of 88% on room air. There is dullness to percussion

76. (*Continued*)

with absent breath sounds in the left hemithorax. A chest radiograph confirms a large left-sided pleural effusion with mediastinal shift to the right. A thoracentesis removes 1.5 L of a milky-appearing fluid. The protein of the fluid is 6.2 mg/dL, LDH is 368 IU/L, and the WBC count is 1500/μL (20% PMNs, 80% lymphocytes). The triglyceride level is 168 mg/dL. Cultures and cytology are negative. Which of the following is the best management for this patient?

A. Placement of a chest tube plus octreotide
B. Placement of a chest tube to wall suction until drainage decreases to less than 100 mL daily
C. Reexploration of the chest with surgical correction of the likely defect
D. Referral for palliative care
E. Repeat thoracentesis for cytologic examination

77. A 28-year-old man presents to the emergency room with acute-onset shortness of breath and pleuritic chest pain on the right that began 2 hours previously. He is generally healthy and has no medical history. He has smoked one pack of cigarettes daily since the age of 18. On physical examination, he is tall and thin with a body mass index of 19.2 kg/m². He has a respiratory rate of 24/min with an oxygen saturation of 95% on room air. He has slightly decreased breath sounds at the right lung apex. A chest x-ray demonstrates a 20% pneumothorax on the right side. Which of the following is TRUE regarding pneumothorax in this patient?

A. A CT scan is likely to show emphysematous changes.
B. If the patient were to develop recurrent pneumothoraces, thorascopy with pleural abrasion has a success rate of nearly 100% for prevention of recurrence.
C. Most patients with this presentation require tube thoracostomy to resolve the pneumothorax.
D. The likelihood of recurrent pneumothorax is about 25%.
E. The primary risk factor for the development of spontaneous pneumothorax is a tall and thin body habitus.

78. The most common cause of a pleural effusion is:

A. Cirrhosis
B. Left ventricular failure
C. Malignancy
D. Pneumonia
E. Pulmonary embolism

79. A patient with mild amyotrophic lateral sclerosis is followed by a pulmonologist for respiratory dysfunction associated with his neuromuscular disease.

79. (*Continued*)

Which of the following symptoms in addition to PaCO₂ of 45 mmHg or greater would necessitate therapy with noninvasive positive pressure ventilation for hypoventilation?

A. Orthopnea
B. Poor quality sleep
C. Impaired cough
D. Dyspnea in activities of daily living
E. All of the above

80. A 27-year-old man with muscular dystrophy is evaluated by his primary care physician for hypoxemia. He reports feeling at his baseline and is not short of breath. On physical examination, finger pulse oximetry is 86% on room air, his lungs are clear, and aside from stigmata of muscular dystrophy, is normal. Chest radiograph shows low lung volumes. Which of the following is most likely the source of his low oxygen saturation?

A. Atelectasis
B. Mucous plug
C. Elevated PaCO₂
D. Pneumonia
E. Methemoglobinemia

81. Patients with chronic hypoventilation disorders often complain of a headache upon wakening. What is the cause of this symptom?

A. Arousals from sleep
B. Cerebral vasodilation
C. Cerebral vasoconstriction
D. Polycythemia
E. Nocturnal microaspiration and cough

82. A 47-year-old woman with idiopathic pulmonary arterial hypertension has failed medical therapy including intravenous epoprostenol. She has advanced right heart failure with severe right ventricular dysfunction on echocardiography and a cardiac index of 1.7 L/min per m². She is referred for lung transplantation. Which of the following statements is true?

A. She will require heart-lung transplantation for her advanced right heart failure.
B. Idiopathic pulmonary arterial hypertension patients have worse 5-year survival than other transplant recipients.
C. Single-lung transplantation is the preferred surgical procedure for idiopathic pulmonary arterial hypertension.
D. Her own right ventricular function will recover after lung transplantation.

82. (*Continued*)

E. She is at risk for recurrent pulmonary arterial hypertension after lung transplantation.

83. A 25-year-old woman with cystic fibrosis is referred for lung transplantation. She is concerned about her long-term outcomes. Which of the following is the main impediment to long-term survival after lung transplantation?

A. Bronchiolitis obliterans syndrome
B. Cytomegalovirus infection
C. Chronic kidney disease
D. Primary graft dysfunction
E. Post-transplant lymphoproliferative disorder

84. A 30-year-old man with end-stage cystic fibrosis undergoes lung transplantation. Three years later, he has a 6-month progressive decline in his renal function. Which of the following medications is the most likely etiology of this?

A. Prednisone
B. Tacrolimus
C. Albuterol
D. Mycophenolate mofetil
E. None of the above

85. A 22-year-old man has cystic fibrosis. He currently is hospitalized about three times yearly for infectious exacerbations. He is colonized with *Pseudomonas aeruginosa* and *Staphylococcus aureus*, but has never had *Burkholderia cepacia* complex. He remains active and is in college studying architecture. He requires 2 L of oxygen with exertion. The most recent pulmonary function tests demonstrate an FEV_1 that is 28% of the predicted value and an FEV_1/FVC ratio of 44%. Measurement of his arterial blood gas or room air is pH 7.38, PCO_2 36 mmHg, and PO_2 62 mmHg. Which of these characteristics is an indication for referral for lung transplantation?

A. Colonization with *Pseudomonas aeruginosa*
B. FEV_1 less than 30% predicted
C. FEV_1/FVC ratio less than 50%
D. PCO_2 less than 40 mmHg
E. Use of oxygen with exertion

86. Clinical trials support the use of noninvasive ventilation in which of the following patients?

A. A 33-year-old man who was rescued from a motor vehicle accident. He is unarousable with possible internal injuries. Room air blood gas is 7.30 (pH), PCO_2 50 mmHg, PO_2 60 mmHg.

86. (*Continued*)

B. A 49-year-old woman with end-stage renal disease admitted with presumed staphylococcal sepsis from her hemodialysis catheter. She is somnolent, blood pressure is 80/50 mmHg, heart rate is 105 beats/min, and room air oxygen saturation is 95%.

C. A 58-year-old woman with a history of cirrhotic liver disease admitted with a presumed esophageal variceal bleed. Her blood pressure is 75/55 mmHg, and she has a heart rate of 110 beats/min. She is awake and alert.

D. A 62-year-old man with a long history of COPD admitted with an exacerbation related to an upper respiratory tract infection. He is in marked respiratory distress but is awake and alert. Chest radiograph only shows hyperinflation. His room air arterial blood gas is pH, 7.28; PCO_2, 75 mmHg; and PO_2, 46 mmHg.

E. A 74-year-old man with cardiogenic shock and an acute ST-segment elevation myocardial infarction. His blood pressure is 84/65 mmHg, heart rate is 110 beats/min, respiratory rate is 24 breaths/min, and room air oxygen saturation is 85%.

87. You are caring for a patient on mechanical ventilation in the intensive care unit. Whenever the patient initiates a breath, no matter her spontaneous respiratory rate, she gets a fixed volume breath from the machine that does not change from breath to breath. After receiving a dose of sedation, she does not initiate any breaths, but the machine delivers the same volume breath at periodic fixed intervals during this time. Which of the following modes of mechanical ventilation is this patient receiving?

A. Assist control
B. Continuous positive airway pressure
C. Pressure control
D. Pressure support
E. Synchronized intermittent mandatory ventilation (SIMV)

88. A 68-year-old woman has been receiving mechanical ventilation for 10 days for community-acquired pneumonia. You are attempting to decide whether the patient is following factors would indicate that the patient is likely to be successfully extubated EXCEPT:

A. Alert mental status
B. PEEP of 5 cmH_2O
C. pH greater than 7.35
D. Rapid shallow breathing index (respiratory rate/tidal volume) greater than 105
E. SaO_2 greater than 90% and FiO_2 less than 0.5

89. A 45-year-old woman with HIV is admitted to the intensive care unit with pneumonia and pneumothorax secondary to infection with *Pneumocystis jiroveci*. She requires mechanical ventilatory support, chest tube placement, and central venous access. The ventilator settings are PC mode; inspiratory pressure, 30 cmH$_2$O, 1.0; and PEEP, 10 cmH$_2$O. An arterial blood gas measured on these settings shows: pH 7.32, 46 mmHg, and 62 mmHg. All of the following are important supportive measures for this patient EXCEPT:

A. Analgesia to maintain patient comfort
B. Daily change of ventilator circuit
C. Gastric acid suppression
D. Nutritional support
E. Prophylaxis against deep venous thrombosis

90. All of the following statements about the physiology of mechanical ventilation are true EXCEPT:

A. Application of PEEP decreases left ventricular preload and afterload.
B. High inspired tidal volumes contribute to the development of acute lung injury caused by overdistention of alveoli with resultant alveolar damage.
C. Increasing the inspiratory flow rate will decrease the ratio of inspiration to expiration (I:E) and allow more time for expiration.
D. Mechanical ventilation provides assistance with inspiration and expiration.
E. PEEP helps prevent alveolar collapse at end-expiration.

91. A 64-year-old man requires endotracheal intubation and mechanical ventilation for chronic obstructive pulmonary disease. He was paralyzed with rocuronium for intubation. His initial ventilator settings were AC mode; respiratory rate 10 breaths/minute; FiO$_2$ 1.0; Vt (tidal volume) 550 mL; and positive end-expiratory pressure 0 cm H$_2$O. On admission to the intensive care unit the patient remains paralzyed; arterial blood gas is pH 7.22, PCO$_2$ 78 mmHg, PO$_2$ 394 mmHg. The FiO$_2$ is decreased to 0.6. Thirty minutes later you are called to the bedside to evaluate the patient for hypotension. Current vital signs are blood pressure 80/40 mmHg, heart rate, 133 beats/min; respiratory rate, 24/minute; and oxygen saturation 92%. Physical examination shows the patient is agitated and moving all extremities, a prolonged expiration with wheezing continuing until the initiation of the next breath. Breath sounds are heard in both lung fields. The high-pressure alarm on the ventilator is triggering. What should be done first in treating this patient's hypotension?

91. (*Continued*)
A. Administer a fluid bolus of 500 mL.
B. Disconnect the patient from the ventilator.
C. Initiate a continuous IV infusion of midazolam.
D. Initiate a continuous IV infusion of norepinephrine.
E. Perform tube thoracostomy on the right side.

92. All of the following are relative contraindications for the use of succinylcholine as a paralytic for endotracheal intubation EXCEPT:

A. Acetaminophen overdose
B. Acute renal failure
C. Crush injuries
D. Muscular dystrophy
E. Tumor lysis syndrome

93. Match the following vasopressors with the statement that best describes their action on the cardiovascular system.

1. Dobutamine
2. Low-dose dopamine (2–4 µg/kg/min)
3. Norepinephrine
4. Phenylephrine
A. Acts solely at α-adrenergic receptors to cause vasoconstriction
B. Acts at β$_1$-adrenergic receptors and dopaminergic receptors to increase cardiac contractility and heart rate; also causes vasodilatation and increased splanchnic and renal blood flow
C. Acts at β$_1$- and, to a lesser extent, β$_2$-adrenergic receptors to increase cardiac contractility, heart rate, and vasodilatation
D. Acts at α- and β$_1$-adrenergic receptors to increase heart rate, cardiac contractility, and vasoconstriction

94. An 86-year-old nursing home resident is brought by ambulance to the local emergency department. He was found unresponsive in his bed immersed in black stool. Apparently, he had not been feeling well for 1–2 days, had complained of vague abdominal pain, and had decreased oral intake; no further history is available from the nursing home staff. His past medical history is remarkable for Alzheimer's dementia and treated prostate cancer. The emergency responders were able to appreciate a faint pulse and obtained a blood pressure of 91/49 mmHg and a heart rate of 120 beats/min. In the emergency department, his pressure is 88/51 mmHg and heart rate is 131 beats/min. He is moaning and obtunded, localizes to pain, and has flat neck veins. Skin tenting is noted. A central venous catheter is placed that reveals CVP less than 5 mmHg, specimens for initial laboratory testing are sent off, and electrocardiogram and chest x-ray are obtained. Catheterization of the bladder yields no urine.

94. (*Continued*)

Anesthesiology has been called to the bedside and is assessing the patient's airway. What is the best immediate step in management?

A. Infuse hypertonic saline to increase the rate of vascular filling.
B. Infuse isotonic crystalloid solution via IV wide open.
C. Infuse a colloidal solution rapidly.
D. Initiate inotropic support with dobutamine.
E. Initiate IV pressors starting with Levophed.

95. In the patient described above, which of the following is true regarding his clinical condition?

A. Loss of 20–40% of the blood volume leads to shock physiology.
B. Loss of less than 20% of the blood volume will manifest as orthostasis.
C. Oliguria is a crucial prognostic sign of impending vascular collapse.
D. Symptoms of hypovolemic shock differ from those of hemorrhagic shock.
E. The first sign of hypovolemic shock is mental obtundation.

96. A 52-year-old man presents with crushing substernal chest pain. He has a history of coronary artery disease and has had two non–ST-segment elevation myocardial infarctions in the past 5 years, both requiring percutaneous intervention and intracoronary stent placement. His electrocardiogram shows ST elevations across the precordial leads, and he is taken emergently to the catheterization laboratory. After angioplasty and stent placement, he is transferred to the coronary care unit. His vital signs are stable on transfer; however, 20 minutes after arrival, he is found to be unresponsive. His radial pulse is thready, extremities are cool, and blood pressure is difficult to obtain; with a manual cuff, it is 65/40 mmHg. The nurse turns to you and asks what you would like to do next. Which of the following accurately represents the physiologic characteristics of this patient's condition?

	CENTRAL VENOUS PRESSURE	CARDIAC OUTPUT	SYSTEMIC VASCULAR RESISTANCE
A.	Decreased	Decreased	Decreased
B.	Decreased	Increased	Decreased
C.	Increased	Increased	Decreased
D.	Increased	Decreased	Increased
E.	Decreased	Decreased	Increased

97. All of the following are factors that are related to the increased incidence of sepsis in the United States EXCEPT:

A. Aging of the population
B. Increased longevity of individuals with chronic disease
C. Increased risk of sepsis in individuals without comorbidities
D. Increased risk of sepsis in individuals with AIDS
E. Increased use of immunosuppressive drugs

98. A 68-year-old woman is brought to the emergency department for fever and lethargy. She first felt ill yesterday and experienced generalized body aches. Overnight, she developed a fever of 39.6°C and had shaking chills. By this morning, she was feeling very fatigued. Her son feels that she has had periods of waxing and waning mental status. She denies cough, nausea, vomiting, diarrhea, and abdominal pain. She has a medical history of rheumatoid arthritis. She takes prednisone, 10 mg daily, and methotrexate, 15 mg weekly. On examination, she is lethargic but appropriate. Her vital signs are blood pressure of 85/50 mmHg, heart rate of 122 beats/min, temperature of 39.1°C, respiratory rate of 24 breaths/min, and oxygen saturation of 97% on room air. Physical examination shows clear lung fields and a regular tachycardia without murmur. There is no abdominal tenderness or masses. Stool is negative for occult blood. There are no rashes. Hematologic studies show a white blood cell count of 24,200/μL with a differential of 82% PMNs, 8% band forms, 6% lymphocytes, and 3% monocytes. Hemoglobin is 8.2 g/dL. A urinalysis has numerous white blood cells with gram-negative bacteria on Gram stain. Chemistries reveal the following: bicarbonate of 16 meq/L, BUN of 60 mg/dL, and creatinine of 2.4 mg/dL. After fluid administration of 2 L, the patient has a blood pressure of 88/54 mmHg and a heart rate of 112 beats/min with a central venous pressure of 18 cmH$_2$O. There is 25 mL of urine output in the first hour. The patient has been initiated on antibiotics with cefepime. What should be done next for the treatment of this patient's hypotension?

A. Dopamine, 3 μg/kg/min IV
B. Hydrocortisone, 50 mg IV every 6 hours
C. Norepinephrine, 2 μg/min IV
D. Ongoing colloid administration at 500–1000 mL/h
E. Transfusion of 2 units of packed red blood cells

99. All of the following statements about the pathogenesis of sepsis and septic shock are true EXCEPT:

99. (*Continued*)

   A. Blood cultures are positive in only 20–40% of cases of severe sepsis.

   B. Microbial invasion of the bloodstream is not necessary for the development of severe sepsis.

   C. Serum levels of TNF-alpha are typically reduced in patients with severe sepsis or septic shock.

   D. The hallmark of septic shock is a marked decrease in peripheral vascular resistance that occurs despite increased plasma levels of catecholamines.

   E. Widespread vascular endothelial injury is present in severe sepsis and is mediated by cytokines and procoagulant factors that stimulate intravascular thrombosis.

100. Which of the following treatments is recommended to improve mortality in septic shock?

   A. Activated protein C (drotrecogin alpha)

   B. Administration of antibiotics within 1 hour of presentation

   C. Bicarbonate therapy for severe acidosis

   D. Erythropoietin

   E. Vasopressin infusion

101. Which of the following statements regarding the distinction between acute lung injury (ALI) and acute respiratory distress syndrome (ARDS) is true?

   A. ALI and ARDS can be distinguished by radiographic testing.

   B. ALI and ARDS can be distinguished by the magnitude of the PaO_2/FiO_2 ratio.

   C. ALI can be diagnosed in the presence of elevated left atrial pressure, but ARDS can not.

   D. ALI is caused by direct lung injury, but ARDS is the result of secondary lung injury.

   E. The risk of ALI but not ARDS increases with multiple predisposing conditions.

102. Which of the following has been demonstrated to reduce mortality in patients with ARDS?

   A. High-dose glucocorticoids within 48 hours of presentation

   B. High-frequency mechanical ventilation

   C. Inhaled nitric oxide

   D. Low tidal volume mechanical ventilation

   E. Surfactant replacement

103. A 38-year-old man is hospitalized in the ICU with ARDS after a motor vehicle accident with multiple long bone fractures, substantial blood loss, and hypotension. By day 2 of hospitalization, he is off vasopressors but is requiring a high FiO_2 and positive end-expiratory pressure (PEEP) to maintain

103. (*Continued*)

adequate oxygenation. His family is asking about the short- and long-term prognosis for recovery. All of the following statements about his prognosis are true EXCEPT:

   A. He has a greater chance of survival than a patient with similar physiology who is older than 70 years old.

   B. His overall mortality from ARDS is approximately 25–45%.

   C. If he survives, he is likely to have some degree of depression or posttraumatic stress disorder.

   D. If he survives, he likely will have normal or near normal lung function.

   E. The most likely cause of mortality is hypoxemic respiratory failure.

104. All of the following statements regarding cardiogenic shock are true EXCEPT:

   A. Approximately 80% of cases of cardiogenic shock complicating acute myocardial infarction are attributable to acute severe mitral regurgitation.

   B. Cardiogenic shock is more common in ST-segment elevation than non–ST-segment elevation myocardial infarction.

   C. Cardiogenic shock is uncommon in inferior wall myocardial infarction.

   D. Cardiogenic shock may occur in the absence of significant coronary stenosis.

   E. Pulmonary capillary wedge pressure is elevated in cardiogenic shock.

105. Aortic counterpulsation with an intra-aortic balloon pump has which of the following as an advantage over therapy with infused vasopressors or inotropes in a patient with acute ST-segment elevation myocardial infarction and cardiogenic shock?

   A. Increased heart rate

   B. Increased left ventricular afterload

   C. Lower diastolic blood pressure

   D. Not contraindicated in acute aortic regurgitation

   E. Reduced myocardial oxygen consumption

106. Which of the following is the most common electrical mechanism to explain sudden cardiac death?

   A. Asystole

   B. Bradycardia

   C. Pulseless electrical activity (PEA)

   D. Pulseless ventricular tachycardia (PVT)

   E. Ventricular fibrillation

107. All of the following statements regarding successful resuscitation from sudden cardiac death are true EXCEPT:

107. (*Continued*)

A. Advanced age does not affect the likelihood of immediate resuscitation, only the probability of hospital discharge.

B. After cardiac out of hospital cardiac arrest, survival rates are approximately 25% if defibrillation is administered after 5 minutes.

C. If the initial rhythm in an out-of-hospital cardiac arrest is pulseless ventricular tachycardia, the patient has a higher probability of survival than asystole.

D. Prompt CPR followed by prompt defibrillation improves outcomes in all settings.

E. The probability of survival from cardiac arrest is higher if the event takes place in a public setting than at home.

108. A 28-year-old woman has severe head trauma after a motor vehicle accident. One year after the accident, she is noted to have spontaneous eye opening and is able to track an object visually at times. She does not speak or follow any commands. She breathes independently but is fed through a gastrostomy tube. She can move all extremities spontaneously but without purposeful movement. What term best describes this patient's condition?

A. Coma
B. Locked-in
C. Minimally conscious state
D. Persistent vegetative state
E. Vegetative state

109. A 52-year-old man is evaluated after a large subarachnoid hemorrhage (SAH) from a ruptured cerebral aneurysm. There is concern that the patient has brain death. What test is most commonly used to diagnose brain death in this situation?

A. Apnea testing
B. Cerebral angiography
C. Demonstration of absent cranial nerve reflexes
D. Demonstration of fixed and dilated pupils
E. Performance of transcranial Doppler ultrasonography

110. Which of the following neurologic phenomena is classically associated with herniation of the brain through the foramen magnum?

A. Third-nerve compression and ipsilateral papillary dilation
B. Catatonia
C. "Locked-in" state
D. Miotic pupils
E. Respiratory arrest

111. A 72-year-old woman is admitted to the intensive care unit after a cardiac arrest at home. She had a witnessed collapse, and her family immediately began to perform cardiopulmonary resuscitation. Emergency medical service arrived within 10 minutes, and the initial cardiac rhythm demonstrated ventricular fibrillation. Spontaneous circulation returned after defibrillation, and the estimated time the patient was without a pulse was 15–20 minutes. The patient is brought to hospital and remains intubated, paralyzed, and sedated in the coronary care unit. She is being treated with medically induced hypothermia and is completely unresponsive to all stimuli 12 hours after the initial event. Her pupils are 3 mm and respond sluggishly to light. She has no cough or gag reflex. Intermittent myoclonic jerks are seen. The family has concerns about her neurologic prognosis after her prolonged cardiac arrest. What advice do you give the family regarding prognosis in this situation?

A. An MRI scan of the brain should be performed before determining neurologic outcome.

B. Apnea testing will be performed at the first opportunity to determine if the patient has suffered brain death.

C. Given the immediate actions of the family to initiate cardiopulmonary resuscitation, the patient has a greater than 50% chance to have good neurologic outcomes.

D. It is impossible to predict the patient's likelihood of neurologic recovery as her examination is unreliable in the face of sedation and hypothermia.

E. No information regarding prognosis can be determined until 72 hours have passed.

112. A 52-year-old man presents to the emergency department complaining of the worst headache of his life that is unresolving. It began abruptly 3 days before presentation and is worse with bending over. It rapidly increased in intensity over 30 minutes, but he did not seek medical care at that time. Over the ensuing 72 hours, the headache has persisted although lessened in intensity. He has not lost consciousness and has no other neurologic symptoms. His vision is normal, but he does report that light is painful to his eyes. His past medical history is notable for hypertension, but he takes his medications irregularly. Upon arrival to the emergency department, his initial blood pressure is 232/128 mmHg with a heart rate of 112 beats/min. No nuchal rigidity is present. A head CT shows no acute bleeding and no mass effect. What is the next best step in the management of this patient?

112. (*Continued*)
    A. Cerebral angiography
    B. CT angiography
    C. Lumbar puncture
    D. Magnetic resonance angiography
    E. Treat with sumatriptan

113. A 56-year-old man is admitted to intensive care with a subarachnoid hemorrhage. Upon admission, he is unresponsive, and his head CT shows evidence of blood in the third ventricle with midline shift. He undergoes successful coiling of an aneurysm of the anterior cerebral artery. All of the following would be indicated in the management of this patient EXCEPT:

    A. Glucocorticoids
    B. Hypernatremia
    C. Nimodipine
    D. Ventriculostomy
    E. Volume expansion

114. A 56-year-old man is admitted to the intensive care unit with a hypertensive crisis after cocaine use. Initial blood pressure is 245/132 mmHg. On physical examination, the patient is unresponsive except to painful stimuli. He has been intubated for airway protection and is being mechanically ventilated, with a respiratory rate of 14 breaths/min. His pupils are reactive to light, and he has normal corneal, cough, and gag reflexes. The patient has a dense left hemiparesis. When presented with painful stimuli, the patient responds with flexure posturing on the right side. Computed tomography (CT) reveals a large area of intracranial bleeding in the right frontoparietal area. Over the next several hours, the patient deteriorates. The most recent examination reveals a blood pressure of 189/100 mmHg. The patient now has a dilated pupil on the right side. The patient continues to have corneal reflexes. You suspect rising intracranial pressure related to the intracranial bleed. All but which of the following can be done to decrease the patient's intracranial pressure?

    A. Administer intravenous mannitol at a dose of 1 g/kg body weight.
    B. Administer hypertonic fluids to achieve a goal sodium level of 155–160 meq/L.
    C. Consult neurosurgery for an urgent ventriculostomy.
    D. Initiate intravenous nitroprusside to decrease the mean arterial pressure (MAP) to a goal of 100 mmHg.
    E. Increase the respiratory rate to 30 breaths/min.

115. A patient is followed closely by her nephrologist for stage IV chronic kidney disease associated with focal segmental glomerulosclerosis. Which of the following is an indication for initiation of maintenance hemodialysis?

    A. Acidosis controlled with daily bicarbonate administration
    B. Bleeding diathesis
    C. BUN greater than 110 mg/dL without symptoms
    D. Creatinine greater than 5 mg/dL without symptoms
    E. Hyperkalemia controlled with sodium polystyrene

116. A 27-year-old woman with chronic kidney disease is undergoing hemodialysis and is found to be hypotensive during her treatment. Which of the following are potential mechanisms for hypotension during hemodialysis?

    A. Antihypertensive agents
    B. Excessive ultrafiltration
    C. Impaired autonomic responses
    D. Osmolar shifts
    E. All of the above

117. A 35-year-old woman with hypertensive kidney disease progresses to end-stage renal disease. She was initiated on peritoneal dialysis 1 year ago and has done well with relief of her uremic symptoms. She is brought to the emergency department with fever, altered mental status, diffuse abdominal pain, and cloudy dialysate. Her peritoneal fluid is withdrawn through her catheter and sent to the laboratory for analysis. The fluid white blood cell count is 125/mm3 with 85% polymorphonuclear neutrophils. Which organism is most likely to be found on culture of the peritoneal fluid?

    A. *C. albicans*
    B. *E. coli*
    C. *M. tuberculosis*
    D. *P. aeruginosa*
    E. *S. aureus*

118. A 45-year-old woman begins hemodialysis for end-stage renal disease associated with diabetes mellitus. Which of the following is the most likely eventual cause of her death?

    A. Dementia
    B. Major bleeding episode
    C. Myocardial infarction
    D. Progressive uremia
    E. Sepsis

119. The "dose" of dialysis is currently defined as:

A. The counter-current flow rate of the dialysate
B. The fractional urea clearance
C. The hours per week of dialysis
D. The number of sessions actually completed in a month

120. Your patient with end-stage renal disease on hemodialysis has persistent hyperkalemia. He has a history of total bilateral renal artery stenosis, which is why he is on hemodialysis. He has electrocardiogram changes only when his potassium rises above 6.0 meq/L, which occurs a few times per week. You admit him to the hospital for further evaluation. Your laboratory evaluation, nutrition counseling, and medication adjustments have not impacted his serum potassium. What is the next reasonable step to undertake for this patient?

A. Adjust the dialysate.
B. Administer a daily dose of furosemide.
C. Perform "sodium modeling."
D. Implant an automatic defibrillator.
E. Perform bilateral nephrectomy.

121. Which of the following statements regarding hemophilia A and B is TRUE?

A. Individuals with factor VIII deficiency have a more severe clinical course than those with factor IX deficiency.
B. Levels of factor VIII or IX need to be measured before administration of replacement therapy in patients presenting with acute bleeding to calculate the appropriate dose of factor.
C. Primary prophylaxis against bleeding is never indicated.
D. The goal level of factor VIII or IX is greater than 50% in the setting of large-volume bleeding episodes.
E. The life expectancy of individuals with hemophilia is about 50 years.

122. A 24-year-old man is admitted to the hospital with circulatory collapse in the setting of disseminated meningococcemia. He is currently intubated, sedated, and on mechanical ventilation. He has received over 6 L of intravenous saline in the past 6 hours but remains hypotensive, requiring treatment with norepinephrine and vasopressin at maximum doses. He is making less than 20 mL of urine each hour. Blood is noted to be oozing from all of IV sites. His endotracheal secretions are blood tinged. His laboratory studies show a white blood cell count of 24,300/μL (82% neutrophils, 15% bands, 3% lymphocytes), hemoglobin of 8.7 g/dL,

122. (*Continued*)
hematocrit of 26.1%, and platelets of 19,000/μL. The international normalized ratio is 3.6, the activated partial thromboplastin time is 75 seconds, and fibrinogen is 42 mg/dL. The lactate dehydrogenase level is 580 U/L, and the haptoglobin is less than 10 mg/dL. The peripheral smear shows thrombocytopenia and schistocytes. All of the following treatments are indicated in this patient EXCEPT:

A. Ceftriaxone 2 g intravenously twice daily
B. Cryoprecipitate
C. Fresh-frozen plasma
D. Heparin
E. Platelets

123. All the following are vitamin K–dependent coagulation factors EXCEPT:

A. Factor X
B. Factor VII
C. Protein C
D. Protein S
E. Factor VIII

124. A 31-year-old man with hemophilia A is admitted with persistent gross hematuria. He denies recent trauma and any history of genitourinary pathology. The examination is unremarkable. Hematocrit is 28%. All the following are treatments for hemophilia A EXCEPT:

A. Desmopressin (DDAVP)
B. Fresh-frozen plasma
C. Cryoprecipitate
D. Recombinant factor VIII
E. Plasmapheresis

125. All of the following statements regarding the lupus anticoagulant (LA) are true EXCEPT:

A. LAs typically prolong the activated partial thromboplastin time.
B. A 1:1 mixing study will not correct in the presence of LAs.
C. Bleeding episodes in patients with LAs may be severe and life threatening.
D. Female patients may experience recurrent midtrimester abortions.
E. LAs may occur in the absence of other signs of systemic lupus erythematosus.

126. All the following cause prolongation of the activated partial thromboplastin time that does not correct with a 1:1 mixture with pooled plasma EXCEPT:

126. (*Continued*)

    A. Lupus anticoagulant

    B. Factor VIII inhibitor

    C. Heparin

    D. Factor VII inhibitor

    E. Factor IX inhibitor

127. You are evaluating a 45-year-old man with an acute upper gastrointestinal (GI) bleed in the emergency department. He reports increasing abdominal girth over the past 3 months associated with fatigue and anorexia. He has not noticed any lower extremity edema. His medical history is significant for hemophilia A diagnosed as a child with recurrent elbow hemarthroses in the past. He has been receiving infusions of factor VIII for most of his life and received his last injection earlier that day. His blood pressure is 85/45 mmHg with a heart rate of 115 beats/min. His abdominal examination is tense with a positive fluid wave. Hematocrit is 21%. Renal function and urinalysis are normal. His activated partial thromboplastin time is minimally prolonged, his international normalized ratio is 2.7, and platelets are normal. Which of the following is most likely to yield a diagnosis for the cause of his GI bleeding?

    A. Factor VIII activity level

    B. *Helicobacter pylori* antibody test

    C. Hepatitis B surface antigen

    D. Hepatitis C RNA

    E. Mesenteric angiogram

128. You are managing a patient with suspected disseminated intravascular coagulopathy (DIC). The patient has end-stage liver disease awaiting liver transplantation and was recently in the intensive care unit with *Escherichia coli* bacterial peritonitis. You suspect DIC based on a new upper gastrointestinal bleed in the setting of oozing from venipuncture sites. Platelet count is 43,000/μL, international normalized ratio is 2.5, hemoglobin is 6 mg/dL, and D-dimer is elevated to 4.5. What is the best way to distinguish between new-onset DIC and chronic liver disease?

    A. Blood culture

    B. Elevated fibrinogen degradation products

    C. Prolonged aPTT

    D. Reduced platelet count

    E. Serial laboratory analysis

129. Which of the following antibiotics inhibit cell wall synthesis?

    A. Ciprofloxacin, metronidazole, and quinupristin/dalfopristin

129. (*Continued*)

    B. Rifampin, sulfamycin, and clindamycin

    C. Tetracycline, daptomycin, and azithromycin

    D. Tobramycin, chloramphenicol, and linezolid

    E. Vancomycin, bacitracin, and penicillin

130. A 23-year-old college student is admitted to the hospital with a fever and painful, erythematous purulent nodules on his forearm. He is an avid weightlifter and other than depression treated with citalopram has been otherwise healthy. These lesions have been present for approximately 1 week, and his primary care physician attempted to treat him with clindamycin as an outpatient. After admission, he develops hypotension and evidence of systemic inflammatory response syndrome, prompting transfer to the medical intensive care unit. There, dopamine is started, linezolid is administered, and hydrocortisone and fludrocortisone are given for possible adrenal insufficiency in the context of septic shock. After 6 hours, he develops an agitated delirium with diaphoresis, tachycardia, a temperature of 103.4°F, and diarrhea. His examination is notable for tremor; muscular rigidity; hyperreflexia; and clonus, especially in the lower extremities. Which of the following drug–drug interactions is most likely the culprit of this clinical syndrome?

    A. Citalopram–dopamine

    B. Citalopram–linezolid

    C. Dopamine–fludrocortisone

    D. Dopamine–linezolid

    E. Fludrocortisone–linezolid

131. All of the following antiviral medications are correctly matched with a significant side effect EXCEPT:

    A. Acyclovir—thrombotic thrombocytopenic purpura

    B. Amantadine—anxiety and insomnia

    C. Foscarnet—acute renal failure

    D. Ganciclovir—bone marrow suppression

    E. Interferon—fevers and myalgias

132. Which of the following fungi is considered dimorphic?

    A. *Aspergillus fumigatus*

    B. *Candida glabrata*

    C. *Cryptococcus neoformans*

    D. *Histoplasma capsulatum*

    E. *Rhizopus* spp.

133. All of the following antifungal medications are available in an oral form EXCEPT:

133. (*Continued*)
   A. Caspofungin
   B. Fluconazole
   C. Griseofulvin
   D. Itraconazole
   E. Posaconazole
   F. Terbinafine

134. All of the following antifungal medications are approved for the treatment of *Candida albicans* fungemia EXCEPT:

   A. Caspofungin
   B. Fluconazole
   C. Micafungin
   D. Posaconazole
   E. Voriconazole

135. Clinically useful serum or urine diagnostic tests exist for all of the following invasive fungal infections EXCEPT:

   A. Aspergillus
   B. Blastomycosis
   C. Coccidioidomycosis
   D. Cryptococcosis
   E. Histoplasmosis

136. A 64-year-old man presents to the emergency department complaining of shortness of breath and facial swelling. He smokes 1 pack of cigarettes daily and has done so since the age of 16 years. On physical examination, he has dyspnea at an angle of 45 degrees or less. His vital signs are heart rate of 124 beats/min, blood pressure of 164/98 mmHg, respiratory rate of 28 breaths/min, temperature of 37.6°C (99.6°F), and oxygen saturation of 89% on room air. Pulsus paradoxus is not present. His neck veins are dilated and do not collapse with inspiration. Collateral venous dilation is noted on the upper chest wall. There is facial edema and 1+ edema of the upper extremities bilaterally. Cyanosis is present. There is dullness to percussion and decreased breath sounds over the lower half of the right lung field. Given this clinical scenario, what would be the most likely finding on CT examination of the chest?

   A. A central mass lesion obstructing the right mainstem bronchus
   B. A large apical mass invading the chest wall and brachial plexus
   C. A large pericardial effusion
   D. A massive pleural effusion leading to opacification of the right hemithorax
   E. Enlarged mediastinal lymph nodes causing obstruction of the superior vena cava

137. In the scenario in question 136, the initial therapy of this patient includes all of the following EXCEPT:

   A. Administration of furosemide as needed to achieve diuresis
   B. Elevation of the head of the bed to 45 degrees
   C. Emergent radiation
   D. Low-sodium diet
   E. Oxygen

138. A 58-year-old woman with known stage IV breast cancer presents to the emergency department with an inability to move her legs. She has had lower back pain for the past 4 days and has found it difficult to lie down. There is no radiating pain. Earlier today, the patient lost the ability to move either of her legs. In addition, she has been incontinent of urine recently. She has been diagnosed previously with metastatic disease to the lung and pleura from her breast cancer but was not known to have spinal or brain metastases. Her physical examination confirms absence of movement in the bilateral lower extremities associated with decreased to absent sensation below the umbilicus. There is increased tone and 3+ deep tendon reflexes in the lower extremities with crossed adduction. Anal sphincter tone is decreased, and the anal wink reflex is absent. What is the most important first step to take in the management of this patient?

   A. Administer dexamethasone 10 mg intravenously.
   B. Consult neurosurgery for emergent spinal decompression.
   C. Consult radiation oncology for emergent spinal radiation.
   D. Perform MRI of the brain.
   E. Perform MRI of the entire spinal cord.

139. A 21-year-old man is treated with induction chemotherapy for acute lymphoblastic leukemia. His initial white blood cell count before treatment was 156,000/μL. All of the following are expected complications during his treatment EXCEPT:

   A. Acute kidney injury
   B. Hypercalcemia
   C. Hyperkalemia
   D. Hyperphosphatemia
   E. Hyperuricemia

140. All of the following would be important for prevention of these complications EXCEPT:

   A. Administration of allopurinol 300 mg/m^2 daily
   B. Administration of intravenous fluids at a minimum of 3000 mL/m^2 daily

140. (*Continued*)

    C. Alkalinization of the urine to a pH of greater than 7.0 by administration of sodium bicarbonate

    D. Frequent monitoring of serum chemistries every 4 hours

    E. Prophylactic hemodialysis before initiating chemotherapy

ANSWERS

1. **The answer is E.**

(*Chap. 1*) An experienced clinician should be able to gain significant insight into the cause of dyspnea or cough in a patient by a thorough pulmonary examination. Wheezes are most commonly high-pitched sounds heard predominantly on expiration and are indicative of obstruction of small airways. The most frequent cause of wheezing is asthma, which results in polyphonic wheezing due to the dynamic variability in airway obstruction throughout the lung fields. However, many other diseases cause wheezing, including congestive heart failure. This so-called "cardiac asthma" is due to peribronchiolar edema that results in narrowing of the adjacent airways. In contrast, rhonchi are caused by obstruction of medium-sized airways and are associated with a lower pitch and more coarse sound. The most common cause of rhonchi is secretions in the airways. Stridor is another breath sound that is commonly labeled as wheezing, but is indicative of upper airway obstruction. When compared to wheezing associated with small airway disease, stridor is loudest during inspiration, although it can be heard during expiration as well.

Crackles (or rales) are predominantly heard during inspiration and are considered a sign of alveolar or interstitial lung disease. A variety of diseases cause crackles including pneumonia, pulmonary edema, and any cause of interstitial lung fibrosis. Some clinicians attempt to distinguish between the "wet" crackles of pulmonary edema or pneumonia compared to the "dry" crackles of interstitial lung disease. However, this is not a reliable finding. A better way to differentiate between the alveolar and interstitial causes of crackles is to test for the presence of egophony. When alveolar filling is present, the "EEE" sound will be heard as a "AH" sound; however, in interstitial lung disease the "EEE" sound will be preserved. Whispered pectoriloquy will also be intensified in alveolar filling processes, but not interstitial lung disease.

The lack of breath sounds is important to note, but can be caused by many factors including severe bullous lung disease, emphysema, pneumothorax, or pleural effusion.

2. **The answer is B.**

(*Chap. 1*) This patient presents with subacute-onset dyspnea and an examination consistent with pleural effusion.

Dullness to percussion can be seen with consolidation, atelectasis, and pleural effusion. With consolidation, voice transmission is increased during expiration so that one may hear whispered pectoriloquy or egophony. However, in both pleural effusion and atelectasis, breath sounds are diminished and there is no augmentation of voice transmission. Although this patient could have either atelectasis or pleural effusion, the lack of tracheal deviation points to pleural effusion. Atelectasis would have to be of many segments to account for these findings, and such significant airway collapse would generally cause ipsilateral tracheal deviation. The clinician would expect to find pleural effusion on chest film, and the most appropriate next management step would be thoracentesis to aid in the diagnosis of the etiology and for symptomatic relief. With a lack of symptoms to suggest infection, antibiotics are not indicated. Similarly, in the absence of wheezing or significant sputum production, bronchodilators and deep suctioning are unlikely to be helpful. Bronchoscopy may be indicated ultimately in the management of this patient, particularly if malignancy is suspected; however, the most appropriate first attempt at diagnosis is by means of thoracentesis.

3. **The answer is D.**

(*Chap. 2*) Shortness of breath, or dyspnea, is a common presenting complaint in primary care. However, dyspnea is a complex symptom and is defined as the subjective experience of breathing discomfort that includes components of physical as well as psychosocial factors. A significant body of research has been developed regarding the language by which a patient describes dyspnea with certain factors being more common in specific diseases. Individuals with airways diseases (asthma, chronic obstructive pulmonary disease [COPD]) often describe air hunger, increased work of breathing, and the sensation of being unable to get a deep breath because of hyperinflation. In addition, individuals with asthma often complain of a tightness in the chest. Individuals with cardiac causes of dyspnea also describe chest tightness and air hunger but do not have the same sensation of being unable to draw a deep breath or have increased work of breathing. A careful history will also lead to further clues regarding the cause of dyspnea. Nocturnal dyspnea is seen in congestive heart failure or asthma, and orthopnea is reported in heart failure, diaphragmatic weakness, and asthma that is triggered by esophageal reflux. When discussing exertional dyspnea, it is important to assess if the dyspnea is chronic and progressive or episodic. Whereas episodic dyspnea is more common in myocardial ischemia and asthma, COPD and interstitial lung diseases present with a persistent dyspnea. Platypnea is a rare presentation of dyspnea in which a patient is dyspneic in the upright position and feels improved with lying flat. On physical examination of a patient with dyspnea, the physician should observe the patient's ability to speak and the use of accessory muscle or preference of the tripod position. As part of vital signs, a pulsus paradoxus may be measured with a value of greater than 10 mmHg common in asthma and COPD. Pulsus paradoxus greater than 10 mmHg may also occur in pericardial tamponade. Lung examination may demonstrate decreased diaphragmatic excursion, crackles, or wheezes that allow one to determine the cause of dyspnea. Further workup may include pulmonary function testing, chest radiography, chest CT, electrocardiography, echocardiography, or exercise testing, among others, to ascertain the cause of dyspnea.

4. The answer is C.

(Chap. 3) Chronic cough is one of the most common causes of referral to pulmonary, allergy, and otolaryngology practices and is frequently encountered in primary care. A cough is classified as chronic when it persists for longer than 8 weeks and has a wide range of differential diagnoses, including cardiac, pulmonary, upper airway, and gastrointestinal diseases. The initial history and physical examination is important in providing clues to the potential etiology, particularly in the setting of a normal chest radiograph and examination. The most common causes of chronic cough in an otherwise normal individual are cough-variant asthma, gastroesophageal reflux disease, postnasal drip, and medications. In this patient, there are clues that should lead one to suspect cough-variant asthma as a potential cause. Asthma can present only with cough. Although this presentation is more common in children, it can present this way in adults as well. This patient does have triggers that include cold air and exercise, both of which can lead to increased bronchoconstriction. In addition, the parasympathetic–sympathetic balance favors bronchoconstriction that is worse in the early morning hours with cough late at night. Although spirometry demonstrating reversible airflow obstruction is typically seen in asthma, asthma has significant clinical variability, and lung function varies over time. In this patient, the spirometry results are normal, and the bronchodilator response is insufficient to diagnose reversibility, which requires a response of at least 12% and an increase of at least 200 mL in either the forced expiratory volume in 1 second (FEV_1) or forced vital capacity (FVC). To establish the diagnosis more definitively, demonstration of a fall in FEV_1 of at least 20% during a bronchoprovocation test with methacholine would be sufficient in this clinical scenario to diagnose asthma and would be safe to perform in this patient with normal pulmonary function at baseline. An alternative approach would be to treat empirically with low-dose inhaled corticosteroids given the clinical history.

In many cases, the cause of chronic cough is multifactorial. This patient has minor symptoms of allergic rhinitis, which may be a contributing factor. Nasal corticosteroids

may also be required, but given the reported triggers, would not be sole treatment. The patient gives no history to suggest GERD, which may be clinically silent. If the cough failed to improve with treatment for asthma, antacid medications may be indicated. Finally, increasing numbers of adults are becoming infected with *Bordetella pertussis* because individual immunity wanes in adulthood, and more parents are electing to forego childhood immunizations. In this scenario, the patient typically gives a history of an upper respiratory infection with a strong cough at the onset of the illness. When the illness has progresses to the recovery phase, diagnosis is typically made by serology, and culture is not useful.

5. The answer is A.

(Chap. 3) Hemoptysis is a relatively common symptom that causes a significant degree of distress in the patient. In most individuals, the hemoptysis is mild and self-limited despite the anxiety that it causes. Worldwide, tuberculosis remains the most common cause of hemoptysis. However, in the United States, the most common cause of hemoptysis is acute bronchitis of viral or bacterial etiology. Given the acute nature of the illness and mild degree of hemoptysis, this patient's presentation would be most consistent with the diagnosis of acute bronchitis. Antiplatelet or anticoagulant agents may increase the risk of bleeding but are not sufficient in the absence of an underlying cause to initiate hemoptysis. Moreover, these agents are typically associated with underlying alveolar rather than airway damage. Most patients who experience hemoptysis fear lung cancer, which can present with acute hemoptysis, but this patient's report of primarily blood-streaked sputum would make this less likely, especially in the face of a normal chest radiograph. Lung abscesses rarely present with hemoptysis, and the typical presentation is one of a prolonged illness.

6. The answer is E.

(Chap. 3) Life-threatening hemoptysis is a medical emergency. Defining *massive hemoptysis* can be difficult but generally should be viewed as any amount of hemoptysis that can lead to airway obstruction because most patients who die of hemoptysis die from asphyxiation and airway obstruction. The immediate management of hemoptysis is to establish a patent airway and establish the site of bleeding. The initial step is to place the patient with the bleeding side in a dependent position. In this patient with a known lesion of the right upper lobe, he should be placed with the right side (not left) in a dependent position. The patient should be intubated with the largest possible endotracheal tube to allow for adequate suctioning. When immediately available, placement of a dual-lumen endotracheal tube can allow selective ventilation of the nonbleeding lung while providing access to continue suctioning from the affected side. Certainly, correction of any underlying coagulopathy would be

important in the management of this patient. If conservative measures fail to stop the bleeding, the first step is to attempt embolization of the bleeding artery, but in rare instances, urgent surgical intervention may be required.

7. The answer is D.

(Chap. 4) When a patient presents for evaluation of hypoxia, it is important to consider the underlying mechanism of hypoxia in order to determine the etiology. The primary causes of hypoxia are related to respiratory disease and include ventilation/perfusion (V/Q) mismatch, hypoventilation, and intrapulmonary right-to-left shunting. Causes of hypoxia outside of the respiratory system include intracardiac right-to-left shunting, high-altitude hypoxia, anemic hypoxia, circulatory hypoxia, and carbon monoxide poisoning. In this patient, the mechanism of hypoxia can be narrowed to two possibilities—intracardiac versus intrapulmonary right-to-left shunting—quite easily because the patient failed to correct his hypoxia in response to 100% oxygen. The history of platypnea and orthodeoxia is suggestive that the likely cause is intrapulmonary rather than intracardiac shunting. The finding of a possible lung nodule on chest radiographs in the lower lung fields also is supportive of a pulmonary cause of shunting through an arteriovenous malformation, which can appear as a lung nodule on chest x-ray. An intracardiac right-to-left shunt is caused by congenital cardiac malformations and Eisenmenger syndrome. If there was an intracardiac cause of shunt, the cardiac examination would be expected to demonstrate a murmur and/or evidence of pulmonary hypertension.

V/Q mismatch is the most common cause of hypoxia and results from perfusion of areas of the lung that receive limited ventilation. Examples of V/Q mismatch include asthma, chronic obstructive pulmonary disease, and pulmonary embolus. Hypoxia caused by V/Q mismatch can be corrected with supplemental oxygen. Hypoventilation can be caused by multiple causes, including acute respiratory depression or chronic respiratory failure with elevations in $PaCO_2$. Hypoxia caused by hypoventilation is also correctable with oxygen but frequently has a normal alveolar–arterial oxygen gradient.

Causes of hypoxia outside the respiratory system are less common. High-altitude hypoxia becomes apparent when individuals travel to elevations greater than 3000 m. Anemic hypoxia is not associated with a decrease in PaO_2, but a decrease in hemoglobin does cause decreased oxygen-carrying capacity in the blood and relative tissue hypoxia if severe. Circulatory hypoxia refers to tissue hypoxia that occurs because of a decrease cardiac output that leads to greater tissue extraction of oxygen. As a result, the venous partial pressure of oxygen is reduced, and there is an increased arterial-mixed venous oxygen gradient.

8. The answer is C.

(Chap. 4) In the evaluation of cyanosis, the first step is to differentiate central from peripheral cyanosis. In central cyanosis, because the etiology is either reduced oxygen saturation or abnormal hemoglobin, the physical findings include bluish discoloration of both mucous membranes and skin. In contrast, peripheral cyanosis is associated with normal oxygen saturation but slowing of blood flow and an increased fraction of oxygen extraction from blood; subsequently, the physical findings are present only in the skin and extremities. Mucous membranes are spared. Peripheral cyanosis is commonly caused by cold exposure with vasoconstriction in the digits. Similar physiology is found in Raynaud's phenomenon. Peripheral vascular disease and deep venous thrombosis result in slowed blood flow and increased oxygen extraction with subsequent cyanosis. Methemoglobinemia causes abnormal hemoglobin that circulates systemically. Consequently, the cyanosis associated with this disorder is systemic. Other common causes of central cyanosis include severe lung disease with hypoxemia, right-to-left intracardiac shunting, and pulmonary arteriovenous malformations.

9. The answer is B.

(Chap. 5) The functional residual capacity of the lung refers to the volume of air that remains in the lung following a normal tidal respiration. This volume of air represents the point at which the outward recoil of the chest wall is in equilibrium with the inward elastic recoil of the lungs. The lungs would remain at this volume if not for the actions of the respiratory muscles. The functional residual capacity is comprised of two lung volumes: the expiratory reserve volume and the residual volume. The expiratory reserve volume represents the additional volume of air that can be exhaled from the lungs when acted upon by the respiratory muscles of exhalation. The residual volume is the volume of air that remains in the lung following a complete exhalation and is determined by the closing pressure of the small airways.

10. The answer is D.

(Chap. 5) This patient presents with subacute dyspnea, stridor, and airflow obstruction, which are consistent with a diagnosis of subglottic stenosis related to his prior prolonged mechanical ventilation. This is confirmed by the finding of fixed obstruction on the flow-volume loop. Flow-volume loops are derived from spirometry. Following a maximum inspiratory effort from residual volume, an individual forces the maximum volume of air from the lungs, and the resultant flows are plotted against the volume. By convention, inspiration is shown on the lower portion of the curve and expiration is on the top. There are characteristic patterns of airflow obstruction that can be evaluated by examining this curve. A fixed central airflow obstruction results in flattening of the flow-volume loop in both inspiration and expiration, yielding the characteristic boxlike effect in this patient. Examples of fixed airflow obstruction include tracheal stenosis and an obstructing central airway tumor. Other patterns of large airway obstruction are a variable intrathoracic obstruction and variable extrathoracic obstruction. In these situations, flattening of the flow-volume curve occurs on only one limb of the flow-volume loop, and the pattern of flattening can be explained by the dynamic changes in pressure that affect the trachea. A variable intrathoracic obstruction causes flattening of the flow-volume curve only on expiration. During inspiration the pleural pressure is more negative than the tracheal pressure, and the trachea remains unimpeded to flow. However, when pleural pressure rises on expiration relative to tracheal pressure, there is collapse of the trachea and flattening of the flow-volume curve. An example of a variable intrathoracic obstruction is tracheomalacia. In contrast, the variable extrathoracic defect leads to flattening of the flow-volume loop on inspiration but not expiration. The relevant pressure acting on airflow in the trachea in an extrathoracic obstruction is atmospheric pressure. During inspiration, the tracheal pressure drops below atmospheric pressure, leading to compromised airflow and the characteristic flattening of the flow-volume loop. However, tracheal pressure rises above atmospheric pressure during expiration, leading to a normal expiratory curve.

11.   The answer is B.

(Chap. 5) Pregnancy is a known risk factor for the development of venous thromboembolic disease and should be suspected in any pregnant patient presenting with acute dyspnea. Determining the need for further testing in a pregnant patient should take into account the potential risks of radiation exposure on the fetus. Unfortunately, the signs and symptoms of pulmonary embolism are often nonspecific. Most chest x-rays are normal, and sinus tachycardia may be the only finding on electrocardiogram. In addition, in the pregnant patient dyspnea is common due to a variety of factors including increased size of the uterus and the effects of progesterone as a central respiratory stimulant. The normal arterial blood gas in pregnancy shows a chronic respiratory alkalosis with a pH ranging as high as 7.47 and $PaCO_2$ between 30 and 32 mmHg. Calculation of the alveolar-arterial gradient (A-a gradient) can be helpful in this situation. It is easy to be fooled by the presence of a normal oxygen saturation and partial pressure of oxygen on arterial blood gas, but the A-a gradient may still be elevated in the presence of respiratory alkalosis. To calculate the A-a gradient, one first must calculate the alveolar oxygen tension with the alveolar gas equation shown below:

$$PaO_2 = PiO_2 - (PaCO_2/R) \text{ where,}$$
$$PiO_2 = \text{inspired partial pressure of oxygen}$$
$$= FiO_2 \times (P_{bar} - P_{H_2O}), \text{ and}$$

$$R = \text{respiratory quotient} = \text{carbon dioxide}$$
$$\text{production/oxygen consumption} = {\sim}0.8$$

In this patient, calculation of the $PaO_2 = (0.21 \times [760 - 47]) - (26/0.8) = 117.23$ mmHg. At the same time the measured arterial partial pressure of oxygen was 85. Thus, the A-a gradient is elevated at 32 mmHg and should prompt the physician to perform further workup for pulmonary embolism. The choice of test for diagnosis of pulmonary embolism in pregnant patients is most commonly CT pulmonary angiography, although ventilation-perfusion scanning may also be used.

12.   The answers are 1. C; 2. B; 3. D; 4. A.

(Chap. 5) Ventilatory function can be easily measured with lung volume measurement and the FEV_1/FVC ratio. A decreased FEV_1/FVC ratio diagnoses obstructive lung disease. Alternatively, low lung volumes, specifically decreased TLC, and occasionally decreased RV diagnose restrictive lung disease. With extensive air trapping in obstructive lung disease, TLC is often increased and RV may also be increased. VC is proportionally decreased. MIP measures respiratory muscle strength and is decreased in patients with neuromuscular disease. Thus, myasthenia gravis will produce low lung volumes and decreased MIP, whereas patients with idiopathic pulmonary fibrosis will have normal muscle strength and subsequently a normal MIP, but decreased TLC and RV. In some cases of pulmonary parenchymal restrictive lung disease, the increase in elastic recoil results in an increased FEV_1/FVC ratio.

13.   The answer is C.

(Chap. 5) In this patient presenting with multilobar pneumonia, hypoxemia is present that does not correct with increasing the concentration of inspired oxygen. The inability to overcome hypoxemia or the lace of a notable increase in PaO_2 with increasing fraction of inspired oxygen to 1.0 physiologically defines a shunt. A shunt occurs when deoxygenated blood is transported to the left heart and systemic circulation without having the capability of becoming oxygenated. Causes of shunt include alveolar collapse (atelectasis), intra-alveolar filling processes, intrapulmonary vascular malformations, or structural cardiac disease leading to right-to-left shunt. In this case, the patient has multilobar pneumonia leading to alveoli that are being perfused but are unable to participate in gas exchange because they are filled with pus and inflammatory exudates. Acute respiratory distress syndrome is another common cause of shunt physiology. Ventilation-perfusion mismatch is the most common cause of hypoxemia and results when there are some alveolar units with low ratios (low ventilation to perfusion) that fail to fully oxygenate perfused blood. When blood is returned to the left heart, the poorly oxygenated blood admixes with blood from normal alveolar units. The resultant hypoxemia is less severe than with shunt and can be corrected with increasing the inspired oxygen concentration. Hypoventilation with or without other causes of hypoxemia is not present in this case as the PaCO$_2$ is less than 40 mmHg, indicating hyperventilation. The acidosis present in this case is of a metabolic rather than a pulmonary source. Because the patient is paralyzed, she is unable to increase her respiratory rate above the set rate to compensate for the metabolic acidosis.

14. The answer is D.

(Chap. 6) This patient presents with a slowly progressive illness manifested by dyspnea on exertion, dry cough, clubbing, and the presence of crackles on examination. In addition, the pulmonary function tests demonstrate restrictive lung disease. This scenario is characteristic of an individual with interstitial lung disease, most commonly idiopathic pulmonary fibrosis in individuals at this age. A more thorough history should be obtained to determine if there are any other exposures or symptoms that could identify other causes of interstitial lung disease. The next step in the evaluation of this patient is to perform a high-resolution computed tomography scan (HRCT) of the chest. The high-resolution technique for CT imaging employs thinner cross-sectional images at approximately 1–2 mm rather than the usual 7–10 mm. This creates more visible details and is particularly useful for recognizing subtle changes of the interstitium and small airways including interstitial lung disease, bronchiolitis, and bronchiectasis. Bronchoscopy with transbronchial biopsy typically does not provide the detail required to adequately diagnose interstitial lung disease. It may be considered if there are specific features on HRCT that would suggest an alternative diagnosis. However, in most instances, the pathologic diagnosis of interstitial lung disease requires a surgical lung biopsy to provide a definitive diagnosis. This patient's symptoms do not suggest coronary artery disease or congestive heart failure. Thus, echocardiography and nuclear stress testing are not indicated.

CT scanning has evolved over the years to offer several different techniques that are useful in a variety of circumstances. Standard CT imaging is most useful for the evaluation and staging of lung masses. Helical CT scanning requires only a single breath hold and provides continuous collection of data with improved contrast enhancement and thinner collimation. Once the data are obtained, the images can be reconstructed into other views including sagittal and coronal planes as well as 3D volumetric representations. A recent use of this technology is employed in the setting of "virtual bronchoscopy" to aid in the planning and performance of bronchoscopy. Multidetector CT scans can obtain multiple slices in a single rotation that are thinner than the usual cuts. Multidetector CT scanners are used in the performance of the CT pulmonary angiogram.

15. The answer is E.

(Chap. 8) The patient in this clinical scenario presents with symptoms typical of asthma, including shortness of breath and wheezing. She also manifests evidence of atopy, the most common risk factor for developing asthma, with sensitivity to outdoor allergens and cats. In addition, the patient has a history of allergic rhinitis and eczema, both of which are commonly seen in individuals with asthma. Indeed, over 80% of asthma patients have a concomitant diagnosis of allergic rhinitis. Atopy is present in 40–50% of the population of affluent countries, but only a small proportion of these individuals develop asthma. Many studies have shown a genetic predisposition via family history and recent genome-wide screens, but no single genetic profile has show high positive predictive value. Overall, the prevalence of asthma in developed countries has increased over the past 30 years, but recently has leveled off with a prevalence of about 15% in children and 10–12% in adults. Asthma deaths remain rare and have decreased in recent decades. In the 1960s, asthma deaths did increase with an overuse of short-acting beta-agonist medications. However, since the introduction of inhaled corticosteroids as maintenance therapy, deaths have declined. Risk factors for fatal asthma include frequent use of rescue inhalers, lack of therapy with inhaled corticosteroids, and prior hospitalizations for asthma. Interestingly, the overall disease severity does not vary significantly within a given patient over the course of the disease. Individuals who have mild asthma typically continue to have mild asthma, whereas as those with severe disease present with severe disease. Diagnosis of asthma can be made by demonstrating airflow obstruction with significant reversibility on bronchodilator administration. In this case, the FEV$_1$/FVC ratio is decreased to 70%, which is low. In addition, the FEV$_1$ increases by 12.4% and 230 mL. This meets the criteria for bronchodilator reversibility of an increase of at least 200 mL and 12%. Bronchoprovocation testing with methacholine may be considered in individuals who have suspected asthma but have normal pulmonary function tests.

16. The answer is B.

(Chap. 8) The pathology of asthma has largely been determined by examining bronchial biopsies of patients with asthma as well as the lungs of individuals who die from asthma. These pathologic changes are centered around the airways with sparing of the alveolar spaces. The airways are infiltrated by eosinophils, activated T lymphocytes, and activated mucosal mast cells. However, the degree of inflammation does not correlate with the severity of asthma. Another common finding in all asthmatics and individuals with eosinophilic bronchitis is thickening of the basement membrane due to collagen deposition in the subepithelium. The airway smooth muscle is hypertrophied as well. Overall, this leads to thickening of the airway wall, which may also exhibit edematous fluid, particularly in those with fatal asthma. In cases of fatal asthma, it is also common to find multiple airways that are occluded by mucous plugs. However,

the disease is limited to the airways, and infiltration of the alveolar spaces by inflammatory cells is not seen.

17. The answer is E.

(Chap. 8) A step up in asthma therapy should be considered when a patient continues to have symptoms after 3 months on appropriate therapy. Symptoms to consider when determining whether asthma therapy should be increased include presence of daily symptoms, nocturnal awakening more than once weekly, and limitations in daily activity. Physicians should also review the use of rescue inhalers and lung function when making decisions to step up therapy. In addition, the use of standard asthma severity questionnaires such as the Asthma Control Score may be helpful. When stepping up therapy in mild persistent asthma, the preferred next step in therapy is increasing to medium-dose inhaled corticosteroids or adding a long-acting beta-agonist. However, an alternate therapy that can be considered is adding a leukotriene antagonist, low-dose theophylline, or the leukotriene synthesis inhibitor zileuton to low-dose inhaled corticosteroids.

18. The answer is C.

(Chap. 8) The preferred method for diagnosing asthma is demonstration of airflow obstruction on spirometry that is at least partially reversible. This is demonstrated in option C with a decreased FEV_1/FVC ratio, decreased FEV_1, and a significant increase in FEV_1 following administration of albuterol. For an individual to be considered responsive to a bronchodilator, the individual should experience an increase in either FEV_1 or FVC of at least 200 mL and 12%. Option A describes someone with postviral cough syndrome, which can persist for several weeks following a viral upper respiratory infection. Option B describes someone with exercise-induced bronchoconstriction (EIB), which, in the absence of other symptoms to suggest asthma, should not be diagnosed as asthma. Isolated EIB lacks the characteristic airway inflammation of asthma and does not progress to asthma. While it is estimated that 80–90% of individuals with asthma experience EIB, many individuals who have EIB do not also have asthma. EIB is caused by hyperventilation with inhalation of cool, dry air that leads to bronchospasm. Option D describes someone with occupational asthma that has occurred after working with animals in the medical laboratory for many years. Symptoms that are characteristic of occupational asthma are symptoms only while at work that improve on the weekends and during holidays. Option E describes a patient with chronic obstructive pulmonary disease (COPD). In COPD, 25–48% of individuals can demonstrate bronchial hyperresponsiveness in response to methacholine.

19. The answer is D.

(Chap. 8) A step-down in asthma therapy can be considered when an individual has been clinically stable for 3–6 months. Factors demonstrating appropriate asthma control include daytime symptoms 2 or fewer times weekly, nighttime symptoms 2 or fewer times monthly, use of rescue inhaler 2 or fewer times weekly, FEV_1 or peak expiratory flow rate at least 80% of personal best, or appropriate control by validated asthma control questionnaires such as the Asthma Control Test or Asthma Therapy Assessment Questionnaire. When stepping down therapy, it is important to review the medications and their dosages. This patient is currently being managed with low-dose inhaled corticosteroids plus a long-acting beta-agonist. At this point, the best course of therapy is to stop the long-acting beta-agonist salmeterol. Since the dose of fluticasone the patient is receiving is already at a low dose, it would not be recommended to decrease it further, and it is never appropriate to treat with a long-acting beta-agonist alone without inhaled corticosteroids. In a large clinical trial, asthma mortality increased in individuals treated with long-acting beta-agonists in the absence of therapy with inhaled corticosteroids. Adding another medication is not indicated as the patient is demonstrating good asthma control.

20. The answer is D.

(Chap. 8) Omalizumab is a blocking antibody that binds to and neutralizes circulating immunoglobulin E (IgE) to inhibit IgE-mediated reactions. Omalizumab therapy can be considered for the outpatient treatment of severe, persistent asthma requiring high-dose inhaled corticosteroids in the presence of sensitivity to an aeroallergen. In clinical trials, treatment with omalizumab has been demonstrated to decrease the number of exacerbations in individual experiences and most individuals are also able to decrease the amount of oral or inhaled corticosteroids they are using. Elevations in serum IgE are frequently seen in asthmatic patients, and omalizumab can be considered in individuals whose IgE ranges from 30 to 700 IU/L. However, the manufacturer recommends not giving omalizumab therapy with marked elevations in IgE (>700 IU/L). Omalizumab is given as an injection every 2–4 weeks and must be given in an office setting because rare anaphylactic reactions can occur. If an individual is experiencing an acute exacerbation of asthma, omalizumab is typically held. However, it is not necessary to normalize lung function or discontinue oral steroids prior to initiating therapy with omalizumab.

21. The answer is C.

(Chap. 9) This patient has an acute presentation with pulmonary infiltrates and a pleural effusion, both of which have an increased percentage of eosinophils. In the United States, drug reactions are the most common cause of pulmonary infiltrates with eosinophilia (PIE syndrome), and among the drugs that can cause eosinophilia, nitrofurantoin is the most common. Nitrofurantoin is known to cause two types of pulmonary drug reaction.

The acute drug reaction occurs within hours to days of starting nitrofurantoin. Patients present with dry cough, dyspnea, and fever. Chest radiograph demonstrates bilateral infiltrates. In a minority of cases, a pleural effusion is seen. Differential cell count demonstrates eosinophilia in both the pleural and bronchoalveolar lavage fluids. Treatment of nitrofurantoin-associated pulmonary eosinophilia consists primarily of stopping the medication. In severe cases, oral corticosteroids can be used as well, but this does not supersede the need to discontinue the nitrofurantoin. High doses of steroids are typically not required for drug-related pulmonary eosinophilia. While pulmonary infections can cause pulmonary eosinophilia, this patient has a typical time course and presentation for nitrofurantoin-associated lung disease. Therefore, one would not wait for cultures before recommending stopping the nitrofurantoin. Multiple drugs have been associated with eosinophilic pulmonary reactions. In addition to nitrofurantoin, they include sulfonamides, NSAIDs, penicillins, thiazides, tricyclic antidepressants, hydralazine, and chlorpropamide, among others. Levothyroxine, however, is not known to cause any lung disease. Both hypo- and hyperthyroidism can be associated with pleural effusions from the primary disease or associated heart failure. However, they are not associated with eosinophilic lung disease, and adjusting the levothyroxine dose is not indicated.

22. The answer is C.

(Chap. 10) Mesothelioma is a rare malignancy of the pleura and peritoneum with almost all cases associated with asbestos exposure. It is notable that the exposure to asbestos could seem almost minimal, but still confer significant risk. Exposures of less than 1–2 years or those that have occurred more than 40 years in the past have been demonstrated to confer an increased risk of mesothelioma. While tobacco smoking in association with asbestos exposure increases the risk of lung cancer several fold, there is no additive or exponential risk of mesothelioma in those who smoke. Mesothelioma most often presents with a persistent unilateral pleural effusion that may mask the underlying pleural tumor. However, the pleura may be diffusely thickened. Even with large effusions, no mediastinal shift is seen on chest radiograph because the pleural thickening associated with the disease leads to a fixed chest cavity size and thoracic restriction. The most difficult diagnostic dilemma in these patients is to differentiate mesothelioma from metastatic lung carcinoma (usually adenocarcinoma), as many patients are at risk for both tumors, and lung cancer is far and away the most common malignancy seen in those individuals with asbestos exposure and cigarette smoking. Pleural fluid cytology is not adequate for the diagnosis of most individuals with mesothelioma, with samples being positive for the disease in less than 50% of individuals. Most often video-assisted thoracoscopy is required to directly

visualize the pleural surfaces and direct biopsy sampling. Unfortunately, there is no proven effective therapy for mesothelioma, and most patients die from local extension of the disease.

23. The answer is E.

(Chap. 10) Silicosis results from the inhalation of free silica (or crystalline quartz) and is associated with mining, stonecutting, foundry work, and quarrying. The chronic form of silicosis has been associated with an increased risk of a variety of diseases. Silica is known to be cytotoxic to alveolar macrophages and thus places patients at increased risk of pulmonary infections that rely on cellular immunity, including *Mycobacterium tuberculosis*, atypical mycobacteria, and fungus. In addition, silicosis is associated with the development of connective tissue disorders including rheumatoid arthritis with rheumatoid nodules (Caplan syndrome) and scleroderma. Finally, silica is listed as a probable lung carcinogen.

24. The answer is D.

(Chap. 10) Occupational lung diseases have been associated with a wide variety of organic and inorganic exposures in the workplace and clinically can range from primarily an airways disease to progressive pulmonary fibrosis. When evaluating a patient for a new pulmonary diagnosis, it is important to perform a detailed occupational history to determine if there is a possibility that the patient's profession may be causing or perpetuating the disease process. Specific clinical syndromes are associated with well-defined clinical exposures. The inorganic dusts include asbestos, silica, coal dust, beryllium, and a variety of other metals. Asbestos and silica are among the most common exposures. Asbestos exposure is associated with mining, construction, and ship repair. In areas near where asbestos mining has occurred, the general population also has shown an increased risk of asbestos-related lung disease. Clinically, asbestos exposure is associated with a range of clinical syndromes including asbestosis, benign pleural plaques and pleural effusions, lung cancer, and mesothelioma. Silica exposure is common among miners, stone masons, and individuals involved in sand blasting or quarrying. A variety of clinical syndromes can occur with silica exposure, the most severe being progressive massive fibrosis with masslike upper-lobe consolidating nodules (>1 cm). Coal mining is also associated with a clinical picture similar to silicosis and progressive massive fibrosis. Beryllium is a lightweight metal that is highly conductive and is used in high-tech industries. The classic disease associated with beryllium exposure is a chronic granulomatous disease similar in clinical appearance to sarcoidosis. Other metals can produce any number of clinical syndromes. Welders of galvanized metal who utilize zinc oxide are susceptible to metal fume fever and present with an acute self-limited influenza-like illness. Organic dusts that can lead to occupational lung disease include cotton dust, grain dust, toxic chemicals, and other agricultural dusts, among many others. Cotton milling and processing can present with a clinical syndrome known as byssinosis, which has asthma-like features. Many of the organic dust exposures also lead to hypersensitivity pneumonitis. Examples of hypersensitivity pneumonitis syndromes related to occupational exposures include farmer's lung, pigeon breeder's lung, and malt worker's lung. Typically, a specific antigen can be identified as the culprit for the development of hypersensitivity pneumonitis. In farmer's lung, the most common cause is thermophilic *Actinomyces* species found in moldy hay.

25. The answer is B.

(Chaps. 8 and 10) The patient presents with typical asthma symptoms; however, the symptoms are escalating and now require nearly constant use of oral steroids. It is of note that the symptoms are worse during weekdays and better on weekends. This finding suggests that there is an exposure during the week that may be triggering the patient's asthma. Often textile workers have asthma resulting from the inhalation of particles. The first step in diagnosing a work-related asthma trigger is to check FEV_1 before and after the first shift of the workweek. A decrease in FEV_1 would suggest an occupational exposure. Skin testing for allergies would not be likely to pinpoint the work-related exposure. Although *A. fumigatus* can be associated with worsening asthma from allergic bronchopulmonary aspergillosis, this would not result in a fluctuation in symptoms throughout the week. The patient does not require further testing to diagnose that he has asthma; therefore, a methacholine challenge is not indicated. Finally, the exercise physiology test is generally used to differentiate between cardiac and pulmonary causes or deconditioning as etiologies for shortness of breath.

26. The answer is D.

(Chap. 10) The patient presents with acute-onset pulmonary symptoms, including wheezing, with no other medical problems. He is a farmer and was recently handling hay. The clinical presentation and radiogram are consistent with farmer's lung, a hypersensitivity pneumonitis caused by *Actinomyces*. In this disorder, spores of actinomycetes in moldy hay are inhaled and produce a hypersensitivity pneumonitis. The disorder is seen most commonly in rainy periods, when the spores multiply. Patients present generally 4–8 hours after exposure with fever, cough, and shortness of breath without wheezing. Chest radiograms often show patchy, bilateral, often upper-lobe infiltrates. The exposure history will differentiate this disorder from other types of pneumonia.

27. The answer is A.

(Chap. 11) Health care–associated pneumonia (HCAP) has emerged as a new category of pneumonia distinct from community-acquired pneumonia (CAP), as individuals at risk of HCAP frequently have multidrug-resistant organisms more typical of hospital-acquired pneumonia (HAP). Several risk factors have been identified for HCAP, and specific organisms are more commonly seen in specific situations. For example, methicillin-resistant *Staphylococcus aureus* (MRSA) has not only been associated with hospitalization for more than 48 hours, but also any hospitalization for 2 or more days in the preceding 3 months, as well as with individuals residing in nursing homes or extended care facilities, chronic dialysis, home infusion therapy, home wound care, or a family member with a multidrug-resistant infection. Antibiotic therapy in the preceding 3 months is not associated with the development of MRSA as a cause of HCAP, but is associated with *Pseudomonas aeruginosa* and multidrug-resistant (MDR) *Enterobacteriaceae* as causes of HCAP.

28. The answer is B.

(Chap. 11) The diagnosis and treatment of community-acquired pneumonia (CAP) often incorporate a combination of clinical, radiographic, and laboratory features to determine the most likely etiology and treatment. In most instances of CAP, outpatient treatment is sufficient, and definitive etiologic diagnosis of the causative organism is not required, nor is it cost-effective. However, the outpatient diagnosis of CAP most often does require confirmation by chest radiograph, as the sensitivity and specificity of the findings on physical examination are about 58% and 67%, respectively. In addition, chest radiograph may identify risk factors for more severe clinical courses such as multifocal infiltrates. Moreover, outside of the 2% of individuals admitted to intensive care for treatment of CAP, there are no data that treatment directed against the specific causative organism is superior to empiric therapy. In some instances, one may decide to attempt to determine a causative organism for CAP, particularly in individuals who have risk factors for resistant organisms or if the patient fails to respond appropriately to initial antibiotic therapy. The most common way CAP is diagnosed is via sputum culture with Gram stain. The primary purpose of the Gram stain is to ensure that the sputum is an adequate lower respiratory sample for culture with fewer than 10 squamous epithelial cells and more than 25 neutrophils per high-powered field. However, at times it can suggest a specific diagnosis based on the appearance. Generally, the yield from sputum culture is 50% or less, even in cases of bacteremic pneumococcal pneumonia. The yield from blood cultures is also low, even when collected prior to initiation of antibiotics, at 5–14%. More recently, antigen tests or polymerase chain reaction (PCR) testing directed against specific organisms has gained favor. The most common antigen test that is performed is for *Legionella pneumophila*, as this organism does not grow in culture unless performed on specific media. Antigen and PCR tests are also available for *Streptococcus pneumoniae* and *Mycoplasma pneumoniae*, but given the costs they are not frequently performed

29. The answer is D.

(Chap. 11) Determining the appropriate empiric coverage for community-acquired pneumonia (CAP) initially requires determining if the severity of illness warrants admission to the hospital. Clinical rules for determining the potential severity of pneumonia have been developed including the Pneumonia Severity Index (PSI) and the CURB-65 criteria. While the PSI has the largest body of research to support its use, the model includes 20 variables, which may be impractical in a busy clinical practice. The CURB-65 criteria include only five variables: (1) **C**onfusion; (2) **U**rea greater than 7 mmol/L; (3) **R**espiratory rate greater than or equal to 30/min; (4) **B**lood pressure less than or equal to 90/60 mmHg; and (5) age of **65** or older. This patient meets none of the criteria for hospitalization and is not hypoxemic or in a high-risk group for complications from CAP. Therefore, he can safely be treated as an outpatient without further diagnostic workup, as his history, physical examination, and chest radiograph are all consistent with the diagnosis of CAP. The empiric antibiotic regimen recommended by the Infectious Diseases Society of America and the American Thoracic Society for individuals who are previously healthy and have not received antibiotics in the prior 3 months is either doxycycline or a macrolide such as azithromycin or clarithromycin. In outpatients with significant medical comorbidities or antibiotics within the prior 3 months, the suggested antibiotic therapy is either a respiratory fluoroquinolone or a beta-lactam plus a macrolide.

30. The answer is E.

(Chap. 11) Ventilator-associated pneumonia (VAP) is a common complication of endotracheal intubation and mechanical ventilation. Prevalence estimates indicate that 70% of patients requiring mechanical ventilation for 30 days or longer will have at least one instance of VAP. However, the epidemiology of VAP has been difficult to accurately study as no single set of criteria is reliably diagnostic of VAP. Generally, it is thought that VAP has a tendency to be overdiagnosed for a variety of reasons, including the high rates of tracheal colonization with pathogenic organisms and the multiple alternative causes of fevers and/or pulmonary infiltrates in critically ill patients. Quantitative cultures have gained favor, as the quantitative nature is thought to discriminate better between colonization and active infection. A variety of approaches have been advocated including endotracheal aspirates yielding more than 106 organisms or protected brush specimens from distal airways yielding more than 103 organisms. However, the quantitative yield of these

tests can be highly influenced by even a single dose of antibiotics, and antibiotic changes are common in critically ill patients, particularly when a new fever has emerged. Thus, the lack of growth on quantitative culture may be difficult to interpret in this setting. More recently, there has been growing use of the Clinical Pulmonary Infection Score (CPIS), which incorporates a variety of clinical, radiographic, and laboratory factors to determine the likelihood of VAP, although its true utility in clinical practice remains to be fully determined.

31. The answer is D.

(Chap. 11) Aspiration can lead to anaerobic infection and chemical pneumonitis. The etiologic differential diagnosis of community-acquired pneumonia (CAP) in a patient with a history of recent travel to the southwestern United States should include *Coccidioides*. *Aspergillus* has a worldwide distribution and is not a cause of CAP syndrome. Alcohol use predisposes patients to anaerobic infection, likely due to aspiration, as well as *S. pneumoniae*. *Klebsiella* is classically associated with CAP in alcoholic patients, but in reality this is rarely seen. Patients with structural lung disease, such as cystic fibrosis or bronchiectasis, are at risk for a unique group of organisms including *P. aeruginosa* and *S. aureus*. Poor dental hygiene is associated with anaerobic infections.

32. The answer is C.

(Chap. 12) Tuberculosis is most commonly transmitted from person to person by airborne droplets. Factors that affect the likelihood of developing tuberculosis infection include the probability of contact with an infectious person, the intimacy and duration of contact, the degree of infectiousness of the contact, and the environment in which the contact takes place. The most infectious patients are those with cavitary pulmonary or laryngeal tuberculosis with about 105 to 107 tuberculous bacteria per milliliter of sputum. Individuals who have a negative acid-fast bacillus smear with a positive culture for tuberculosis are less infectious but may transmit the disease. However, individuals with only extrapulmonary (e.g., renal, skeletal) tuberculosis are considered noninfectious.

33. The answer is D.

(Chap. 12) Aging, chronic disease, and suppression of cellular immunity are risk factors for developing active tuberculosis in patients with latent infection. (See Table 12-1.) The greatest absolute risk factor for development of active tuberculosis is HIV positivity. The risk of developing active infection is greatest in those with the lowest CD4 counts; however, having a CD4 count above a threshold value does not negate the risk of developing an active infection. The reported incidence of developing active tuberculosis in HIV-positive individuals with a positive purified protein derivative result is 10% per year compared with a lifetime risk of 10% in immunocompetent individuals.

Whereas malnutrition and severe underweight confer a two-fold greater risk of developing active tuberculosis, IV drug use increases the risk 10 to 30 times. Silicosis also increases the risk of developing active tuberculosis 30 times. Although the risk of developing active tuberculosis is greatest in the first year after exposure, the risk also increases in elderly adults. Coal mining has not been associated with increased risk independent of other factors, such as tobacco smoking.

34. The answer is A.

(Chap. 12) The chest radiograph shows a right upper lobe infiltrate with a large cavitary lesion. In this man from an endemic area for tuberculosis, this finding should be treated as active pulmonary tuberculosis until proven otherwise. In addition, this patient's symptoms suggest a chronic illness with low-grade fevers, weight loss, and temporal wasting that would be consistent with active pulmonary tuberculosis. If a patient is suspected of having active pulmonary tuberculosis, the initial management should include documentation of disease while protecting health care workers and the population in general. This patient should be hospitalized in a negative-pressure room on airborne isolation until three expectorated sputum samples have been demonstrated to be negative. The samples should preferably be collected in the early morning because the burden of organisms is expected to be higher on a more concentrated sputum. The sensitivity of a single sputum for the detection of tuberculosis in confirmed cases is only 40% to 60%. Thus, a single sputum sample is inadequate to determine infectivity and the presence of active pulmonary tuberculosis. Skin testing with a purified protein derivative of the tuberculosis mycobacterium is used to detect latent infection with tuberculosis and has no role in determining whether active disease is present. The cavitary lung lesion shown on the chest imaging could represent malignancy or a bacterial lung abscess, but because the patient is from a high-risk area for tuberculosis, tuberculosis would be considered the most likely diagnosis until ruled out by sputum testing.

35. The answer is A.

(Chap. 12) Initial treatment of active tuberculosis associated with HIV disease does not differ from that of a non–HIV-infected person. The standard treatment regimen includes four drugs: isoniazid, rifampin, pyrazinamide, and ethambutol (RIPE). These drugs are given for a total of 2 months in combination with pyridoxine (vitamin B6) to prevent neurotoxicity from isoniazid. After the initial 2 months, patients continue on isoniazid and rifampin to complete a total of 6 months of therapy. These recommendations are the same as those of non–HIV-infected individuals. If the sputum culture remains positive for tuberculosis after 2 months, the total course of antimycobacterial therapy is increased from 6 to 9 months. If an individual is already on antiretroviral

therapy (ART) at the time of diagnosis of tuberculosis, it may be continued, but often rifabutin is substituted for rifampin because of drug interactions between rifampin and protease inhibitors. In individuals not on ART at the time of diagnosis of tuberculosis, it is not recommended to start ART concurrently because of the risk of immune reconstitution inflammatory syndrome (IRIS) and an increased risk of medication side effects. IRIS occurs as the immune system improves with ART and causes an intense inflammatory reaction directed against the infecting organism(s). There have been fatal cases of IRIS in association with tuberculosis and initiation of ART. In addition, both ART and antituberculosis drugs have many side effects. It can be difficult for a clinician to decide which medication is the cause of the side effects and may lead unnecessarily to alterations in the antituberculosis regimen. ART should be initiated as soon as possible and preferably within 2 months. Three-drug regimens are associated with a higher relapse rate if used as a standard 6-month course of therapy and, if used, require a total of 9 months of therapy. Situations in which three-drug therapy may be used are pregnancy, intolerance to a specific drug, and in the setting of resistance. A five-drug regimen using Rifampin, Isoniazide, Pyrazinamide, Ethambutol (RIPE) plus streptomycin is recommended as the standard retreatment regimen. Streptomycin and pyrazinamide are discontinued after 2 months if susceptibility testing is unavailable. If susceptibility testing is available, the treatment should be based on the susceptibility pattern. In no instance is it appropriate to withhold treatment in the setting of active tuberculosis to await susceptibility testing.

36. The answer is B.

(Chap. 12) The aim of treatment of latent tuberculosis is to prevent development of active disease, and the tuberculin skin test (purified protein derivative [PPD]) is the most common means of identifying cases of latent tuberculosis in high-risk groups. To perform a tuberculin skin test, 5 tuberculin units of PPD are placed subcutaneously in the forearm. The degree of induration is determined after 48 to 72 hours. Erythema only does not count as a positive reaction to the PPD. The size of the reaction to the tuberculin skin test determines whether individuals should receive treatment for latent tuberculosis. In general, individuals in low-risk groups should not be tested. However, if tested, a reaction larger than 15 mm is required to be considered as positive. School teachers are considered low-risk individuals. Thus, the reaction of 7 mm is not a positive result, and treatment is not required. A size of 10 mm or larger is considered positive in individuals who have been infected within 2 years or those with high-risk medical conditions. The individual working in an area where tuberculosis is endemic has tested newly positive by skin testing and should be treated as a newly

infected individual. High-risk medical conditions for which treatment of latent tuberculosis is recommended include diabetes mellitus, injection drug use, end-stage renal disease, rapid weight loss, and hematologic disorders. PPD reactions 5 mm or larger are considered positive for latent tuberculosis in individuals with fibrotic lesions on chest radiographs, those with close contact with an infected person, and those with HIV or who are otherwise immunosuppressed. There are two situations in which treatment for latent tuberculosis is recommended regardless of the results on skin testing. First, infants and children who have had close contact with an actively infected person should be treated. After 2 months of therapy, a skin test should be performed. Treatment can be discontinued if the skin test result remains negative at that time. Also, individuals who are HIV positive and have had close contact with an infected person should be treated regardless of their skin test results.

37. The answer is C.

(Chap. 12) T-lymphocyte release of interferon-gamma in response to highly specific tuberculosis antigen stimulation is the basis for the commercially available interferon-gamma release assays (IGRAs). IGRAs are more specific than tuberculin skin testing caused by less cross-reactivity with non-mTB organisms, including Bacillus Calmette-Guérin and nontuberculous mycobacteria. The absolute sensitivity of IGRAs is not clearly known because of the difficulty in establishing a gold standard, but most studies demonstrate superior performance in detecting latent tuberculosis in low-incidence settings. They also are more user friendly because there is no administration expertise, interpretation is less subjective, and results do not require a second visit. The results are far less clear in settings of high tuberculosis or HIV burden. The tuberculin skin testing booster phenomenon, a spurious conversion caused by serial testing, does not occur with IGRAs; however, a tuberculin skin test may cause a false-positive IGRA result. In the United States, IGRA is preferred for most persons older than 5 years of age being screened for latent tuberculosis.

38. The answer is E.

(Chap. 12) Bacillus Calmette-Guérin (BCG) is derived from an attenuated strain of *Mycobacterium bovis*. It has been available since 1921. Many vaccines are available, but they vary in efficacy from 0% to 80% in clinical trials. The vaccine protects infants and young children from serous forms of tuberculosis, including meningitis and miliary disease. Side effects from the vaccine are rare, but BCG dissemination (BCGitis) may occur in patients with severe combined immunodeficiency or advanced HIV-induced immune suppression. BCG cross-reacts with tuberculin skin testing, but the size of the response wanes with time. BCG vaccination is currently recommended in countries with a high TB prevalence. It is not

recommended in the United States because of the low prevalence of disease and cross-reactivity with tuberculin skin testing. Infants with unknown HIV infection status, infants of mothers with known HIV infection, and HIV-infected individuals should not receive BCG vaccination.

39. The answer is D.

(Chap. 14) This patient presents with symptoms of the common cold with a self-limited illness characterized by rhinorrhea and sore throat. The most common viruses causing the common cold are rhinoviruses, which are implicated in as many as 50% of common colds. Rhinoviruses are small single-stranded RNA viruses of the Picornaviridae family. There are three genetic species of rhinoviruses with 102 serotypes identified. Rhinoviruses grow preferentially at the temperature of the nasal passages (33° to 34°C) rather than the temperature of the lower airways (37°C). Although rhinovirus infections occur year round, there are seasonal peaks of the infection in the early fall and spring in temperate climates. Overall, the rates of rhinovirus infection are highest in infants and young children and decrease with age. The virus is most often introduced into families through young children in preschool or grade school. After the index infection, secondary infections occur in other family members 25% to 70% of the time. Rhinovirus spreads through direct contact with infected secretions, which can occur through respiratory droplets or hand-to-hand contact. It can also be transmitted through large or small particle aerosols. Finally, the virus can be isolated from plastic surfaces from 1 to 3 hours after inoculation, raising the possibility that the virus can also be transmitted through environmental contact.

40. The answer is C.

(Chap. 14) Acute viral respiratory illnesses are the most common illness worldwide, and a wide variety of viruses have been implicated as causes. Rhinoviruses are the most common virus causing the common cold and are found in about 50% of cases. The second most commonly isolated viruses are coronaviruses. These viruses are more common in the late fall, winter, and early spring, primarily at times when rhinoviruses are less active. Other causes of common cold in children are adenoviruses, whereas these viruses are uncommon in adults with the exception of outbreaks in individuals living in close quarters such as military recruits. Although human respiratory syncytial virus characteristically causes pneumonia and bronchiolitis in young children, the virus can cause common cold and pharyngitis in adults. Parainfluenza virus is another virus classically associated with croup in children, but it causes common cold in adults. Enteroviruses most often cause an undifferentiated febrile illness.

41. The answer is A.

(Chap. 14) The common viruses causing respiratory infections often have specific associated clinical syndromes. Rhinoviruses are primarily responsible for the common cold. Coronaviruses are also commonly associated with colds. However, in 2002 to 2003, there was an outbreak of a coronavirus-associated illness that originated in China and spread to 28 countries in Asia, Europe, and North and South America. This illness was named severe acute respiratory syndrome (SARS) and caused severe lower respiratory illness and acute respiratory distress syndrome. Overall, the case-fatality rate was 9.5%. Human respiratory syncytial virus is the primary agent responsible for lower respiratory disease and bronchiolitis in infants and young children. Another virus primarily associated with childhood illness is parainfluenza virus. This virus is a frequent cause of croup in young children characterized by a febrile illness with a barking cough and stridor. Adenovirus often causes a febrile illness with the common cold and pharyngitis in children. In adults, it is associated with outbreaks of respiratory illness in military recruits. Herpes simplex virus is associated gingivostomatitis in children and pharyngotonsillitis in adults.

42. The answer is C.

(Chap. 14) In infants, human respiratory syncytial virus (HRSV) is frequently associated with lower respiratory infections in 25% to 40% of infections. This can present as pneumonia, tracheobronchitis, or bronchiolitis. In cases of lower respiratory infections, tachypnea, wheezing, and hypoxemia are common and can progress to respiratory failure. Treatment is primarily supportive with hydration, suctioning of secretions, and administration of humidified oxygen. Bronchodilators are also used to treat wheezing and bronchospasm. In more severe cases, aerosolized ribavirin has been demonstrated to modestly improve the time to resolution of respiratory illness. The American Academy of Pediatrics states that aerosolized ribavirin may be considered in infants who are seriously ill or who are at high risk of complications, including bronchopulmonary dysplasia and congenital heart disease and those who are immunosuppressed. However, no benefit has been demonstrated with use of standard intravenous immunoglobulin or HRSV-specific immunoglobulin.

43. The answer is E.

(Chap. 13) Pandemic strains of influenza emerge through genetic reassortment of RNA segments between viruses that affect different species, including humans, swine, and birds. This process is also called antigenic shift during which a new strain of influenza emerges to which very few people have immunity. Antigenic shift only occurs with influenza A because it is the only influenza that crosses between species. Antigenic drift is the result of point mutations in the hemagglutinin or neuramidase proteins. Antigenic drift occurs frequently and is responsible for the interpandemic influenza outbreaks.

44. The answer is A.

(Chap. 13, www.cdc.gov/flu) This patient is presenting with an influenza-like illness during the typical flu season. Hospital infection control practices in this setting are to treat all patients presenting with an influenza-like illness as if they have influenza until proven otherwise. This includes institution of droplet precautions to prevent spread to other individuals as well as performing testing to confirm influenza diagnosis. This is most commonly done via a nasopharyngeal swab but can also be done on throat swab, sputum, nasotracheal aspirates, or bronchoscopic specimens if available. If influenza diagnosis is confirmed, assessment of close household contacts for individuals who may be candidates for chemoprophylaxis against influenza is important, particularly individuals who would be high risk of complications from influenza infection. This group includes children younger than 4 years old, pregnant women, individuals age 65 years or older, individuals with heart or lung disease, individuals with abnormal immune systems, and individuals with chronic metabolic diseases or renal disease.

As far as treatment is concerned, clearly, oxygen should be given to individuals who are hypoxemic. Other appropriate supportive care should also be administered, including intravenous fluids and respiratory therapy support to manage secretions. In general, treatment with antiviral medications has been demonstrated to decrease the duration of symptoms by 1 to 1.5 days when initiated within the first 48 hours after the onset of symptoms. However, the Centers for Disease Control and Prevention (CDC) recommends treatment with antiviral medications as early as possible in patients hospitalized with severe pneumonia. Some evidence indicates that use of antiviral therapy might be effective in decreasing morbidity and mortality in individuals who are hospitalized with severe pneumonia even when given more than 48 hours after the onset of symptoms. The preferred class of antiviral therapy is the neuraminidase inhibitors, which have efficacy against both influenza A and B. In addition, resistance is much lower among this class of medications. This class includes the drugs zanamivir, oseltamivir, and peramivir. Of these, oseltamivir is most commonly used because it is an oral medication with limited side effects. Zanamivir is given by inhalation and can cause bronchoconstriction in individuals with asthma. Peramivir is currently an investigational medication that is administered intravenously.

The adamantine agents include amantadine and rimantadine. These medications have no efficacy against influenza B and also have a high degree of antiviral resistance (>90%) in North America to H3N2 strains of influenza A. It is important to know the resistance patterns to antiviral agents during the local flu season. The CDC currently does not recommend amantadine as first-line therapy for severe influenza. Antibacterial therapy should be reserved for individuals with suspected bacterial complications of influenza.

45. The answer is A.

(Chap. 13, www.cdc.gov/flu) The intranasal influenza vaccine contains a cold-adapted, live-attenuated influenza virus. Because of this, its use is more limited than intramuscular inactivated influenza vaccine. It is currently only recommended for healthy individuals between the ages of 2 and 49 years. Contraindications to the use of the live-attenuated intranasal influenza vaccine include pregnancy, chronic pulmonary or cardiovascular conditions, immunosuppressed patients, individuals with a history of Guillain-Barré syndrome, and individuals with a history of severe egg allergy. In addition, individuals who regularly are in contact with immunosuppressed people should not receive the intranasal vaccine, or if it is given, they should avoid contact with severely immunosuppressed patients for 7 days after receipt of the vaccine. In young children, a history of asthma precludes the use of intranasal influenza vaccination because the vaccine can precipitate episodes of wheezing. The Centers for Disease Control and Prevention recommends avoiding the use of the live-attenuated vaccine in individuals whose parents report an episode of wheezing within the past 12 months regardless of whether asthma is a chronic diagnosis. A final caveat in the use of the live-attenuated intranasal influenza vaccine is its use in individuals who are actively taking antiviral medications as chemoprophylaxis against influenza because antiviral medications interfere with the immune response to the live-attenuated influenza vaccine. The current recommendations are that live-attenuated influenza vaccination not be administered for 48 hours after antiviral medications have been stopped and that antiviral medications not be given for 2 weeks after receipt of the live-attenuated influenza vaccine. However, the immune response to the intramuscular inactivated vaccine is not affected by coadministration with antiviral drugs.

46. The answer is D.

(Chap. 13) The majority of influenza infections are clinically mild and self-limited. Treatment with over-the-counter cough suppressants and analgesics such as acetaminophen is often adequate. Patients who are younger than the age of 18 years are at risk of developing Reye's syndrome if they are exposed to salicylates such as aspirin. The neuraminidase inhibitors oseltamivir and zanamivir have activity against influenza A and B. They can be used within 2 days of symptom onset and have been shown to reduce the duration of symptoms by 1 or 2 days. This patient has had symptoms for more than 48 hours, so neither drug is likely to be effective. The patient's history of asthma is an

additional contraindication to zanamivir because this drug can precipitate bronchospasm. The M2 inhibitors amantadine and rimantadine have activity against influenza A only. However, since 2005, more than 90% of A/H3N2 viral isolates demonstrated resistance to amantadine, and these drugs are no longer recommended for use in influenza A.

47. The answer is C.

(Chap. 15) Patients receiving biologic agents, including the tumor necrosis factor antagonists infliximab and etanercept, are at increased risk of multiple with most people exposed before 5 years of age. Airborne transmission has been demonstrated in animal studies, and epidemiologic studies suggest person-person transmission in nosocomial settings. Patients with defects in cell and humoral immunity are at risk for developing pneumonia. Most cases are in HIV-infected patients with CD4 counts less than 200/μL. Others at risk include patients receiving immunosuppressive agents (particularly glucocorticoids) for cancer or organ transplantation, children with immunodeficiency, premature malnourished infants, and patients receiving biologic immunomodulating agents. Pneumocystis pneumonia typically presents in non–HIV-infected patients with several days of dyspnea, fever, and nonproductive cough. Often symptoms develop during or soon after a glucocorticoid taper. Pneumocystis is associated with a reduced diffusing capacity on pulmonary function that typically causes mild hypoxemia and significant oxygen desaturation with exertion. Chest radiography often shows bilateral diffuse infiltrates without pleural effusion. Early in the disease, the radiograph may be unremarkable, but chest computed tomography (CT) will show diffuse ground glass infiltrates as in this case. Patients receiving biologic agents are at risk of pneumonia caused by tuberculosis (the patient was on prophylaxis in this case), *Aspergillus* spp., and *Nocardia* spp. *Aspergillus* spp., *Nocardia* spp., and septic emboli typically appear as nodules on chest CT. Rheumatoid nodules would be unlikely in the context of improving joint disease.

48. The answer is D.

(Chap. 15) Prophylaxis is effective in decreasing the risk of *Pneumocystis* pneumonia. It is clearly indicated in HIV-infected patients with oropharyngeal candidiasis or CD4 count below 200/μL and in HIV-infected or non–HIV-infected patients with a history of prior *Pneumocystis* pneumonia. Prophylaxis may be discontinued in HIV-infected patients who respond to therapy after the CD4 count has risen more than 200/μL for more than 3 months. Indications for primary prophylaxis for at-risk non-HIV infected patients without prior pneumocystis pneumonia (e.g., patients receiving induction chemotherapy or high-dose corticosteroids) are less clear. Trimethoprim–sulfamethoxazole remains the drug of

choice for primary and secondary prophylaxis. It also provides protection from opportunistic toxoplasmosis and some bacterial infections.

49. The answer is E.

(Chap. 15) Pneumocystis jiroveci lung infection is known to worsen after initiation of treatment, likely caused by lysis of organisms and immune response to their intracellular contents. It is thought that adjunct administration of glucocorticoids may reduce inflammation and subsequent lung injury in patients with moderate to severe pneumonia caused by P. jiroveci. Adjunct administration of glucocorticoids in patients with moderate to severe disease as determined by a room air below 70 mmHg or an A –a gradient greater than 35 mmHg has been shown to decrease mortality. Glucocorticoids should be given for a total duration of 3 weeks. Patients often do not improve until many days into therapy and often initially worsen; steroids should be used early in the course of illness rather than waiting for lack of improvement. Pneumothoraces and adult respiratory distress syndrome (ARDS) are common feared complications of Pneumocystis infection. If patients present with ARDS caused by Pneumocystis pneumonia, they meet the criterion for adjunct glucocorticoids because of the severe nature of disease. The use of glucocorticoids as adjunctive therapy in HIV-infected patients with mild disease or in non–HIV-infected patients remains to be evaluated.

50. The answer is D.

(Chap. 16) Bronchiectasis occurs when there is irreversible dilation of the distal airways and can occur in a focal or diffuse fashion. The most common cause of diffuse bronchiectasis worldwide is prior granulomatous infection due to Mycobacterium tuberculosis. In the developed world, tuberculosis is a less common cause of bronchiectasis, with nontuberculous mycobacteria such as Mycobacterium avium-intracellulare complex being a more common cause, particularly in the midlung fields. Other potential etiologies of diffuse bronchiectasis include cystic fibrosis, postradiation pneumonitis, immunoglobulin deficiency, end-stage fibrotic lung disease, and recurrent aspiration. However, despite extensive workup, as many as 25–50% of cases remain idiopathic.

51. The answer is C.

(Chap. 16) Bronchiectasis is a disorder with a variable presentation depending on cause. In inherited disorders such as cystic fibrosis, the symptoms of bronchiectasis most often begin in early childhood. However, in general, the incidence of bronchiectasis increases with age, typically affecting women more than men. The primary clinical symptom of bronchiectasis is a daily productive cough. Classically, the sputum is described as large volume with a thick tenacious character. Hemoptysis

may also occur in association with bronchiectasis. The physical examination may demonstrate crackles or wheezing with mild to moderate airflow obstruction on pulmonary function testing. In more advanced cases, digital clubbing may be seen. The diagnosis of bronchiectasis is often suspected based on clinical symptoms, but confirmation of diagnosis on high-resolution CT imaging of the chest is recommended. The chest radiograph may show tram tracking, but is frequently normal and is of insufficient sensitivity to definitively make the diagnosis. On high-resolution chest CT imaging, bronchiectatic airways appear dilated more than 1.5 times the size of the adjacent pulmonary artery. In addition, the airways fail to taper in the periphery, and airways may be identifiable within 1 cm of the pleural surface, which is clearly abnormal. Bronchial wall thickening and inspissated secretions may also be seen. Contrast administration is not necessary to visualize bronchiectasis. Once bronchiectasis is confirmed as the etiology of the patient's chronic cough, workup for the underlying etiology of the bronchiectasis should be performed and would likely include sputum cultures for mycobacteria and bacteria, serum immunoglobulin, and $\alpha 1$ antitrypsin levels, among others.

52. The answer is A.

(Chap. 16) This patient presents with a clinical history that is consistent with a polymicrobial lung abscess with infection by anaerobic bacteria. Often individuals present with an indolent course and nonspecific symptoms including fever, fatigue, and weight loss. Cough with a foul-smelling sputum production may also be seen. Individuals presenting with lung abscess often have risk factors for aspiration and evidence of periodontal infection. In more advanced cases, the lung abscess can erode into the pleura, creating an empyema with associated pleuritic chest pain. Although chest radiograph often demonstrates a cavitary lesion, a CT may be performed to determine the extent of the disease and whether there are associated lesions. Bacterial, mycobacterial, and fungal cultures should be performed, but this should not delay treatment of the most likely cause of the lung abscess. A sputum culture on an expectorated sample will only detect aerobic organisms, and the detection of anaerobes would be confounded by the presence of multiple oral anaerobes that could contaminate an expectorated specimen. Initial treatment should be directed primarily at anaerobic organisms. Recommended antibiotics are clindamycin IV 600 mg four times daily or a β-lactam/β-lactamase inhibitor combination (ampicillin-sulbactam, amoxicillin-clavulanic acid). Metronidazole is not recommended because it has poor activity against the microaerophilic streptococci that commonly infect lung abscesses. The duration of treatment is not well defined. Some experts recommend continuing therapy until the abscess has entirely healed.

Persistence of fever beyond 5–7 days should prompt the clinician to investigate further. Potential complications include development of empyema or a bronchopleural fistula. In addition, one should consider performing bronchoscopy to rule out an obstructing lesion. Percutaneous or surgical intervention is generally not required unless the patient fails to respond to antibiotic therapy or has a lung abscess greater than 6 cm.

53. The answer is D.

(Chap. 16) The combination of infertility and recurrent sinopulmonary infections should prompt consideration of an underlying disorder of ciliary dysfunction that is termed primary ciliary dyskinesia. These disorders account for approximately 5–10% of cases of bronchiectasis. A number of deficiencies have been described, including malfunction of dynein arms, radial spokes, and microtubules. All organ systems that require ciliary function are affected. The lungs rely on cilia to beat respiratory secretions proximally and subsequently to remove inspired particles, especially bacteria. In the absence of this normal host defense, recurrent bacterial respiratory infections occur and can lead to bronchiectasis. Otitis media and sinusitis are common for the same reason. In the genitourinary tract, sperm require cilia to provide motility. Kartagener's syndrome is a combination of sinusitis, bronchiectasis, and situs inversus. It accounts for approximately 50% of patients with primary ciliary dyskinesia. Cystic fibrosis is associated with infertility and bilateral upper-lobe infiltrates. It causes a decreased number of sperm or absent sperm on analysis because of the congenital absence of the vas deferens. Sarcoidosis, which is often associated with bihilar adenopathy, is not generally a cause of infertility. A water balloon–shaped heart is found in those with pericardial effusions, which one would not expect in this patient.

54. The answer is E.

(Chap. 17) Cystic fibrosis (CF) is a common autosomal-recessive disorder that affects 1 out of every 3000 live births in the Caucasian population of North America and Europe. There have been more than 1500 mutations identified in the gene for the cystic fibrosis transmembrane conductance regulator (CFTR)—the abnormal protein identified in CF. This protein is a large transmembrane protein involved in the transport of chloride and other ions, and abnormalities of the CFTR lead to abnormalities of salt and water transport. The primary clinical manifestations of CF are due to the effects of the mutated CFTR in the lungs, gastrointestinal tract, and pancreas. In the lungs, abnormal CFTR leads to thick, sticky mucus with abnormal mucociliary clearance. A patient will have recurrent respiratory infections with development of cystic bronchiectasis over time. The presenting manifestation in infancy is often meconium ileus and can lead to constipation and distal intestinal obstruction in adults. Failure of the CFTR in the pancreas prevents appropriate release of pancreatic enzymes to allow for proper digestion of food, especially fatty foods, with resultant malnutrition and steatorrhea. While most patients with CF present in infancy or childhood, about 5% of all individuals with CF will not be diagnosed until adulthood. Presenting symptoms in adulthood can be myriad and often result from minor mutations of the CFTR gene. These symptoms can include recurrent lung and sinus infections, malnutrition, sinus disease, and infertility, especially absence of the vas deferens in men. The standard test for the diagnosis of CF is the sweat chloride test. Elevated values are pathognomonic for CF, with a cutoff of greater than 70 meq/L in adults being diagnostic. Values greater than approximately 35 meq/L fall within the indeterminate range. DNA analysis for common CF mutations is often performed, and one would want to demonstrate two alleles known to cause CF before making the diagnosis, as the disease is autosomal recessive. Identification of only one allele only identifies the carrier state. In some individuals, the diagnosis can remain elusive. In such cases, referral to a tertiary center for nasal potential difference (PD) testing can be helpful, as CF patients demonstrate an elevated baseline nasal PD with failure to respond to stimulation with beta-agonists. Presence of *Pseudomonas aeruginosa* is common in adults with CF, but is not specific for the diagnosis of the disease as bronchiectasis from any cause can lead to *P. aeruginosa* colonization.

55. The answer is C.

(Chap. 17) Individuals with cystic fibrosis (CF) experience recurrent pulmonary and sinus infections. In childhood, the most commonly isolated organisms are *Haemophilus influenzae* and *Staphylococcus aureus*. However, over time, most adults demonstrate *Pseudomonas aeruginosa*. It is now recognized that chronic colonization with *Pseudomonas*, especially multidrug-resistant organisms, is associated with a more rapid decline in lung function. The Cystic Fibrosis Foundation recommends quarterly office visits with a physician, with assessment of respiratory cultures at each visit. When *Pseudomonas* is initially detected, attempts to eradicate the organism should be undertaken. Clinical trials have not definitively determined the best regimen for eradicating *Pseudomonas*, but the most common utilized treatment is the aminoglycoside antibiotic tobramycin given as a nebulized solution twice daily every other month with follow-up cultures at the next office visit to determine if the therapy should be continued. For all patients chronically colonized with *Pseudomonas*, inhaled tobramycin every other month should be continued on an indefinite basis. In addition, azithromycin 500 mg three times weekly or 250 mg daily is also utilized. Whether azithromycin primarily exerts its beneficial effect through anti-inflammatory or antimicrobial actions is not definitively known at the present time. As the patient is clinically well without any symptoms of acute exacerbation, the use of intravenous antibiotics

is not required. Chest wall oscillation and hypertonic saline are both mechanisms to improve airway clearance. By history and lung function, the patient is achieving adequate airway clearance at the present time, so escalation of care in this area is not required.

56. The answer is B.

(Chap. 17) Patients with cystic fibrosis are at risk for colonization and/or infection with a number of pathogens, and in general these infections have a temporal relationship. In childhood, the most frequently isolated organisms are *Haemophilus influenzae* and *Staphylococcus aureus*. As patients age, *Pseudomonas aeruginosa* becomes the predominant pathogen. Interestingly, *Aspergillus fumigatus* is found in the airways of up to 50% of cystic fibrosis patients. All these organisms merely colonize the airways but occasionally can also cause disease. *Burkholderia* (previously called *Pseudomonas*) *cepacia* can occasionally be found in the sputum of cystic fibrosis patients, where it is always pathogenic and is associated with a rapid decline in both clinical parameters and pulmonary function testing. Atypical mycobacteria can occasionally be found in the sputum but are often merely colonizers. *Acinetobacter baumannii* is not associated with cystic fibrosis; rather, it is generally found in nosocomial infections.

57. The answer is D.

(Chap. 18) Chronic obstructive pulmonary disease (COPD) affects more than 10 million Americans and is currently the fourth leading cause of death in the United States. Worldwide, COPD is also increasing as cigarette smoking, the primary risk factor for the development of COPD, is increasing in prevalence throughout the world. While cigarette smoking is clearly identified as a risk factor for COPD, other factors have also been identified to contribute to the risk of COPD. In many developing countries, the prevalence of smoking among women remains low. However, the incidence of COPD is increasing in women as well as men. In many developing countries, this increased incidence of COPD in women is attributable to the use of biomass fuels in poorly ventilated areas for heat and cooking. In addition, passive cigarette smoke exposure may also contribute. Occupational exposures also lead to an increased risk of COPD. While some exposures such as cotton textile dust and gold mining have not been definitively associated with COPD, coal dust exposure is a risk factor for emphysema in both smokers and nonsmokers. Inherent properties of the airways also affect the risk of COPD. Airway hyperresponsiveness increases the risk of lung function decline and is a risk factor for COPD. While there is much interest in the role of chronic or recurrent infections as a risk factor for COPD, there has been no proven link.

58. The answer is B.

(Chap. 18) Chronic obstructive pulmonary disease (COPD) is a disease process encompassing the clinical entities of emphysema and chronic bronchitis. COPD is defined pathophysiologically by the presence of irreversible airflow obstruction with hyperinflation and impaired gas exchange. The airflow obstruction occurs for several reasons including decreased elastic recoil of the lungs, increased airway inflammation, and increased closure of small airways due to loss of tethering in emphysematous lungs. This leads to early closure of airways in expiration with air trapping and hyperinflation. Finally, the loss of alveoli in emphysematous lungs leads to a progressive decline in gas exchange with alterations of ventilation-perfusion relationships. On pulmonary function testing, these pathophysiologic changes result in a typical pattern, with the primary characteristic of COPD being a decrease in the FEV_1/FVC ratio and FEV_1. The severity of airflow obstruction is graded by the degree of decline in the percentage predicted FEV_1. The FVC may or may not be decreased. With hyperinflation, the total lung capacity increases with a concomitant increase in residual volume. Finally, the diffusion capacity for carbon monoxide is also characteristically decreased in most cases of COPD. Some patients with pure chronic bronchitis without any emphysematous component may have a preserved carbon monoxide diffusing capacity (DLCO). This same pattern of pulmonary function testing can be seen in asthma with the exception of the DLCO, which is normal or increased in asthma.

59. The answer is D.

(Chap. 18) This patient has a known diagnosis of chronic obstructive pulmonary disease (COPD) with worsening symptoms and pulmonary function testing consistent with a moderate degree of disease. By the Global Initiative for Lung Disease (GOLD) criteria, the patient would have stage II disease. He is currently undermanaged with a short-acting beta-agonist only in the setting of limiting symptoms. Unfortunately, there is no medical therapy that alters mortality or definitively decreases the rate of decline in lung function in COPD, with the exception of smoking cessation, oxygen for chronic hypoxemia, and lung volume reduction surgery in a small subset of highly selected patients. Therefore, the goal of therapy in COPD is to improve symptoms and quality of life. The best initial medication for this patient would be to add a long-acting bronchodilator in the form of the antimuscarinic agent tiotropium. In large randomized controlled trials, tiotropium has been demonstrated to improve symptoms and decrease exacerbations in COPD. Ipratropium, a short-acting anticholinergic medication, also improves symptoms, but has not been similarly shown to decrease exacerbation rate. Combinations of long-acting beta-agonists and inhaled glucocorticoids have also been shown to decrease exacerbations and improve quality of life in those with COPD. The largest trial of these medications to date has demonstrated a trend toward improved mortality.

Currently the recommendation for initiation of long-acting beta-agonist and inhaled glucocorticoid combinations is to consider starting the medication if the patient has two or more exacerbations yearly or demonstrates significant acute bronchodilator reactivity on pulmonary function testing. At one time, physicians considered prescribing long-term oral glucocorticoids if a patient demonstrated significant improvement in lung function in response to a trial of oral steroids. However, long-term treatment with steroids has an unfavorable risk–benefit ratio including weight gain, osteoporosis, and increased risk of infection, especially pneumonia. Oxygen therapy improves outcomes in individuals who are hypoxemic at rest or have borderline hypoxemia with evidence of end-organ damage (pulmonary hypertension, polycythemia, etc.). While oxygen may be prescribed for individuals with isolated exercise or nocturnal hypoxemia, research to date has not demonstrated any change in outcomes with oxygen in these settings.

60. The answer is E.

(Chap. 18) Acute exacerbations of chronic obstructive pulmonary disease (COPD) are marked by an increase in dyspnea, an increase in sputum, and a change in sputum color. Acute exacerbations of COPD account for more than $10 billion in health care expenditures annually in the United States, with a significant morbidity and mortality associated with these exacerbations. Prompt treatment can improve symptoms and decrease hospitalizations and mortality in this setting. In patients presenting with hypercarbic respiratory failure in the setting of an acute exacerbation, the treatment that has demonstrated the strongest reduction in mortality is noninvasive positive pressure ventilation (NIPPV) when compared to traditional mechanical ventilation. NIPPV also decreases the need for endotracheal intubation, complications, and length of stay in the hospital. Antibiotics, bronchodilators, and glucocorticoids are all cornerstones of therapy in the treatment of acute exacerbations in COPD, but have not been demonstrated in clinical trials to have similar mortality benefits in the situation of acute hypercarbic respiratory failure. Specifically, no benefit is demonstrated for intravenous versus oral corticosteroids. Likewise, the choice of antibiotic should be made based on local susceptibility patterns, and the need for broad-spectrum antibiotics that cover *Pseudomonas* is not typically indicated.

61. The answer is C.

(Chap. 18) The only therapies that have been proven to improve survival in patients with COPD are smoking cessation, oxygen in patients with resting hypoxemia, and lung volume reduction surgery in a very small subset of highly selected patients. This patient probably has resting hypoxemia resulting from the presence of an elevated jugular venous pulse, pedal edema, and an elevated hematocrit.

Theophylline has been shown to increase exercise tolerance in patients with COPD through a mechanism other than bronchodilation. Oral glucocorticoids are not indicated in the absence of an acute exacerbation and may lead to complications if they are used indiscriminately. Atenolol and enalapril have no specific role in therapy for COPD but are often used when there is concomitant hypertension or cardiovascular disease.

62. The answer is E.

(Chap. 19) Usual interstitial pneumonia is the pathologic hallmark of idiopathic pulmonary fibrosis (IPF), but can occur in rheumatologic disorders or secondary to exposures. If no other cause is identified on history or serologic workup, then the patient is given the diagnosis of IPF. IPF is a disease that typically presents with progressive dyspnea on exertion and dry cough in an older individual. It is rare in individuals younger than 50. On physical examination, inspiratory crackles and clubbing are common. Pulmonary function tests demonstrate restrictive ventilatory defect with a low DLCO. High-resolution chest CT shows interstitial fibrosis that is worse in the bases and begins in the subpleural areas. Bronchoscopy is insufficient for histologic confirmation, and a surgical lung biopsy is required for definitive diagnosis. The natural history of IPF is one of continued progression of disease and a high mortality rate. Acute exacerbations also occur with a rapid progression of symptoms associated with a pattern of diffuse ground-glass opacities on CT. These are associated with a high mortality. Unfortunately, no therapy has been found to be effective for the treatment of IPF. Referral for lung transplantation or participation in clinical trials should be considered in all patients with a diagnosis of IPF.

63. The answer is C.

(Chap. 19) In many cases of interstitial lung disease, bronchoscopy can offer some clues to the cause of the disease. Diffuse alveolar hemorrhage (DAH) is a pathologic process that can occur in many diseases including vasculitis, Goodpasture's syndrome, systemic lupus erythematosus, crack cocaine use, mitral stenosis, and idiopathic pulmonary hemosiderosis, among many others. On bronchoscopy, one would expect to see a progressively increasing bloody return on sequential aliquots of lavage fluid. Microscopic examination would show hemosiderin-laden macrophages and red blood cells. Atypical hyperplastic type II pneumocytes are seen in diffuse alveolar damage or cases of drug toxicity. Ferruginous bodies and dust particles are found in asbestos-related pulmonary disease. Lymphocytosis is common to hypersensitivity pneumonitis and sarcoidosis. Hypersensitivity pneumonitis has a low CD4:CD8 ratio, whereas sarcoidosis has an elevated CD4:CD8 ratio. The bronchoalveolar lavage fluid in pulmonary alveolar proteinosis has a milky appearance with foamy macrophages.

64 and 65. The answers are E and E, respectively.
(*Chap. 19*) Pulmonary alveolar proteinosis (PAP) is a rare disorder with an incidence of approximately one per million. The disease usually presents in those between the ages of 30 and 50 and is slightly more common in men. Three distinct subtypes have been described: congenital, acquired, and secondary (most frequently caused by acute silicosis or hematologic malignancies). Interestingly, the pathogenesis of the disease has been associated with antibodies to granulocyte-macrophage colony-stimulating factor (GM-CSF) in most cases of acquired disease in adults. The pathobiology of the disease is failure of clearance of pulmonary surfactant. These patients typically present with subacute dyspnea on exertion with fatigue and low-grade fevers. Associated laboratory abnormalities include polycythemia, hypergammaglobulinemia, and increased LDH levels. Classically, the CT appearance is described as "crazy pavement" with ground-glass alveolar infiltrates in a perihilar distribution and intervening areas of normal lung. Bronchoalveolar lavage is diagnostic, with large amounts of amorphous proteinaceous material seen. Macrophages filled with periodic acid–Schiff (PAS)-positive material are also frequently seen. The treatment of choice is whole-lung lavage through a double-lumen endotracheal tube. Survival at 5 years is higher than 95%, although some patients will need a repeat whole-lung lavage. Secondary infection, especially with *Nocardia*, is common, and these patients should be followed closely.

66. The answer is E.
(*Chap. 19*) This patient's clinical presentation and CT imaging are consistent with the diagnosis of idiopathic pulmonary fibrosis (IPF), which is manifested histologically as usual interstitial pneumonitis (UIP). On microscopic examination, UIP is characterized by a heterogeneous appearance on low magnification with normal-appearing alveoli adjacent to severely fibrotic alveoli. There is lymphocytic infiltrate and scattered foci of fibroblasts within the alveolar septae. End-stage fibrosis results in honeycombing with loss of all alveolar structure. The typical clinical presentation of IPF/UIP is slowly progressive exertional dyspnea with a nonproductive cough. Clinical examination reveals dry crackles and digital clubbing. Patients with IPF are usually older than 50 years, and more than two-thirds have a history of current or former tobacco use. In the typical clinical situation of an older individual, a high-resolution CT scan of the chest can be diagnostic and shows subpleural pulmonary fibrosis that is greatest at the lung bases. As disease progresses, traction bronchiectasis and honeycombing are characteristic on CT scan. The cause of UIP is unknown, and no therapies have been shown to improve survival in this disease, with the exception of lung transplantation.

The presence of a dense, amorphous material in alveolar spaces that is periodic acid–Schiff positive is characteristic of pulmonary alveolar proteinosis. Pulmonary alveolar proteinosis is an interstitial lung disease that presents with progressive dyspnea, and CT imaging shows characteristic "crazy paving" with ground-glass infiltrates and thickened alveolar septae. Fibrosis is not present. Alveolar destruction with emphysematous changes would be seen in chronic obstructive pulmonary disease (COPD). The presence of crackles without wheezing or hyperinflation on examination does not suggest COPD. Furthermore, clubbing is not typically seen in COPD. Diffuse alveolar damage is seen in acute interstitial pneumonitis and acute respiratory distress syndrome (ARDS). These disorders present with a rapid, acute course that is not present in this case. The formation of noncaseating granulomas is typical of sarcoidosis, a systemic disease that usually presents in younger individuals. It is more common in those of African-American race. A typical CT in sarcoidosis would show interstitial infiltrates and hilar lymphadenopathy. End-stage disease may result in pulmonary fibrosis, but it is greatest in the upper lobes. Poorly formed granulomas may be seen in hypersensitivity pneumonitis.

67. The answer is A.
(*Chap. 19*) Pulmonary complications are common in patients with systemic lupus erythematosus (SLE). The most common manifestation is pleuritis with or without effusion. Other possible manifestations include pulmonary hemorrhage, diaphragmatic dysfunction with loss of lung volumes (the so-called shrinking lung syndrome), pulmonary vascular disease, acute interstitial pneumonitis, and bronchiolitis obliterans organizing pneumonia. Other systemic complications of SLE also cause pulmonary complications, including uremic pulmonary edema and infectious complications. Chronic progressive pulmonary fibrosis is not a complication of SLE. Cavitary lung nodules are typical of Wegener's granulomatosis but may also be seen in a variety of necrotizing lung infections.

68. The answer is E.
(*Chap. 19*) This patient with rheumatoid arthritis (RA) is presenting with pulmonary symptoms, and the biopsy shows a pattern of cryptogenic organizing pneumonia (COP), a known pulmonary manifestation of rheumatoid arthritis. COP (formerly bronchiolitis obliterans organizing pneumonia, BOOP) usually presents in the fifth or sixth decade with a flulike illness. Symptoms include fever, malaise, weight loss, cough, and dyspnea. Inspiratory crackles are common, and late inspiratory squeaks may also be heard. Pulmonary function testing reveals restrictive lung disease. The typical pattern on high-resolution chest CT is patchy areas of airspace consolidation, nodular opacities, and ground-glass opacities that occur more frequently in the lower lung zones. Pathology shows the presence of granulation tissue plugging

airways, alveolar ducts, and alveoli. There is frequently chronic inflammation in the alveolar interstitium. Treatment with high-dose steroids is effective in two-thirds of individuals, with most individuals being able to be tapered to lower doses over the first year. Azathioprine is an immunosuppressive therapy that is commonly used in interstitial lung disease due to usual interstitial pneumonitis. While it may be considered in COP that is unresponsive to glucocorticoids, it would not be a first-line agent used without concomitant steroid therapy. RA has multiple pulmonary complications. However, therapy with infliximab or methotrexate, which is useful for severe RA, is not used in the treatment of COP. Methotrexate also has pulmonary side effects and may cause pulmonary fibrosis. Hydroxychloroquine is frequently useful for joint symptoms in autoimmune disorders. Its major side effect is retinal toxicity, and it is not known to cause COP.

69. The answer is B.
(Chap. 20) The D-dimer measured by enzyme-linked immunosorbent assay (ELISA) is elevated in the setting of breakdown of fibrin by plasmin, and the presence of a positive D-dimer can prompt the need for additional imaging for deep venous thrombosis and/or pulmonary embolus in specific clinical situations where the patient would be considered to have an elevation in D-dimer. However, one must be cautious about placing value on an elevated D-dimer in other situations where there can be an alternative explanation for the elevated level. Of the scenarios listed in the question, the only patient who would be expected to have a negative D-dimer would be the patient with calf pain and recent air travel. The presence of a normal alveolar-arterial oxygen gradient cannot reliably differentiate between those with and without pulmonary embolism. In all the other scenarios, elevations in D-dimer could be related to other medical conditions and provide no diagnostic information to inform the clinician regarding the need for further evaluation. Some common clinical situations in which the D-dimer is elevated include sepsis, myocardial infarction, cancer, pneumonia, the postoperative state, and the second and third trimesters of pregnancy.

70. The answer is B.
(Chap. 20) Clinically, individuals with massive pulmonary embolus present with hypotension, syncope, or cyanosis. The hypotension and syncope occur due to acute right ventricular overload, and elevated troponin or NT-pro-brain natriuretic peptide can result from this right ventricular strain. Both elevated troponin and NT-pro-brain natriuretic peptide predict worse outcomes in pulmonary embolism. Further prognostic signs of massive pulmonary embolism include the presence of right ventricular enlargement on CT of the chest or right ventricular hypokinesis on echocardiogram. The presence

of hemoptysis, pleuritic chest pain, or cough in association with pulmonary embolism most commonly indicates a small peripheral lesion.

71. The answer is B.
(Chap. 20) For many years, ventilation-perfusion imaging (V-Q) was the standard for the diagnosis of pulmonary embolism (PE). Determination of abnormal V-Q imaging can be difficult. To call a V-Q scan a high-probability scan, one needs to see two or more segmental perfusion defects in the setting of normal ventilation. In patients with underlying lung disease, however, ventilation is frequently abnormal, and most patients with PE do not actually have high-probability V-Q scans. When there is a high-probability V-Q scan, the likelihood of PE is 90% or greater. Alternatively, patients with normal perfusion imaging have a very low likelihood of PE. Most patients fall into either the low or intermediate probability of having a PE by V-Q imaging. In this setting, 40% of patients with a high clinical suspicion of PE are determined by pulmonary angiography to indeed have a PE despite having a low-probability V-Q scan. At the present time, V-Q scanning is largely supplanted by multidetector-row spiral CT angiography of the chest. When compared to conventional CT scanning with intravenous contrast, the multidetector spiral CT can provide evaluation of the pulmonary arteries to the sixth-order branches, a level of resolution that is as good as or exceeds that of conventional invasive pulmonary angiography. In addition, the CT allows evaluation of the right and left ventricles as well as the lung parenchyma to provide additional information regarding prognosis in acute PE or alternative diagnosis in the patient with dyspnea. Magnetic resonance angiography is a rarely used alternative to the above modalities in patients with contrast dye allergy. This technique provides the ability to detect large proximal PEs, but lacks reliability for segmental and subsegmental PE.

72. The answer is E.
(Chap. 20) This patient is presenting with massive pulmonary embolus with ongoing hypotension, right ventricular dysfunction, and profound hypoxemia requiring 100% oxygen. In this setting, continuing with anticoagulation alone is inadequate, and the patient should receive circulatory support with fibrinolysis if there are no contraindications to therapy. The major contraindications to fibrinolysis include hypertension greater than 180/110 mmHg, known intracranial disease or prior hemorrhagic stroke, recent surgery, or trauma. The recommended fibrinolytic regimen is recombinant tissue plasminogen activator (rTPA), 100 mg IV over 2 hours. Heparin should be continued with the fibrinolytic to prevent a rebound hypercoagulable state with dissolution of the clot. There is a 10% risk of major bleeding with fibrinolytic therapy, with a 1–3% risk of intracranial hemorrhage. The only

indication approved by the U.S. Food and Drug Administration for fibrinolysis in pulmonary embolus (PE) is for massive PE presenting with life-threatening hypotension, right ventricular dysfunction, and refractory hypoxemia. In submassive PE presenting with preserved blood pressure and evidence of right ventricular dysfunction on echocardiogram, the decision to pursue fibrinolysis is made on a case-by-case basis. In addition to fibrinolysis, the patient should also receive circulatory support with vasopressors. Dopamine and dobutamine are the vasopressors of choice for the treatment of shock in PE. Caution should be taken with ongoing high-volume fluid administration, as a poorly functioning right ventricle may be poorly tolerant of additional fluids. Ongoing fluids may worsen right ventricular ischemia and further dilate the right ventricle, displacing the interventricular septum to the left to worsen cardiac output and hypotension. If the patient had contraindications to fibrinolysis and was unable to be stabilized with vasopressor support, referral for surgical embolectomy should be considered. Referral for inferior vena cava filter placement is not indicated at this time. The patient should be stabilized hemodynamically as a first priority. The indications for inferior vena cava filter placement are active bleeding, precluding anticoagulation, and recurrent deep venous thrombosis on adequate anticoagulation.

73. The answer is E.

(*Chap. 20*) Warfarin should not be used alone as initial therapy for the treatment of venous thromboembolic disease (VTE) for two reasons. First, warfarin does not achieve full anticoagulation for at least 5 days, as its mechanism of action is to decrease the production of vitamin K–dependent coagulation factors in the liver. Second, a paradoxical reaction that promotes coagulation may also occur upon initiation of as it also decreases the production of the vitamin K–dependent anticoagulants protein C and protein S, which have shorter half-lives than the procoagulant factors. For many years, unfractionated heparin delivered IV was the treatment of choice for VTE. However, it requires frequent monitoring of activated partial thromboplastin time (aPTT) levels and hospitalization until therapeutic international normalized ratio (INR) is achieved with warfarin. There are now several safe and effective alternatives to unfractionated heparin that can be delivered SC. Low-molecular-weight heparins (enoxaparin, tinzaparin) are fragments of unfractionated heparin with a lower molecular weight. These compounds have a greater bioavailability, longer half-life, and more predictable onset of action. Their use in renal insufficiency should be considered with caution because low-molecular-weight heparins are renally cleared. Fondaparinux is a direct factor Xa inhibitor that, like low-molecular-weight heparins, requires no monitoring of anticoagulant effects and has been demonstrated to be safe and effective in treating both deep venous thrombosis and pulmonary embolism.

74. The answer is E.

(*Chap. 21*) Parapneumonic effusions are one of the most common causes of the exudative pleural effusion. When an effusion is identified in association with pneumonia, it is prudent to perform a thoracentesis if the fluid can be safely accessed. One way to know if there is enough fluid for thoracentesis is to perform a lateral decubitus film and observe if there is 10 mm of free flowing fluid along the chest wall-pleural interface. However, if the fluid does not layer, this may indicate that it is a complex loculated fluid. A loculated effusion often indicates an infected effusion and may require chest tube drainage or surgical intervention. Other factors that are associated with the need for more invasive procedures include pleural fluid pH less than 7.20, pleural fluid glucose less than 60 mg/dL (<3.3 mmol/L), positive Gram stain or culture of the pleural fluid, and presence of gross pus in the pleural space (empyema). Fluid recurrence following initial thoracentesis does indicate a complicated pleural effusion, but a repeat thoracentesis should be performed to ensure that no concerning features have developed.

75. The answer is A.

(*Chap. 21*) The characteristics of the pleural fluid in this patient are consistent with an exudate by Light's criteria. These criteria are as follows: pleural fluid protein/serum protein greater than 0.5, pleural fluid LDH/serum LDH greater than 0.6, and pleural fluid LDH more than two-thirds of the upper limit of normal serum values. If one of the criteria is met, then the effusion would be classified as an exudate. This patient clearly meets the criteria for an exudate. Exudative pleural effusions occur when there are alterations in the local environment that change the formation and absorption of pleural fluid. The most common causes of exudative pleural effusion are infection and malignancy. Other less common causes include pulmonary embolism, chylothorax, autoimmune diseases, asbestos exposure, drug reactions, hemothorax, and postoperative cardiac surgery or other cardiac injury, among others. Unfortunately, 25% of transudative effusions can be incorrectly identified as exudates by these criteria. Most often this occurs when the effusion has an increased number of cells to cause an elevation in the LDH or has been treated with diuretics to cause an increase in pleural fluid protein. Transudative effusions are most often caused by heart failure, but can also be seen in cirrhosis, nephrotic syndrome, and myxedema.

76. The answer is A.

(*Chap. 21*) The pleural fluid characteristics are typical of a chylothorax, which occurs when there has been an injury to the thoracic duct leading to accumulation of chyle in the pleural space. The most common cause of chylothorax is traumatic disruption of the thoracic duct, especially following surgeries. The surgeries that have been associated most often with chylothorax are esophagectomy and correction of congenital heart disease. The patient often presents with rapidly progressive shortness of breath within a few weeks of the surgery and has large pleural effusions. The appearance of a milky fluid on thoracentesis should alert one to the possibility of chylothorax and prompt measurement of triglyceride levels of the pleural fluid. A triglyceride level of more than 110 mg/dL (1.2 mmol/L) is characteristic of chylothorax. The treatment of chylothorax is placement of a chest tube with administration of octreotide, a somatostatin analogue. While it is not entirely clear why this is effective, the hypothesis is that octreotide decreases splanchnic blood flow and thereby decreases triglyceride production and thoracic duct flow. Patients are often also asked to stop all oral intake to further decrease chyle production. If conservative measures fail, the thoracic duct ligation can be performed. Prolonged chest tube drainage is contraindicated, however, as the high protein content in the drained fluid can lead to malnutrition and increased infection risk.

77. The answer is B.

(Chap. 21) A primary spontaneous pneumothorax occurs in the absence of trauma to the thorax. Most individuals who present with a primary spontaneous pneumothorax are young, and primary spontaneous pneumothorax occurs almost exclusively in cigarette smokers, with cigarette smoking being the primary risk factor. Primary spontaneous pneumothorax is also more common in men and has been associated with a tall, thin body habitus. The primary cause is the rupture of small apical pleural blebs or cysts, and the CT scan of the chest is often normal. About half of individuals will experience more than one primary spontaneous pneumothorax. The initial treatment is simple needle aspiration, which is most commonly done with ultrasound or CT guidance. Oxygen is given simultaneously to speed resorption of the residual air in the pleural space. If conservative treatment fails, tube thoracostomy can be performed. Pneumothoraces that fail to resolve or are recurrent often require thoracoscopy with stapling of blebs and pleural abrasion, a treatment that is effective in almost 100% of cases.

78. The answer is B.

(Chap. 21) The most common cause of pleural effusion is left ventricular failure. Pleural effusions occur in heart failure when there are increased hydrostatic forces increasing the pulmonary interstitial fluid and the lymphatic drainage is inadequate to remove the fluid. Right-sided effusions are more common than left-sided effusions in heart failure. Thoracentesis would show a transudative fluid. Pneumonia can be associated with a parapneumonic effusion or empyema. Parapneumonic effusions are the most common cause of exudative pleural effusions and are second only to heart failure as a cause of

pleural effusions. Empyema refers to a grossly purulent pleural effusion. Malignancy is the second most common cause of exudative pleural effusion. Breast and lung cancers and lymphoma cause 75% of all malignant pleural effusions. On thoracentesis, the effusion is exudative. Cirrhosis and pulmonary embolus are far less common causes of pleural effusions.

79. The answer is E.

(Chap. 22) Patients with amyotrophic lateral sclerosis (ALS) often develop hypoventilation due to involvement of their respiratory pump muscles, e.g., diaphragm, intercostal muscles, and sternocleidomastoids. Noninvasive positive pressure ventilation (NIPPV) has been used successfully in the therapy of patients with hypoventilation such as ALS. Nocturnal NIPPV can improve daytime hypercapnia, prolong survival, and improve health-related quality of life. Current ALS guidelines are to institute NIPPV if symptoms of hypoventilation exist and $PaCO_2$ is 45 mmHg or greater, nocturnal desaturation to less than 89% is documented for 5 consecutive minutes, maximal inspiratory pressure is less than 60 cmH$_2$O, or FVC is less than 50% predicted. Symptoms of hypoventilation are not particular to ALS and may include the following: dyspnea during activities of daily living, orthopnea in diseases that affect diaphragm function, poor quality sleep, daytime hypersomnolence, early morning headaches, anxiety, and impaired cough in neuromuscular disease.

80. The answer is C.

(Chap. 22) The patient has muscular dystrophy and is at risk for the development of hypoventilation. Many patients with hypoventilation are relatively asymptomatic or only endorse symptoms after pointed questions about sleep quality, morning headache, or orthopnea due to diaphragmatic weakness if present. The patient described here has asymptomatic hypoxemia and a normal chest radiograph aside from low lung volumes. Ventilation–perfusion mismatch and shunt are unlikely to be present without infiltrates, thus atelectasis, mucous plug, and pneumonia are not the correct answers. The patient has no risk factors described for methemoglobinemia. The most likely explanation is the presence of hypoventilation with alveolar hypoxia due to elevated $PaCO_2$ through the alveolar gas equation. An arterial blood gas measurement would confirm this with elevation in $PaCO_2$, depressed PaO_2, and a normal A–a gradient.

81. The answer is B.

(Chap. 22) The physiologic effects of hypoventilation are typically magnified during sleep because of a further reduction in central respiratory drive. Hypercapnia causes cerebral vasodilation, which manifests as headache upon wakening. The headache typically resolves soon after awakening as cerebral vascular tone returns to normal with

increased ventilation. Patients with frequent nocturnal arousals from sleep and patients with nocturnal hypoventilation commonly complain of daytime somnolence and may also exhibit confusion and fatigue. Hypoventilation causes an increase in PCO_2 and an obligatory fall in PO_2. The hypoxemia can stimulate erythropoiesis and result in polycythemia. With central hypoventilation disorders, patients may also have impaired cranial nerve reflexes or muscular function, causing aspiration.

82. The answer is D.

(Chap. 24) Common indications for lung transplantation include chronic obstructive pulmonary disease, idiopathic pulmonary fibrosis, suppurative lung disease such as cystic fibrosis, and pulmonary arterial hypertension. Five-year survival is similar for all indications for lung transplantation at approximately 50%. For most indications, double-lung transplantation is the preferred procedure, and it is mandatory for patients with suppurative lung disease like cystic fibrosis. In general, in patients with idiopathic pulmonary arterial hypertension, double-lung transplantation is preferred because of concern of overcirculation in the low-resistance vascular bed of the transplanted lung when a native lung is present with markedly elevated pulmonary vascular resistance. It is very rare for the primary disease to recur after transplantation, and this has not been described in idiopathic pulmonary arterial hypertension. The right ventricle is highly plastic and will generally recover function after elevated pulmonary vascular resistance is removed by lung transplantation. Subsequently, it is rare to perform heart-lung transplantation in pulmonary arterial hypertension patients unless there is concomitant complex congenital heart disease that cannot be repaired at the time of lung transplantation.

83. The answer is A.

(Chap. 24) The long-term complications of lung transplantation are multisystem and range from the diseases that affect the lung and are complications of a foreign body in the chest to distant organ disease, either due to infections or complications of immunosuppressive therapy. Although osteoporosis, post-transplant lymphoproliferative disorders, and chronic kidney disease are important complications of steroids, calcineurin inhibitors, and other agents used for immunosuppression, the major complications post-transplant are in the lung. Primary graft dysfunction is a form of acute lung injury immediately after lung transplantation and is relatively rare, with severe disease occurring in only 10–20% of cases. Airway complications such as anastomotic dehiscence or stenosis have similar occurrence rates, but can usually be managed bronchoscopically with good survival. Rejection of transplanted organ is very common and is the main limitation to better medium- and long-term outcomes. Rejection occurs as acute cellular rejection often presenting with

cough, low-grade fever, dyspnea, infiltrates on radiographs, and declining lung function. In contrast, chronic rejection typically presents with advancing obstruction on pulmonary function testing, no infiltrates, and worsening dyspnea on exertion. This constellation in post-transplant patients is termed bronchiolitis obliterans syndrome. Fifty percent of lung transplant patients have some degree of bronchiolitis obliterans syndrome, and it is the main impediment to better long-term survival. Therapy is often with augmented immunosuppression, although there is no consensus of how to do this or the duration of this augmentation.

84. The answer is B

(Chap. 24) Chronic kidney disease is a common finding in patients after lung transplantation and is associated with poorer outcomes. While rarely patients may have hemolytic-uremic syndrome underlying the kidney disease, it is usually acute, and the most common etiology of gradually progressive decline in renal function is calcineurin inhibitor neuropathy. Cyclosporine and tacrolimus are calcineurin inhibitors commonly used in immunosuppressive regimens after lung transplantation. The exact mechanism of this toxicity is unclear but may include a direct toxicity of inhibition of the calcineurin-NFAT system within the kidney, alteration in glomerular blood flow, and host/environment interactions within the kidney with calcineurin inhibitors. Prednisone, albuterol, and mycophenolate mofetil are not known to be nephrotoxic.

85. The answer is B.

(Chap. 24) The optimal timing for lung transplantation is critical to improve survival and add quality-adjusted life years. Individuals with cystic fibrosis should be considered for lung transplantation when the FEV_1 is less than 30% predicted or is rapidly falling. Other indications for lung transplantation in cystic fibrosis include oxygen-dependent respiratory failure, hypercapnia, and pulmonary hypertension.

86. The answer is D.

(Chap. 26) Noninvasive ventilation (NIV) has been gaining more acceptance because it is effective in certain conditions, such as acute and chronic respiratory failure, and is associated with fewer complications, namely, pneumonia and tracheolaryngeal trauma. The major limitation to its widespread application has been patient intolerance because the tight-fitting mask required for NIV can cause both physical and emotional discomfort. In addition, NIV has had limited success in patients with acute hypoxemic respiratory failure, for whom endotracheal intubation and conventional mechanical ventilation remain the ventilatory method of choice. The most important group of patients who benefit from a trial of NIV are those with acute exacerbations of chronic obstructive pulmonary disease (COPD) leading to respiratory acidosis (pH <7.35). Experience from several well-conducted randomized trials has shown that in patients with ventilatory failure characterized by blood pH levels between 7.25 and 7.35, NIV is associated with low failure rates (15–20%) and good outcomes (intubation rate; length of stay in intensive care; and in some series, mortality rates). In more severely ill patients with pH below 7.25, the rate of NIV failure is inversely related to the severity of respiratory acidosis, with greater failure as the pH decreases. In patients with milder acidosis (pH >7.35), NIV is not better than conventional therapy that includes controlled oxygen delivery and pharmacotherapy for exacerbations of COPD (systemic corticosteroids; bronchodilators; and, if needed, antibiotics). The contraindications to NIV are listed in the Table 26-1.

87. The answer is A.
(Chap. 26) Modes of ventilation differ in how breaths are triggered, cycled, and limited. All modes allow determination of either the pressure or volume limit. Assist control and synchronized intermittent mandatory ventilation (SIMV) are volume cycled, in which a fixed volume is delivered to the patient by the machine using the necessary inspiratory pressure. Pressure control and pressure support are pressure cycled, in which a known pressure limit is imposed and volume delivered by the machine may vary. Continuous positive airway pressure does not alter pressure or deliver a fixed volume to the patient. Assist control and SIMV differ by the response to patient initiated breaths. Both will deliver a fixed volume when the patient does not initiate a breath. However, with SIMV, if the patient is breathing at a rate greater than set on the machine, each spontaneous breath is dependent completely on patient effort. On assist control, each patient initiated breath above the set rate is supported by the machine by delivering the set rate. In patients with a high respiratory rate, this can result in hyperventilation, and intrinsic PEEP because of inadequate time for exhalation of the full tidal volume. In the patient described, because each breath that is either initiated by the patient or the machine is at a set rate and a fixed volume, this is most consistent with the assist control mode of mechanical ventilation.

88. The answer is D.
(Chap. 26) Determining when an individual is an appropriate candidate for a spontaneous breathing trial is important for the care of mechanically ventilated patients. An important initial step in determining if a patient is likely to be successfully extubated is to evaluate the mental status of the patient. This can be difficult if the patient is receiving sedation, and it is recommended that sedation be interrupted on a daily basis for a short period to allow assessment of mental status. Daily interruption of sedation has been shown to decrease the duration of mechanical ventilation.

If the patient is unable to respond to any commands or is completely obtunded, the individual is at high risk for aspiration and unlikely to be successfully extubated. In addition, the patient should be hemodynamically stable and the lung injury stable or improving. If these conditions are met, the patient should be on minimal ventilatory support. This includes the ability to maintain the pH between 7.35 and an SaO_2 greater than 90% while receiving an FiO_2 of 0.5 or less and a PEEP of 5 cmH_2O or less. The presence of rapid shallow breathing during a spontaneous breathing trial identifies patients who are less likely to be extubated successfully.

89. The answer is B.
(Chap. 26) Patients initiated on mechanical ventilation require a variety of supportive measures. Sedation and analgesia with a combination of benzodiazepines and narcotics are commonly used to maintain patient comfort and safety while mechanically ventilated. Recent studies have shown the utility of minimizing sedation in critically ill patients. However, adequate pain control is an essential component of patient comfort. In addition, patients are immobilized and are thus at high risk for development of deep venous thrombosis and pulmonary embolus. Prophylaxis with unfractionated heparin or low-molecular-weight heparin should be administered subcutaneously. Prophylaxis against diffuse gastrointestinal mucosal injury is also indicated, particularly in individuals with neurologic insult and those with severe respiratory failure and adult respiratory distress syndrome. Gastric acid suppression can be managed with H2-receptor antagonists, proton pump inhibitors, and sucralfate. It is also recommended that individuals who are expected to be intubated for more than 72 hours receive nutritional support. Prokinetic agents are often required. Frequent positional changes and close surveillance for skin breakdown should be instituted in all intensive care units to minimize development of decubitus ulcers. In the past, frequent ventilator circuit changes had been studied as a measure for prevention of ventilator-associated pneumonia, but they were ineffective and may even have increased the risk of ventilator-associated pneumonia.

90. The answer is D.
(Chap. 26) Mechanical ventilation is frequently used to support ventilation in individuals with both hypoxemic and hypercarbic respiratory failure. Mechanical ventilators provide warm, humidified gas to the airways in accordance with preset ventilator settings. The ventilator serves as the energy source for inspiration, but expiration is a passive process, driven by the elastic recoil of the lungs and chest wall. PEEP may be used to prevent alveolar collapse on expiration. The physiologic consequences of PEEP include decreased preload and decreased afterload. Decreased preload occurs because

PEEP decreases venous return to the right atrium and may manifest as hypotension, especially in an individual who is volume depleted. In addition, PEEP is transmitted to the heart and great vessels. This complicated interaction leads to a decrease in afterload and may be beneficial to individuals with depressed cardiac function. When using mechanical ventilation, the physician should also be cognizant of other potential physiologic consequences of the ventilator settings. Initial settings chosen by the physician include mode of ventilation, respiratory rate, fraction of inspired oxygen, and tidal volume if volume-cycled ventilation is used or maximum pressure if pressure-cycled ventilation is chosen. The respiratory therapist also has the ability to alter the inspiratory flow rate and waveform for delivery of the chosen mode of ventilation. These choices can have important physiologic consequences for the patient. In individuals with obstructive lung disease, it is important to maximize the time for exhalation. This can be done by decreasing the respiratory rate or decreasing the inspiratory time (decrease the inspiration-to-expiration ratio, prolong expiration), which is accomplished by increasing the inspiratory flow rate. Care must also be taken in choosing the inspired tidal volume in volume-cycled ventilatory modes because high inspired tidal volumes can contribute to development of acute lung injury caused by overdistention of alveoli.

91.   The answer is B.

(*Chap. 26*) Patients intubated for respiratory failure because of obstructive lung disease (asthma or chronic obstructive pulmonary disease) are at risk for the development of intrinsic positive end-expiratory pressure (auto-PEEP). Because these conditions are characterized by expiratory flow limitation, a long expiratory time is required to allow a full exhalation. If the patient is unable to exhale fully, auto-PEEP develops. With repeated breaths, the pressure generated from auto-PEEP continues to rise and impedes venous return to the right ventricle. This results in hypotension and increases the risk for pneumothorax. Both of these conditions should be considered when evaluating this patient. However, because breath sounds are heard bilaterally, pneumothorax is less likely, and tube thoracostomy is not indicated at this time. Development of auto-PEEP has most likely occurred in this patient because the patient is currently agitated and hyperventilating as the effects of the paralytic agent wear off. In AC mode ventilation, each respiratory effort delivers the full tidal volume of 550 mL, and there is a decreased time for exhalation, allowing auto-PEEP to occur. Immediate management of this patient should include disconnecting the patient from the ventilator to allow the patient to fully exhale and decreasing the auto-PEEP. A fluid bolus may temporarily increase the blood pressure but would not eliminate the underlying cause of the hypotension. After treatment of the auto-PEEP

by disconnecting the patient from the ventilator, sedation is important to prevent further occurrence of auto-PEEP by decreasing the respiratory rate to the set rate of the ventilator. Sedation can be accomplished with a combination of benzodiazepines and narcotics or propofol. Initiation of vasopressor support is not indicated unless other measures fail to treat the hypotension and it is suspected that sepsis is the cause of hypotension.

92.   The answer is A.

(*Chap. 26*) To obtain a stable airway for invasive mechanical ventilation, patients must safely undergo endotracheal intubation. In most patients, paralytic agents are used in combination with sedatives to accomplish endotracheal intubation. Succinylcholine is a depolarizing neuromuscular blocking agent with a short half-life and is one of the most commonly used paralytic agents. However, because it depolarizes the neuromuscular junction, succinylcholine cannot be used in individuals with hyperkalemia because the drug may cause further increases in the potassium level and potentially fatal cardiac arrhythmias. Some conditions in which it is relatively contraindicated to use succinylcholine because of the risk of hyperkalemia include acute renal failure, crush injuries, muscular dystrophy, rhabdomyolysis, and tumor lysis syndrome. Acetaminophen overdose is not a contraindication to the use of succinylcholine unless concomitant renal failure is present.

93.   The answers are 1–C; 2–B; 3–D; 4–A.

(*Chaps. 27, 28, and 30*) A variety of vasopressor agents are available for hemodynamic support. The effects of these medications depend on their effects on the sympathetic nervous system to produce changes in heart rate, cardiac contractility, and peripheral vascular tone. Stimulation of $\alpha 1$ adrenergic receptors in the peripheral vasculature causes vasoconstriction and improves MAP by increasing systemic vascular resistance. The $\beta 1$ receptors are located primarily in the heart and cause increased cardiac contractility and heart rate. The $\beta 2$ receptors are found in the peripheral circulation and cause vasodilatation and bronchodilation. Phenylephrine acts solely as an α-adrenergic agonist. It is considered a second-line agent in septic shock and is often used in anesthesia to correct hypotension after induction of anesthesia. Phenylephrine is also useful for spinal shock. The action of dopamine depends on the dosage used. At high doses, dopamine has high affinity for the α receptor, but at lower doses (<5 µg/kg/min), it does not. In addition, dopamine acts at $\beta 1$ receptors and dopaminergic receptors. The effect on these receptors is greatest at lower doses. Norepinephrine and epinephrine affect both α and $\beta 1$ receptors to increase peripheral vascular resistance, heart rate, and contractility. Norepinephrine has less $\beta 1$ activity than epinephrine or dopamine and thus has less associated tachycardia. Norepinephrine and dopamine are the recommended first-line therapies for septic shock. Epi-nephrine is the drug of choice for anaphylactic shock. Dobutamine is primarily a β1 agonist with lesser effects at the β2 receptor. Dobutamine increases cardiac output through improving cardiac contractility and heart rate. Dobutamine may be associated with development of hypotension because of its effects at the β2 receptor causing vasodilatation and decreased systemic vascular resistance.

94 and 95. The answers are B and C, respectively.
(Chap. 27) Hypovolemic shock is the most common form of shock and occurs either because of hemorrhage or loss of plasma volume in the form of gastrointestinal, urinary, or insensible losses. Symptoms of hemorrhagic and nonhemorrhagic shock are indistinguishable. Mild hypovolemia is considered to be loss of less than 20% of the blood volume and usually presents with few clinical except save for mild tachycardia. Loss of 20–40% of the blood volume typically induces orthostasis. Loss of more than 40% of the blood volume leads to the classic manifestations of shock, which are marked tachycardia, hypotension, oliguria, and finally obtundation. Central nervous system perfusion is maintained until shock becomes severe. Oliguria is a very important clinical parameter that should help guide volume resuscitation. After assessing for an adequate airway and spontaneous breathing, initial resuscitation aims at reexpanding the intravascular volume and controlling ongoing losses. Volume resuscitation should be initiated with rapid IV infusion of isotonic saline or Ringer's lactate. In head-to-head trials, colloidal solutions have not added any benefit compared with crystalloid and in fact appeared to increase mortality for trauma patients. Hemorrhagic shock with ongoing blood losses and a hemoglobin of 10 g/dL or less should be treated with transfusion of packed red blood cells (PRBCs). After hemorrhage is controlled, transfusion of PRBCs should be performed only for hemoglobin of 7 g/dL or less. Patients who remain hypotensive after volume resuscitation have a very poor prognosis. Inotropic support and intensive monitoring should be initiated in these patients. An algorithm for the resuscitation of a patient in shock is shown in Figure 27-3.

96. The answer is D.
(Chap. 27) The patient is in cardiogenic shock from an ST-elevation myocardial infarction. Shock is a clinical syndrome in which vital organs do not receive adequate perfusion. Understanding the physiology underlying shock is a crucial factor in determining appropriate management. Cardiac output is the major determinant of tissue perfusion and is the product of stroke volume and heart rate. In turn, stroke volume is determined by preload, or ventricular filling, afterload, or resistance to ventricular ejection, and contractility of the myocardium. In this patient,

the hypoxic and damaged myocardium has suddenly lost much of its contractile function, and stroke volume will therefore decrease rapidly, dropping cardiac output. Systemic vascular resistance will increase in order to improve return of blood to the heart and increase stroke volume. Central venous pressure is elevated as a consequence of increased vascular resistance, decreased cardiac output and poor forward flow, and neuroendocrine-mediated vasoconstriction. The pathophysiology of other forms of shock is shown in Table 27-4 as a comparison.

97. The answer is C.
(Chap. 28) The annual incidence of sepsis has increased to >700,000 individuals yearly in the United States, and sepsis accounts for more than 200,000 deaths yearly. Approximately two-thirds of the cases of sepsis occur in individuals with other significant comorbidities, and the incidence of sepsis increases with age and preexisting comorbidities. In addition, the incidence of sepsis is thought to be increasing as a result of several other factors. These include increased longevity of individuals with chronic disease, including AIDS, and increased risk for sepsis in individuals with AIDS. The practice of medicine has also influenced the risk of sepsis, with an increased risk of sepsis related to the increased use of antimicrobial drugs, immunosuppressive agents, mechanical ventilation, and indwelling catheters and other hardware.

98. The answer is B.
(Chap. 28) Sepsis is a systemic inflammatory response that develops in response to a microbial source. To diagnose the systemic inflammatory response syndrome (SIRS), a patient should have two or more of the following conditions: (1) fever or hypothermia; (2) tachypnea; (3) tachycardia; or (4) leukocytosis, leukopenia, or greater than 10% band forms. This patient fulfills the criteria for sepsis with septic shock because she meets these criteria for SIRS with the presence of organ dysfunction and ongoing hypotension despite fluid resuscitation. The patient has received 2 L of intravenous colloid and now has a central venous pressure of 18 cmH₂O. Ongoing large-volume fluid administration may result in pulmonary edema as the central venous pressure is quite high. At this point, fluid administration should continue but at a lower infusion rate. In this patient, who is receiving chronic glucocorticoids for an underlying inflammatory condition, stress-dose steroids should be administered because adrenal suppression will prevent the patient from developing the normal stress response in the face of SIRS. If the patient fails to respond to glucocorticoids, she should be started on vasopressor therapy. The diagnosis of adrenal insufficiency may be very difficult in critically ill patients. Whereas a plasma cortisol level of less than 15 μg/mL indicates adrenal insufficiency (inadequate production of cortisol), many experts now feel

that the adrenocorticotropic hormone stimulation test is not useful for detecting less profound degrees of corticosteroid deficiency in patients who are critically ill. A single small study has suggested that norepinephrine may be preferred over dopamine for septic shock, but these data have not been confirmed in other trials. The "Surviving Sepsis" guidelines state that either norepinephrine or dopamine should be considered as a first-line agent for the treatment of septic shock. Transfusion of red blood cells in critically ill patients has been associated with a higher risk for development of acute lung injury, sepsis, and death. A threshold hemoglobin value of 7 g/dL has been shown to be as safe as a value of 10 g/dL and is associated with fewer complications. In this patient, a blood transfusion is not currently indicated, but it may be considered if the central venous oxygen saturation is below 70% to improve oxygen delivery to tissues. An alternative to blood transfusion in this setting is the use of dobutamine to improve cardiac output.

99. The answer is C.

(Chap. 28) Sepsis occurs as a result of the inflammatory reaction that develops in response to an infection. Microbial invasion of the bloodstream is not necessary for the development of severe sepsis. In fact, blood culture results are positive in only 20–40% of cases of severe sepsis and in only 40–70% of cases of septic shock. The systemic response to infection classically has been demonstrated by the response to lipopolysaccharide (LPS) or endotoxin. LPS binds to receptors on the surfaces of monocytes, macrophages, and neutrophils, causing activation of these cells to produce a variety of inflammatory mediators and cytokines, most notably tumor necrosis factor α (TNF-α). TNF-α stimulates leukocytes and vascular endothelial cells to release other cytokines (as well as additional TNF-α), to express cell-surface molecules that enhance neutrophil–endothelial adhesion at sites of infection, and to increase prostaglandin and leukotriene production. Whereas blood levels of TNF-α are not elevated in individuals with localized infections, they increase in most patients with severe sepsis or septic shock. Moreover, IV infusion of TNF-α can elicit the characteristic abnormalities of SIRS. Although TNF-α is a central mediator, it is only one of many proinflammatory molecules that contribute to innate host defense. Chemokines, most prominently interleukin-8 (IL-8) and IL-17, attract circulating neutrophils to the infection site. These and other proinflammatory cytokines probably interact synergistically with one another and with additional mediators to promote the process of complement activation and increase in procoagulant factors, cellular injury, and intravascular thrombosis. The nonlinearity and multiplicity of these interactions have made it difficult to interpret the roles played by individual mediators in both tissues and blood. This process is meant to wall off invading microorganisms to prevent infection from spreading to other tissues, but in cases of severe sepsis, this leads to tissue hypoxia and ongoing cellular injury. In addition, systemic hypotension develops as a reaction to inflammatory mediators and occurs despite increased levels of plasma catecholamines. Physiologically, this is manifested as a marked decrease in systemic vascular resistance despite evidence of increased sympathetic activation. Survival in sepsis has improved in the past decades largely because of advances in supportive care in the intensive care unit.

100. The answer is B.

(Chap. 28) As the mortality from sepsis has increased over the past 20 years, more research has been performed to attempt to limit mortality. Antimicrobial chemotherapy should be started as soon as samples of blood and other relevant sites have been obtained for culture. A large retrospective review of patients who developed septic shock found that the interval between the onset of hypotension and the administration of appropriate antimicrobial chemotherapy was the major determinant of outcome; a delay of as little as 1 hour was associated with lower survival rates. Empiric antibiotics should have broad coverage of gram-positive and -negative organisms. In general, combination therapy has no advantage over monotherapy with broad-spectrum antibiotics. Use of inappropriate antibiotics, defined on the basis of local microbial susceptibilities and published guidelines for empirical therapy, was associated with fivefold lower survival rates even among patients with negative culture results. Specific therapies have been developed to target the inflammatory response to sepsis, particularly the effect of the inflammatory response on the coagulation system. Unfortunately, none of the pathophysiologically oriented therapies has shown consistent benefit in sepsis. Recently, activated protein C (drotrecogin-α), which had been approved by the U.S. Food and Drug Administration for the treatment of septic shock, was removed from the market by its manufacturer after the European PROWESS-SHOCK trial failed to show a survival benefit. Bicarbonate therapy is commonly used when severe metabolic acidosis (pH <7.2) is present in septic shock. However, there is no evidence that bicarbonate improves hemodynamics, response to vasopressors, or outcomes in septic shock. In patients with septic shock, plasma vasopressin levels increase transiently but then decrease dramatically. Early studies found that vasopressin infusion can reverse septic shock in some patients, reducing or eliminating the need for catecholamine vasopressors. More recently, a randomized clinical trial that compared vasopressin plus norepinephrine with norepinephrine alone in 776 patients with pressor-dependent septic shock found no difference between treatment groups in the primary study outcome, 28-day mortality. Although some patients with sepsis may benefit from red blood cell transfusion, erythropoietin is not used to treat anemia in sepsis.

101. The answer is B.

(Chap. 29) ALI and ARDS are both characterized by diffuse lung injury, bilateral radiographic infiltrates, and hypoxemia in the absence of left atrial hypertension. ALI is considered a less severe form of diffuse lung injury that may evolve to ARDS or warrant intensive therapy to forestall the progression. The distinction between ALI and ARDS is made by the magnitude of the PaO_2/FiO_2 ratio with ARDS defined as a ratio of 200 mmHg or below and ALI 300 mmHg or below. Many medical and surgical illnesses are associated with the development of ALI and ARDS, but most cases (>80%) are caused by a relatively small number of clinical disorders, namely, severe sepsis syndrome and bacterial pneumonia (40–50%), trauma, multiple transfusions, aspiration of gastric contents, and drug overdose. Among patients with trauma, pulmonary contusion, multiple bone fractures, and chest wall trauma or flail chest are the most frequently reported surgical conditions in ARDS, but head trauma, near drowning, toxic inhalation, and burns are rare causes. The risks of developing ARDS are increased in patients with more than one predisposing medical or surgical condition (e.g., the risk for ARDS increases from 25% in patients with severe trauma to 56% in patients with trauma and sepsis). Several other clinical variables have been associated with the development of ARDS. These include older age, chronic alcohol abuse, metabolic acidosis, and severity of critical illness.

102. The answer is D.

(Chap. 29) To date, despite intensive investigation of multiple pathophysiologically based therapies, the only intervention that decreased mortality in patients with ARDS was a low tidal volume (6 mL/kg ideal body weight) mechanical ventilation strategy. The rationale for this intervention is that overdistension of normal alveoli in patients with ARDS promotes further lung injury. Maintaining a normal or low left atrial filling pressure is also recommended therapy for patients with ARDS. It minimizes pulmonary edema and prevents further decrements in arterial oxygenation and lung compliance, improves pulmonary mechanics, and shortens intensive care unit stay and the duration of mechanical ventilation. Numerous studies have demonstrated that placing the patient in the prone position may improve oxygenation, but there has been no consistent mortality benefit. Other "lung protective" strategies of mechanical ventilation (high-frequency ventilation, high positive end-expiratory pressure, pressure-volume curve measurement) are under investigation. Inflammatory mediators and leukocytes are abundant in the lungs of patients with ARDS. Many attempts have been made to treat both early and late ARDS with glucocorticoids to reduce this potentially deleterious pulmonary inflammation. Few studies have shown any benefit. Current evidence does *not* support the use of high-dose glucocorticoids in the care of ARDS patients.

Similarly, ARDS is characterized by a surfactant deficiency, but administration of exogenous surfactant has not yielded clinical results (in contrast to the dramatic benefit in neonatal lung injury). See Table 29-3.

103. The answer is E.

(Chap. 29) Recent mortality estimates for ARDS range from 26–44%. The mortality rate in ARDS is largely attributable to nonpulmonary causes, with sepsis and nonpulmonary organ failure accounting for more than 80% of deaths. Mortality caused by hypoxemic respiratory failure is not typical. The degree of hypoxemia during ARDS is also not a strong predictor of outcome. The major risk factors for ARDS mortality include age, preexisting chronic medical conditions or organ dysfunction, and severity of critical illness (number of organ failures). Patients with ARDS from direct lung injury (including pneumonia, pulmonary contusion, and aspiration) have nearly twice the mortality rate of those with indirect causes of lung injury, but surgical and trauma patients with ARDS, especially those without direct lung injury, have a better survival rate than other ARDS patients. The majority of patients recover nearly normal lung function with 1 year. One year after endotracheal extubation, more than one-third of ARDS survivors have normal spirometry values and diffusion capacity, and most of the remaining patients have only mild abnormalities in their pulmonary function. Unlike the risk for mortality, recovery of lung function is strongly associated with the extent of lung injury in early ARDS. When caring for ARDS survivors, it is important to be aware of the potential for a substantial burden of emotional and respiratory symptoms. There are significant rates of depression and posttraumatic stress disorder in ARDS survivors.

104. The answer is A.

(Chap. 30) Cardiogenic shock (CS) is characterized by systemic hypoperfusion caused by severe depression of the cardiac index (<2.2 L/min/m^2) and sustained systolic arterial hypotension (<90 mmHg) despite an elevated filling pressure (pulmonary capillary wedge pressure >18 mmHg). It is associated with in-hospital mortality rates above 50%. Acute myocardial infarction (MI) with left ventricular dysfunction is the most common cause of cardiogenic shock. Other complications of acute MI such as mitral regurgitation or free wall rupture are far less common. CS is the leading cause of death of patients hospitalized with MI. Early reperfusion therapy for acute MI decreases the incidence of CS. Shock typically is associated with ST-segment elevation MI and is less common with non–ST-segment elevation MI. In patients with acute MI, older age, female sex, prior MI, diabetes, and anterior MI location are all associated with an increased risk of CS. Shock associated with a first inferior MI should prompt a search for a mechanical cause. Reinfarction soon after MI increases the risk of CS.

Two-thirds of patients with CS have flow-limiting stenoses in all three major coronary arteries, and 20% have stenosis of the left main coronary artery. CS may rarely occur in the absence of significant stenosis, as seen in LV apical ballooning/Takotsubo's cardiomyopathy.

105. The answer is E.

(Chap. 30) In patients with acute myocardial infarction and cardiogenic shock, percutaneous coronary intervention can improve mortality rate and outcomes. Stabilizing the patient in cardiogenic shock is an important first maneuver. Initial therapy is aimed at maintaining adequate systemic and coronary perfusion by raising systemic blood pressure with vasopressors and adjusting volume status to a level that ensures optimum left ventricular filling pressure. Decreased diastolic blood pressure is detrimental because it reduces coronary blood flow. However, vasopressor and inotropic agents have the potential to exacerbate the ischemic process by raising myocardial oxygen consumption, increasing heart rate, or increasing left ventricular afterload. Norepinephrine is associated with fewer adverse events, including arrhythmias, compared with dopamine. Dobutamine has greater inotropic than chronotropic action but may cause a reduction in blood pressure due to vasodilation. Aortic counterpulsation with an intraaortic balloon pump (IABP) is helpful in rapidly stabilizing patients because it is capable of augmenting both arterial diastolic pressure and cardiac output. The balloon is automatically inflated during early diastole, augmenting coronary blood flow, and it collapses in early systole, reducing the left ventricular afterload. IABP improves hemodynamic status temporarily in most patients with cardiogenic shock. In contrast to vasopressors and inotropic agents, myocardial O_2 consumption is reduced, ameliorating ischemia. IABP is contraindicated if aortic regurgitation is present or aortic dissection is suspected.

106. The answer is E.

(Chap. 31) The most common electrical mechanism for cardiac arrest is ventricular fibrillation, which is responsible for 50–80% of cardiac arrests. Severe persistent bradyarrhythmias, asystole, and pulseless electrical activity (PEA: organized electrical activity, unusually slow, without mechanical response, formerly called electromechanical dissociation) cause another 20–30%. Pulseless sustained ventricular tachycardia (a rapid arrhythmia distinct from PEA) is a less common mechanism. Acute low cardiac output states, having a precipitous onset also may present clinically as a cardiac arrest. These hemodynamic causes include massive acute pulmonary emboli, internal blood loss from a ruptured aortic aneurysm, intense anaphylaxis, and cardiac rupture with tamponade after myocardial infarction. Sudden deaths from these causes are not typically included in the category of sudden cardiac death.

107. The answer is A.

(Chap. 31) The probability of achieving successful resuscitation from cardiac arrest is related to the interval from onset of loss of circulation to institution of resuscitative efforts, the setting in which the event occurs, the mechanism (ventricular fibrillation, ventricular tachycardia, PEA, asystole), and the clinical status of the patient before the cardiac arrest. Return of circulation and survival rates as a result of defibrillation decrease almost linearly from the first minute to 10 minutes. After 5 minutes, survival rates are no better than 25–30% in out-of-hospital settings. Settings in which it is possible to institute prompt cardiopulmonary resuscitation (CPR) followed by prompt defibrillation provide a better chance of a successful outcome. However, the outcome in intensive care units (ICUs) and other in-hospital environments is heavily influenced by the patient's preceding clinical status. The immediate outcome is good for cardiac arrest occurring in ICUs in the presence of an acute cardiac event or transient metabolic disturbance, but survival among patients with far-advanced chronic cardiac disease or advanced noncardiac diseases (e.g., renal failure, pneumonia, sepsis, diabetes, cancer) is low and not much better in the in-hospital than in the out-of-hospital setting. Survival from unexpected cardiac arrest in unmonitored areas in a hospital is not much better than that it is for witnessed out-of-hospital arrests. Because implementation of community response systems, survival from out-of-hospital cardiac arrest has improved, although it still remains low under most circumstances. Survival probabilities in public sites exceed those in the home environment. This may be because many patients with at home cardiac arrest have severe underlying cardiac disease. The success rate for initial resuscitation and survival to hospital discharge after an out-of-hospital cardiac arrest depends heavily on the mechanism of the event. Most cardiac arrests that are caused by ventricular fibrillation (VF) begin with a run of nonsustained or sustained ventricular tachycardia (VT), which then degenerates into VF. When the mechanism is pulseless VT, the outcome is best, VF is the next most successful, and asystole and PEA generate dismal outcome statistics. Advanced age also adversely influences the chances of successful resuscitation as well as outcomes after resuscitation.

108. The answer is D.

(Chap. 34) Alterations in consciousness are among the most common reasons for admission to the hospital and occur frequently in seriously ill patients. When evaluating a patient with an alteration in consciousness, one must have a framework for understanding the spectrum of arousability one may encounter. *Coma* is a frequently misunderstood term that refers to a deep, sleeplike state from which a patient cannot be aroused. A stuporous patient can be aroused briefly with noxious stimuli, and drowsiness refers to a patient who can be aroused easily

with maintenance of attention for brief periods. Other conditions that alter the ability of a patient to respond appropriately to stimuli and are often confused with coma. A vegetative state is an awake but unresponsive condition that can occur in a patient who has emerged from a coma and is associated with extensive bilateral cerebral damage. A patient in a vegetative state can open the eyes spontaneously and often track objects. In addition, the patient has retention of respiratory and autonomic functions as well as spontaneous movement of extremities. However, meaningful responses to stimuli do not occur, and a vegetative state is sometimes referred to as an "awake coma." This patient would be characterized as being in a persistent vegetative state because the duration of the vegetative state has been 1 year. At this point, the likelihood of meaningful recovery of mental faculties is almost zero. A minimally conscious state is a less severe manifestation of bilateral cerebral injury. A patient in a minimally conscious state may have rudimentary vocal or motor behaviors and minimal responses to external stimuli. Other conditions that may be misinterpreted as a coma include akinetic mutism, catatonia, abulia, and locked-in syndrome.

109. The answer is A.

(Chap. 34) Brain death occurs when all cerebral function has ceased but the patient continues to have cardiac activity while supported by artificial means. If an individual is determined to have brain death, life-sustaining therapies are withdrawn. Although this can occur without the consent of the family, certainly it is important to have open communication with the family to allow the withdrawal of care without conflict. Most hospitals have developed specific protocols to diagnose a patient with brain death. Three essential elements should be demonstrated for the diagnosis of brain death. First, the patient should widespread cortical damage with complete absence of response to all external stimuli. Second, the patient should have no evidence of brainstem function with loss of oculovestibular and corneal reflexes and absent pupillary reaction to light. Finally, there should be no evidence of medullary activity manifested by apnea. When a brain death examination is performed, the patient should not be receiving any medications that could alter consciousness. The bedside examination will confirm absence of responsiveness to stimuli and lack of brainstem function. Apnea testing is the final examination in the performance of the brain death examination. This test is important for documenting the absence of medullary function. For an apnea test result to be accurate, the carbon dioxide must be allowed to rise to a level that would stimulate respiration. When performing the test, the patient is preoxygenated with 100% oxygen, which is sustained throughout the test. At this point, ventilator support is stopped. In the absence of any respiration, carbon dioxide rises by 2–3 mmHg/min, and it is necessary for arterial partial pressure of carbon

dioxide to rise to between 50–60 mmHg. If the patient has a normal $PaCO_2$ before beginning the apnea test, the test would typically need to continue for at least 5 minutes to be valid. The patient is observed for respiratory effort, and a $PaCO_2$ level is often measured at the end of the test to document that the rise in carbon dioxide is adequate to stimulate respiration. Some patients may have cardiovascular instability that makes the performance of apnea testing risky because one does not wish for the apnea test to lead to cardiovascular collapse. In this setting, an electroencephalogram demonstrating absence of electrical activity is used as an adjunctive diagnostic test. Newer methods of testing, including radionuclide brain scanning, cerebral angiography, and transcranial Doppler ultrasonography, may be used, but these tests are less well validated. In most cases, clinical evidence of brain death must be sustained for 6–24 hours before withdrawal of care.

110. The answer is E.

(Chap. 34) Foraminal herniation, which forces the cerebellar tonsils into the foramen magnum, leads to compression of the medulla and subsequent respiratory arrest. Central transtentorial herniation occurs when the medial thalamus compresses the midbrain as it moves through the tentorial opening; miotic pupils and drowsiness are the classic clinical signs. A locked-in state is usually caused by infarction or hemorrhage of the ventral pons; other causes include Guillain-Barré syndrome and use of certain neuromuscular blocking agents. Catatonia is a semi-awake state seen most frequently as a manifestation of psychotic disorders such as schizophrenia. Third-nerve palsies arise from an uncal transtentorial herniation in which the anterior medial temporal gyrus herniates into the anterior portion of the tentorial opening anterior to the adjacent midbrain. Coma may occur because of compression of the midbrain.

111. The answer is D.

(Chap. 35) Clinicians caring for critically ill individuals are often asked to determine prognosis after events that lead to anoxic-ischemic brain injury, including prolonged cardiac arrest, shock, and carbon monoxide poisoning. Lack of cerebral circulation for longer than 3–5 minutes most often results in at least minor permanent cerebral damage, which can be difficult to predict. In the early hours after an anoxic-ischemic event, family members often ask for guidance regarding prognosis, and the clinical examination over a period of 72 hours provides important clues to whether any meaningful recovery of cerebral function may occur. However, before performing the examination, the patient must be in a stable clinical state without medications or other clinical factors that would prevent an appropriate examination. In recent years, clinical trials have supported the use of induced hypothermia to improve neurologic outcomes

after cardiac arrest, and current clinical practice is to lower body temperature to 33°C for 12–24 hours. To ensure patient comfort during induced hypothermia and prevent elevation in body temperature from shivering, the patient is heavily sedated and often paralyzed for the duration of the hypothermia and through the rewarming process. Given that this patient is hypothermic, sedated, and paralyzed, the clinical examination cannot be used to provide any prognostic information to the family at the present time.

If the patient were not hypothermic, paralyzed, or sedated, the initial examination should assess for the presence of brainstem function to determine if brain death is present. If brainstem function was present, other clinical signs of poor prognosis in the first 1–3 days include the presence of status epilepticus, frequent myoclonus, lack of response on somatosensory evoked potentials, or a serum neuron specific enolase level greater than 33 μg/L. After 72 hours, the patient is often reassessed for the response to noxious stimuli and corneal or pupillary response. The absence of response or an extensor motor response only at this point in time predicts a 0–3% long-term likelihood of neurologic recovery.

112. The answer is C.

(Chap. 35) When a patient presents to the emergency department with a severe headache, the most immediately life-threatening diagnosis is SAH. The most common cause of SAH outside of trauma is rupture of a saccular aneurysm, and some patients may experience a sentinel bleed from a small rupture, providing a window of opportunity to definitively treat the aneurysm before a more substantial bleed.

The most common symptom of a SAH is a severe headache that is abrupt in onset (thunderclap headache). About 50% of individuals experience a sudden loss of consciousness caused by a rapid increase in intracranial pressure that is followed by the severe headache upon regaining consciousness. Other common characteristics associated with SAH are worsening of pain with exertion or bending forward, neck stiffness, and vomiting. In 95% of cases, blood in the subarachnoid space is visible on a noncontrasted CT scan of the head. However, if the event occurred more than 3 days previously as in this case, blood may not be seen. In this situation, the patient should undergo lumbar puncture to determine if red blood cells are present in the CSF without clearing. At this stage, the red blood cells will likely have undergone some degree of lysis with a resultant discoloration of the CSF to a characteristic yellow color called xanthochromia. The peak intensity of xanthochromia is at 48 hours, but it persists for 1–4 weeks. If the lumbar puncture demonstrates xanthochromia, then further evaluation would most likely consist of a conventional four-vessel cerebral angiography to localize the aneurysm

and provide a potential method of treatment via endovascular techniques. CT angiography may be used as an alternative for localization but does not provide the opportunity for intervention. Lumbar puncture will also evaluate for meningitis and encephalitis, which are also possible in this case. Appropriate culture and polymerase chain reaction diagnostic tests should be included in the diagnostic evaluation.

113. The answer is A.

(Chap. 35) This patient presents with an SAH caused by a ruptured anterior cerebral artery and has evidence of increased intracranial pressure with midline shift on a CT scan of the head. He has undergone aneurysm repair, and the care now should focus on the medical management of SAH. Some of the principles of the medical management of SAH include treatment of intracranial hypertension, management of blood pressure, prevention of vasospasm, and prevention of rebleeding. A patient who is unresponsive with evidence of intracranial hypertension should immediately undergo emergent ventriculostomy, which allows measurement of intracranial pressure (ICP) and can treat elevated ICP. Other strategies for treatment of elevated ICP include hyperventilation, mannitol, sedation, and hypernatremia. If a patient survives the initial aneurysmal bleed and the aneurysm is treated, the leading cause of morbidity and mortality after SAH is development of cerebral vasospasm. Vasospasms occur in about 30% of patients after SAH, typically between day 4 and 14, peaking at day 7. Efforts to prevent vasospasm include administration of nimodipine 60 mg orally every 4 hours. The mechanism of action is not clear. It may act to limit vasospasm but also likely prevents ischemia–induced cerebral injury as well. When administering the calcium channel blocker, it is important to prevent hypotension. Concurrent administration of vasopressors may be required. In addition, most patients also receive volume expansion. This therapy has commonly been known as "triple H" therapy for hypertension, hypervolemia, and hemodilution. Glucocorticoids are not used in the treatment of SAH. There is no evidence that they reduce cerebral edema or have a neuroprotective effect.

114. The answer is D.

(Chap. 35) This patient has evidence of ICP and needs to be managed urgently. A variety of maneuvers may decrease ICP acutely. Hyperventilation causes vasoconstriction, reducing cerebral blood volume and decreasing ICP. However, this can be used only for a short period because the decrease in cerebral blood flow is of limited duration. Mannitol, an osmotic diuretic, is recommended in cases of increased ICP resulting from cytotoxic edema. Hypotonic fluids should be avoided. Instead, hypertonic saline is given to elevate sodium levels and prevent worsening of edema. A more definitive treatment to

decrease ICP is to have a ventriculostomy placed by which excessive pressure can be relieved by draining CSF. Further decreases in MAP may worsen the patient's clinical status. The patient already has had more than a 20% reduction in MAP, which is the recommended reduction in cases of hypertensive emergency. In addition, the patient is exhibiting signs of increased ICP, which indicates that cerebral perfusion pressure (MAP − ICP) has been lowered. Paradoxically, the patient may need a vasopressor agent to increase MAP and thus improve cerebral perfusion. Finally, in cases of increased ICP, nitroprusside is not a recommended intravenous antihypertensive agent because it causes arterial vasodilation and may decrease cerebral perfusion pressure and worsen neurologic function.

115. The answer is B.

(Chap. 36) The commonly accepted criteria for initiating patients on maintenance dialysis include the presence of uremic symptoms, the presence of hyperkalemia unresponsive to conservative management, persistent extracellular volume expansion despite diuretics, acidosis refractory to medical therapy, bleeding diathesis, or a creatinine clearance or estimated GFR below 10 mL/min per 1.73m². BUN or creatinine values alone are inadequate to initiate dialysis.

116. The answer is E.

(Chap. 36) Hypotension is the most common complication of hemodialysis. There are many potential etiologies of hypotension including antihypertensive use, excessive ultrafiltration, impaired vasoactive or autonomic responses, impaired cardiac reserve, and osmolar shifts. Less common causes include dialyzer reactions and high-output heart failure related to large arteriovenous (AV) fistulae. Manipulation of buffer for dialysate, alterations of timing of ultrafiltration, and midodrine may be used to improve hemodynamic tolerance to hemodialysis. Patients with unexpected or new hypotension during stable dialysis should also be evaluated for graft infection and bacteremia.

117. The answer is E.

(Chap. 36) The major complication of peritoneal dialysis therapy is peritonitis, though other complications include catheter-associated non-peritonitis infections, weight gain, metabolic derangements, and residual uremia. Peritonitis is usually a result from a failure of sterile technique during the exchange procedure. Transvisceral infection from the bowel is much less common. Because of the high dextrose used in dialysate, the environment is conducive for the development of bacterial infection. This can be diagnosed by the presence of more than 100/mm³ leukocytes with more than 50% polymorphonuclear cells on microscopy. Cloudy dialysate and abdominal pain are the most common symptoms.

The most commonly isolated bacteria are skin flora such as *Staphylococcus*. Gram-negative organisms, fungi, and mycobacteria have also been described. A recent Cochrane review (Wiggins KJ et al: Treatment for peritoneal dialysis-associated peritonitis. *Cochrane Database of Systematic Reviews* 2008, Issue 1. Art. No.: CD005284. DOI: 10.1002/14651858.CD005284.pub2) concluded that intraperitoneal administration of antibiotics was more effective than intravenous administration, and that adjunctive treatment with urokinase or peritoneal lavage offers no advantage. Intraperitoneal vancomycin is common initial empiric therapy.

118. The answer is C.

(Chap. 36) The most common cause of mortality in patients with end-stage renal disease is cardiovascular disease (stroke and myocardial infarction). Although the underlying mechanisms driving this association are under active investigation, the shared risk factors of diabetes, hypertension, and dyslipidemia in addition to specific risks such as increased inflammation, hyperhomocysteinemia, anemia, and altered vascular function are thought to play an important role. Inefficient or inadequate dialysis is a risk for patients with difficult vascular access or poor adherence to therapy. Patients receiving hemodialysis are at risk and often develop neurologic, hematologic, and infectious complications. Nevertheless, the biggest risk to survival in these patients is also the most common cause of death in the general population.

119. The answer is B.

(Chap. 36) Although the dose is currently defined as a derivation of the fractional urea clearance, factors that are also important include patient size, residual kidney function, dietary protein intake, comorbid conditions, and the degree of anabolism/catabolism. The efficiency of dialysis depends on the counter-current flow rate of the dialysate. The number of hours/sessions prescribed for a patient is derived from the dialysis dose and is individualized.

120. The answer is A.

(Chap. 36) The potassium concentration of dialysate is usually 2.5 meq/L but may be varied depending on the predialysis serum potassium. This patient may need a lower dialysate potassium concentration. Sodium modeling is an adjustment of the dialysate sodium that may lessen the incidence of hypotension at the end of a dialysis session. Aldosterone defects, if present, are not likely to play a role in this patient since his kidneys are not being perfused. Therefore, nephrectomy is not likely to control his potassium. Similarly, since the patient is likely anuric, there is no efficacy in utilizing loop diuretics to effect kaluresis. This patient has no approved indications for implantation of a defibrillator.

121. The answer is D.

(*Chap. 39*) The hemophilias are X-linked inherited disorders that cause deficiency of factor VIII (hemophilia A) or factor 9 (hemophilia B). The hemophilias affect about one in 10,000 males worldwide with hemophilia A responsible for 80% of cases. Clinically, there is no difference between hemophilia A and B. The disease presentation largely depends on the residual activity of factor VIII or factor IX. Severe disease is typically seen when factor activity is less than 1%, and moderate disease appears when the levels range between 1% and 5%. The clinical manifestation of moderate and severe disease is commonly bleeding into the joints, soft tissues, and muscles that occurs after minimal trauma or even spontaneously. When factor activity is greater than 25%, bleeding would occur only after major trauma or surgery, and the diagnosis may not be made unless a prolonged activated partial thromboplastin time is seen on routine laboratory examination. To make a definitive diagnosis, one would need to measure specific levels of factor VIII and IX. Without treatment, life expectancy is limited, but given the changes in therapy since the 1980s, life span is about 65 years. Early treatment of hemophilia required the use of pooled plasma that was used to make factor concentrates. Given the large number of donors required to generate the factor concentrates and the frequent need for transfusion in some individuals, bloodborne pathogens such as HIV and hepatitis C are among the leading cause of death in patients with hemophilia. In the 1990s, recombinant factor VIII and IX were developed. Primary prophylaxis is given to individuals with baseline factor activity levels of less than 1% to prevent spontaneous bleeding, especially hemarthroses. Although this strategy is highly recommended, only about 50% of eligible patients receive prophylactic therapy because of the high costs and need for regular intravenous infusions. When an individual is suspected of having a bleed, the treatment should begin as soon as possible and not delayed until factor activity levels return. Factor concentrates should be given to raise the activity level to 50% for large hematomas or deep muscle bleeds, and an individual may require treatment for a period of 7 days or more. For milder bleeds, including uncomplicated hemarthrosis, the goal factor activity level is 30% to 50% with maintenance of levels between 15% and 25% for 2 to 3 days after the initial transfusions. In addition to treatment with factor concentrates, care should be taken to avoid medications that inhibit platelet function. DDAVP, a desmopressin analogue, can be given as adjunctive therapy for acute bleeding episodes in hemophilia A because this may cause a transient rise in factor VIII levels and von Willebrand factor because of release from endothelial cells. This medication is typically only useful in mild to moderate disease. Antifibrinolytic drugs such as tranexamic acid or ε-amino caproic acid are helpful in promoting hemostasis for mucosal bleeding.

122. The answer is D.

(*Chap. 39*) Disseminated intravascular coagulation (DIC) is a consumptive coagulopathy that is characterized by diffuse intravascular fibrin formation that overcomes the body's natural anticoagulant mechanisms. DIC is most commonly associated with sepsis, trauma, or malignancy or in obstetric complications. The pathogenesis of DIC is not completely elucidated, but it involves intravascular exposure to phospholipids from damaged tissue, hemolysis, and endothelial damage. This leads to stimulation of procoagulant pathways with uncontrolled thrombin generation and microvascular ischemia. A secondary hyperfibrinolysis subsequently occurs. The primary clinical manifestations of DIC are bleeding at venipuncture sites, petechiae, and ecchymoses. Severe gastrointestinal and pulmonary hemorrhage can occur. The clinical diagnosis of DIC is based on laboratory findings in the appropriate clinical setting, such as severe sepsis. Although there is no single test for DIC, the common constellation of findings is thrombocytopenia (<100,000/μL), elevated prothrombin time and activated partial thromboplastin time, evidence of microangiopathic hemolytic anemia, and elevated fibrin degradation productions and D-dimer. The fibrinogen level may be less than 100 mg/dL but often does not decrease acutely unless the DIC is very severe. The primary treatment of DIC is to treat the underlying cause, which in this case would be antibiotic therapy directed against *Neisseria meningitidis*. For patients such as this one who are experiencing bleeding related to the DIC, attempts to correct the coagulopathy should be undertaken. Platelet transfusions and fresh-frozen plasma (FFP) should be given. In addition, cryoprecipitate is indicated as the fibrinogen level is less than 100 mg/dL. In general, 10 U of cryoprecipitate are required for every 2 to 3 units of FFP. In acute DIC, heparin is not been demonstrated to be helpful and may increase bleeding. Low-dose heparin therapy (5–10 U/kg) is used for chronic low-grade DIC such as that seen in acute promyelocytic leukemia or removal of a dead fetus.

123. The answer is E.

(*Chap. 39*) Vitamin K is a fat-soluble vitamin that plays an essential role in hemostasis. It is absorbed in the small intestine and stored in the liver. It serves as a cofactor in the enzymatic carboxylation of glutamic acid residues on prothrombin-complex proteins. The three major causes of vitamin K deficiency are poor dietary intake, intestinal malabsorption, and liver disease. The prothrombin complex proteins (factors II, VII, IX, and X and protein C and protein S) all decrease with vitamin K deficiency. Factor VII and protein C have the shortest half-lives of these factors and therefore decrease first. Therefore, vitamin K deficiency manifests with prolongation of the prothrombin time first. With severe deficiency, the activated partial thromboplastin time will be prolonged as well. Factor VIII is not influenced by vitamin K.

124. The answer is E.

(Chap. 39) Hemophilia A results from a deficiency of factor VIII. Replacement of factor VIII is the centerpiece of treatment. Cessation of aspirin or nonsteroidal anti-inflammatory drugs is highly recommended. Fresh-frozen plasma (FFP) contains pooled plasma from human sources. Cryoprecipitate refers to FFP that is cooled, resulting in the precipitation of material at the bottom of the plasma. This product contains about half the factor VIII activity of FFP in a tenth of the volume. Both agents are therefore reasonable treatment options. DDAVP (desmopressin) causes the release of a number of factors and von Willebrand factor from the liver and endothelial cells. This may be useful for patients with mild hemophilia. Recombinant or purified factor VIII (i.e., Humate P) is indicated in patients with more severe bleeding. Therapy may be required for weeks, with levels of factor VIII kept at 50%, for postsurgical or severe bleeding. Plasmapheresis has no role in the treatment of patients with hemophilia A.

125. The answer is C.

(Chap. 39) Lupus anticoagulants (LAs) cause prolongation of coagulation tests by binding to phospholipids. Although most often encountered in patients with systemic lupus erythematosus, they may also develop in normal individuals. The diagnosis is first suggested by prolongation of coagulation tests. Failure to correct with incubation with normal plasma confirms the presence of a circulating inhibitor. Contrary to the name, patients with LA activity have normal hemostasis and are not predisposed to bleeding. Instead, they are at risk for venous and arterial thromboembolisms. Patients with a history of recurrent unplanned abortions or thrombosis should undergo lifelong anticoagulation. The presence of LAs or anticardiolipin antibodies without a history of thrombosis may be observed because many of these patients will not go on to develop a thrombotic event.

126. The answer is D.

(Chap. 39) The activated partial thromboplastin time (aPTT) involves the factors of the intrinsic pathway of coagulation. Prolongation of the aPTT reflects either a deficiency of one of these factors (factor VIII, IX, XI, XII, and so on) or inhibition of the activity of one of the factors or components of the aPTT assay (i.e., phospholipids). This may be further characterized by the "mixing study" in which the patient's plasma is mixed with pooled plasma. Correction of the aPTT reflects a deficiency of factors that are replaced by the pooled sample. Failure to correct the aPTT reflects the presence of a factor inhibitor or phospholipid inhibitor. Common causes of a failure to correct include the presence

of heparin in the sample, factor inhibitors (factor VIII inhibitor being the most common), and the presence of antiphospholipid antibodies. Factor VII is involved in the extrinsic pathway of coagulation. Inhibitors to factor VII would result in prolongation of the prothrombin time.

127. The answer is D.

(Chap. 39) This patient presents with a significant upper gastrointestinal (GI) bleed with a prolonged prothrombin time (PT). Hemophilia should not cause a prolonged PT. This and the presence of ascites raise the possibility of liver disease and cirrhosis. The contamination of blood products in the 1970s and 1980s resulted in widespread transmission of HIV and hepatitis C virus (HCV) within the hemophilia population receiving factor infusions. It is estimated in 2006, that more than 80% of hemophilia patients older than 20 years old are infected with HCV. Viral inactivation steps were introduced in the 1980s, and recombinant factor VIII and IX were first produced in the 1990s. HCV is the major cause of morbidity and the second leading cause of death in patients exposed to older factor concentrates. Patients develop cirrhosis and complications that include ascites and variceal bleeding. End-stage liver disease requiring a liver transplant is curative for the cirrhosis and the hemophilia (the liver produces factor VIII). Hepatitis B was not transmitted in significant numbers to patients with hemophilia. Diverticular disease or peptic ulcer disease would not explain the prolonged PT. Patients with inadequately repleted factor VIII levels are more likely to develop hemarthroses than GI bleeds, and the slightly prolonged activated partial thromboplastin time makes this unlikely.

128. The answer is E.

(Chap. 39) The differentiation between disseminated intravascular coagulation (DIC) and severe liver disease is challenging. Both entities may manifest with similar laboratory findings, which are elevated fibrinogen degradation products, prolonged activated partial thromboplastin time and prothrombin time, anemia, and thrombocytopenia. When suspecting DIC, these tests should be repeated over a period of 6 to 8 hours because abnormalities may change dramatically in patients with severe DIC. In contrast, these test results should not fluctuate as much in patients with severe liver disease. Bacterial sepsis with positive blood cultures is a common cause of DIC but is not diagnostic.

129. The answer is E.

(Chap. 40) All bacteria, both gram negative and gram positive, have rigid cell walls that protect bacterial intracellular hyperosmolarity from the host environment. Peptidoglycan is the present in both gram-negative and gram-positive bacteria, but only gram-negative bacteria have an additional outer membrane external to peptidoglycan. Many antibiotics

target cell wall synthesis and thus lead to inhibition of growth or cell death. These antibiotics include bacitracin, glycopeptides such as vancomycin, and β-lactam antibiotics. Macrolides such as azithromycin, lincosamides (clindamycin), linezolid, chloramphenicol, aminoglycosides such as tobramycin, mupirocin, and tetracycline all inhibit protein synthesis. Sulfonamides and trimethoprim interrupt cell metabolism. Rifampin and metronidazole alter nucleic acid synthesis. The quinolones, such as ciprofloxacin, and novobiocin inhibit DNA synthesis. Finally, polymixins, gramicid, and daptomycin disrupt the cellular membrane.

130. The answer is B.

(Chap. 40) The patient presents with evidence of methicillin-resistant *Staphylococcus aureus*–associated soft tissue infection that has failed therapy with clindamycin. Linezolid is an appropriate choice for antibiotic coverage in this situation. Subsequent development of neurologic symptoms, including agitated delirium, evidence of autonomic instability coupled with tremor, muscular rigidity, hyperreflexia, and clonus, suggests serotonin syndrome. Because linezolid is a monoamine oxidase inhibitor, it interacts with selective serotonin reuptake inhibitors and can cause serotonin syndrome. Other potential triggers include tyramine-rich foods and sympathomimetics such as phenylpropanolamine. The other drug–drug combinations in the answer choices are not described to be associated with serotonin syndrome.

131. The answer is A.

(Chap. 41) Compared with the large number of antimicrobials directed against bacterial, antiviral therapies have been fewer, and advances in antiviral therapy have come more slowly. However, in recent years, a large number of antiviral medications have been introduced, and it is generally important to be familiar with the common side effects of these medications. Acyclovir and valacyclovir are most commonly used for the treatment of herpes simplex viruses I and II as well as varicella–zoster virus. Acyclovir is generally a well-tolerated drug, but it can crystallize in the kidneys, leading to acute renal failure if the patient is not properly hydrated. Valacyclovir is an ester of acyclovir that significantly improves the bioavailability of the drug. It is also well tolerated but has been associated with thrombotic thrombocytopenic purpura or hemolytic uremic syndrome when used at high doses. Ganciclovir and foscarnet are medications used to treat cytomegalovirus (CMV) infection. Ganciclovir is primarily given intravenously because the oral bioavailability is less than 10%. Ganciclovir is associated with bone marrow suppression and can cause renal dysfunction. Foscarnet is used for ganciclovir-resistant CMV infections. Renal impairment commonly occurs with its use and causes hypokalemia, hypocalcemia, and hypomagnesemia. Thus, careful monitoring of electrolytes and renal function is warranted with foscarnet use. Amantadine is an antiviral

medication used for the treatment of influenza A. It has been demonstrated to have a variety of central nervous system (CNS) side effects, including dizziness, anxiety, insomnia, and difficulty concentrating. Although initially used as an antiviral drug, the CNS effects of amantadine have led to its use in Parkinson's disease. Interferons are a group of cytokines produced endogenously in response to a variety of pathogens, including viruses and bacteria. Therapeutically, interferons have been studied extensively in the treatment of patients with chronic hepatitis B and C. Interferons lead to a host of systemic effects, including symptoms of a viral syndrome (fevers, chills, fatigue, and myalgias) as well as leukopenia.

132. The answer is D.

(Chap. 42) The classification of fungal infections is typically based on anatomic location of infection and epidemiology of the organism. Additionally, it is important to know the descriptive characteristics of fungi in culture because that information may be useful clinically. Endemic mycoses (e.g., coccidioidomycosis, blastomycosis) are infections that are caused by fungi that are not typically part of human microbial flora. Opportunistic mycoses (e.g., *Candida*, *Aspergillus*) are infections that are caused by fungi that are commonly part of the human microbial flora. Yeasts (*Candida*, *Cryptococcus*) are seen microscopically as single cells or rounded organisms. Molds (*Aspergillus*, *Rhizopus*) grow as filamentous forms (hyphae) at room temperature and in tissue. *Dimorphic* is the term to describe fungi that exist as yeasts or large spherical structures in tissue but in filamentous forms in the environment. Blastomycosis, histoplasmosis, paracoccidioidomycosis, coccidioidomycosis, and sporotrichosis are typically dimorphic. *Candida* may exist as a yeast or filamentous form in tissue infection, with the exception of *Candida glabrata*, which only exists as a yeast in tissue infection.

133. The answer is A.

(Chap. 42) The azole antifungals (fluconazole, itraconazole, voriconazole, and posaconazole) all have oral formulations. The azoles inhibit ergosterol synthesis in the fungal cell wall. Compared with amphotericin B, they are considered fungistatic but do not cause significant renal toxicity. Fluconazole is effective for *Candida albicans* and coccidioidomycosis. Voriconazole has broader spectrum against *Candida* spp., including *Candida glabrata* and *Candida krusei*. Itraconazole is the drug of choice for mild to moderate histoplasmosis and blastomycosis. Posaconazole is approved in immunocompromised patients as prophylaxis against *Candida* and *Aspergillus* infection. Studies of posaconazole have suggested efficacy for zygomycosis, *Aspergillus*, and cryptococcal infections. It also has activity against fluconazole-resistant *Candida*. The echinocandins (caspofungin,

anidulafungin, micafungin) only have intravenous formulations at this time. They are considered fungicidal for *Candida* and fungistatic for *Aspergillus*. Griseofulvin is an oral medication used historically primarily for ringworm infection. Terbinafine is more effective than griseofulvin for ringworm and onychomycosis.

134. The answer is D.

(Chap. 42) All patients with *Candida* fungemia should be treated with systemic antifungals. Fluconazole has been shown to be an effective agent for candidemia with equivalence to amphotericin products and caspofungin. Voriconazole is also active against *Candida albicans* but has many drug interactions that make it less desirable against this pathogen. However, it has broader activity against *Candida* spp. including *Candida glabrata* and *Candida krusei*. No trials of posaconazole for candidemia have yet been reported. The echinocandins, including micafungin and caspofungin, have broad activity, are fungicidal against *Candida* spp., and have low toxicity. They are among the safest antifungal agents.

135. The answer is B.

(Chap. 42) The definitive diagnosis of an invasive fungal infection generally requires histologic demonstration of fungus invading tissue along with an inflammatory response. However, *Coccidioides* serum complement fixation, cryptococcal serum and cerebrospinal fluid antigen, and urine/serum *Histoplasma* antigen are all tests with good performance characteristics, occasionally allowing for presumptive diagnoses before pathologic tissue sections can be examined or cultures of blood or tissue turn positive. Serum testing for galactomannan is approved for the diagnosis of *Aspergillus* infection. However, false-negative test results may occur. Multiple serial tests may decrease the incidence of false-negative test results. There is no approved urine or serologic test for blastomycosis.

136 and 137. The answers are E and C, respectively.

(Chap. 43) This clinical scenario describes an individual with superior vena cava (SVC) syndrome, which is an oncologic emergency. Eighty-five percent of cases of SVC syndrome are caused by either small cell or squamous cell cancer of the lung. Other causes of SVC syndrome include lymphoma, aortic aneurysm, thyromegaly, fibrosing mediastinitis, thrombosis, histoplasmosis, and Behçet's syndrome. The typical clinical presentation is dyspnea, cough, and facial and neck swelling. Symptoms are worsened by lying flat or bending forward. As the swelling progresses, it can lead to glossal and laryngeal edema with symptoms of hoarseness and dysphagia. Other symptoms can include headaches, nasal congestion, pain, dizziness, and syncope. In rare cases, seizures can occur from cerebral edema, although this is more commonly associated with brain metastases. On physical examination, dilated neck veins with collateralization on the anterior chest wall are frequently seen. There is also facial and upper extremity edema associated with cyanosis. The diagnosis of SVC syndrome is a clinical diagnosis. A pleural effusion is seen in about 25% of cases, more commonly on the right. A chest CT scan would demonstrate decreased or absent contrast in the central veins with prominent collateral circulation and would help elucidate the cause. Most commonly this would be mediastinal adenopathy or a large central tumor obstructing venous flow. The immediate treatment of SVC syndrome includes oxygen, elevation of the head of the bed, and administration of diuretics in combination with a low-sodium diet. Conservative treatment alone often provides adequate relief of symptoms and allows determination of the underlying cause of the obstruction. In this case, this would include histologic confirmation of cell type of the tumor to provide more definitive therapy. Radiation therapy is the most common treatment modality and can be used in an emergent situation if conservative treatment fails to provide relief to the patient.

138. The answer is A.

(Chap. 43) This patient presents with symptoms of spinal cord compression in the setting of known stage IV breast cancer. This represents an oncologic emergency because only 10% of patients presenting with paraplegia regain the ability to walk. Most commonly, patients develop symptoms of localized back pain and tenderness days to months before developing paraplegia. The pain is worsened by movement, cough, or sneezing. In contrast to radicular pain, the pain related to spinal cord metastases is worse with lying down. Patients presenting with back pain alone should have a careful examination to attempt to localize the lesion before development of more severe neurologic symptoms. In this patient with paraplegia, there is a definitive level at which sensation is diminished. This level is typically one to two vertebrae below the site of compression. Other findings include spasticity, weakness, and increased deep tendon reflexes. In those with autonomic dysfunction, bowel and bladder incontinence occur with decreased anal tone, absence of the anal wink and bulbocavernosus reflexes, and bladder distention. The most important initial step is the administration of high-dose intravenous corticosteroids to minimize associated swelling around the lesion and prevent paraplegia while allowing further evaluation and treatment. MRI should be performed of the entire spinal cord to evaluate for other metastatic disease that may require therapy. Although a brain MRI may be indicated in the future to evaluate for brain metastases, it is not required in the initial evaluation because the bilateral nature of the patient's symptoms and sensory level clearly indicate the spinal cord as the site of the injury. After an MRI has been performed, a definitive

treatment plan can be made. Most commonly, radiation therapy is used with or without surgical decompression.

139 and 140. The answers are B and E, respectively.
(Chap. 43) Tumor lysis syndrome occurs most commonly in individuals undergoing chemotherapy for rapidly proliferating malignancies, including acute leukemias and Burkitt's lymphoma. In rare instances, it can be seen in chronic lymphoma or solid tumors. As the chemotherapeutic agents act on these cells, there is massive tumor lysis that results in release of intracellular ions and nucleic acids. This leads to a characteristic metabolic syndrome of hyperuricemia, hyperphosphatemia, hyperkalemia, and hypocalcemia. Acute kidney injury is frequent and can lead to renal failure, requiring hemodialysis if uric acid crystallizes within the renal tubules. Lactic acidosis and dehydration increase the risk of acute kidney injury. Hyperphosphatemia occurs because of the release of intracellular phosphate ions and causes a reciprocal reduction in serum calcium. This hypocalcemia can be profound, leading to neuromuscular irritability and tetany. Hyperkalemia can become rapidly life threatening and cause ventricular arrhythmia.

Knowing the characteristics of tumor lysis syndrome, one can attempt to prevent the known complications from occurring. It is important to monitor serum electrolytes very frequently during treatment. Laboratory studies should be obtained no less than three times daily, but more frequent monitoring is often needed. Allopurinol should be administered prophylactically at high doses. If allopurinol fails to control uric acid to less than 8 mg/dL, rasburicase, a recombinant urate oxidase, can be added at a dose of 0.2 mg/kg. Throughout this period, the patient should be well hydrated with alkalinization of the urine to a pH of greater than 7.0. This is accomplished by administration of intravenous normal or ½ normal saline at a dose of 3000 mL/m² daily with sodium bicarbonate. Prophylactic hemodialysis is not performed unless there is underlying renal failure before starting chemotherapy.

INDEX

Bold page number indicates the start of the main discussion of the topic. Page numbers with "f" or "t" refer to figures and tables, respectively.

573